FOR REFERENCE

Do Not Take From This Room

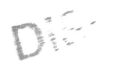

MRI of the Musculoskeletal System

FIFTH EDITION

MRI of the Musculoskeletal System

FIFTH EDITION

EDITOR

■ **THOMAS H. BERQUIST, MD, FACR**

Consultant, Department of Diagnostic Radiology
Mayo Clinic
Jacksonville, Florida
Professor of Diagnostic Radiology
Mayo Clinic College of Medicine
Director of Education
Mayo Foundation
Rochester, Minnesota

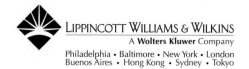

LIPPINCOTT WILLIAMS & WILKINS
A **Wolters Kluwer** Company

Philadelphia • Baltimore • New York • London
Buenos Aires • Hong Kong • Sydney • Tokyo

Acquisitions Editor: Lisa McAllister
Developmental Editor: Louise Bierig
Project Manager: Bridgett Dougherty
Senior Manufacturing Manager: Ben Rivera
Marketing Manager: Angela Panetta
Design Coordinator: Terry Mallon
Production Services: Laserwords Private Limited
Printer: Edwards Brothers

5th Edition
© 2006 by Lippincott Williams & Wilkins
530 Walnut Street
Philadelphia, PA 19106
4/e-2001 LWW

Library of Congress Cataloging-in-Publication Data

MRI of the musculoskeletal system / editor, Thomas H. Berquist. — 5th ed.
    p. ; cm.
  Includes bibliographical references and index.
  ISBN 0-7817-5502-6
  1. Musculoskeletal system—Magnetic resonance imaging.
 I. Berquist, Thomas H. (Thomas Henry), 1945- .
  [DNLM: 1. Musculoskeletal Diseases—diagnosis. 2. Magnetic
Resonance Imaging—methods. 3. Musculoskeletal System—anatomy
& histology. WE 141 M9389 2005]
  RC925.7.M34 2005
  616.7'07548—dc22

                              2005014571

Care has been taken to confirm the accuracy of the information presented and to describe generally accepted practices. However, the authors, editors, and publisher are not responsible for errors or omissions or for any consequences from application of the information in this book and make no warranty, expressed or implied, with respect to the currency, completeness, or accuracy of the contents of the publication. Application of this information in a particular situation remains the professional responsibility of the practitioner.

The authors, editors, and publisher have exerted every effort to ensure that drug selection and dosage set forth in this text are in accordance with current recommendations and practice at the time of publication. However, in view of ongoing research, changes in government regulations, and the constant flow of information relating to drug therapy and drug reactions, the reader is urged to check the package insert for each drug for any change in indications and dosage and for added warnings and precautions. This is particularly important when the recommended agent is a new or infrequently employed drug.

Some drugs and medical devices presented in this publication have Food and Drug Administration (FDA) clearance for limited use in restricted research settings. It is the responsibility of health care providers to ascertain the FDA status of each drug or device planned for use in their clinical practice.

The publishers have made every effort to trace copyright holders for borrowed material. If they have inadvertently overlooked any, they will be pleased to make the necessary arrangements at the first opportunity.

To purchase additional copies of this book, call our customer service department at (800) 639-3030 or fax orders to (301) 824-7390. International customers should call (301) 714-2324. Lippincott Williams & Wilkins customer service representatives are available from 8:30 am to 6:00 pm, EST. Visit Lippincott Williams & Wilkins on the Internet at http://www.lww.com.

10 9 8 7 6 5 4 3 2 1

How do you thank someone who had so much influence on your life? Someone who took the time to meet with you at 5:00 AM every week for an entire semester so that you could learn the writing skills you would need to become an author of medical textbooks? I dedicate the Fifth Edition of *MRI of the Musculoskeletal System* to Dr. Walther Prausnitz of Concordia College, Moorhead, Minnesota, for his contributions to my career.

Contents

Preface

The Fourth Edition of this text was published in 2001. Since that time, new magnet configurations (extremity, open) and higher field strengths (3 T) have begun to impact the practice for musculoskeletal magnetic resonance (MR) imaging. Coupled with improvements in software, pulse sequences, and examination techniques, the musculoskeletal applications for MR imaging have expanded dramatically. Gadolinium use for intravenous, intraarticular, and angiographic imaging has become routine. Spectroscopy in the clinical setting is also more commonly employed, though not to the level of more conventional imaging techniques.

The Fifth Edition of *MRI of the Musculoskeletal System* provides significant updates on principles, techniques, and applications for musculoskeletal imaging. Chapter 1 reviews basic principles of physics, pulse sequences, and terminology, using an approach that is easy to read and comprehend. Chapter 2 provides essentials of interpretation with many new images and pulse sequences to explain the signal changes of pathologic tissues compared to signal intensity of normal tissue. Chapter 3 discusses safety issues, sedation, patient selection, patient positioning, coil selection, pulse sequences, and the uses of gadolinium for musculoskeletal imaging.

Chapters 4 through 11 are anatomically oriented, with new anatomic MR images in each chapter. Improved images using new techniques and the expanded applications are reviewed in each chapter. Pediatric applications are included in these anatomic chapters as appropriate.

A thorough discussion of musculoskeletal neoplasms and neoplasm-like conditions is included in Chapter 12. Chapter 13 is dedicated to musculoskeletal infections, including soft tissue, osseous, articular, spondylopathy, and postoperative infections. Chapter 14 provides in-depth coverage of diffuse marrow diseases, and Chapter 15 is designed to review miscellaneous and evolving MR imaging applications. The final chapter, Chapter 16, updates clinical uses of spectroscopy.

New technology has led to a significant increase in the utility of MRI for evaluation of the musculoskeletal system. This edition provides a thorough review of anatomy, techniques, and applications, with many new images. This text will be of use to physicians, residents, students, and other health professionals who perform or request MR imaging examinations.

Acknowledgments

Preparation of this text required the support of my clinical colleagues; our musculoskeletal fellow, Dr. Elizabeth Ann Kelley; and our dedicated MR technical staff. A special thank you to Lisa Broddle, Lynn Hill, and Tony Schroeder for their assistance with special pulse sequences and MR anatomy.

I am especially thankful for the assistance in preparing the manuscript provided by Linda Downie, Pamela Chirico, Samantha Lehman, and Diane Anderson. John Hagen was responsible for the anatomic drawings and artwork. I have been fortunate to enlist John's help for all of my textbooks.

Finally, I would like to thank the staff at Lippincott Williams & Wilkins, Lisa McAllister, Kerry Barrett, Louise Bierig, and Bridgett Dougherty, for their assistance in the development and editing of this text.

Contributors

LAURA W. BANCROFT, MD Assistant Professor of Diagnostic Radiology, Mayo Clinic College of Medicine, Jacksonville, Florida; Consultant, Department of Diagnostic Radiology, Mayo Clinic, Jacksonville, Florida

THOMAS H. BERQUIST, MD, FACR Professor of Diagnostic Radiology, Mayo Clinic College of Medicine, Jacksonville, Florida; Consultant, Department of Diagnostic Radiology, Mayo Clinic, Jacksonville, Florida

DANIEL F. BRODERICK, MD Assistant Professor of Diagnostic Radiology, Mayo Clinic College of Medicine, Rochester, Minnesota; Consultant, Department of Diagnostic Radiology, Mayo Clinic, Jacksonville, Florida

MARK S. COLLINS, MD Assistant Professor of Diagnostic Radiology, Mayo Clinic College of Medicine, Rochester, Minnesota; Consultant, Department of Diagnostic Radiology, Mayo Clinic, Rochester, Minnesota

RICHARD L. EHMAN, MD Professor of Diagnostic Radiology, Mayo Clinic College of Medicine, Rochester, Minnesota; Consultant, Department of Diagnostic Radiology, Mayo Clinic, Rochester, Minnesota

JOEL P. FELMLEE, PHD Professor of Diagnostic Radiology, Mayo Clinic College of Medicine, Rochester, Minnesota; Consultant, Department of Diagnostic Radiology, Mayo Clinic, Rochester, Minnesota

CLYDE A. HELMS, MD Professor, Department of Diagnostic Radiology; Head of Musculoskeletal Section, Duke University, Durham, North Carolina

ELIZABETH ANN KELLEY, MD Musculoskeletal Radiologist, Carolina Radiology, Myrtle Beach, South Carolina

MARK J. KRANSDORF, MD Professor of Diagnostic Radiology, Mayo Clinic College of Medicine, Rochester, Minnesota; Chief, Department of Diagnostic Radiology, Mayo Clinic, Jacksonville, Florida

KARL N. KRECKE, MD Assistant Professor of Diagnostic Radiology, Mayo Clinic College of Medicine, Rochester, Minnesota; Consultant, Division of Neuroradiology; Mayo Clinic, Rochester, Minnesota

JOHN I. LANE, MD Assistant Professor of Diagnostic Radiology, Mayo Clinic College of Medicine, Rochester, Minnesota; Consultant, Division of Neuroradiology, Mayo Clinic, Rochester, Minnesota

GARY MICHAEL MILLER, MD Associate Professor of Radiology, Mayo Clinic College of Medicine, Rochester, Minnesota; Consultant, Department of Diagnostic Radiology, Mayo Clinic, Rochester, Minnesota

RICHARD L. MORIN, MD Professor of Diagnostic Radiology, Mayo Clinic College of Medicine, Rochester, Minnesota; Consultant in Medical Physics, Mayo Clinic, Jacksonville, Florida

WILLIAM A. MURPHY, JR, MD Professor of Radiology, Department of Diagnostic Radiology, University of Texas, MD Anderson Cancer Center, Houston, Texas

JEFFREY JAMES PETERSON, MD Assistant Professor of Diagnostic Radiology, Mayo Clinic College of Medicine, Rochester, Minnesota

ROBERT A. POOLEY, PHD Instructor of Radiologic Physics, Mayo Clinic College of Medicine, Rochester, Minnesota; Consultant, Department of Diagnostic Radiology, Mayo Clinic, Jacksonville, Florida

JAMES B. VOGLER, III, MD Clinical Associate Professor of Radiology, Department of Radiology, University of Florida College of Medicine, Gainesville, Florida; Co-Director, Invision Outpatient Imaging Center, North Florida Regional Medical Center, Gainesville, Florida

ROBERT J. WITTE, MD Assistant Professor of Diagnostic Radiology, Mayo Clinic College of Medicine, Rochester, Minnesota; Consultant, Division of Neuroradiology, Mayo Clinic, Rochester, Minnesota

Basic Principles and Terminology of Magnetic Resonance Imaging

Robert A. Pooley   *Joel P. Felmlee*
Richard L. Morin

This chapter is presented to acquaint those new to magnetic resonance imaging (MRI) with the fundamental concepts and basic principles responsible for the nuclear magnetic resonance (NMR) phenomenon and MRI. At the outset, it is important to understand that this chapter is intended to be tutorial in nature. In addition to the fundamental concepts of the physical phenomenon of NMR itself, techniques relevant to clinical imaging are discussed in the context of a tutorial presentation of fundamentals for those new to MRI. It is important to appreciate that the physics principles associated with MRI often take a while to assimilate. There are many approaches to the discussion and presentation of the fundamental physics of MRI. Technical details and in-depth coverage can be found in MRI texts and review articles (1–5). The appendix lists terms that have been selected from the American College of Radiology glossary of MR terms (6) and are provided for the sake of completeness and reference.

A chronology of the historical development of MRI is listed in Table 1-1. The principle of NMR was first elucidated in the late 1940s by Professor Bloch at Stanford and Professor Purcell at Harvard. In 1952, they shared the Nobel Prize in physics for their work. The importance of this technique lies in the ability to define and study the molecular structure of the sample under investigation. In the 1970s, the principle of NMR was utilized to generate cross-sectional images similar in format to x-ray computed tomography (CT). By 1981, clinical research was underway.

The intense enthusiasm for and the rapid introduction of MRI into the clinical environment stem from the abundance of diagnostic information present in MR images. Although the image format is similar to CT, the fundamental principles are quite different; in fact, an entirely different part of the atom is responsible for the image formation. In MRI it is the *nucleus* that provides the signal used in generating an image. We note that this differs from conventional diagnostic radiology in which the *electrons* are responsible for the imaging signal. Furthermore, it is not only the nucleus of the atom but also its structural and biochemical environment that influence the signal.

Currently, fast imaging techniques are increasing as important clinical methods. Echo planar imaging (EPI), as well as fast spin-echo and gradient-echo based acquisitions,

allows image acquisition in the sub-second to breathhold (15 second) range. These techniques hold the potential for high-resolution studies acquired quickly, thereby "freezing" many physiologic motions. Using these fast acquisition techniques, encoding functional and flow information into the image are areas of clinical interest and research.

Throughout this discussion we illustrate the underlying physics principles with analogies and discuss the nature of the physics from a "classical" rather than a "quantum mechanical" point of view. Both approaches result in accurate explanations of the NMR phenomenon; however, they differ in their mathematical constructs and visualization of the underlying physical principles.

THE NUCLEAR MAGNETIC RESONANCE EXPERIMENT

When certain nuclei (those with an odd number of protons, an odd number of neutrons, or an odd number of both) are placed in a strong magnetic field, they align themselves with the magnetic field and begin to rotate at a precise rate or frequency (Larmor frequency). If a radio transmission is made at this precise frequency, the nuclei will absorb the radio frequency (RF) energy and become "excited." After termination of the radio transmission, the nuclei will calm down (or relax) with the emission of radio waves. The emission of RF energy as the nuclei relax is the source of the NMR signal. The ability of a system to absorb energy that is "packaged" in a particular kind of way is termed *resonance*. This condition is analogous to the pushing of a child on a swing. If the child is pushed at the highest point of return, then the maximum amount of energy is transmitted to the swing. Attempting to push the child at the midpoint of return results in a low transfer of energy, and in this sense would be *off-resonance*. Hence, the resonance condition in this case is the timing of pushes with the exact frequency of the pendulum movement of the swing.

The precession of nuclei about a magnetic field is similar in concept to the precession of a spinning top in the presence of a gravitational field, as illustrated in Fig. 1-1. This type of rotation occurs whenever a spinning motion interacts with another force. Nuclei with an odd number of protons or neutrons or both possess a property of "spin," which in this case interacts with the magnetic field, thereby inducing precession of the nuclei about the magnetic field. The precessional or Larmor frequency is determined by the individual nuclei and the magnetic field strength [given in the SI unit Tesla (T) or the centimeter-gram-second unit gauss (G), where 1 T = 10,000 G]. The mathematical definition of the Larmor frequency is given by

$$\omega = \gamma B_o$$

where ω is the Larmor frequency, B_o is the static magnetic field strength, and γ is the gyromagnetic ratio (a constant that is different for each nucleus). Larmor frequencies for

TABLE 1-1
HISTORICAL DEVELOPMENT OF MRI

1946	Elucidation of NMR phenomena and technique—Bloch, Purcell
1951	Single dimension spatial localization—Gabillard
1952	Nobel Prize to Bloch and Purcell
1959	Blood flow by NMR—Singer
1971	*In vitro* cancer detection by NMR—Damadian
1972	*In vivo* cancer detection by NMR—Weisman
1972	NMR imaging—Damadian
1973	NMR zeugmatography—Lauterbur
1975	Commercial development
1981	Clinical trials with prototypes

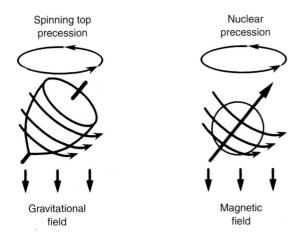

Figure 1-1 Illustration of precession. (Adapted from Fullerton GD. Basic concepts for nuclear magnetic resonance imaging. *Magn Reson Imaging* 1982;1:39–55, with permission.)

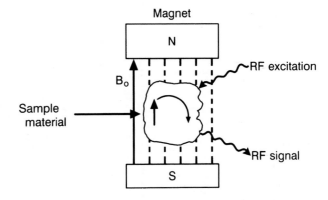

Figure 1-2 Basics of NMR measurements. Here the magnetization is nutated 90° by the RF excitation. (Adapted from Fullerton GD. Basic concepts for nuclear magnetic resonance imaging. *Magn Reson Imaging* 1982;1:39–55, with permission.)

various nuclei and field strengths are given in Tables 1-2 and 1-3. For protons at a field strength of 1.5 T, the Larmor frequency is 64 MHz, which is the same frequency used for transmitting the television signal of channel 3.

In summary, the fundamentals of the NMR experiment are illustrated in Fig. 1-2 and consist of three steps: (a) placing a sample in a magnetic field, thereby inducing a nuclear precession, (b) transmitting an RF pulse at the Larmor frequency, and (c) "listening" for the returning NMR signal. Note that the frequency of the transmitted RF and the returning signal are dependent upon both the nuclei of interest and the magnetic field strength B_o.

THE NUCLEAR MAGNETIC RESONANCE SIGNAL

The form of the RF signal produced by the NMR experiment depends on the number of nuclei present (spin density) and the time it takes for the nuclei to relax (T1 and T2). The parameter T1 (spin-lattice relaxation time) measures the

rate of return of the nuclei to alignment with the static magnetic field (B_o) and reflects the chemical environment of the proton. T2 (spin-spin relaxation time) measures the dephasing of the nuclei in the transverse plane and reflects the relationship of the proton to the surrounding nuclei. These processes are illustrated in Fig. 1-3. The degree to which the NMR signal depends on spin density, T1 or T2, is determined by the pulse sequence, which we shall discuss later. The nature of this signal and its decay due to relaxation are of fundamental importance and we shall discuss this process in detail.

The form of the basic NMR signal [free induction decay (FID)] is shown in Fig. 1-4. The signal is a time oscillating waveform that is detected in the *x–y*, or transverse, plane, defined by the coordinate system for the experiment as shown in Fig. 1-5. Note that after a 90° rotation, the magnetization vector is in the "transverse" plane. The received signal is oscillating because we measure it from the transverse plane as the magnetization vector rotates about the longitudinal axis. Hence, a rotating signal is translated into a sinusoidal time-varying voltage.

It is important to understand that we can only measure the macroscopic magnetization vector, that is, the algebraic summation of all nuclear spins under investigation (see Fig. 1-6). In reality, not all nuclear spins in a sample

TABLE 1-2	
LARMOR (RESONANCE) FREQUENCIES FOR HYDROGEN	
Field Strength (T)	**Resonance Frequency (MHz)**
0.15	6.4
0.35	14.9
0.50	21.3
1.00	42.6
1.50	63.9
2.00	85.2
4.00	170.3

TABLE 1-3	
LARMOR (RESONANCE) FREQUENCIES AT 1.0 T	
Nucleus	**Larmor Frequency (MHz)**
^{1}H	42.6
^{13}C	11.0
^{14}N	3.0
^{31}P	17.1

H, hydrogen; C, carbon; N, nitrogen; P, phosphorus.

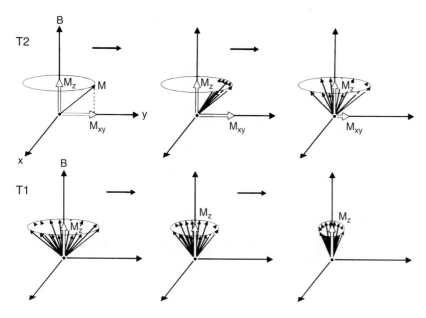

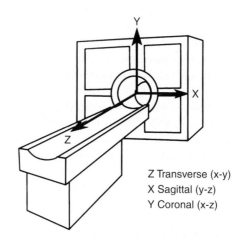

Figure 1-3   Diagram of T2 (spin-spin, transverse) relaxation and T1 (spin-lattice, longitudinal) relaxation after a 90° nutation pulse.

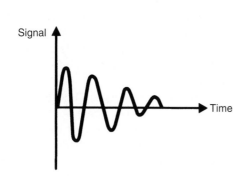

Figure 1-4   Plot of free induction decay (FID), the basic NMR signal.

Figure 1-5   MRI coordinate system.

Z Transverse (x-y)
X Sagittal (y-z)
Y Coronal (x-z)

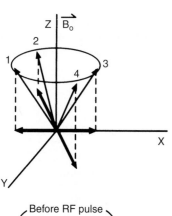

Before RF pulse
Macroscopic
magnetization
vector = 0

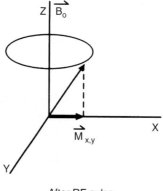

After RF pulse
Macroscopic
magnetization
vector = $\vec{M}_{x,y}$

Figure 1-6   Illustration of the macroscopic magnetic vector formed by individual nuclei. **A:** Individual nuclei 1, 2, 3, and 4 precessing about the magnetic field B_o. The measured macroscopic magnetization vector is zero due to the algebraic summation of x and y components of the randomly oriented nuclei. **B:** Macroscopic magnetization vector formed by the phasing of individual nuclei 1, 2, 3, and 4. The macroscopic magnetization vector formed by the phasing of individual nuclei 1, 2, 3, and 4. The macroscopic magnetization vector measured is the component in the transverse plane (i.e., $M_{x,y}$).

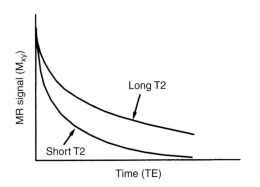

Figure 1-7 Plot of the loss of magnetization in the transverse (*xy*) plane following cessation of RF transmission.

precess at the same frequency. Each individual nucleus is influenced by a slightly different magnetic field due to the interactions of electrons that surround individual nuclei or the movements of adjacent molecules. The first process that occurs upon RF transmission is the phasing of individual nuclear spins to create the macroscopic magnetization vector M_{xy} (similar to the military command "fall in" given to a group of soldiers). This ensemble of phased nuclear spins then changes its orientation with regard to the *z*-axis. The rotation of this phased macroscopic magnetic vector is the property that we detect causing an oscillatory MR signal with time.

The decay of the signal as shown in Fig. 1-4 occurs because following cessation of the radio RF transmission, the nuclear spins dephase. Since magnetization is a vector quantity, dephasing causes the macroscopic magnetic vector to decrease in magnitude. Since this activity takes place in the *x*–*y*, or transverse, plane, this process is also called *transverse relaxation*. In a chemical sense, this relaxation is due to interactions that occur between adjacent nuclei and is therefore termed *spin-spin relaxation*. The effect of T2 relaxation for substances with different T2 values is illustrated in Fig. 1-7.

As the above-mentioned dephasing or T2 relaxation is occurring, the entire ensemble of nuclei are returning to

alignment with the main magnetic field B_o, which is oriented along the *z* axis. Hence, the longitudinal or *z* component of the macroscopic magnetic vector "grows" or increases with time, as the protons realign with B_o and return to an equilibrium value. Since this T1 recovery occurs along the direction of the longitudinal axis, it is termed *longitudinal relaxation*. In a chemical sense, this process is governed by the strength with which an individual nucleus is bound to its chemical backbone (water, lipid, protein, etc.) and hence this process is often termed *spin-lattice relaxation*. The effect of T1 relaxation is represented in Fig. 1-8 for substances of different T1 values.

MAGNETIC RESONANCE IMAGING

An illustration of an MRI system is shown in Fig. 1-9. To conduct the NMR experiment, a strong magnet, radio transmitter, and radio receiver are necessary. To produce MR images, additional magnetic coils (gradient coils) are necessary to encode the signal and thus allow its origin to be determined. In addition, a computer system is necessary to control the sequencing of the RF, gradients, data collection, and operations and to perform the final image reconstruction.

In the most common type of MRI, spatial localization is obtained using additional magnetic fields superimposed on the main magnetic field. The key to understanding this phenomenon lies in the Larmor equation. Recall that the precessional frequency is directly related to magnetic field strength. If a spatially varying magnetic field is superimposed on the main magnetic field, then precessional frequencies will be related to a location in space, analogous to the frequency obtained by the specific location of keys on a piano. This translation between frequency and spatial location is shown in Fig. 1-10.

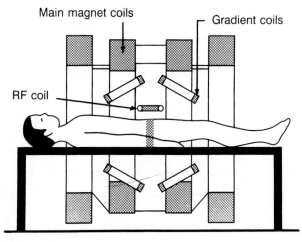

Figure 1-9 Diagram of MRI system. (Adapted from Fullerton GD. Basic concepts for nuclear magnetic resonance imaging. *Magn Reson Imaging* 1982;1:39–55, with permission.)

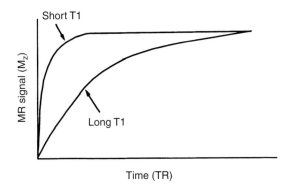

Figure 1-8 Plot of recovery of magnetization in the longitudinal (*z*) direction.

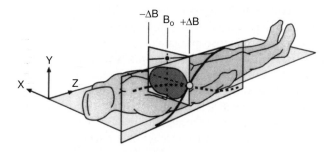

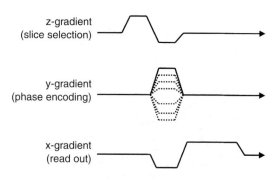

Figure 1-10 Diagram of spatial encoding of MR signal by super-position of magnetic field gradients (different resonance frequencies correspond to different positions along the gradient).

Figure 1-11 Gradient activation versus time for MRI acquisition of a single transverse slice. For this case, slice selection is in the craniocaudal (C-C) direction, phase encoding in the anteroposterior (A-P) direction, and frequency encoding in the right-left (R-L) direction.

The most common imaging technique [two-dimensional Fourier transform (2DFT)] (7–9) involves the use of three such gradient fields to localize a point in space. It is important to understand that all three gradients will be turned on and off at different times. The particular application and relative timing of the x, y, and z gradients determines which axis (x, y, or z) is being localized. In general, signals will be localized by selective application of slice selection, phase encoding, and frequency encoding gradients. A schematic diagram of the timing of these gradients is given in Fig. 1-11. We describe each in detail for the acquisition of a transverse slice.

The slice is first selected by applying a gradient along the z-axis while applying a RF pulse with a narrow frequency range. This excites the nuclei only in the slice of interest so that they are all precessing at the same frequency and phase (Fig. 1-10). However, the signal we detect is from the entire slice, so at this point it is not possible to form an image.

Next, the relative phase of spin precession is modified by applying a gradient in the y direction. This gradient causes the atoms at different locations along y to precess at different frequencies while the y gradient is applied (see Fig. 1-12). If no gradient is present, the nuclei precess at the Larmor frequency corresponding to the main magnetic field strength. If a slightly higher magnetic field is superimposed with a gradient, as shown in Fig. 1-12, the nuclei in row 1 precess at a slightly higher frequency than those in row 2; likewise for rows 2 and 3. When the gradient is turned off, all the

rows will once again precess at the same frequency. However, since row 1 was previously precessing at a slightly higher frequency than row 2, all the nuclei in row 1 will be slightly ahead of those in row 2; that is, they will be precessing at the same frequency but at different phases. Likewise, each successive row will precess at the same frequency but at a slightly different phase. To obtain discrimination in the phase encoding direction, this process must be repeated many (e.g., 256) times. This result of increased phase encoding is shown pictorially in Fig. 1-13 for a coronal image with phase encoding in the anteroposterior direction (10).

The precessing nuclei are frequency encoded by the application of a magnetic gradient in the x direction. This gradient causes the atoms to precess at different frequencies (see Fig. 1-14) and is usually applied while the MR signal is being collected (hence, it is sometimes called the readout gradient).

The MR signal is digitized and stored on the acquisition workstation (in "k-space") for subsequent Fourier reconstruction to form the clinical image. Each point in k-space represents a different spatial frequency in the object being imaged. The strength of the MR signal (and thus the value of a data point in k-space) indicates the degree to which that spatial frequency is represented in the object. Lower spatial frequencies are located near the center of k-space and contain information related to image contrast. Higher

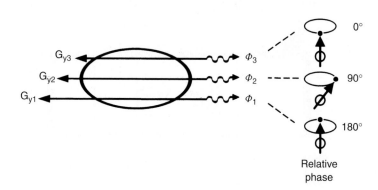

Figure 1-12 Phase encoding in the y direction. Here the gradient increases from top to bottom.

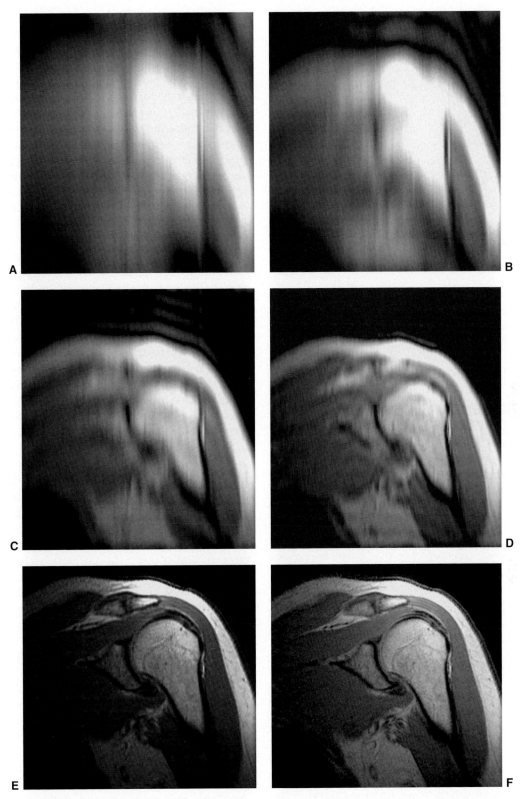

Figure 1-13   MRI phase encoding (10). All images are from the same acquisition (TR = 500, TE = 20, 2 excitation, 5 mm slice, 256 phase encoding steps). The original raw data were truncated to demonstrate the effect of phase encoding. **A:** 2 steps. **B:** 8 steps. **C:** 16 steps. **D:** 32 steps. **E:** 64 steps. **F:** 256 steps.

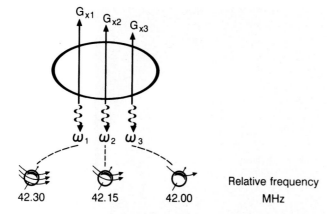

Figure 1-14   Frequency encoding in the x direction. Here the gradient decreases from *left* to *right*.

spatial frequencies are located at the periphery of k-space and contain information related to image sharpness. This is demonstrated in Fig. 1-15 by viewing k-space and the clinical images reconstructed from the center or periphery of k-space.

MAGNETIC RESONANCE IMAGING PULSE SEQUENCES

MRI pulse sequences are basically the recipe for the application of RF pulses, the sequencing of gradient pulses in the x, y, and z direction, and the acquisition of the resultant MR signal.

The most basic component of a pulse sequence is the specification of the RF excitation and subsequent signal detection. Timing diagrams for two pulse sequences [inversion recovery (IR) and spin echo (SE)] are given in Figs. 1-16 and 1-17. We discuss each sequence in detail.

The schematic diagram for the IR pulse sequence is shown in Fig. 1-16. This sequence is characterized by the application of a RF pulse of sufficient power to tip the nuclei through 180°, an inversion time (TI), and the subsequent application of a 90° pulse (to rotate the magnetization into the transverse plane), followed by signal detection. This pulse sequence can be used to measure the longitudinal recovery of magnetization (see Fig. 1-18). Because the range of measured magnetization for this pulse sequence varies from $-M_z$ to $+M_z$, if phase-sensitive image reconstruction is employed, the magnitude of measured differences for a sample due to T1 relaxation may be larger with the IR sequence than those with the spin-echo technique below (in which the longitudinal magnetization varies from 0 to $+M_z$). These differences may not be as pronounced with magnitude reconstruction (Fig. 1-18). Hence, image contrast due to T1 differences can be greater with IR. Example images acquired using this pulse sequence and magnitude reconstruction are given in Fig. 1-19.

The pulse diagram for the SE pulse sequence is shown in Fig. 1-17. The spin-echo pulse sequence is characterized by the application of a 90° pulse, which therefore tips the nuclei into the transverse or x–y plane. This is followed by successive 180° pulses, separated by the delay period TE, which causes the formation of successive signals for detection, termed spin echoes. The entire pulse sequence is repeated following the delay interval TR. The formation of spin echoes is demonstrated in Fig. 1-20. The fundamental characteristic of this sequence lies in the fact that the nuclei are dephasing following the 90° pulse. If this dephasing spin system is rotated through 180°, individual spins will now be traveling toward one another instead of away from one another. When all spins meet, a spin echo is produced. Following that moment in time, the spin system once again will be dephasing and can be refocused or rephased with another 180° pulse. Depending on the acquisition TE and TR, this sequence can be useful in demonstrating differences due to either T1 or T2 relaxation time as shown in Fig. 1-21. Example images acquired using this pulse sequence are given in Fig. 1-22. In summary, the spin density, T1, and T2 represent inherent properties of tissues. TE and TR are properties of the image acquisition that are under operator control. The TE and TR of an image acquisition can be manipulated such that the difference between signals from tissues (which ultimately determines the image contrast) is weighted by tissue spin density, T1, or T2 relaxation.

The previous discussion dealt with pulse sequences that were concerned only with RF excitation and signal detection. Hence, this discussion would be germane to spectroscopy as well as imaging. For MRI, the pulse sequence must also identify the timing information associated with the gradients necessary to prepare or localize the signal for image reconstruction.

An example of an MRI pulse sequence is shown in Figs. 1-11 and 1-23. We note that the gradients are labeled as slice selection, phase encoding, and readout (or frequency encoding). The reason for this specification is that slice selection can be along the transverse, coronal, or sagittal planes, with phase and readout gradients along the other two orthogonal planes. The dotted lines indicating progression of phase encoding implies that this pulse sequence will be repeated many times, with a differing amount of phase encoding at each repetition. The rest of the sequence (RF, Gx, and Gz) will remain exactly the same with each repetition.

It is the variation in timing and relative temporal placements of the three magnetic gradient sequences that are largely responsible for the plethora of the imaging sequences currently available. We use such diagrams in later sections to understand the differences and consequences of employing various pulse sequences. An understanding of the effects of frequency shifts and dephasing effects are of central importance to understanding image characteristics and artifacts in MRI. Because this is a currently active area of

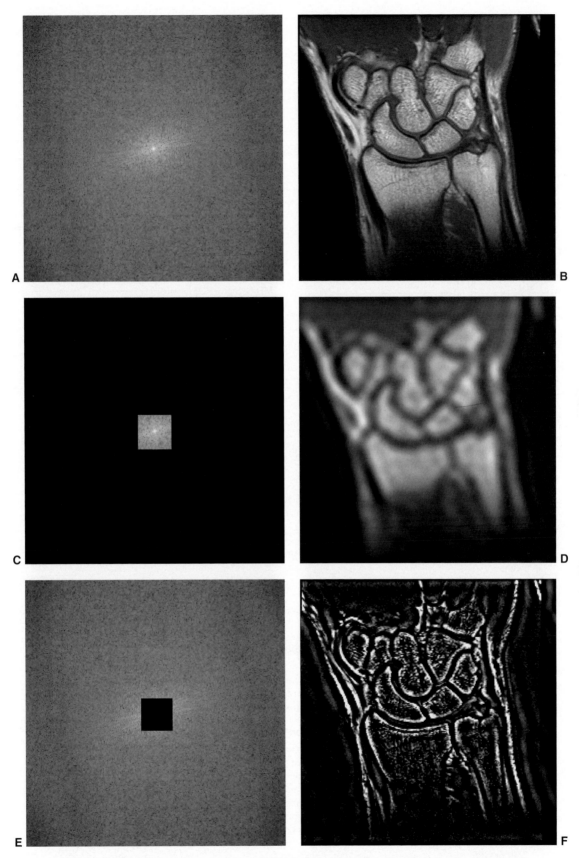

Figure 1-15   Reconstruction of k-space. **A:** Original k-space data. **B:** Image data reconstructed from **A**, showing good image contrast and spatial resolution. **C:** Center portion of k-space. **D:** Image data reconstructed from **C**, showing good image contrast but poor spatial resolution. **E:** Peripheral portion of k-space. **F:** Image data reconstructed from **E**, showing poor image contrast but good spatial resolution (*edges*).

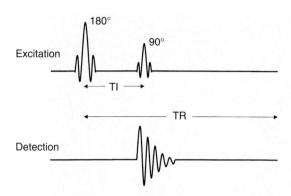

Figure 1-16   Inversion recovery pulse sequence.

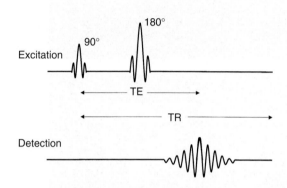

Figure 1-17   Spin-echo pulse sequence.

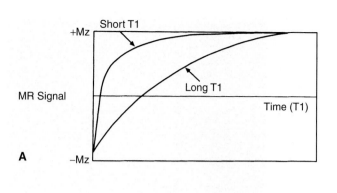

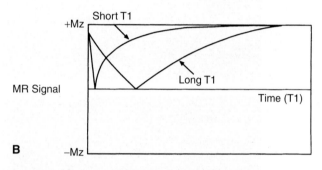

Figure 1-18   Recovery of magnetization for inversion recovery pulse sequence. **A:** Phase sensitive image reconstruction. **B:** Magnitude image reconstruction.

TABLE 1-4

MOTION-ARTIFACT-REDUCTION TECHNIQUES

Acronym	Description	Vendor
A. Spatial Presaturation to Reduce MR Signal Intensity in Specific Locations		
SAT	Saturation or Presaturation	GE, Hitachi, Shimadzu, Siemens
REST	Regional saturation technique	Philips
B. Spectral Presaturation to Reduce MR Signal Intensity of Fat		
FATSAT	Fat saturation	GE, Siemens
SPIR	Spectral presaturation with inversion recovery	Philips
ChemSat	Chemical saturation	GE
C. Reduction of Motion-Induced Phase Shifts During TE		
GMR	Gradient motion reduction	Siemens
GMN	Gradient moment nulling	GE
FLOW COMP	Flow compensation	GE, Toshiba
CFAST	Cerebrospinal-fluid-artifact suppression technique	Toshiba
FLAG	Flow-adjustable gradients	Philips
FC	Flow compensation	GE, Philips, Siemens
GR or GRE	Gradient rephrasing	Hitachi

Adapted from Acronyms common to MRI. *JMR*, 1992; 2(Suppl.). *SMRI MR research guide*, 1992–1993 edition.

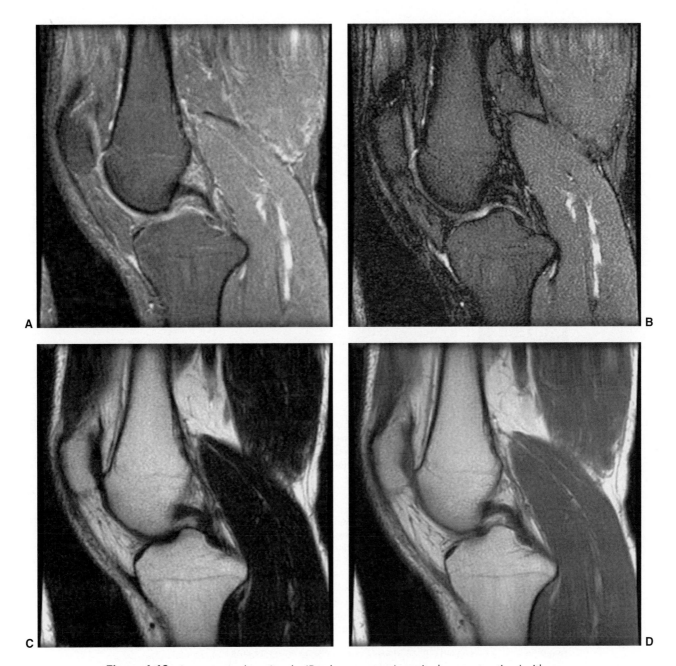

Figure 1-19   Image examples using the IR pulse sequence (magnitude reconstructions) with varying TI (TE = 14, 256 × 192, TR = 1500, 24 cm, 5 mm, 0.75 NEX, SAT on). **A:** TI = 100. **B:** TI = 170. **C:** TI = 400. **D:** TI = 800.

development, similar techniques have been developed by different sources, resulting in different acronyms for essentially the same procedure.

It is important to note that although essentially similar results have been accomplished by various investigational groups and vendors, hardware and software differences in the exact realization may result in subtle but sometimes important image variation. Tables 1-4 and 1-5 present a compilation of the acronyms for similar imaging techniques (11,12). These acronyms represent in some cases broad classifications provided by various manufacturers, yet they are routinely used in the literature. For more information about

any of these techniques, the reader is referred to the technical representatives of the particular vendor of interest.

FLOW AND MOTION COMPENSATION TECHNIQUES

Any movement of structures during MRI data acquisition can cause artifacts ranging from image "unsharpness" (as experienced in other modalities) to intense streaks that totally obscure the image. Such movements in patients can be caused by fluid flow or physiologic motion. Because the

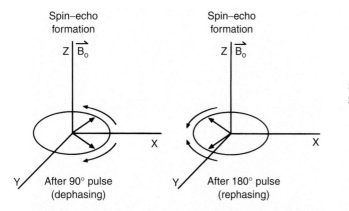

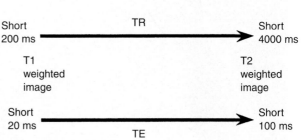

Figure 1-20 Spin-echo formation. **A:** Individual nuclei are precessing away from one another following 90° RF pulse. **B:** Individual nuclei are precessing toward one another following 180° (rephasing) RF pulse.

Figure 1-21 Nomogram for contrast dependence using the spin-echo sequence.

TABLE 1-5
ACRONYMS FOR FAST MRI

Acronym	Definition
Spin-Echo Based Techniques	
FSE/TSE	Fast Spin-Echo/Turbo Spin-Echo. Uses series of 180° pulses to generate multiple spin echoes, each of which is used to fill lines of k-space.
RARE	Rapid Acquisition with Relaxation Enhancement. Phase encodes between multiple 180° pulses to reduce acquisition time (rather than collecting multiple echoes).
Gradient-Echo Based Techniques	
FAST	Also called FISP or GRASS. An SFP sequence that refocuses only in the phase-encoding direction (enhances T1/T2 effects).
FISP	Fast Imaging with Steady-state free Precession—see FAST.
FLASH	Fast-Low Angle single-SHot imaging. Dephases transverse magnetization prior to next RF pulse. Signal depends on T1 and $T2^*$.
FSPGR	Fast SPGR. Uses fractional RF pulses and fractional echoes (data collected from only a portion of the echo) to decrease imaging time.
GRASS	GRAdient-recalled Steady State—see FAST.
GFE	Gradient Field Echo imaging. Fast GFE is also known as FGFE or FFE.
SFP	Steady-state Free Precession.
SPGR	SPoiled GRadient echo. Uses RF pulse to spoil (dephase) residual signal, may be used in 2D or 3D mode.
SSFP	Another widely used short form for SFP.
TRUE FISP	An SFP experiment that rephases in both read and phase encoding. Signal varies with T1/T2 and $T2^*$. Also called FIESTA and Balanced Fast Field Echo.
VIBE	Volume Interpolated Breath-hold Examination. FLASH technique optimized for 3D abdominal imaging.
General Techniques	
EPI	Echo-Planar Imaging. Fast read-out technique which includes BLIP-EPI when gradient pulses between read intervals are applied and SEPI when spiral EPI is used.
HALF FOURIER	Any technique that uses only one-half of the usual number all steps had been used. Also implemented as fractional or partial Fourier.
SMASH	Parallel imaging technique in which k-space data from multiple coils is interpolated to form an image
SENSE	Parallel imaging technique in which image domain data from multiple coils is "unwrapped" to reconstruct a larger field-of-view.

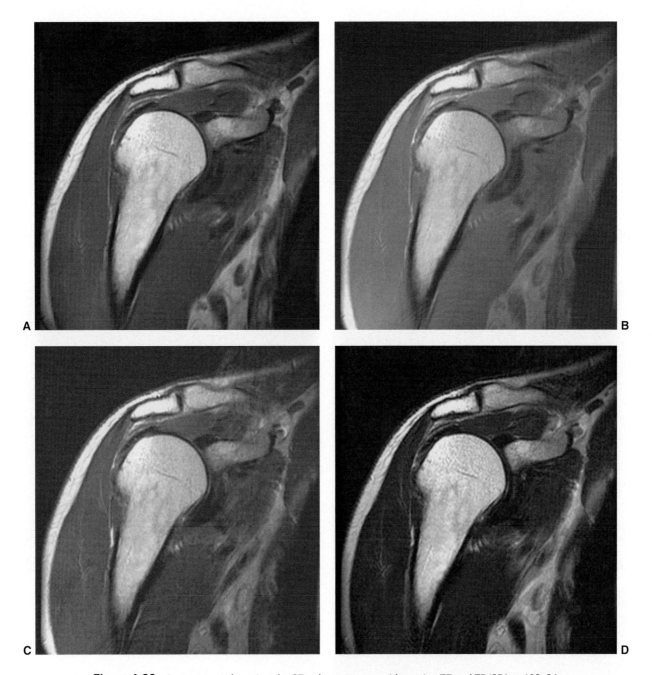

Figure 1-22 Image examples using the SE pulse sequence with varying TE and TR (256 × 192, 24 cm, 5 mm, 2 NEX). **A:** T1 weighted, TR = 500, TE = 20. **B:** Proton density weighted, TR = 2000, TE = 20. **C:** T2 weighted, TR = 2000, TE = 60. **D:** T2 weighted, fast spin echo, TR = 3000, TE (effective) = 90.

total sampling time in the phase encoding direction (TR × number of phase encoding steps) is substantially greater than the sampling time in the frequency encoding direction (~10 ms time frame), the amount of movement is much greater in the phase encoding direction. Image artifacts generally appear as linear bands in the phase encoding direction. Although the fundamental principles of physical movement during data acquisition are the same for both fluid flow and physiologic motion, the nature of each produces different artifacts and,

therefore, different strategies are needed for motion artifact compensation.

Flow artifacts, such as those shown in Fig. 1-24, occur because the spins in the flowing blood accrue phase due to their movement in the presence of the gradient (13). Since the flow is not constant, the amount of accrued phase varies from view to view. The 2DFT image reconstruction translates this view-to-view phase variation to a distribution of intensities extending along the phase encoding direction (flow artifacts). Two approaches are often used to

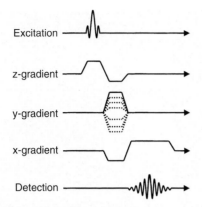

Figure 1-23 An MRI pulse sequence.

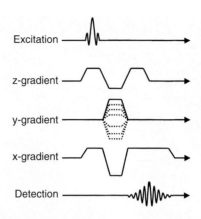

Figure 1-25 Pulse sequence that illustrates gradient moment nulling. Extra applications of the slice selection (*z*) and frequency encoding (*x*) gradients are utilized to compensate for flow.

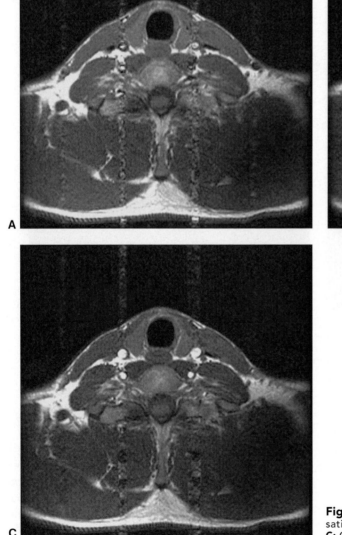

Figure 1-24 Flow artifact compensation. **A:** No flow compensation. **B:** Compensation using spatial presaturation. **C:** Compensation using gradient moment nulling.

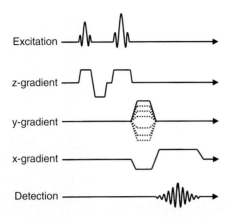

Figure 1-26 Pulse sequence that illustrates spatial presaturation. An extra RF pulse and application of the z-gradient is used for presaturation in the superior-inferior direction.

eliminate flow artifacts: gradient moment nulling (GMN) and spatial presaturation (SAT). Both techniques involve changes in the basic pulse sequence yet provide different corrections. GMN (14) essentially eliminates the phase accrual due to movement of spins, thereby decreasing the artifact and producing an image in which the vessel is of high intensity. SAT (15) eliminates the high signal due to the inflow of fresh spins and produces an image with vessels of low intensity. The pulse sequences for each technique are given in Figs. 1-25 and 1-26. As demonstrated, GMN is accomplished by variation in the slice selection and frequency encoding gradients. SAT is accomplished by the addition of a 90° RF pulse and a localization gradient that is repeated for each slice of a multiple slice acquisition. The effects of flow compensation are shown in Fig. 1-24. Table 1-4 contains a summary of artifact reduction techniques and the acronyms used by various vendors.

ANGIOGRAPHIC TECHNIQUES

While flow compensation techniques are used to suppress unwanted signals from flowing blood, other techniques can be used to create images of flowing blood to visualize vascular structure. The three primary techniques currently in use are *time-of-flight* (TOF), *phase contrast* (PC), and *contrast-enhanced* MR angiography.

TOF techniques are based on gradient-echo pulse sequences with flow compensation and take advantage of a "flow-related enhancement" phenomenon to distinguish between moving and stationary spins. Because TOF pulse sequences use short TR values, the net magnetization from stationary spins does not have time to recover fully. The signal produced by these spins is low and results in dark pixel values in the image. Blood flowing into the tissue contains "fresh" spins that have not experienced the repeated RF pulses. The signal produced by these spins results in bright pixel values in the image. To optimize this flow-related signal enhancement, image slices are oriented

perpendicular to the direction of blood flow, as shown in Fig. 1-27A. The stack of slices from the imaging volume may then be reformatted (e.g., using a *maximum intensity projection* technique) to visualize the vascular structure as shown in Fig. 1-27B.

The PC technique takes advantage of the phase differences of spins moving during the application of bipolar (positive and negative) gradients. For stationary tissue, the application of bipolar gradients will have no net effect on the phase of the spins. Spins that have moved during the application of the bipolar gradients will experience a different amount of positive and negative phase accumulation, resulting in a net phase difference. This phase difference is used to distinguish between moving and stationary tissue (see Fig. 1-27C).

The third method commonly used for visualizing vascular structure in MR is contrast-enhanced angiography (CE-MRA). This method utilizes the T1 shortening properties of a paramagnetic contrast agent (e.g., a gadolinium chelate) to enhance the signal from blood after contrast injection. The imaging pulse sequence will be a rapid T1 weighted sequence optimized to acquire the center of k-space (image contrast information) during the time when the peak concentration of contrast agent passes through the vascular structure of interest (see Fig. 1-27D,E). CE-MRA may also be used with multi-stage volume acquisitions to create images of the peripheral vasculature with a single contrast injection (see Fig. 1-27F).

FAST SCANNING TECHNIQUES

In general, the fundamental limit on image resolution in MRI is motion unsharpness due to physiologic movement within the patient. Accordingly, techniques have been developed (12,16,17) to acquire MRI data in very short time periods. One popular technique uses an approach to limit the flip angle of RF excitation (less than the usual 90°) and thereby decrease the time necessary to wait for recovery. Hence, the repetition time can be decreased, allowing faster acquisitions. The concept of limited flip angle is illustrated in Fig. 1-28. The signal that is acquired is most often an echo, as described earlier, except that the echo is produced not by successive 180° RF pulses but by reversal of the gradient field. The pulse sequence for this technique of gradient recalled echo (GRE) or field echo (FE) imaging is shown in Fig. 1-29. The principle of GRE imaging lies in the fact that the application of a gradient actually dephases the spins due to a difference in field strength which is dependent upon position. By reversing the direction of the gradients (−G to +G), the effect is to rephase the spins that were initially dephased (see Fig. 1-30). The contrast weighting dependencies in GRE imaging are given in Table 1-6.

Another technique uses multiple spin echoes to acquire different lines of k-space data (views), rather than to create multiple images. Acquiring eight echoes in this manner

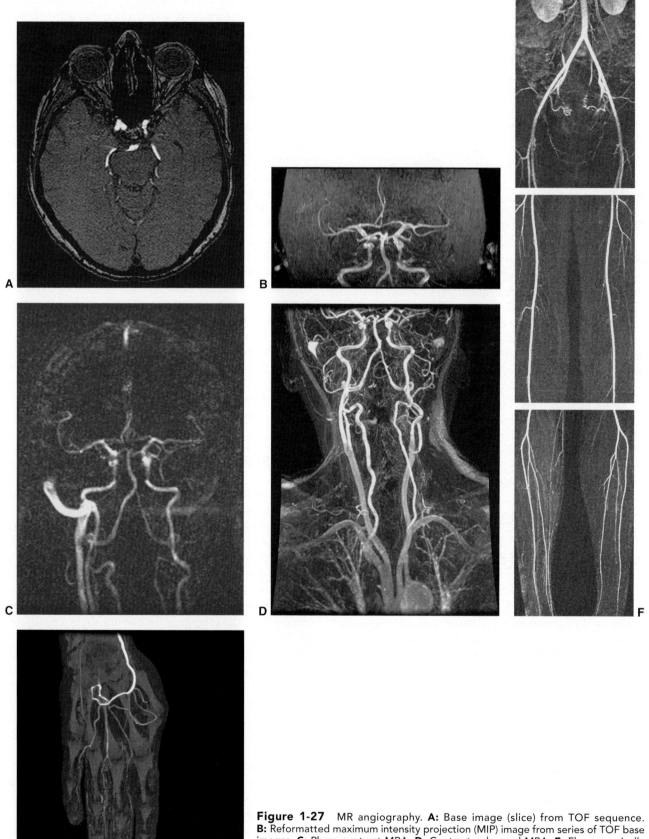

Figure 1-27 MR angiography. **A:** Base image (slice) from TOF sequence. **B:** Reformatted maximum intensity projection (MIP) image from series of TOF base images. **C:** Phase contrast MRA. **D:** Contrast-enhanced MRA. **E:** Fluoroscopically triggered contrast-enhanced MRA of the hand. **F:** Multi-stage peripheral MRA with single contrast injection.

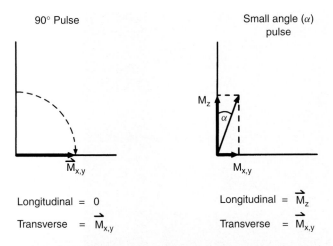

Figure 1-28 Limited flip angle RF excitation showing the presence of longitudinal magnetization following excitation.

decreases the scan time by a factor of eight, but slice throughput and image contrast issues are also important. In general, useful image contrast and resolution are obtained in shorter acquisition time when compared to the standard (one view per TR) acquisition. A compilation of various fast scanning techniques is presented in Table 1-5 (12). Echo planar techniques acquire image data in a short period of time, as short as 40 ms. Often this requires special hardware, although interleaved versions of EPI can be used on standard imager hardware. These techniques acquire the image data using multiple "shots" or acquisitions. This results in breathhold acquisition times for a single image of 1 to 20 seconds, depending upon the number of interleaves and desired image resolution.

PARALLEL IMAGING TECHNIQUES

Receiver coils placed at the patient's surface have a nonuniform signal response with depth as shown in Fig. 1-31A. This phenomenon can be exploited to decrease image

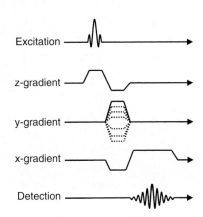

Figure 1-29 Pulse sequence diagram that illustrates gradient recalled echo formation. Extra application of the frequency encoding gradient (x) causes rephasing and hence echo production.

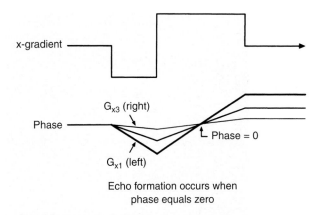

Figure 1-30 The production of echoes by gradient reversal. G × 1 and G × 3 refer to Figure 1-14.

acquisition time or increase image resolution. The signal at a single location within the image is measured by each of multiple coils. This data redundancy can be used to fill k-space lines, allowing a complete image to be reconstructed from fewer phase encoding steps (resulting in scan time reduction as shown in Fig. 1-31B), or added to the standard data acquisition to provide higher image resolution with no time penalty. It should be noted that the resulting image will have decreased SNR in comparison to the original acquisition.

CHEMICAL SHIFT IMAGING TECHNIQUES

The principle involved in the phenomenon described as "chemical shift" relates to the difference in Larmor frequencies for spins at different field strengths. The magnetic field actually experienced by a nucleus will depend on the molecular configuration of the chemical backbone to which the nucleus is attached. This depends on the configuration of electrons about the atom, which results in slight changes of the magnetic field at the nucleus due to the shielding effects of the electrons. Hence, at a constant field strength, the precessional frequency of fat is different from the precessional frequency of water (e.g., by about 220 Hz at 1.5 T). Therefore,

TABLE 1-6
CONTRAST DEPENDENCE USING THE GRADIENT-ECHO SEQUENCE (GRASS)

TR	TE	Flip Angle (α)	Contrast
Long (300 ms)	Short (13 ms)	High (60)	T1
Long (300 ms)	Long (30 ms)	Low (10)	T2*
Short (30 ms)	Short	High (60)	T2*
Long (300 ms)	Short	Low (10)	Proton density

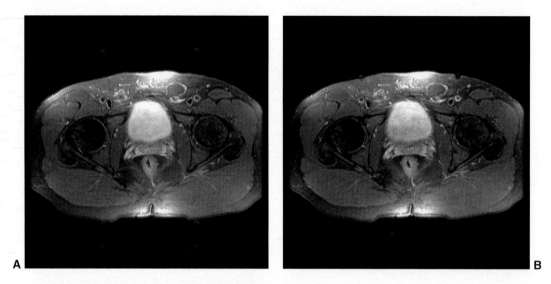

Figure 1-31 Parallel imaging in MRI. **A:** Original image acquired with an acquisition time of 2:36. **B:** Image acquired using parallel imaging technique and an acquisition time of 1:28.

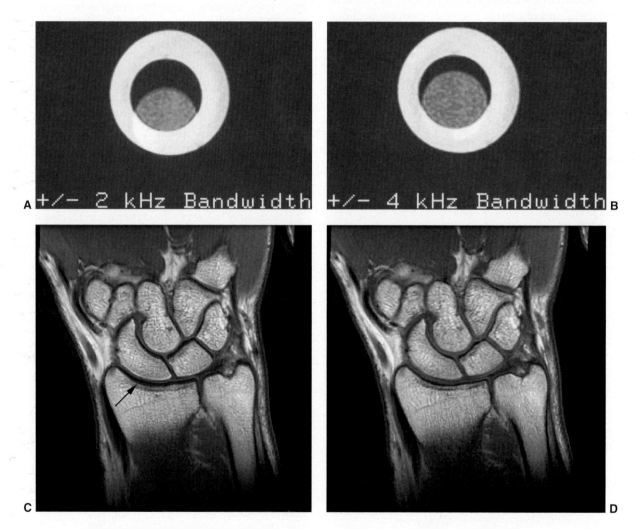

Figure 1-32 Chemical shift in MRI. The frequency encoding axis is vertical in these images. Note that the image displacement is more pronounced when using a narrow receive bandwidth. For these images the receive bandwidth equals +/− 2kHz (**A**), +/− 4kHz (**B**), +/− 10 kHz (**C**), and +/− 32 kHz (**D**).

the "shift" refers to the precessional frequency that results from the "chemical" environment of the nuclei.

The chemical shift can defeat the image reconstruction process and result in a spatial shift in the image. The images in Fig. 1-32 A and B show coronal images of a vial of mineral oil within a cylinder of water. The central oil displaces along the frequency encoding direction, by an amount determined by the chemical shift (3.4 ppm at 1.5 T = 220 Hz) and the acquisition receive bandwidth. The receive bandwidth defines the range of frequencies that comprise the image field of view along the frequency encoding axis. As the range of frequency narrows (bandwidth decreases), the 220 Hz chemical shift becomes associated with a larger distance. For example, an acquisition bandwidth of 32 kHz and frequency encoding resolution of 256 results in 125 Hz frequency range for each pixel in the image (32,000 Hz/256 pixels). The shift within the image due to chemical shift in this scenario is 1.76 pixels (220 Hz divided by 125 Hz/pixel). For a 4 kHz bandwidth, the chemical shift is 14 pixels (220 Hz/16 Hz/pixel), as shown in Table 1-7. This shift is also observed by comparing Fig. 1-32 C and D, as noted by the apparent increase in radial cortical thickening (arrow).

The chemical shift phenomenon can also be exploited to obtain images that suppress either the fat or water signals. The technique, first reported by Dixon (18), uses the SE pulse sequence shown in Fig. 1-33 or gradient-echo images acquired at specific TE values. As demonstrated in Fig. 1-34, due to differences in precessional frequencies, the fat and water signals can be obtained when the two are either together (in phase) or opposite (opposed). Algebraic combination of these images results in the suppression of one or the other signal, as demonstrated in Fig. 1-35.

Other techniques are also useful to suppress "unwanted" signal intensities. Fat suppression can be accomplished using the STIR (19) pulse sequence as illustrated in Fig. 1-36, and shown in Fig. 1-37. Here a short inversion time (TI) is used to create an image where the net longitudinal magnetization of fat is minimal. Spectral presaturation (fat sat) is often accomplished by application of an RF pulse designed to saturate only fat based spins prior to application of the imaging pulse sequence. A third technique designated as "classic" fat

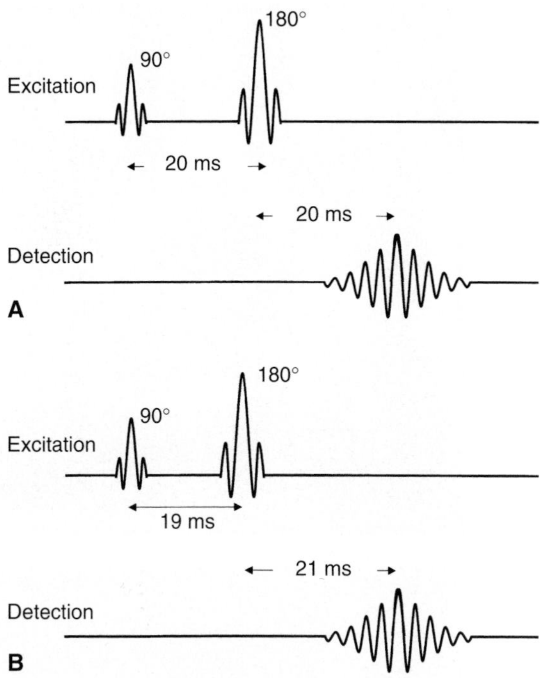

Figure 1-33 Pulse sequences for chemical shift imaging. **A:** Equal timing to acquire in-phase images for a spin-echo sequence. **B:** Unequal timing to acquire an opposed image in a spin-echo sequence.

suppression or water excitation excites a narrow range of proton frequencies centered on water. The fat protons that are not excited will not contribute to the MR signal. These techniques decrease the intensity of fat anywhere within the image, and are dependent on the RF homogeneity, which can result in nonuniform fat suppression around surface coils, for example.

MAGNETIC RESONANCE IMAGING ARTIFACTS

Artifacts in MRI can come from many sources (20–22). In general, the primary sources of artifacts are those that affect

TABLE 1-7	
CHEMICAL SHIFTS ASSOCIATED WITH ACQUISITION BANDWIDTH AT 1.5 T (256 PIXEL RESOLUTION ALONG THE FREQUENCY ENCODING AXIS)	

Receive Bandwidth (kHz)	No. of Shifted Pixels Associated with 220 Hz Chemical Shift (1.5T)
±16 (32)	1.76
±8 (16)	3.50
±4 (8)	7.00
±2 (4)	14.00

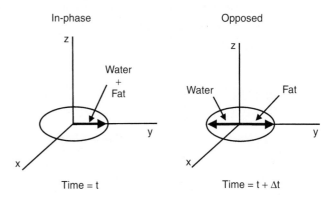

Figure 1-34 Precessional behavior for water and fat. Water precesses faster than fat.

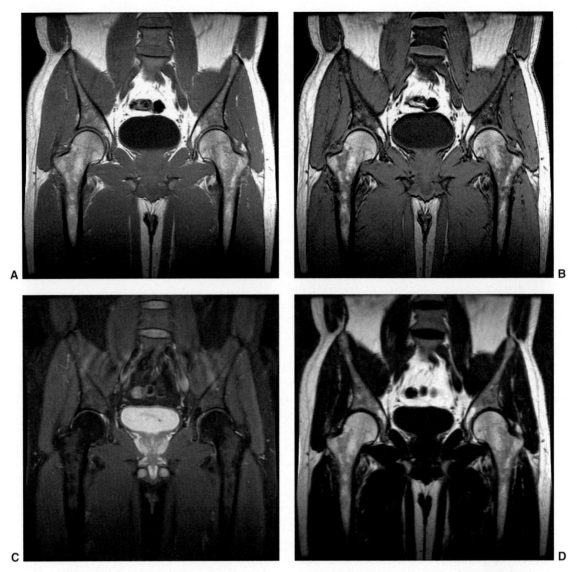

Figure 1-35   Chemical shift images. **A:** In-phase image. **B:** Opposed image. **C:** Water image. **D:** Fat image.

the frequency or phase dispersion of the spin system. Recall that, fundamentally, the signal strength at a particular frequency is interpreted to reside at a particular point in space. Hence, anything that changes the frequency or adds signal at a particular frequency will result in a displacement or addition of intensity in the direction of the frequency encoding gradient. In an analogous fashion, something that changes the relative order of the phase of the spin precession (either during or between views) will produce artifacts in the phase encoding direction. The sources of such artifacts are wide-ranging, such as data sampling problems, electromagnetic noise, patient motion, magnetic field inhomogeneities, magnetic susceptibility, computer malfunctions, and chemical shift (20–22). A listing of some common artifacts and their effects is given in Table 1-8. Examples of several of these artifacts are demonstrated in Fig. 1-38. It is also important to understand that particular types of artifacts may be associated with specific types of imaging procedures (e.g., spin-echo imaging versus GRE imaging).

TABLE 1-8
MRI ARTIFACTS

Frequency Effects	Phase Effects
Chemical Shift	Wrap-around/aliasing
Susceptibility	Gibbs
Magnetic field inhomogeneity	Motion

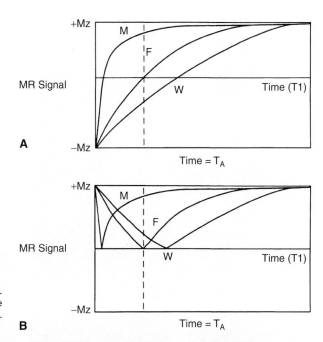

Figure 1-36 The effect obtained with short TI inversion recovery. By gathering data at time T_A, signal from tissue F will be zero where both other tissues of shorter and longer T_1 will be enhanced. **A:** Phase sensitive reconstruction. **B:** Magnitude reconstruction.

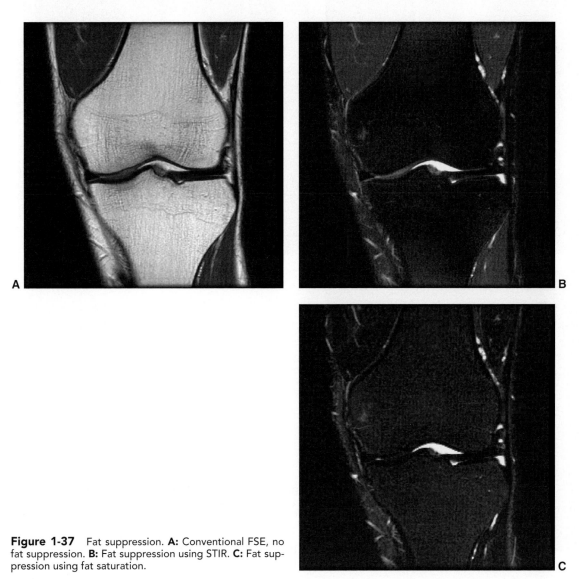

Figure 1-37 Fat suppression. **A:** Conventional FSE, no fat suppression. **B:** Fat suppression using STIR. **C:** Fat suppression using fat saturation.

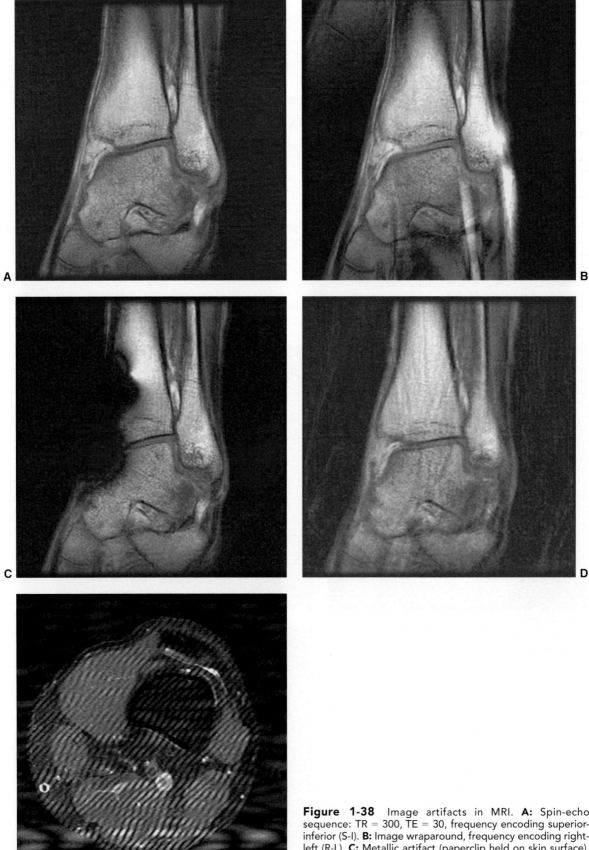

Figure 1-38 Image artifacts in MRI. **A:** Spin-echo sequence: TR = 300, TE = 30, frequency encoding superior-inferior (S-I). **B:** Image wraparound, frequency encoding right-left (R-L). **C:** Metallic artifact (paperclip held on skin surface). **D:** Patient motion (slow rocking of ankle during acquisition). **E:** RF artifact (interference from another nearby MR scanner).

RECEIVER COIL INTENSITY/ UNIFORMITY CORRECTION

As presented in the parallel imaging section, receiver coils (including arrays of multiple coils) have the highest signal near the coil, which falls off with depth. This effect is apparent with individual surface coils as well as coil arrays as shown in Fig. 1-39A. The high signal at the surface is artifactual, a direct result of coil positioning and geometry. Algorithms and techniques can be employed to correct this bright signal located near the coils. The uniformity-corrected image shown in Fig. 1-39B retains the image resolution showing the underlying anatomy while also preserving the image contrast weighting associated with the original acquisitions.

PRACTICAL ASPECTS OF MAGNETIC RESONANCE IMAGING

Biologic Effects

Three areas have received attention in terms of the biologic effects of MRI: high static magnetic fields (B_o), time-varying magnetic fields (gradients), and radio frequency (RF) irradiation (23–25).

The first area concerned the use of strong static magnetic fields (B_o). The primary theoretical concerns had to do with the effects of the magnetic field on the protons and electrons within molecules that could affect chemical bonding or biochemical reactions. Experiments have been conducted both *in vitro* as well as *in vivo* for cellular preparations, tissues, and organisms (26–28). The conclusion

from these data is that no deleterious biologic effects have been demonstrated for magnetic field strengths commonly found in MRI. Currently, 8 T is accepted as the limit below which no deleterious biologic effects have been demonstrated.

The second area of concern centered on the use of time-varying magnetic fields (gradient fields). Changing magnetic fields can induce electric currents in biologic tissues. The two tissues of primary concern are the heart and the nervous system. In addition, it is possible to stimulate the retina with an appropriate gradient. Current induction is dependent upon the rate of magnetic field change (dB/dt) and the duty cycle (the relationship of pulse width and the interpulse delay). In the systems studied, the thresholds for these biological effects are sufficiently high that a biological stimulation does not occur for the gradient fields typically found in MRI, usually less than 400 T/s. Since peripheral nerve stimulation represents a sensation and not a deleterious biologic effect, it can be used as a safe level of operation. With this in mind, dB/dt change at levels below discomfort or pain are allowed.

EPI and fast spin-echo based acquisitions that can use gradients that easily exceed 40 T/s are currently under development. These are promising imaging techniques, and the effects of these high dB/dt levels are areas of current research.

The third area of concern centered on the biological effects associated with the use of radio frequency radiation. This field of investigation has been the subject of scientific inquiry (apart from MRI) for quite a long time. The primary biologic effect of interest is that of heating due to the oscillation of the atoms and molecules stimulated by the radio frequency radiation. The amount of heating is

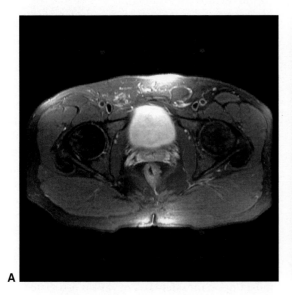
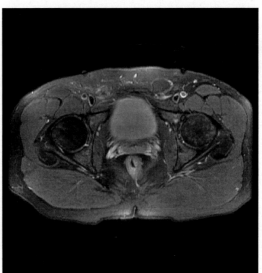

A   **B**

Figure 1-39   Receiver coil intensity-uniformity correction. **A:** Original image with no correction. **B:** Corrected image. Both images are displayed at the same window width and level.

dependent on several factors, including the RF frequency, the absorption of the RF energy, and the thermoregulatory mechanisms within humans.

The quantity used to characterize the RF absorption is the specific absorption rate (SAR), which is a measure of power deposition in watts per unit mass. This absorption is essentially dependent on the conductivity and density of the patient, and the electric field strength of the RF radiation. The SAR is related to the RF pulse height, the RF pulse width, the interpulse delay, and the absorption properties of the patient. Most current MRI systems require an input of patient weight and calculate the SAR for a given pulse sequence. This calculation in general is an overestimate of the RF heating because most current models do not account for the astoundingly efficient thermoregulatory mechanism of healthy humans (29). Although a rise in body temperature is possible, it is usually not a problem in patients whose cardiovascular or thermoregulatory systems are not compromised. Hence, RF heating is not deemed a contraindication for the use of routine clinical MRI.

The U.S. Food and Drug Administration (FDA) has developed guidelines for nonsignificant risk (30) regarding the strength of static, time-varying, and RF fields for MRI. The current guidelines are listed in Table 1-9. At the present time, all clinical MRI systems operate within these guidelines.

Safety

The MRI environment is different from other imaging areas. The following highlights the main issues associated with patient and occupational safety in the MRI environment. The safety risks are minimized with diligence and ongoing personnel training. Routine review of established safety procedures for medical emergencies and fire is recommended. The safety procedures used in the MRI environment are

designed to protect everyone in the scan room. It is important to train and support the individuals who are responsible for safety at your MRI suite.

The following are important points regarding your patient's safety that should be considered before entering the MRI environment.

1. It is important to verify the safety of any questionable device prior to MRI. No one with a pacemaker should enter the MR scan room. Also, various models of aneurysm clips and catheters may not be allowed in the MR scanner. Dental implants held by magnets may be damaged by the strong magnetic field. A list of contraindications should also be reviewed with the patient prior to MRI.
2. All equipment entering the scan room must be verified to be MR safe. Even equipment that is moved in and out of the scan room often must be checked.
3. Verify that any catheters or wires that may be involved in the care of your patient are MR safe. This is especially important if surface coils or electrocardiographic monitoring is used for the examination.
4. Electrocardiogram leads must be placed down the center of the magnet bore as much as possible. Do not allow the leads to touch the magnet bore wall.
5. Whenever possible, position the patient away from any wires and the sides of the bore. Generally the MR technologist will work to position the patient for imaging by centering the region of clinical interest.
6. Because of the magnetic and RF fields, special equipment is used in and around MR imagers. If you have equipment that you are interested in, verify that it is MR compatible prior to use.

With regard to occupational safety, keep the following important points in mind when entering and working within the MR environment.

1. The magnet is always on! Any ferromagnetic material can become a projectile with the potential to cause harm.
2. No one with a pacemaker should enter the MR scan room. The MR technologist must also be informed of any aneurysm clips, catheters, cochlear implants, vascular filters, or dental implants held by magnets.
3. You should empty your pockets prior to entering the scan room to minimize the chance of a projectile.
4. Again, any equipment entering the scan room must be verified to be MR safe. Even equipment that is moved in and out of the scan room often must be checked—you may be unaware that someone has placed a pair of scissors on top of your MR safe equipment, for example.

To date, no deleterious effects have been demonstrated from working within a clinical MRI environment. The most important safety risk of MRI is associated with metal objects inadvertently entering the scan room and being attracted to the magnet. Where noise from some scanning

TABLE 1-9
FDA SAFETY PARAMETER ACTION LEVELS

Static magnetic field (B_o)	8 T or less
Specific absorption rate (SAR)	4 W/kg or less (whole body) averaged over 15 min 3 W/kg or less (head) averaged over 10 min 8 W/kg in 1g (head/torso), or 12 W/kg in 1 g (extremities) over 5 min
Changing gradient fields (dB/dt)	Below threshold of severe discomfort or painful nerve stimulation
Acoustic noise	140 dB or less (peak unweighted sound pressure level), or 99 dB [A-weighted root-mean-square (rms) sound pressure level with hearing protection]

sequences is an issue, earplugs or other MR safe hearing protection is recommended. The RF field used for imaging can result in slight patient heating. However, tolerable limits for patient RF exposure have been set by the FDA. RF exposure outside of the magnet bore is decreased by a factor of 1,000,000 at 3 ft and it would take more than 100 years of continuous RF exposure at 3 ft to equal that of 1 hour in the magnet. You will not experience an increase in temperature due to occupational RF exposure during a clinical MRI exam. Helpful MR safety-related resources include references (31) and (32).

Operational Aspects

As with other imaging systems, the detailed operational procedures for any MRI system are dependent, to a large extent, on factors related to the operation of the department and institution. However, some general observations regarding operational parameters unique to MRI can be made.

Security issues are more important for MRI than most other imaging systems. Magnetic field strengths of 1 to 4 T have sufficient power to lift a wheelchair off the ground and pull it to the magnet. Hence, it is important that the entrance to the magnet room be limited and under the control of appropriate personnel. Many facilities also restrict access such that maintenance personnel, emergency teams, and even firefighters are denied access to the magnet room. Since pacemakers may change pacing modes in fields of 5 g or greater, general access should be restricted in those areas where the field is greater than 5 g. Metallic objects should be tested with a strong, small magnet to determine if they contain any ferromagnetic material prior to placing them in the magnetic room. This is particularly true for equipment that may leave the room for servicing or modification.

There are many patient and personnel safety issues that must be discussed and decided upon during the design and installation of the MRI system (31). MRI is contraindicated for some patients due to the presence of certain biomedical implants. A determination must be made by the facility as to which devices, if present, would constitute a contraindication for an MRI exam (33).

The emergency procedures must be explicit. Significant harm can come to both personnel and patient if the emergency resuscitation team were to enter the magnet room. It is important that both visual and audio contact be provided for both patient comfort and assurance of patient safety. Both respiratory and cardiac monitoring must be available if any critically ill patients are to be scanned.

With regard to personnel, it is useful to bring all alarm systems (scan room oxygen, patient oxygen, computer room temperature, cryogen storage, smoke detectors, halon release, etc.) to one panel so that the technologist may locate the source of an alarm quickly and easily. Many facilities also utilize a lock for the magnet room door with only authorized personnel (normally MRI technologists) having access to the key. It is also useful to install a warning device, such as a photo-optical or infrared chime system, to alert the MRI technologist that someone is approaching the magnet room door.

MR safe air packs can be purchased and made available at each site in the unlikely event of a quench with the release of helium into the magnet room. This is a situation with a low probability of occurrence yet catastrophic consequences. A technologist rushing into the magnet room during such an event to assist the patient may quite likely die of asphyxia before the patient is withdrawn from the room.

In facilities experiencing their initial encounter with MRI, it is essential that the radiology staff as well as support staff, engineers, security personnel, custodial personnel, and fire department personnel receive adequate safety training prior to routine operation of MRI system.

Perhaps of greatest importance from an operational sense is the design and implementation of acquisition protocols to optimize the diagnostic capability of MRI. With the vast armament of scan sequences and scan parameters available, a balance must be made between the number and type of scans that are performed and the amount of time available to scan an individual patient.

Siting Requirements

The placement of MRI systems within a hospital is significantly different from other imaging modalities. Today, many systems use superconducting magnets and operative field strengths between 0.2 and 4 T. Depending upon the design, these systems may require RF and magnetic shielding for clinical operation. The RF shield is used to attenuate environmental RF radiation transmission and contain the RF generated by the imager.

The primary purpose of magnetic shielding is to shield the environment from stray magnetic fields that may have deleterious effects on all types of electronic equipment. In addition, it is necessary to maintain a high degree of magnetic field homogeneity. Recall that precessional frequencies are related to magnetic field strengths and, therefore, uniform stimulation requires a uniform magnetic field. Large masses of ferrous metal adjacent to the magnet will deform the magnetic field. However, the effects of environmental metal can be counteracted with a process of "shimming." This is performed by placing pieces of metal within the magnet (passive shimming) and by the use of additional magnetic coils (shim coils) to produce small magnetic fields that increase or decrease the observed field to produce a uniform field (active shimming). Therefore, the primary concern is not large, stationary metallic objects but moving metallic structures such as elevators or heavy traffic.

New technology and emphasis on magnet design has provided a range of magnet designs of varying field strength, size, and magnetic shielding. New magnet designs can include "active" magnetic shielding that can decrease the magnetic "footprint." This technique uses additional magnet windings to oppose the external fringe field. In this manner, an actively shielded magnet may require minimal external magnetic shielding. Careful review of the magnetic fringe field and equipment planned for adjacent areas will determine the need for room shielding. Vibration analysis of the site may become important, as well; verify the importance of this with your equipment vendor. On-site measurements to establish the vibration levels due to building, traffic, air handling equipment, and other sources, which may affect the stability of your imager, must be part of the site planning process.

Currently, RF and magnetic shielding are not obstacles to siting of MRI systems. Equipment suppliers often will provide the planning details necessary to design and construct the appropriate shielding.

For superconducting magnet systems, a structure must be provided to allow for the escape of large quantities of helium gas should the magnet lose its superconductive state (quench). Also, appropriate accessibility must be provided for the replenishment of cryogenic coolants.

It may be important to consider hospital gas (O_2, air, suction) access and a designated code area near the MRI suite. Cardiac defibrillators generally do not work above 25 G, and additional lighting, electrical power, and space may be needed in an emergency. One design incorporates these features into the hallway/entry wall leading to the MR imager suite.

SUMMARY

MRI is a technique that makes use of both magnetic and RF fields to produce images of the internal structures of the body. The fundamentals of the technique involve placing the patient in a strong magnetic field, stimulation of the atomic nuclei with a radio transmission, and the detection of a radio transmission from the nuclei as they return to their prestimulation state. The technique uses nonionizing electromagnetic radiation for stimulation and detection. The available tissue contrast (due primarily to differences in relaxation times) is currently the highest among all medical imaging modalities. The technique is noninvasive and at present demonstrates no untoward biological effect. The placement and operation of MRI systems are markedly different from conventional imaging systems and demand a greater level of attention and forethought.

REFERENCES

1. Fullerton GD. Basic concepts for nuclear magnetic resonance imaging. *Magn Reson Imaging* 1982;1:39–55.
2. Partains CL, Price RR, Patton JA, et al. Nuclear magnetic resonance imaging. *Radiographics.* Volume 4, Special Edition, January 1984;4:5–25.
3. Young SW. *Nuclear magnetic resonance imaging: basic principles.* New York: Raven Press, 1984.
4. Balter S. An introduction to the physics of magnetic resonance imaging. *Radiographics* 1987;7:371–383.
5. Fullerton GD. Magnetic resonance imaging signal concepts. *Radiographics* 1987;7:579–596.
6. American College of Radiology. *Glossary of MR terms,* 2nd ed. Reston, VA: American College of Radiology, 1986.
7. Kumar A, Welti D, Ernst RR. NMR Fourier zeugmatography. *J Magn Reson* 1975;18:69–83.
8. Edelstein WA, Hutchison JMS, Johnson G, et al. Spin warp NMR imaging. *Phys Med Biol* 1980;25:751–756.
9. Hutchison J. NMR scanning: the spin-warp method. In: Witcofski RL, Karstaedt N, Partain CL, eds. *NMR imaging,* Winston-Salem, NC: Bowman-Gray School of Medicine, 1982: 77–80.
10. Felmlee JP, Morin RL, Salutz JR, et al. Magnetic resonance imaging phase encoding: a pictorial essay. *Radiographics* 1989;9: 717–722.
11. Acronyms common to MRI. *J Magn Res Imaging* 1992; 2(Suppl.). *SMRI MR research guide,* 1992–1993 edition.
12. Haacke EM. Editorial. *Magn Reson Imaging* 1988;6:353–354.
13. Hinks RS, Quencer RM. Motion artifacts in brain and spine MR. *Radiol Clin North Am* 1988;26:737–753.
14. Glover GH, Pelc NJ. A rapid gated cine MRI technique. In: Kressel HY, ed. *Magnetic resonance annual,* New York: Raven Press, 1988: 299–333.
15. Felmlee JP, Ehman RL. Spatial presaturation: a method for suppressing flow artifacts and improving depiction of vascular anatomy in MR imaging. *Radiology* 1987;164:559–564.
16. Haase A, Frahm J, Matthaei D, et al. FLASH imaging: rapid NMR imaging using low flip angle pulses. *J Magn Reson* 1986;67: 258–266.
17. Mansfield P. Multi-planar image formation by NMR. *J Phys (E)* 1977;10:L55.
18. Dixon WT. Simple proton spectroscopic imaging. *Radiology* 1984;153:189–194.
19. Dwyer AJ, Frank JA, Sank VJ, et al. Short-TI inversion-recovery pulse sequence: analysis and initial experience in cancer imaging. *Radiology* 1988;168:827–836.
20. Bellon ER, Haacke EM, Coleman PE, et al. MR artifacts: a review. *Am J Roentgenol* 1986;147:1271–1281.
21. Pusey E, Lufkin RB, Brown RKJ, et al. MRI artifacts: mechanism and clinical significance. *Radiographics* 1986;6:891–911.
22. Hahn FJ, Chu WK, Coleman PE, et al. Artifacts and diagnostic pitfalls on magnetic resonance imaging: a clinical review. *Radiol Clin North Am* 1988;26:717–735.
23. Persson BBR, Stahlberg F. *Health and safety of clinical NMR examination.* Boca Raton, FL: CRC Press, 1989.
24. NRPB advisory group on NMR clinical imaging. Revised guidance on acceptable limits of exposure during nuclear magnetic resonance clinical imaging. *Br J Radiol* 1983;56:974–977.
25. McRobbie D, Foster MA. Thresholds for biological effects of time-varying magnetic fields. *Clin Phys Physiol Meas* 1984; 5:67–78.
26. Budinger TF. Thresholds for physiological effects due to RF and magnetic fields used in NMR imaging. *IEEE Trans Nucl Sci* 1979;NS-26:2812–2815.
27. Paptheofanis FJ. A review on the interaction of biological systems with magnetic fields. *Physiol Chem Phys Med NMR* 1984;16: 251–255.
28. Jehenson P, Duboc D, Lavergne T, et al. Change in human cardiac rhythm induced by a 2-T static magnetic field. *Radiology* 1988;166:227–230.
29. Pavlicek W, Salem D, Horton J. Comparative measurements of RF absorbed power using 0.15, 0.6, and 1.5 Tesla magnets. *Radiology* 1984;153(P):98.
30. Food and Drug Administration. Magnetic resonance diagnostic device: panel recommendation and report on petitions for MR reclassification. *Fed Reg* 1988;53:7575–7579.
31. Kanal E, Borgstede JP, Barkovich AJ, et al. American College of Radiology white paper on MR safety. *AJR* 2002;178:1335.
32. Shellock FG, ed. *Magnetic resonance procedures: health effects and safety.* Boca Raton, FL:CRC Press, 2001
33. Shellock FG, Crues JV. High-field-strength MR imaging and metallic biomedical implants: an ex vivo evaluation of deflection forces. *AJR Am J Roentgenol* 1988;151:389–392.

APPENDIX

(Glossary of MRI Terms Adapted from Reference 6)

Aliasing   Consequence of sampling in which any components of signal that are at a higher frequency than the Nyquist limit will be "folded" in the spectrum so that they appear to be at a lower frequency. In Fourier transform imaging, this can produce an apparent wrapping around to the opposite side of the image of a portion of the object that extends beyond the edge of the reconstructed region.

Artifacts   False features in the image produced by the imaging process. The random fluctuation of intensity due to noise can be considered separately from artifacts.

Attenuation   Reduction of power, for example, due to passage through a medium or electrical component. Attenuation in electrical systems is commonly expressed in decibels (dB).

B_o   A conventional symbol for the constant magnetic field in an NMR system (units of Tesla).

B_1   A conventional symbol for the radio frequency magnetic field used in an MR system. It is useful to consider it as composed of two oppositely rotating vectors, usually in a plane transverse to B_o. At the Larmor frequency, the vector rotating in the same direction as the precessing spins will interact strongly with the spins.

Bandwidth   A general term referring to a range of frequencies (e.g., contained in a signal or passed by a signal processing system).

Chemical shift   The change in the Larmor frequency of a given nucleus when bound at different sites in a molecule, due to the magnetic shielding effects of the electron orbitals. Chemical shifts make possible the differentiation of different molecular compounds and different sites within the molecules in high-resolution NMR spectroscopy. The amount of the shift is proportional to magnetic field strength and is usually specified in parts per million (ppm) of the resonance frequency relative to a standard. The actual frequency measured for a given spectral line may depend on environmental factors such as effects on the local magnetic field strength due to variations of magnetic susceptibility.

Chemical shift imaging   A magnetic resonance imaging technique that provides mapping of the regional distribution of intensity (images) of a restricted range of chemical shifts, corresponding to individual spectral lines or groups of lines.

Chemical shift spatial offset   Image artifact of apparent spatial offset of regions with different chemical shifts along the direction of the frequency encoding gradient (see Fig. 1-32).

Coherence   Maintenance of a constant phase relationship between rotating or oscillating waves or objects. Loss of phase coherence of the spin results in a decrease in the transverse magnetization and hence a decrease in the MR signal.

Contrast enhanced angiography   A technique for visualizing vascular structure in which a T1 shortening paramagnetic contrast agent is injected into the blood and used to enhance the signal from blood during a rapid T1 weighted imaging pulse sequence. The bolus injection must be timed such that the peak concentration of contrast agent passes through the vascular structure of interest during the acquisition of the center of k-space.

Echo planar imaging (EPI)   A technique of planar imaging in which a complete planar image is obtained from one selective excitation pulse. The FID is observed while periodically switching the *y*-magnetic field gradient field in the presence of a static *x*-magnetic field gradient field. The Fourier transform of the resulting spin-echo train can be used to produce an image of the excited plane.

Flip angle   Amount of rotation of the macroscopic magnetization vector produced by an RF pulse, with respect to the direction of the static magnetic field.

Flow-related enhancement   The increase in intensity that may be seen for flowing blood or other liquids with some MRI techniques, due to the inflow of unsaturated spins from outside of the image slice.

Fourier transform imaging   MRI techniques in which at least one dimension is phase encoded by applying variable gradient pulses along that dimension before "reading out" the MR signal with a magnetic field gradient perpendicular to the variable gradient. The Fourier transform is then used to reconstruct an image from the set of encoded MR signals. One imaging technique of this type is spin warp imaging. A commonly used technique is two-dimensional Fourier transform (2DFT) imaging.

Free induction decay (FID)   If transverse magnetization of the spins is produced, for example, by a 90° pulse, a transient MR signal results that decays toward zero with a characteristic time constant T2 (or T2*); this decaying signal is the FID. In practice, the first part of the FID is not observable due to residual effects of the powerful exciting RF on the electronics of the receiver and the receiver dead time.

Frequency encoding   Encoding the distribution of sources of MR signals along a direction by detecting the signal in the presence of a magnetic field gradient along that direction so that there is a corresponding gradient of resonance frequencies along that direction. In the absence of other position encoding, the Fourier transform of the resulting signal is a projection profile of the object.

Gauss (G)   A unit of magnetic flux density in the older centimeter-gram-second system. The earth's magnetic field is approximately 0.5 to 1 G, depending on location. The currently preferred (SI) unit is the Tesla (T) (1 T = 10,000 G).

Gradient echo Spin echo produced by reversing the direction of a magnetic field gradient or by applying balanced pulses of magnetic field gradient before and after a refocusing RF pulse so as to cancel out the position-dependent phase shifts that have accumulated due to the gradient. In the latter case, the gradient echo is generally adjusted to be coincident with the RF spin echo.

Gradient magnetic field A magnetic field that changes in strength in a certain given direction. Such fields are used in MRI with selective excitation to select a region for imaging and also to encode the location of MR signals received from the object being imaged. Measured in Tesla per meter (T/m).

Gyromagnetic ratio The ratio of the magnetic moment to the angular momentum of a particle. This is a constant for a given nucleus.

Image acquisition time Time required to carry out an MRI procedure comprising only the data acquisition time. The total image acquisition time will be equal to the product of the repetition time, TR, the number of excitations, and the number of different signals (encoded for position) to be acquired for use in image reconstruction. The additional image reconstruction time will also be important to determine how quickly the image can be viewed. In comparing sequential plane imaging and volume imaging techniques, the equivalent image acquisition time per slice must be considered, as well as the actual image acquisition time.

Interpulse time Times between successive RF pulses used in pulse sequences. Particularly important are the inversion time (TI) in inversion recovery, and the time between 90° pulse and the subsequent 180° pulse to produce a spin echo, which will be approximately one-half the spin-echo time (TE). The time between repetitions of the pulse sequence is the repetition time (TR).

Inversion recovery A pulse NMR technique that can be incorporated into MRI, wherein the nuclear magnetization is inverted at the beginning of the pulse sequence. The resulting partial T1 relaxation of the spins within different structures being imaged can be used to produce an image that depends strongly on T1. This may bring out differences in the appearance of structures with different T1 relaxation times. Note that this weighted by T1 relaxation and does not directly produce an image of T1. T1 in a given region can be calculated from the change in the NMR signal from the region due to the inversion pulse compared to the signal with no inversion pulse or an inversion pulse with a different inversion time (TI).

K-space Comprised of the digitized MR signal. Data points in k-space represent different spatial frequencies in the object being imaged and are reconstructed via Fourier transformation to form the clinical image.

Longitudinal magnetization (M_z) Component of the macroscopic magnetization vector along the direction of the static magnetic field. Following excitation by a RF pulse, M_z will approach its initial value M_0, with a characteristic time constant T1.

Longitudinal relaxation Return of longitudinal magnetization to its equilibrium value after excitation; requires exchange of energy between the nuclear spins and the lattice. The rate of return is characterized by the T1 time.

Macroscopic magnetization vector Net magnetic moment per unit volume (a vector quantity) of a sample in a given region, considered as the integrated effect of all the individual microscopic nuclear magnetic moments.

Magnetic field gradient A magnetic field that changes in strength given direction. Such fields are used in NMR imaging with selective excitation to select a region for imaging and also to encode the location of NMR signals received from the object being imaged. This gradient is measured in millitesla per meter (mT/m) or gauss per centimeter (G/cm).

Magnetic resonance (MR) Resonance phenomenon resulting in the absorption and/or emission of electromagnetic energy by nuclei or electrons in a static magnetic field, after excitation by a suitable RF magnetic field. The peak resonance frequency is proportional to the magnetic field and is given by the Larmor equation.

Magnetic susceptibility Measure of the ability of a substance to become magnetized. A difference in susceptibility between tissues can therefore lead to a difference in stimulation and the resultant signal.

Maximum intensity projection A technique used to reformat images of blood vessel cross-sections to visualize vascular structure. The technique projects the brightest pixel in a row onto a plane perpendicular to the viewing angle. Projections may be created at different angles to view the vasculature at those angles.

Phase In a periodic function (such as rotational or sinusoidal motion), the position relative to a particular part of the cycle.

Phase contrast angiography A technique for visualizing vascular structure in which moving spins from flowing blood are distinguished from surrounding stationary tissue by the differences in phase accumulation during the application of bipolar gradients.

Phase encoding Encoding the distribution of sources of MR signals along a direction in space with different phases, by applying a pulsed magnetic field gradient along that direction prior to detection of the signal. In general, it is necessary to acquire a set of signals with a suitable set of different phase encoding gradient pulses to reconstruct the distribution of the sources along the encoded direction.

Precession Comparatively slow gyration of the axis of a spinning body so as to trace out a cone; caused by the application of a torque tending to change the direction of the rotation axis, and continuously directed at right angles to the plane of the torque. The magnetic moment of a nucleus with spin will experience such a torque when inclined at an angle to the magnetic field, resulting in precession at the Larmor frequency. A familiar example is the effect of gravity on the motion of a spinning top or gyroscope.

Pulse sequences   The timing of RF (and/or gradient) magnetic field pulses to produce NMR images. A "shorthand" designation of interpulse times used to generate a particular image is to list the repetition time (TR), the echo time (TE), and, if using inversion recovery, the inversion time (TI), with all items given in milliseconds (ms). For example, 2,500/30/1,000 would indicate an inversion recovery pulse sequence with RT of 2,500 ms, TE of 30 ms, and TI of 1,000 ms. If using multiple spin echoes, as in CPMG, the number of the spin echo used should be stated.

Rephasing gradient   Magnetic field gradient applied for a brief period after a selective excitation pulse, of opposite polarity to the gradient used for the selective excitation. The result of the gradient reversal is a rephasing of the spins (which will have gotten out of phase with each other along the direction of the selection gradient), forming a gradient echo and improving the sensitivity of imaging after the selective excitation process.

Resonance   A large amplitude vibration in a mechanical or electrical system caused by a relatively small periodic stimulus with a frequency at or close to a natural frequency of the system; in NMR apparatus, resonance can refer to the NMR itself or to the tuning of the RF circuitry.

Spatial frequency   The rate at which an object or signal occurs in some distance. For example, a resolution test pattern may include lines (objects) that occur at a spatial frequency of 10 lines per cm. In MRI, low spatial frequencies of the object being imaged are located near the center of k-space and carry information related to image contrast. High spatial frequencies are located near the periphery of k-space and carry information related to image sharpness.

Spin   The intrinsic angular momentum of an elementary particle or system of particles, such as a nucleus, that is also responsible for the magnetic moment; or, a particle or nucleus possessing such a spin. The spins of nuclei have characteristic fixed values. Pairs of neutrons and protons align to cancel out each other's spins, so that nuclei with an odd number of neutrons and/or protons will have a nonzero rotational component characterized by an integer or half integer quantum "nuclear spin number."

Spin echo   Reappearance of an NMR signal after the FID has apparently died away, as a result of the effective reversal of the dephasing of the spins (refocusing) by techniques such as specific RF pulse sequences, for example, Carr-Purcell sequence (RF spin-echo), or pairs of magnetic field gradient pulses (gradient echo), applied in times shorter than or on the order of T2. Unlike RF spin echoes, gradient echoes will not refocus phase differences due to chemical shifts or inhomogeneities of the magnetic field.

Spin-echo imaging (SE)   Any of many MRI techniques in which the spin echo is used rather than the FID. Can be used to create images that depend strongly on T2 if TE has a value on the order of or greater than T2 of the relevant image details. Note that spin-echo imaging does not directly produce an image of T2 distribution. The spin echoes can be produced as a train of multiple echoes, for example, using the CPMG pulse sequence.

T1   Spin-lattice or longitudinal relaxation time; the characteristic time constant for spins to tend to align themselves with the external magnetic field. Starting from zero magnetization in the z direction, the z magnetization will grow to 63% of its final maximum value in a time T1.

T2   Spin-spin or transverse relaxation time; the characteristic time constant for loss of phase coherence among spins oriented at an angle to the static magnetic field, due to interactions between the spins. Starting from a nonzero value of magnetization in the xy plane, the xy magnetization will decay so that it loses 63% of its initial value in a time T2.

T2* ("T-two-star")   The observed time constant of the FID due to loss of phase coherence among spins oriented at an angle to the static magnetic field, commonly due to a combination of magnetic field inhomogeneities and spin-spin (T2) relaxation. This results in rapid loss of transverse magnetization and NMR signal.

TE   Echo time. Time between the RF pulse and center of the readout gradient used for echo production.

Tesla (T)   The preferred (SI) unit of magnetic flux density. One Tesla is equal to 10,000 gauss.

TI   Inversion time. In inversion recovery, time between middle of inverting (180°) RF pulse and middle of the subsequent exciting (90°) pulse to detect amount of longitudinal magnetization.

Time-of-flight angiography   A technique for visualizing vascular structure in which moving spins from flowing blood (which have not experienced repeated RF pulses) contribute higher signal than the stationary spins of surrounding tissue (that have experienced repeated RF pulses).

TR   Repetition time. The period of time between the beginning of a pulse sequence and the beginning of the succeeding (essentially identical) pulse sequence.

Interpretation of Magnetic Resonance Images

2

Mark S. Collins   Richard L. Ehman

Magnetic resonance imaging (MRI) is a powerful and versatile diagnostic tool utilized by radiologists and clinicians to provide definitive diagnoses for a wide range of musculoskeletal pathology. Compared to conventional radiographs, nuclear medicine studies, musculoskeletal computer tomography (CT), and ultrasound, MRI provides the best combined sensitivity and specificity for clinical differential diagnostic considerations, which include a broad spectrum of osseous, cartilage, and soft tissue pathology. The goals of the musculoskeletal imager include providing images that demonstrate excellent spatial resolution to evaluate complex soft tissue anatomy while still maintaining maximal signal-to-noise ratio. Most importantly, the

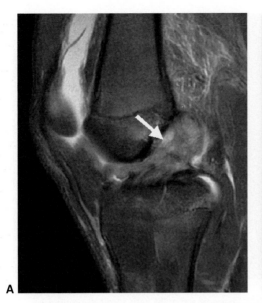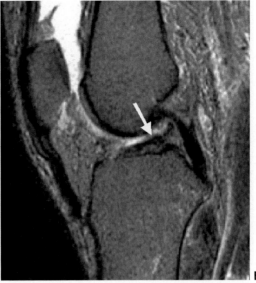

Figure 2-1 **A:** Fat-suppressed, T2-weighted fast spin echo–XL (FSE-XL) image of a patient with acute anterior cruciate ligament (ACL) disruption (*arrow*) that demonstrates abnormal morphology (indistinct, discontinuous ligament fibers and mass effect) and abnormal increased signal intensity (due to intrasubstance hemorrhage and edema). **B:** Fat-suppressed, T2-weighted FSE-XL image of a patient with chronic ACL tear (*arrow*) with abnormal morphology (ligament discontinuity, attenuation and laxity) but normal signal intensity.

ultimate goal is to demonstrate excellent conspicuity of pathology as compared to normal background structures to assist in making confident imaging diagnoses. This is accomplished by tailoring the imaging sequences to do the best evaluation of clinical diagnostic considerations and may include the use of intravenous or intraarticular gadolinium.

This chapter provides an overview of basic interpretation techniques that establish a confident imaging diagnosis. These techniques take into account inherent properties of normal and pathologic musculoskeletal tissues that are emphasized by MR tissue characterization. These physical properties may be accentuated by tailoring the MR examination to demonstrate the conspicuity of pathologic processes by applying the best combination of a multitude of available MR sequences. There are certainly many individual preferences utilized by experienced musculoskeletal imagers that may differ due to different magnet systems, coil design, and uniquely developed sequences appropriate for those systems. Regardless, the goal is the same: obtaining the most accurate diagnosis possible, utilizing superior imaging techniques and thorough interpretation patterns.

BASIC IMAGE INTERPRETATION

Interpretation of MR images initially begins with differentiation of normal structures from pathologic processes. Pathologic processes of the musculoskeletal system are identified at MRI by abnormal morphology, abnormal signal characteristics, or the combination of both. An acute disruption of the anterior cruciate ligament of the knee is demonstrated by the presence of abnormal morphology

(discontinuous or indistinct fibers, ligamentous laxity, and mass effect) and abnormal signal intensity (due to intrasubstance hemorrhage or edema) (see Fig. 2-1A). A chronic tear of a ligament may demonstrate abnormal morphology (ligament attenuation and laxity) with normal signal intensity (see Fig. 2-1B). Figure 2-2 demonstrates a partial thickness intrasubstance tear of the supraspinatus tendon, which has abnormal signal but grossly normal morphology.

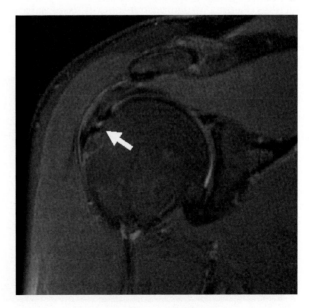

Figure 2-2 Fat-suppressed, T2-weighted FSE-XL image of a patient with surgically confirmed, partial thickness, undersurface tear of the distal supraspinatus tendon (*arrow*). There is focal abnormal T2 signal at the tear site; however, the tendon morphology is grossly normal.

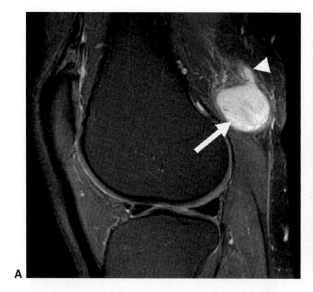
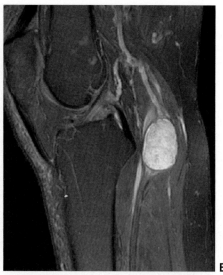

Figure 2-3   A: Fat-suppressed, T2-weighted FSE-XL image of a patient with surgically confirmed peripheral nerve sheath tumor (PNST) of the tibial nerve within the upper popliteal fossa (*arrow*). The imaging morphology allows a confident imaging diagnosis, in this case demonstrating continuity with a traversing nerve structure (*arrowhead*). **B:** Fat-suppressed, T2-weighted FSE-XL image of a different patient with surgically confirmed PNST of the tibial nerve within the lower popliteal space with typical findings of a fusiform mass contiguous with the traversing nerve.

Most nonlipomatous, solid, soft tissue masses have relatively nonspecific MR features that do not allow tissue-specific diagnoses. However, on occasion, careful evaluation of the morphology and internal signal characteristics of soft tissue masses can provide a definitive prebiopsy histologic diagnosis. Figure 2-3 demonstrates two different cases of peripheral nerve sheath tumors, which are characterized by their fusiform shape and continuity with traversing nerve structures. Figure 2-4 demonstrates a soft tissue sarcoma with internal signal characteristics that allow a unique and accurate diagnosis. Some soft tissue masses have unique morphology, signal characteristics, and anatomic location, which allow a confident MR diagnosis. Figure 2-5 demonstrates the classic MR appearance of benign elastofibroma dorsi. The characteristic imaging appearance of this mass precludes the need for biopsy.

It is advantageous to interpret MR images in conjunction with other available images, such as radiographs, scintigraphy, ultrasound, or CT. As a general rule, musculoskeletal MR cases should always be evaluated with a corresponding,

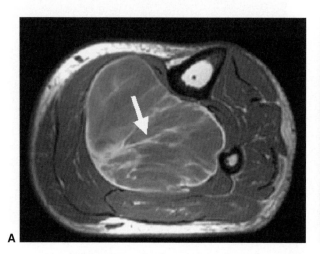
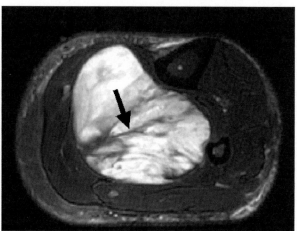

Figure 2-4   Axial T1- **(A)** and T2-weighted **(B)** images of a surgically confirmed myxoid liposarcoma of the deep posterior compartment of the lower calf. Careful assessment of the internal architecture of the mass demonstrates linear, fatty strands that confirm the diagnosis (*arrow*). Most soft tissue sarcomas have a nonspecific MR appearance that does not allow a definitive diagnosis as in this case.

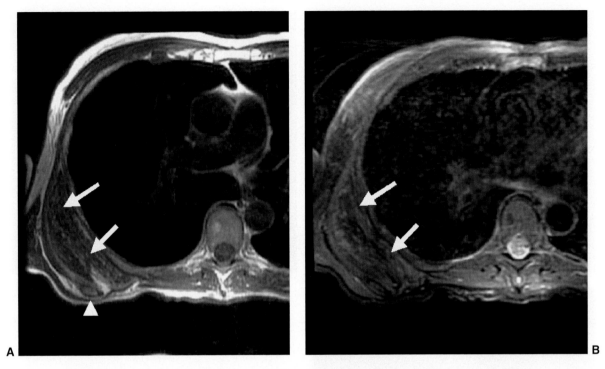

Figure 2-5 Axial T1- (**A**) and T2-weighted (**B**) images of the upper torso demonstrate the typical location and appearance of an elastofibroma dorsi (*arrows*). The elliptical shaped, fibro-fatty mass is located deep to the serratus muscle and inferior margin of the scapula (*arrowhead*).

current radiograph. Figure 2-6 demonstrates a case of evolving myositis ossificans traumatica. Without identifying the characteristic zonal, peripheral mineralization pattern on the radiograph, the MR could be misinterpreted as representing a soft tissue neoplasm or infectious etiology. Unfortunately, if a percutaneous biopsy were to be performed in this case, the histopathology could suggest soft tissue sarcoma, which would clearly lead to inappropriate and aggressive clinical management.

These cases present just a few examples of the application of basic interpretation techniques in analyzing musculoskeletal pathology. Multiple additional examples will be included throughout the remaining chapters of the text that more specifically deal with targeted anatomic locations.

TISSUE CHARACTERIZATION

The process of extracting information about tissue type and pathology by MR techniques has been called "tissue characterization." This description has often been applied specifically to the use of quantitative measurements of relaxation times. Many studies of tissue characterization by *in vivo* measurement of relaxation times have appeared in the literature (1–8). These have generally not demonstrated a strong clinical role for "tissue characterization," although it is fair to say that the hypothesis that accurate measurement of tissue relaxation times may be clinically useful has not yet been adequately tested.

Given the expanded definition for tissue characterization described above, what are the properties that are important in clinical imaging? A key word in this question is "imaging." Some of the tissue properties that are important in this context are unique to the imaging process. This includes anatomic detail, which can demonstrate a lesion solely by its effect on morphology (see Fig. 2-7). Another similar property is tissue texture: mass lesions in muscle are often characterized by their homogeneous texture, compared to the reticulated texture of normal muscle (see Fig. 2-8) (9). As we shall see, even some of the classical tissue characterization parameters have special meanings in the imaging context.

MR images basically reflect the distribution of mobile hydrogen nucleii. The brightness of each image pixel depends on, among other things, the density of mobile protons in the corresponding volume element and on the way that these protons respond to the externally superimposed static and fluctuating magnetic fields (see Chapter 1). This response depends on the chemical and biophysical environment of the protons and is described concisely by the relaxation times T1 and T2.

The spin-lattice relaxation time, T1, is an exponential time constant that describes the gradual increase in magnetization that takes place when a substance is placed in a strong magnetic field (see Fig. 2-9). T1 predicts the time that it will take for nearly two-thirds (actually about 63%) of the longitudinal magnetization to be restored after it has been tipped 90° by a radio frequency (RF) pulse. The spin-lattice relaxation time of water protons in tissue depends in a

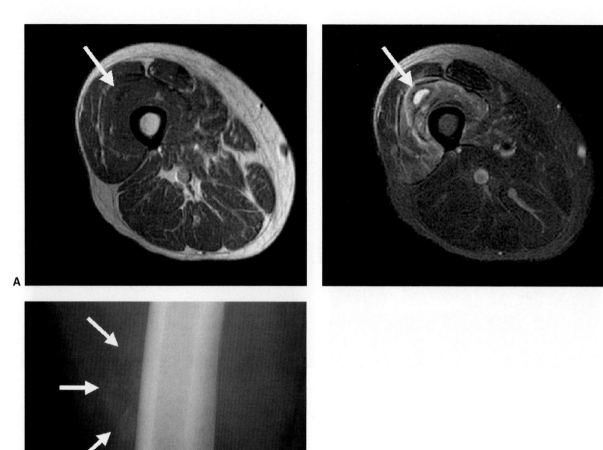

Figure 2-6 Axial T1- **(A)** and T2-weighted **(B)** images of the thigh in an adult male patient with a palpable mass following incidental trauma. Study demonstrates an ill-defined region of reticulated and hazy abnormal increased T2 signal and mass effect in the vastus intermedius that contains an irregular central fluid collection (*arrow*). Corresponding AP radiograph **(C)** demonstrates faint, peripheral mineralization in a zonal pattern, which confirms the diagnosis of evolving myositis ossificans traumatica.

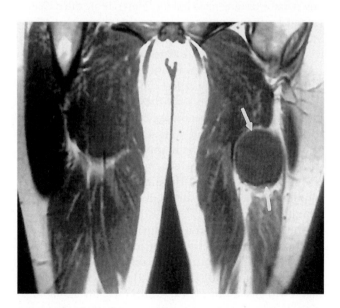

Figure 2-7 Malignant soft tissue tumor (*arrows*), which is differentiated from adjacent muscle by its mass effect and homogeneity rather than by a signal intensity difference.

complex fashion on rotational, vibrational, and translational motions and on the way that these are modified by proximity to macromolecules.

The spin-spin relaxation time, T2, is a time constant that describes the rate of exponential decay of transverse magnetization that would occur if the field was perfectly homogeneous (see Fig. 2-10). Thus, for a spin-echo sequence, the net transverse magnetization at an echo delay time of TE = T2 will be approximately two-thirds (actually 63%) less than what was present immediately after the 90° pulse. The transverse magnetization is the component that creates a signal in MRI. Like T1, the spin-spin relaxation time depends on the natural motions of molecules. It is also affected by other processes that will be described later in this chapter.

It is difficult to accurately measure *in vivo* relaxation times with most MR imagers. These difficulties result from the necessity of irradiating a large but well-defined volume with RF energy and performing the steps required to create an image. Slice-selective 90° and 180° RF pulses, for instance, tend to be inaccurate near the boundaries of the section (10). The signal obtained from tissue that is irradiated with

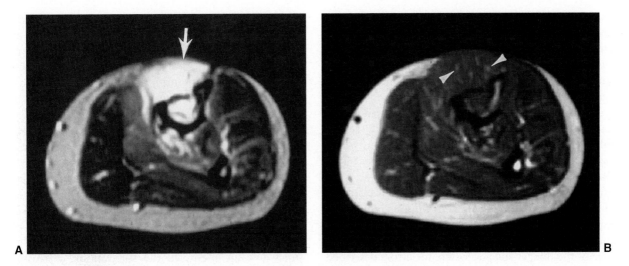

Figure 2-8 A: A T2-weighted image of a patient who previously underwent surgical resection of a sarcoma from the anterior aspect of the leg demonstrates a mass with high signal intensity (*arrow*) that suggests tumor recurrence. **B:** A T1-weighted image of the same area demonstrates tiny streaks of fat (*arrowheads*) within the mass, typical of muscle, which effectively rules out tumor. The mass was a muscle flap that was placed in the tumor bed at the time of initial resection.

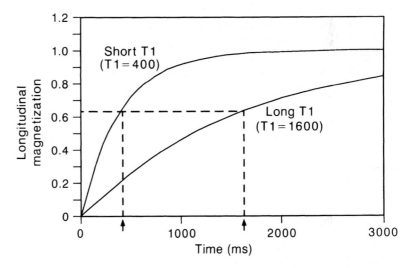

Figure 2-9 The T1 relaxation time describes the regrowth of longitudinal magnetization after it is reduced to zero by a 90° RF pulse.

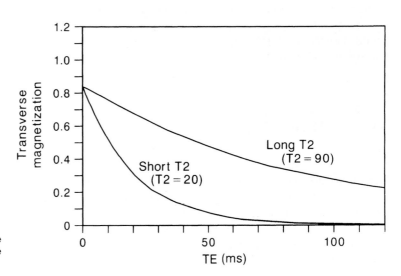

Figure 2-10 The T2 relaxation time describes the exponential decay of magnetization in the transverse plane after it is placed there by a 90° RF pulse.

inaccurate RF pulses will not be the same as what would be obtained with ideal pulses. Relaxation times calculated from such measurements will be correspondingly incorrect. Other problems include the effects of applied field gradients, motion, and the small number of data points that are typically acquired.

In spite of these problems, properly performed *in vivo* relaxation time measurements are surprisingly reproducible with the same imager when they are performed on tissues that are stationary (11,12). On the other hand, physiological motion can produce large random and systematic errors in relaxation times calculated from image data (13). Relaxation times obtained with one type of MR imager are usually not directly comparable to data obtained for the same tissue with another imager. This is because of the imager-specific systematic errors described above and the fact that relaxation times are field strength dependent. The T1 of muscle tissue, for instance, is nearly twice as long at 1.5 T (Tesla) as it is at 0.15 T (14,15).

Given these problems, it is not surprising that clinical applications requiring quantitative measurement of tissue relaxation times have been slow to emerge. Nevertheless, it is essential to understand the relative relaxation time relationships of tissues and pathological processes, because this is the key to understanding the highly variable gray scale of MRI.

Spin density (mobile proton density, hydrogen density) is another important property that determines the appearance of tissue in magnetic resonance images. Few *in vivo* measurements of tissue spin density have been reported. This is probably because absolute measurements are difficult to perform with imagers. The derived spin densities are relative values that can only be compared within the same image. Nevertheless, spin density differences are an important source of image contrast in some tissues. There are large differences between the spin density of adipose tissue and muscle, for instance (16).

Many other physical properties can potentially be measured or monitored by MR techniques to noninvasively characterize tissue. These include measuring the diffusion rate of water protons (17–20) and differentiating between groups of protons on the basis of the characteristic chemical shift in their resonant frequency (3,21–31).

SIGNIFICANCE OF TISSUE RELAXATION TIMES

A detailed discussion of the physical mechanisms that determine relaxation time in biological systems is beyond the scope of this chapter. Indeed, these processes are as yet relatively poorly understood. Nevertheless, some of the concepts in the current view of this area are useful for understanding the appearance of normal and pathological tissue in clinical images.

Relaxation times describe the time course of the bulk magnetization of resonating protons following the application of perturbing RF pulses. The bulk magnetization is a vector quantity (i.e., having a magnitude and direction) that is the sum of the minute magnetic contributions of each of the resonating protons in tissue. The magnetic behavior of individual protons is quantum mechanical in nature, but the process of summing huge numbers of protons results in a bulk magnetization vector that can assume a continuous range of magnitudes and orientations.

As already noted, the spin-lattice relaxation time (T1) describes the *restoration* of the longitudinal component of magnetization after it has been destroyed or reduced by an RF pulse. For this to happen, some of the protons that have been boosted into a higher energy level by the RF pulse must give up energy to the surrounding environment (sometimes called the "lattice"). This corresponds to reorienting individual proton magnetic moments from a direction that is roughly opposite to that of the main field to one that is, on average, in the same direction.

This process depends on interaction between the excited protons and neighboring nuclei in the lattice (32). The protons are subjected to a rapidly varying perturbation by the magnetic fields of adjacent nuclei. The frequency with which they vary is determined by the tumbling and translational motions of the protons and their neighbors. The perturbing motions are most effective for stimulating spin-lattice relaxation when they fluctuate at the Larmour frequency of the system.

The characteristic length of time during which the magnetic field of a proton interacts with that of an adjacent nucleus with a magnetic moment is called the correlation time, τ (32). Essentially, this quantity is proportional to the period (i.e., inversely proportional to the frequency) of the cyclic field fluctuations caused by motion. Each mode of molecular motion has a characteristic correlation time. For tumbling motion, the correlation time is proportional to the period of rotation (see Fig. 2-11). For translational motion, the correlation time can be regarded as proportional to the

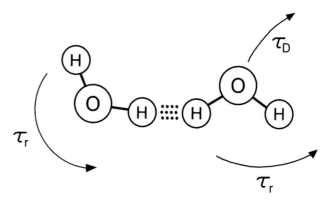

Figure 2-11 As water molecules tumble and randomly jump in Brownian motion, the dipole moments of protons interact with a characteristic period that is called the correlation time.

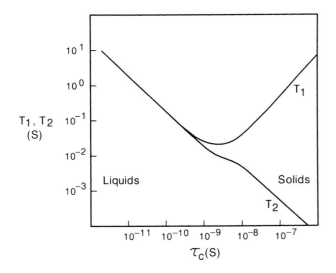

Figure 2-12   Relationship between correlation time and the T1 and T2 relaxation times.

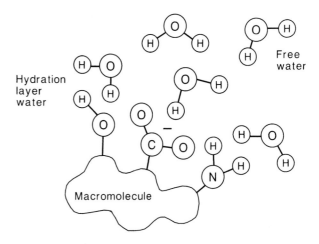

Figure 2-13   Two-state model for organization of water in cytoplasm.

average time between the Brownian "jumps." The combined correlation time is the parallel sum of the individual τ values associated with each of the perturbing motions:

$$1/\tau_c = 1/\tau_r + 1/\tau_d \qquad [1]$$

As shown in Fig. 2-12, the spin-lattice relaxation time decreases to a minimum as correlation time is lengthened, and then increases again. The position of the minimum of this curve is dependent on the Larmour frequency and, thus, the strength of the B_o field (33). Free water has a short correlation time of about 10^{-12} seconds and thus it has a long spin-lattice relaxation time.

The spin-spin or T2 relaxation time of protons is also dependent on correlation times. It is also strongly affected by slowly varying and static magnetic fields at the molecular level (32). Such fields form gradients that cause moving protons to process at rates that have a small, random variation with time. Thus, they do not stay in phase with each other for as long as they would without the static field gradients, and this is reflected as a reduction in the T2 relaxation time (Chapter 1). Figure 2-12 shows that in contrast to the T1 relaxation time, T2 continues to shorten as correlation times become longer and longer. Thus, the proton T1 and T2 relaxation times of solids, which have very slow molecular motion and longer correlation times, will be long and short respectively.

Although pure water has long T1 and T2 relaxation times of more than 2 seconds, much shorter relaxation times are typically observed in tissue. This is a result of the hydrophylic properties of many macromolecules. These molecules, which include proteins and polynucleic acids, have electric dipole and ionic sites that allow hydrogen bonding with water molecules in solution (see Fig. 2-13) (34–36). The water in this hydration layer is less mobile than free water, and thus the correlation time is longer

$(\tau_c = 10^{-9} \text{ s})$. As a result, the T1 and T2 of hydration water are much shorter than that of free water.

The residence time of individual water molecules in the hydration layer of macromolecules is transient. Thus, individual water protons may alternately experience conditions that are favorable and unfavorable for relaxation as they exchange back and forth between bound and free states, respectively. Under these "fast exchange" conditions, the observed relaxation time of water protons will be an average of the relaxation times in the bound and free states, weighted by the fraction in each state (34).

$$1/T1_o = (1 - F_b)/T1_f + F_b/T1_b \qquad [2]$$

where $T1_o$ is the observed T1, $T1_f$ and $T1_b$ are the relaxation times in the free and bound states, respectively, and F_b is the fraction of bound protons. The equation for T2 is similar. More complex models have been created to explain tissue relaxation behavior (14), but this simple, two-state, fast exchange model is very helpful for understanding clinical images. The T1 relaxation time of free water is approximately 2,500 ms, while that of hydration water is less than 100 ms. The model predicts that relaxation times of tissues with higher bound water fractions will be shorter than tissues that have a larger percentage of free water.

Tissue water proton relaxation times depend on many other factors. Field strength is one of the most important of these (14,15,37,38). The trough of the T1 relaxation time curve in Fig. 2-12 moves upward and to the left as field strength increases (33). This means that the relaxation times of protons with correlation times in this range (bound water protons, for instance) will be longer at higher field strengths. It follows that the T1 relaxation time of most tissues increases with field strength because of the influence on the bound water component. In contrast, the T2 relaxation times of most tissues are relatively independent of field strength, except for a clinically important exception described below.

Paramagnetic contrast agents like Gd-DTPA can strongly affect tissue relaxation times when they are present (39). These are substances with very strong magnetic moments that can enhance the relaxation of neighboring protons by perturbing them in a manner analogous to the way that proton fields interact with other protons. Many of these agents are paramagnetic by virtue of the presence of an unpaired orbital electron. The magnetic dipole moment generated by the unopposed electron is about 700 times stronger than the magnetic moment of a proton. The proton relaxation enhancement effect of these molecules is correspondingly intense.

When a sufficient amount of paramagnetic agent is added to an aqueous solution, the T1 and T2 relaxation times are shortened. The effect can be represented by the following equations:

$$1/T1_o = 1/T1_d + 1/T1_p \qquad [3]$$

$$1/T2_o = 1/T2_d + 1/T2_p \qquad [4]$$

where $T1_o$ and $T2_o$ are the new observed relaxation times, $T1_d$ and $T2_d$ are the (diamagnetic) relaxation times of the solution or tissue without the paramagnetic agent, and $T1_p$ and $T2_p$ represent the extra relaxation process provided by the addition of the paramagnetic material. These latter quantities depend on the concentration of paramagnetic material:

$$1/T1_p = K1 \, [P] \qquad [5]$$

$$1/T2_p = K2 \, [P] \qquad [6]$$

where [P] is the concentration of the paramagnetic material and K1 and K2 are constants that depend on the type of paramagnetic agent and on the characteristics of the tissue or solution.

Paramagnetic material may be endogenous in origin or it may be exogenously administered as a contrast agent for MRI. Endogenous paramagnetic materials are not believed to be present in sufficient concentration to affect the relaxation behavior of most normal human tissues significantly, but they do have a substantial effect in some pathological states such as transfusional hemosiderosis (40).

RELAXATION TIMES OF MUSCULOSKELETAL TISSUES

Tables of quantitative *in vivo* relaxation time measurements (14) are of limited clinical usefulness because they are dependent on the field strength and on technical details of the imager and measurement method. Nevertheless, a general understanding of the relative relaxation characteristics of normal and pathological tissues is absolutely essential for competent interpretation of clinical magnetic resonance imagery. This task is relatively easy for the musculoskeletal system because the number of different tissues is small.

TABLE 2-1

RELATIVE RELAXATION TIMES OF MUSCULOSKELETAL TISSUES

Tissue	T1	T2
Muscle	Medium	Short
Adipose tissue	Short	Medium
Nerve	Medium	Medium
Other soft tissue	Medium to long	Medium to long
Tendon, bone	—	Very short

At the field strengths commonly used for proton imaging (0.15 T to 1.5 T), the T1 relaxation times of most soft tissues range between 250 and 1200 ms. The range of T2 values for most soft tissues is between approximately 25 and 120 ms. Fluids and fibrous tissue depart from this range. The relative relaxation times of musculoskeletal tissues are summarized in Table 2-1.

These relationships can be summarized in a simple relaxation time map (see Fig. 2-14). This figure shows that most musculoskeletal soft tissues fall into three distinct classes. Adipose tissue is characterized by its short T1 relaxation time in comparison to most other tissues, which dominates its appearance with most common MRI techniques. Healthy skeletal muscle has a short T2 relaxation time that is characteristic. Most other soft tissues, including tumors, have T1 relaxation times that are longer than that of adipose tissue and T2 relaxation times that are longer than that of muscle. The mobile proton density of bone, tendon, and dense fibrous tissue is low so that these tissues have low intensity in most MR images. These relationships form the basis for understanding and manipulating contrast in clinical MR of the musculoskeletal system.

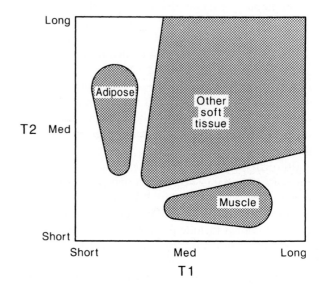

Figure 2-14 Relaxation time map for musculoskeletal tissues.

EFFECT OF PATHOLOGY ON TISSUE RELAXATION TIMES

The relaxation times of many musculoskeletal tissues change in rather distinctive ways when they are affected by specific pathological processes (41). The significance and basic biophysical mechanisms for these changes are relatively poorly understood and few clinical applications have been demonstrated for their quantitative measurement. But they do result in diagnostically useful changes in the signal intensity and contrast of tissues in MR images. The general trend of the relaxation time changes for some important musculoskeletal disease processes is summarized in Table 2-2.

Inflammation

Inflammatory processes are generally characterized by prolongation of T1 and T2 relaxation times (42). The presence of edema seems to be the most likely mechanism to explain these changes. Accumulation of extracellular and possibly intracellular water causes an increase in the total water content of tissue. The previously described two-state, fast exchange model is helpful for understanding how even a small change in water content can result in a large alteration in relaxation times. Since water protons freely diffuse between the intracellular and extracellular spaces and the number of macromolecular binding sites is relatively fixed, the increased water content represents an increase in the fraction of free water.

Figure 2-15 shows theoretically expected tissue T1 values for various free water fractions, calculated using Eq. 2. The relaxation times $T1_f$ and $T1_b$ were assigned values of 2,500 and 50 ms, respectively. The resulting T1 relaxation time rapidly increases as the fraction of free water increases above 85%. Note, for instance that a 1% increase in free water from 91% to 92% causes a 10% increase in relaxation time.

Neoplasms

With certain exceptions, most solid neoplasms are characterized by relaxation times that are prolonged relative to their host tissues. Many studies of this phenomenon have appeared in the literature (43). Some studies have demonstrated increases in tissue water content that correlate with

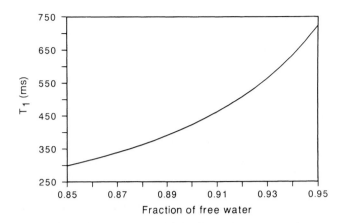

Figure 2-15 Relationship between spin-lattice relaxation time and fraction of unbound or free water with a fast exchange, two-state model for tissue relaxation times.

the degree of relaxation time prolongation, while others have not (34). The changes probably reflect an alteration in the ratio of free to bound water in tumor tissue, possibly related to changes in the way that water is ordered within and adjacent to the hydration layer of macromolecules.

Although the elevation of T1 and T2 relaxation times in neoplastic tissue is usually less than that resulting from inflammation, there is considerable overlap, and distinction between these processes must usually be made on the basis of morphology and history.

Fibrosis

As noted above, the mobile spin density of predominantly fibrous tissue is low, thus providing little MR signal. Diffuse fibrosis of parenchymal tissues may be difficult to detect until it is well advanced and a substantial amount of the tissue has been replaced. The T2 relaxation time of mature fibrotic tissue is often reduced. In contrast, the T2 relaxation time of immature fibrosis in granulation tissue is usually long, causing high intensity in T2-weighted images.

Fatty Infiltration

Fatty infiltration of muscles and other musculoskeletal tissues causes a shortening of *in vivo* T1 relaxation times because of the very short T1 of fat. A distinguishing feature between this and most other spin-lattice relaxation time changes related to disease is that the relaxation curves are not uniexponential (44). This is because there is little exchange between the protons in fat and those in the host tissue. The relaxation is therefore biexponential, with a fast component due to fat protons and a slower component due to water protons in the host tissue. Most *in vivo* methods for measuring T1 are incapable of resolving the biexponential nature of the recovery curve and simply show that the relaxation time is short.

TABLE 2-2

RELAXATION TIMES FOR COMMON MUSCULOSKELETAL DISORDERS

Disease Process	T1	T2
Inflammation	Increased	Increased
Neoplasia	Increased	Increased
Fibrosis	—	Decreased
Fatty infiltration	Decreased	—
Interstitial hemorrhage	Increased	Increased

Hematoma

Interstitial hemorrhage in muscle and other tissues usually causes prolongation of both T1 and T2 relaxation times, probably due to the presence of inflammation and edema (45,46).

The relaxation time characteristics of hematomas (confluent collections of extravasated blood) are much more variable. They are strongly influenced by formation of paramagnetic substances (46–48). Oxygenated hemoglobin contains iron in a "low spin" ferrous state that is not paramagnetic. Thus, the proton relaxation times of stationary oxygenated blood are mainly determined by the concentration of protein (albumin and hemoglobin), which determines the fraction of water protons that are in the bound, fast relaxing state. The T1 and T2 relaxation times of fresh oxygenated blood are medium or long in comparison to most solid tissues. Deoxygenation of hemoglobin has little effect on the relaxation time of hematomas at imager fields of less than 1.0 T. Deoxyhemoglobin contains iron in a "high spin" ferrous state, which is paramagnetic, but the area of the unpaired electron is relatively inaccessible to water protons because of the conformation of the molecule. Thus, the T1 relaxation of water protons is not enhanced because they are unable to interact with the paramagnetic center.

As time passes, oxidative denaturation of deoxyhemoglobin causes formation of methemoglobin, which contains iron in a ferric form and is strongly paramagnetic. Water molecules have relatively free access to the paramagnetic site, and thus the relaxation times are shortened. The T1 relaxation time of the hematoma is typically reduced more than T2 by the presence of methemoglobin. This can be rationalized by noting that the T2 of acute hematoma is short compared to its T1 relaxation time even though it is long in comparison to solid tissue. Even if $T1_p$ and $T2_p$ are relatively long, corresponding to a low concentration of methemoglobin, Eqs. 3 and 4 show that $T1_o$ will be affected more than $T2_o$. For instance, if the $T1_d$ and $T2_d$ values of an acute hematoma are 600 and 150 ms, respectively, and after a period of time a small amount of methemoglobin is formed to yield paramagnetic contributions ($T1_p$ and $T2_p$) on the order of 1,000 ms, then the observed $T1_o$ and $T2_o$ values of the hematoma will be 375 and 130 ms, respectively. In a T1-weighted image, this would result in a substantial increase in signal intensity.

At higher field strengths (>1.0 T), an additional physical process begins to affect the relaxation times of hematogenous material. Empirical observations have shown that the T2 relaxation time of hematomas can be extremely short at high field strength (1.5 T), while it is long in comparison to soft tissue at low and medium field strengths (48). The explanation relates to the fact that while deoxyhemoglobin is not an effective proton relaxation enhancer, it does cause the magnetic susceptibility of the erythrocyte cytoplasm to differ significantly from that of plasma. When a substance is placed in a magnetic field, the strength of the local magnetization typically differs from the external field strength by a proportionality factor called the bulk magnetic susceptibility.

The difference in magnetic susceptibility between plasma and cytoplasm results in a small difference in the field strength between the interior and exterior of erythrocytes. This field gradient is only one or two ten-thousandths of 1% of the main magnetic field ($1-2$ ppm), but that is enough to shorten the T2 relaxation at high field (49). The mechanism is due to diffusion of water protons through the field gradients near the erythrocyte membrane (see Fig. 2-16). Protons moving in such a fashion accumulate phase differences that would not have been present if the field gradients were absent, resulting in more rapid decay of the transverse magnetization. The phase errors are proportional to the square of the gradient. Since the gradient is proportional to the field strength, this means that the effect is much more pronounced at high field strength.

It is interesting to note that this T2 relaxation enhancement effect is operative only when erythrocyte membranes are intact. On lysis, deoxyhemoglobin is distributed uniformly and the local field gradients abolished. Figure 2-17 shows a simple experiment in which two samples of diluted deoxygenated blood were imaged at 0.15 T and 1.5 T. The sample on the right in the images was osmotically lysed. Note that both samples have identical intensity in a T2-weighted image at 0.15 T, while the tube containing intact cells was dramatically reduced in intensity in a similar image at 1.5 T. The measured T2 relaxation times of both tubes at 0.15 T and the lysed tube at 1.5 T were greater than 150 ms. The T2 of the intact cells at 1.5 T was less than 45 ms.

Similar field-dependent T2 proton relaxation effects can also occur at the periphery of old hemorrhagic lesions due

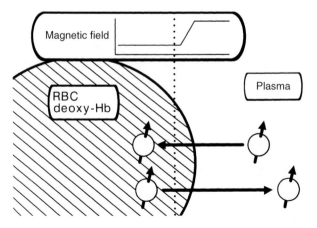

Figure 2-16 Water protons diffusing near the cell membranes of erythrocytes containing deoxyhemoglobin experience a tiny shift in their resonant frequency due to the presence of a field gradient. This causes selective reduction of T2 relaxation time at high field strengths.

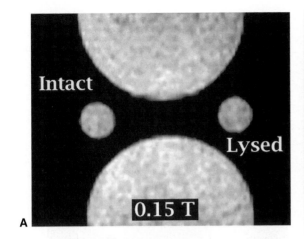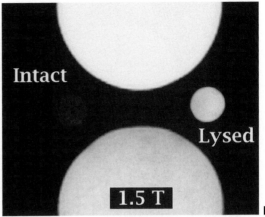

Figure 2-17   **A:** Low field T2-weighted image of two vials (small diameter disks) containing blood. The image demonstrates no intensity difference between lysed blood in the tube on the right of the picture and intact cells in the left. The two large disks are reference standards. **B:** High field T2-weighted image of same vials as in **(A)** demonstrates striking reduction in the intensity of the non-lysed blood.

to susceptibility gradients in the vicinity of hemosiderin-laden macrophages (48).

In summary, the relaxation times of hematomas are affected by many factors, including protein concentration, formation of paramagnetic methemoglobin, and T2 proton relaxation enhancement by local heterogeneity in magnetic susceptibility at high field strength.

OTHER PHENOMENA THAT AFFECT TISSUE RELAXATION TIMES

The apparent T2 relaxation time of some tissues depends on their orientation with respect to the static magnetic field. This phenomenon occurs in tissues such as tendon, which are composed of spatially oriented macromolecules. The highly ordered molecules restrict the motion and orientation of hydration water protons. The resulting effect on dipolar interactions leads to alterations in the observed T2 relaxation times of such materials, depending on their orientation to the static magnetic field. Investigators have demonstrated this phenomenon in experimental and clinical MRI (50–52). In tendons and ligaments, T2 prolongation is greatest when they are oriented approximately 55° to the static magnetic field. This angle is commonly referred to as the "magic angle" (51). Tendons oriented at the magic angle will have higher signal intensities due to T2 prolongation. The increased signal intensity is usually most apparent in T1 and spin density-weighted sequences. In musculoskeletal imaging, it is important not to confuse magic angle affects with tendon pathology. Magic angle effects can be minimized by changing the course of the anatomic structure or by relying on longer TE sequences for accurate interpretation (see Figs. 2-18 and 2-19).

INFLUENCE OF RELAXATION TIMES AND PULSE SEQUENCE PARAMETERS ON CONTRAST

The appearance of tissue in clinical magnetic resonance images depends on tissue properties and on the parameters of the pulse sequence. As already noted, the most important tissue properties in this context are the relaxation times T1 and T2 and the spin density N(H). The most important pulse sequence parameters are the pulse repetition time (TR) and the echo delay time (TE) for the spin-echo sequence. The inversion recovery sequence has an additional important parameter: inversion time (TI). In the discussion that follows, we will concentrate on spin-echo methods, because these are the most frequently used techniques in current clinical MRI. A few unique features of gradient-echo imaging are outlined in a subsequent section.

The importance of understanding the influence of these tissue properties and pulse sequence parameters on the contrast between tissues cannot be overemphasized. It provides a basis for characterizing tissue in clinical images. It also provides guidance for selecting appropriate MRI techniques from the huge number of possible parameter combinations so that the examination can be tailored to individual diagnostic problems.

Typical MR images are displayed in such a way that the brightness of each pixel is dependent on the MR signal that is obtained from each corresponding voxel (volume element) within the patient (see Fig. 2-20). The precessing magnetization vector in each volume element has a certain magnitude and phase angle with respect to the magnetization vectors in neighboring voxels. These two quantities are dependent on the relaxation times, spin density, and motion of the protons within the volume element and on details of the magnetic resonance technique. The phase

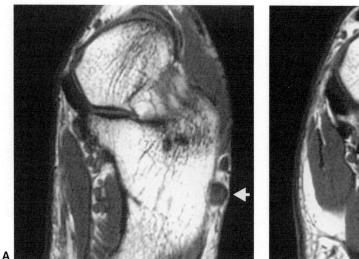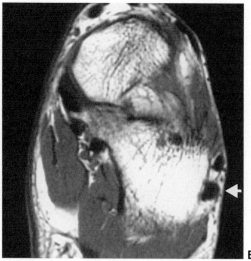

Figure 2-18 Affect of tendon orientation on MRI appearance. T1-weighted SE images (TR = 500/TE = 13) were obtained at identical window and level settings. **A:** An oblique axial image through the ankle tendons with the foot in neutral position demonstrates increased signal within the peroneus longus tendon (*arrow*) and the peroneus brevis tendon. **B:** Oblique axial image through the ankle tendons at the same level as in **A**, now with the foot in plantar flexion, demonstrates low signal within the peroneus longus tendon (*arrow*) and the peroneus brevis tendon. The tendons are oriented near the "magic angle" in relation to the main magnetic field with the foot in neutral position and are nearly parallel to the main magnetic field when the foot is in plantar flexion.

angle is usually used to determine the spatial location of the magnetic resonance signals. The magnitude of the magnetization vector in each volume element determines the brightness of each corresponding pixel in the final image.

It is useful to study a simplified model for the intensity of spin-echo signals from tissue:

$$\text{Intensity} = N(H)\, e^{-TE/T2}(1 - e^{-TR/T1}) \qquad [7]$$

where N(H) is the spin density; T1 and T2 are the spin-lattice and spin-spin relaxation times, respectively; TR is the pulse repetition time; and TE is the echo delay time. This model ignores many important factors that affect the spin-echo signal, such as the presence of motion, flow, diffusion, and the technical details of the pulse sequence and imager. Nevertheless, it is helpful for understanding the basis for image contrast.

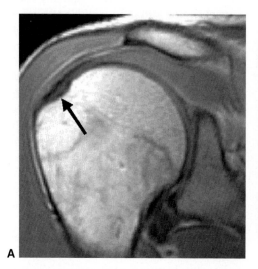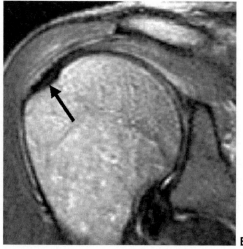

Figure 2-19 Affect of TE on MRI appearance of magic angle. Dual spin-echo oblique-coronal image **(A)** of the curved supraspinatus tendon (*arrow*) demonstrates intermediate signal on the proton density images (TR = 2,000/TE = 20). At this same location on the T2-weighted image **(B)** (TR = 2,000/TE = 60), the signal decreases slightly, characteristic of magic angle effect.

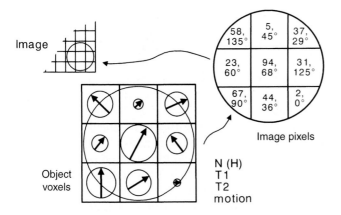

Figure 2-20 Relationship between image pixels and object voxels.

Note first that the intensity of the signal is proportional to the spin density, and this is true for images with any combination of TR and TE. The dependence of intensity on T2 is governed by the first exponential in this equation, and the dependence on T1 is modeled by the terms within the parentheses.

The behavior of the portion of the Eq. 7 that is within the parentheses is shown in Fig. 2-9. A spin-echo sequence begins with a 90° RF pulse, which tips the magnetization that is parallel to the main magnetic field (longitudinal magnetization) into the transverse plane. The amount of longitudinal magnetization that is available is dependent on the time that has passed since the previous 90° pulse. Spin-echo sequences with TR values that are long in comparison to the T1 of tissue will have large amounts of magnetization to tip into the transverse plane, while short TR values will cause the amount of available longitudinal magnetization to be reduced. When TR is at least three times as long as the T1 of the tissue, then the amount of longitudinal magnetization will be more than 95% of what would be present with an infinite waiting time. If TR is the same as T1, then the magnetization that is available will be about 63% of the maximum value. As TR is further reduced, the available magnetization becomes less and less. The latter condition is called a state of "partial saturation." Note that a spin-echo sequence with a given TR may cause partial saturation of one tissue with a long T1, while some other tissue that has a short T1 may not be partially saturated.

Once the longitudinal magnetization is flipped into the transverse plane by the 90° RF pulse, a spin-echo signal is created at time TE by a 180° RF pulse applied at time TE/2. Equation 7 shows that the intensity or strength of the spin-echo signal depends on an exponential decay function that is governed by the ratio of TE/T2. Clearly, sequences with short echo delay times will produce stronger spin echoes than those with long TE values in relation to the transverse relaxation time T2. As shown in Fig. 2-10, tissues with long T2 relaxation times will yield spin echoes with higher intensity than those with short T2 values, all other factors being equal.

The significance of all of this is that TR is a user-selectable parameter that determines the maximum signal that a given tissue will yield (dependent on the rate of growth of longitudinal magnetization; i.e., T1). The selection of TE governs the exponential T2 decay of the potential signal before a spin echo is created. Given a pair of tissues with different relaxation times, it is possible to select TR and TE in such a way as either to minimize or maximize the intensity difference (contrast) between the two tissues.

Note that Eq. 7 indicates that if the T1 of a tissue is increased, its spin-echo intensity will be reduced. As shown in Fig. 2-9, this is because less longitudinal magnetization is available for flipping into the transverse plane and later creation of a spin echo. The reverse condition applies for T2. If the T2 relaxation time of a tissue is increased, its spin-echo intensity will increase because less transverse decay will occur before a spin echo is formed, as shown in Fig. 2-10.

T1- AND T2-WEIGHTED SEQUENCES

The concept of T1- and T2-weighted sequences is very useful for selecting sequences and understanding the gray scale of MR images. Consider a hypothetical case in which we wish to provide contrast between two tissues on the basis of their different T2 relaxation times. This means that it is desirable to select a sequence that is relatively insensitive to differences in T1 while yielding large intensity differences between tissues with different T2 values. The first goal can be achieved by selecting a TR time that is long in comparison to all of the tissues. This will ensure that there is enough recovery time between 90° pulses so that full longitudinal magnetization develops in all tissues, regardless of the particular T1 relaxation time. The second goal is facilitated by selecting a TE that is relatively long so that there is a large difference in spin-echo intensity between tissues with slow and fast T2 decay.

A T2-weighted spin-echo sequence is therefore one in which the TR is long in relation to the T1 of the tissues of interest, and the TE is also relatively long. The freedom from T1 influence is dependent on the long TR, while the sensitivity to T2 differences is determined by TE. Although the relative intensity difference between tissues with differing T2 values increases with TE, there is a practical limit to the allowable maximum echo delay time. This is imposed by the fact that the absolute magnitude of the signals decrease with echo delay time so that at some point the ratio of signal to noise in the image is degraded so much that further enhancement of relative contrast is useless.

Consider a second case in which we wish to differentiate between tissues on the basis of T1 differences. In order to minimize T2-dependent intensity differences, it is necessary to make TE as short as possible. By also selecting a short TR, tissues will be placed in a state of partial saturation, depending on their T1 relaxation time. Tissues with long T1 values will fail to remagnetize as much as those with shorter T1 times between 90° pulses, and thus their spin-echo signals will be reduced.

A T1-weighted spin-echo sequence is therefore one with a relatively short TR and short TE. In practice, very short TE values are technically difficult to achieve in spin-echo sequences. The extent to which TR can be shortened in spin-echo sequences is also limited, because this progressively reduces the longitudinal magnetization, resulting in lower signal-to-noise.

T1- and T2-weighted sequences are very useful for a number of reasons. They allow qualitative recognition of the relaxation time characteristics of lesions in relation to adjacent tissues, which can be very helpful diagnostically. But the most important reason for employing such sequences is that they are most likely to provide lesion contrast. Many pathological processes, including inflammation, neoplasia, and parenchymal hemorrhage, are characterized by parallel increases in both T1 and T2 relaxation times. As already noted, these tend to produce opposite changes in spin-echo intensity, so that for certain combinations of TR and TE the contrast between a lesion and adjacent normal tissue may be low. Isointensity between tumors and other soft tissue is particularly common with spin-echo sequences that are neither T1- or T2-weighted by the above criteria, especially spin-echo techniques with TR values of 500 to 1,500 and TE values in the range of 20 to 40 ms. Figure 2-21 shows such a situation. The frequency of such problems can be reduced by employing strongly T1- or T2-weighted sequences. In general, the best practice is to image the same area with at least two combinations of TR and TE.

One way to evaluate the weighting of particular MRI techniques is to determine the magnitude and direction of the change in image intensity that would result if the T1 and T2 of a particular tissue are changed by a small amount simultaneously. For example, if T1 and T2 were both increased, then a T1-weighted sequence would register a reduction of intensity and a T2-weighted sequence would show an increase. Mixed or unweighted techniques would yield small or no change of tissue intensity. By this standard, most long TR and long TE spin-echo sequences may be regarded as strongly T2-weighted. On the other hand, it is difficult to obtain a strongly T1-weighted spin-echo image without using very short TE times (10–15 ms). Strongly T1-weighted techniques can easily be obtained using inversion recovery sequences.

Lesion conspicuity in MRI is not solely a function of contrast as measured by the relative or absolute intensity differences. Noise is an important additional factor that must be considered. This includes thermal noise and coherent noise (e.g., motion artifacts). It is tempting to try to find methods for "optimizing" the contrast-to-noise ratio for particular lesions (53,54). In practice, these approaches have limited value because the relaxation times of pathological and surrounding tissues are rarely known with sufficient precision to make such procedures worthwhile. In addition, the process of optimizing contrast may compromise the clarity of other tissue interfaces. Clearly, the important goal is simply to display the lesion with enough contrast so that it can be detected. This goal is best achieved by imaging with several different MRI techniques, at least some of which should be strongly T1- or T2-weighted.

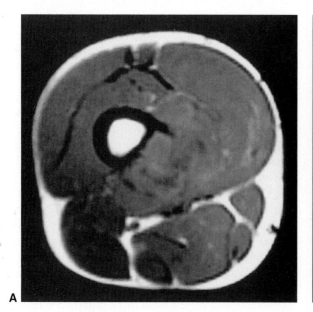
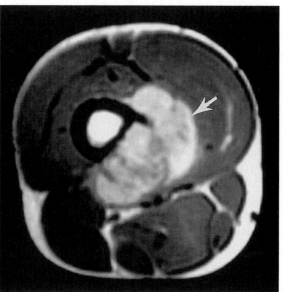

A

B

Figure 2-21 **A:** Proton density-weighted spin-echo image of a patient with chondrosarcoma does not allow easy delineation of margins between the tumor and surrounding muscle. **B:** T2-weighted spin-echo image provides good contrast between tumor and adjacent muscle (*arrow*).

CONTRAST IN GRADIENT-ECHO SEQUENCES

Gradient-echo techniques (Chapter 1) have seen increasing use for musculoskeletal imaging applications, especially for joint imaging (35,55–59). They provide interesting capabilities in terms of image contrast and acquisition speed. They permit practical use of high-resolution three-dimensional acquisition techniques, which would require prohibitively long acquisition times with conventional spin-echo sequences. Gradient echo sequences add an additional parameter to the list of settings that affect image contrast, namely the tip angle, which is usually represented by the symbol α. Several features distinguish gradient-echo sequences from spin-echo sequences. One of the most important of these is that gradient-echo sequences can utilize very short pulse repetition times, thereby permitting rapid image acquisition. Such short TR times are possible because the low nutation angle RF pulses destroy only a fraction of the longitudinal magnetization in each pulse repetition cycle. This is in contrast to the spin-echo technique, in which longitudinal magnetization is reduced in each repetition cycle by the initial 90° RF pulse.

Gradient-echo techniques can be broadly divided into "steady state" sequences such as gradient-recalled steady state (GRASS) and fast imaging with steady state precession (FISP), and "spoiled" sequences such as fast low-angle single-shot (FLASH) imaging and spoiled gradient echo (55,60). The concept of "residual transverse magnetization" is central to this classification. When short TR times are utilized with gradient-echo sequences, transverse magnetization created by each RF pulse may not have dephased appreciably before the next RF pulse is applied. This is especially likely to occur in tissues with long T2 relaxation times. If such transverse magnetization is present at the time of the next RF pulse, a portion of it will be rotated back into the longitudinal direction. The next RF pulse can then convert a portion of this same magnetization back into transverse magnetization. In this way, magnetization can be "recycled" back and forth between the longitudinal and transverse directions. This steady state magnetization contributes to the signal generated in each gradient echo.

The sequences in the "steady state" category employ various methods to preserve and enhance the contribution of steady state magnetization to the gradient-echo signal. The intensity of fluid and other materials with long T2 relaxation times is increased by this contribution in GRASS and FISP images. As a consequence, these images often have contrast characteristics reminiscent of T2-weighted spin-echo images.

The "spoiled" gradient-echo sequences, of which FLASH is the prototype, employ methods to eliminate the contribution of steady state magnetization. This tends to reduce the intensity of structures with long T2 relaxation times. Spoiled gradient sequences are well suited for providing T1-weighted contrast characteristics.

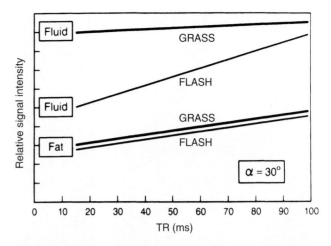

Figure 2-22 Comparison of contrast characteristics of a "steady state" type gradient-echo sequence with a "spoiled" type gradient-echo sequence. The differences are most apparent for materials with long T2 relaxation times (i.e., fluid), and at short pulse repetition times. The behavior illustrated here makes steady state sequences suitable for providing T2-weighted contrast characteristics and spoiled sequences best for providing T1-weighted contrast.

The differences between steady state and spoiled gradient-echo sequences tend to be reduced for sequences with long pulse repetition times because the longer time between successive RF pulses allows the transverse magnetization to die away (see Fig. 2-22).

The contrast characteristics of gradient-echo sequences are more complex than spin-echo sequences. Gradient echo images are strongly affected by a number of technical and tissue variables that tend to make the gray scale characteristics somewhat less predictable and consistent compared with spin-echo sequences. Gradient echo sequences are more strongly affected by field inhomogeneity, magnetic susceptibility effects, and motion effects than spin-echo sequences. The magnetic susceptibility effects of gradient-echo sequences may be utilized in making accurate tissue diagnoses. Figure 2-23 demonstrates a case of pigmented villonodular synovitis of the knee. The paramagnetic effects of hemosiderin contained within the synovial masses are well demonstrated on the gradient recalled echo (GRE) sequences. This phenomenon has been referred to as "blooming artifact." Also, gradient-echo sequences are markedly degraded by metallic susceptibility artifact.

APPROACH FOR SELECTING MRI TECHNIQUES

Certain clinical problems in musculoskeletal MRI can serve as examples to clarify the rationale for selecting sequences and interpreting images. These problems include detection of primary soft tissue neoplasms, recurrent soft tissue tumors after surgery, and identification of hematomas.

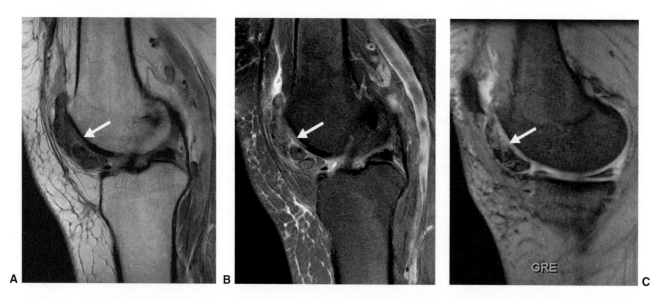

Figure 2-23 Female patient with knee pain and recurrent effusion due to surgically proven pigmented villonodular synovitis. Proton density- **(A)** and T2-weighted FSE-XL images **(B)** demonstrate a lobulated intra-articular mass with low signal intensity (*arrows*). On the gradient-echo image **(C)**, the mass decreases in signal due to the paramagnetic effects of hemosiderin.

In Chapter 12, one of the most successful applications of MRI is delineation of soft tissue tumors of the musculoskeletal system (61). Often these lesions are surrounded by muscle, and it is this situation that will be examined first. The ground rules are simple: most malignant lesions have T1 and T2 relaxation times that are longer than muscle. Healthy skeletal muscle tissue has a remarkably short T2 relaxation time in comparison to almost any other soft tissue, and certainly it is much shorter than most malignant soft tissue tumors. Given these facts, consider the expected time course of longitudinal magnetization that is shown in Fig. 2-24. The longer T1 of tumor means that its longitudinal magnetization will be less than that of muscle, particularly with a short TR such as 500 ms.

Figure 2-24B shows the time course of the transverse magnetization that would occur after the 180° RF pulse in a sequence with a relatively short TR. The shorter T2 of muscle causes its transverse magnetization to decay more quickly than that of the tumor so that the curves cross. In Fig. 2-24C, the transverse magnetization is traced for the case in which a longer TR is used. Note that the starting transverse magnetization is stronger and that the initial difference between tumor and muscle is smaller. Because tumor and muscle differ markedly in their T2 relaxation times, a T2-weighted sequence is able to display the interface with a high degree of contrast. The T1-weighted spin-echo sequence provides a lower degree of contrast in this case because of its "mixed" response to both T1 and T2 differences.

Tumors are not always completely surrounded by a single tissue, and in these situations several different MRI techniques may be necessary to delineate the borders of

the lesion completely. Figure 2-25 shows T1 and T2-weighted images from a patient with a metastatic tumor in the wrist region. It is necessary to use both images to completely delineate the boundaries of lesion. Figure 2-26 shows T1- and T2-weighted images from a patient with an osteogenic sarcoma of the distal femur with cortical destruction and soft tissue extension. The tumor margins within the medullary canal are best demonstrated on the T1-weighted images given the excellent contrast between the mass and the normal high signal intensity marrow fat. The fat-suppressed T2-weighted images better delineate the extraosseous soft tissue component and areas of central necrosis within the mass. The majority of the mass is low to intermediate in signal intensity on the T2-weighted images due to the heavy matrix mineralization that is present.

Adipose tissue has a T1 relaxation time that is dramatically shorter than almost any other soft tissue, as shown in Fig. 2-14. The T2 relaxation times of fat and tumor can overlap. Figure 2-27A demonstrates that the longitudinal magnetization that is available in fat is large even with a short TR. In Fig. 2-27B the transverse magnetization is traced in fat and tumor for a T1-weighted spin-echo sequence. Note that this sequence provides high contrast at short echo delay times. Although transverse magnetization is stronger when the TR is long as shown in Fig. 2-27C, the contrast between fat and tumor is poor.

T1-weighted spin-echo sequences are therefore very helpful for differentiating fatty tissue from other tissues. Although they are not particularly T1-weighted, the very short T1 of fat provides sufficient T1-dependent contrast. The margins between tumor and adipose tissue are delineated in the T1-weighted spin-echo image in Fig. 2-25A,

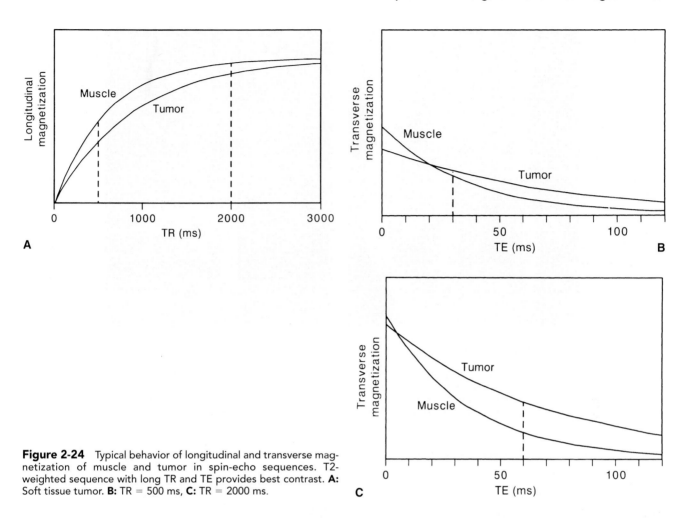

Figure 2-24 Typical behavior of longitudinal and transverse magnetization of muscle and tumor in spin-echo sequences. T2-weighted sequence with long TR and TE provides best contrast. **A:** Soft tissue tumor. **B:** TR = 500 ms, **C:** TR = 2000 ms.

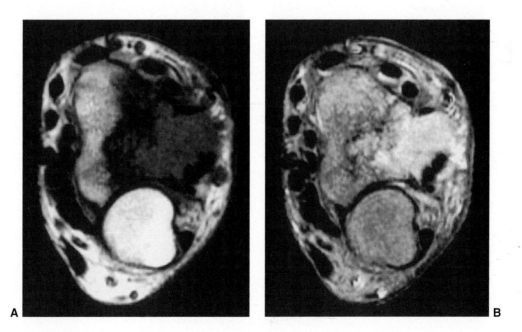

Figure 2-25 **A:** T1-weighted spin echo and **B:** T2-weighted sequences are both needed to adequately trace the borders of this metastatic melanoma in the wrist region.

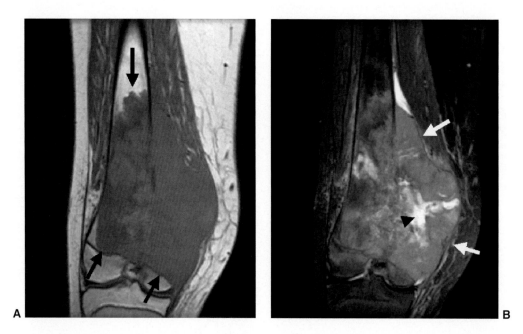

Figure 2-26   Coronal T1- **(A)** and fat-suppressed T2-weighted **(B)** images of the distal femur in an adolescent male patient with osteogenic sarcoma. The T1-weighted image **A** provides excellent contrast between the intramedullary extent of the tumor and adjacent fatty marrow (*black arrows*). The T2-weighted image **B** demonstrates better contrast between the soft tissue component of the mass and adjacent normal structures (*white arrows*). Central necrosis is present (*arrowhead*). The tumor has relatively low signal intensity on the T2 images due to matrix mineralization.

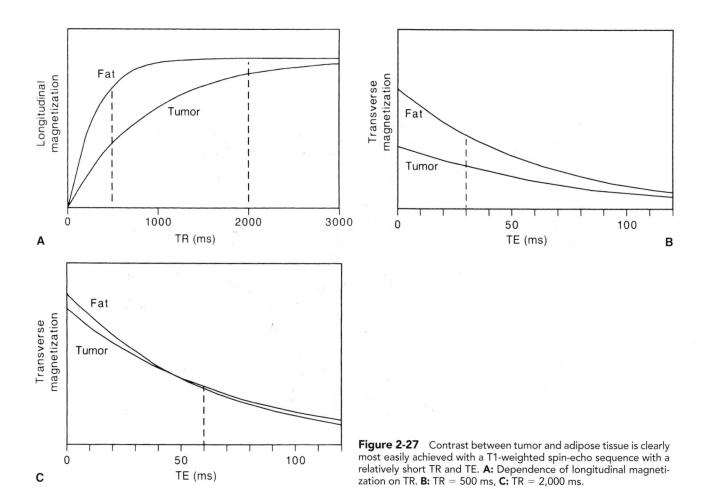

Figure 2-27   Contrast between tumor and adipose tissue is clearly most easily achieved with a T1-weighted spin-echo sequence with a relatively short TR and TE. **A:** Dependence of longitudinal magnetization on TR. **B:** TR = 500 ms, **C:** TR = 2,000 ms.

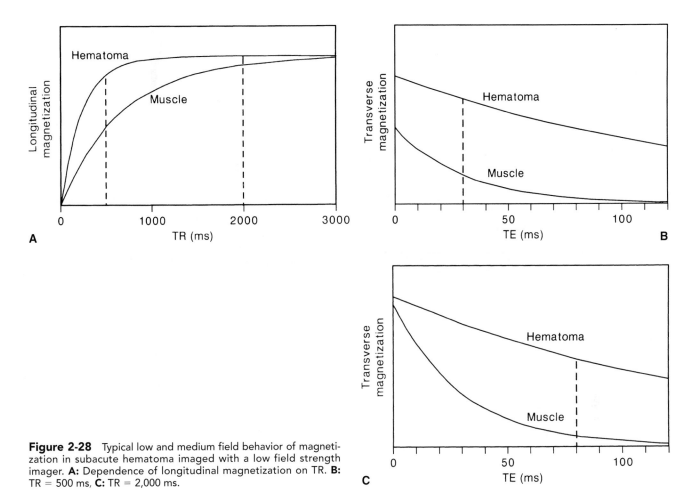

Figure 2-28 Typical low and medium field behavior of magnetization in subacute hematoma imaged with a low field strength imager. **A:** Dependence of longitudinal magnetization on TR. **B:** TR = 500 ms, **C:** TR = 2,000 ms.

but those with muscle are difficult to identify. The T2-weighted image provides just the reverse.

As described in a previous section, hematomas can have a variety of different appearances because of the unique physical processes that can affect their relaxation times. Some of these are diagnostic. The T1 relaxation times of hematomas may be short at all field strengths due to the proton relaxation enhancement effect of methemoglobin. A second effect that may be characteristic is the selective T2 proton relaxation enhancement produced at high field by deoxyhemoglobin in intact erythrocytes. As demonstrated in Fig. 2-28, such lesions are of high intensity in both T1- and T2-weighted images at low and medium field strengths. At high field strength, the selective T2 shortening effect comes into play so that the hematoma may have a very low intensity in both T2-weighted and T1-weighted spin-echo sequences as shown diagrammatically in Fig. 2-29. A clinical example is shown in Fig. 2-30.

These examples have shown how it is possible to tailor the contrast of MRI sequences by choosing appropriate acquisition parameters. Coupled with a general knowledge of tissue relaxation behavior, this provides a useful qualitative tissue characterization capability, which goes one step beyond morphologic imaging.

CONTRAST PROVIDED BY OTHER MAGNETIC RESONANCE IMAGING SEQUENCES

Since MRI was introduced into clinical practice in the early 1980s, researchers have introduced a steady stream of new pulse sequences and imaging techniques. Some of these sequences have provided improved (or at least different) kinds of contrast. Others have provided decreased imaging time. Radiologists now have an almost bewildering array of MRI sequences to choose from in their clinical practice.

In musculoskeletal MRI, the motivation for using these alternative techniques may include the need to reduce physiologic motion effects, to improve scanner efficiency, to obtain higher spatial resolution or to provide a particular kind of tissue contrast.

A sequence that has been widely adopted in the last several years is known as "fast spin-echo" (FSE; also called "turbo spin-echo" by some vendors) (62–64). This sequence is based on a technique called rapid acquisition with relaxation enhancement (RARE), which was originally described in 1986. The most important feature of the FSE sequence is that it can provide T2-weighted images in a much shorter acquisition time than conventional spin-echo methods.

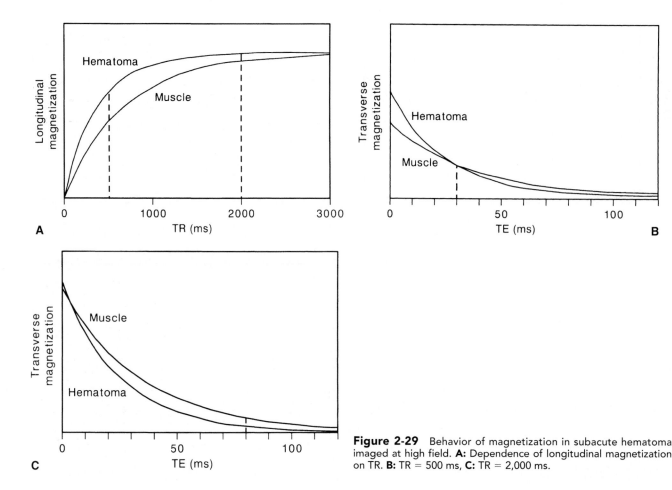

Figure 2-29 Behavior of magnetization in subacute hematoma imaged at high field. **A:** Dependence of longitudinal magnetization on TR. **B:** TR = 500 ms, **C:** TR = 2,000 ms.

FSE sequences acquire multiple views per TR cycle by applying different phase encoding gradients to each echo in a spin-echo train. If 16 echoes, for instance, are acquired in each repetition of a sequence, then the total acquisition time for a complete image will be reduced by a factor of 16. FSE images are reconstructed from data obtained at many different TE times. In practice, the contrast behavior of FSE images is usually described in terms of an average or effective TE value. It turns out that it is possible to change the effective TE of a sequence by adjusting the order in which the phase encoding views are collected.

FSE images may have poorer contrast characteristics compared to conventional spin-echo images, which can make reliable assessment of ligament, tendon, and meniscal tears more difficult. If conventional spin-echo sequences are not included in routine examinations such as the knee or shoulder, careful assessment of the menisci and rotator cuff tendon morphology is necessary to avoid missing pathology due to decreased contrast. FSE sequences may also be less reliable in detecting and characterizing musculoskeletal masses. The problem is that for musculoskeletal tissues, the sequence does not always seem to provide the reliable contrast characteristics that are so important in these tasks. The relative insensitivity of FSE sequences to susceptibility contrast can occasionally be a disadvantage in detecting hemorrhagic lesions.

Although FSE sequences may have poorer lesion contrast compared to conventional spin-echo sequences, the technique can be useful to depict morphology with relatively high-resolution T2-weighted images. The potential shorter acquisition times of FSE sequences allow for higher resolution imaging by increasing the matrix size or the number of excitations. When trying to produce high-resolution images, it is important to recognize that FSE sequences can be prone to degradation by blurring, which is most pronounced when using short effective TEs and long echo train lengths. Consequently, the echo train length may need to be shortened when using short effective TE FSE sequences. Using longer effective TEs can allow for relatively higher spatial resolution, because the peripheral reconstruction space is filled with high signal-to-noise short TE echoes.

The clinical applications of the FSE technique have included head, spine, pelvic, musculoskeletal, and abdominal MRI examinations. Generally, the sequence is used as an alternative to conventional T2-weighted spin-echo sequences. In head and spine studies, FSE images often appear almost indistinguishable from conventional spin-echo images, with a considerable acquisition time advantage. Figure 2-31 compares a sagittal T2-weighted spin-echo image, which required 8 min, 46 s of imaging time, with a FSE image that required only 1 min, 6 s for acquisition.

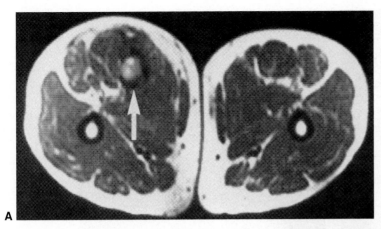

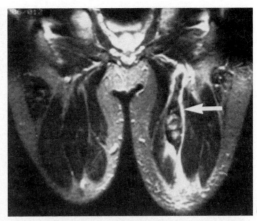

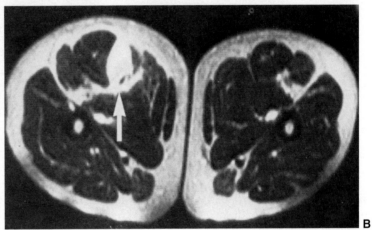

Figure 2-30 A: Subacute hematoma imaged at low field (0.15 T) with a strongly T1-weighted sequence. Image demonstrates a halo of low intensity (*arrow*), surrounding a central area of increased intensity. The low intensity is due to prolongation of T1. The area of high intensity is due to T1 shortening caused by a paramagnetic product of oxydative denaturation of hemoglobin. **B:** The hematoma has a high intensity in T2-weighted images at low field strength because of its long T2 relaxation time. **C:** This coronal T2-weighted image of the same hematoma was acquired on the same date but with a high field imager (1.5 T). The peripheral areas which had the highest intensities with the same sequence in **(B)** are of low intensity here because of dramatic T2 shortening at high field.

As high-resolution techniques continue to develop and evolve, FSE sequences are becoming increasingly utilized for musculoskeletal applications. FSE images may be T1, Proton Density or T2-weighted depending on the designated TR and effective TE. As compared to conventional spin-echo sequences, fat and water tend to have higher signal intensity on the FSE images. Therefore, it is advantageous to employ some sort of fat suppression technique to increase the conspicuity of pathology on T2-weighted images. Figure 2-32 demonstrates a case of patellofemoral

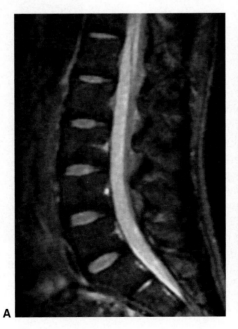

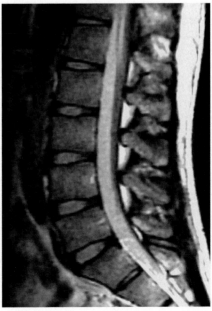

Figure 2-31 Comparison of lumbar spine images. **A:** Conventional T2-weighted spin-echo sequence with an 8 min 46 s acquisition time. **B:** Fast spin-echo sequence which required only 1 min 6 s of acquisition time.

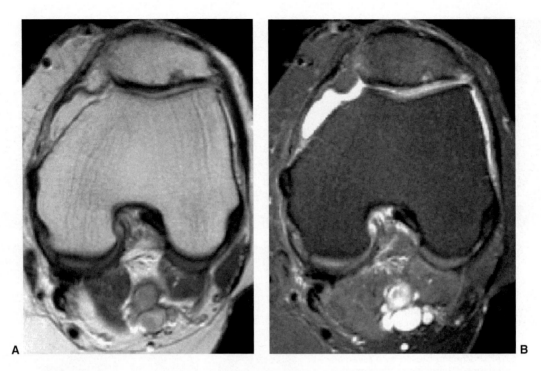

Figure 2-32 T2-weighted FSE images of a patient with chondromalacia patella, without **(A)** and with **(B)** fat suppression. Fat has higher signal on FSE images versus conventional spin echo.

chondromalacia with comparison axial T2-weighted FSE images without and with fat suppression. Many musculoskeletal imagers utilize "hybrid" (intermediate between proton density and T2 weighting) FSE sequences with long TRs and effective TE times of approximately 40 and 50 ms. It is important to account for the presence of magic angle artifact in curved tendons and ligaments when utilizing sequences with effective TEs less than 40 ms. Because of the excellent contrast between joint fluid and hyaline articular cartilage, fat-suppressed hybrid and T2-weighted FSE sequences are very useful in the evaluation of chondral injury and degeneration providing an MR "arthrographic" appearance. Figure 2-33 demonstrates a case of posttraumatic chondral injury in a young athlete.

As previously stated, FSE sequences are probably most useful in their ability to provide high-resolution detail of complex anatomic structures of the peripheral joints. Figure 2-34 demonstrates a case of a clinically proven complex ligamentous injury of the ankle in a soccer player that was obtained with a specialized foot and ankle coil on a 1.5 T strength magnet. Figure 2-35 demonstrates exquisite detail of wrist osseous, cartilage, and ligament anatomy utilizing a high resolution, fat-suppressed T2-weighted FSE sequence. The images were obtained with a highly specialized wrist coil and a 3 T strength magnet that maximizes the signal-to-noise ratio. The 3 T magnet also allows for decreased time of imaging.

FSE images are less degraded by artifact from implanted metal than comparable conventional spin echo and GRE images. Metallic artifact can be further diminished by broadening the receiver bandwidth. Also, FSE-IR images with broadened receiver bandwidth tend to provide a further decrease in metal artifact and a more uniform fat suppression on T2-weighted images (see Fig. 2-36).

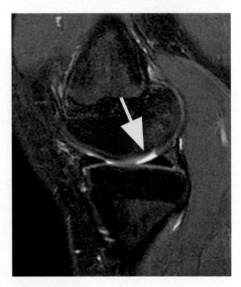

Figure 2-33 Sagittal high-resolution fat suppressed T2-weighted FSE-XL image demonstrates an acute, posttraumatic chondral defect (*arrow*) of the medial femoral condyle.

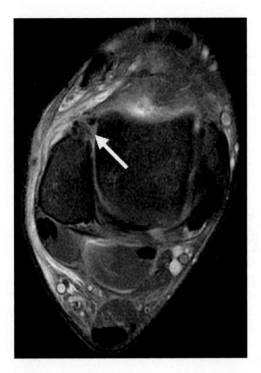

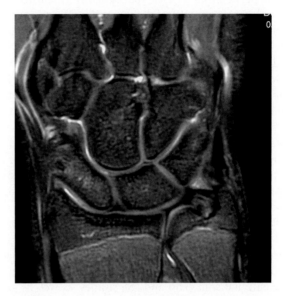

Figure 2-34 Axial high-resolution fat suppressed T2-weighted FSE-XL image demonstrates disruption of the anterior inferior tibiofibular ligament (*arrow*) in a young athlete.

Figure 2-35 Coronal high-resolution fat suppressed T2-weighted FSE-XL images of the wrist obtained with a specialized wrist coil on a 3 T magnet demonstrate exquisite anatomical detail of the osseous, cartilage, and ligamentous anatomy in an asymptomatic patient.

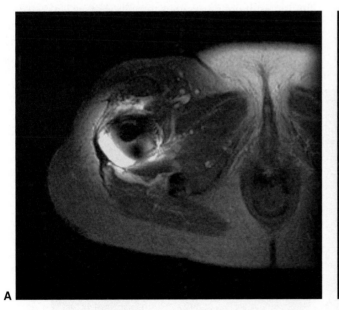

A

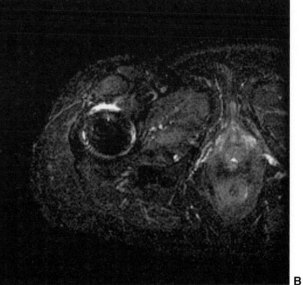

B

Figure 2-36 **A:** Fat-suppressed T2-weighted FSE images obtained with a broadened receiver bandwidth diminish some of the metallic artifact in this patient with hip pain. **B:** The metallic artifact is further diminished and the fat suppression is more uniform utilizing an FSE-IR sequence with broadened receiver bandwidth and a TI of 130 ms.

MISCELLANEOUS TECHNIQUES

A great deal of attention has been directed at the possibility of performing *in vivo* spectroscopy of proton and phosphorus resonances to characterize tissue at a biochemical level (5,22,28–30,32,65–68). These techniques offer potentially exciting prospects but they have yet to find wide use in clinical practice.

Many additional techniques for tissue characterization are possible with MRI. Some of the simplest ones are most intriguing and seem to be particularly suitable for musculoskeletal problems. A good example is computation of special-purpose images from standard MR images. Calculated maps of T1, T2, and spin density can be produced, and from them it is possible to generate supplementary images that can depend on any arbitrary function of T1, T2, and N(H) (69).

Fat-suppression techniques are widely used in musculoskeletal MRI, most commonly to increase lesion conspicuity on T2-weighted images. Perhaps the most useful method is spectral presaturation, which is applicable to conventional spin echo and FSE studies, as well as gradient-echo and contrast-enhanced imaging. This fat-suppression technique is most uniform when images are obtained at the isocenter of the magnet. Fat suppression may be nonuniform, with imaging obtained out of isocenter, or at curved soft-tissue and air interfaces as occur at the shoulder and heel. FSE-IR sequences may provide more reliable fat suppression in these cases (see Fig. 2-37).

Intravenous or intra-articular gadolinium is utilized in some musculoskeletal MR cases to provide additional diagnostic information. Intravenous gadolinium is most useful in establishing whether a soft tissue or intra-osseous lesion is solid or cystic (see Fig. 2-38). Other indications for intravenous gadolinium include the assessment of soft tissue infections, inflammatory arthropathies, osteonecrosis and ischemia, mechanical stenosing tenosynovitis, and defining complex postoperative fluid collections. Intra-articular gadolinium is useful in assessing joint soft tissue pathology such as labral tears of the shoulder and hip (see Fig. 2-39). Occasionally, it is utilized in the assessment of osteochondral injuries of the knee and talar dome and in detecting occult ligamentous injuries of the wrist and elbow.

APPEARANCE OF VASCULAR STRUCTURES IN MAGNETIC RESONANCE IMAGING

Arteries and veins of varying size can be identified in most musculoskeletal MR images. These vessels are of great intrinsic interest. It is important to define the relationship of major vessels to musculoskeletal tumors if surgery is planned. Many of the primary effects and complications of trauma can affect the vascular supply and drainage of an extremity. Atherosclerosis and deep venous thrombosis represent very important primary vascular diseases that affect extremities.

In most MR images, the appearance of normal arteries and veins is quite variable. The lumens of vessels may be of low intensity, high intensity, or mixed intensity. This is disturbing because it hinders reliable identification of such important lesions as venous thrombosis (see Fig. 2-40).

To select examination techniques that facilitate diagnosis of vascular disease and to interpret the images, it is important to have a basic understanding of the physical

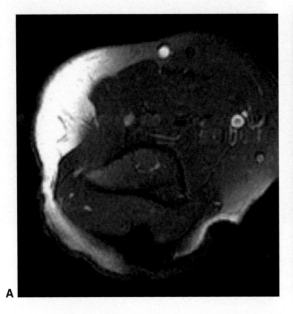
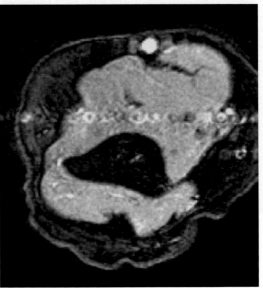

Figure 2-37   Axial fat-suppressed T2-weighted images (**A** and **B**) of the elbow obtained out of isocenter demonstrate inhomogeneous fat suppression. Use of FSE-IR sequences in this same patient provided uniform fat suppression as in **B**.

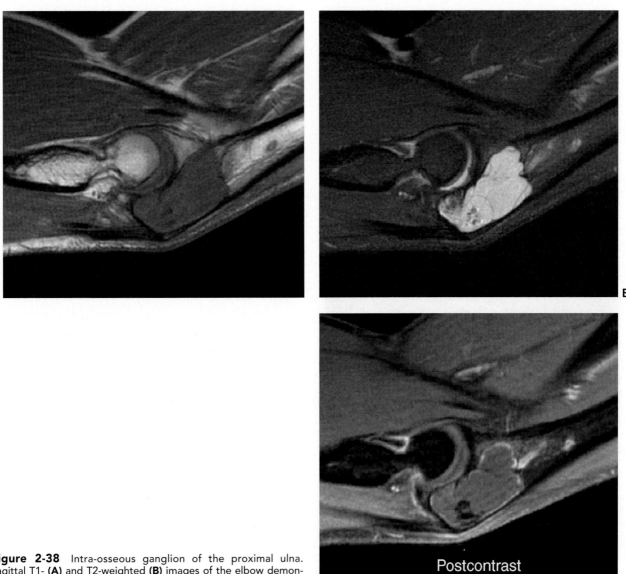

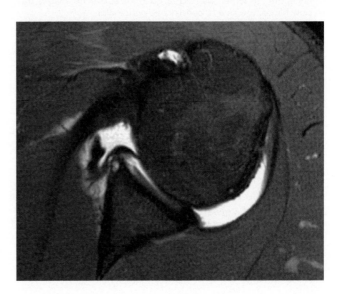

Figure 2-38 Intra-osseous ganglion of the proximal ulna. Sagittal T1- **(A)** and T2-weighted **(B)** images of the elbow demonstrate a juxta-articular lesion within the proximal ulna. The use of intravenous gadolinium **(C)** confirms the cystic nature of the lesion.

Figure 2-39 MR arthrogram of the shoulder with dilute gadolinium demonstrates a posttraumatic tear of the anterior glenoid labrum with a cartilage defect.

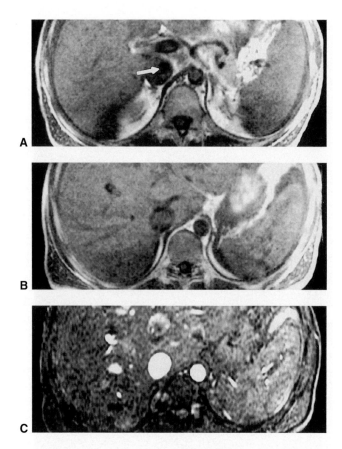

Figure 2-40   **A:** This patient had a diagnosis of thrombosis of the inferior vena cava (IVC) on the basis of a prior MRI examination. In this follow-up T1-weighted spin-echo image, the IVC (*arrow*) again demonstrates the lack of a low intensity "flow void," except for an area of apparent recanalization. **B:** A section obtained more superiorly also shows intraluminal signal in a generous-sized lumen suggestive of thrombosis of the IVC. **C:** In contrast to the spin-echo findings, gradient-echo images obtained at same levels demonstrate flow enhancement throughout the IVC lumen, ruling out thrombosis. Further MRI demonstrated pericardial thickening, consistent with constrictive pericarditis. The patient was treated with partial pericardiectomy. This case emphasizes the importance of caution in attributing the lack of a typical "flow void" in spin-echo images to vascular thrombosis. Here, the increased intraluminal signal in the IVC lumen was increased in the spin-echo images due to slow blood flow due to constrictive pericarditis.

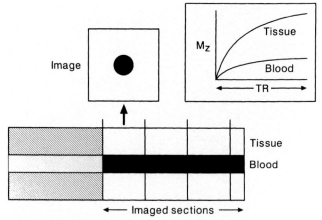

Figure 2-41   Liquid blood has a longer T1 relaxation time than many tissues, especially perivascular fat. Disregarding the effect of flow, it tends to have a lower intensity than surrounding tissue in T1-weighted images because it is more saturated.

processes that govern the appearance of moving blood in MRI (70–72). For simplicity, this discussion will only consider vessels that are perpendicular to the plane of section.

The signal intensity of flowing blood is governed by three basic processes: saturation, spin phase, and washout effects. Saturation effects (see Fig. 2-41) depend on the fact that the T1 relaxation time of fluid blood is longer than most soft tissues. Thus, the intensity of intravascular blood would be expected to be lower than adjacent tissue if the T1 weighting of a given pulse sequence is sufficient.

The saturation effect is often counteracted by a mechanism called "flow-related enhancement" (see Fig. 2-42). This results from flow of blood from outside the image volume in the interval between 90° RF pulses. These "fresh"

spins carry full longitudinal magnetization because they have not been partially saturated by previous exposure to RF pulses. They can therefore provide more spin-echo signal. This is the main cause of the bright intraluminal signals that are often present in MRIs of blood vessels. Naturally, the effect is most pronounced in the sections that are closest to the entry point of the vessel into the image volume. Flow-related enhancement (and the flow artifacts that often accompany it) can be reduced by a technique called "spatial presaturation" (SAT) (73,74).

Two other effects tend to decrease the intensity of flowing blood. One of these is known as the "spin dephasing" effect. Figure 2-43 demonstrates that the volume element corresponding to a single image pixel can be conceptually broken down into smaller volume elements that are called

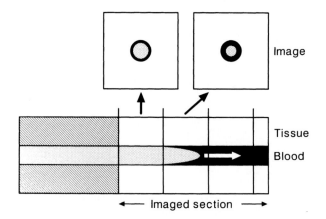

Figure 2-42   Flow-related enhancement counteracts the effect of saturation on blood in the vessel lumen. Spins that have not recently been irradiated with RF flow into the plane of section between repetitions. They yield more signal because they are unsaturated. The effect is more pronounced in sections close to the nonirradiated volume.

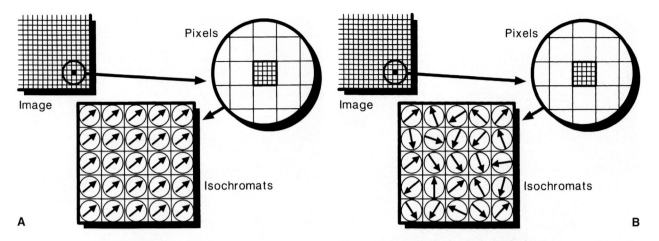

Figure 2-43 The contents of a voxel can be conceptually divided into smaller elements called isochromats. The spin-echo signal from each isochromat is a vector quantity, having a magnitude and phase (direction). If the phase angles of most isochromats are similar **(A)**, then the vectors add constructively. If the varied phase angles are present **(B)**, then the net signal from the volume element will be reduced.

"isochromats." The net magnetization vector of the entire volume element is the vector sum of the individual magnetizations of the isochromats. If the phase angles of the isochromats are not identical, then the magnitude of their vector sum will be reduced. This is the basic principle for spin-phase effects. The moving spins in flowing blood are subjected to magnetic field gradients in the course of imaging. These field gradients cause isochromats to accumulate phase differences with respect to stationary spins in tissue. The amount of phase shift depends on the velocity of the individual isochromats and the strength and duration of the field gradients. At the time of the spin echo, the magnetization isochromats with varying phase angles adds together in an incoherent fashion so that signal intensity is reduced (see Fig. 2-44).

Dephasing effects can reduce the intensity of blood so that any flow-related enhancement that may have been present is masked. A technique called "gradient moment nulling" (GMN) or "flow compensation," can counteract the dephasing effects of gradients so that intensity is restored (see Fig. 2-45) (75). This technique is employed to reduce blood flow artifacts in gradient-echo images, as well as tissue motion and cerebrospinal fluid flow artifacts in T2-weighted spin-echo images (76). A phenomenon called "even echo rephasing" sometimes causes a similar effect in images of even-numbered echos in multiple spin-echo sequences.

The most important mechanism that reduces the MRI intensity of flowing blood has not yet been described here. This is the "washout effect," shown in Fig. 2-46. Protons must receive both 90° and 180° RF pulses to yield a spin-echo signal. In most imagers, these pulses are "slice selective" so that their effects are spatially limited to the confines of imaged sections. Flowing protons that escape the plane of section in the time interval between 90° and 180° RF pulses will not produce a signal. This establishes a

"cutoff velocity" for blood flow, above which no intraluminal signal can be present. This velocity can be calculated by dividing the section thickness by time interval between the 90° and 180° RF pulses. Note that the washout effect is not operative in gradient-echo imaging, because only a single RF pulse is employed.

In spin-echo imaging, it is often valuable to use techniques that will depict patent vessels with reliable flow voids. Such flow voids are promoted by avoiding flow-related enhancement through the use of SAT, avoiding

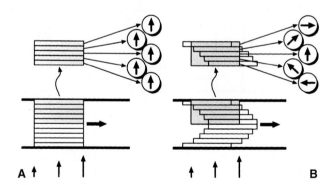

Figure 2-44 **A:** "Plug flow," which is a model for flow that assumes that the velocity of fluid is the same near the center of the lumen as it is at the sides. Thus, each isochromat has the same velocity. The *vertical arrows* along the base of the vessel represent the strength of the local magnetic field at each point. This gradient causes the phase angle of each isochromat to change as it flows along the vessel, but since the velocities are identical the phase angles of all the isochromats in the volume element will be the same at the time of the spin echo. **B:** "Laminar flow," a situation in which the velocity has a parabolic profile across the lumen of the vessel. In this case, the phase errors accumulated by isochromats as they flow through the magnetic field gradient are variable because the velocities are different. Thus, the net signal intensity from a voxel is reduced at the time of spin-echo creation because the isochromats do not add constructively. This has been called the "dephasing effect."

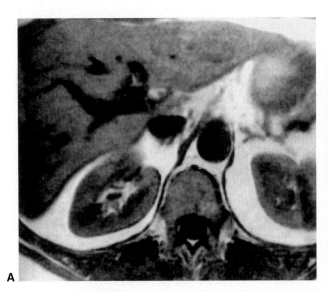
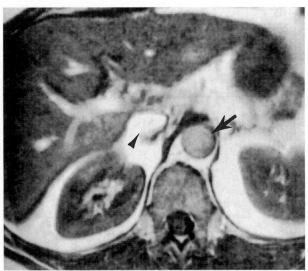

A

B

Figure 2-45 Effect of eliminating intravoxel dephasing. **A:** A T1-weighted image of the upper abdomen. The aorta, inferior vena cava, and intrahepatic blood vessels have low signal intensity. **B:** Image was acquired with identical parameters, but with the addition of gradient moment nulling ("flow compensation"), a pulse sequence technique that eliminates intravoxel dephasing. The signal intensity of the aorta, inferior vena cava, and intrahepatic blood vessels is markedly increased in comparison to **A.** The elimination of intravoxel dephasing has "unmasked" flow-related enhancement, which was present in **A** but was suppressed by dephasing effects. Note that the signal intensity of the aorta (*arrow*) is lower than that of the inferior vena cava (*arrowhead*). This is due to the "washout effect" described in Fig. 2-46, which is more prominent in vessels with high blood flow velocity.

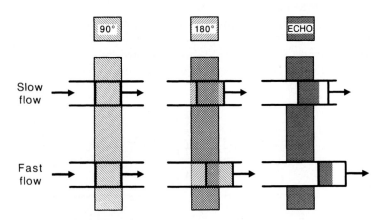

Figure 2-46 "Washout effect." Flowing spins that move out of the section in the time between 90° and 180° pulses will not yield a spin-echo signal. The amount of signal loss due to washout increases with flow velocity. With very fast flow, all of the blood in the segment of lumen may be replaced so that the spin-echo signal will be zero. The minimum velocity that replaces all spin in such a fashion is called the "cutoff velocity."

GMN, and using a slightly longer echo delay if needed to permit more washout. An alternative approach is to depict patent vessels with high intensity. This method typically employs gradient-echo sequences (which are not subject to the washout effect) and GMN to reduce dephasing.

Many different flow effects can be observed in MRI, but the principles that have been described here can be used to explain the majority of them.

REFERENCES

1. Agartz I, Saaf J, Wahlund L-O, et al. T1 and T2 relaxation time estimates in the normal human brain. *Radiology* 1991;181:537–543.
2. Dooms GC, Hricak H, Moseley ME, et al. Characterization of lymphadenopathy by magnetic resonance relaxation times: preliminary results. *Radiology* 1985;155:691–697.
3. Keller PJ, Hunter WW Jr, Schmalbrock P. Multisection fat water imaging with chemical shift selective presaturation. *Radiology* 1987;164:539–541.
4. McSweeney MB, Small WC, Cerny V, et al. Magnetic resonance imaging in the diagnosis of breast disease: use of transverse relaxation times. *Radiology* 1984;153:741–744.
5. Ohtomo K, Itai Y, Furui S, et al. Hepatic tumors: differentiation by transverse relaxation time (T2) of MR resonance imaging. *Radiology* 1985;155:421–423.
6. Pettersson H, Slone RM, Spanier S, et al. Musculoskeletal tumors: T1 and T2 relaxation times. *Radiology* 1988;167:783–785.
7. Schmidt HC, Tscholakoff D, Hricak H, et al. MR image contrast and relaxation times of solid tumors in the chest, abdomen, and pelvis. *J Comput Assist Tomogr* 1985;9:738–748.
8. Wehrli FW, MacFall JR, Shutts D, et al. Mechanisms of contrast in NMR imaging. *J Comp Assist Tomogr* 1984;8(3):369–380.
9. Biondetti PR, Ehman RL. Soft-tissue sarcomas: use of textural patterns in skeletal muscle as a diagnostic feature in postoperative MR imaging. *Radiology* 1992;183:845–848.

10. Joseph PM, Axel L. Potential problems with selective pulses in NMR imaging systems. *Med Phys* 1984;11:772–777.
11. Kjos BO, Ehman RL, Brandt Zawadzki M. Reproducibility of T1 and T2 relaxation times calculated from routine MR imaging sequences: phantom study. *AJNR* 1985;6:277–283.
12. Kjos BO, Ehman RL, Brant Zawadzki M, et al. Reproducibility of relaxation times and spin density calculated from routine MR imaging sequences: clinical study of the CNS. *AJNR* 1985;6:271–276.
13. Ehman RL, McNamara MT, Brasch RC, et al. Influence of physiological motion on the appearance of tissue in MRI. *Radiology* 1986;143:1175–1182.
14. Bottomley PA, Foster TH, Argersinger RE, et al. A review of normal tissue hydrogen NMR relaxation times and relaxation mechanisms from 1 to 100 MHz: dependence on tissue type, NMR frequency. *Med Phys* 1984;11(4):425–448.
15. Johnson GA, Herfkins RJ, Brown MA. Tissue relaxation time: in vivo field dependence. *Radiology* 1985;156:805–810.
16. Ehman RL, Kjos BO, Hricak H, et al. Relative intensity of abdominal organs in magnetic resonance images. *J Comp Assist Tomogr* 1985;9:315–319.
17. Posse S, Cuenod CA, Le Bihan D. Human brain: proton diffusion MR spectroscopy. *Radiology* 1993;188:719–725.
18. Sevick RJ, Kanda F, Mintorovitch J, et al. Cytotoxic brain edema: assessment with diffusion-weighted MR imaging. *Radiology* 1992;185:687–690.
19. Wesbey GE, Moseley M, Ehman RL. Translational molecular self diffusion in magnetic resonance imaging: effects on observed spin spin relaxation. *Invest Radiol* 1984;19:484–490.
20. Wesbey GE, Moseley M, Ehman RL. Translational molecular self diffusion in magnetic resonance imaging: measurement of the self diffusion coefficient. *Invest Radiol* 1984;19:491–498.
21. Ballon D, Jakubowski A, Gabrilove J. et al. In vivo measurements of bone marrow cellularity using volume-localized proton NMR spectroscopy. *Magn Res Med* 1991;19:85–95.
22. Barany M, Lander BG, Glick RP. et al. In vivo H 1 spectroscopy in humans at 1.5 T. *Radiology* 1988;167:839–844.
23. de Kerviler E, Leroy-Willig A, Jehenson P, et al. Exercise-induced muscle modifications: study of healthy subjects and patients with metabolic myopathies with MR imaging and P-31 spectroscopy. *Radiology* 1991;181:259–264.
24. Dixon WT. Simple proton spectroscopic imaging. *Radiology* 1984;153:189–194.
25. Frahm J, Haase A, Hanicke W, et al. Chemical shift selective MR imaging using a whole body magnet. *Radiology* 1985;156:441–444.
26. Fraser DD, Frank JA, Dalakas MC. Inflammatory myopathies: MR imaging and spectroscopy. *Radiology* 1991;179:341–342.
27. Karczmar GS, Meyerhoff DJ, Boska MD, et al. P-31 spectroscopy study of response of superficial human tumors to therapy. *Radiology* 1991;179:149–153.
28. Narayana PA, Hazle JD, Jackson EF, et al. In vivo 1H spectroscopic studies of human gastrocnemius muscle at 1.5 T. *Magn Reson Imaging* 1988;6:481–485.
29. Narayana PA, Jackson EF, Hazle JD, et al. In vivo localization proton spectroscopic studies in human gastrocnemius muscle. *Magn Reson Med* 1988;8:151–159.
30. Pykett IL, Rosen BR. Nuclear magnetic resonance in vivo proton chemical shift imaging. *Radiology* 1983;149:197–201.
31. Rosen BR, Fleming DM, Kushner DC, et al. Hematologic bone marrow disorders: quantitative chemical shift MR imaging. *Radiology* 1988;169:799–804.
32. Farrar TC, Becker ED *Pulse and Fourier transform NMR: introduction to theory and methods.* New York: Academic Press, 1971.
33. Bloembergen EM, Purcell EM, Pound RV. Relaxation effects in nuclear magnetic resonance absorption. *Phys Rev* 1948;73:679–712.
34. De Vre RM. Biomedical implications of the relaxation behavior of water related to NMR imaging. *Br J Radiol* 1984;57:955–976.
35. Fullerton GD, Potter JL, Dornbluth NC. NMR relaxation of protons in tissues. *Magn Reson Imaging* 1982;1:209–228.
36. Hazelwood CF. A view of the significance and understanding of the physical properties of cell associated water. In: Drost Hansen W, Clegg J, eds. *Cell associated water,* New York: Academic Press, 1979:165–260.
37. Crooks LE, Arakawa M, Hoenninger J, et al. Magnetic resonance imaging: effects of magnetic field strength. *Radiology* 1984;151:127–133.
38. Fullerton GD, Cameron IL, Ord VA. Frequency dependence of magnetic resonance spin lattice relaxation of protons in biological materials. *Radiology* 1984;151:135–138.
39. Brasch RC. Work in progress: methods of contrast enhancement for NMR imaging and potential applications. *Radiology* 1983;147:781–788.
40. Brasch RC, Wesbey GE, Gooding CA, et al. Magnetic resonance imaging of transfusional hemosiderosis complicating thalassemia major. *Radiology* 1984;150:767–771.
41. Mitchell DG, Burk DL Jr, Vinitski S, et al. Biophysical basis of tissue contrast in extracranial MR imaging. *AJR* 1987;149:831–837.
42. Herfkins R, Davis PL, Crooks LE, et al. Nuclear magnetic resonance imaging of the abnormal live rat and correlations with tissue characteristics. *Radiology* 1981;141:211–218.
43. Beall PT, Amtey SR, Kasturi SR. *NMR data handbook for biomedical applications.* New York: Pergamon, 1984.
44. Fullerton GD, Cameron IL, Hunter K, et al. Proton magnetic resonance relaxation behavior of whole muscle with fatty inclusions. *Radiology* 1985;155:727–730.
45. Dooms GC, Fisher MR, Hricak H, et al. MR imaging of intramuscular hemorrhage. *JCAT* 1985;9:908–913.
46. Swenson SJ, Keller PL, Berquist TH, et al. Magnetic resonance imaging of hemorrhage. *AJR* 1985;145:921–927.
47. Bradley WG, Schmidt PG. Effect of methemoglobin formation on the appearance of subarachnoid hemorrhage. *Radiology* 1985;156:99–103.
48. Gomori JM, Grossman RI, Goldberg HI, et al. Intracranial hematomas: imaging by high field MR. *Radiology* 1985;157:87–93.
49. Thulborn KR, Waterton JC, Matthews PM, et al. Oxygenation dependence of the transverse relaxation time of water protons in whole blood at high field. *Biochem Biophys Acta* 1982;714(2):265–270.
50. Berendsen HJC. Nuclear magnetic resonance study of collagen hydration. *J Chem Phys* 1962;36:3297–3305.
51. Erickson SJ, Cox IH, Hyde JS, et al. Effect of tendon orientation on MR imaging signal intensity: a manifestation of the magic angle phenomenon. *Radiology* 1991;181:389–392.
52. Fullerton GD, Cameron IL, Ord VA. Orientation of tendons in the magnetic field and its effect on T2 relaxation times. *Radiology* 1985;155:433–435.
53. Kurtz D, Dwyer A. Isosignal contours and signal gradients as an aid to choosing MRI imaging techniques. *J Comput Assist Tomogr* 1984;8:819–828.
54. Richardson ML, Amparo EG, Gillespy T, et al. Theoretical considerations for optimizing intensity differences between primary musculoskeletal tumors and normal tissue with spin echo MRI. *Invest Radiol* 1985;20:492–497.
55. Harms SE, Flamig DP, Fisher CF, et al. New method for fast MR imaging of the knee. *Radiology* 1989;173:743–750.
56. Konig H, Sauter R, Deimling M, et al. Cartilage disorders: comparison of spin echo CHESS, and FLASH sequence MR images. *Radiology* 1987;164:753–758.
57. Siemens Medical Systems. FLASH and FISP gradient echo pulse sequences, 1989.
58. Solomon SL, Totty WG, Lee JKT. MR imaging of the knee: comparison of three dimensional FISP and two dimensional spin echo pulse sequences. *Radiology* 1989;173:739–742.
59. Wehrli FW, Perkins TG, Shimakawa A, et al. Chemical shift induced amplitude modulations in images obtained with gradient refocusing. *Magn Res Imaging* 1987;5:157–158.
60. General Electric Medical Systems. *Introduction to fast scan magnetic resonance.* Milwaukee, WI: General Electric, 1986:72–99.
61. Ehman RL, Berquist TH, McLeod RA. MR imaging of the musculoskeletal system: a 5 year appraisal. *Radiology* 1988;166:313–320.
62. Hennig J, Nauerth A, Friedburg H. RARE imaging: a fast imaging method for clinical MR. *Magn Reson Med* 1986;3:823–833.
63. Melki PS, Mulkern RV, Lawrence PP, et al. Comparing the FAISE method with conventional dual-echo sequences. *JMRI* 1991;1:319–326.

64. Mulkern RV, Wong STS, Winalski C, et al. Contrast manipulation and artifact assessment of 2D and 3D RARE sequences. *Magn Reson Imaging* 1990;8:557–566.
65. Lenkinski RE, Holland GA, Allman T, et al. Integrated MR imaging and spectroscopy with chemical shift imaging of P 31 at 1.5 T: initial clinical experience. *Radiology* 1988;169:201–206.
66. Nidecker AC, Muller S, Aue WP. Extremity bone tumors: evaluation by p31 spectroscopy. *Radiology* 1985;157:167–174.
67. Redmond OM, Stack JP, Dervan PA, et al. Osteosarcoma: use of MR imaging and MR spectroscopy in clinical decision making. *Radiology* 1989;172:811–815.
68. Zochodne DW, Thompson RT, Driedger AA, et al. Metabolic changes in human muscle denervation: topical 31P NMR spectroscopy studies. *Magn Reson Med* 1988;7:373–383.
69. Ortendahl DA, Hylton N, Kaufman L, et al. Analytical tools for magnetic resonance imaging. *Radiology* 1984;153:479–488.
70. Axel L. Blood flow effects in magnetic resonance imaging. *AJR* 1984;143:1157–1166.
71. Bradley WG, Waluch V. Blood flow: magnetic resonance imaging. *Radiology* 1985;154:443–450.
72. Wehrli FW, MacFall JR, Axel L, et al. Approaches to in plane and out of plane flow imaging. *Noninvasive Med Imaging* 1984;1: 127–136.
73. Edelman RR, Atkinson DJ, Silver MS, et al. FRODO pulse sequences: a new means of eliminating motion, flow, and wraparound artifacts. *Radiology* 1988;166:231–236.
74. Felmlee JP, Ehman RL. Spatial presaturation: a method for suppressing flow artifacts and improving depiction of vascular anatomy in MR imaging. *Radiology* 1987;164:559–564.
75. Pattany PM, Phillips JJ, Chiu LC, et al. Motion artifact suppression technique (MAST) for MR imaging. *J Comput Assist Tomogr* 1987;11:369–377.
76. Ehman RL, Felmlee JP. Flow artifact reduction in MRI: a review of the roles of gradient moment nulling and spatial presaturation. *Magn Reson Med* 1990;14:293–307.

General Technical Considerations in Musculoskeletal MRI

3

Thomas H. Berquist

Magnetic resonance imaging (MRI) is an excellent technique for evaluation of the musculoskeletal system (1–8). Respiratory motion, often a significant problem in the chest and upper abdomen, is generally not a problem in the pelvis and extremities (1,9). Images can be obtained in the coronal, sagittal, transaxial, and oblique planes. Radial (multiple oblique planes radiating from a central localization point) imaging techniques are also possible. Three-dimensional techniques are also available and particularly suited to areas where anatomy is complex (10–13).

New coil technology, faster pulse sequences, and increased utilization of contrast agents have expanded the musculoskeletal applications of MRI (14–19). Arthrographic and angiographic techniques are now commonly employed (17,20–34). Spectroscopy is used more frequently, but it is still not commonly used in day-to-day practice (35–38).

New magnet designs, including higher field strengths [up to 8 Tesla (T)], open systems, and extremity systems, are also available (see Fig. 3-1) (36,39,40). Dedicated extremity units are less expensive and easily sited. Field strengths vary from 0.2 to 1.0 T. Positioning can be a problem with some patients, and the field of view (FOV) is limited.

As a rule, higher field strengths provide superior spatial and contrast resolution (1,39,41). Experience with 3 T

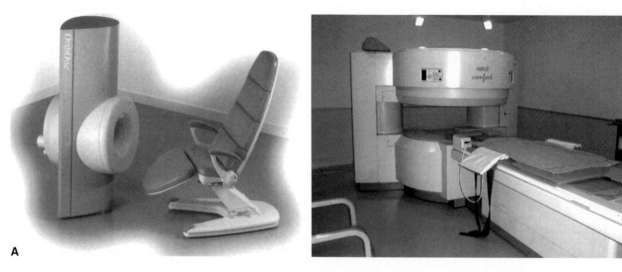

Figure 3-1   Photographs of an extremity magnet **(A)** (Courtesy of ONI Medical Systems, Inc. Willingham, MA) and an open magnet **(B)** (Courtesy of Hitachi Medical Systems, Inc. Twinsburg, OH).

imaging is increasing. Signal-to-noise (S/N) ratios increase in a linear fashion with field strength. Therefore, the S/N ratio at 3 T is twice that at 1.5 T. This allows increased spatial resolution without increasing imaging time. Chemical shift artifact is increased at 3 T, but this may be compensated for by increasing the bandwidth. Fat suppression is also more uniform at 3 T compared to 1.5 T.

MRI examinations must be conducted differently than radiographic or computed tomography (CT) examinations. Patient selection, positioning, coil selection, pulse sequences, and use of intravenous or intraarticular contrast agents must all be considered prior to the examination to optimize image quality and properly characterize pathologic lesions. This section will discuss practical clinical concepts for musculoskeletal MR imaging. More specific techniques and applications will be discussed in the anatomic chapters that follow.

PATIENT SELECTION

MR images are produced using a static magnetic field, magnetic gradients, and radio frequency (RF) pulses (see Chapter 1). No ionizing radiation is used. To date, no untoward biologic effects have been identified at commonly used field strengths ($\leq$2 T) (42,43).

PATIENT SCREENING — SAFETY ISSUES

Prior to considering MRI as the method for imaging patients, certain screening issues and patient safety factors must be considered. The Safety Committee of the International Society for Magnetic Resonance in Medicine (ISMRM) recommends that each site or facility develop a standard policy for patient screening (44–46).

The screening methods may vary depending upon the type of facility, patient population (i.e., metal or construction workers, children, etc.), and allied health workers' knowledge of MR imaging and potential risk factors (41,45).

Most agree that a written questionnaire with specific but easily answered questions (Table 3-1) should be completed by patients and further verbal discussions be held as the patient is being prepared for the examination. This should prevent overlooking obvious risk factors such as cardiac pacemakers, cerebral aneurysm clips, metallic foreign bodies, or electrical devices that may place the patient at risk during the examination. When metallic foreign bodies are suspected, radiographs or, in some cases, CT should be obtained to confirm or exclude these potential problems. Boutin et al. (45) reviewed safety data from 205 institutions and noted that 85% of departments used radiographs for screening (specifically for suspected foreign bodies in the orbit), 41% used CT, and 12% used metal detectors as a part of their patient screening program (46–49).

Magnetic fields may affect certain metal implants and electrical devices (1,41,60,61,71). In many situations, the exact metallic content of the implant cannot be determined (59). Though evaluations are still in progress, many reports have defined a number of implants that may be potentially dangerous to the patient or affect image quality (1,54–57,59,62,65–68,72). Synchronous pacemakers convert to the asynchronous mode when placed in MR imagers. The pacemaker power pack may change its orientation in the magnetic field. In addition, significant image degradation may occur if the power pack is in the region being examined. Numerous heart valves have been studied at field strengths of 0.35 to 1.5 T. The artifacts created by most values are negligible, and it has been concluded that patients with these prosthetic values can be safely imaged (65,69). However, movement or torque was demonstrated with certain valves

TABLE 3-1
SAFETY SCREENING QUESTIONNAIRE

	Yes	No
Suggested Questions: (check one)		
1. Have you had previous surgery?	___	___
If yes, list operations.	___	___
2. Are you aware of any previous metal		
injuries (bullets, BBs, wire or metal fragments)?	___	___
If yes, list location.		
3. Do you work with metal in your occupation	___	___
(machinist, welder, etc.)?		
4. Do you have any of the following metals in your body?	___	___
Cardiac pacemaker or defibrillator	___	___
Heart valves	___	___
Aneurysm clips	___	___
Ear implants	___	___
Eye implants	___	___
Dental implants	___	___
Magnetic implants	___	___
Metallic foreign bodies	___	___
Orthopaedic implants (total joints, plates, screws,	___	___
wires, cables)		
Eyelid tattoo	___	___
Drug patches	___	___
Catheters or tubes	___	___
Penile or genitourinary prostheses	___	___
5. Do you have any allergies? If yes, please list.	___	___

From references 9, 45, 46, 48, and 50–70.

(Table 3-2). In spite of this response to the static magnetic field, the deflection is minimal and not considered a contraindication (65). Patients with heart valves typically also have sternotomy wires. Patients with sternotomy wires and retained epicardial pacemaker wires can be safely examined with MRI (73).

Most surgical clips at our institution are nonferromagnetic or contain minimal ferromagnetic material. However, a significant number of aneurysm clips (19 of 32) (Table 3-3) are ferromagnetic and may twist or turn in a magnetic environment (62,65,75–77). Brown et al. (52) demonstrated that the strongest torque and most significant image artifacts were present with clips made of 17-7HP stainless steel. Titanium and tantalum clips showed the least attractive force and minimal image distortion. We do not examine patients with cerebral aneurysm clips or pacemakers. However, hemostasis clips are usually not a significant problem in musculoskeletal imaging (see Fig. 3-2).

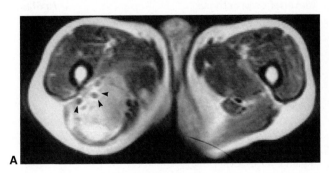

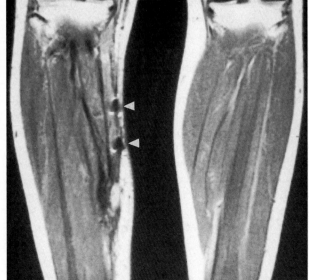

Figure 3-2 MR artifacts created by hemostasis clips. **A:** 0.15 T SE 500/20 image in a patient with a partially resected liposarcoma. Note the focal areas of no signal with small bright halos (*black arrowheads*) caused by the surgical clip artifacts. **B:** 1.5 T SE 500/20 coronal images of the calves. Note the surgical clip artifacts (*white arrowheads*) in the right calf medially.

TABLE 3-2

HEART VALVES DEMONSTRATING TORQUE OR DEFLECTION WITH STATIC MAGNETIC FIELD

Beall (Coratonic, Indiana, PA)
Bjork-Shiley (universal/spherical) (Shiley)
Bjork-Shiley, model MBC (Shiley)
Bjork-Shiley, model 25 MBRC 11030 (Shiley)
Carpentier-Edwards, model 2650 (American Edwards)
Carpentier-Edwards (porcine) (American Edwards)
Hall-Kaster, model A7700 (Medtronic, Minneapolis, MN)
Hancock I (porcine) (Johnson & Johnson, Anaheim, CA)
Hancock II (porcine) (Johnson & Johnson)
Hancock extracorporeal, modes 242R (Johnson & Johnson)
Hancock extracorporeal, model M 4365-33 (Johnson & Johnson)
Ionescu-Shiley (Universal ISM)
Lillehi-Kaster, model 300S (Medical, Inver Grove Heights, MN)
Lillehi-Kaster, model 5009 (Medical)
Medtronic-Hall (Medtronic)
Medtronic Hall, model A7700-D-16 (Medtronic)
Omnicarbon, model 3523 (Medical)
Omniscience, model 6522 (Medical)
Smeloff-Cutter (Cutter Laboratories, Berkeley, CA)
Starr-Edwards, model 1260 (American Edwards)
Starr-Edwards, model 2320 (American Edwards)
Starr-Edwards, model Pre 6000 (American Edwards)
Starr-Edwards, model 6520 (American Edwards)
St. Jude, model A 101 (St. Jude Medical)
St. Jude, model M 101 (St. Jude Medical)

From references 47, 54, 66, and 74.

TABLE 3-3

ANEURYSM AND HEMOSTASIS CLIPS EXHIBITING TORQUE IN MAGNETIC FIELD

Drake (DR14, DR24) (Edward Weck, Triangle Park, NJ)
Drake (DR 16) (Edward Weck)
Drake (301 SS) (Edward Weck)
Downs multipositional (17-7PH)
Heifetz (17-7PH) (Edward Weck)
Housepian
Kapp (405 SS) (V. Mueller, McGaw Park, IL)
Kapp curved (404 SS) (V. Mueller)
Kapp straight (404 SS) (V. Mueller)
Mayfield (301 SS) (Codman & Shurtleff, Randolph, MA)
Mayfield (304 SS) (Codman & Shurtleff)
McFadden (301 SS) (Codman & Shurtleff)
Pivot (17-7PH) (V. Mueller)
Scoville (EN58J) (Downs Surgical, Decatur, GA)
Sundt-Kees (301 SS) (Downs Surgical)
Sundt-Kees Multi-Angle (17-7PH) (Downs Surgical)
Vari-Angle (17-7PM SS) (Codman & Shurtleff)
Vari-Angle Spring (17-7PM SS) (Codman & Shurtleff)

From references 38, 52, 75, and 78.

Other nonorthopaedic metallic devices, including dental materials, ear implants, vascular filters and coils, genitourinary prostheses, ocular implants, and intrauterine devices, have also been investigated (53,56,61,65,70). Some removable dental plates are ferromagnetic and cause significant local artifact (Table 3-4) (53,66). These materials should be removed prior to MR imaging (53). Permanent appliances such as braces may contain ferromagnetic material, but patients can be studied safely (66). The facial region is not included on most musculoskeletal MR images. Therefore, artifacts from dental appliances usually are not a problem. We do not examine patients with permanent dental prostheses held in with magnetic posts as it is not yet clear what effect the magnetic field will have on these components (41).

To date, the only ear implants that may be contraindicated are cochlear implants (3M/House and 3M/Vienna) that deflect *in vitro* when placed in MR imagers. Patients with intraocular lens implants and copper intrauterine devices can be examined safely with MRI (65).

Genitourinary (GU) prostheses and vascular filters and coils, because of their location, are more likely to create artifacts and need to be considered carefully (see Fig. 3-3). Most penile implants and GU sphincter prostheses do not contain significant ferromagnetic material. An exception is the Omni Phase (Dacomed) that contains significant amounts of metal (65). Shellock (65,67) and Teitelbaum et al. (72) studied vascular coils, stents, and filters *in vitro* and *in vivo* (Table 3-5) (65,72). Their data indicate that artifact and torque are most significant with vascular appliances constructed with 304 and 316 stainless steel. Though

TABLE 3-4

DENTAL APPLIANCES: MR IMAGE ARTIFACTS

Material or prosthesis	Artifact
Dental amalgam	No
Soft tissue conditioning material	No
Orthodontic wire	Yes
Type III gold	Yes
Type IV gold	Yes
Porcelain fixed to gold	No
Crown and bridge acrylic resin	No
Titanium implants	Yes
Polyurethane	No
Fixed partial denture, type III gold	Yes
Metal ceramic crown	Yes
Maxillary removable partial obturator	Yes

From Carr AB, Gibilisco JA, Berquist TH. Magnetic resonance imaging of the temporomandibular joint: preliminary work. *J Craniomandib Disord* 1987;1(2):89–96; and Shellock FG, Myers SM, Kimble KJ. Monitoring heart rate and oxygen saturation with a fiber-optic pulse oximeter during MR imaging. *AJR* 1992;158:663–664.

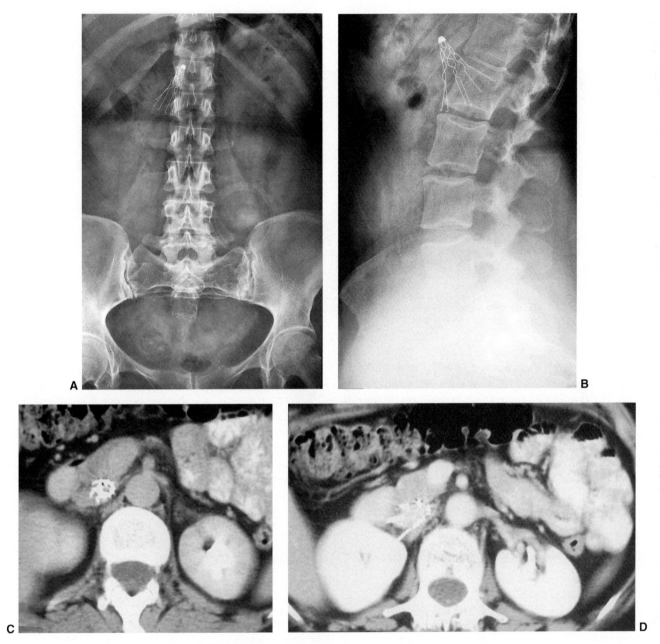

Figure 3-3 Kimray-Greenfield vena cava filter. Anteroposterior (AP) **(A)** and lateral **(B)** radiographs of the lumbar spine demonstrate the caval filter at L1–L2. CT images **(C-E)** demonstrate some streak artifact. Sagittal SE 500/20 MR image **(F)** demonstrates artifact (*arrowheads*) with trapped thrombus.

the latter is not ferromagnetic in its original form, it does appear to undergo some change during configuration of appliances (i.e., Palmaz endo stent). Materials creating minimal artifact include the appliances made with Beta-3 titanium, Elgiloy, nitinol, and mP32-N alloys (72). Despite their magnetic susceptibility and the degree of artifact created (Table 3-5), patients with these devices generally can be imaged safely. The ferromagnetic devices (Greenfield filter, constructed of 316L stainless steel) did not displace or

perforate the inferior vena cava (IVC) (79). The position of devices containing ferromagnetic material [Gianturco embolization coil, Gianturco bird nest filter, Gianturco zigzag stent, Greenfield filter (316L stainless steel) and retrievable IVC filter, and Palmaz endovascular stent] should be confirmed radiographically prior to examination. If the device is perpendicular to the magnetic field or immediately adjacent to the area of interest, the examination maybe inadequate and patient risk (due to change in

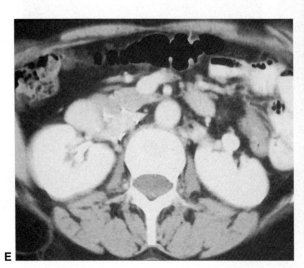

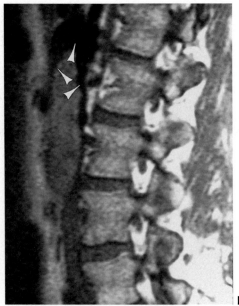

Figure 3-3 (*continued*)

position) is more significant (72,80). More recently, Shellock and Shellock (78) evaluated ten endovascular stents. They concluded there was no significant interaction (motion or heating) with stents made of Elgiloy (cobalt, chromium, nickel, iron, and molybdenum), platinum-nickel, or tantalum.

A potentially more difficult problem exists in patients with nonmedical foreign bodies or ferromagnetic material.

Patients with shrapnel or other metal foreign bodies may not be aware that this material is present (see Fig. 3-4). In this setting there is little that can be done until an artifact is detected during the examination. If the patient expresses concern over a potential foreign body, one should consider a radiograph or CT (orbital foreign bodies) of the area or, if clinically indicated, cancel the examination (45,82). If an object is detected in the extremity and it is not near a nerve

TABLE 3-5
VASCULAR APPLIANCES: CONSTRUCTION MATERIAL AND ARTIFACTS

Device	Material	Company	Artifact
Greenfield filter	a) 316L stainless steel	Meditech, Watertown, MA	Significant
	b) Beta-3 titanium	Ormco, Glendora, CA	Minimal–none
Mobin-Uddin IVC Umbrella	Elginoy and silicone Rubber	American Edwards, Santa Ana, CA	Mild
Amplatz retrievable IVC filter	MP 32N alloy	Cook, Bloomington, IN	Mild
Gunther retrievable IVC filter	304 stainless steel	William Cook, Europe	Severe
Gianturco bird nest IVC filter	304 stainless steel	William Cook, Europe	Severe
Retrievable filter	304 stainless steel	Thomas Jefferson Univ., Philadelphia, PA	Severe
Cragg nitinol spiral IVC filter			Mild
Maass helical IVC filter	Mediloy stainless steel	Medinvent, Lausanne, Switzerland	Moderate
Maass endovascular	Mediloy stainless steel	Medinvent, Lausanne, Switzerland	Moderate
Palmaz endo stent	316 stainless steel	Ethicon, Summerville, NJ	Severe
GEC coil	304 stainless steel	Cook, Bloomington, IN	Severe

From Shellock FG, Myers SM, Kimble KJ. Monitoring heart rate and oxygen saturation with a fiber-optic pulse oximeter during MR imaging. *AJR* 1992;158:663–664; Teitelbaum GP, Ortega HV, Vinitski S, et al. Low-artifact intravascular devices: MR imaging evaluation. *Radiology* 1988;168:713–719; and Theumann NH, Pfirrmann CWA, Antonio GE, et al. Extrinsic carpal ligaments: normal MR arthrographic appearance in cadavers. *Radiology* 2003;226:171–179.

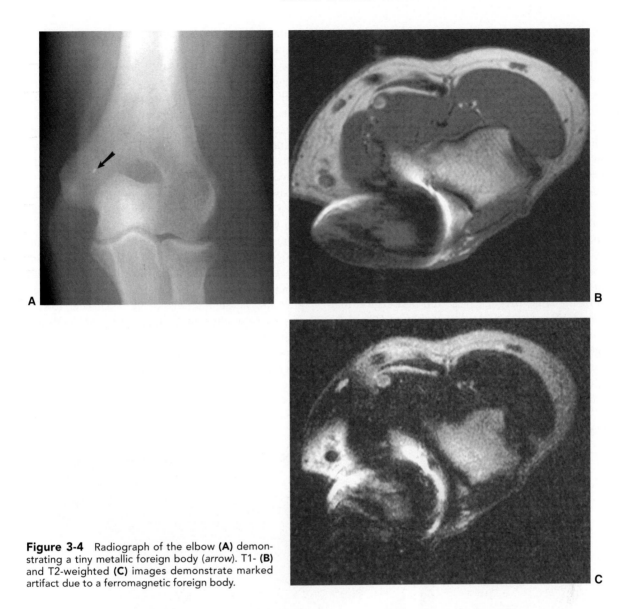

Figure 3-4 Radiograph of the elbow **(A)** demonstrating a tiny metallic foreign body (*arrow*). T1- **(B)** and T2-weighted **(C)** images demonstrate marked artifact due to a ferromagnetic foreign body.

or in a region where its motion could cause damage, the examination can be performed with close monitoring (technologist in the room, questioning the patient during and between pulse sequences). If the object has been present for 6 months or more, it will likely be fixated by scar tissue that reduces the risk of motion. Pigments in facial makeup (eyeliner, mascara, eye shadow) and certain tattoos may also contain ferromagnetic material (brown-ferric sulfate, flesh-color iron oxide, blue-cobalt chloride) and cause local heating and cutaneous inflammation (57,64). Patients with tattooed eyeliner are particularly susceptible. These factors should be considered, and avoiding these examinations may be indicated.

Manufacturers of orthopaedic appliances (plates, screws, joint prostheses, etc.) generally use high-grade stainless steel, cobalt-chromium, titanium, or multiphase alloys (1,41). These materials are usually not ferromagnetic but may contain minimal ferromagnetic impurities. All of the orthopaedic appliances at our institution have been tested for magnetic properties (torque or twisting in the magnet) and heating. No heating or magnetic response could be detected (1,83). Davis et al. (54) also studied the effects of RF pulses and changing magnetic fields on metal clips and prostheses. No heating could be detected with small amounts of metal. Heating was demonstrated with two adjacent hip prostheses in a saline medium. However, it was concluded that metal heating in patients should not be a problem even with a large prostheses (59,83). Heating and skin burns have occurred with looped or improperly positioned electrocardiogram (ECG) leads.

Metal materials can cause significant beam hardening artifacts on CT images (1,54,61,84). Recently, reconstruction methods have been introduced to reduce metal artifacts on CT images (84).

Nonferromagnetic metal materials may cause less significant artifacts on MR images and, if small enough, the insignificant area of signal void may be overlooked. The extent of metal susceptibility artifact created depends upon the size, shape, magnetic susceptibility, and field strength of the imager (1,8,85). On low field systems, some local distortion (see Fig. 3-5) may be seen. The extent of artifact is usually more obvious on high field (≥1 T) systems (see Fig. 3-6). Many artifacts noted on MR images are due to local magnetic field distortions caused by both ferromagnetic and nonferromagnetic appliances. The degree of artifact is greater with the former. These distortions result in signal amplitude reduction near the metal surface (70). The artifacts generally is oriented in the direct of the frequency readout gradient (55,86,87).

The artifacts created by orthopaedic devices varies significantly. When imaging a hip prosthesis, more artifact is created by the large, irregular head and neck region than the more regular and smaller femoral stem (Fig. 3-5). There is also more artifacts from metal screws and Harrington rods (see Fig. 3-7) (1,59). This may be due to the irregular contour (threads and ridges), screw position, or increased amounts of ferromagnetic impurities. Even small amounts of ferromagnetic materials can cause significant artifact (88). For example, histological evidence has demonstrated metal debris in histiocytes around screw tracts, suggesting that small amounts of ferromagnetic material are present in screws used for internal fixation. Drill bit fragments may also contribute to screw tract artifacts. A fibrohistiocytic response normally occurs around these screws if they are left in place for a significant length of time (>3 months). This phenomenon may allow artifacts to occur even though no significant metal can be detected on routine radiographs (Fig. 3-7).

In recent years, multiple MRI parameter changes have been tested to reduce metal artifact (85). As 120,000 total hip procedures are performed each year in the United States, much of the effort has been directed at imaging of patients with hip arthroplasty (see Fig. 3-8) (8,89–93). Misregistration artifact is proportional to the field inhomogeniety and inversely proportional to the frequency encoding gradient strength (Fig. 3-8). Therefore, increasing the frequency encoding gradient strength decreases the artifact (8). Also, aligning the frequency encoding direction along the device reduces artifact (8,91). Increasing the number of pixels in the frequency encoding direction also serves to reduce diffusion related signal intensity loss (8).

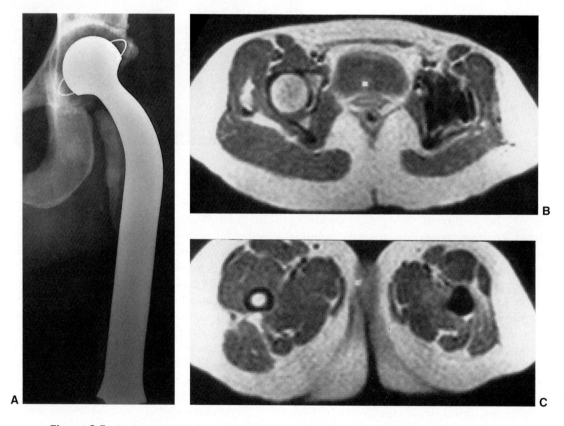

Figure 3-5 Radiograph **(A)** of a custom total hip arthroplasty demonstrating a large amount of metal in the hip and upper femur. Low field (0.15 T) MR image **(B)** at the femoral head level shows local distortion due to the size and configuration of the metal. In the region of the smaller smoother femoral stem there is no significant artifact on the low field MR image **(C)**.

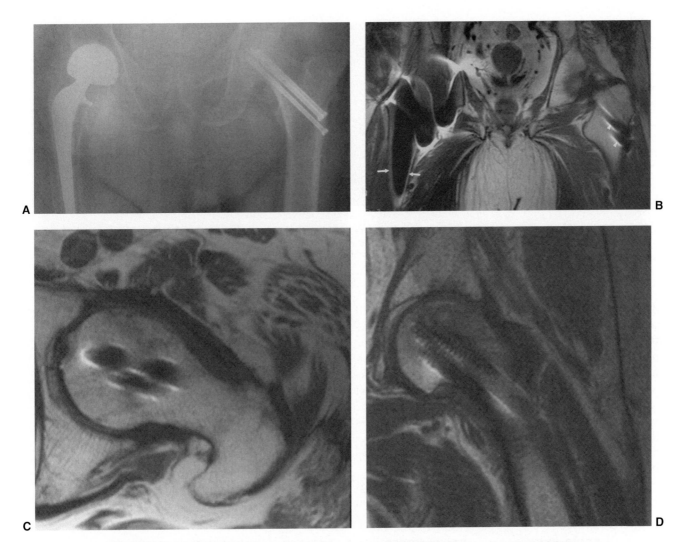

Figure 3-6   A: AP radiograph of the pelvis demonstrates a bipolar implant on the right and three cannulated hip screws on the left. Coronal T1-weighted image **(B)** demonstrates marked artifact (compare to **Fig. 3-5B** at 0.15 T) in the region of the femoral head, but bone is clearly seen along the smoother femoral stem (*arrows*). There is less artifact along the smooth portion of the screws (*arrowheads*). There is slightly more artifact on the axial **(C)** and coronal **(D)** images along the threaded portion of the screws.

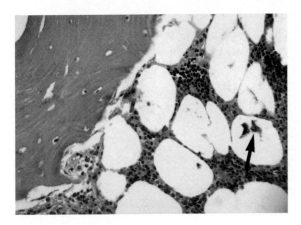

Figure 3-7   Histologic specimen of a screw tract with metal debris (*arrow*). (Courtesy of Les Wold, M.D., Department of Surgical Pathology, Mayo Clinic, Rochester, MN.)

Proper selection of pulse sequences is also important. Fast spin-echo (FSE) and fast short TI inversion recovery (STIR) sequences serve to increase signal intensity near the metal implant (see Fig. 3-9) (8,91). Also, use of water excitation instead of fat suppression not only reduces artifact but reduces imaging time by up to 50% (89). Increasing the bandwidth (Fig. 3-10) also reduces metal artifact (91).

Methyl methacrylate is used to fill medullary cavities as well as to cement components. With the former, artifacts are not created on MR images. Methacrylate is seen as a dark area of no signal, but there is no image distortion (see Fig. 3-11).

External fixation devices may be bulky, but most are not ferromagnetic as the materials are similar to those used in internal fixateurs (1,41). Magnetic properties can be easily checked with a hand-held magnet prior to the

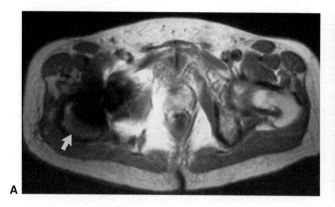
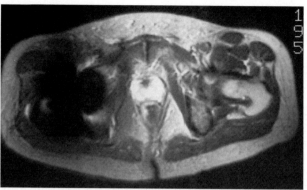

Figure 3-8 Axial images of the hip in a patient with a total hip arthroplasty. The artifact created at 1.5T using SE 2000/30 **(A)** is significant, but the fluid collection around the hip can still be identified (*arrow*). The artifact on the second echo SE 2000/60 **(B)** is significantly greater, obscuring the pathology.

MR examination. The extent of image degradation will vary with the magnetic susceptibility. Recently, manufacturers of fixateurs have begun to use nonferromagnetic material (86). Table 3-6 lists the materials used for external fixation devices in order of increasing artifact production on MR images (50). In addition to the artifact potential, coil selection may also be restricted due to the size of these fixation systems. This can result in a decreased signal-to-noise ratio (SNR) and reduced image quality. However, most patients can be examined using the head or body coils.

Evaluation of patients with casts and bulky dressings (Robert-Jones, etc.) is also possible with MRI. Though coil

TABLE 3-6

ARTIFACTS ON MR IMAGES DUE TO EXTERNAL FIXATION DEVICES

Composition	Artifact
Graphite	None–minimal
Titanium	Minimal
Aluminum	Mild–moderate
Stainless steel	Moderate–severe

From Ballock RT, Hajek PC, Byrne TP, et al. The equality of magnetic resonance imaging as affected by the composition of halo orthosis. *J Bone Joint Surg* 1979;71A:431–434.

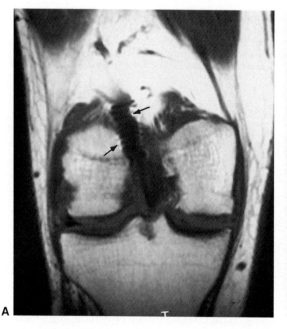
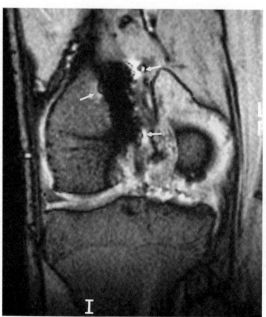

Figure 3-9 Coronal MR images after anterior cruciate ligament repair with interference screw in the femur. The artifact (*arrows*) is less significant on the spin-echo (SE 500/20) image **(A)** than the gradient-echo image **(B)**.

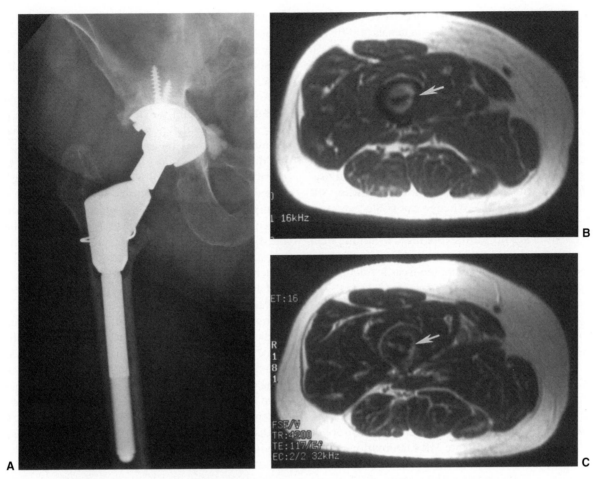

Figure 3-10 **A:** AP radiograph of the hip with a custom right hip arthroplasty. Note the difference in image quality (*arrow*) when increasing the bandwidth from 16 kHz **(B)** to 32 kHz **(C)**.

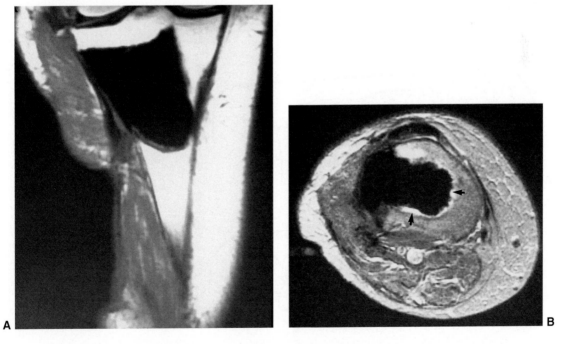

Figure 3-11 MR images of the upper tibia in a patient who had curettage of giant cell tumor with insertion of methyl methacrylate. **A:** Coronal SE 500/20 image shows no signal in the region of the methyl methacrylate, but there is no artifact or image distortion. The axial T2WI (SE 2000/60) **(B)** shows a similar area with no signal. There is reactive edema (*arrows*) in the adjacent marrow.

selection is more restrictive, we have not detected any reduction in image quality because of these materials (1,90).

PATIENT MONITORING AND SEDATION

The patient's age, clinical status, and type and length of MR examination must be considered prior to determining if sedation, anesthesia, or pain medication will be required. Monitoring of physiologic parameters such as blood pressure, heart rate, skin temperature, respiratory rate, and oxygen saturation can all be evaluated safely during MR examinations (9,41,58,94). Whenever possible, examinations are performed without medication.

Most high-field MRI gantries are more confining than a conventional fluoroscopic unit or CT scanner. New short-bore, high-field systems are more easily tolerated by most patients. Mid- and low-field systems (0.02 to 0.5 T) with open gantries and extremity systems (Fig. 3-1) allow easier patient access and increased flexibility for patient positioning (5,41). These systems are better suited for claustrophobic and heavy patients. Patients are positioned in the center of the cylindrical or open-bore magnet chamber during the examination (see Fig. 3-12). Despite the confined feeling that patients experience, sedation is only required in 3% to 4% of patients because of claustrophobia (41,95–97). Patients with claustrophobic tendencies seem to tolerate MR examinations more readily if they are in the prone position (Fig. 3-12). Gantry noise may also create patient anxiety (97). Music provided by nonmetallic headsets is preferred by some patients. Both adults and children may tolerate the examination more easily if a friend or family member is allowed to sit near the gantry and talk or read to the patient during the examination (41). It is important to remember that such persons must also be screened for personal safety. Oral or intravenous sedation is indicated in some cases, especially children (41,98).

Anxious patients or patients with significant pain or inability to maintain the necessary positions may not be able to tolerate the potentially lengthy examinations. Premedication may be useful in some cases (98). Young children (<6 years) may not be able to cooperate sufficiently to obtain an optimal examination. A parent or friend can be in the examination suite adjacent to the gantry and talk with patients during the examination. When this technique is not possible, sedation may be indicated. Use of sedation requires appropriate selection of the safest and most efficient method and monitoring the patient during the examination. Appropriate observation and discharge techniques are also required (51).

Patients should be screened for risk factors. These include respiratory (chronic lung disease, asthma, etc.), cardiovascular, neurologic, gastrointestinal, and other systemic conditions. The American Society of Anesthesiology also has devised a classification scheme to identify underlying diseases. Class 1 patients are healthy; Class 2 patients have mild systemic diseases; Class 3 patients have severe systemic disease; Class 4, severe life-threatening systemic disease; and Class 5 patients are terminal with ≤24-hour survival. Sedation should be reserved for Class 1 and 2 patients with some exceptions (99,100).

Sedation may be divided into several categories depending on the patient's status and type of sedation required. Conscious sedation is a pharmacologically induced state of depressed consciousness that still permits

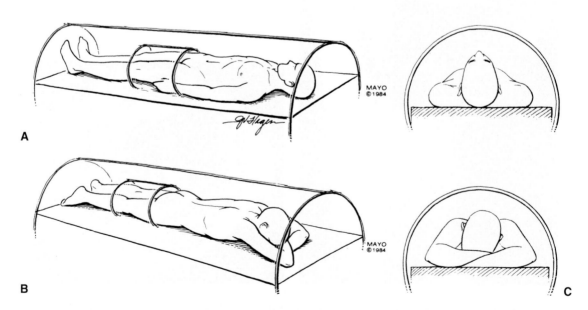

Figure 3-12 Illustrations of patients positioned supine (**A**) and prone (**B**) in the gantry of an MR imager. **C:** Patient viewed from one end.

the patient to respond to verbal commands. Deep sedation is similar to general anesthesia, reducing the ability to communicate with the patient (99). The medication selected is based upon clinical status and the level of sedation required (98–101).

When possible, oral sedation is preferred. Chloral hydrate is an effective oral sedation for children, especially for those under 2 years of age (41,98). Chloral hydrate can be administered incrementally. In patients older than 1 year of age, oral hydroxyine can be added. In patients 2 to 4 years of age, some pediatricians recommend meperidine intramuscularly when the above approaches fail (99,100,102). Greenberg et al. (98) reported excellent results when combining chloral hydrate (50 to 100 mg per kg 30 minutes prior to the examination) with thioridazine (2 to 4 mg per kg 2 hours prior to examination) in pediatric patients who were difficult to sedate.

Mason et al. (101) obtained successful sedation in 94% to 98% of children with intravenous pentobarbital. This technique may be unsuccessful in 1% to 2%, have a paradoxical effect in 1.2%, and cause adverse reactions in 6%. In patients who are difficult to sedate, fentanyl citrate and midazolam hydrochloride can be added (101).

Intravenous sedation or pain medications require patient monitoring, but the onset and effects are more predictable. We use Versed, fentanyl, and, for the elderly, Benadryl for intravenous sedation. The type of intravenous sedation used varies with the patient's status, length of examination, and physician preference (41,99,102).

Initially, there was concern that patient monitoring could not be effectively performed during MR examinations (94,103). Ferromagnetic anesthesia equipment cannot be moved into the magnet room or near the gantry without creating potential safety hazards or affecting the image quality. Our experience shows that critically ill patients or patients requiring general anesthesia can be monitored successfully without interfering with image quality. Initially, we studied 20 patients requiring cardiac and respiratory support. Patients were monitored with a blood pressure cuff with plastic connectors, an Aneuroid Chest Bellows for respiratory rate, and a Hewlett-Packard ECG telemetry system. The respiratory rate and ECG were monitored on a Saturn monitor. Certain problems were encountered during the study. RF pulses caused ECG artifacts, especially if short repetition times were used. This problem was overcome by using a Doppler system to monitor the pulse during the imaging sequences. Satisfactory monitoring was achieved in all patients, and equipment used did not affect image quality (94).

Today there are multiple devices available to monitor blood pressure, heart rate, and oxygen saturation safely (104). Patients can be monitored by trained staff (nurses, nurse anesthetists, trained technologists, radiologists, or anesthesiologists). Patients who are being monitored for their illnesses or patients given intravenous sedation or general anesthesia should be monitored (66,104).

When monitoring patients receiving intravenous sedation or general anesthesia, care must be taken when placing monitor leads to avoid burns. Boutin et al. (45) reported that 9 of 14 MR injuries were related to burns. Burns generally occur due to current created when in coils, in ECG wires, or other conductive material present in the magnet during examination. Most problems, in our experience, are related to large patients and patients under general anesthesia or who are otherwise unable to communicate, who have coiled or improperly positioned ECG leads near the magnet base (41,66).

Patients who have been sedated, specifically those in deep sedation, must be observed following the procedure. Prior to discharge, patients should be stable, easily aroused, have reflexes intact, and be able to communicate accurately (51,99). Children can be dismissed to a parent or guardian. Adults should not be allowed to drive for 24 hours. Therefore, they must be accompanied by another adult if they must travel after the procedure.

Optimally, a written policy similar to the safety questionnaire discussed earlier should be available for patients and referring physicians. This will allow proper preparation (i.e., driver to accompany the patient, etc.). If sedation becomes a consideration (not prearranged) and the patient is alone, the examination may have to be rescheduled if transportation cannot be made available (51).

PATIENT POSITIONING AND COIL SELECTION

Patient positioning considerations include size, body part or anatomic region to be examined, and expected examination time. The patient should be studied with the most closely coupled coil possible (smallest coil that covers the anatomy) to achieve the maximum SNR and the best spatial resolution (1,95,105,106). The body coil is used to evaluate the trunk and thigh region (see Fig. 3-13). Patients can be positioned either supine or prone. The prone position should be used when pathology is suspected in the posterior soft tissues. This will prevent compression of soft tissues and anatomic distortion. The body coil may also be used for tumors in the lower extremity. Though the image quality is superior with surface coils, the body coil facilitates examination of the entire structure. In this way, one can perform the examination quickly and avoid overlooking skip lesions (Fig. 3-13) (41).

The head coil, if open at both ends, can be used for children and when comparison of the calves is required. Again, in this setting the patient should be positioned prone to avoid compressing the posterior soft tissues (see Fig. 3-14).

Care should be taken when marking the area of interest with vitamin E tablets. Compression of tissues in the area of interest distorts the anatomy and may cause misdiagnosis (see Fig. 3-15).

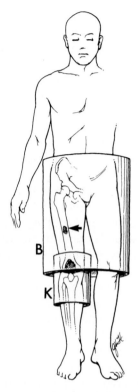

Figure 3-13 Illustration of patient with a neoplasm in the distal femur. Using the knee coil (*K*) would provide superior image quality. However, the skip lesion (*arrow*) would be missed if the torso coil (*B*) was not selected.

Many musculoskeletal examinations in the extremities are performed using surface coils. Surface coils can improve SNR four to six times compared to head and body coils (16,105–107). The type of coil used depends on the anatomic site and whether motion studies may be indicated (41). As a rule, one should match the sensitivity of the coil to the needed FOV to maximize image quality (108,109). Most peripheral structures are imaged using an 8 to 16m FOV. Surface coils (flat coils) are usually receive-only coils and minimally contoured. The depth of view is equal to approximately half the radius of the coil. This results in exaggeration of fat signal adjacent to the coil and signal decrease as the distance from the coil increases (see Fig. 3-16). Though this has been a problem, new software programs are now available to create more uniform signal

intensity throughout the image volume. Despite problems with uniformity of signal, flat coils or coupled flat coils offer advantages in positioning and allow more motion for cine studies (see Fig. 3-17) (41,79).

The lack of uniformity with surface coils can be corrected with whole or partial volume coils (1,110). Partial volume coils include Helmholtz pairs or contoured coils. These coils partially surround the part to be examined (109,111). Whole volume coils are circumferential and provide uniform signal (Fig. 3-17) but restrict positioning to some degree (108,109,111).

Newer coil developments, including dual switchable coils for examining both extremities simultaneously and multiple coil arrays, will facilitate examinations and patient throughput (14,18,108,112). Multiple coil arrays allow use of multiple coils simultaneously to increase the SNR. The examination time can also be reduced with this technique (41,109).

Positioning of patients for lower extremity examinations is not difficult. Structures can be positioned near the midline, which allows optimal use of surface coils with small or reduced fields of view. Motion studies for the knee, foot, and ankle can be easily accomplished. Positioning of the upper extremity is more difficult. This is especially true with large patients. Problems with image quality can be partially overcome by rotating the patient to bring the elbow, wrist, or shoulder closer to the midline (see Fig. 3-18). If this is not possible, the extremity may be placed above the head during the examination (see Fig. 3-19). This position is uncomfortable and cannot be maintained for significant time periods. Motion artifact degrades images in patients positioned with the arm above the head in up to 25% of cases. More specific information on coil selection and positioning will be provided in later chapters as they apply to specific clinical problems (1,41).

PULSE SEQUENCES AND SLICE SELECTION

Chapters 1 and 2 discussed basic principles of MR pulse sequences and tissue characterization. Use of different pulse sequences [spin-echo (SE), FSE, inversion recovery (IR), STIR, gradient-recalled echo (GRE) sequences, etc.]

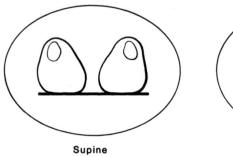

Supine

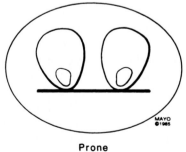

Prone

Figure 3-14 Illustration of supine and prone positioning and the compression effect created on the calves when the patient is supine. The head or torso coil is useful when comparison is needed.

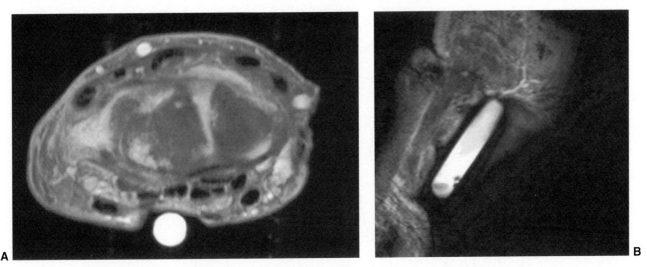

Figure 3-15 Axial **(A)** and coronal **(B)** T2-weighted images with compression of the area of interest by a large vitamin E capsule.

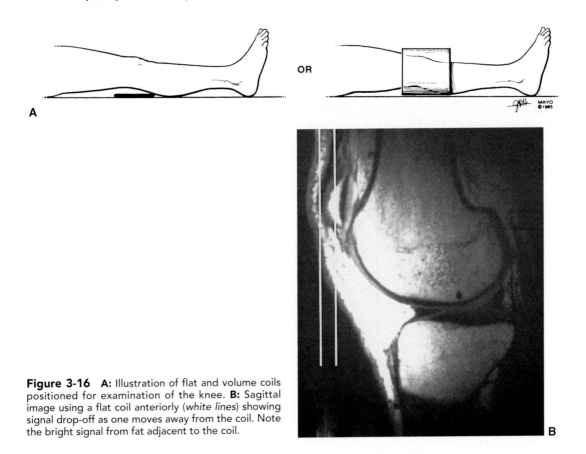

Figure 3-16 **A:** Illustration of flat and volume coils positioned for examination of the knee. **B:** Sagittal image using a flat coil anteriorly (*white lines*) showing signal drop-off as one moves away from the coil. Note the bright signal from fat adjacent to the coil.

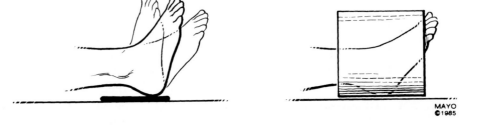

Figure 3-17 Illustration of flat and volume coils for examination of the ankle. The flat coil permits more flexibility in positioning. The foot must be plantar flexed when the volume coil is used.

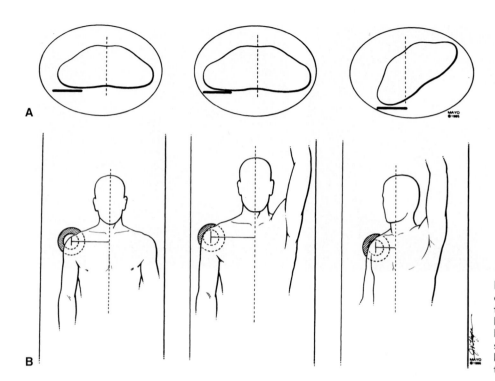

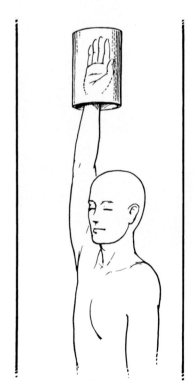

Figure 3-18 Illustrations of upper extremity positioning. **A:** Rotating the patient can bring the body part being examined closer to the midline so the arm can remain at the side. As an alternative, **(B)** the arm to be examined can be placed above the head.

and the many available TE and TR selections at first may be confusing (4,61,70,103,113–118). Additional parameters such as fat suppression or water excitation must also be considered (41,89,119). Echo planar and perfusion-diffusion imaging are not commonly employed for musculoskeletal studies (120,121).

Figure 3-19 Illustration of patient positioned for wrist examination with the arm above the head, using a volume coil.

However, current experience indicates that in most situations, selection of a T1-weighted and T2-weighted or STIR sequence will provide the necessary diagnostic information (2,41,61,122,123). Today, one must consider optimizing techniques with appropriate pulse sequences, intravenous or intraarticular gadolinium, and MR angiography (10,11,20,21,24,31,41,124,125).

There have been numerous changes in pulse sequences over the years in attempts to reduce examination time and improve lesion detection and characterization (41,121,126,127). Spin-echo sequences with short TE and repetition time (TR) (TE 12 to 17, TR 450 to 550) and IR sequences are T1 weighted (contrast due primarily to T1 recovery). Short TE/TR spin-echo sequences provide excellent image quality and can be performed quickly due to the short TR [scan time = TR × number of acquisitions × number of phase encoding steps (128 to 512)]. The average examination time for conventional T1-weighted SE sequences is 4 to 5 minutes. The short TR (450 to 550 ms) allows these sequences to be performed more than four times as fast as most conventional T2 -weighted (TR 2,000 to 2,500) and IR sequences. Repetition times commonly used with IR are in the 1,500 to 2,100 ms range. Conventional IR sequences are rarely used today. Abnormal tissues and fluid collections (long T1 relaxation time) have low signal intensity (dark) using T1-weighted sequences. Therefore, T1-weighted sequences provide excellent contrast differentiation between normal marrow and fat (see Fig. 3-20). However, lesions may be nearly the same signal intensity as muscle using short TE/TR (SE 500/20 sequences) (see Fig. 3-21). Thus, T2-weighted sequences (contrast primarily due to T2 relaxation) are also required. Spin-echo sequences with long TE and TR (TE ≥60, TR ≥2,000) are T2-weighted.

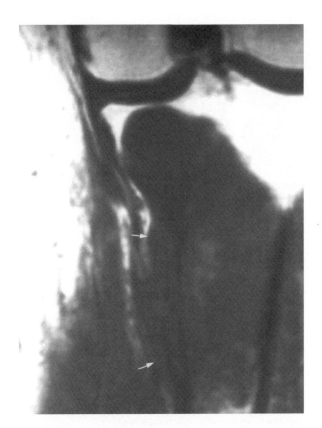

Figure 3-20 Coronal SE 500/15 image of the tibia shows a low intensity neoplasm in the marrow. This clearly demonstrates the abnormal signal of the tumor compared to the fat signal of the normal marrow. The ability to demonstrate cortical break through (*arrows*) is more difficult on T1-weighted images.

Abnormal tissues (long T2 relaxation time) have increased signal intensity, allowing differentiation from muscle (see Fig. 3-22), cortical bone, and fibrous structures (ligaments, tendon, scar tissue). Joint fluid (in fact, most fluid) has high signal intensity on T2-weighted SE and T2*-weighted gradient-echo images (see Fig. 3-23) (41). We typically use a double echo sequence (TE 20 to 30/60 to 80, TR 2,000) that provides an excellent anatomic display with the first echo (SE 2000/20 to 30). And on the second echo (SE 2,000/60 to 80), T2-weighting causes increased intensity in tissues

with long T2 relaxation times and suppresses the signal intensity of fat (Figs. 3-22 and 3-23) (1,41).

Using conventional SE sequences normal tissues have characteristic MR appearance. With short SE sequences (SE 450 to 550/12 to 17), fat and marrow have high signal intensity and appear bright on MR images (Table 3-7). Muscle has intermediate signal intensity, neural tissue has slightly lower signal intensity than muscle, and cortical bone, ligaments, tendons, and fibrocartilage have low (black) signal intensity. The signal intensity of hyaline cartilage appears gray or between muscle and fat. It has been suggested that the difference in appearance of hyaline and fibrocartilage may be due to variation in the type of collagen fibers and water content of these structures (128). The water content of hyaline cartilage (articular cartilage) is 75% to 80% higher than fibrocartilage (menisci). Fibrocartilage, ligaments, and tendons are composed of predominantly Type I collagen (articular cartilage is Type II) and contain less water (124,126).

The signal intensity of normal tissues is similar, with the exception of fat, on long TE/TR SE sequences (Table 3-7). Signal intensity of fat is suppressed on the second echo of long TE SE sequences (see Fig. 3-24).

Typically, flowing blood does not produce signal; hence vessels appear as low signal-intensity structures on MR images. This phenomenon is due to the fact that the moving protons are not stimulated along with stationary tissue or leave prior to signal collection (129–135). However, flow factors and pulse sequences can cause significant problems related to both interpretation and artifact creation. The signal intensity in blood vessels (Table 3-7) depends upon the flow velocity, orientation of the vessel in the image plane (perpendicular or oblique), the presence of turbulence, pulse sequence selection, and single or multislice format (129–133,136). Phenomena have been clearly described that explain certain signal changes noted in blood vessels (see Chapter 2). In large arteries, the flow is more rapid, with most flow occurring in systole. Velocity is decreased in branch vessels. Flow is also faster in the lumen than along vessel walls. Venous flow is slower than arterial flow, but inconsistent velocity is present due

TABLE 3-7

SIGNAL INTENSITY OF MUSCULOSKELETAL TISSUES

	SE 450-550/12-17	SE PD 2000/20	SE T2 2000/80
Fat	High (white)	Intermediate	Low intensity
Marrow	High (white)	Intermediate/white	Low intensity
Hyaline cartilage	Intermediate	Intermediate	High
Muscle	Intermediate	Intermediate	Intermediate
Nerves	Intermediate (slightly<muscle)	Intermediate (slightly<muscle)	Intermediate (slightly<muscle)
Fibrocartilage	Low (black)	Low (black)	Low (black)
Ligaments – tendons	Low (black)	Low (black)	Low (black)
Blood vessels	Low (black)	Low (black)	Low or high

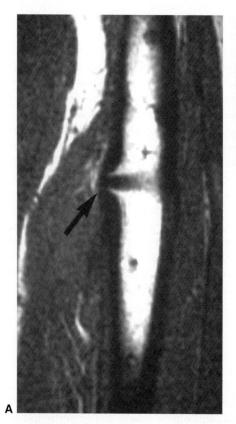

A

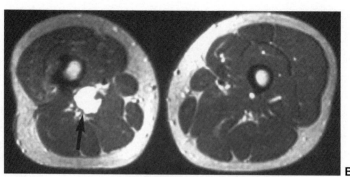

B

Figure 3-21 **A:** Sagittal T1-weighted sequence of the thigh shows a pin tract in the femur (*arrow*), but a mass is not visible. **B:** T2-weighted axial image clearly defines the posttraumatic neuroma (*arrow*).

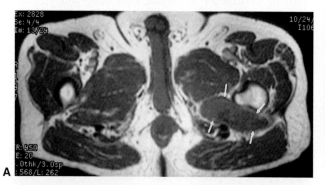

A

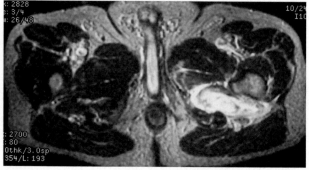

B

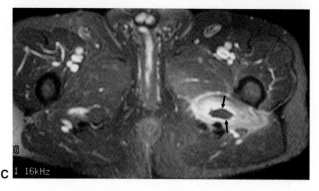

C

Figure 3-22 Axial images of the gluteal region in a patient with a soft tissue sarcoma. **A:** SE 450/20 image shows excellent soft tissue anatomy, but the mass is isointense to muscle and only visible due to the differences in size, (*arrows*) compared to the opposite side. **B:** SE 2000/80 image clearly demonstrates the high signal intensity tumor. Note the decreased signal intensity of fat and marrow. **C:** Postgadolinium, fat-suppressed T1-weighted image shows tumor enhancement except the central necrotic area (*arrows*).

to respiratory changes, transmitted pulsations, and muscle pressure (129). As noted above, flowing blood produces signal void if flow is rapid enough or there are areas of turbulence. Increased signal in vessels is seen with thrombosis (19,134). In this setting, especially venous thrombosis, the

vessel lumen is often dilated (see Fig. 3-25). Increased signal in vessels can also be noted with "flow-related enhancement" when unsaturated spins (those not stimulated) enter the image plane. This usually occurs with slow flow and is common in veins. Increased signal may also be

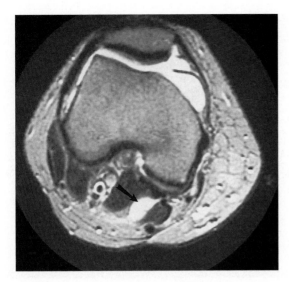

Figure 3-23 Axial SE 2000/80 image through the knee demonstrating a distended suprapatellar bursa with high signal intensity fluid. There is also fluid in a small popliteal cyst (*arrow*).

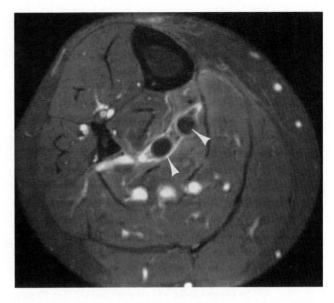

Figure 3-25 Contrast enhanced image of the calf demonstrates no flow in two large veins (*arrowheads*) due to thrombosis.

noted with even echo rephasing. For example, for a dual echo sequence, the signal on the SE 2,000/60 images may be brighter than that seen on the first echo (SE 2,000/20) image. This should not be confused with thrombosis (41,131–133,135). Similarly, signal may increase in vessels during diastole due to the reduced flow rates. This is termed diastolic pseudogating (41,129,131–133).

An additional flow-related problem is the linear artifact created, usually by arteries, when using two-dimensional Fourier transform formats (see Fig. 3-26). The artifact occurs in the phase encoding direction. Two methods can be used to solve this problem. First, if the site of suspected pathology is known, one can change the phase encoding direction to prevent the artifact from obscuring the region of interest. Second, spatial presaturation may be used to saturate spins entering the slice. This is also effective in reducing flow artifact (see Chapter 2) (136).

Continuous development in the type and flexibility of pulse sequences has improved patient throughput, increased contrast of pathologic versus normal tissues, and permitted refinement in MR angiography (see Fig. 3-27) (1,2,24,89,121). FSE sequences are commonly used to replace conventional SE T1, proton density, and T2-weighted sequences (13,123,127,137,138). T1-weighted sequences can be performed in 4 to 5 minutes (e.g., 568/15, 256 × 256, one acquisition = 4 min, 55 s). FSE T1-weighted sequences can be done in about half the time (example: 663/12, ET 3, 256 × 256, one acquisition = 1 min, 57 s) and image quality is comparable. In our practice we still use conventional T1-weighed SE sequences for most musculoskeletal examinations except the spine (see Fig. 3-28).

Double echo (PD and T2) T2-weighted sequences take 8 to 13 minutes to perform using conventional SE techniques (example: 2,000/20, 80, 256 × 256, 1 acquisition =

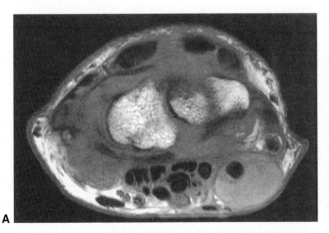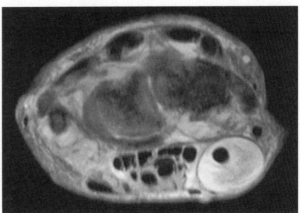

Figure 3-24 Axial proton density (**A**) and T2-weighted (**B**) fast spin-echo sequences in a patient with rheumatoid arthritis and extensive synovitis. The signal intensity of the fluid increases on the second echo and fat signal is suppressed.

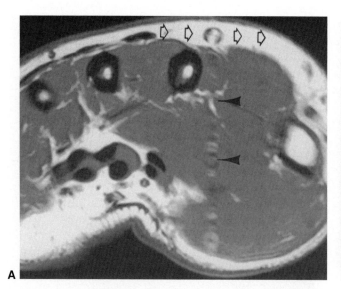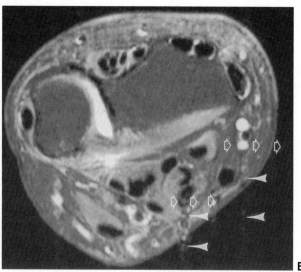

A   B

Figure 3-26 Proton density **(A)** and T2-weighted **(B)** images demonstrate flow artifact (*arrow-heads*). Swapping the phase direction (*open arrows*) would change the direction of the artifacts moving them out of the area of interest.

8 min, 53 s). FSE sequences using proton density or T2-weighting can be performed in fewer than 4 minutes (e.g., FSE T2 with fat suppression — 4,000/92, ETL 8, 256 × 256, 1 acquisition = 3 min, 39 s). Fat suppression or water excitation are commonly, if not routinely, used with FSE sequences (13,89,123,139). Fat suppression is used to emphasize water sensitivity on proton density and T2-weighted sequences. Fat signal is suppressed along with chemical shift artifact (89,91). Also, the contrast effect of gadolinium is enhanced on T1-weighted images (88,89). Fat suppression with FSE sequences is accomplished with frequency-selective fat saturation. Fat saturation is sensitive to tissue inhomogeniety or magnetic susceptibility. Uniform fat suppression can be difficult to attain (see Fig. 3-29) (89). Also, additional time is required to incorporate the fat saturation pulse into the imaging parameters (88,89,123).

Water excitation is an alternative to fat suppression. With this technique, only water is excited using spectral spatial pulses. The examination time can be reduced by up to 50% compared to fat suppression T1-weighted sequences. Similar savings cannot be accomplished with proton density and T2-weighted sequences. Fat suppression is more uniform with water excitation. Metal artifact is also reduced using water excitation compared to fat suppression (89).

Both techniques have been used with proton density and T2-weighted sequences to evaluate articular cartilage (7,13,89,123,140). Fat-suppressed proton density FSE sequences may be preferable to water excitation in this setting (123).

STIR is a second technique for fat suppression (89). Instead of the usual TI of 600 to 700 ms, a TI of 100 to 150 ms is used with an echo time of 30 ms and a TR of 1,500 ms (115,141). Today, most institutions use fast STIR techniques that can be accomplished in 4 to 5 minutes. STIR sequences enhance lesion conspicuity, especially when

there are only subtle changes in marrow signal intensity on conventional sequences (see Fig. 3-30) (115).

GRE uses reduced flip angles and short repetition times (131,142). SE sequences use pairs of RF pulses, while GRE sequences are produced by single radiofrequency RF pulses in conjunction with gradient field reversals (47). The mechanisms and terms used by vendors vary (e.g., FISP, fast imaging with steady precession; FLASH, fast low-angle shot; GRASS, gradient reduced acquisition in steady state; and GRIL, GRASS interleaved) but the image appearances are similar (see Chapter 1) (132,143). GRE sequences can be used instead of conventional SE sequences to reduce examination time and reduce motion artifact when examining difficult patients. These sequences are particularly useful in the upper extremity where motion artifact is a more significant problem (41). Cine-video studies can be easily performed using these fast sequences (41,47,103,144). Fast scan techniques are also useful for three-dimensional imaging (103). We use a three-dimensional gradient-echo technique termed DESS (dual echo steady state) for evaluating articular cartilage (126). Two different gradient echoes are obtained during the TR. The first is a strongly T2-weighted PSIF (time inverted FISP), and the second is a FISP (Fig. 3-31).

Early experience with echo-planar pulse sequences has been encouraging. This fast pulse sequence permits images to be obtained in no more than 20 ms. The faster image time is accomplished by obtaining the spatial-encoding data with a single RF pulse (2). This technique shows promise for motion studies and vascular imaging (2).

Diffusion/perfusion sensitive imaging has become a useful tool for neurological imaging (120,121). Applications for this technique have not been commonly evaluated for musculoskeletal imaging except to differentiate benign from malignant vertebral compression fractures. It has been reported that signal attenuation is obvious in benign

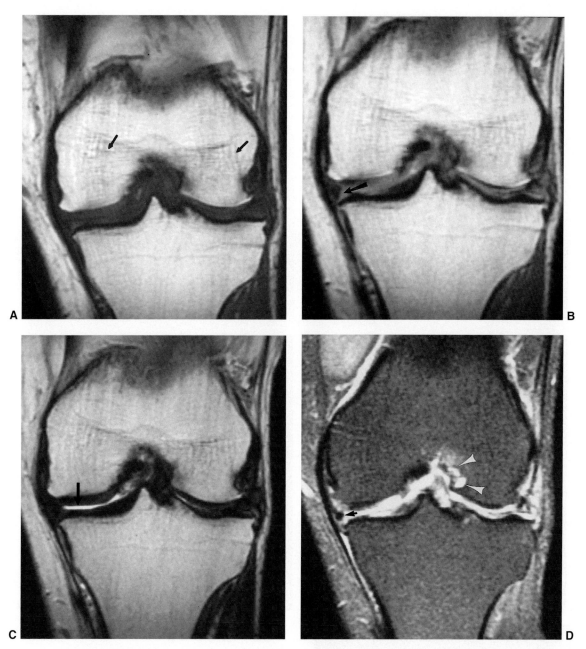

Figure 3-27   MR images of the knee using different pulse sequences. **A:** Coronal SE 500/20, 256 × 256 matrix, 1 acquisition (NEX), 16 cm FOV. Bone marrow and subcutaneous fat have similar signal intensity due to yellow marrow content. The bone trabeculae are seen as a low intensity lattice (*black arrows*). Joint fluid and menisci are not clearly separated due to similar signal intensity. **B:** Proton density coronal image using SE 2000/20, 256 × 256 matrix, 1 NEX, 16 cm FOV. Contrast between joint fluid (intermediate signal intensity) and menisci and ligaments (low signal intensity) permits structures and pathology to be more clearly defined. Marrow and subcutaneous fat have slightly lower signal intensity than the T1-weighted spin-echo sequence in **A**. Note the truncated medial meniscus (*arrow*). **C:** FSE T2 sequence 4800/98, 256 × 192, 1 NEX, 16 cm FOV. Joint fluid has high signal intensity (*arrow*) but there is less fat suppression compared to conventional SE T2W sequences. The meniscal tear (see **C**) is not clearly defined. **D:** Fat-suppressed T2W sequence (SE 2500/80), 256 × 256 matrix, 16 cm FOV. The signal intensity of marrow and subcutaneous fat is suppressed and joint fluid and vessels are high intensity. The meniscal tear (*arrow*) and intercondylar erosions (*arrowheads*) are easily seen. **E, F:** Gradient echo (MPGR) 700/12 **E** and 700/31 with 25° flip angle, 256 × 256 matrix, 1 NEX, 16 cm FOV. The meniscal tear (*arrow*) and erosive changes (*arrowheads*) are clearly demonstrated. **G, H:** Axial SE 500/16 T1 weighted **G** and spoiled GRASS 55/5, 45° flip angle **H** image demonstrating the dramatic difference in signal intensity of articular cartilage using these sequences. **I:** Axial fat-suppressed FSE image shows increased signal in the patellar articular cartilage with erosions (*black arrows*), patellar tilt, and a large effusion.

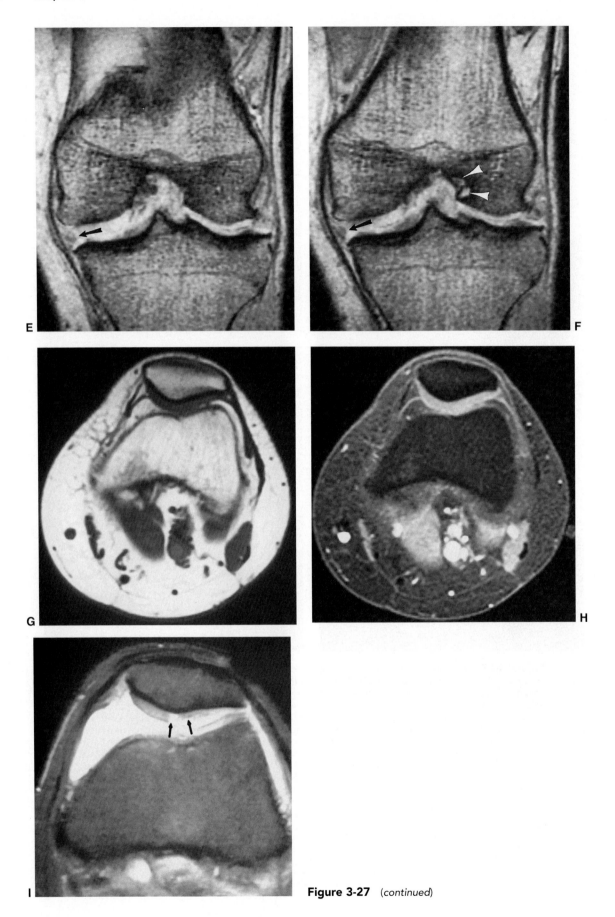

Figure 3-27 (continued)

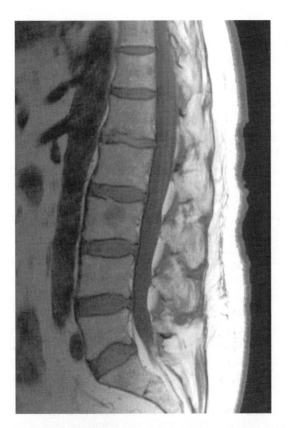

Figure 3-28 Sagittal fast spin-echo T1-weighted image of the spine. Image quality compares to conventional spin-echo sequences. Note the metastatic lesion in L3.

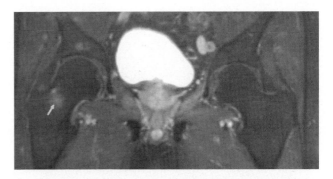

Figure 3-30 Coronal fast STIR image shows excellent fat suppression in the marrow and soft tissues. The insufficiency fracture in the right femoral neck (*arrow*) is clearly demonstrated.

compression fractures and slight in malignant compression fractures using diffusion weighted imaging (121). In theory, this is due to edema and hemorrhage in benign fractures increasing water mobility while tumor cells packed in a malignant compression fracture reduce water mobility. The apparent diffusion coefficient is statistically higher in benign compared to malignant fractures (121).

Specific use of pulse sequences and other imaging parameters will be discussed in more detail in specific anatomic and pathologic chapters that follow (1,145). However, use of gadolinium and MR angiographic techniques will be discussed more completely in this section to avoid redundancy in subsequent chapters.

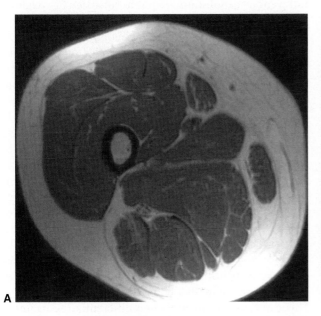
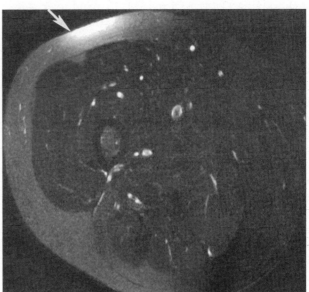

A   B

Figure 3-29 Nonuniform fat suppression. **A:** Axial T1-weighted image of the thigh demonstrating high signal intensity fatty tissue. **B:** Axial T2-weighted fast spin-echo with fat suppression. Fat signal intensity varies near the coil (*arrow*) and from left to right.

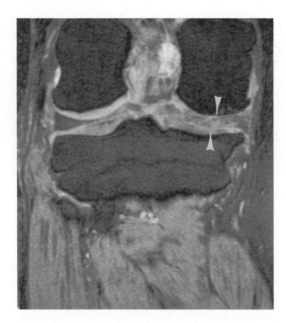

Figure 3-31 Coronal DESS image of the knee. Note the high signal intensity of articular cartilage and fat-suppressed marrow. There is marked loss of the articular cartilage (*arrowheads*) medially compared to the lateral compartment.

Gadolinium

Intravenous and intraarticular contrast enhanced studies have become routine in recent years (21,25,31,40,41, 146–150). Gadolinium is a paramagnetic metal ion with seven unpaired electrons that has gained popularity in MRI due to its relative lack of side effects and efficiency for shortening T1 (41,82,151,152). To avoid toxic side effects, gadolinium has been chelated with several substances, including dimeglumine (gadopentatate dimeglumine), tetra-azacyclodatecane tetra-acetic acid, and diethylenetriamine penta-acetic acid (19,82,148,152). Side effects and T1 relaxation effects vary to some degree depending upon the compound used, but in most situations, 0.1 mmol per kg of these substances is used in the clinical setting. Nephrotoxicity is less than iodinated contrast agents (153).

Intravenous Injections

Intravenous gadolinium remains intravascular for a short period of time and is quickly distributed to intracellular fluid. Areas of increased vascularity (neoplasms, inflammation, etc.) enhance rapidly and retain contrast longer than normal tissue (82,152). Techniques for intravenous injection vary with suspected pathology. However, in most cases, precontrast images are obtained using T1- and T2-weighted sequences followed by postcontrast T1-weighted or gradient-echo images (82,154). GRE and FSE sequences are also used with dynamic gadolinium studies (32,154). Fat-suppression techniques are commonly employed when T1-weighted sequences are used after contrast injection (see Fig. 3-32) (119,155).

Dynamic scan techniques have been advocated for evaluating musculoskeletal neoplasms with regard to tumor type (benign vs. malignant) and response to therapy (32,149). In 1988, Erleman et al. (3) demonstrated a specific technique for musculoskeletal tumors. Using a 1.5 T MR unit, preinjection images were followed by a series of three images per minute using a TR/TE of 40/10 and a 90 degree flip angle GRE sequence. Signal intensity curves for malignant lesions had a steeper slope compared to benign lesions and normal tissue. However, in our experience, more work is required, as tumors may behave differently and lesion characterization is not always accurate (see Fig. 3-33) (41). Also, the characteristic appearance of certain tumors based on conventional sequences may be confused by using gadolinium (see Fig. 3-34).

In recent years, new dynamic techniques have been employed using bolus or power injection (0.1 to 0.2 mmol per kg at 2 to 4 mmol per second) with fast scan images every 3 to 7 seconds. This technique, like that described above, permits images to demonstrate early intravascular and interstitial accumulation of contrast. Early phases of enhancement occur in the initial 5 to 6 seconds after arterial enhancement. Patterns of enhancement (no enhancement, peripheral enhancement, diffuse homogeneous, or inhomogeneous) are useful in characterizing pathology and improve differentiation of benign versus malignant lesions (1,149). Dynamic images should be obtained over 3 to 5 minutes (40,149).

Vanel et al. (149) used dynamic contrast subtraction MRI to evaluate recurrence of aggressive and malignant lesion. T1- and T2-weighted images were followed by bolus intravenous gadolinium. Rapid acquisition T1-weighted images were obtained at 45 seconds, 1.5 minutes, and 5 minutes following injection. All but one recurrence in 21 patients undergoing surgery was identified on precontrast T2-weighted images. On the basis of these data, dynamic scanning might be reserved for selected or equivocal non-contrast studies (149).

Intravenous gadolinium can also be used to study internal derangement and other articular disorders (3,152,156). Enhancement of synovium occurs with arthropathies (see Chapter 15) and synovial fluid enhances as early as 10 minutes following injection. Enhancement increases over time, so joint images can be obtained for up to 1 hour after injection. This technique provides images similar to intraarticular injection (3,152,156). Synovial changes and pannus volume can be used to monitor response to therapy for conditions such as rheumatoid arthritis (see Fig. 3-35). Inflamed periarticular structures may also enhance using this technique. This can cause confusion when differentiating ligament and tendon tears from inflammation.

Intraarticular Gadolinium

Use of intraarticular gadolinium has increased in recent years. The technique is most commonly used for shoulder,

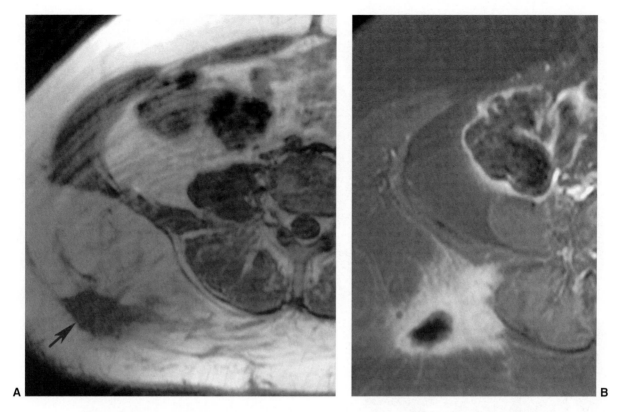

Figure 3-32 Pre- and post-gadolinium images in a patient with a soft tissue abscess in the gluteal region. **A:** T1-weighted image demonstrates an irregular low-intensity lesion in the soft tissues. **B:** Postcontrast fat-suppressed T1-weighted image demonstrates an abscess with no central enhancement and surrounding inflammation.

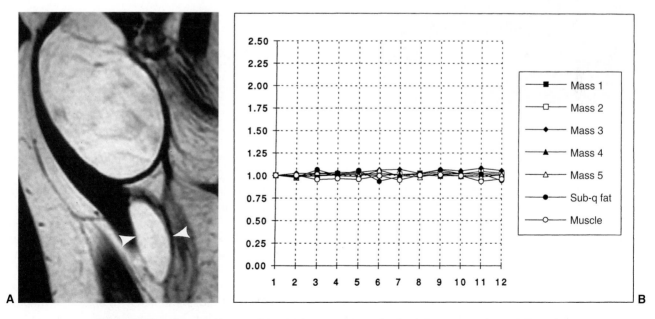

Figure 3-33 **A:** Sagittal image of the thigh in a patient with a large liposarcoma (low grade) and small typical lipoma (*arrowheads*) just below the larger lesion. The lesion was studied with dynamic gadolinium and slopes plotted for five regions in the liposarcoma **(B).** The slope (signal intensity vs. time) was flat and comparable to normal muscle and fat. There were no changes in slope to suggest malignancy.

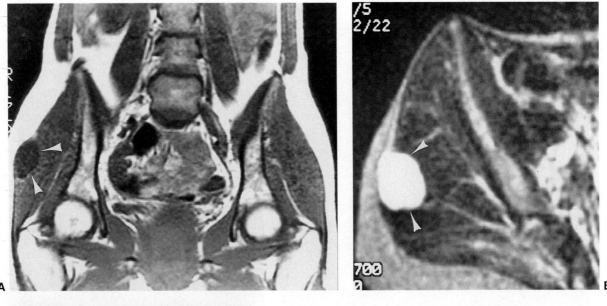

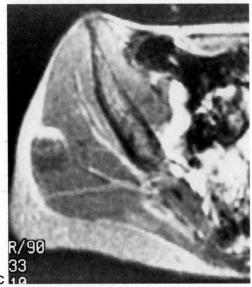

Figure 3-34 Coronal SE 500/20 image **(A)** and axial SE 2700/80 image **(B)** of a benign myxoma with typical well-marginated homogeneous signal intensity (*arrowheads*). The postgadolinium MPGR 33/10, flip angle of 90° image **(C)** shows inhomogeneous enhancement that could be confused with a more aggressive lesion.

elbow, wrist, hip, and knee MR arthrography (26,31,147, 157,158–160). We use intraarticular injections routinely to define certain articular disorders such as articular cartilage loss, partial ligament or tendon tears, and labral tears in the shoulder and hip. Though the technique is only minimally invasive, it does require scheduling modifications, cost and time for examinations are increased, and informed consent or institutional review board approval is required.

Dilution levels of gadolinium, dilution solutions, and safety for intraarticular use have been documented (17,78,151). Brown et al. (151) found normal saline, iodinated contrast, and lidocaine could be safely mixed with gadolinium without concern for dissociation that could result in free gadolinium, which may cause adverse effects. Iodinated contrast is an important dilution solution as it can

be used to confirm needle position is intra-articular. Schulte-Altedorneburg et al. (17) reviewed clinical trials of intra-articular gadolinium from 1987 to 2001. Intraarticular injection was safe and efficacious at a concentration of 2 mmol/L. Though the U.S. Food and Drug Administration has not approved gadolinium for intraarticular use, most institutions employ MR arthrography with approval of the institutional review board.

Specific arthrographic technique for each articulation will be discussed more completely in anatomic chapters that follow. However, basic concepts deserve mention here. Most authors agree that a mixture of 0.2 mL of gadolinium with 50 mL of saline provides optimal intra-articular contrast (148,159). We use a 50/50 mixture of marcaine and iodinated contrast to dilute the gadolinium. This ensures accurate needle position. Images should be

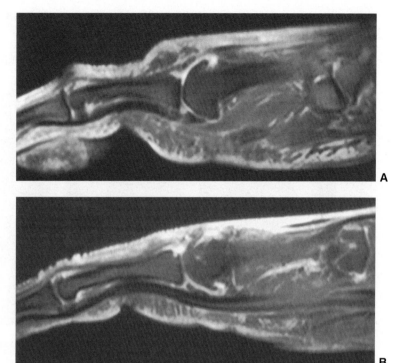

Figure 3-35 Sagittal fat-suppressed T1-weighted images **(A,B)** after contrast enhancement demonstrate osteophytes and synovial enhancement in the metacarpophalangeal and proximal interphalangeal joints.

obtained within 30 minutes of injection to optimize contrast benefit. Fat-suppressed, T1-weighted images are optimal for intra-articular detail. However, FSE proton density and T2-weighted sequences with fat suppression are useful for evaluating periarticular pathology (31,159). Perilabral cysts in the shoulder and hip may not fill with contrast injected into the joint. Therefore, T2-weighted sequences may be the only method to define these abnormalities (see Fig. 3-36).

MAGNETIC RESONANCE ANGIOGRAPHY

MRI studies can provide valuable information regarding vascular structures (arteries, veins, lymphatics) (see Fig. 3-37) (21,23,29,74,161). Over the last several years, there has been significant progress made in MR angiography (11,12,24,25, 27,28,30,125,162–164).

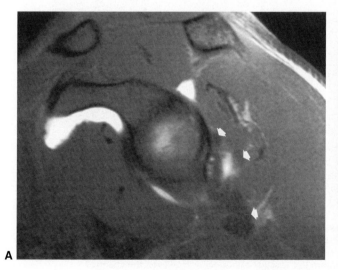
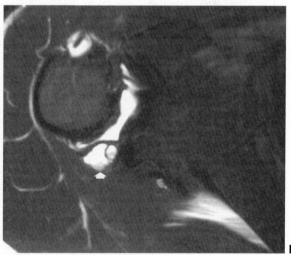

Figure 3-36 Shoulder arthrogram. **A:** Sagittal fat-suppressed T1-weighted image demontrates contrast in the joint, but the low signal intensity complex paralabral cyst (*arrows*) does not fill. **B:** Axial fat-suppressed T2-weighted fast spin-echo image clearly demonstrates the high signal intensity cyst (*arrow*).

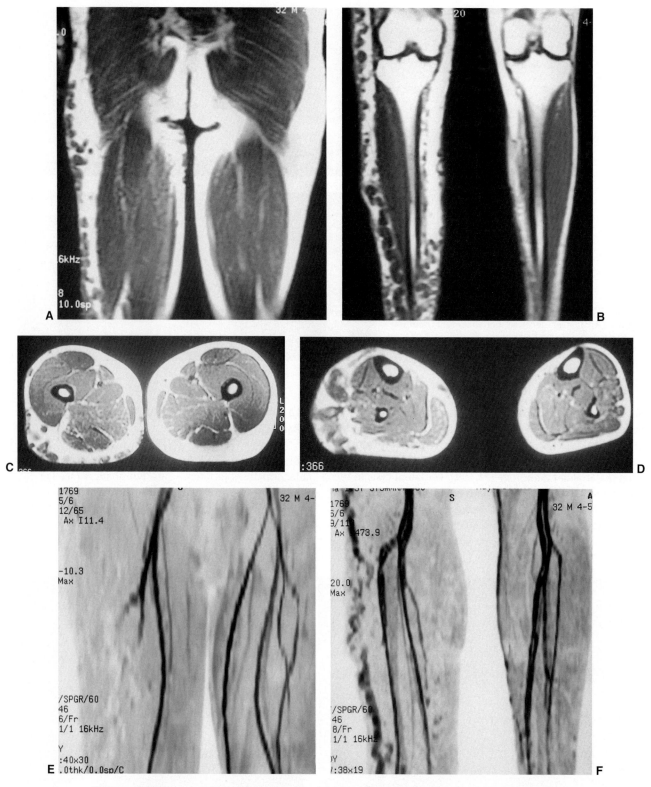

Figure 3-37   Coronal SE 366/17 T1 weighted images of the thighs **(A)** and calves **(B)** and axial images **(C)** and **(D)** clearly demonstrate a subcutaneous vascular malformation. Note the compression of the posterior soft tissues in **C, D** due to supine positioning. Time-of-flight TOF MR angiographic images of the thigh **(E)** and legs **(F)** confirm the vascular abnormality. However, the changes in the thigh are not as well seen as on T1-weighted images **A, C**.

Both noncontrast and gadolinium bolus injection techniques have been developed. Initially, most angiographic techniques were employed in the head and neck (165). However, aortic and peripheral applications have expanded due to improved imaging approaches (11,12,21,25,125,162–164). TOF and phase contrast techniques were used early in an attempt to match the accuracy of conventional angiography (33,34,165).

Two-dimensional TOF sequences maximize flow signal using flow-related enhancement combined with suppression of signal intensity from stationary tissue. Flow-related enhancement is maximized with section planes perpendicular to flow. Therefore, axial images are most often used in the extremities (33,34). Though contrast between stationary tissues and arterial flow is increased with higher flip angles, there is also associated loss of vascular signal intensity. Thus, short TE, short TR, and reduced flip angles (≤60 degrees) are most often used for clinical imaging (33,34). Suggested TOF sequences may include TR of 33 ms, TE of 4 to 6 ms, flip angle of 60°, inferior presaturation, one acquisition, 2-mm-thick sections, 16- to 24-cm FOV, matrix of 256 × 256 or 256 × 128, and flow compensation technique (27,28,30). Selective venous imaging can be accomplished by using presaturation pulses above the image slices to eliminate signal from arterial flow (33,34, 163,165). Kaufman et al. (27) described pitfalls experienced with two-dimensional TOF MR angiography. One of the most common artifacts is due to in-plane flow when a vessel is in the section plane (see Fig. 3-38A). This may result in irregularity or loss of flow that can simulate stenosis or occlusion. Other causes of signal loss include turbulence, saturation of slow flow, and collateral vessels. Flow signal may also be distorted by adjacent bowel gas or metal. Pulsatile artifacts (see Fig. 3-38B) may be seen in the phase encoding direction (27,29).

Phase contrast sequences can be performed using two- and three-dimensional and cine phase contrast (161,165, 166). Phase contrast techniques are less sensitive to bulk motion and pulsatile flow compared to TOF techniques. Flow is detected and imaged based upon the shifts in phase that occur as a substance changes position in the presence of a magnetic field gradient.

The vessels imaged are determined by using flow encoding velocity sensitive gradients. Arterial flow is faster, so velocities greater than 80 cm per second are typically selected. Stronger phase encoding gradients are used for slow flow and weaker gradients for high velocity flow (165). Cine phase contrast sequences can be performed using cardiac gating (33,34,165).

Newer approaches use two- and three-dimensional technique with bolus injections of gadolinium. Contrast injection techniques have proven to be superior to two-dimensional TOF MR angiography (28). Multiple imaging approaches have been described (11,12,28,162–164).

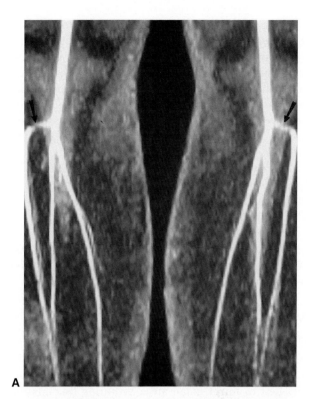

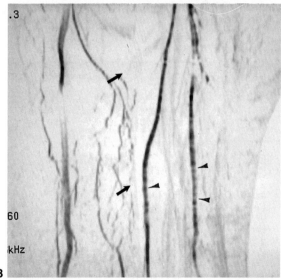

Figure 3-38   A: Lower extremity MR angiogram with signal reduction and irregularity of the proximal anterior tibial arteries (*arrows*) due to in plane flow saturation. **B:** Two-dimensional time-of-flight angiogram demonstrates pulsatile artifacts (*arrowheads*), artifactual flow voids in collaterals (*arrows*).

Contrast enhanced three-dimensional techniques can be performed on most MRI systems (11). Gradient-echo breath-hold techniques are useful in the abdomen and pelvis. Three-dimensional technique with a TR 6.4 to 13.5 millisecond, TE of 1.6 to 3.5 ms, and flip angle of 60° can be used for the abdominal aorta. This technique was 97% sensitive and 92% specific for arterial stenosis greater than 50% (10,25,125).

Bolus chase MR angiography is effective for studies of the abdominal aorta and lower extremities. This technique is performed using a bolus of 15 to 20 mL of gadolinium with a step table and coil holder, which permits images to be obtained synchronously as contrast moves peripherally into the extremities. The major arteries can be accurately displayed in less than 1 minute. The exact parameters of this technique are completely described by Meaney et al. (162) and Wang et al. (164).

Bilecen et al. (21) improved MR angiography for the hand and wrist by using a subsystolic blood pressure cuff during imaging to reduce venous overlay (see Fig. 3-39). This technique could also be utilized in the foot and ankle.

MR angiography can provide valuable information regarding anatomy and primary vascular pathology or vascular abnormalities in lesions such as musculoskeletal neoplasms (9,11,27,30).

Miscellaneous Parameters

Slice selection will vary depending upon the volume of tissue to be studied, size of the suspected pathology, and type of coil (body vs. closely coupled or surface coil). It is usually best to image small areas, requiring fine anatomic detail, with thin (1- to 3-mm) sections. Larger areas can be

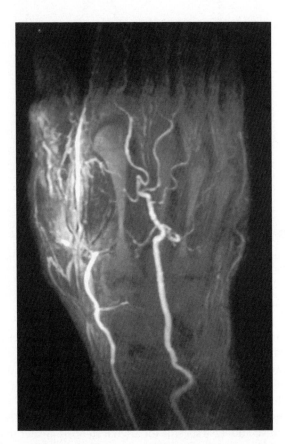

Figure 3-39 MR angiogram of the hand and wrist in a patient with vasculitis and multiple areas of occlusion and narrowing.

studied with 0.4- to 1.0-cm-thick slices. This slice thickness is especially useful for screening examinations with FSE T2-weighted sequences. When using T2-weighted sequences, an interslice gap is important to avoid unintentional stimulation of adjacent slices. This phenomenon can affect contrast and signal of adjacent slices. We typically use a gap equal to 13% of the slice width with T2-weighted sequences. Contrast is less critical with typically anatomic T1-weighted sequences, so using interslice gaps is less critical (9,167).

It is also important to select the optimal FOV. This is especially important when using surface coils on the peripheral extremities. A smaller FOV improves spatial resolution significantly. However, SNRs decrease with smaller FOV (168).

Additional parameters that not only affect image quality but also affect image time are the matrix size and number of excitations or acquisitions. An increase in spatial resolution or pixel size reduction is accomplished with matrixes of 256 or 512, but this results in increased image time. The number of acquisitions is also a factor. Increasing the acquisitions improves the SNR and image quality but also increases image time. Image time is dependent upon repetition time, the number of acquisitions, and the matrix chosen. For example, a T2-weighted SE sequence takes 8.53 minutes. FSE T2-weighted sequences can be performed in 3 to 5 minutes. Contrast and lesion conspicuity may be reduced in some cases (169).

One must consider the image quality, examination time, and use of other parameters such as flow compensation techniques, respiratory compensation (pelvis and trunk), presaturation, and compensation for phase or frequency wrap when setting up an MR examination (170,171). All imaging factors will be discussed more completely in later chapters as they apply to specific anatomic regions and pathologic conditions (41,172).

COMMON ARTIFACTS

Certain MRI artifacts have been discussed previously (metal, flow, etc.). In this section, common artifacts and correction techniques will be reviewed.

Motion Artifacts

Motion problems from patient discomfort or positioning were described earlier. However, respiratory motion and peristalsis may also cause problems with image quality when imaging the chest wall and the abdomen and upper and mid-pelvis. These artifacts occur because the phase encoding gradient cannot properly encode moving structures. Therefore, moving structures are reconstructed repeatedly in the phase encoding direction (see Fig. 3-40). Similar ghost artifacts can be created by cardiac motion, flow, or even motion of cerebrospinal fluid (91). Respiratory and cardiac gating can be used to reduce these artifacts. Flow compensation or presaturation techniques can reduce flow

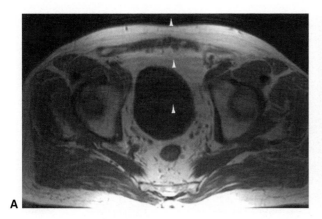
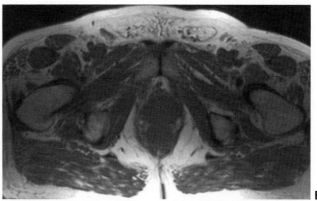

Figure 3-40   Axial T1-weighted images of the pelvis at the hip level (**A**) and trochanteric level (**B**). There is respiratory motion artifact in **A** (*arrowheads*) but not in **B**.

artifacts (91,129,136). In the peripheral extremities, blood pressure cuffs can be used to reduce venous overlay in MR angiography (21). Glucagon is useful in reducing artifacts created by peristalsis. This is commonly used in abdominal imaging, but we rarely use glucagon for examinations of the pelvis and hips.

Chemical Shift

Chemical shift artifact is a misregistration artifact resulting in high signal intensity where fat and water protons overlap and low signal intensity where fat and water protons separate. The artifact is more obvious on high field-strength magnets (>1.5 T) (91,122). In musculoskeletal imaging the artifact can be encountered in several situations. Perhaps the simplest example is a ganglion cyst surrounded by fatty

tissue (see Fig. 3-41). The artifact has been used to advantage in lipid-containing lesions in the central nervous system and body (focal fat in the liver, accentuating visceral margins) (122). Chemical shift artifact can be reduced by changing frequency and phase encoding directions or increasing the bandwidth (91).

Saturation Artifact

Saturation artifacts cause signal loss due to overlapping of adjacent image slices. In musculoskeletal imaging this can be created when image planes are aligned in the plane of the intervertbral discs (see Fig. 3-42) or when radial imaging is used (see Fig. 3-43). The artifact can be reduced by removing the image section overlays or by using gradient-echo sequences with reduced flip angles (91).

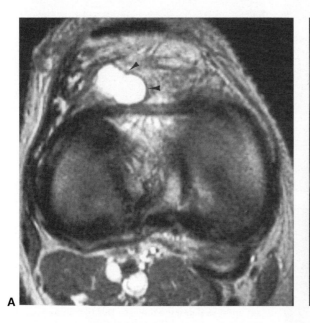
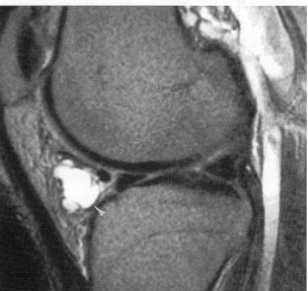

Figure 3-41   Ganglion cyst in the infrapatellar fat. Axial (**A**) and sagittal (**B**) T2-weighted images demonstrate low signal intensity margins (*arrowheads*) due to chemical shift artifact.

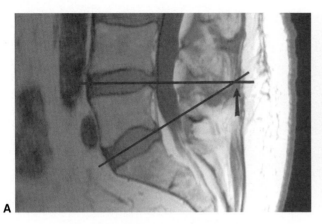
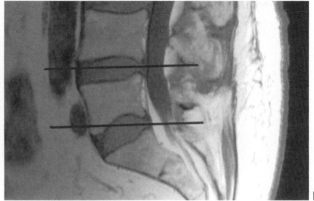

Figure 3-42   A: Sagittal image of the lumbar spine with sections selected in the plane of the discs. There would be loss of signal in the crossover area (*arrow*) on the axial images. **B:** Image planes corrected by using parallel sections.

Aliasing Artifacts

Aliasing artifacts or wraparound artifacts fold part of the region of interest to the opposite side of the image. This artifact is created by using a too-small FOV, such that the phase-encoded signal outside the FOV is incorporated inside the FOV (see Fig. 3-44) (91). This can be corrected by increasing the FOV, which may decrease image quality if the change is too great (i.e., 8 to 16 cm). Oversampling doubles the phase encoding steps and doubles the FOV in the phase encoding direction. This also doubles the scan time, which can be compensated for by reducing the number of

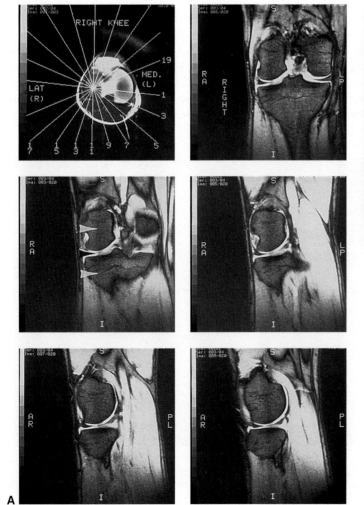

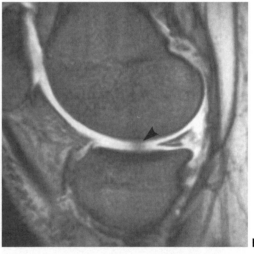

Figure 3-43   A: Radial GRIL images of the right knee set up to evaluate the menisci. This technique provides tangential views of the menisci. There is a band of no signal (*arrowheads*) at the crossover point. **B:** Close up saggital image demonstrates signal void (*arrowhead*) where the image planes intersect.

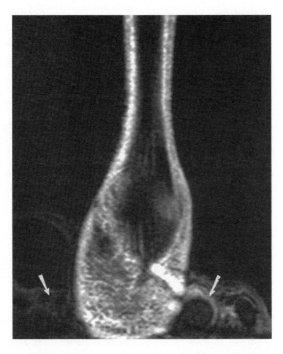

Figure 3-44   Aliasing artifact. Coronal DESS image of the ankle shows the foot superimposed (*arrows*).

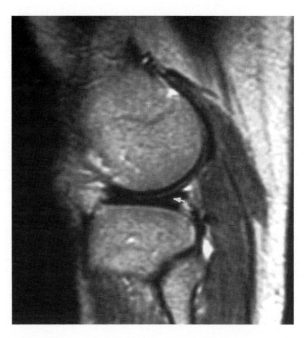

Figure 3-45   Truncation artifact. Sagittal image of the knee demonstrates a linear density (*arrow*) in the posterolateral menicus due to truncation artifact.

acquisitions by 50%. Image quality is maintained and aliasing is eliminated (173). Using a rectangular FOV also reduces aliasing artifacts (91,173).

Truncation Artifacts

Truncation artifacts look like parallel striations and are most apparent in regions where tissues of significantly different signal intensity are adjacent to each other (170,173) (see Fig. 3-45). Cartilage imaging or menisci with adjacent fluid are examples in musculoskeletal imaging. The artifact has been most commonly described in the spine. This artifact is created by undersampling in the phase encoding direction. Each sample is equivalent to a phase encoding step that fills one Fourier line in the k space. Truncation artifact occurs when there are too few Fourier lines in the

k space. This can be corrected by increasing the matrix in the phase encoding direction (91,170,173).

Nonuniform Fat Suppression

Fat-suppression techniques are commonly employed in musculoskeletal imaging to increase lesion conspicuity in the marrow and soft tissues. This technique is also important after intravenous or intraarticular gadolinium injections (89,155). Fat suppression is usually accomplished with frequency selective fat saturation (155). Uneven fat suppression occurs with abrupt changes in tissue such as the craniocervical junction and the distal extremities (Fig. 3-29). Fat suppression is also less uniform in patients with metal implants (8,91,92) (see Fig. 3-46). More uniform fat suppression can be obtained by using water bags around

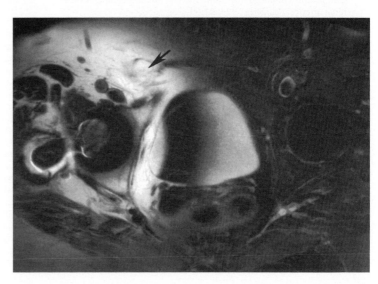

Figure 3-46   Axial fat-suppressed fast spin-echo T2-weighted sequence in a patient with a right hip arthroplasty. There is no fat suppression (*arrow*) around the implant.

the extremity to improve field uniformity or by selecting certain pulse sequences or imaging parameters (91,110). STIR sequences or water excitation may provide more uniform fat suppression (89,155).

RELAXATION TIMES/SPECTROSCOPY

Specificity of MR data such as T1 and T2 relaxation times has been disappointing thus far. However, recent data indicate that 1.5 T imagers can measure T1 and T2 with a precision of around 5% (6,113,171). Spectroscopy has not yet achieved widespread clinical use. However, muscle diseases, tumor therapy response, and transplant rejection appear to lead early applications (see Chapter 16) (36,125,174,175).

REFERENCES

1. Berquist TH. Magnetic resonance techniques in musculoskeletal diseases. *Rheum Dis Clin North Am* 1991;17(3):599–615.
2. DeLaPaz RL. Echo-planar imaging. *Radiographics* 1994;14: 1045–1058.
3. Drape J, Thelen P, Gay-Depassier P, et al. Intra-articular diffusion of Gd-DOTA after intravenous injection in the knee: MR imaging evaluation. *Radiology* 1993;188:227–234.
4. Evans RG, Evans RG Jr. Economic and utilization analysis of MR imaging units in the United States in 1987. *Radiology* 1988; 166:27–30.
5. Jackson JG, Acker JD. Permanent eyeliner and MR imaging (letter). *AJR* 1987;149:1080.
6. LeBlanc A, Evans H, Schonfeld E, et al. Relaxation times of normal and atrophied muscle. *Med Phys* 1986;13:514–517.
7. Vasnawala SS, Pauly JM, Nishimura DG, et al. MR imaging of knee cartilage with FEMR. *Skeletal Radiol* 2002;31:574–580.
8. White LM, Kim JK, Mehta M, et al. Complications of total hip arthroplasty: MR imaging-initial experience. *Radiology* 2000;215: 254–262.
9. Bellon EM, Haacke EM, Coleman PE, et al. MR artifacts. A review. *AJR* 1986;147:1271–1281.
10. Hahn U, Miller S, Nägele T, et al. Renal MR angiography at 1.0T: three-dimensional (3D) phase-contrast techniques versus gadolinium-enhanced 3D fast low-angle shot breath-hold imaging. *AJR* 1998;172:1501–1508.
11. Hany TF, Schmidt M, Davis CP, et al. Diagnostic impact of four post-processing techniques in evaluating contrast-enhanced three-dimensional MR angiography. *AJR* 1998;170:907–912.
12. Lee VS, Rofsky NM, Kruisky GA, et al. Single-dose breath-hold gadolinium-enhanced three-dimensional MR angiography of the renal arteries. *Radiology* 1999;211:69–78.
13. Mohr A. The value of water-excitation 3D flash and fat saturated PDw TSE MR imaging for detecting and grading articular cartilage lesions of the knee. *Skeletal Radiol* 2003;32:396–402.
14. Hardy CJ, Katzberg RW, Frey RL, et al. Switched surface coil system for bilateral MR imaging. *Radiology* 1988;167:835–838.
15. Mattery RF. Perfluorooctylbromide: a new contrast agent for CT, sonography and MR imaging. *AJR* 1989;152:247–252.
16. Schenck JR, Hart HR, Foster TH, et al. High field surface coil magnetic resonance imaging of localized anatomy. *Am J Neuroradiol* 1985;6:193–196.
17. Schulte-Altedorneburg G, Gebhard M, Wohlgemuth WA, et al. MR arthrography: pharmacology, efficacy and safety in clinical trials. *Skeletal Radiol* 2003;32:1–12.
18. Totterman SM, Heberger R, Miller R, et al. Two-piece wrist surface coil. *AJR* 1991;156:343–344.
19. Wesbey GE. Magnetopharmaceuticals. In: Wehrlie FW, Shaw D, Kneeland JB, eds. *Biomedical magnetic resonance imaging,* Weinheim, Germany: VCH, 1988:157–183.
20. Bergin D, Schweitzer ME. Indirect magnetic resonance arthrography. *Skeletal Radiol* 2003;32:551–558.
21. Bilecen D, Aschwander M, Heidecker HG, et al. Optimized assessment of hand vascularization on contrast enhanced MR angiography with a subsystolic continuous compression technique. *AJR* 2004;182:180–182.
22. Brenner ML, Morrison WB, Carrino JA, et al. Direct MR arthrography of the shoulder: is exercise prior to imaging beneficial or detrimental. *Radiology* 2000;215:491–496.
23. Dumoulin CL, Hart HR. Magnetic resonance angiography. *Radiology* 1986;161:717–720.
24. Forster BB, Houston G, Machan LS, et al. Comparison of two-dimensional time-of-flight dynamic magnetic resonance angiography with digital subtraction angiography in popliteal artery entrapment syndrome. *Can Assoc Radiol J* 1997;48:11–18.
25. Gilfeather M, Yoon H-C, Siegelman ES, et al. Renal artery stenosis: evaluation with conventional angiography versus gadolinium-enhanced MR angiography. *Radiology* 1999;210:367–372.
26. Haims A, Katz LD, Busconi B. MR arthrography of the hip. *Magn Reson Imaging Clin N Am* 1998;6:871–883.
27. Kaufman JA, McCarter D, Geller Sc, et al. Two-dimensional time-of-flight MR angiography of the lower extremities: artifacts and pitfalls. *AJR* 1998;171:129–135.
28. Lee HM, Wang Y, Schwartz LH, et al. Distal lower extremity arteries: Evaluation with two-dimensional MR digital subtraction angiography. *Radiology* 1998;207:505–512.
29. McCauley TR, Monik A, Dickey KW, et al. Peripheral vascular disease: accuracy and reliability of time-of-flight MR angiography. *Radiology* 1994;192:351–357.
30. Quinn SF, Dunlow TA, Hallin RW, et al. Femoral MR angiography versus conventional angiography: preliminary results. *Radiology* 1993;189:181–184.
31. Steinbach LS, Palmer WE, Schweitzer ME. MR arthrography. *Radiographics* 2002;22:1223–1246.
32. Verstr<e KL, Dierick A, DeDeene Y, et al. First pass images of musculoskeletal Lesions: a new useful diagnostic application of dynamic contrast enhanced MRI. *Magn Reson Imaging* 1994;12: 687–702.
33. Yucek EK, Dumoulen CL, Waltman AC. MR angiography of lower extremity arterial disease: preliminary experience. *J Magn Reson Imaging* 1992;2:303–309.
34. Yucek EK, Kaufman JA, Geller SC, et al. Time-of-flight MR angiography in evaluation of lower extremity arterial occlusive disease. *Radiology* 1992;185(P):132.
35. Bárány M, Langer BG, Glick RP, et al. In vivo H-1 spectroscopy in humans at 1.5T. *Radiology* 1988;167:839–844.
36. Barfuss H, Fischer H, Hentschel D, et al. Whole-body MR imaging and spectroscopy with a 4-T system. *Radiology* 1988;169: 811–816.
37. Breger RK, Rimm AA, Fischer ME, et al. T1 and T2 measurements on a 1.5T commercial MR imager. *Radiology* 1989;1:273–276.
38. Ng TC, Majors AW, Vijayakumar S, et al. Human neoplasm pH and response to radiation therapy: P-31 MR spectroscopic studies in situ. *Radiology* 1989;170:875–878.
39. Magee T, Shapiro M, Williams D. Comparison of high-field-strength versus low-field-strength MRI of the shoulder. *AJR* 2003;181:1211–1215.
40. Parkkola RK, Mattila KT, Heikkila JT, et al. Dynamic contrast-enhanced MR imaging and MR-guided bone biopsy on a 0.23 T open imager. *Skeletal Radiol* 2001;30:620–624.
41. Berquist TH. Magnetic resonance imaging: preliminary experience in orthopedic radiology. *Magn Reson Imaging* 1984;2:41–52.
42. Saunders RD. Biological effects of NMR clinical imaging. *Appl Radiol* 1982;11:43–46.
43. Schwartz JL, Crooks LE. NMR imaging produces no observable mutations or cytotoxicity in mammalian cells. *AJR* 1982;139: 583–585.
44. Bottomley PA. Human in vivo NMR spectroscopy in diagnostic medicine: clinical tool or research probe? *Radiology* 1989;170: 1–15.
45. Boutin RD, Briggs JE, Williamson MR. Injuries associated with MR imaging: survey of safety records and methods used to screen patients for metallic foreign bodies before imaging. *AJR* 1994;162:189–194.
46. Elster AD, Link KM, Carr JJ. Patient screening prior to MR imaging: a practical approach synthesized from protocols at 15 U.S. medical centers. *AJR* 1994;162:195–199.

47. Elster AD. Gradient-echo MR imaging: techniques and acronyms. *Radiology* 1993;186:1–8.
48. Giradot C, Hazebroucq VG, Fery-Lemonmer E, et al. MR imaging and CT of surgical materials currently used in ophthalmology. In vitro and in vivo studies. *Radiology* 1994;191:433–439.
49. Taljanovic M, Hunter TB, Fitzpatrick KA, et al. Musculoskeletal magnetic resonance imaging: importance of radiography. *Skeletal Radiol* 2003;32:403–411.
50. Ballock RT, Hajek PC, Byrne TP, et al. The equality of magnetic resonance imaging as affected by the composition of halo orthosis. *J Bone Joint Surg* 1989;71A:431–434.
51. Berlin L. Sedation and analgesia in MR imaging. *AJR* 2001;177:293–296.
52. Brown MA, Carden JA, Coleman RE, et al. Magnetic field effects on surgical ligation clips. *Magn Reson Imaging* 1987;5:443–453.
53. Carr AB, Gibilisco JA, Berquist TH. Magnetic resonance imaging of the temporomandibular joint: preliminary work. *J Craniomandib Disord* 1987;1(2):89–96.
54. Davis PL, Crooks L, Arakawa M, et al. Potential hazards of MR imaging: heating and effects of changing magnetic fields and RF fields on small metallic implants. *AJR* 1981;7:857–860.
55. Harris R, Wesby G. Artifacts in magnetic resonance imaging. *Magn Reson Annu* 1988;71–112.
56. Huston J III, Ehman RL. Comparison of time-of-flight and phase-contrast MR neuroangiographic techniques. *Radiographics* 1993;13:5–19.
57. Kanal E, Shellock FG, Talagala L. Safety considerations in MR imaging. *Radiology* 1990;176:593–606.
58. Kanal E, Borgstede JP, Barkovich AJ, et al. American College of Radiology white paper on MR safety: 2004 update and revisions. *AJR* 2004;182:1111–1114.
59. Lackman RW, Kaufman B, Han JS, et al. MR imaging in patients with metallic implants. *Radiology* 1985;157:711–714.
60. Mechlin M, Thickman D, Kressel HY, et al. Magnetic resonance imaging of postoperative patients with metallic implants. *AJR* 1984;143:1281–1284.
61. Merritt CRB. Magnetic resonance imaging - a clinical perspective: image quality, safety and risk management. *Radiographics* 1987;7:1001–1016.
62. New PF, Rosen BR, Brady TJ, et al. Potential hazards and artifacts of ferromagnetic and nonferromagnetic surgical and dental materials and devices in nuclear magnetic resonance imaging. *Radiology* 1983;147:137–148.
63. Porter BA, Hastrup W, Richardson ML, et al. Classification and investigation of artifacts in magnetic resonance imaging. *Radiographics* 1987;7:271–287.
64. Sacco DC, Steiger DA, Bellon EM, et al. Artifacts caused by cosmetics in MR imaging of the head. *AJR* 1987;148:1001–1004.
65. Shellock FG, Kanal E. 5 MRI report: Policies, guidelines and recommendations for MR imaging safety and patient management. *J Magn Reson Imaging* 1991;1:97–101.
66. Shellock FG, Myers SM, Kimble KJ. Monitoring heart rate and oxygen saturation with a fiber-optic pulse oximeter during MR imaging. *AJR* 1992;158:663–664.
67. Shellock FG, Slump G. Halo vest for cervical spine fixation during MR imaging. *AJR* 1990;154:631–632.
68. Shellock FG. MR imaging of metallic implants and materials: a compilation of the literature. *AJR* 1988;151:811–814.
69. Soulen RL, Budinger TF, Higgins CB. Magnetic resonance imaging of prosthetic heart valves. *Radiology* 1985;154:705–707.
70. Teitelbaum GP, Bradley WG Jr, Klein BD. MR imaging artifacts, ferromagnetism and magnetic torque of intravascular filters, stents and coils. *Radiology* 1988;166:657–664.
71. Pusey E, Lufkin RB, Brown RKJ, et al. Magnetic resonance imaging artifacts: mechanism and clinical significance. *Radiographics* 1986;6:891–911.
72. Teitelbaum GP, Ortega HV, Vinitski S, et al. Low-artifact intravascular devices: MR imaging evaluation. *Radiology* 1988;168:713–719.
73. Hartnell GG, Spence L, Hughes LA, et al. Safety of MR imaging in patients who have retained metallic materials after cardiac surgery. *AJR* 1997;168:1157–1159.
74. Spritzer CE, Sussman SK, Blurder RA, et al. Deep venous thrombosis evaluation with limited flip angle, gradient refocused MR imaging: preliminary experience. *Radiology* 1988;166:371–375.
75. Dujovny M, Gundamraj NR, Alp MS, et al. Aneurysm clip testing for ferromagnetic properties. Clip variability issues. *Radiology* 1997;202:637–639.
76. Dujovny M, Kossovsky N, Kossowsky R. Aneuyssm clip motion during magnetic resonance imaging: in vivo experimental study with metallurgical factor analysis. *Neurosurgery* 1985;17:543–548.
77. Kanal E, Shellock FG. Patient monitoring during clinical MR imaging. *Radiology* 1992;185:623–629.
78. Shellock FG, Shellock VJ. Metallic stents: Evaluation of MR imaging safety. *AJR* 1999;173:543–547.
79. Rubin JB, Enzmann DR. Optimizing conventional MR imaging of the spine. *Radiology* 1987;163:777–783.
80. Liebman CE, Messersmith RN, Levin DN, et al. MR imaging of inferior vena caval filters: Safety and artifacts. *AJR* 1988;150:1174–1176.
81. Theumann NH, Pfirrmann CWA, Antonio GE, et al. Extrinsic carpal ligaments: normal MR arthrographic appearance in cadavers. *Radiology* 2003;226:171–179.
82. Beltran J, Chandnani V, McGhee RA, et al. Gadopentetate dimeglumine-enhanced MR imaging of the musculoskeletal system. *AJR* 1991;156:457–466.
83. Herman LJ, Beltran J. Pitfalls in MR imaging of the knee. *Radiology* 1988;167:775–781.
84. Robertson DD, Magid D, Poss R, et al. Enhanced computed tomographic techniques for the evaluation of total hip arthroplasty. *J Arthroplasty* 1989;4:271–276.
85. Suh J-S, Jeong E-K, Shin K-H, et al. Minimizing artifacts caused by metallic implants at MR imaging: experimental and clinical studies. *AJR* 1998;171:1207–1213.
86. Malko JA, Hoffman JC, Jarrett PJ. Eddy-current-induced artifacts caused by an "MRI-compatible" halo device. *Radiology* 1989;3:563–564.
87. Tkach JA, Haacke EM. A comparison of fast spin echo and gradient field echo sequences. *Magn Reson Imaging* 1988;6:373–389.
88. Pavlicek W, Geisinger M, Castle L, et al. The effects of nuclear magnetic resonance on patients with cardiac pacemakers. *Radiology* 1983;147:149–153.
89. Hauger O, Dumont E, Chateil J-F, et al. Water excitation as an alternative to fat saturation in MR imaging: preliminary results in musculoskeletal imaging. *Radiology* 2002;224:657–663.
90. Major NM, Banks MC. MR imaging of complications of loose surgical tacks in the shoulder. *AJR* 2003;180:377–380.
91. Peh WCG, Chan JHM. Artifacts in musculoskeletal magnetic resonance imaging: identification and correction. *Skeletal Radiol* 2001;30:179–191.
92. Sugimoto H, Hirose I, Miyaoka E, et al. Low-field –strength MR imaging of failed hip arthroplasty: association of femoral periprosthetic signal intensity with radiographic, surgical and pathologic findings. *Radiology* 2003;229:718–723.
93. Twair A, Ryan M, O'Connell M, et al. MRI of failed total hip replacement caused by abductor muscle avulsion. *AJR* 2003;181:1547–1550.
94. Roth JL, Nugent M, Gray JE, et al. Patient monitoring during magnetic resonance imaging. *Anesthesiology* 1985;62:80–83.
95. Bloomfield EL, Masaryk TJ, Caplin A, et al. Intravenous sedation for MR imaging of the brain and spine in children: pentobarbital versus propofol. *Radiology* 1993;18b:93–97.
96. Brummett RE, Talbot JM, Charuhas P. Potential hearing loss resulting from MRI imaging. *Radiology* 1988;169:539–540.
97. Quirk ME, Letendre AJ, Ciottone RA, et al. Anxiety in patients undergoing MR imaging. *Radiology* 1989;170:463–466.
98. Greenberg SB, Faeber EN, Radke JL, et al. Sedation of difficult to sedate children undergoing MR imaging. Value of thioridazine as an adjunct to chloral hydrate. *AJR* 1994;163:165–168.
99. Frush DP, Bissett GS III. Sedation of children in radiology: time to wake up. *AJR* 1995;165:913–914.
100. Vade A, Sukhani R, Dolenga M, et al. Chloral hydrate sedation of children undergoing CT and MR imaging: safety as judged by the American Academy of Pediatrics guidelines. *AJR* 1995;105:905–909.
101. Mason KP, Zurakowski D, Karian VE, et al. Sedatives used in pediatric imaging: comparison of IV pentobarbital with midazolam added. *AJR* 2001;177:427–430.

102. Frush DP, Bissett GS III, Hall SC. Pediatric sedation in radiology: the practice of safe sleep. *AJR* 1996;167:1381–1387.
103. Haacke EM, Tkac JA. Fast MR imaging: techniques and clinical applications. *AJR* 1990;155:951–964.
104. Kanal E, Shellock FG. MR imaging of patients with intracranial aneurysm clips. *Radiology* 1993;187:612–614.
105. Arakaw M, Crooks LE, McCarten B, et al. A comparison of saddle shaped and solenoidal coils for magnetic resonance imaging. *Radiology* 1985;154:227–228.
106. Fisher MR, Barker B, Amparo EG, et al. MR imaging using specialized coils. *Radiology* 1985;157:443–447.
107. Jack CR Jr, Berquist TH, Miller GM, et al. Field strength in neuro-MR imaging: comparison of 0.5T and 1.5T. *J Comput Assist Tomogr* 1990;14:505–513.
108. Kneeland JB, Hyde JS. High-resolution MR imaging with local coils. *Radiology* 1989;171:1–7.
109. Kneeland JB, Knowles RJR, Cahill PT. Magnetic resonance imaging systems: optimization in clinical use. *Radiology* 1984;153:473–478.
110. Smith DK, Wright J. Waterbags: an inexpensive method for improving fat suppression in MR imaging of the extremities. *AJR* 1994;162:1252–1253.
111. Reiman TH, Heiken JP, Totty WG, et al. Clinical MR imaging with a Helmholtz-type surface coil. *Radiology* 1988;169:564–566.
112. Wright SM, Wright RM. Bilateral MR imaging with switched mutually coupled receiver coils. *Radiology* 1989;170:249–255.
113. Hood MN, Ho VB, Smirniotopoulos JG, et al. Chemical shift: the artifact and clinical tool revisited. *Radiographics* 1999;19: 357–371.
114. Rosen BR, Fleming DM, Kushner DC, et al. Hematologic bone marrow disorders: quantitative chemical shift MR imaging. *Radiology* 1988;169:799–804.
115. Shuman WP, Baron RL, Peters MJ, et al. Comparison of STIR and spin echo MR imaging at 1.5T in 90 lesions of the chest, liver and pelvis. *AJR* 1989;152:853–859.
116. Tyrell RL, Gluckert K, Pathria M, et al. Fast three-dimensional MR imaging of the knee: comparison with arthroscopy. *Radiology* 1988;166:865–872.
117. van der Meulen P, Groen JP, Tinus AMC, et al. Fast field echo imaging: an overview and contrast calculations. *Magn Reson Imaging* 1988;6:355–368.
118. Wismer GL, Rosen BR, Buxton R, et al. Chemical shift imaging of bone marrow: preliminary experience. *AJR* 1985;145:1031–1037.
119. Delfaut RM, Beltran J, Johnson G, et al. Fat suppression in MR imaging: techniques and pitfalls. *Radiographics* 1999;19:373–382.
120. Crawley AP, Pooublanc J, Ferrari P, et al. Basics of diffusion and perfusion MRI. *Appl Radiol* 2003;32:13–23.
121. Maeda M, Sakuma H, Maier SE, et al. Quantitative assessment of diffusion abnormalities in benign and malignant vertebral compression fractures by scan diffusion-weighted imaging. *AJR* 2003;181:1203–1209.
122. Hovsepain DM, Amis ES. Penile prosthetic implants. a radiographic atlas. *Radiographics* 1989;9:707–716.
123. Sonin AH, Pensy RAA, Mulligan ME, et al. Grading articular cartilage of the knee using fast spin-echo proton density-weighted MR imaging without fat suppression. *AJR* 2002;179:1159–1166.
124. Alley MT, Shifrin RY, Pelc NJ, et al. Ultrafast contrast-enhanced three-dimensional MR angiography: state of the art. *Radiographics* 1998;18:273–285.
125. Bakker J, Beek FJA, Bentler JJ, et al. Renal artery stenosis and accessory renal arteries: accurancy of detection and visualization with gadolinium-enhanced breath-hold MR angiography. *Radiology* 1998;207:497–504.
126. McCauley TR, Disler DG. MR imaging of articular cartilage. *Radiology* 1998;206:629–640.
127. Potter HG, Linklater JM, Allen AA, et al. Magnetic resonance imaging of articular cartilage in the knee. An evaluation with use of fast-spin-echo imaging. *J Bone Joint Surg* 1998;80A:1276–1284.
128. King CL, Henkelman RM, Poon PY, et al. MR imaging of the normal knee. *J Comput Assist Tomogr* 1984;8:1147–1154.
129. Axel L. Blood flow effects in magnetic resonance imaging. *AJR* 1984;143:1157–1166.
130. Bradley WG Jr, Waluch V, Lai KS, et al. The appearance of rapidly flowing blood on magnetic resonance images. *AJR* 1984;143:1167–1174.
131. Bradley WG Jr, Waluch V. Blood flow: magnetic resonance imaging. *Radiology* 1985;154:443–450.
132. Bradley WG Jr. Flow phenomena in MR imaging. *AJR* 1988;160:983–994.
133. Bradley WG. When should GRASS be used? *Radiology* 1988;169:574–575.
134. Erdman WA, Weinreb JC, Cohen JM, et al. Venous thrombosis: clinical and experimental MR imaging. *Radiology* 1986;161:233–238.
135. White EM, Edelman RR, Wedeen VJ, et al. Intravascular signal in MR imaging. Use of phase display for differentiation of blood-flow signal from intraluminal disease. *Radiology* 1986;161:245–249.
136. Felmlee JP, Ehman RL. Spatial presaturation: a method for suppressing flow artifacts and improving depiction of vascular anatomy in MR imaging. *Radiology* 1987;164:559–564.
137. Carrino JA, Morrison WB, Zou KH, et al. Noncontrast MR imaging and MR arthrography of the ulnar collateral ligament of the elbow: prospective evaluation of two-dimensional pulse sequences for detection of complete tears. *Skeletal Radiol* 2001;30:625–632.
138. Eustace S, Hentzen P, Adams J, et al. Comparison of conventional and turbo spin-echo T1-weighted MR imaging in acute knee trauma. *AJR* 1999;172:1393–1395.
139. Eustace S, Jara H, Goldberg R, et al. A comparison of conventional spin-echo and turbo spin-echo imaging of soft tissues adjacent to orthopedic hardware. *AJR* 1998;70:455–458.
140. Wayne JS, Kraft KA, Shields KJ, et al. MR imaging of normal and matrix depleted cartilage: correlation with biomechanical function and biomechanical composition. *Radiology* 2003;228: 493–499.
141. Dwyer AJ, Frank JA, Sank VJ, et al. Short-TI inversion-recovery pulse sequence: analysis and initial experience in cancer imaging. *Radiology* 1988;168:827–836.
142. Gullberg GT, Wehril FW, Shimakawa A, et al. MR vascular imaging with a fast gradient refocusing pulse sequence and reformatted images for transaxial sections. *Radiology* 1987;165:241–246.
143. König H, Sauter R, Deimling M, et al. Cartilage disorders: comparison of spin-echo, CHESS, and FLASH sequence MR images. *Radiology* 1987;164:753–758.
144. Heuck AF, Steiger P, Stoller DW, et al. Quantification of knee fluid volume by MR imaging and CT using 3-D data processing. *J Comput Assist Tomogr* 1989;13:287–293.
145. Ruel L, Brugieres P, Luciani A, et al. Comparison of in vitro and in vivo MRI of the spine using parallel imaging. *AJR* 2004;182:749–755.
146. Binkert CA, Zanetti M, Gerber C, et al. MR arthrography of the glenohumeral joint: two concentrations of gadoteridol versus ringer solution as the intraarticulat contrast material. *Radiology* 2001;220:219–224.
147. Funke M, Kopka L, Vosshenrich R, et al. MR arthrography in diagnoses of rotator cuff tears: standard spin-echo alone or with fat suppression. *Acta Radiol* 1996;37:627–632.
148. Hajek PC, Sartoris DJ, Neumann CH, et al. Potential contrast agents for MR arthrography: in vitro evaluation and practical observations. *AJR* 1987;149:97–104.
149. Vanel D, Shapeero LG, Tardivon A, et al. Dynamic contrast-enhanced MRI with subtraction of aggressive soft tissue tumors after resection. *Skeletal Radiol* 1998;27:505–510.
150. Wolf GL. Current status of MR imaging contrast agents. A special report. *Radiology* 1989;172:709–710.
151. Brown RB, Clarke DW, Daffner RH. Is a mixture of gadolinium and iodinated contrast material safe during MR arthrography? *AJR* 2000;175:1087–1090.
152. Winalski S, Aliabadi P, Wright RJ, et al. Enhancement of joint fluid with intravenously administered gadopenetate dimeglumine: techniques, rationale, and implications. *Radiology* 1993;187:179–185.
153. Prince MR, Arnoldus C, Frisoli JK. Nephrotoxicity of high-dose gadolinium compared with iodinated contrast. *J Magn Reson Imaging* 1996;6:162–166.
154. Erleman R, Reiser M, Peters PE, et al. Time dependent changes in signal intensity in neoplastic and inflammatory lesions of the musculoskeletal system following intravenous administration of Gd-DTPA. *Radiology* 1988;28:269–276.

155. Maas M, Dijkstra PF, Akkerman EM. Uniform fat suppression in hands and feet through the use of two-pound Dixon chemical shift MR imaging. *Radiology* 1999;210:189–193.

156. Vahlensieck M, Peterfly CG, Wischer T, et al. Indirect MR arthrography: optimization and clinical applications. *Radiology* 1996;200:249–254.

157. Chandani VP, Ho C, Chu P, et al. Knee hyaline cartilage evaluated with MR imaging: a cadaveric study involving multiple imaging sequences and intra-articular injection of gadolinium and saline solution. *Radiology* 1991;178:557–561.

158. Haims A, Schweitzer ME, Morrison WB, et al. Internal derangement of the wrist: indirect MR arthrography versus unenhanced MR imaging. *Radiology* 2003;227:701–707.

159. Kramer J, Scheurecher A, Mohr E, et al. Magnetic resonance arthrography: benefits and indications. *Adv MRI Contrast* 1997;4:104–119.

160. Recht MP, Kramer J, Petersilge CA, et al. Distribution of normal and abnormal fluid collections in the glenohumeral joint: implications for MR arthrography. *J Magn Reson Imaging* 1994;4:173–177.

161. Keller PG, Drayer BD, Fram EK, et al. MR angiography with two-dimensional acquisition and three-dimensional display. *Radiology* 1989;173:527–532.

162. Meaney JFM, Ridgway JP, Chakravety S, et al. Stepping-table gadolinium-enhanced digital subtraction MR angiography of the aortic and lower extremity arteries: preliminary experience. *Radiology* 1999;211:59–67.

163. Moody AR, Pollock JG, O'Connor AR, et al. Lower limb deep venous thrombosis: direct MR imaging of the thrombus. *Radiology* 1998;209:349–355.

164. Wang Y, Lee HM, Khilnani NM, et al. Bolus-chase MR digital subtraction angiography in the lower extremity. *Radiology* 1998;207:263–269.

165. Hyde JS, Kneeland JB. High resolution methods using surface coils. In: Wehrlie FW, Shaw D, Kneeland JB, eds. *Biomedical magnetic resonance imaging.* Weinheim: VCH, 1988:189–222.

166. Lenz GW, Haacke EM, Masaryk TJ, et al. In-plane vascular imaging: pulse sequence design and strategy. *Radiology* 1988;166:875–882.

167. Schwaighofer BS, Yu KK, Mattery RF. Diagnostic significance of interslice gap and imaging volume in body MR imaging. *AJR* 1989;153:629–632.

168. Miller RG, Carlson PJ, Moussavi RS, et al. The use of magnetic resonance spectroscopy to evaluate muscle fatigue and human muscle disease. *Appl Radiol* 1989;18(3):33–38.

169. des Plantes BGZ, Falke THM, den Boer JA. Pulse sequences and contrast in magnetic resonance imaging. *Radiographics* 1984;4:869–883.

170. Frank LR, Brossmann J, Buxton RB, et al. MR imaging truncation artifacts can create a false laminar appearance in cartilage. *AJR* 1997;168:547–554.

171. Kuno S, Katsuta S, Inouye T, et al. Relationship between MR relaxation time and muscle fiber composition. *Radiology* 1988;169:567–568.

172. Lufkin RB, Pusey E, Stark DD, et al. Boundary artifact due to truncation errors in MR imaging. *AJR* 1986;147:1283–1287.

173. Arena L, Morehouse HT, Safir J. MR imaging artifacts that simulate disease. How to recognize and eliminate them. *Radiographics* 1995;15:1373–1394.

174. Bodne D, Quinn SF, Cochran CF. Imaging foreign glass and wooden bodies of the extremities with CT and MR. *J Comput Assist Tomogr* 1988;12:608–611.

175. Lenkinski RE, Holland GA, Allman T, et al. Integrated MR imaging and spectroscopy with chemical shift imaging of P-31 at 1.5 T: Initial clinical experience. *Radiology* 1988;169:201–206.

The Temporomandibular Joint

Thomas H. Berquist   *Clyde A. Helms*

Magnetic resonance imaging (MRI) of the temporomandibular joint (TMJ) has rapidly replaced arthrography and computed tomography (CT) as the imaging modality of choice for evaluating internal derangement (1–9). MRI can directly visualize the disc, accurately determine the disc position, and evaluate condylar motion in a noninvasive manner (10–13). MRI also provides information on the state of hydration and morphology of the disc that may be helpful in staging internal derangement (14–18). Although it will not rival the resolution of CT in examining bony detail, MRI provides an accurate picture of most bony abnormalities (19,20). In addition, MRI demonstrates other intraarticular and periarticular abnormalities (13,21,22).

Ultrasound has been evaluated as a screening technique in recent years. However, this technique requires considerable experience by the examiner (23). To date, sonography is not frequently utilized to evaluate internal derangement of the TMJ.

ANATOMY

The TMJ is a synovial joint divided into superior and inferior compartments by a fibrous disc (24,25). The two compartments do not communicate unless there is a perforation of the disc. The joint is formed by the mandibular condyle and articular fossa of the temporal bone (see Fig. 4-1) (24,26).

The disc is normally biconcave with three distinct segments (see Fig. 4-2). The thickest portion of the disc is the posterior band. The posterior band is separated from the anterior band by a thin, intermediate zone, thus the concave or "bow-tie" appearance (24,25,27). Disc stability is provided by multiple attachments. Posteriorly, a ligament, also referred to as the bilaminar zone, serves to attach the disc and capsule to the condylar margin and temporal bone (24,25). The posterior attachment contains a rich vascular supply and neural elements that innervate the disc (25,27,28).

The disc attaches to the superior belly of the lateral pterygoid muscle anteriorly (Fig. 4-1) (21,22,24). The muscle tension is balanced by the elastic fibers in the bilaminar zone (24,25,29). The pterygoid muscles course medially to insert on the pterygoid plates. Therefore, anteriorly displaced discs tend to lie somewhat anteromedially. There

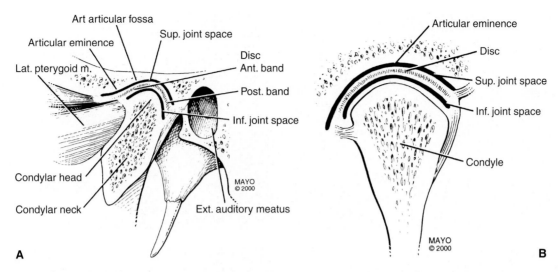

Figure 4-1   Illustration of the temporomandibular joint in the sagittal **(A)** and coronal **(B)** planes.

are also additional capsular attachments anteriorly, medially, and laterally (25).

When the mouth is in the closed position, the posterior band (Fig. 4-2) is normally at the apex of the mandibular condyle (24,25,30). The inferior concave portion of the disc rests on the curved surface of the mandibular condyle. With opening of the mouth, the condyle moves forward and the normal disc remains centered over the condyle (24,30). In the fully open position, the thin intermediate zone rests between the condyle and articular eminence of the temporal bone (Fig. 4-2) (25). During normal motion in the sagittal plane, the disc moves in a convex path over a distance of 10 mm (31,32).

IMAGING TECHNIQUES

Many different imaging protocols have been proposed for evaluating the TMJ (18,33–37). Most rely upon sagittal images in the closed and open positions, though coronal images, motion studies, and intravenous or intraarticular gadolinium studies have also been advocated (38–41). Ideally, examinations should be tailored based on clinical findings and the philosophy of the referring physician or dentist (41–43).

Certain basic parameters are necessary for examination efficiency and optimal image quality. A small (3- to 5-in) surface coil is mandatory to provide sufficient signal-to-noise to

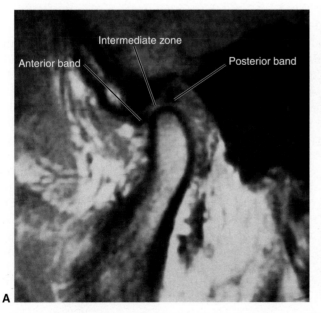
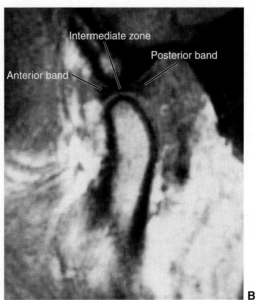

Figure 4-2   Sagittal T1-weighted MR images in the closed **(A)** and open **(B)** positions. The posterior band is normally above the condyle in the closed position **A**. In the open mouth position **B**, the disc is more easily appreciated. The thin intermediate zone rests between the condyle and eminence of the temporal bone.

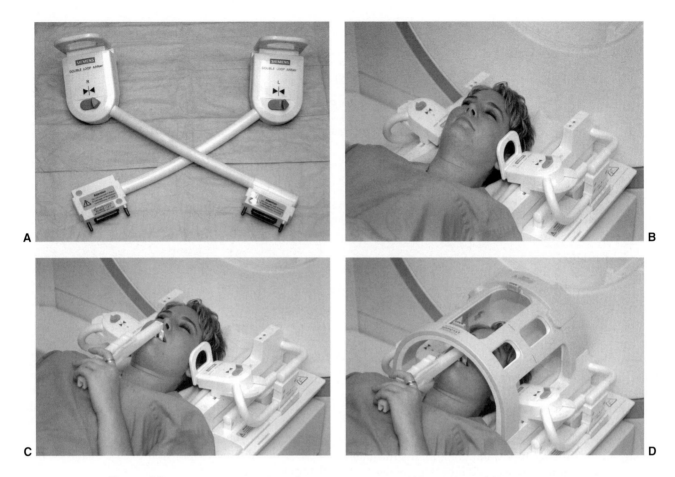

Figure 4-3 Coils and opening device for TMJ imaging. **A:** Dual loop array coils. **B:** Patient positioned with dual coils for bilateral TMJ imaging. **C:** Patient positioned with dual coils and opening device used for cine imaging. **D:** Patient positioned with dual TMJ coils and head coil in place. Opening device for cine images.

assure high image quality. Bilateral coupled coils (see Fig. 4-3A and C) are most commonly used. This permits both TMJs to be studied in the same time required for unilateral examinations (3,34,44). Newer scanners allow the dual coils to be used with the head coil, which adds versatility to the examination (see Fig. 4-3D). A small field of view (FOV) (10-14cm), 256 × 256 or 256 × 192 matrix, and one to three excitations are most often used (37,39,44). However, some authors prefer 512 × 512 matrix when using gradient-echo sequences (45).

IMAGE PLANES AND PULSE SEQUENCES

A double localizer (axial and sagittal) scout image is obtained (SE 20/5, FOV 28 cm, 126 × 50 matrix, three to four 1-cm sections through palpated TMJ region, one excitation, scan time <10 seconds) to select image planes for sagittal and, if needed, coronal images (see Fig. 4-4) (Table 4-1). The condyles are oriented about 30 degrees medially on the axial view. Though controversial, most institutions orient the image planes obliquely for sagittal and coronal studies (Fig. 4-4A and D). Whether one selects direct or oblique sagittal images, most institutions use 2- to 4-mm-thick sections (34,37,39,44,46,47).

Several approaches have been suggested for sagittal imaging (Table 4-1). Basic anatomy and disc position can be evaluated using T-1 weighted spin-echo sequences in the open and closed positions (47–51). Parameters include TE 10 to 11, TR 400 to 500, 256 × 256 or 256 × 192 matrix, 4-mm-thick sections, one excitation, and a FOV of 12 to 14 cm. No attempt is made to obtain a full open-mouth image unless specifically requested by the clinician. In the closed-mouth images, the condyle is seated in the glenoid fossa with the disc interposed between the condylar head and the glenoid (see Fig. 4-5). Because the disc is predominantly low in signal and is tightly placed between two low signal areas of cortex, it can be very difficult to visualize adequately in many instances. If the patient assumes a partial open-mouth position, the condylar head moves slightly out of the glenoid fossa, allowing the disc to be separated from the bony surfaces so it is more easily seen in its entirety (Fig. 4-2B).

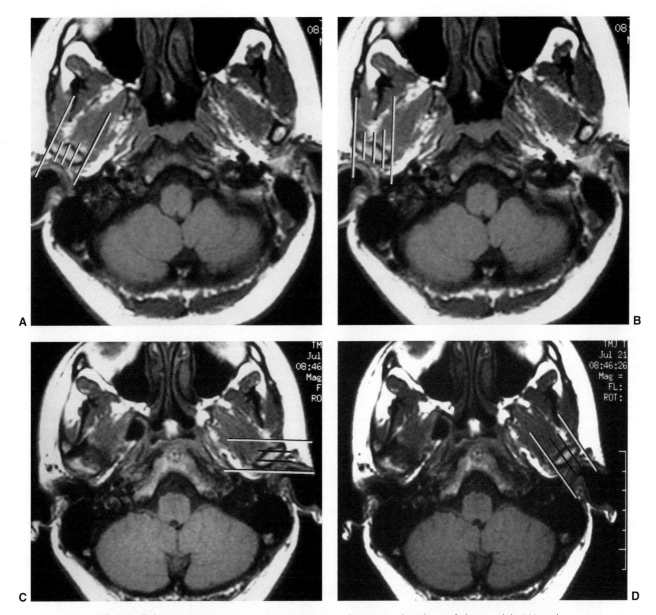

Figure 4-4 Axial scout images demonstrating selection in the plane of the condyle **(A)** and straight sagittal images **(B)**. Straight coronal **(C)** and oblique coronal in the plane of the condyle **(D)**.

In the partial open-mouth position, the disc often is in a normal position, having reduced from an anteriorly displaced position. Hence, many false negative studies could result if the partial open-mouth images are relied on for diagnosing disc position. It is important to judge the disc position on the closed-mouth images and rely on the partial open-mouth images to note the size, shape, and signal characteristics (Figs. 4-2 and 4-5). The information obtained on the partial open-mouth images concerning the disc size and shape can then be applied to the closed-mouth images to locate the disc position more confidently (Figs. 4-2 and 4-5). If the closed-mouth images alone are used, a small but significant number of cases will be almost nondiagnostic (34,36).

Other approaches to sagittal imaging have also become popular in recent years. T2-weighted spin echo,

fat-suppressed fast spin-echo, or turbo spin-echo sequences in the open and closed positions have proved useful for identifying joint effusions (15,42,43,52–54). Conventional spin-echo sequence parameters include SE 2,000/20,80, 256 × 192 matrix, one excitation, 3- to 4-mm sections with 0.5 mm gap and 12 cm FOV. Fast or turbo spin-echo T2-weighted sequences have largely replaced conventional spin-echo sequences to reduce scan time (44,51) (Table 4-1). Proton density sequences (Table 4-1) are useful in evaluating disc morphology in a similar fashion to meniscal pathology in the knee (see Chapter 7). Gradient-echo sequences have also been used in both closed and open positions or with multiple small increments to produce a cine-loop motion study (7,55). Roditi et al. (7) found gradient-echo images using 512 × 512 matrix were superior to fast spin-echo sequences.

TABLE 4-1

IMAGING PARAMETERS FOR THE TEMPOROMANDIBULAR JOINT

Image Plane	Pulse Sequence	Slice Thickness	Field of View (FOV)	Matrix	Acquisitions	Scan Time
Scout axial/sagittal	2D localizer 20/5/40° FA	10 mm	280 mm	256 × 128	1	9.2 s
Axial Closed	SE 416/17	3 mm	120 mm	256 × 256	1	1:03 min
Sagittal Oblique Open left	TSE 300/19	3 mm	120 mm	256 × 256	3	1:57 min
Sagittal Oblique Open right	TSE 459/19	3 mm	120 mm	256 × 256	3	2:58 min
Sagittal Cine	TSE 459/19	3 mm	120 mm	256 × 256	3	2:58 min
Sagittal Left Cine	80/11/30° FA	4 mm	140 mm	256 × 256	1	7:06 min
Sagittal Right	80/11/30° FA	4 mm	140 mm	256 × 256	1	7:06 min
[a]Sagittal proton density	TSE 1,500/19	3 mm	120 mm	256 × 192	1	2:27 min
[a]Coronal proton density	TSE 1,500/19	3 mm	120 mm	256 × 192	1	2:27 min
[a]Oblique axial	TSE 1,500/19	3 mm	120 mm	256 × 192	1	2:27 min

FA, flip angle; TSE, turbo spin echo.
[a] Optional.

A cine technique employing fast gradient-echo images (Table 4-1) has been used in conjunction with a device that will incrementally open the mouth in 1- to 3-mm steps for each image (Fig. 4-3) (14,56,57). A dozen or more images are obtained, each one in a different jaw position from fully closed to open position (58). Using the cine technique demonstrated in Table 4-1, the examination takes 7:06 minutes for each TMJ. When played as a video "loop," this shows condylar translation and disc movement, including disc reduction, if it occurs (see Fig. 4-6). The physiology and

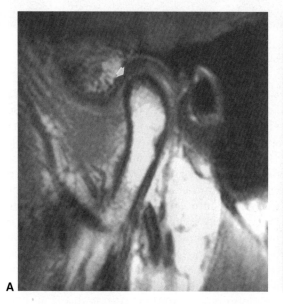

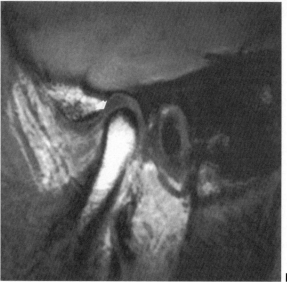

Figure 4-5 T-1 weighted sagittal images in the closed position. **A:** The disc (*arrow*) is tightly placed between the condyle and eminence. **B:** The disc is better visualized (*arrow*). Note the intermediate areas of signal intensity indicating normal hydration.

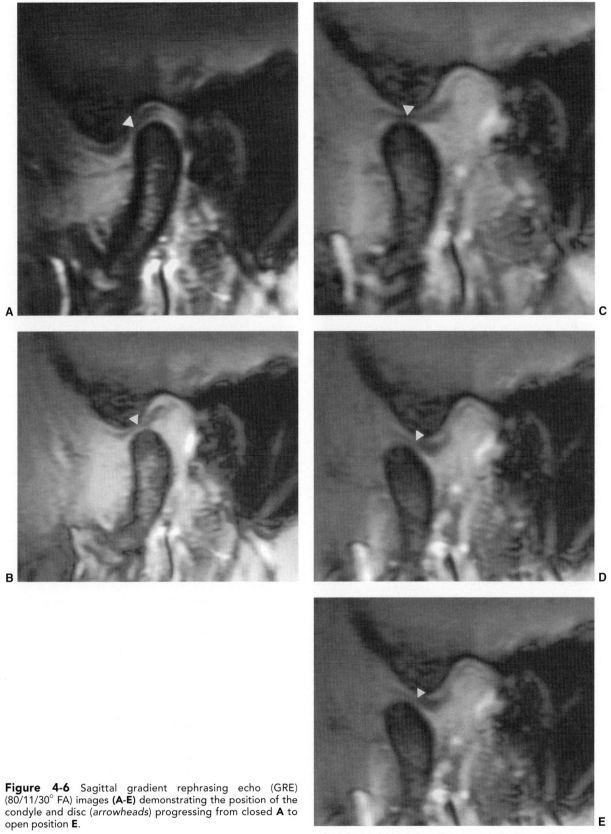

Figure 4-6 Sagittal gradient rephrasing echo (GRE) (80/11/30° FA) images **(A-E)** demonstrating the position of the condyle and disc (*arrowheads*) progressing from closed **A** to open position **E**.

biomechanics can be distorted because the technique relies on an external device to force mouth opening rather than the patient's intrinsic musculature. Also, since the dynamics of the TMJ can and do change quite frequently, any motion study, whether an arthrogram, CT, or MRI, must be viewed as a temporary set of events.

Cine-looped imaging provides additional information to data gained with the study of condylar and disc motion as the condylar moves from the closed to open position (Fig. 4-6) (31,42,58–60). Morphology and abnormalities such as "stuck disc" may be more easily appreciated (31,60).

Coronal images (oblique preferred; Fig. 4-4) are useful to evaluate medial and lateral disc displacements (51,61). Proton density sequences display disc position in the fossa and over the condyle (see Fig. 4-7).

More recently, Chen et al. (33) described an oblique axial image plane to demonstrate the disc–condyle relationship better in patients with anterior disc displacement. A sagittal image is used to determine the slope of the eminence at the level of the outer third of the condyle (see Fig. 4-8A). Oblique axial images are obtained in a plane perpendicular to the slope of the eminence. This approach demonstrates the medial or lateral displacement of the disc more clearly than conventional coronal images when anterior disc displacement is present (see Fig. 4-8B to D) (33).

Three-dimensional volume acquisitions have also been useful (25,62). This allows a volume of tissue to be rapidly imaged, rather than a slice, that can then be viewed as thin slices in the desired plane. In the TMJ, the images would be sagittally oriented and could be as thin as 1 mm through each condylar head. It has been shown that smaller flip angles (around 20°) result in better disc visualization with longer flip angles (25).

CONTRAST ENHANCED MAGNETIC RESONANCE IMAGING

Finally, some centers use intravenous or intraarticular gadolinium in selected situations (35,36,38,41). Anatomy, posterior detachments, and marrow lesions may be more easily appreciated when intravenous gadolinium is used in conjunction with fat-suppressed T1-weighted images (35, 36,38). Early synovial inflammation is more easily identified with intravenous contrast. Ogasawara et al. (38) described contrast enhancement using intravenous injection of 0.1 mmol per kg of gadolinium. Images were obtained in the oblique sagittal plane with the mouth open and closed. T1-weighted fat-suppressed and T1-weighted fast spin-echo sequences were obtained after injection.

Suenaga et al. (40) used a rapid bolus injection with T1-weighted fat-suppressed oblique sagittal images at 2, 4, 6, and 10 minutes to evaluate early synovial inflammation. In our practice, we rarely use intravenous gadolinium except in patients with rheumatoid arthritis or other early inflammatory arthropathies (see Fig. 4-9). We have not used MR

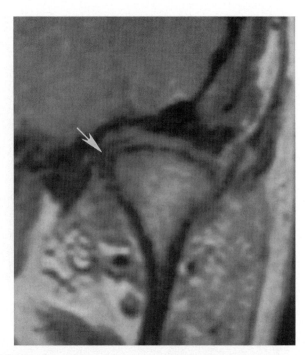

Figure 4-7 Coronal proton density (TSE 1,500/19) demonstrating a deformed disc with medial displacement (*arrow*).

arthrography due to the time, cost, and difficulty that may occur with this invasive approach. However, MR arthrography does provide more information regarding adhesions, perforation, and posterior detachment (41).

Toyama et al. (41) evaluated 13 joints in 11 patients with MR arthrography. Needle position was confirmed with a small amount of iodinated contrast. A gadolinium solution (0.3 to 1.0 mL of 0.25 mmol/L) was injected into the lower (0.3 mL) and upper (0.5 mL) compartments. If a perforation was present, about 1 mL was injected to fill both compartments. Gadolinium was slowly injected into both the upper and lower compartments to avoid capsular rupture.

A perforation or posterior detachment was diagnosed when contrast flowed from one compartment to the next. Adhesions were diagnosed by incomplete filling of the injected compartment (see Fig. 4-10). Surgical correlation was 100% for perforations. Accuracy for adhesions was 85% in the lower compartment and 77% in the upper compartment (41).

INTERNAL DERANGEMENT

Internal derangement has been defined as an abnormal relationship or position of the disc in relation to the mandibular condyle and articular eminence (25,27,63). The etiology is uncertain; however, the condition is three to five times more common in females, and symptoms typically become evident by the fourth decade (25,63,64). Suggested etiologies include trauma, primary osseous abnormalities, malocclusion, bruxism, hypermobility, stress, and absence of the posterior teeth (21,65,66).

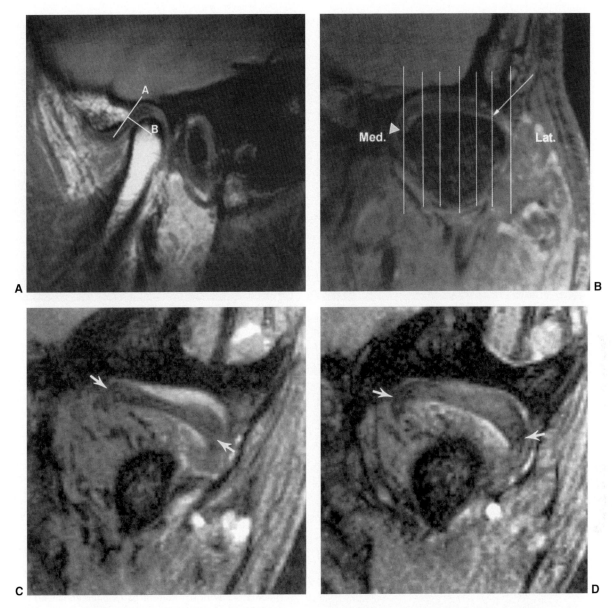

Figure 4-8 Axial-oblique technique. **A:** Sagittal image taken at the outer third of the condyle. Images (line *B*) are taken perpendicular to the slope of the eminence (line *A*). **B:** The condyle is divided into six parts. The lateral margin of the disc (*arrow*) is medial to the lateral sixth of the condyle so the disc is medially displaced. The disc can also be seen (*arrowhead*) extending beyond the medial condylar margin (**C,D**). Axial images clearly demonstrate the disc and the lateral and medial margins (*arrows*). (Fig. 4-8, B to D, courtesy of Chen YJ, Gallo LM, Meier D, et al. Individualized oblique-axial magnetic resonance imaging for improved visualization of mediolateral TMJ disc displacement. *J Orofacial Pain* 2000;14(2):128–139.)

Normally, the disc is positioned such that the bilaminar zone is at 12 o'clock in the closed mouth position (Fig. 4-2A) (67). However, some degree of anterior, medial, or lateral displacement may be evident in up to 34% of asymptomatic patients (51,61).

The mandibular condyle (see Fig. 4-11A) is centered to slightly posterior in the condylar fossa. The normal condyle is 6.41 mm (range 4.2 to 8.2 mm) in the sagittal plane (68,69). Reduction in condylar size as measured on the axial images may also play a role in internal

derangement. Kurita et al. (70) demonstrated an association between condylar size, especially medial to lateral, and internal derangement (see Fig. 4-11B). Fossa size and shape are also important, as changes in configuration may play a role in disc displacement (30,68,71). Changes in morphology in one joint may also effect the contralateral TMJ (30,68).

Internal derangement is a progressive process. Initially, anterior, medial, or lateral displacement may be evident in the closed position that reduces with opening. As the elastic

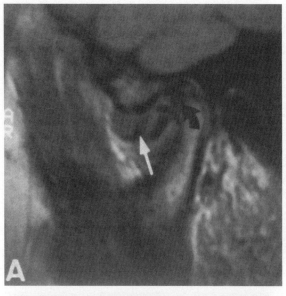

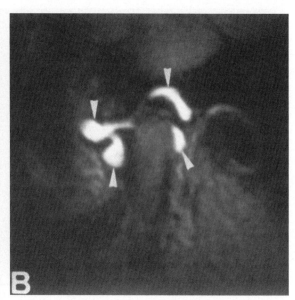

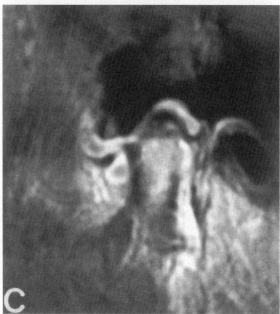

Figure 4-9 Contrast enhanced evaluation of the TMJ in a patient with rheumatoid arthritis. **A:** T1-weighted sagittal non contrast image in the closed position demonstrates anterior disc displacement (*straight arrow*) and condylar erosion (*curved arrow*). **B:** T2-weighted oblique sagittal image demonstrates joint effusions in the upper and lower joint spaces (*arrowheads*). **C:** Contrast enhanced T1-weighted sagittal demonstrates synovial enhancement without fluid enhancement. (From Suenaga S, Ogura T, Matsuda T, et al. Severity of synovium and bone marrow abnormalities of the temporomandibular joint in early rheumatoid arthritis. Role of gadolinium enhanced fat-suppressed T1-weighted spin echo MRI. *J Compt Assist Tomogr* 2000; 24(3):461–465.)

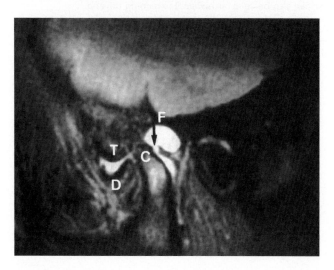

Figure 4-10 MR arthrogram of the TMJ in a female with anterior disc displacement without reduction and osteoarthritis. Sagittal arthrogram image demonstrates posterior detachment (*arrow*). *C*, condyle; *D*, disc; *F*, fossa; *T*, temporal eminence. (From Toyama M, Kurita K, Koga K, et al. Magnetic resonance arthropathy of the temporomandibular joint. *J Oral Maxillofacial Surg* 2000;58(9):978–983.)

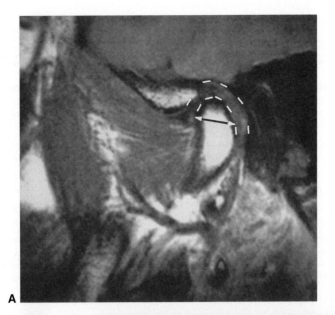

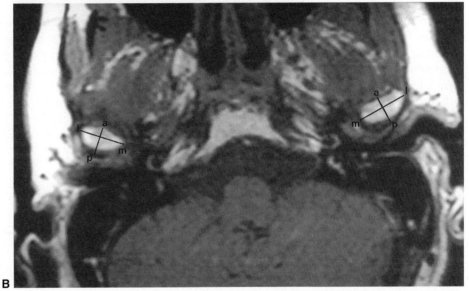

Figure 4-11 Condylar size and joint space measurements. **A:** Sagittal T1-weighted image demonstrating condylar width (*double arrow*) (normal 6.41 mm; range 4.2 to 8.2 mm) and joint space (*parallel lines*) regions to evaluate. **B:** Axial image through the condyles. Normal anteroposterior and mediolateral measurements on the left with reduced dimensions and internal derangement on the right AP, anteroposterior; ml, medial–lateral.

fibers in the posterior laminar zone (Fig. 4-1) become lax, the disc no longer reduces with opening or condylar translation. Over time, the disc becomes deformed, secondary osseous and articular changes occur, and perforations may develop in the disc (25,32,44,51,69,72–76).

Wilkes (66) described the clinical stages of internal derangement in 1989 (Table 4-2). During the early stage there is "clicking" with early opening or later with the closing phase, with no pain or decreased motion. Clicking is often the most common complaint, occurring in 53% of patients (52). Over time, there is progressive increase in symptoms, with reduced motion, pain, joint tenderness, and crepitation on physical examination (12,25,66).

Shellhas (63) correlated the image and histologic features of internal derangement similar to the clinical and surgical correlation provided by Wilkes (66) (Table 4-3). As expected, the morphologic features of the disc and joint changes correlate closely with the clinical and histologic features of internal derangement (8,25,63). As the process progresses, the image features become more dramatic with disc deformity, joint changes, condylar deformity, and avascular necrosis (AVN) (63).

MRI studies should be tailored to the suspected extent (clinical stage I to V) and site (unilateral vs. bilateral) of involvement. In our practice, we generally evaluate both joints as changes and often bilateral (80% to 90%) and

TABLE 4-2

INTERNAL DERANGEMENT: CLINICAL AND PATHOLOGIC FEATURES, WILKES CLASSIFICATION

Stage	Clinical Features	Pathologic Features
I	Clicking during opening or late closing; no pain or reduced motion	Normal morphology
II	Increased clicking; occasional locking or catching; episodes of pain, tenderness, headaches	Anteriorly displaced, early deformity, well-defined intermediate zone
III	Multiple episodes of pain, headaches, and joint tenderness; major mechanical symptoms	Displaced with marked deformity, variable adhesions, no osseous changes
IV	Chronic symptoms, reduced motion, undulating course	Increased deformity, bone changes, osteophytes, multiple adhesions in anterior, lateral, and posterior recesses
V	Decreased motion, reduced function, crepitation on examination	Gross degenerative changes in disc and articular surfaces, erosions, adhesions, subchondral cysts

From Wilkes CH. Internal derangements of the temporomandibular joint. Pathological variations. *Arch Otolaryngol Head Neck Surg* 1989;115:469–477.

comparison can be useful (25,51,77). Sagittal, coronal, and cine motion studies are usually obtained (Table 4-1). MR findings must be correlated with clinical features, as up to 34% of patients may have some degree of displacement without symptoms (27,44,61).

Evaluation of MR images should begin with a review of the disc morphology and position with the mouth open and closed. In some cases, the anatomy is only clearly presented on motion studies. This is especially true when the disc is deformed or medially or laterally displaced. This may cause confusion on sagittal images. Coronal proton density images (Table 4-1) should be added in this setting.

As noted above, the disc normally has a "bow-tie" or drumstick appearance, with the posterior band slightly larger than the anterior band (Figs. 4-2, 4-5, and 4-6). On T1-weighted images, a small amount of signal should be present with the overall appearance of the disc being low signal intensity (63,78). The disc is made up of proteoglycans somewhat like the nucleus pulposis in the spine. Therefore, it should be expected to have some degree of hydration; this is seen best in the posterior band as intermediate signal on T1-weighted images and high signal on T2- or T2*-weighted images (see Fig. 4-12) (63,78). As internal derangement progresses, the disc loses its normal hydration, and normal signal intensity seen on T1-weighted images is no longer apparent. This is believed to be due to disc desiccation and correlates with the duration of the patient's symptoms and the presence of degenerative joint disease (1,79). In addition to signal intensity, the shape of the disc should be evaluated. Disc configurations have been described as biconcave, biplanar, hemiconvex, biconvex, or folded (markedly deformed) (see Figs. 4-2 and 4-13) (27,80).

Tasaki et al. (51) described a classification system for disc displacement. Eight categories of disc displacement were described in addition to normal and indeterminate.

In some patients, the type of displacement could not be determined due to large perforations, previous surgery, or poor image definition (see Fig. 4-14) (51). Disc displacement may be anterior, in which case the posterior band is anterior to the condyle without associated medial or lateral displacement (Fig. 4-14B). The disc may also be partially displaced in the lateral part of the joint anteriorly (Fig. 4-14C) or medial joint anteriorly (Fig. 4-14D).

TABLE 4-3

IMAGE FEATURES OF INTERNAL DERANGEMENT

Stage	MR Features
I	Anterior displacement, normal disc morphology, reduces with opening
II	Disc displacement and deformity reduces with opening ± signal changes in disc ± effusions
III	Disc displacement and deformity No reduction with opening ± effusion
IV	Severe disc deformity and displacement No reduction with opening Effusion Osseous changes
V	Severe deformity and no reduction Perforation at attachment Progressive osseous deformity (avascular necrosis, osteochondritis, sclerosis)

Adapted from Schellhas KP. Internal derangement of the temporomandibular joint: radiologic staging with clinical, surgical, and pathological correlation. *Magn Reson Imaging* 1989;7:495–515; and Wilkes CH. Internal derangements of the temporomandibular joint. Pathological variations. *Arch Otolaryngol Head Neck Surg* 1989;115:469–477.

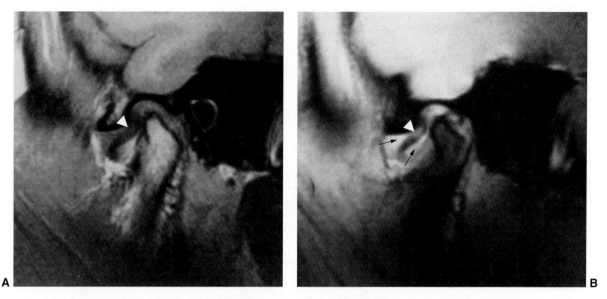

Figure 4-12 Sagittal T1-weighted **(A)** and gradient-echo **(B)** images demonstrate anterior disc displacement. There is intermediate signal (*arrowhead* in **A**) and high signal (*arrowhead* in **B**) due to normal disc hydration. There is fluid (*small arrows*) in the upper and lower joint space.

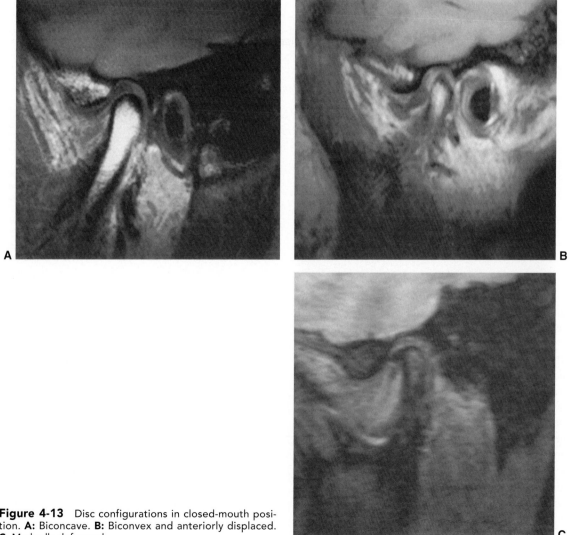

Figure 4-13 Disc configurations in closed-mouth position. **A:** Biconcave. **B:** Biconvex and anteriorly displaced. **C:** Markedly deformed.

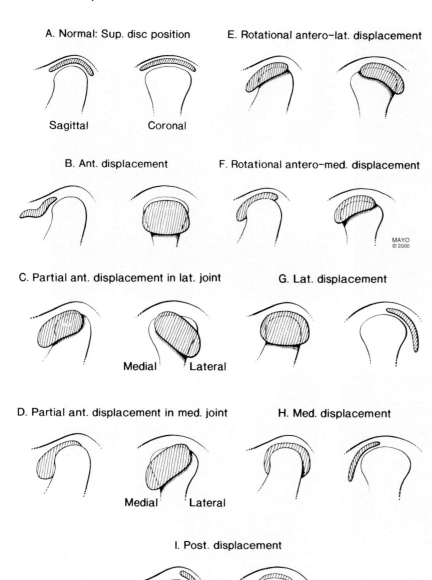

A. Normal: Sup. disc position

Sagittal   Coronal

B. Ant. displacement

C. Partial ant. displacement in lat. joint

Medial   Lateral

D. Partial ant. displacement in med. joint

Medial   Lateral

E. Rotational antero-lat. displacement

F. Rotational antero-med. displacement

MAYO
© 2000

G. Lat. displacement

H. Med. displacement

I. Post. displacement

MAYO
© 2000

Figure 4-14 Illustration of the disc displacement classification. **A:** Normal. **B:** Anterior displacement. **C:** Partial anterior displacement in lateral joint. **D:** Partial anterior displacement in medial joint. **E:** Rotational anterolateral displacement. **F:** Rotational anteromedial displacement. **G:** Lateral displacement. **H:** Medical displacement. **I:** Posterior displacement.

Rotational displacement in the anterolateral (Fig. 4-14E) and anteromedial (Fig. 4-14F) joints may also occur. The superior component of the disc does have sideways rotation with rotational displacements. The disc may also be displaced lateral to the lateral pole of the condyle, medial to the condyle, and rarely, posteriorly (Fig. 4-14, G to I). Anterior and anterolateral displacement were most common (46%) in this group of 300 patients (51). Of 57 symptom-free volunteers, the disc was in the normal superior position in 70% (51).

More than 90% of nondeformed anteriorly displaced discs reduced with opening (see Fig. 4-15). If the disc was distorted (Fig. 4-13, B and C), more than 76% did not reduce in the open position (27).

The incidence of each type of disc displacement varies depending on the study. Foucart et al. (44) reported a large series with data from 732 TMJs. Seventy-eight percent of discs were anteriorly displaced (52% reduced with opening, 26% did not reduce) (see Fig. 4-16). Discs in these patients also demonstrated rotational displacement (34% of discs without reduction and 53% of discs that reduced with opening). The remaining categories of displacement were seen less frequently (11% partial anterior displacement, 5% medial or lateral displacement, 4% "stuck discs"). In this series, MRI was 95% accurate for disc position and classification and 93% accurate for demonstrating osseous abnormalities. Both sagittal and coronal images were obtained that assist in defining rotational, medial,

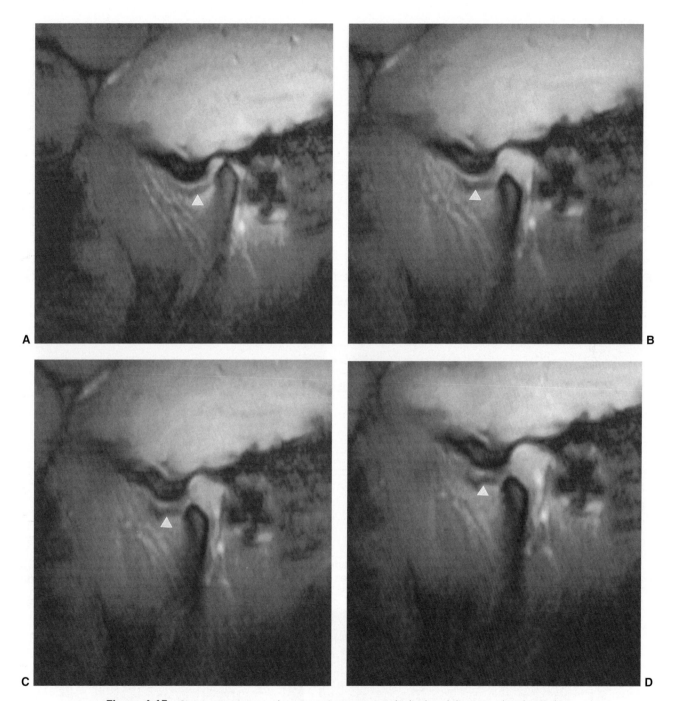

Figure 4-15 Cine motion images demonstrating an anteriorly displaced disc (*arrowheads*) **(A)** that buckles with opening **(B** to **E)** and demonstrates late reduction **(F)**.

and lateral displacement (see Figs. 4-17 and 4-18) (44,47,48,81).

The "stuck disc" deserves separate mention as conventional MR imaging in the sagittal plane may not be adequate, especially if the disc is not clearly visualized. Normally, there is disc motion with the condyle with recapture in patients with anterior displacement with reduction (10,44,47,59,74,80). In some cases (4%–11%),

the disc remains fixed in normal or displaced position when the condyle moves from the closed to open position (47,60,82). In this setting, cine studies are useful to define disc location and confirm lack of motion (32,83). Recognition of this condition is important because it may alter patient management (47).

Most simple MR classifications do not include the "stuck disc" or posterior displacement (47,51,82).

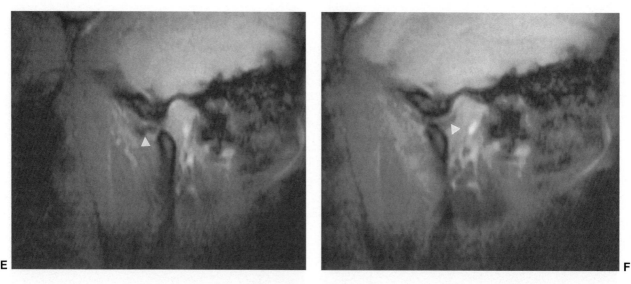

E

F

Figure 4-15 *(continued)*

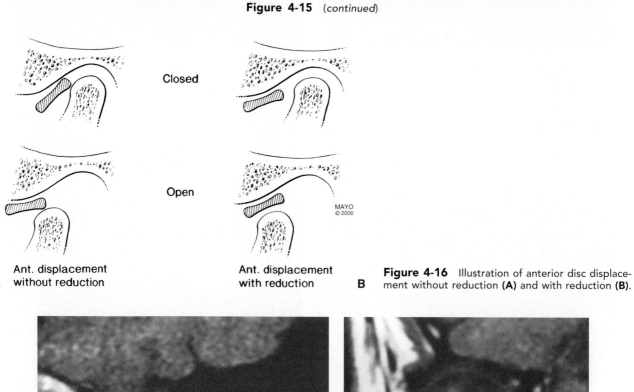

Closed

Open

Ant. displacement
A   without reduction

Ant. displacement
B   with reduction

MAYO
© 2000

Figure 4-16 Illustration of anterior disc displacement without reduction **(A)** and with reduction **(B)**.

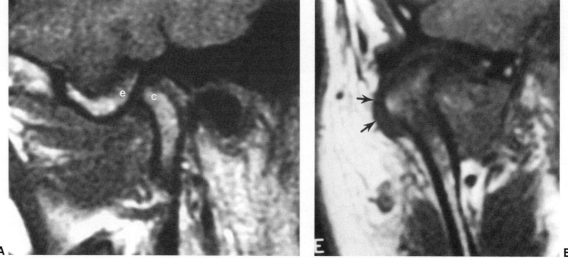

A

B

Figure 4-17 Patient with chronic symptoms of internal derangement. The sagittal image **(A)** does not clearly demonstrate the disc between the condyle (*c*) and eminence (*e*). **(B)** Coronal image demonstrates lateral displacement (*arrows*).

or lateral rotation in 50% of these patients, reemphasizing the utility of coronal images (61,84).

A grading system for internal derangements has been proposed that grades the severity of the internal derangement according to the morphology of the disc (78). An anteriorly displaced disc that maintains its normal bow-tie or drumstick configuration is considered grade 1. An anteriorly displaced disc that does not have a normal morphology is grade 2 (Fig. 4-13B and C).

In a study of more than 200 joints, 17% of the grade 1 joints had degenerative joint disease (DJD), while 95% of the grade 2 joints had DJD (4,34,78,79). The duration of symptoms and the presence of increased joint noise for the grade 2 joints were significantly greater than that of the grade 1 or normal joints. Since the long-term sequelae of an internal derangement is known to be DJD, it would appear that this grading system correlates with the severity of the disease process. Most of the grade 2 joints had discs that were irreparable at surgery, while virtually all of the grade 1 joints had disc repair attempted. The decreased signal seen with disc desiccation was not incorporated into the grading scale, as it was felt to be too subjective and dependent on too many variables, such as window and level setting. Nevertheless, decreased disc signal was found to be statistically significant in its association with DJD and duration of symptoms (4,34,79). Surgeons and anatomists have reported that the normal disc is flexible and pliable and proceeds to a more stiff, inflexible state following internal derangement (43,85). The end result of a long-term or severe internal derangement is disc derangement and maceration with secondary bony changes of DJD (see Fig. 4-20) (84,86–88).

Other MR features may also be useful for evaluating internal derangement. The presence of an effusion is a useful finding. Fluid is seen as high signal intensity on T2-weighted images (Figs. 4-9B and 4-12B). This is most commonly identified with stage IV disc internal derangement (Tables 4-1 and 4-2). Effusions may also be evident in 46% of patients with clicking (1) (Table 4-4). MRI is

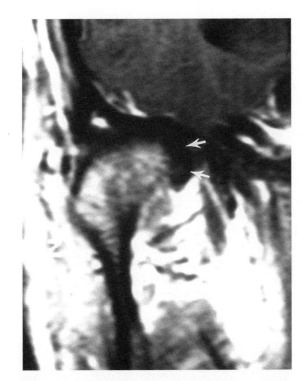

Figure 4-18 Coronal image demonstrating medial disc displacement (*arrows*).

Though rare, Westesson et al. (84) noted posterior displacement in 32 of 3,200 patients (1%). In 26 cases, the disc was flattened and extended posterior to the condyle. In three patients, the entire disc was located posteriorly, and in the remaining three cases there was a central perforation with a large portion of the disc posterior to the condyle (see Fig. 4-19) (84). There was associated medial

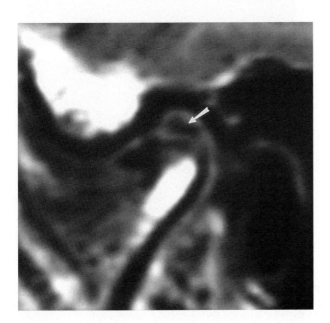

Figure 4-19 Sagittal T1-weighted image demonstrating a large perforation with a large posterior fragment (*arrow*) in the joint space.

TABLE 4-4
SECONDARY FINDINGS OF INTERNAL DERANGEMENT OF THE TEMPOROMANDIBULAR JOINT
Joint effusion
Joint space asymmetry
Condylar size
Condylar erosion
Condylar marrow edema
Eminence deformities
Hypermobility
Lateral pterygoid abnormalities
Capsular/ligament laxity

From references 19–22, 25, 30, 68, 70, 71, 80, 89, and 90.

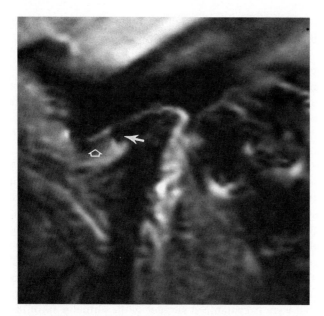

Figure 4-20 Sagittal gradient-echo image demonstrates flattening of the condyle with an anterior osteophyte (*arrow*) and a deformed anteriorly displaced disc (*open arrow*).

also useful for evaluating other osseous and soft tissue abnormalities.

Articular and extraarticular soft tissue abnormalities may contribute to internal derangement and disc displacement. Laxity of joint capsules, ligaments, and lateral pterygoid pathology are associated with hypermobility and internal derangement (21,22). Patients present with clicking, locking, and myofacial pain (21). Hypermobility can be measured on sagittal images. The condition is present when the condyle passes greater than 30° beyond the eminence (see Fig. 4-21) (21).

Yang et al. (32) described lateral pterygoid abnormalities (hypertrophy, atrophy, contracture) on MRI in 77% of

patients with hypermobility (Fig. 4-21). In this same group of patients, 40% had disc displacement. In those patients with no displacement there was condylar pressure on the disc.

In another report, Yang et al. (22) found MR abnormalities in the lateral pterygoid in 75% of patients with anterior disc displacement with reduction. The superior belly of the pterygoid is most often involved, the inferior belly less frequently, and both were involved in 30% of patients (22).

Osseous changes may involve the eminence or mandibular condyle. Certain changes occur after severe internal derangement, while others are felt to predispose to the condition (71,80,89,90).

Changes in the eminence include flattening, shape variation (box, sigmoid), and articular deformity (see Fig. 4-22) (71,90). Flattening may be a precursor to disc displacement, but it has definitely been described following

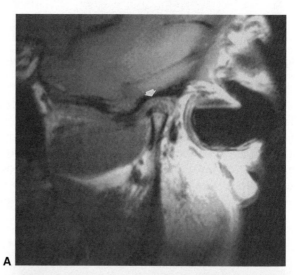

A

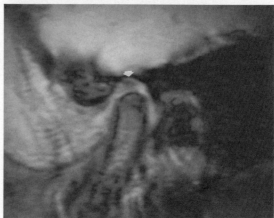

B

Figure 4-22 A: Sagittal T1-weighted image with anterior displacement and flattening of the temporal fossa (*arrow*). **B:** Sagittal gradient-echo image demonstrating normal depth of the temporal fossa (*arrow*).

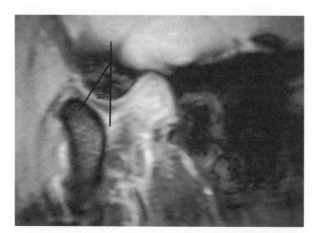

Figure 4-21 Sagittal gradient-echo image demonstrates condylar motion greater than 30°, indicating hypermobility. The disc has reduced.

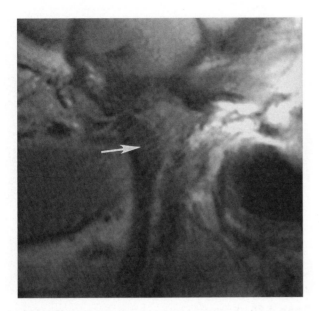

Figure 4-23 Sagittal T1-weighted image demonstrates low signal intensity in the proximal mandible (*arrow*) due to marrow edema.

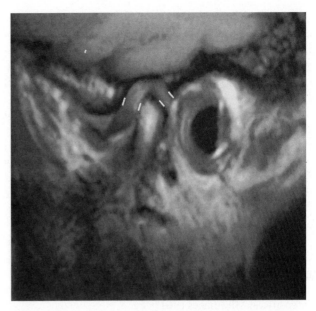

Figure 4-24 Sagittal T1-weighted image with anterior disc displacement. The anterior joint space is wider than the posterior joint space (*lines*).

long term internal derangement (90). There was disc displacement associated with a steeper slope (sigmoid) in the eminence compared to box and flat configurations. Other deformities were too infrequent to obtain adequate data (90).

Joint space symmetry and changes in the mandibular condyle have also been evaluated (19,20,30,68,70,80,89). Condylar changes include size, shape (Fig. 4-11), erosions, edema, AVN, osteochondritis dissecans, and osteophytes (Fig. 4-20). Edema and shape are likely precursors, with the other etiologies occurring either prior to or after significant internal derangement (see Fig. 4-23) (19,20,70,80,89).

The anterior joint space (see Fig. 4-24) is typically increased and the posterior decreased compared to normal controls in patients with anterior disc displacement (30,68).

Bone marrow edema (Fig. 4-23) is demonstrated in the mandibular condyle in patients with disc displacement as well as patients with advanced degenerative disc disease or early AVN (20,89). The condyle has low signal intensity on T1-weighted sequences, high signal intensity on T2-weighted sequences, and there is enhancement on post contrast images (Fig. 4-23) (20).

The size of the mandibular condyle has also been evaluated as it relates to disc displacement. Kurita et al. (70) measured the condyle (medial to lateral, and anterior to posterior) and found correlation between disc displacement and reduced transverse (medial to lateral) condylar dimensions (Fig. 4-11B) (70). Resorption of the superior lateral pole of the condyle was demonstrated in 37% of patients with disc displacement (19). This feature is most obvious on coronal or axial MRI.

As mentioned, DJD occurs with long-standing or severe internal derangements (Tables 4-1 and 4-2). Bone sclerosis is low signal intensity on T1- and T2-weighted images. Marrow edema is low on T1- and high intensity on T2-weighted images (91). Although the MR appearance of condylar head AVN has been reported (80), this is not widely agreed upon and remains controversial. Typically, there is an effusion with condylar marrow replaced by fibrous tissue and sclerotic bone (low signal intensity) (25).

Disc perforations cannot currently be demonstrated with conventional MR studies unless they are extremely large (Fig. 4-10) (79,34). Up to 67% of perforations are missed when MRI and surgical correlation are tabulated (55). This is not a serious drawback for most clinicians, however, as very few surgeons use disc perforation as a criteria to operate and no definitive treatment regimen is currently advocated for patients with disc perforations. Currently, conventional arthrograms or MR arthrography must be performed to diagnose a disc perforation (35, 36,91,92).

POSTOPERATIVE JOINTS

Clinical and imaging analysis is critical to plan proper conservative and surgical approaches to internal derangement (12,93). Up to 70% of patients with anterior displacement with reduction respond to disc repositioning therapy (12,77,94). Surgical procedures include condylar ostectomy (17), modified condylotomy (95), disc repositioning (94), discectomy without replacement, and replacement procedures (17,47). Replacement procedures are generally performed to prevent progression of DJD and relieve pain. Several approaches to disc replacement have been used with either autogenous grafts (fascia, dermal, rib) or allografts (Teflon, silicone, silastic) (17,47,96).

MRI is useful for evaluating conservative and surgical treatment results. Patients with disc repositioning splints may be studied to determine condylar position and whether there is disc recapture with opening (94). Imaging results are most satisfactory if ceramic brackets are used anteriorly and direct bonding tubes are used on the molars. When stainless steel implants are used posteriorly, artifact may impact image quality significantly (93).

Some patients are treated with discectomy without replacement. In this setting, MRI is useful to evaluate progressive osseous changes. In addition, there is frequent tissue that fills the disc void that is intermediate to high intensity on MR images (96).

MRI is also useful for monitoring results in patients with autogenous and artificial disc replacements.

Artificial implants may include silastic and proplast/Teflon implants (16,77,97). These implants have a signal void with a linear appearance on sagittal T1-weighted images (see Fig. 4-25). MRI can show the position of the prosthesis and whether or not it is fractured. Images also demonstrate the amount of giant-cell tissue reaction and scar surrounding the prosthesis that can interfere with function and may require prosthesis removal (see Fig. 4-26) (47,96–98). T2-weighted images, postintravenous gadolinium, or MR arthrograms are superior for evaluating effusions, synovitis, and other complications (35,36,41). Other

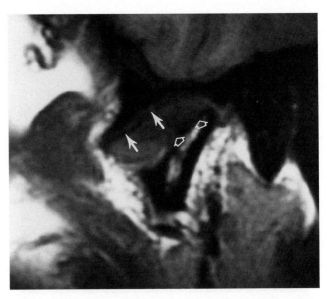

Figure 4-26   Fractured implant with exuberant granulation tissue. The patient had placement of a proplast/Teflon graft (*arrows*), which is seen as a linear low intensity structure. Note the large area of intermediate signal intensity due to granulation tissue. The condyle (*open arrows*) is deformed.

complications include graft displacement, epithelial inclusions, infection, and joint remodeling (96).

MISCELLANEOUS CONDITIONS

MRI of the TMJ is less commonly performed to evaluate trauma or other arthropathies (40,92,99,100). However, the technique may be of value in selected cases.

The TMJ may be involved with rheumatoid arthritis (Fig. 4-9), gout, calcium pyrophosphate dihydrate deposition disease, synovial chondromatosis, pigmented villonodular synovitis (see Fig. 4-27), ankylosing spondylitis, and infection (18, 29,99–101). Forty-five percent of patients with rheumatoid arthritis have TMJ involvement (15,40). Patients with juvenile chronic arthritis have TMJ involvement in 28% to 63% of cases (102). Though rare, osteochondromatosis (see Fig. 4-28), loose bodies, and neoplasms may also involve the TMJ (101,103).

MRI examination in patients with these conditions can be performed similar to studies for internal derangement. However, early synovial disease may be more effectively evaluated after intravenous gadolinium using fat-suppressed T1-weighted sequences (40,92).

PITFALLS

Though there is generally good interobserver data for MR interpretations, several pitfalls must be kept in mind (103). Technical factors and poor image quality are obvious problems. In some patients, the degree of internal derangement

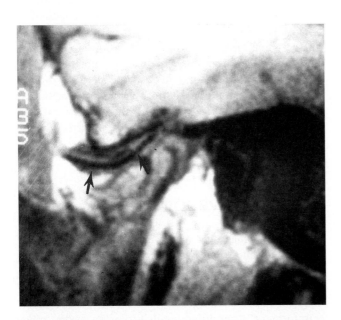

Figure 4-25   Normal silastic implant. The patient has had placement of a silastic implant (*arrows*) that is of uniform low signal intensity. It is sutured to the glenoid fossa and covers the condyle during condylar translation.

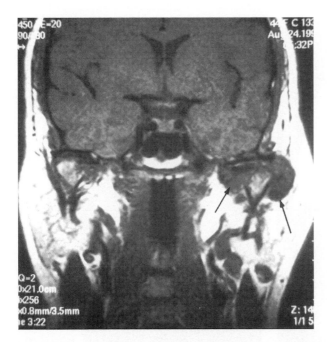

Figure 4-27 Coronal T1-weighted image demonstrates extensive soft tissue proliferation (*arrows*) due to pigmented villonodular synovitis. (From Kisnisci RS, Tuz HH, Gunhan O, et al. Villonodular synovitis of the temporomandibular joint: case report. *J Oral Maxillofacial Surg* 2001;59(12):1482–1484.)

and disc deformity may cause confusion in accurately defining the disc position (1,59,47). Several other pitfalls have been described. Crabbe, et al. (104) described a low-intensity density posterior to the mandibular condyle

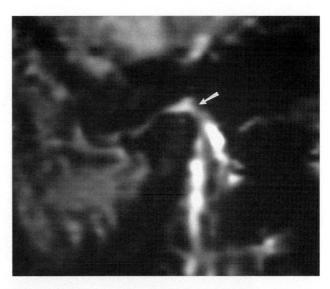

Figure 4-29 Sagittal gradient-echo image demonstrates a low intensity ovoid structure posteriorly (*arrow*) due to flow phenomenon in the superficial temporal artery.

caused by a flow phenomenon of the superficial temporal artery on gradient-echo images. This should not be confused with a loose body or posterior disc displacement (see Fig. 4-29).

Pneumatization of the temporal bone is symmetrical in 72% to 99% of patients (105). This process begins in the perinatal period and progresses to adulthood. Pneumatized areas in the temporal bone should not be confused with

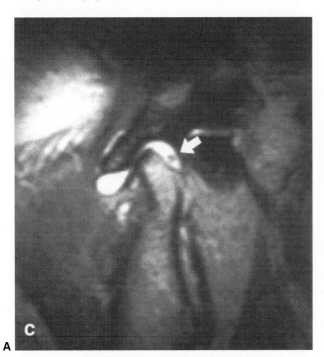

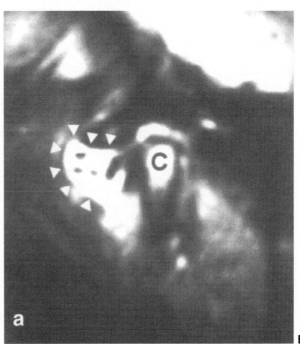

Figure 4-28 Synovial chondromatosis. Sagittal T2-weighted images demonstrate a joint effusion with a small posterior loose body (*arrow*) in **A** and capsular distention (*arrowheads*) with multiple loose bodies in **B**. *C*, condyle (From Kim HG, Park KH, Hah JK, et al. Magnetic resonance imaging characteristics of synovial chondromatosis of the temporomandibular joint. *J Orofacial Pain* 2002;16(2):148–153.)

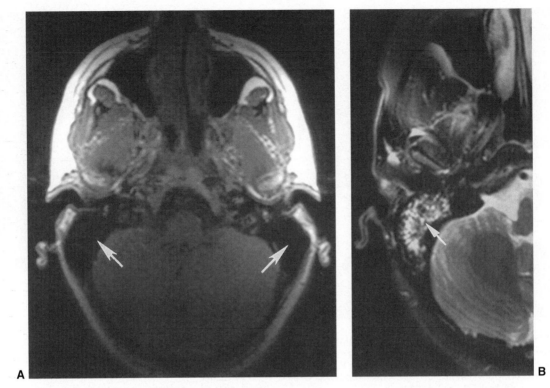

Figure 4-30 Temporal bone pneumatization. **A:** Axial T1-weighted scout image shows low intensity in the temporal bone (*arrows*) due to normal pneumatization. **B:** T2-weighted axial image shows diffuse high signal intensity in the mastoids (*arrow*) due to mastoiditis.

abnormal bone sclerosis (105). When there is concern, a routine radiograph or CT will solve the problem (see Fig. 4-30).

REFERENCES

1. Adame CG, Monje F, Munoz M, et al. Effusion in magnetic resonance imaging of the temporomandibular joint: a study of 123 joints. *J Oral Maxillofac Surg* 1998;56:314–318.
2. Carr AB, Gibilisco JA, Berquist TH. MRI of the temporomandibular joint: preliminary work. *J Craniomandib Disord* 1987; 1: 89–96.
3. Harms SE, Wilk RM, Wolford LM, et al. The temporomandibular joint: magnetic resonance imaging using surface coils. *Radiology* 1985;157:133–136.
4. Helms CA, Doyle GW, Orwig D, et al. Staging of internal derangements of the TMJ with magnetic resonance imaging: preliminary observations. *J Craniomandib Disord* 1989;3:93–99.
5. Katzberg RW, Laskin DM. Commentary. Radiographic and clinical significance of temporomandibular joint alloplastic disk implants. *AJR* 1988;151:736–738.
6. Major P, Ramos-Remus C, Suarez-Almajon ME, et al. Magnetic resonance imaging and clinical assessment of temporomandibular joint pathology in analyzing spondylitis. *J Rheumatol* 1999; 26:616–621.
7. Roditi GH, Duncan KA, Needham G, et al. Temporomandibular joint MRI: A 2-D gradient-echo technique. *Clin Radiol* 1997;52: 441–444.
8. Westesson PL. Structural hard-tissue changes in temporomandibular joints with internal derangement. *Oral Surg Oral Med Oral Pathol* 1985;59:220–224.
9. Westesson P-L, Bronstein SL, Liedberg JL. Internal derangement of the temporomandibular joint: morphologic description with correlation to function. *Oral Surg Oral Med Oral Pathol* 1985; 59:323–331.
10. Aoyama S, Kino K, Amagasa T, et al. Clinical and magnetic resonance imaging study of unilateral sideways disc displacements of the temporomandibular joint. *J Med Dent Sci* 2002;49:89–94.
11. Chossegros C, Cheynet F, Guyot L, et al. Posterior disc displacement of the TMJ: MRI evidence in two cases. *J Craniomandibular Pract* 2001;9(4):289–293.
12. Emshoff R, Brandlmaier I, Bertram S, et al. Comparing methods for diagnosing temporomandibular joint disc displacement without reduction. *J Am Dent Assoc* 2002;133(4):442–451.
13. Westesson PL, Katzberg RW, Tallents RH, et al. Temporomandibular joint: comparison of MR images with cryosectional anatomy. *Radiology* 1987;164:59–64.
14. Bell KA, Miller KD, Jones JP. Cine MR imaging of the temporomandibular joint: ochsner experience. *Radiology* 1989;173:101.
15. Celiher R, Gokce-Kutsal Y, Eryilmaz M. Temporomandibular joint involvement in rheumatoid arthritis. *Scand J Rheumatol* 1995;24:22–25.
16. Chuong R, Piper MA, Boland TJ. Recurrent grant cell reaction to residual proplast in the temporomandibular joint. *Oral Surg Oral Med Oral Pathol* 1993;76:16–19.
17. Santler G, Kärcher H, Simbrunner J. MR imaging of the TMJ: MR diagnosis and intra operative findings. *J Craniomaxillofac Surg* 1998;21:284–288.
18. Westesson P, Katzberg RW, Tallents RH, et al. CT and MR of the temporomandibular joint: comparison with autopsy specimens. *AJR Am J Roentgenol* 1987;148:1165–1171.
19. Kurita H, Ohtsuka A, Kobayashi H, et al. Resorption of the lateral pole of the mandibular condyle in temporomandibular disc displacement. *Dentomaxillofac Radiol* 2001;39(2):88–91.
20. Sano T, Westesson PL, Larheim TA, et al. The association of temporomandibular joint pain with abnormal bone marrow in the mandibular condyle. *J Oral Maxillofac Surg* 2000;58(3): 254–257.
21. Yang X, Pernu H, Pyhtinen J, et al. MRI findings concerning the lateral pterygoid muscle in patients with symptomatic TMJ hypermobility. *Cranio* 2001;19(4):260–268.

22. Yang X, Pernu H, Pyhtinen J, et al. MR abnormalities of the lateral pterygoid muscle in patients with nonreducing disc displacement of the TMJ. *Cranio* 2002;20(3):209–221.

23. Emshoff R, Jank S, Bertram S, et al. Disc displacement of the temporomandibular joint: sonography versus MR imaging. *AJR* 2002;178:1557–1562.

24. Kamelchuk L, Baker C, Major P. Adolescent TMJ tomography and magnetic resonance imaging: a comparative analysis. *J Orofac Pain* 1997;11(4):321–327.

25. Rao VM, Vinitski S, Barbaria A. Comparison of SE and short TE three-dimensional gradient-echo imaging of the temporomandibular region. *Radiology* 1989;173:99.

26. Katzberg RW, Bessette RW, Tallents RH. Normal and abnormal temporomandibular joint: MR imaging with surface coil. *Radiology* 1986;158:183–189.

27. Nebbe B, Brooks SL, Hatcher D, et al. Interobserver reliability on quantitative MRI assessment of temporomandibular joint disc status. *Oral Surg Oral Med Oral Pathol Oral Radiol Endod* 1998; 86:746–750.

28. Griffin CJ, Sharpe CJ. Distribution of elastic tissue in the human temporomandibular meniscus especially in respect to "compression" areas. *Aust Dent J* 1962;7:72.

29. Katzberg RW, Schenck J, Roberts D, et al. Magnetic resonance imaging of the temporomandibular joint meniscus. *Oral Surg Oral Med Oral Pathol* 1985;59:332–335.

30. Rammelsberg P, Jager L, Duc JM. Magnetic resonance imaging-based joint space measurements in temporomandibular joints with disc displacements and in controls. *Oral Surg Oral Med Oral Pathol Oral Radiol Endod* 2000;90(2):240–248.

31. Perrini F, Tallents RH, Katzberg RW, et al. Generalized joint laxity and temporomandibular disorders. *J Orofac Pain* 1997;11: 215–221.

32. Yustin DC, Rieger MR, McGucken RS, et al. Determination of the existence of huge movements of the temporomandibular joint during normal opening by cine-MRI and computer digital addition. *J Prosthodont* 1993;2:190–195.

33. Chen YJ, Gallo LM, Meier D, et al. Individualized oblique-axial magnetic resonance imaging for improved visualization of mediolateral TMJ disc displacement. *J Orofac Pain* 2000;14(2): 128–139.

34. Helms CA, Kaban L, McNeill C, et al. Temporomandibular joint MR: morphology and signal characteristics of the disc. *Radiology* 1989;172:817–820.

35. Takaku S, Yoshida M, Sano T, et al. Magnetic resonance images in patients with acute traumatic surgery of the temporomandibular joint. A preliminary report. *J Craniomaxillofac Surg* 1996;24:173–177.

36. Tasaki MM, Westesson P-L. Temporomandibular joint. Diagnostic accuracy of sagittal and coronal MR imaging. *Radiology* 1993;186: 723–729.

37. Taylor DB, Babyn P, Blaser S, et al. MR evaluation of the temporomandibular joint in juvenile rheumatoid arthritis. *J Comput Assist Tomogr* 1993;17:449–454.

38. Ogasawara T, Kitagawa Y, Ogawa T, et al. Inflammatory change in the upper joint space in temporomandibular joint with internal derangement on gadolinium-enhanced MR imaging. *Int J Oral Maxillofac Surg* 2002;31:252–256.

39. Suenaga A, Abiyama K, Noikura T. Gadolinium-enhanced MR imaging of temporomandibular disorders: Improved lesion detection of posterior disk attachment on T1-weighted images obtained with fat suppression. *AJR Am J Roentgenol* 1998;171:511–517.

40. Suenaga S, Ogura T, Matsuda T, et al. Severity of synovium and bone marrow abnormalities of the temporomandibular joint in early rheumatoid arthritis: Role of gadolinium-enhanced fat-suppressed T1-weighted spin-echo MRI. *J Comput Assist Tomogr* 2000;24(3):461–465.

41. Toyama M, Kurite K, Koga K, et al. Magnetic resonance arthrography of the temporomandibular joint. *J Oral Maxillofac Surg* 2000;58(9):978–983.

42. Gibbs SJ, Simmons C. A protocol for magnetic resonance imaging of temporomandibular joints. *Cranio* 1998;16:236–241.

43. Tanaka T, Morimoto Y, Masumi S, et al. Utility of frequency-selective fat saturation T2-weighted MR images for detection of joint effusion in the temporomandibular joint. *Dentomaxillofac Radiol* 2002;31:303–312.

44. Foucart J-M, Carpenter P, Pajoni D, et al. MR of 732 TMJs: anterior, rotational, partial and sideways disc displacements. *Eur J Radiol* 1998;28:86–94.

45. Sanroman JF, Gonzalez JMG, Del Hoyo JA, et al. Morphometric and morphological charges in the temporomandibular joint after orthognathic surgery: a magnetic resonance imaging and computed tomographic prospective study. *J Craniomaxillofac Surg* 1997;25:139–148.

46. Hollener L, Barclay P, Maravilla K, et al. The depiction of the bilaminar zone of the temporomandibular joint by magnetic resonance imaging. *Dentomaxillofacial Radiol* 1998;27:45–47.

47. Ribeiro RF, Tallents RH, Katzberg RW, et al. The prevalence disc replacement in symptomatic and asymptomatic volunteers aged 6 to 25 years. *J Orofac Pain* 1997;11:37–47.

48. Brady AP, McDevitt L, Stack JP, et al. A technique for magnetic resonance imaging of the temporomandibular joint. *Clin Radiol* 1993;47:127–133.

49. Chen J, Buckwalter K. Displacement analysis of the temporomandibular condyle from magnetic resonance images. *J Biomech* 1993;26:1455–1462.

50. Ozawu S, Tanne K. Diagnostic accuracy of sagittal condylar movement patterns for identifying internal derangement of the temporomandibular joint. *J Orofac Pain* 1997;11:222–231.

51. Tasaki MM, Westesson P-L, Isberg AM, et al. Classification and prevalence of temporomandibular joint disk replacement in patients and symptom-free volunteers. *Am J Orthod Dentofacial Orthop* 1996;109:249–262.

52. Cholitgul W, Nishiyama H, Sasai T, et al. Clinical and magnetic resonance imaging findings in temporomandibular joint disc displacement. *DentoMaxilloFac Radiol* 1997;26(3):183–188.

53. Liedberg J, Panmekrate J, Petersson A, et al. Evidence-based evaluation of three imaging methods of the temporomandibular disc. *Dentomaxillofac Radiol* 1995;25(5):234–241.

54. Orsini MG, Kuboki T, Terada S, et al. Diagnostic value of 4 criteria to interpret temporomandibular joint disc position on magnetic resonance images. *Oral Surg Oral Med Oral Pathol Oral Radiol Endod* 1998;86:489–497.

55. Scapino RP. Histopathology associated with malposition of the human temporomandibular joint disc. *Oral Surg* 1983; 55:382.

56. Burnett K, Davis CL, Read J. Dynamic display of the TMJ meniscus by using "Fast-Scan" MRI. *AJR Am J Roentgenol* 1987;149:959–962.

57. Schellhas KP, Wilkes CH, El Deeb M, et al. Permanent proplast temporomandibular joint implants: MR imaging of destructive complications. *AJR* 1988;151:731–735.

58. Dorsay TA, Youngberg RA. Cine MRI of the TMJ: need for critical closed mouth images without the burnett device. *J Comput Assist Tomogr* 1995;9(1):163–164.

59. Behr M, Held P, Leibrock A, et al. Diagnostic potential of pseudodynamic MRI (cine mode) for evaluation of internal derangement of the TMJ. *Eur J Radiol* 1996;28:212–215.

60. Benito C, Casares G, Benito C. TMJ static disk: correlation between clinical findings and pseudodynamic magnetic resonance images. *Cranio* 1998;16(4):242–251.

61. Haiter-Neto F, Hollender L, Barclay P, et al. Disk position and the bilaminar zone of the temporomandibular joint in asymptomatic young individuals by magnetic resonance imaging. *Oral Surg Oral Med Oral Path Oral Rad Endod* 2002;94(3): 372–378.

62. Chu SA, Suvinen TI, Clement JG, et al. The effect of interocclusal appliances on temporomandibular joints as asserted by 3-D reconstruction of MRI scans. *Aust Dent J* 2001;46(1):18–23.

63. Schellhas KP. Internal derangement of the temporomandibular joint: Radiologic staging with clinical, surgical, and pathological correlation. *Magn Reson Imaging* 1989;7:495–515.

64. Janzen DL, Connell DG, Murk PL. Current imaging of temporomandibular joint abnormalities: a pictorial essay. *Can Assoc Radiol J* 1998;49(1):21–34.

65. Tallents RH, Macher DJ, Kyrkanides S, et al. Prevalence of missing posterior teeth and intra articular temporomandibular joint disorders. *J Prosthet Dent* 2002;87(1):45–50.

66. Wilkes CH. Internal derangements of the temporomandibular joint. Pathological variations. *Arch Otolaryngol Head Neck Surg* 1989;115:469–477.

67. Orwig DS, Helms CA, Doyle GW. Optimal mouth position for magnetic resonance imaging of the disc. *J Craniomandib Disord* 3:138–142.

68. Pullinger AG, Seligman DA, John MT, et al. Multifactorial modeling of temporomandibular anatomic and orthopedic relationships in normal versus undifferentiated disc displacement joints. *J Proth Dent* 2002;87(3):289–297.

69. Rammelsberg P, Pospiech PR, Jager L, et al. Variability of disk position in asymptomatic volunteers and patients with derangements of the TMJ. *Oral Surg Oral Med Oral Pathol Oral Radiol Endod* 1997;83:393–399.

70. Kurita H, Ohtsuka A, Kobayashi H, et al. Alteration of the horizontal mandibular condyle size associated with temporomandibular joint internal derangement in adult females. *Dentomaxillofac Radiol* 2002;31(6):373–378.

71. Kurita H, Ohtsuka A, Kobayashi H, et al. Is the morphology of the articular eminence of the temporomandibular joint a predisposing factor for disc displacement. *Dentomaxillofac Radiol* 2000;29(3):159–162.

72. Miller-Leisse C, Augthum M, Bayer W, et al. Anterior disc displacement without reduction in temporomandibular joint: MRI and associated clinical findings. *J Magn Reson Imaging* 1996;6:169–774.

73. Murakami J, Takahashi A, Nishiyama H. Magnetic resonance evaluation of temporomandibular joint disc position and configuration. *Dentomaxillofac Radiol* 1993;22:205–207.

74. Rao VM. Imaging of the temporomandibular joint. *Semin Ultrasound CT MR* 1995;16(6):513–526.

75. Schellhas KP, Wilkes CH, Fritts HM, et al. MR of osteochondritis and avascular necrosis of the mandibular condyle. *AJR Am J Roentgenol* 1989; 152:551–560.

76. Stack BC Jr., Stack BC. Underutilization of MRI: a suggested protocol. *Cranio* 1998;16(3):131–132.

77. Kurita H, Kuraschina K, Baba H, et al. Evaluation of disk capture with a splint repositioning appliance: clinical and critical assessment with MR imaging. *Oral Surg Oral Med Oral Pathol Oral Radiol Endod* 1998;85(4):377–380.

78. Blaustein DI, Scapino RP. Remodeling of the temporomandibular joint disk and posterior attachment in disk displacement specimens in relation to glycosaminoglycan content. *Plast Reconstr Surg* 1986;78:756–764.

79. Helms CA, Gillespy T III, Sims RE, et al. Magnetic resonance imaging of internal derangements of the temporomandibular joint. *Radiol Clin North Am* 1986;24:189–192.

80. Milano V, Desiate A, Bellin R, et al. Magnetic resonance imaging of temporomandibular disorders: classification, prevalence, interpretation of disc displacement and deformation. *Dentomaxillofac Radiol* 2000;29(6):352–361.

81. Brooks SL, Westesson P-L. Temporomandibular joint: value of coronal MR images. *Radiology* 1993;188:317–321.

82. Rao VM, Liem MD, Favola A, et al. Elusive "stuck" disk in the temporomandibular joint: Diagnosis with MR imaging. *Radiology* 1993;189:823–827.

83. Gaggl A, Schultes G, Santler H, et al. Clinical and magnetic resonance findings in the temporomandibular joints of patients before and after orthognatic surgery. *Br J Oral Maxillofacial Surg* 1999;37:41–45.

84. Westesson P-L, Rohlin M. Internal derangement related to osteoarthrosis in temporomandibular joint autopsy specimens. *Oral Surg* 1984;57:17–22.

85. Isberg A, Hagglund M, Paesani D. The effect of age and gender on the onset of symptomatic temporomandibular joint disk displacement. *Oral Surg Med Oral Pathol Oral Radiol Endod* 1998; 85:252–257.

86. Blackwood HJ. Arthritis of the mandibular joint. *Br Dent J* 1963;115:317–324.

87. Katzberg RW, Westesson P, Tallents RH, et al. Temporomandibular joint: assessment of rotational and sideways disk displacements. *Radiology* 1988;169:741–748.

88. Westesson P-L, Larheim TA, Tanaka H. Posterior disk displacement in the temporomandibular joint. *J Oral Maxillofac Surg* 1998;56:1266–1273.

89. Emshoff R, Brandlmaier I, Schmid C, et al. Bone marrow edema of the mandibular condyle related to internal derangement, osteoarthrosis and joint effusion. *J Oral Maxillofac Surg* 2003; 61(1):35–40.

90. Kurita H, Ohtsuka A, Kobayashi H, et al. Flattening of the articular eminence correlates with progressive internal derangement of the temporomandibular joint. *Dentomaxillofac Radiol* 2000; 29(5):277–279.

91. Liebereman JM, Gardner CL, Motta AO, et al. Prevalence of bone marrow signal abnormalities observed in the temporomandibular joint using magnetic resonance imaging. *J Oral Maxillofac Surg* 1996;54:434–439.

92. Takebayashi S, Takarma T, Okada S, et al. MRI of the TMJ disc with intravenous administration of gadopentetate dimeglumine. *J Comput Assist Tomogr* 1997;21:209–215.

93. Okano Y, Yamashiro M, Kaneda T, et al. Magnetic resonance imaging diagnosis of the temporomandibular joint in patients with orthodontic appliances. *Oral Surg Oral Med Oral Pathol Oral Radiol Endod* 2003;95:255–263.

94. Gökalp H, Türkkahvaman H. Change in position of the temporomandibular joint disc and condyle after disc repositioning appliance therapy: A functional examination and magnetic resonance imaging study. *Angle Orthod* 2000;70(5):400–408.

95. McKenna SJ, Cornella F, Gibbs SJ. Long-term follow-up of modified condylotomy for internal derangement of the temporomandibular joint. *Oral Surg Oral Med Oral Pathol Oral Radiol Endod* 1996;81(5):509–515.

96. Takaku S, Sano T, Yoshida M. Long-term magnetic resonance imaging after temporomandibular joint discectomy without replacement. *J Oral Maxillofac Surg* 2000;58(7):739–745.

97. Schmolke C, Hugger A. The human temporomandibular joint region in different positions of the mandible. *Ann Anat* 1999; 181:61–64.

98. Katzberg RW, Westesson P, Tallents RH, et al. Orthodontics and temporomandibular joint derangement. *Am J Orthod Dentofacial Orthop* 1996;109(5):515–520.

99. Kim HG, Park KH, Huh JK, et al. Magnetic resonance imaging characteristics of synovial chondromatosis of the temporomandibular joint. *J Orofac Pain* 2002;16(2):148–153.

100. Kisnisci RS, Tuz HH, Gunhan O, et al. Villonodular synovitis of the temporomandibular joint: case report. *J Oral Maxillofac Surg* 2001;59(12):1482–1484.

101. Ercoli C, Boncan RB, Tallents RH, et al. Loose bodies of the temporomandibular joint: a case report. *Clin Orthod Res* 1998; 1:62–67.

102. Küseler A, Pedersen TK, Herlin T, et al. Contrast-enhanced magnetic resonance imaging as a method to diagnose early inflammatory changes in the temporomandibular joint in children with juvenile rheumatoid arthritis. *J Rheumatol* 1998; 25:1406–1412.

103. Nomoto M, Nagao K, Nurnata T, et al. Synovial osteochondromatosis of the temporomandibular joint. *J Laryngol Oto* 1993; 107:742–745.

104. Crabbe JP, Brooks SL, Lillie JH. Gradient-echo MR imaging of the temporomandibular joint: diagnostic pitfall caused by the superficial temporal artery. *AJR Am J Roentgenol* 1995;164:451–454.

105. Haynes RC, Amy JR. Asymmetric temporal bone pneumatization: an MR imaging pitfall. *AJNR Am J Neuroradiol* 1988;9:169.

Spine

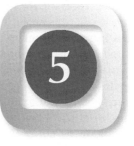

**Robert J. Witte   John I. Lane   Gary Michael Miller
Karl N. Krecke**

When multimodality imaging is available, the clinical uses of each modality tend to spread from a single niche. Magnetic resonance (MR), the only modality that directly images the spinal cord, is unique because no other invasive or noninvasive technique possesses this capability. Spinal MR accounts for approximately 35% of our practice.

A variety of considerations, including clinical, technical, and anatomical factors, influence MR imaging (MRI). Unlike the head, where a survey examination may be adequate to delineate many clinical disorders, a survey examination of the spine is apt to be less rewarding. Instead, spinal imaging requires clinical expertise, special equipment, specific imaging sequences, and perhaps imager interaction to obtain adequate examinations. The application of multispecialty expertise seems essential to exploit MR's versatility. Translation of the clinical characterization and localization of neurologic disorders potentiates MR's effectiveness. The same thorough neurologic and neurosurgical evaluation that is key to an accurate clinical diagnosis is equally crucial in optimizing MR scanning sequences because confirmation of the diagnosis is often possible with MR. Additional consultation between radiologists and their clinical colleagues is sometimes important in handling those patients who have painful disorders or convoluted clinical problems.

TECHNICAL CONSIDERATIONS

Imaging of the spine is complex. In contrast to the head, where the volume and composition of its tissues are almost constant, the spine is less predictable. The length of the spinal column, its dorsal location, and the small size of the intraspinal content preclude effective imaging by a volume coil such as a body coil. To improve image quality, surface coils must be used to increase the signal-to-noise ratio, whereas smaller fields of view (FOVs; 16 to 24 cm) are often needed to improve spatial resolution. As a result, multiple coil placements are necessary for a complete study of the entire spine unless multicoil technology is available. When coupled with the desire to obtain more than one imaging sequence to detect or characterize pathology, the examination is prolonged to such an extent that the patient may be unable to cooperate.

As expected, motion—both patient and physiologic—obscures anatomic and pathologic detail. Sedatives may be necessary in children, whereas analgesics are sometimes needed in patients who are evaluated for a painful condition. If patient motion can be obviated, physiologic motion due to the proximity of the spine to the heart, great vessels, diaphragm, and aerodigestive system becomes a problem. Motion from the beating heart, flowing blood, diaphragmatic excursion, normal swallowing, and cerebrospinal fluid (CSF) pulsation create artifacts that simulate or obscure significant pathology (1). This is particularly true on T2-weighted and gradient-echo sequences where internal motion results in artifacts from the spatial mismapping of the signal intensities present (2,3). This lowers the contrast resolution between the CSF and spinal cord and causes areas of decreased signal in the CSF and corresponding areas of increased signal in the spinal cord parenchyma (see Fig. 5-1). On T1-weighted sequences, these artifacts are less apparent but can result in areas of increased signal in the CSF (see Fig. 5-2). Because of this, a variety of motion compensation mechanisms, including flow compensation gradients, presaturation pulse sequences, phase and frequency gradient direction reversal, and cardiac/respiratory gating (4–7) are used to reduce the effect of physiologic internal motion, to maximize the contrast between CSF and spinal cord, and to minimize misregistration artifacts. Most vendors have many of these options available, and one or several must be used to reduce artifacts and enhance visualization of either pathology or normal anatomy.

Another artifact that can obscure pathology or simulate intramedullary lesions is the truncation artifact or Gibb phenomenon (8–10). This is a sampling-related effect that occurs at high contrast boundaries such as the CSF spinal cord interface. It is most apparent when the object imaged is small relative to the pixel size used, resulting in alternating bands of high and low signal that parallel the high contrast interface. It is best seen on sagittal sequences where it can simulate a syrinx. This artifact can be reduced by using small FOVs, small slice thicknesses, and a 192 or greater matrix.

The presence of spinal fixation hardware poses unique problems in spinal imaging. The resultant susceptibility artifacts can result in uninterpretable examinations. With careful selection of imaging parameters, compromised but interpretable examinations can be obtained. These artifacts are reduced by the multiple 180° refocusing pulses in rapid

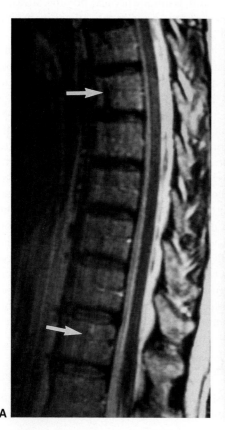
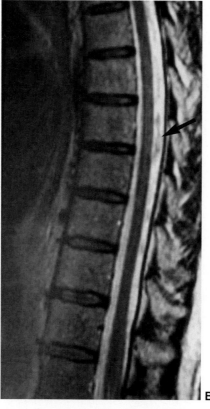

A   B

Figure 5-1 Phase misregistration artifact from cardiac motion. **A:** When the phase encoding direction is anterior to posterior (AP) linear areas of increased and decreased signal are seen (*arrows*). The cerebrospinal fluid–cord and extradural interfaces are blurred (T2-weighted fast spin echo). **B:** The phase encoding direction has been reversed from AP in **A** to superior-inferior, which improves the image. Mild cerebrospinal fluid pulsation artifact persists (*arrow*) (T2-weighted fast spin echo).

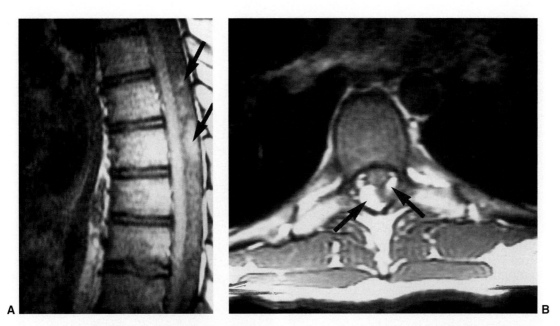

Figure 5-2 Cerebrospinal fluid pulsation artifact. **A:** Unusual ill-defined high signal intensity structures can be identified posterior to the thoracic spinal cord (*arrows*) (T1-weighted). **B:** These "lesions" are also present in the axial plane (*arrows*) (T1-weighted).

acquisition with relaxation enhancement (RARE) imaging. Further reduction occurs when using a high receiver bandwidth (32 KHz) and smaller pixel size (512 × 512 matrix), at the expense of reduced signal-to-noise ratio (see Figs. 5-3 and 5-4) (11,12).

Body habitus, spinal curvature, and the size of the intraspinal components play a significant role and compound the technical difficulty of obtaining an adequate examination. Some patients exceed the weight limitations of the table, whereas others will not fit within the

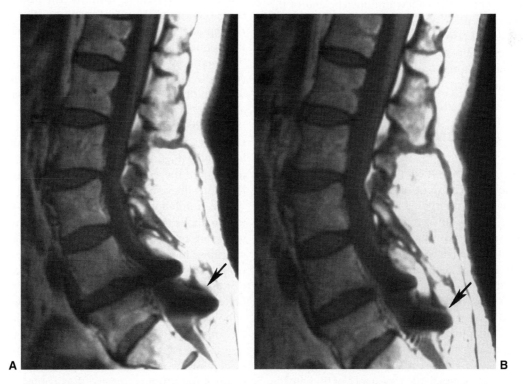

Figure 5-3 Metal artifact reduction, lumbar spine. **A:** Severe susceptibility distortion of the thecal sac by pedicle screws (*arrow*) (TE 20 ms, TR 450 ms, matrix 256 × 192, bandwidth 16 kHz). **B:** The artifact is reduced (*arrow*) and the disc-thecal sac interface better delineated by using a RARE sequence (echo train length 4) and increasing the receiver bandwidth (32 kHz).

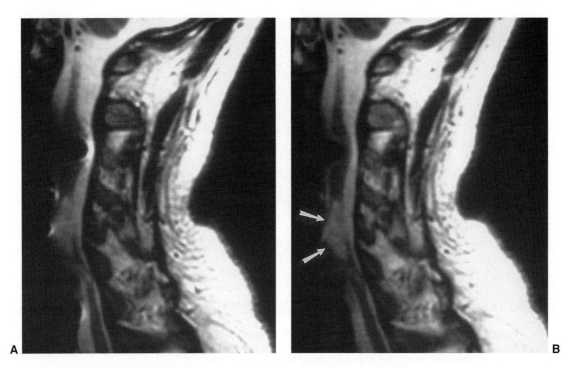

Figure 5-4   Metal artifact reduction, cervical spine. **A:** Severe metallic susceptibility artifact from spinal fusion prevents evaluation of the cervical cord (TR 3,000 ms, TE 100 ms, echo train length 8, bandwidth 16 kHz). **B:** The cervical cord and a small syrinx (*arrows*) are better seen by increasing the receiver bandwidth (32 kHz), and echo train length 16.

bore of the magnet. The size of the spinal cord, which measures about 1 cm in diameter; of parenchymal pathology, which is no more than a few millimeters; and of the nerve roots, which are 1 mm or less, demands excellent contrast and spatial resolution. As a result, even the most powerful commercially available magnets are taxed if the duration of the examination is not compatible with reasonable patient comfort.

NORMAL ANATOMY

The anatomy of the spine is complex, being composed of multiple tissue types. The vertebral bodies provide mechanical support, whereas interposed intervertebral discs cushion motion. A variety of ligaments link these structures together. The spinal cord, which is bathed in the CSF, lies within the protective environment of the spinal column. At each segment, a pair of spinal nerves exits through the neural foramen. An extensive vascular network is also present, with arteries segmentally supplying the bones, muscles, meninges, and cord, and a network of draining veins that extends within the spinal canal and surrounds the vertebral bodies. Each of these structures has different signal characteristics depending on pulse sequences selected. Figures 5-5 to 5-13 illustrate the normal MR appearance of the spine in a variety of commonly used imaging planes and pulse sequences.

Spinal Column

There are 33 vertebrae, with the usual distribution being seven cervical, 12 thoracic, five lumbar, five sacral, and four coccygeal segments, but this may only be present in 20% of the population. The sacrum and coccyx are usually fused. Vertebral numbers can vary between 32 and 35, with the cervical region most constant and coccygeal region most variable (13). Various methods have been proposed to accurately determine vertebral levels.

Identifying the location of the right renal artery on sagittal images has been shown to be located at the L1 to L2 disc level in the majority of cases (14). However, identifying the position of the C2 vertebral body on a large FOV sagittal localizing image may be the most accurate (15).

The morphology of each vertebra is similar, with individual variations in each region (16). The first two cervical vertebrae are an exception because they are highly specialized structures. In general, each vertebra is composed of a body, which is located anteriorly, and a posterior arch. The posterior arch is formed by two pedicles that extend from the body to an articular mass or pars interarticularis. Projections of bone extend above and below each articular mass to form the superior and inferior facets. They articulate with the corresponding facet of the adjacent vertebral bodies at a synovial joint. Two laminae extend posteriorly where they fuse to form the spinous process, thus completing a ring and forming the spinal canal. Laterally, transverse processes extend from the posterior arches that, together with the

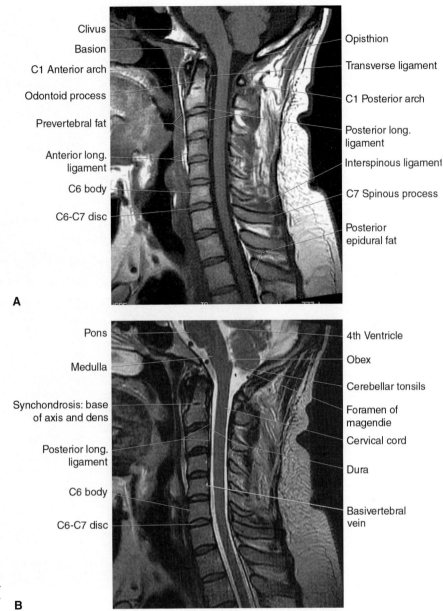

Clivus
Basion
C1 Anterior arch
Odontoid process
Prevertebral fat
Anterior long. ligament
C6 body
C6-C7 disc

Opisthion
Transverse ligament
C1 Posterior arch
Posterior long. ligament
Interspinous ligament
C7 Spinous process
Posterior epidural fat

A

Pons
Medulla
Synchondrosis: base of axis and dens
Posterior long. ligament
C6 body
C6-C7 disc

4th Ventricle
Obex
Cerebellar tonsils
Foramen of magendie
Cervical cord
Dura
Basivertebral vein

B

Figure 5-5 Normal cervical spine—sagittal plane. **A:** T1-weighted. **B:** T2-weighted fast spin echo.

spinous processes, act as levers for the attachment of many skeletal muscles. In addition to the synovial facet joints, an additional articulation is found in the cervical region. A lateral ridge of bone, the uncinate process, extends from the superior surface of each cervical vertebral body that articulates with a notch in the inferior aspect of the vertebral body above, forming the uncovertebral joints of Lushka (16). This is not a true joint but rather is thought to represent the lateral extension of the intervertebral disc, which has partially degenerated by adulthood.

The spinal nerves course through the neural foramina at each vertebral body level. In the cervical region, the neural foramina can be elongated, forming a canal that is bordered by the pedicles of adjacent vertebrae above and below (17,18). The anterior margin of the foramen or canal is the posterior vertebral body and uncinate process. The articular masses and facet joints form the posterior margin. The ventral and dorsal roots are located within the inferior portion of the foramen, at and below the disc level (18). In the lumbar region, the superior and inferior borders of the neural foramen are again formed by the pedicles. The posterior vertebral body above and the posterior disc margin below form the anterior margin. The facet joint and a small portion of the ligamentum flavum form the posterior border. The lumbar nerve roots are located within the superior portion of the foramen above the disc level.

The first two cervical vertebrae, the atlas and the axis, are different in morphology because of their specialized function of holding up the head and allowing for a variety of rotational and tilting motions (16). The atlas, or C1, is

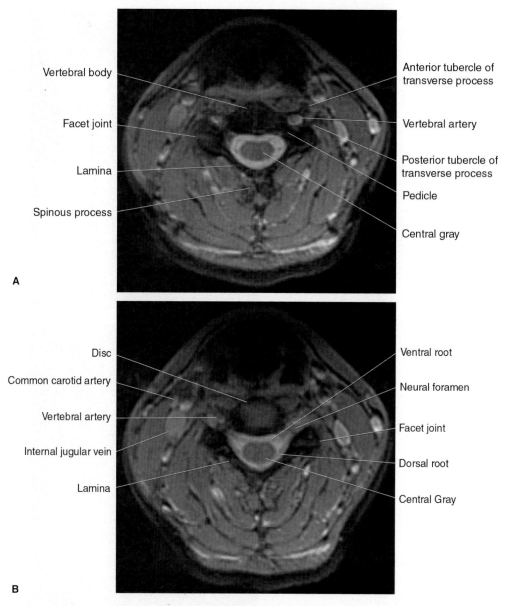

Figure 5-6   Normal cervical spine—axial plane. **A** and **B:** Gradient echo. **C:** T1-weighted. **D:** Three-dimensional constructive interference at steady state (3 T) (TR 8.9 ms, TE 4.4 ms, 35-degree flip angle).

ring-shaped and lacks a well-formed vertebral body. It has an anterior arch and a posterior arch connected by a lateral mass on each side. The superior articulating facets articulate with the occipital condyle at the base of the skull, and the inferior articular facets articulate with the superior articulating facets of the axis. A long process extends from the superior surface of the body of the axis, which is called the odontoid process or the dens. It forms a synovial joint at its articulation with the posterior aspect of the anterior arch of C1; is held in place by a set of strong ligaments, which is discussed later; and provides a pivot on which the atlas and skull can rotate (16).

The signal intensity of the vertebral bodies depends on the amount and type of marrow present. Normally, the proportion of red to yellow marrow is high so that the vertebral bodies show medium to high signal with T1-weighted and RARE sequences, intermediate to low signal with T2-weighted, and low signal on gradient-echo sequences. The signal pattern may be homogeneous or inhomogeneous, depending on the distribution of marrow fat and fibrous tissue. The endplates demonstrate low signal on T1-weighted, T2-weighted, and partial flip angle sequences because of a combination of the composition (cortical bone covered with cartilage) and chemical shift artifact (19). The articular cartilage lining the facet joints usually demonstrates low signal intensity on T1- and T2-weighted sequences and is difficult to distinguish from cortical bone (20). However, it demonstrates increased signal

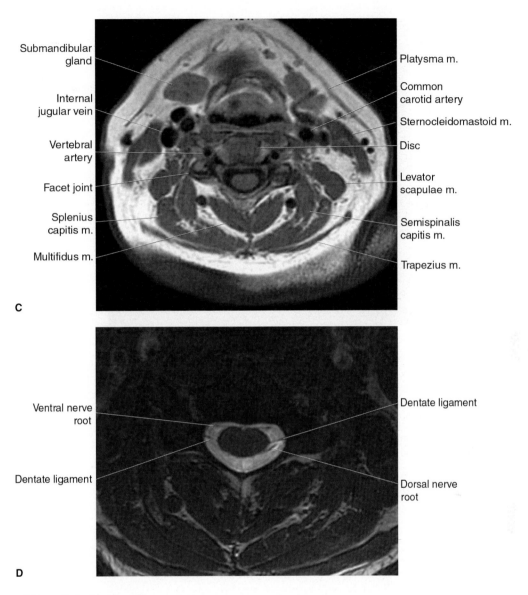

Submandibular gland

Internal jugular vein

Vertebral artery

Facet joint

Splenius capitis m.

Multifidus m.

Platysma m.

Common carotid artery

Sternocleidomastoid m.

Disc

Levator scapulae m.

Semispinalis capitis m.

Trapezius m.

C

Ventral nerve root

Dentate ligament

Dentate ligament

Dorsal nerve root

D

Figure 5-6 (*continued*)

Intervertebral Discs

The intervertebral discs are interposed between adjacent vertebral bodies and hydrostatically cushion the mechanical forces present. The disc consists of a central gelatinous nucleus pulposus that is believed to be the remnant of the primitive notochord and peripheral fibrocartilage (19,21). This fibrocartilage is arranged in a concentric lamellar pattern that forms the anulus fibrosis and is designed to withstand radial tension. Superiorly and inferiorly, collagenous (Sharpey) fibers insert into the ring apophysis of the vertebral body endplates. The superior and inferior portions of

on gradient-echo sequences, distinct from the bone. After radiation therapy, the vertebral bodies become brighter in intensity on T1-weighted sequences when fat replaces the marrow elements (see Fig. 5-14).

the disc are at least partially covered by a thin hyaline cartilage that is continuous with the cartilage over the adjacent vertebral body endplates (16). Although these components are histologically separate in a normal disc, discrete border zones are not identified at pathology. Rather, the nucleus pulposus blends imperceptibly with the anulus fibrosis.

The MR appearance of the intervertebral disc reflects its water content. Normal discs demonstrate low signal on T1-weighted sequences and high signal on T2-weighted and gradient-echo sequences. The decline in T2 signal radially from the nucleus pulposus out to the periphery of the disc parallels the normal decrease in water content seen at pathology. The water content, varying from 85% to 90% in the nucleus to 70% to 80% in the innermost anulus, falls to its lowest concentration in the most peripheral portions of the disc (22). On MR, the outermost anular fibers show

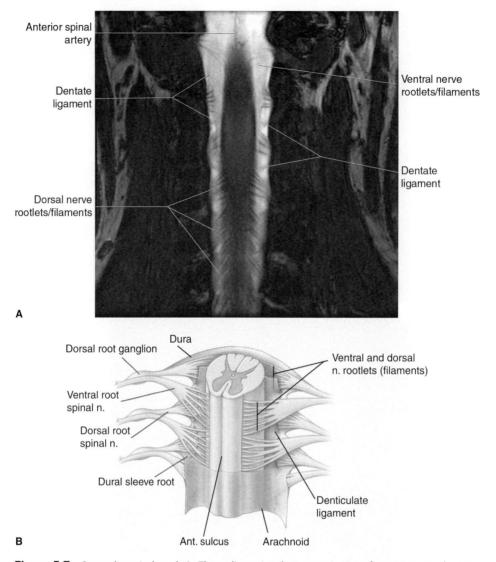

Anterior spinal artery

Dentate ligament

Dorsal nerve rootlets/filaments

Ventral nerve rootlets/filaments

Dentate ligament

A

Dorsal root ganglion

Dura

Ventral and dorsal n. rootlets (filaments)

Ventral root spinal n.

Dorsal root spinal n.

Dural sleeve root

Denticulate ligament

B   Ant. sulcus   Arachnoid

Figure 5-7   Coronal cervical cord. **A:** Three-dimensional constructive interference at steady state (3 T). **B:** Illustration.

low signal on T1-weighted and T2-weighted sequences, so distinction from the anterior and posterior longitudinal ligaments or the vertebral body endplates is not possible. The transition zone from nucleus pulposus to anulus fibrosis is relatively sharp in the young but becomes less distinct with aging. A horizontal band of low signal on T2-weighted sequences may be seen within the central portion of the disc on sagittal images, which can vary from a small notch to a complete partition (19,22–24). Its etiology is unclear. Some authors describe anular-like tissue in the region of the cleft at pathology that is believed to represent degenerative fibrosis (23,24). Other researchers have failed to find a pathologic correlate (19).

With aging, there is progressive loss of water content in the nucleus pulposus and anulus fibrosis. Also, the biochemical structure of the nucleus pulposus changes with replacement of the gelatinous matrix by disorganized fibrocartilage (21,22). Eventually, the degenerated nucleus blends imperceptibly with the anulus fibrosis on imaging and at pathology. The result is a progressive decrease in signal on T2-weighted sequences, as the disc becomes a desiccated, degenerated structure that is mostly fibrocartilage.

Spinal Ligaments

The vertebral bodies and intervertebral discs are linked together by a variety of ligaments (16). The anterior longitudinal ligament extends from the base of the skull to the sacrum and is adherent to the anterior vertebral bodies and the anterior disc margins. A corresponding ligament, the posterior longitudinal ligament, extends from C2 to the sacrum. This ligament is firmly attached to the vertebral body endplates and posterior disc margins but is separated from the midposterior vertebral body to allow room for the anterior internal epidural venous plexus and basivertebral veins. The anatomy of this more patulous portion of

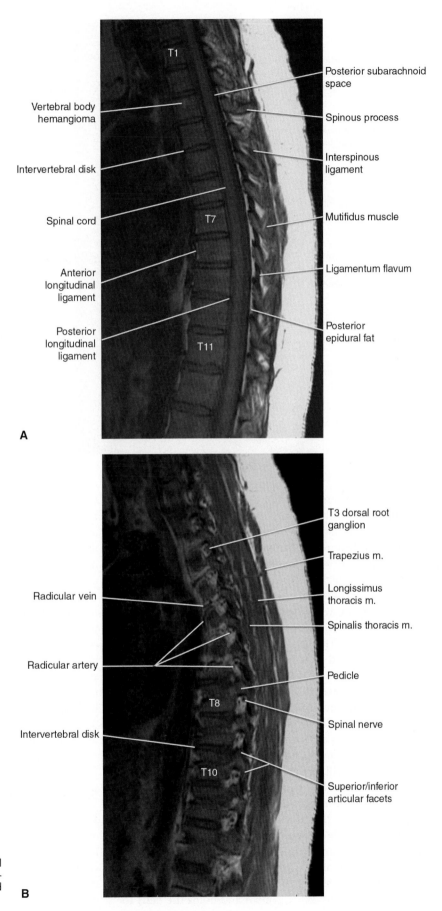

Vertebral body hemangioma

Intervertebral disk

Spinal cord

Anterior longitudinal ligament

Posterior longitudinal ligament

T1

T7

T11

Posterior subarachnoid space

Spinous process

Interspinous ligament

Mutifidus muscle

Ligamentum flavum

Posterior epidural fat

A

Radicular vein

Radicular artery

Intervertebral disk

T8

T10

T3 dorsal root ganglion

Trapezius m.

Longissimus thoracis m.

Spinalis thoracis m.

Pedicle

Spinal nerve

Superior/inferior articular facets

B

Figure 5-8 Normal thoracic spine—sagittal plane. **A:** T1-weighted, midline. **B:** T1-weighted, lateral to midline. **C:** T2-weighted fast spin echo.

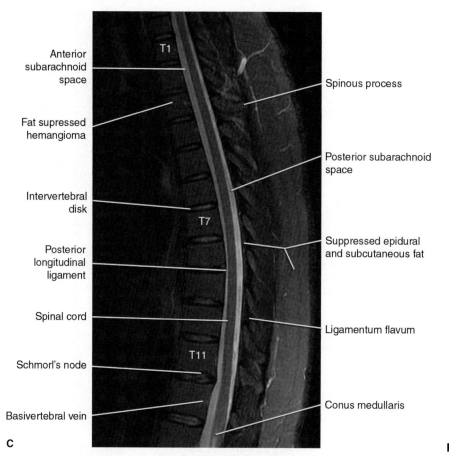

Anterior subarachnoid space

Fat supressed hemangioma

Intervertebral disk

Posterior longitudinal ligament

Spinal cord

Schmorl's node

Basivertebral vein

Spinous process

Posterior subarachnoid space

Suppressed epidural and subcutaneous fat

Ligamentum flavum

Conus medullaris

T1

T7

T11

C

Figure 5-8 (continued)

the anterior epidural space at the level of the vertebral body has been further defined. A midline septum anchors the posterior longitudinal vertebral body to the posterior longitudinal ligament. Thin membranes extend laterally from the posterior longitudinal ligament, dividing this space. These structures result in predictable patterns of involvement by neoplasms and infection (25).

The superior extension of the posterior longitudinal ligament is the tectorial membrane that extends from C2 to the lower clivus. The laminae of each vertebral body are segmentally joined by the ligamentum flavum, named for its yellow color noted at surgery. The ligamentum flavum extends posterolaterally to merge with the facet joint. The interspinous ligament segmentally connects the spinous processes and the supraspinous ligament extends along the tips of the spinous processes.

Additional ligaments are present at the craniovertebral junction that stabilizes the atlantoaxial and cranial cervical junction. The anterior atlantooccipital membrane extends from the anterior margin of the foramen magnum to the anterior arch of the atlas. A corresponding posterior atlantooccipital membrane extends from the posterior margin of the foramen magnum to the posterior arch of the atlas. An important ligament is the cruciform ligament, named for its crosslike shape. It has a horizontal portion that forms the transverse ligament and holds the dens to

the ring of C1 and a vertical portion that, together with the tectorial membrane, attaches to the lower clivus. The apical ligament extends from the tip of the dens to the anterior margin of the foramen magnum, and the alar ligaments extend laterally from the dens to each occipital condyle (16).

On MR, most ligaments, with the exception of the ligamentum flavum, demonstrate low signal intensity, similar to bone, on all imaging sequences because of their high collagen content (20,26). The ligaments blend imperceptibly with cortical bone, the outer fibers of the anulus fibrosis, and the dura. The ligamentum flavum demonstrates intermediate signal on T1- and T2-weighted sequences and high signal on gradient-echo sequences. The reason for this discrepancy is presumably related to its different biochemical composition. The ligamentum flavum contains only 20% collagen and 80% elastin (20,27).

Spinal Cord and Nerves

The spinal cord begins as the caudal extension of the medulla oblongata at the level of the foramen magnum. Its distal extent is more variable and age dependent. The spinal cord and vertebral column are equal in length until the third fetal month. Thereafter, because of discordant growth between the cord and the spinal column, the tip

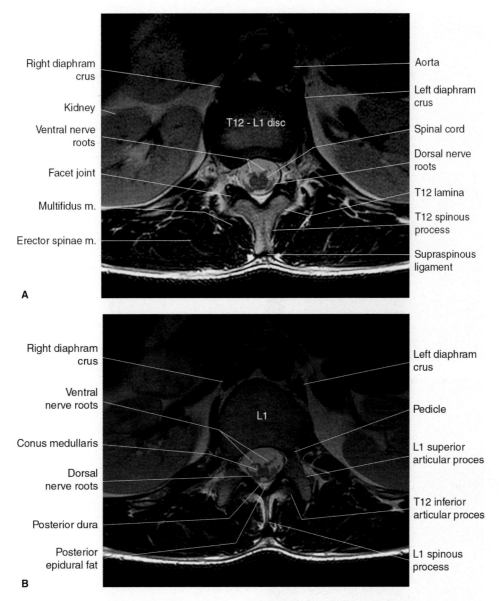

Right diaphram crus
Kidney
Ventral nerve roots
Facet joint
Multifidus m.
Erector spinae m.

Aorta
Left diaphram crus
Spinal cord
Dorsal nerve roots
T12 lamina
T12 spinous process
Supraspinous ligament

T12 - L1 disc

A

Right diaphram crus
Ventral nerve roots
Conus medullaris
Dorsal nerve roots
Posterior dura
Posterior epidural fat

Left diaphram crus
Pedicle
L1 superior articular proces
T12 inferior articular proces
L1 spinous process

L1

B

Figure 5-9 Normal thoracic spine—axial plane, T2-weighted fast spin echo. **A:** At the distal spinal cord. **B:** At the conus.

of the conus "ascends" to lie opposite of the L1 vertebral body in the adult, with a range from the eleventh thoracic interspace to the second lumbar interspace (28). The conus terminates in the filum terminale, which is less than 2 mm in diameter and extends to the first coccygeal segment (28).

The spinal cord varies in size depending on its level within the spinal canal. It is widest at the cervical enlargement (C5 to C6), narrowest at the mid thoracic region (T5 to T9), and enlarges again in the lumbar region from T10 to the conus (28). The anteroposterior diameter of the cord remains relatively constant at 9 to 10 mm throughout its length.

Small nerve rootlets emerge from posterior and anterior lateral sulci along the length of the spinal cord to form the dorsal and ventral nerve roots. The union of the

dorsal sensory and the ventral motor roots form the spinal nerves. There are eight pairs of cervical nerve roots but only seven cervical vertebral bodies. The first seven cervical nerves exit above the pedicles of their corresponding vertebral body level. For example, the C5 nerve root exits at the fourth cervical interspace above the C5 pedicle. The C8 nerve root exits below the C7 pedicle at the seventh cervical interspace. Below T1, the remaining nerve roots exit inferior to their corresponding vertebral body levels so that T1 nerve root exits at the first thoracic interspace, T2 nerve root exits at the second thoracic interspace, and so on. In the cervical region, the nerve roots course relatively horizontal to exit their neural foramen. Because of the discrepancy between the length of the spinal cord and vertebral column, the course of the nerve roots becomes progressively more vertical throughout the thoracic region. Below

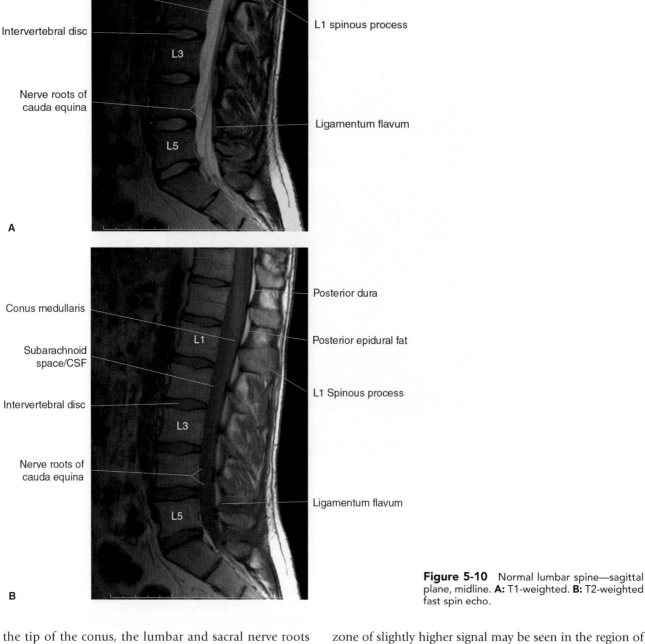

Conus medullaris

Subarachnoid
space/CSF

Intervertebral disc

Nerve roots of
cauda equina

Posterior dura

Posterior epidural fat

L1 spinous process

Ligamentum flavum

A

Conus medullaris

Subarachnoid
space/CSF

Intervertebral disc

Nerve roots of
cauda equina

Posterior dura

Posterior epidural fat

L1 Spinous process

Ligamentum flavum

B

Figure 5-10 Normal lumbar spine—sagittal plane, midline. **A:** T1-weighted. **B:** T2-weighted fast spin echo.

the tip of the conus, the lumbar and sacral nerve roots have a rather long, parallel, vertical course that forms the cauda equina (16).

On MR, the spinal cord has intermediate signal on T1-weighted sequences and low signal on T2-weighted and gradient echo sequences. On high-resolution studies at high field strength, some internal architecture can be seen on T2-weighted and gradient echo sequences. This is particularly apparent on axial images where an "H"-shaped

zone of slightly higher signal may be seen in the region of a central gray matter surrounded by the slightly lower signal of the white matter tracts (Fig. 5-6). A corresponding longitudinal stripe of slightly higher signal is seen within the mid spinal cord on the sagittal T2-weighted and gradient-echo sequences (29). This distinction between white and gray matter is thought to be secondary to a combination of the differences in water content between white and gray matter, the differences in relaxation times, and the

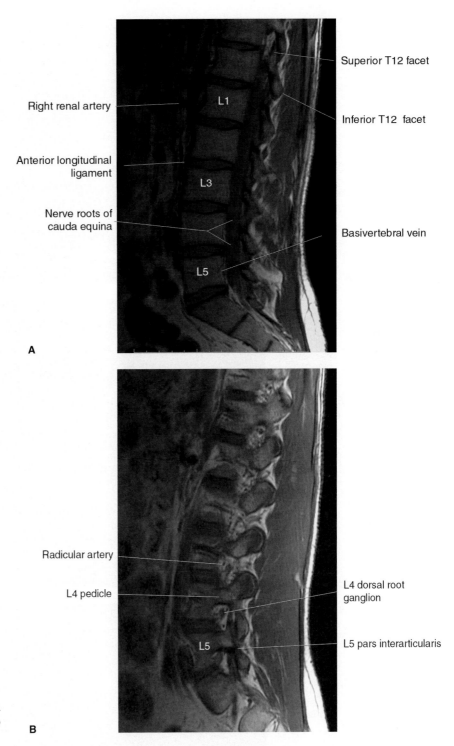

Right renal artery

Anterior longitudinal
ligament

Nerve roots of
cauda equina

L1

L3

L5

Superior T12 facet

Inferior T12 facet

Basivertebral vein

A

Radicular artery

L4 pedicle

L5

L4 dorsal root
ganglion

L5 pars interarticularis

Figure 5-11 Normal T1-weighted lumbar spine—sagittal plane. **A:** Lateral to midline. **B:** Far lateral to midline.

B

presence or absence of myelin (29). These changes are not apparent on T1-weighted sequences. Individual nerve roots and rootlets can sometimes be resolved with high-resolution imaging at high field strengths (Figs. 5-6 and 5-7).

Dural Coverings

The dural coverings of the spinal cord and nerve roots are in continuity with those in the cranial cavity. The dura and the arachnoid are closely adherent, with only a potential space between the two. They form the outer boundary of the subarachnoid space. The inner boundary is formed by the pia mater, which is closely adherent to the spinal cord and nerve roots. The pia mater is attached to the dura on both sides of the spinal cord by pointed processes known as the denticulate (dentate) ligaments. CSF circulates within the subarachnoid space and freely communicates with the cranial CSF spaces. It demonstrates low signal

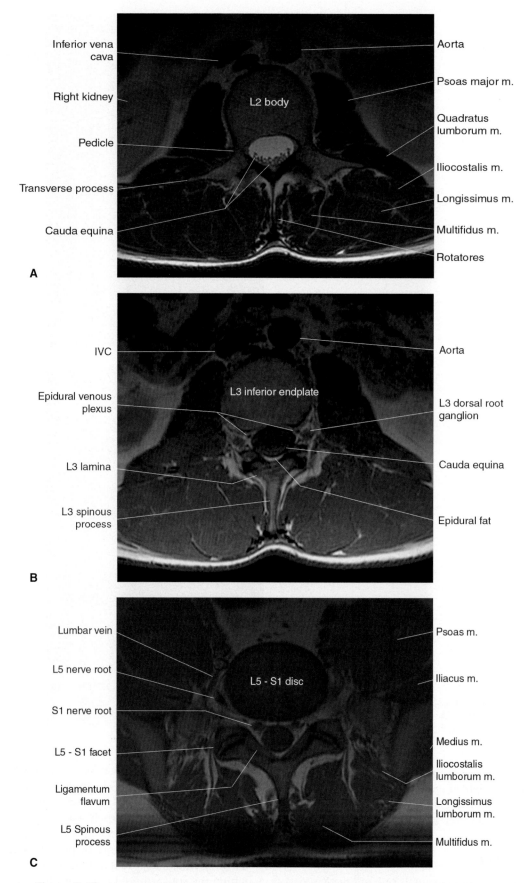

Figure 5-12   Normal lumbar spine—axial plane. **A:** T2-weighted fast spin echo at the L2 body. **B:** T1-weighted at the L3 inferior endplate. **C:** T1-weighted at the L5 interspace.

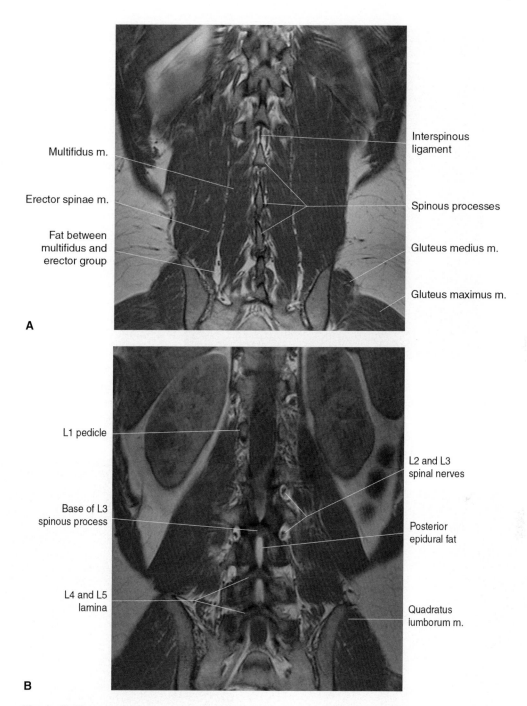

Multifidus m.

Erector spinae m.

Fat between multifidus and erector group

A

Interspinous ligament

Spinous processes

Gluteus medius m.

Gluteus maximus m.

L1 pedicle

Base of L3 spinous process

L4 and L5 lamina

B

L2 and L3 spinal nerves

Posterior epidural fat

Quadratus lumborum m.

Figure 5-13 Normal T1-weighted lumbar spine—coronal plane. **A:** Far posterior at the spinous processes. **B:** Posterior at the lamina. **C:** At the vertebral body/pedicle.

intensity (lower than spinal cord) on T1-weighted sequences and cannot be distinguished from the dura or posterior longitudinal ligament. On gradient-echo and T2-weighted sequences, the CSF becomes high in signal, much greater than the spinal cord.

Vascular

The blood supply to the spinal cord is via a larger anterior spinal artery that supplies the anterior two thirds to four fifths of the spinal cord and two small posterior spinal arteries that supply the remainder of the cord (16). The anterior and posterior spinal arteries are asymmetrically and variably supplied at a few levels by medullary branches of the radiculomedullary arteries that arise from the vertebral arteries, aortic intercostal arteries, and lumbar arteries. At the skull base, the junction of paired medullary branches of the intracranial vertebral arteries forms the anterior spinal artery. Additional arterial contribution is seen at two or three other cervical levels. The upper thoracic cord is poorly

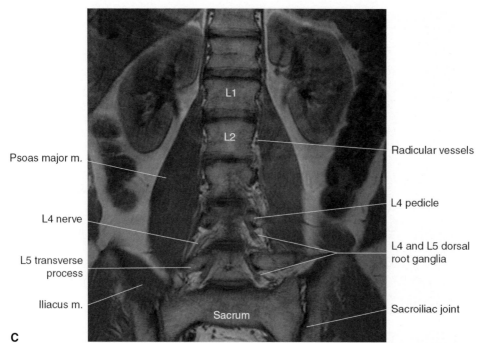

Psoas major m.

Radicular vessels

L4 nerve

L4 pedicle

L5 transverse process

L4 and L5 dorsal root ganglia

Iliacus m.

Sacrum

Sacroiliac joint

C

Figure 5-13 *(continued)*

supplied with a watershed zone at approximately T4. The predominant arterial supply to the thoracolumbar region is the great anterior medullary artery, the artery of Adamkiewicz. It arises on the left side 75% of the time and usually between T9 and L2 (85%) (28). It makes a characteristic hairpin bend as it forms the ascending and descending anterior spinal artery (see Fig. 5-15). The venous system roughly mirrors the arterial system, with multiple medullary veins draining into pial veins that communicate with the prominent posterior

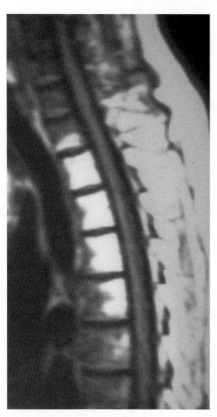

Figure 5-14 Radiation changes, T1-weighted sagittal. High marrow fat signal is seen within the upper thoracic vertebral bodies.

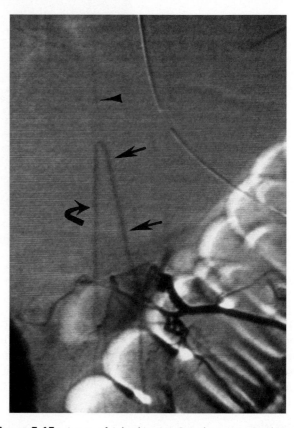

Figure 5-15 Artery of Adamkiewicz. Spinal arteriogram demonstrating the characteristic hairpin bend of Adamkiewicz (*arrows*), giving rise to the ascending (*arrowhead*) and descending (*curved arrow*) branches.

spinal vein and smaller anterior spinal veins (16). Radicular veins coursing with the nerve roots at variable levels drain the pial veins into the internal vertebral venous plexus that is in the epidural space surrounded by fat (30). The internal vertebral venous plexus drains into the external vertebral venous plexus either via the basivertebral vein through the vertebral body or via paired anterior longitudinal epidural veins that drain through the neural foramen (16). The external vertebral venous plexus ultimately empties into the azygos system.

EXAMINATION TECHNIQUE

Surface coils are used for the evaluation of the spine because of the need for high signal-to-noise ratio and resolution. Only one segment of the spine can be optimally imaged, as these coils have a limited FOV. They come in a variety of shapes and configurations, including special coils for the neck. In the cervical region, a special posterior neck coil works well. It is shaped to conform to the cervical lordotic curve and is quite comfortable for the patient to lie on. If this is not available, a 7- by 11-in rectangular "license plate" coil or a 5-in round circular coil may be used. In general, at least three coil placements are necessary for evaluation of the spinal canal from the foramen magnum to the upper sacrum.

Various multicoil array systems are available that function by combining signals from multiple surface coils assembled in series along the spinal axis (see Fig. 5-16). This versatile system gives the operator the choice of high-resolution imaging of the entire spinal axis or small spinal segments. The result is improved image quality in a shorter time because the need to move the patient or a single surface coil is eliminated (31,32). Software advances have further improved the ability to quickly survey the entire spinal axis by combining separate high-resolution data sets into a single composed image (see Fig. 5-17). Pediatric multicoil array systems are particularly advantageous in this patient population, because these patients are often sedated (see Fig. 5-18).

A T1-weighted sagittal sequence is initially performed. RARE (i.e., fast spin-echo, turbo spin-echo) T2-weighted sagittal sequences are used instead of standard T2-weighted or gradient recalled echo sequences because they produce high-resolution, heavily T2-weighted sequences in a fraction of the imaging time. In the evaluation of degenerative disc disease, axial sequences are performed next, with the axial sections parallel to the interspaces (see Fig. 5-19). In the lumbar region, T1-weighted axial sequences are utilized to take advantage of the sharp contrast between intraspinal fat and disc material, nerve roots, and bone. The axial images are then repeated using fast spin echo to differentiate disc from CSF. Gradient-echo axials are used in the cervical region as they tend to differentiate spinal cord, dural sac, disc material, and bone (33–35) and are free from the confusing flow artifact often seen with fast spin-echo axial

sequences. Axial gradient-echo sequences can often confirm and further characterize intradural or intramedullary lesions seen on the sagittal sequences (36). Intravenous contrast is administered and T1-weighted sagittal and/or axial sequences are repeated if intradural pathology is found or if the clinical indication suggests a meningeal process or a spinal vascular malformation.

Patients with scoliosis require special imaging considerations. Only small portions of the spinal canal and cord are imaged on each slice. Intradural pathology may be obscured, with the pathology mimicking volume averaging. Repeating the T1-weighted sequences in the coronal plane usually provides additional information. Also, the coronal and sagittal planes may be angled to allow imaging of a larger portion of the spine on any one slice. Scoliosis often precludes the possibility of visualizing the intraspinal structures on a single or few adjacent scans. A curved reformatting feature is available on some scanning systems and most workstations, which can be helpful in evaluating pathology or the disc–spinal canal interface in these problematic spines (see Fig. 5-20). Contrast may be used more liberally to increase the conspicuity of intradural lesions in a patient with a documented myelopathy.

There is no one correct way to image the spine. Multiple pulse sequences and imaging options are available. Presaturation pulses are routinely applied anteriorly to minimize artifacts from normal physiologic motion of the heart and great vessels, chest wall, and abdomen. Other motion compensation mechanisms (respiratory compensation, cardiac gating) may be used, but not all options are available on each imager. The choice of repetition times, echo times, and flip angles to achieve optimum contrast between spinal cord and CSF on T2-weighted, RARE, or gradient-echo sequences may vary depending on the motion compensation mechanisms available and the type of magnet. A sample protocol is included in Table 5-1. A "screening" examination is often supplemented with additional pulse sequences, discussed in other sections of this chapter. Each request for a spinal MR examination needs to be carefully reviewed to assure the optimal pulse sequences are being used to answer the proposed clinical question.

MAGNETIC RESONANCE CONTRAST AGENTS

There are currently five MR contrast agents approved for use to evaluate spinal disease: Magnevist (gadopentetate dimeglumine, Berlex Laboratories, Wayne, NJ), Omniscan (gadodiamide, Amersham Health Inc., Princeton, NJ), ProHance (gadoteridol) and MultiHance (gadobenate dimeglumine, Bracco Diagnostics, Princeton, NJ), and OptiMARK, (gadoversetamide, Mallinckrodt Inc., St. Louis, MO). All are gadolinium complexes. Gadolinium was chosen because it has strong paramagnetic properties.

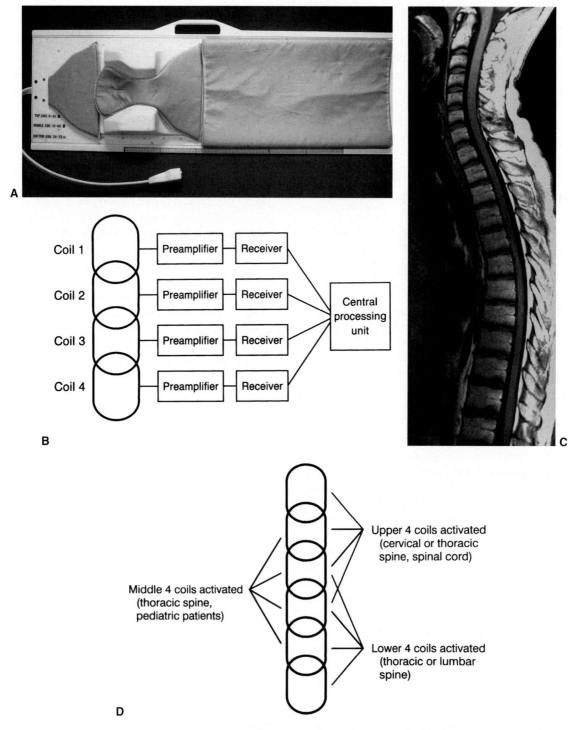

Figure 5-16   Phased array multicoil (General Electric, Milwaukee, WI). **A:** Six coil array spine multicoil. **B:** Schematic representation of multicoil hardware modifications. **C:** T1-weighted large-field-of-view image made by combining the signal generated by each coil element. **D:** Schematic representation of the six-coil array. The MR operator chooses which four coils are active during scanning.

In contrast to conventional iodinated material where the agent itself is imaged, paramagnetic materials themselves do not produce signals. Rather, they alter the molecular environment of the tissue in which they reside, thus affecting the signal of the hydrogen nuclei present (37,38).

The magnetic moment of a paramagnetic agent is considerably greater than the moment of the nearby hydrogen nuclei, due to the presence of unpaired electrons. Paramagnetic agents are also designed to bind water molecules. The large magnetic moment of a paramagnetic

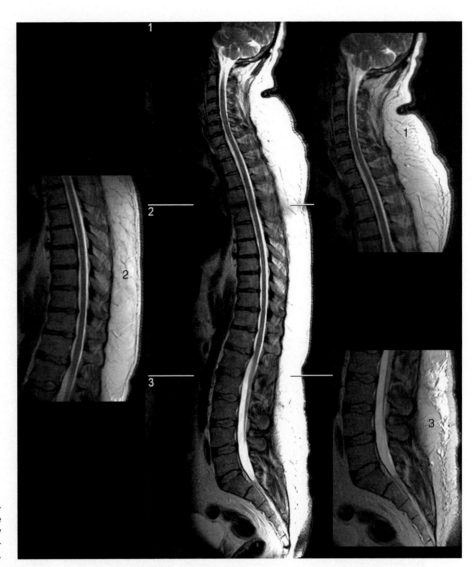

Figure 5-17 T2-weighted fast spin-echo composite image. This image was generated at a workstation by using a tool that combines three small-field-of-view, high-resolution images.

TABLE 5-1

MAGNETIC RESONANCE SPINAL PULSE SEQUENCES

	Plane	TR (ms)	TE (ms)	Pulse Sequence	Other	Views/ NEX	Thickness/ Skip (mm)	Field of View (cm)	Time (min.)
Cervical	SAG	400	16	SE	—	192/3	3.5/0.5	22	4
	SAG	3,275	105	frfsexL	ETL = 17	256/4	3.5/0.5	22	3
	AXIAL	400	17	fgre	20° flip	192/2	4/0	20	5
Thoracic	SAG	475	16	SE	—	256/2	3.5/0.5	28	4
	SAG	2,800	105	frfsexL	ETL = 17	256/4	3.5/0.5	28	3
	AXIAL	350	17	MPGR	20° flip	192/4	4/0	20	4.5
Lumbar	SAG	475	16	SE	—	256/2	4/1	28	4
	SAG	2,800	102	frfsexL	ETL = 17	256/4	4/1	28	3
	AXIAL	470	17	SE	—	192/2	5/interleaved	18	6
	AXIAL	2,800	105	frfsexL	—	256/3	5/interleaved	18	5
Multilevel	SAG	500	16	SE	—	512/2	3.5/0.5	48	4
	SAG	3,000	105	frfsexL	ETL = 17	256/2	3.5/0.5	22	3

NEX, number of excitations; ETL, echo train length; frfsexL, fast recovery fast spin echo; RARE, rapid acquisition relaxation enhancement; MPGR, multiplanar gradient echo; fgre, fast gradient echo; SE, spin echo.

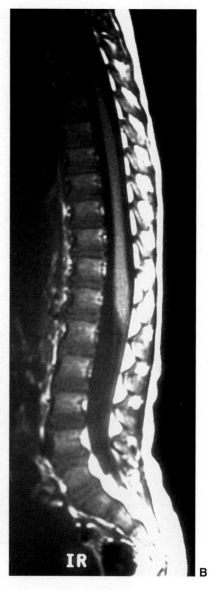

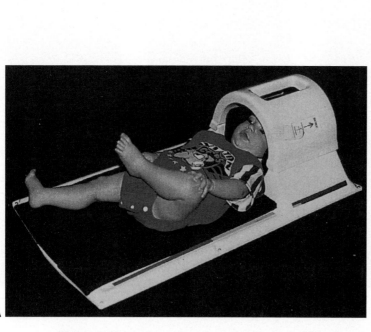

Figure 5-18 Pediatric phased array multicoil. **A:** Toddler positioned on the integrated head and spine coil. **B:** Sagittal T1-weighted image of the majority of the thoracolumbar spine obtained by selecting the middle and lower spinal portions of the array.

agent enhances relaxation or shortens the relaxation time of the bound water protons that are continually exchanging with free water. They enhance both the T1 and T2 relaxation. At the clinically effective dosage used the T1 relaxation effect predominates, resulting in an area of increased signal on T1-weighted sequences wherever the agent has accumulated (37,38).

The volume of distribution of gadolinium compounds in the central nervous system (CNS) is similar to that of iodinated agents. Blood supply to the tissue and blood–brain barrier breakdown are required to allow accumulation of the agent. Gadolinium is excreted unchanged in the urine. Eighty percent is excreted within the first 6 hours, with 90% being eliminated by 24 hours. The biologic half-life is about 90 minutes (39).

Gadolinium is a safe agent with few side effects (40) and is safer than iodinated contrast. It is helpful or essential in the diagnosis and characterization of intraspinal neoplasms, meningeal abnormalities, inflammatory conditions, and postoperative failed back syndromes (41).

PATHOLOGIC CONDITIONS

Degenerative Disease

To facilitate clear communication of imaging and surgical findings, the American Society of Neuroradiology, the American Society of Spine Radiology, and the North American Spine Society developed a consensus nomenclature and classification of lumbar disc pathology (42).

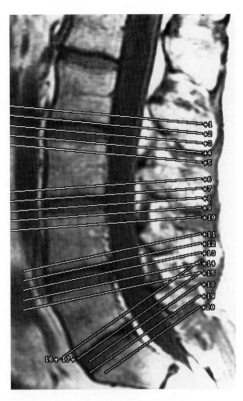

Figure 5-19 This scout view from a lumbar spine exam demonstrates the orientation of the axial slices.

The definitions are based on anatomy and pathology and are not intended to imply etiology, relationship to symptoms, or need for specific treatment. This system of nomenclature and classification is used herein. The terminology was developed specifically for the lumbar spine; it may be reasonably extrapolated to describe similar anatomy and pathology in the cervical and thoracic regions.

Incidental MR findings are a major confounder in the evaluation of patients with spinal pain. MR imaging commonly demonstrates degenerative interspace, disc, and facet joint abnormalities in asymptomatic persons, including high prevalence of herniated disc (20% to 70%), bulging disc (20% to 81%), degenerative disc (46% to 93%), anular tear (14% to 56%), and advanced spinal canal narrowing (1% to 21%), dependent on study population and definition of specific abnormalities (43). Teresi et al. have observed asymptomatic "significant" cervical spinal cord impingement in 16% to 26% of patients referred for MR examinations of the larynx (44). These studies underscore the importance of careful correlation of the anatomic abnormalities with the specific clinical syndrome. Because of the ease in obtaining an MRI examination and its noninvasive nature, the MR examination may be performed in lieu of a detailed neurologic examination in patients with nonspecific symptoms. Caution is advised in interpreting MRI studies to avoid subjecting patients to unnecessary,

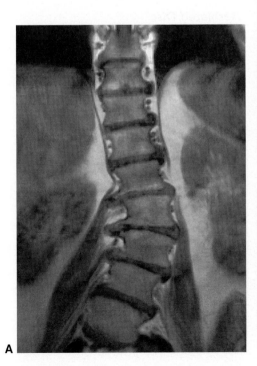

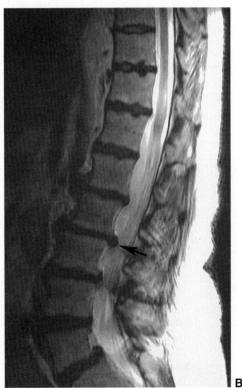

Figure 5-20 Scoliosis with curved reformatting. **A:** Coronal T1-weighted image demonstrating lumbar scoliosis. **B:** A small disc herniation (*arrow*) is demonstrated on a curved reformatted image, generated from a sagittal T2-weighted fast spin-echo series.

potentially invasive therapies. To be most efficacious, spinal MRI for pain must be designed and interpreted in the context of the individual patient's clinical syndrome.

American College of Radiology Appropriateness Criteria include guidelines for imaging patients with chronic neck pain (45) and acute low back pain (46). Despite the exquisite display of spinal anatomy, MR examination for these syndromes is best reserved for patients with clear neurologic signs or symptoms, warning signs of serious systemic disease, or evidence of bone or disc destruction on conventional radiographs.

Disc Disease (Nonsurgical)

Anular Degeneration

The most common finding for MR of the spine at our institution is degenerative disc disease. Age- and activity-related degeneration of the disc spaces and facet joints is inevitable. Disc degeneration begins early in life as a loss of hydration resulting in loss of interspace height and diffuse bulging of the disc and anulus. Tears, or fissures, develop in the anulus fibrosis with three distinct types identified at autopsy: concentric, radial, and transverse (47,48). Concentric and transverse tears are thought to have no clinical significance. The significance of radial tears remains controversial. Radial tears are defined as fissures extending through all layers of the anulus between the nucleus pulposus and the disc surface without herniation of the nucleus pulposus. Leakage of irritative nuclear material into the anulus fibrosis and epidural space has been implicated as a cause of chronic low back pain that has been termed "discogenic" pain (48). Small, discrete areas of increased T2 signal within the anulus fibrosis of cadavers have correlated with radial tears (48) and similar areas of gadolinium enhancement in living patients have corresponded to vascularized granulation tissue within radial tears at surgery (49). Studies addressing

the clinical relevance of these findings are lacking. It is important to note that the common usage of the term "anular tear" does not imply traumatic etiology.

Vertebral Body Marrow Changes

Vertebral body marrow changes are reactive modifications associated with active or chronic disc inflammation and degenerative disease. Three types of marrow signal patterns are classified by Modic et al. (50). Type 1 changes are characterized by decreased signal intensity on T1-weighted images and by increased signal intensity on T2-weighted images indicating marrow edema associated with acute or subacute inflammation and granulation tissue (see Fig. 5-21). The granulation tissue will typically enhance with intravenous gadolinium administration. Type 2 changes are characterized by increased signal on T1-weighted images and isointense or increased signal intensity on T2-weighted images indicating reactive replacement of typical bone marrow with yellow fat (see Fig. 5-22). Type 3 refers to decreased T1 and T2 signal due to chronic reactive osteosclerosis (see Fig. 5-23). Both type 2 and type 3 findings indicate chronic vertebral changes and may be seen as sequelae to type 1 changes. While Modic changes are uncommon in asymptomatic patients, the significance in patients with spine pain is uncertain (51). These signal changes can be quite exuberant and it is important to recognize the degenerative etiology rather than neoplastic or infectious origins.

Disc Disease (Surgical)

Herniated Disc

Focal disc herniations result from rupture of the anulus fibrosis with protrusion or extrusion of the nuclear material into or through the anulus. In the lumbar region, herniations are most commonly posterior into the spinal

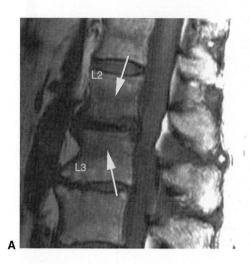
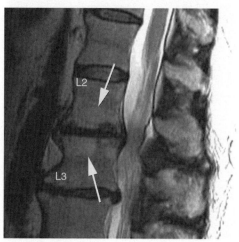

Figure 5-21   Type 1 vertebral marrow changes (Modic). **A:** Decreased T1 signal in the inferior aspect of *L2* vertebral body and the superior aspect of *L3* body. **B:** Corresponding T2 signal increase is seen on the T2-weighted fast spin-echo image.

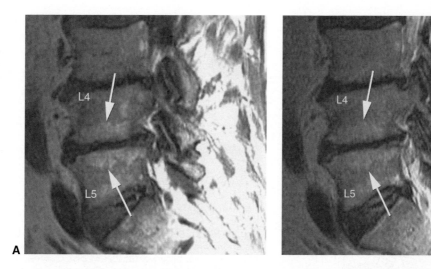

Figure 5-22 Type 2 vertebral marrow changes (Modic). **A:** Increased T1 signal in inferior aspect of the *L4* vertebral body and superior aspect of *L5* body. **B:** Corresponding T2 signal increase is seen on the T2-weighted fast spin-echo image.

canal, where they may be midline in location or paramedian to the right or left. Midline disc herniations are often asymptomatic, distorting the ventral surface of the thecal sac without impingement on individual nerve roots. Occasionally, large midline herniations will compromise the spinal canal, resulting in a cauda equina syndrome. Symptomatic posterior disc herniations typically are centered to the right or left of midline and distort the nerve root exiting the spinal canal at the next vertebral body segment. Irritation of the nerve roots results in radiculopathy. Ten percent to 15% of all disc herniations are lateral, with extension of disc material within or beyond the neural foramen (28). These herniations can be subtle and may be confused with diffuse bulging of the anulus fibrosis. Close inspection of the neural foramina and paraspinal fat

immediately lateral to the foramen may increase sensitivity. Lateral disc herniations typically cause a radiculopathy of the nerve root of the same vertebral body segment. Other locations of herniations include intravertebral herniations with extension of disc material into adjacent vertebral bodies (Schmorl nodes) (see Fig. 5-24) and anterior locations with extension of disc material anterior to the vertebral bodies (52,53). Whether or not these herniations are clinically or surgically significant remains controversial. Currently, intravertebral and anterior herniations have no surgical significance.

The term *herniated disc* refers to localized displacement of nucleus, cartilage, fragmented apophyseal bone, or fragmented anular tissue beyond the intervertebral disc space. The disc space is defined by the vertebral body endplates

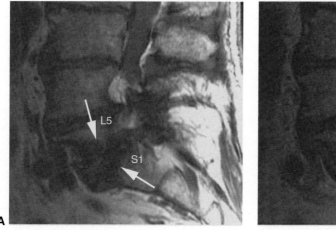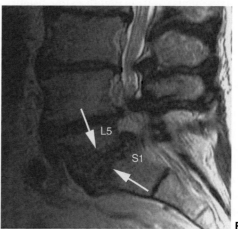

Figure 5-23 Type 3 vertebral marrow changes (Modic). **A:** Decreased T1 signal in the inferior aspect of *L5* vertebral body and superior aspect of *S1* body. **B:** Corresponding T2 signal decrease is seen on the T2-weighted image, characteristic of osteosclerosis.

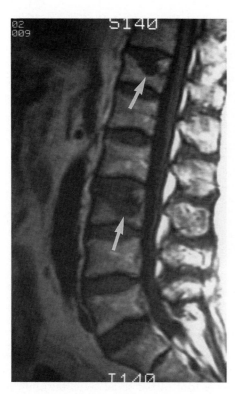

Figure 5-24 Schmorl node, T1-weighted. Note the central herniation of disc material through the superior endplates of T12 and L3 (*arrows*).

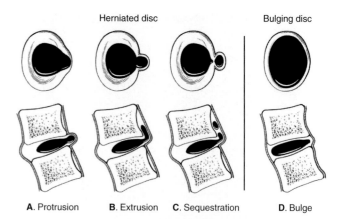

A. Protrusion   **B**. Extrusion   **C**. Sequestration   **D**. Bulge

Figure 5-25 Schematic of disc herniation and bulging anulus based on consensus nomenclature. **A:** Disc protrusion, defined as relatively short, broad extension of disc material into the anulus fibrosis. **B:** Disc extrusion, defined as a taller, more narrow extension of disc material through the radial thickness of the anulus. **C:** Disc sequestration, defined as a migrated fragment of extruded disc that has lost continuity with the disc of origin. **D:** Disc bulge, defined as broad expansion of the circumference of the disc due to shortening of the interspace height and radial spreading of the nucleus and anulus.

and by the edges of the vertebral ring apophyses, exclusive of osteophyte formations. To be considered *herniated*, disc material must be displaced from its native location in association with disruption of the anulus, or in the case of intravertebral herniation, an acquired defect of the vertebral body endplate. Subcategorization of herniation into *protrusion* or *extrusion* is based on the geometry of the displaced disc material. A disc is considered *protruded* (see Fig. 5-25A) if the greatest distance between the edge of the native disc margin and the edge of the displaced disc material is smaller than the distance between the edges at the base of the herniation. The term *extruded* disc (see Fig. 5-25B) is reserved for herniations in which the extension of displaced disc material beyond the native disc margin is greater than the width of the base of the herniation in any plane. *Migrated* disc material is extruded disc that is displaced away from the site of extrusion, typically cranially or caudally in the anterior epidural space. A *sequestered* or "free" disc fragment (see Fig. 5-25C) is migrated disc material that has no evident continuity with the parent disc.

The term *bulge* refers to generalize extension of disc tissues beyond the native edges of the ring apophyses (see Fig. 5-25D). Bulging of the anulus involves at least 50% of the disc circumference and extends a few millimeters beyond the apophyses in a relatively uniform manner. By definition, bulging is not a herniation because there is no radial disruption of the anulus fibrosis.

Not all disc herniations are surgical lesions (54). Anular tears and disc protrusions are frequent findings in asymptomatic patients. Disc extrusions, sequestrations, and nerve root compression are uncommon in asymptomatic volunteers (51,55,56). To be considered a true positive finding, the herniated disc must be large enough and in the correct location to distort or compress the specific nerve root or roots that correspond to the clinical syndrome.

On MR, lumbar disc herniations may be suspected on sagittal images but must be confirmed on axial sequences. Posterior disc herniations result in a focal bulge in the disc contour, resulting in compression of epidural fat and mass effect upon the adjacent thecal sac or traversing nerve root sleeves. Herniations are visible typically as foci of decreased T1 and decreased T2 signal effacing the bright epidural fat on T1-weighted images and distorting the bright CSF on T2-weighted images (see Fig. 5-26). Relatively acute disc extrusions (see Fig. 5-27) may demonstrate signal intensity isointense or brighter than the parent disc on T2-weighted sequences, presumably secondary to local inflammatory response (57). Postcontrast T1-weighted axial images may better delineate the herniated disc fragment from dural sac as the peripheral portion of the disc may enhance, presumably secondary to ingrowth of new vessels in an attempt at repair. However, administration of intravenous gadolinium is not standard practice in the evaluation of the unoperated spine (58). Lateral disc herniations are more challenging to detect. Sagittal or axial views often show a soft tissue mass within, or lateral to, the neural foramen that obliterates the perineural fat plane (see Fig. 5-28). MR has been shown to be equal to computed tomography (CT) myelography in the diagnosis of disc herniations in the lumbar region (59). However, MR examinations can be

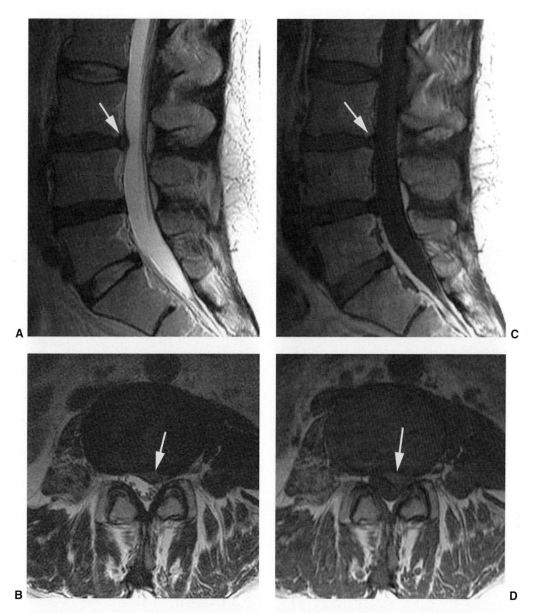

Figure 5-26   Lumbar disc protrusion. L3 disc herniation with the base of the herniation wider than the distance away from the parent disc. The protrusion is evident principally as a distortion of the cerebrospinal fluid-containing thecal sac on the T2-weighted images (**A** and **B**) and as effacement of the epidural fat on the T1-weighted images (**C** and **D**).

suboptimal for a number of reasons, including patient motion, body habitus, and asymmetric positioning. Also, patients with moderate or advanced degenerative changes typically have effacement of epidural fat, making disc herniation more difficult to recognize against a background of similar signaling structures. Up to 20% of clinically significant herniations may escape detection and a CT myelogram may be indicated in a patient with a clear radiculopathy and a discordant MR examination (60).

Effective MRI of degenerative disease in the cervical spine and spinal canal is a greater challenge. Structures are smaller, there is limited soft tissue contrast because of a relative lack of epidural fat, and patient swallowing motion

requires relatively short scan times. Image quality is a struggle between spatial and contrast resolution and time. In the cervical region, many studies show MR to be more or less equal to CT myelography in diagnosing disc herniations, particularly if the herniated fragment is large or has a midline component (see Fig. 5-29) (61–63). However, due to the small size of the structures being imaged, small slice thicknesses and small FOV are necessary to evaluate the neural foramina. This pushes the technique to the limits of its resolution, so that small disc herniations may be overlooked or overdiagnosed. While CT myelography suffers from similar limitations, the spatial resolution is higher and the combination of a cervical myelogram and high-resolution CT

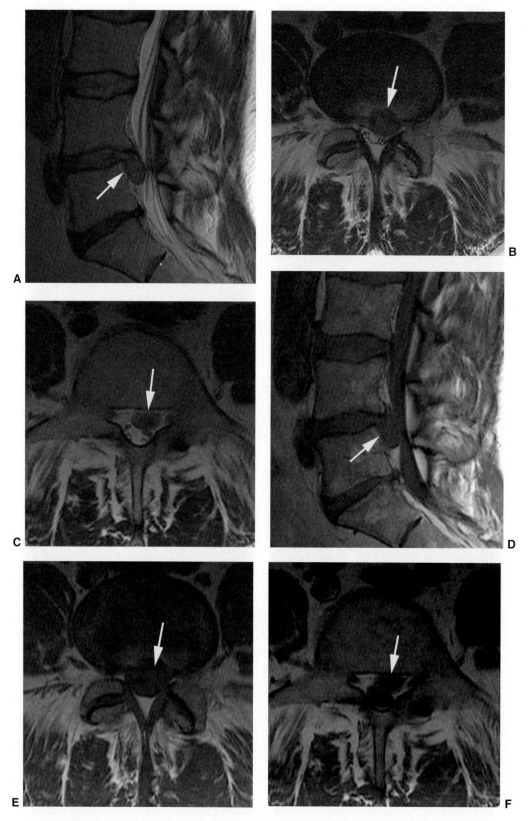

Figure 5-27   Lumbar disc extrusion. L-4 disc herniation with the distance from the edge of the extruded fragment greater than the width of the base. Inferior migration of disc material caudal to the superior endplate of L5. **A** and **D:** The disc material has T2 and T1 signal intensities similar to the parent disc. Axial views establish the central and left central location of the extrusion with distortion of the thecal sac and left L5 root sleeve origin on the T2-weighted images (**B** and **C**) and effacement of epidural fat on the T1 weighted images (**E** and **F**).

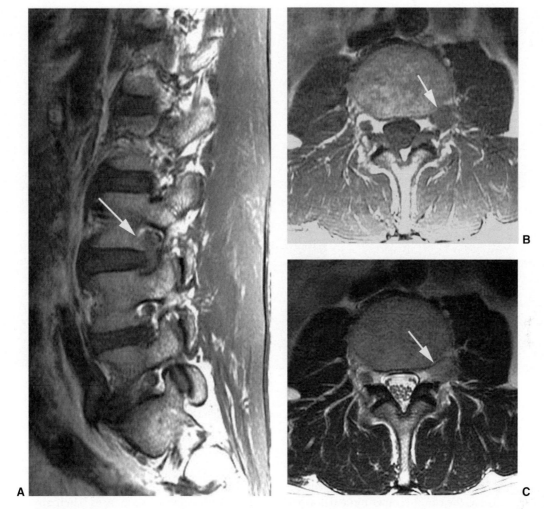

Figure 5-28 Lateral disc extrusion. **A:** Sagittal T1-weighted image shows abnormal soft tissue mass in left L3 foramen (*arrow*). **B:** Axial T1-weighted image immediately cranial to L3 endplate shows abnormal soft tissue effaces the normal fat plane surrounding the L3 nerve root sleeve (*arrow*). **C:** Axial T2-weighted image at the same level as B shows the extruded disc material (*arrow*) between edge of the L3 end-plate and displaced L3 nerve root (*white arrow*).

can afford the best opportunity to diagnose clinically significant small cervical herniations. In the cervical spine, simple disc herniation is less common than in the lumbar regions. Osteophytes and disc–osteophyte complexes are the more common cause of nerve root irritation and radiculopathy.

Disc herniations may also occur in the thoracic region. Many of these lesions have no clinical or surgical significance, unless large and causing spinal cord compression and myelopathy symptoms (64). Similar imaging criteria, as used in the cervical or lumbar region, are applied here (65). Axial views are necessary to determine the degree of cord compression.

Spinal Stenosis

Loss of interspace height associated with degenerative disc disease may result in mal-alignment and altered mechanical stresses upon the facet joints and ligaments. Reactive

remodeling of the interfaces can result in bone hypertrophy manifested as ridges of very low-signal cancellous bone and redundancy of the ligamentum flavum. Facet joint hypertrophy and diffuse bulging of the anulus fibrosis can result in narrowing of the spinal canal, lateral recesses, or neural foramina. This process may affect multiple levels and may progress to spinal cord or cauda equina compression, resulting in the clinical syndrome known as spinal stenosis. These degenerative changes are manifested on MRI as ventral and dorsolateral extradural impressions at the level of the interspaces (see Fig. 5-30). Axial T1-weighted and T2-weighted images, preferably parallel to the interspaces in question, are essential for characterizing the degree of spinal canal narrowing as sagittal images can be misleading. T1-weighted sequences tend to underestimate the degree of spinal and foraminal narrowing while T2-weighted or gradient-echo images tend to overestimate it. Similar changes occur in the cervical region, and rarely

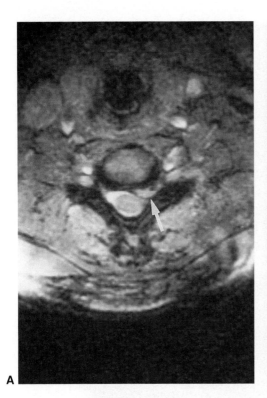
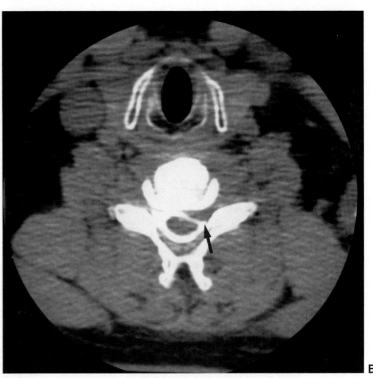

Figure 5-29   Cervical disc extrusion. **A:** Gradient-echo axial image showing a focal disc extrusion at C6 on the left effaces the subarachnoid space and partially fills the neural foramen (*arrow*). **B:** Postmyelogram computed tomography at the same level confirms these findings.

in the thoracic region, which can be asymptomatic or cause a compressive myelopathy (see Fig. 5-31). The incidence of myelopathy increases as the cord becomes more deformed and compressed (66). As in the lumbar spine, these changes usually involve multiple levels and predominantly involve the mid and lower cervical interspaces. In acute or subacute cord compression, edema may be seen as an increase in T2 signal closely related to the level of cord distortion with indistinct transition to normal cord signal above and below the compression. With chronic compression, relatively shorter segments of increased T2 signal and cord atrophy may be demonstrated representing cystic necrosis and volume loss from myelomalacia (67,68). This finding has prognostic significance as patients with myelomalacia respond less favorably to surgical or medical management than those without (68). These patients have a poor prognosis regardless of management. When the imaging findings do not correlate with the patient's specific signs and symptoms, a CT myelogram may provide valuable additional information.

Synovial Cyst

Synovial cysts arise from periarticular tissues and may arise in any joint, including the facet joints of the spine. They are typically associated with facet joint degeneration and are an uncommon cause of radiculopathy or spinal stenosis syndromes. Synovial cysts present as a posterolateral epidural mass, intimately associated with the ligamentum flavum, with signal similar to CSF on T1- and T2-weighted sequences. Their appearance is variable because the cysts may contain calcium, air, or hemorrhage byproducts (see Fig. 5-32) (69–71).

Cervical juxtafacet cysts are a rare cause of radiculopathy and myelopathy associated with degenerative disease. Unlike synovial cysts in the lumbar spine, many do not have a true synovial lining. They are most frequently located posterolateral in the spinal canal adjacent to the facet joint at C7–T1. Also, unlike lumbar synovial cysts, they are typically isointense to the ligamentum flavum on T1-weighted images and isointense to hypointense on T2-weighted images (see Fig. 5-33) (72).

Postoperative Evaluation

Causes of persistent pain following surgery, the failed back syndrome, include mechanical low back pain from altered stresses and spinal instability, arachnoiditis, dural scarring, and recurrent disc herniation. Often, these conditions cannot be differentiated clinically. Imaging evaluation of the postlaminectomy patient with recurrent pain is difficult but clinically important because patients with recurrent disc herniation may benefit from reoperation. Whereas in the other conditions listed, symptoms may actually worsen because further laminectomy may make

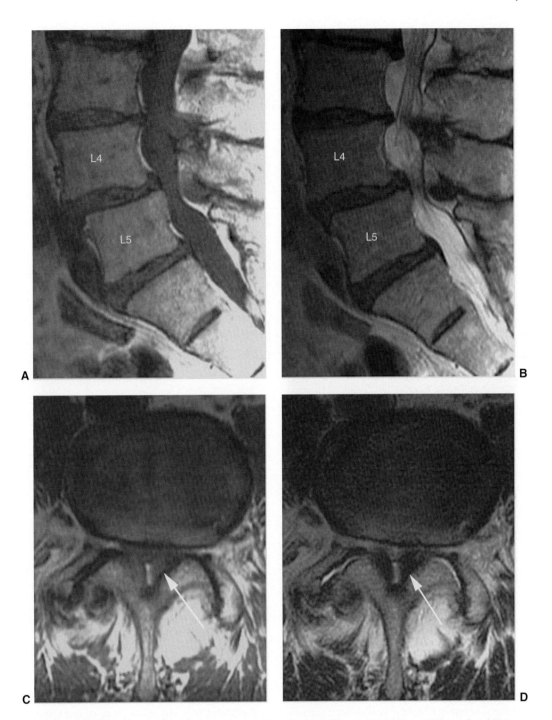

Figure 5-30 Advanced lumbar canal narrowing. Sagittal T1-weighted **(A)** and T2-weighted **(B)** images show anterior subluxation of *L4* on *L5*. Axial T1-weighted **(C)** and T2-weighted **(D)** images show advanced degenerative enlargement of the facet joints with redundancy of the ligamentum flavum (*arrows*) combine to cause advanced narrowing of the lumbar spinal canal in a patient with pseudoclaudication.

the spine more unstable and increase the amount of arachnoiditis and dural scarring. MRI has been shown to be useful in the differentiation of recurrent disc from dural scarring (73–80).

In arachnoiditis, the nerve roots of the cauda equina either clump together or migrate to the periphery of the dural sac where they become incorporated into the dural wall resulting in a thick rind of dura, nerve roots, and scar tissue. The MR appearance of arachnoiditis has been described in the literature (81). The findings are best seen on T2-weighted axial images and are similar to those on the CT myelogram as clumping of nerve roots, peripheral migration to the edges of the dural sac, and thickening of the dura (see Fig. 5-34).

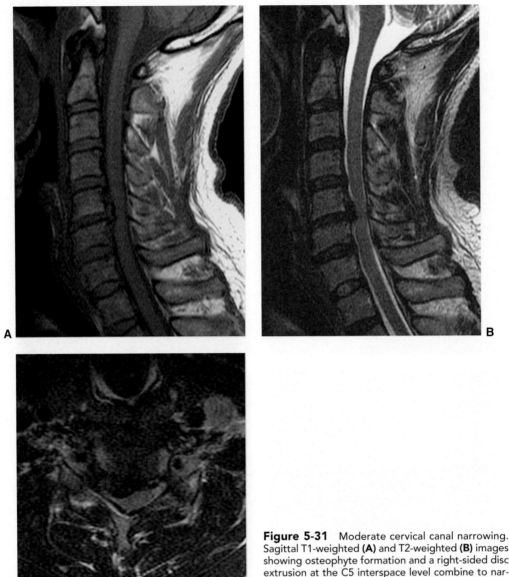

A

B

C

Figure 5-31 Moderate cervical canal narrowing. Sagittal T1-weighted **(A)** and T2-weighted **(B)** images showing osteophyte formation and a right-sided disc extrusion at the C5 interspace level combine to narrow the cervical spinal canal. **C:** Axial gradient-echo image shows the spinal cord being displaced posterior and to the left in this asymptomatic patient.

Postcontrast MR is useful in differentiating recurrent disc herniation from dural scarring (76,78). This differentiation has always been difficult because not even a CT myelogram or a contrast-enhanced CT can reliably distinguish between the two (82–84). In both conditions, a soft tissue mass may be present at the level of the interspace, resulting in obliteration of the epidural fat and nonvisualization of the nerve root or roots on the noncontrast MR image. This soft tissue may or may not be continuous with the laminectomy site. Sometimes the signal of the tissue may be different than the dural sac, disc margin, and nerve roots on T1- or T2-weighted sequences, so a diagnosis of scar tissue can be made with confidence. More often, the signal of the soft tissue cannot be differentiated from normal neural structures.

Intravenous gadolinium administration has been most valuable in this situation. Scar tissue enhances because it is vascular (76–78). Although disc material is avascular, contrast will diffuse from the endplates into the disc over time (85).

As a result, T1-weighted axial sequences should be performed immediately following contrast infusion to differentiate scar tissue from the dural sac, nerve roots, and disc material. If the epidural soft tissue enhances and the traversing or exiting nerve root can be well-visualized and not displaced, a confident diagnosis of dural scarring can be made (see Fig. 5-35). If a nonenhancing anterior soft tissue mass persists that displaces or compresses the nerve root, a recurrent disc herniation is suspect. Some combination of

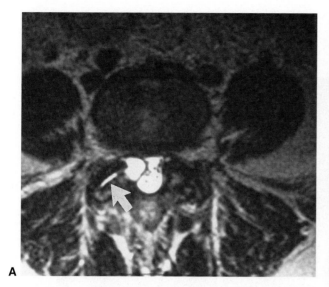

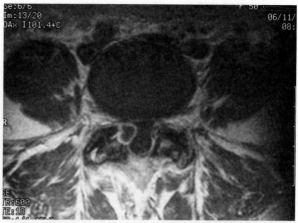

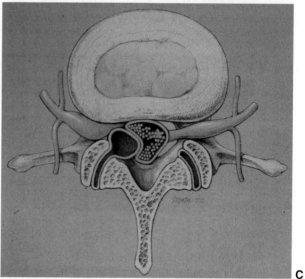

Figure 5-32 Synovial cyst. **A:** The cyst signals similar to cerebrospinal fluid on an axial T2-weighted fast spin-echo image. Note the fluid within the L4 facet joint (*arrow*). **B:** The periphery of the cyst enhances with contrast on an axial T1-weighted image. **C:** Artist drawing of a synovial cyst compressing the posterolateral aspect of the dural sac.

enhancing scar and nonenhancing disc material is usually present (see Fig. 5-36). Despite optimal technique, confusion sometimes still exists if there is soft tissue enhancement and mass effect with displacement of the nerve roots. We have observed enhancement of surgically proven disc fragments as well as nerve roots being tethered and displaced by dural scar.

Neoplasms

Spinal neoplasms are best characterized by their location relative to the dural sac and spinal cord. Three main compartments can be identified: extradural, intradural extramedullary, and intramedullary (28). The extradural compartment contains the spinal column and ligaments, epidural space and venous plexus, and the intervertebral discs. The pia, arachnoid, CSF, blood vessels, and nerve roots comprise the intradural extramedullary compartment. The intramedullary compartment includes the spinal

cord parenchyma and the filum terminale. The differential diagnosis of spinal neoplasms depends on the compartment in which the neoplasm arises because characteristic lesions are seen at each location.

Extradural Lesions

Extradural neoplasms may be primary bone tumors (chordoma, sarcoma), focal or diffuse marrow infiltrative disorders (multiple myeloma, lymphoma), or, more commonly, metastatic lesions. Extradural extension can also occur from paraspinal neoplasms such as lymphomas or sarcomas. Unlike CT or plain films, MR studies do not directly image the bone but rather the bone marrow. Bone neoplasms are best identified on T1-weighted sequences because they replace the normal marrow fat signal (see Fig. 5-37). Increased signal on T2-weighted or gradient-echo sequences may be seen (86–89). The neoplasm may be indistinguishable from normal bone marrow on fast spin-echo T2-weighted sequences because the bone marrow normally

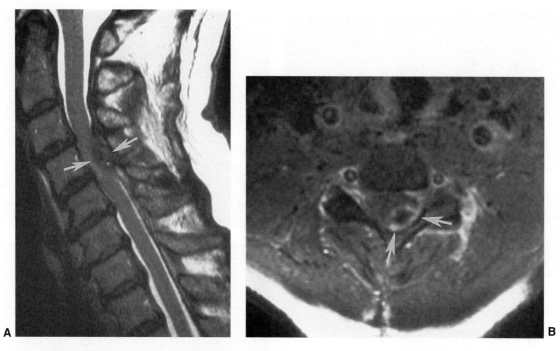

Figure 5-33 Cervical juxtafacet cyst. The juxtafacet cyst (*arrows*) is hypointense on the sagittal T2-weighted fast spin-echo image **(A)**, and isointense with peripheral enhancement on axial, the T1-weighted image with fat suppression **(B)**.

has high signal. Fat-suppression techniques are useful in these cases. Short TI inversion recovery (STIR) sequences provide fat suppression with the improved sensitivity to the prolonged T1 and T2 of abnormal tissues (90,91). By combining with RARE techniques (i.e., fast spin-echo,

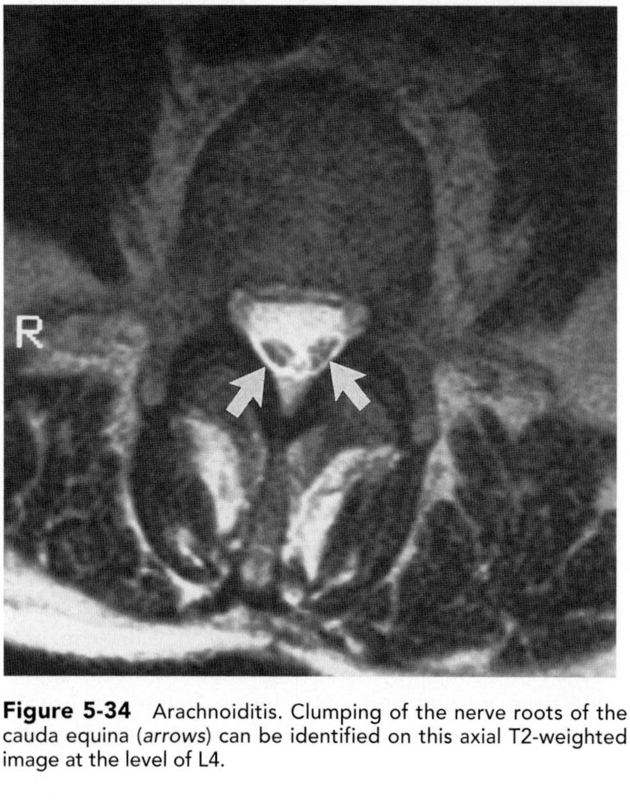

turbo STIR) the imaging times have been significantly reduced (see Fig. 5-38). MRI is more sensitive than a radionuclide bone scan in the detection of spinal metastasis (86,88).

The benign cavernous hemangioma is the only lesion that shows increased signal relative to normal marrow on T1-weighted sequences and variable signal (increased, decreased, isointense) relative to normal marrow on T2-weighted or gradient echo sequences (see Fig. 5-39). Spinal involvement, even in advanced multiple myeloma, can be difficult to detect on MRI. Some patients will demonstrate focal vertebral body lesions or diffuse marrow abnormalities. However, many will have normal-appearing marrow with benign-appearing compression fractures (92,93). The differential diagnosis of bone neoplasms and marrow infiltrative disorders will be discussed in more detail in Chapters 12 and 14, respectively.

One major advantage of MRI compared with CT, plain films, and myelography is the ability of MRI to noninvasively image epidural extension of neoplasm directly (94,95). Spinal cord or nerve root compromise can be identified and the levels of involvement determined for surgical or radiation therapy planning (see Fig. 5-40). These patients often have difficulty holding still because of severe pain, which makes it difficult to obtain diagnostic images. In a prospective study comparing MRI to myelography in cancer patients with suspected epidural disease, Quint et al. (95) found that 40% of the MR exams were nondiagnostic despite sedatives. The multicoil array and faster T2-weighted pulse sequences (RARE with fat saturation) can significantly shorten the examination time. If MR-compatible monitoring systems are

Figure 5-34 Arachnoiditis. Clumping of the nerve roots of the cauda equina (*arrows*) can be identified on this axial T2-weighted image at the level of L4.

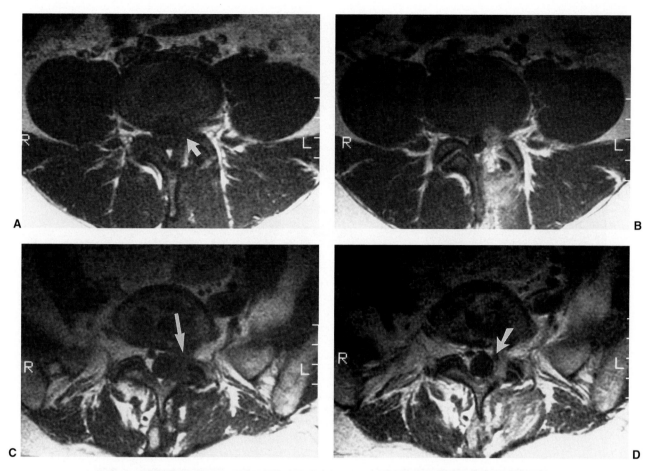

Figure 5-35 Dural scar. **A:** Axial T1-weighted image showing obliteration of the epidural fat on the left (*arrow*) and a soft tissue mass, which is suspicious for a recurrent disc herniation. **B:** Postcontrast image at the same level demonstrates enhancing scar tissue only. **C:** Axial T1-weighted image in another patient is indeterminate for recurrent disc herniation (*arrow*). **D:** This proved to be enhancing scar which surrounds the left S1 nerve root (*arrow*).

available, anesthesia support can reduce the number of non-diagnostic exams.

Contrast may provide additional information in the evaluation of extradural neoplasm. Fat suppression improves lesion conspicuity and detection of epidural extension, because extradural and vertebral neoplasms often enhance to a similar intensity to normal marrow on T1-weighted images without fat suppression (see Figs. 5-41 and 5-42) (96,97). Although MR has been helpful, differentiating benign (osteoporotic) from malignant compression fractures remains a difficult imaging problem. Homogeneous and diffuse vertebral signal abnormality, a convex vertebral border, complete pedicle involvement (unilateral or bilateral), and a cervical or lumbar location favor a malignant etiology (98).

Although the pattern of vertebral enhancement has been shown to be useful by some, others have found considerable overlap (99). The application of newer pulse sequences such as diffusion-weighted imaging in the spine may help to differentiate benign from malignant compression fractures (100). Ultimately, a followup study (2 to 3 months) or biopsy is necessary (101).

Spinal Angiolipomas

Angiolipomas are benign neoplasms composed of adipose and vascular elements. They are most common in the extremities and subcutaneous tissues. Spinal angiolipomas are uncommon and account for only about 0.14% of spinal axis tumors (102).

They are epidural tumors (very rarely intramedullary) that are more common in women, and often present in the fifth decade. The clinical presentation often includes back pain with progressive paraparesis, and lower extremity sensory changes. The more typical noninfiltrating (encapsulated) type is usually located in the posterior epidural space of the thoracic spine. The less common infiltrating (nonencapsulated) type is generally in the anterior epidural space.

The MR appearance predominantly reflects the fatty component of these tumors. They are hyperintense on T1-weighted images, with varying degrees of heterogeneity due to differing amounts of vascular elements (103). Flow voids are usually not seen since the vascular components consist of primarily capillaries and small venous channels

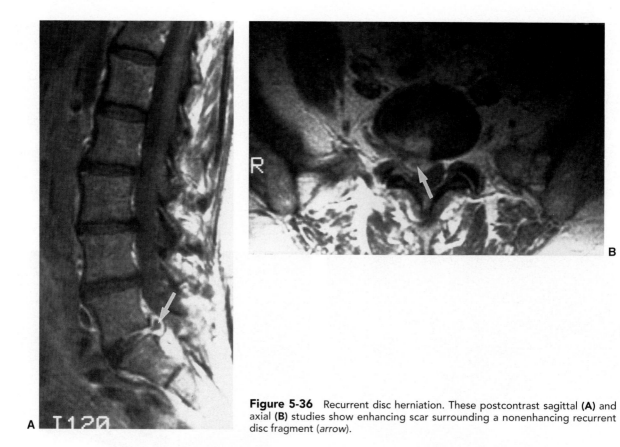

Figure 5-36 Recurrent disc herniation. These postcontrast sagittal **(A)** and axial **(B)** studies show enhancing scar surrounding a nonenhancing recurrent disc fragment (*arrow*).

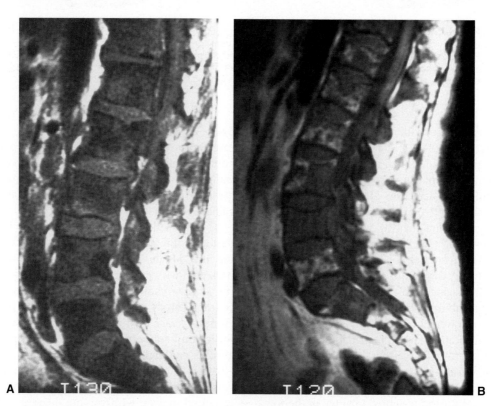

Figure 5-37 Metastasis. The bone marrow signal on T1-weighted imaging is abnormal in three patients with **(A)** metastatic prostate carcinoma, **(B)** multiple myeloma, and **(C)** metastatic hepato-cellular carcinoma. Compare this appearance to the normal marrow signal in Fig. 5-8.

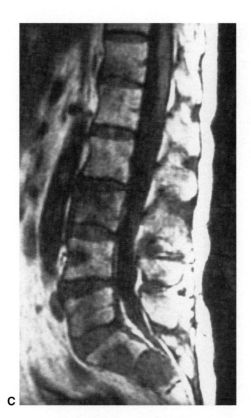

Figure 5-37 (continued)

without shunting. Characteristic contrast enhancement is best seen when using fat suppression (see Fig. 5-43).

Lymphoma

Spinal lymphoma commonly involves paravertebral lymph nodes. Extension may then occur to vertebral bodies, or to the epidural space through adjacent neural foramen. Occasionally, there is exclusive vertebral or epidural space involvement. MRI best demonstrates all of the above areas of involvement (see Fig. 5-44) (104). Any tumor that involves the paraspinous soft tissues can potentially gain access to the epidural space through the neural foramen (see Fig. 5-45).

Intradural Extramedullary Lesions

Meningiomas and neurogenic tumors (neurilemoma and neurofibroma) are the most common intradural extramedullary neoplasms encountered. Less common lesions include lipomas, intradural cysts, and intradural metastases.

Meningioma

Meningiomas most commonly occur in the thoracic region in middle-age females, lie posterior to the spinal cord, and compress the posterior columns. A few may be located anteriorly. Typically, they present as a well-circumscribed thoracic intradural mass that is separate from the spinal cord.

Figure 5-38 Metastatic breast carcinoma. **A:** There are numerous hypointense metastases on a sagittal T1-weighted image. Note bright signal in the uninvolved vertebral bodies from prior radiation. **B:** The lesions are bright on STIR images when the fat is homogeneously suppressed (TI 150 ms; TR 2,000; TE 120; echo train length 8).

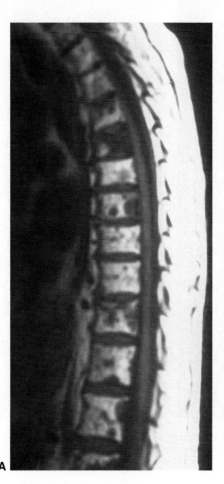

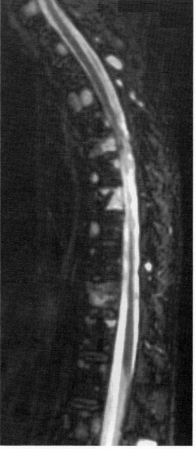

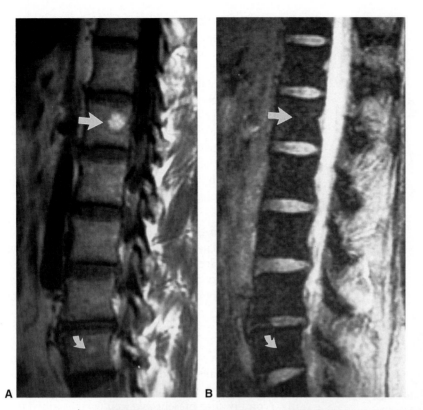

Figure 5-39 Cavernous hemangioma. **A:** A well-circumscribed lesion of increased T1 signal is identified within L1 vertebral body (*arrow*). There is a similar but smaller lesion within L5 (*small curved arrows*). **B:** They become isointense to normal bone marrow on this with T2-weighted gradient echo image. (TR 350 ms, TE 20 ms, 12° flip angle).

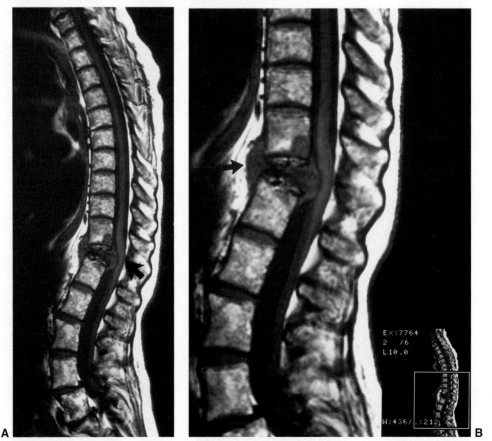

Figure 5-40 Metastasis with cord compression. **A:** T1-weighted image showing a pathologic fracture of T12 from breast carcinoma metastasis. Epidural extension of neoplasm compresses the thoracic cord (*arrow*). **B:** This is better seen on a 2 × magnification view. Note the paraspinal mass (*arrow*).

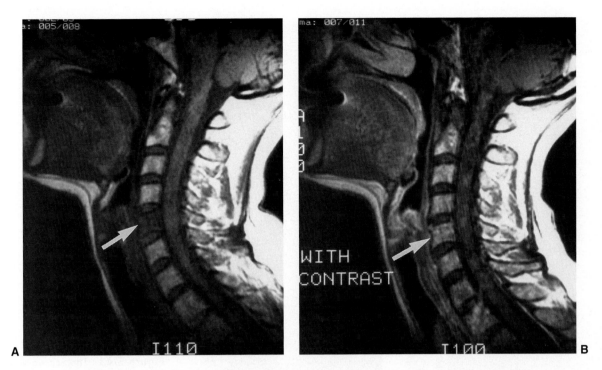

Figure 5-41 Enhancing metastasis. **A:** Note the loss of the normal T1 marrow fat signal of C5 from a breast carcinoma metastasis (*arrow*). **B:** The metastasis is difficult to identify after contrast is administered, because it enhances similar to normal bone marrow (*arrow*). (From Miller GM, Forbes GS, Onofrio BM. Magnetic resonance imaging of the spine. *Mayo Clin Proc* 1989;64:986–1004.)

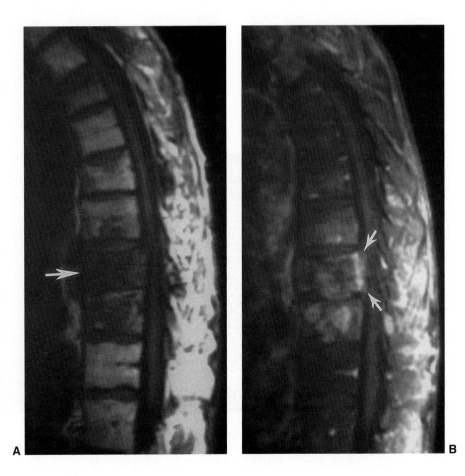

Figure 5-42 Metastatic carcinoid. **A:** Carcinoid metastasis to the thoracic spine including complete involvement of the T9 vertebral body (*arrow*). **B:** Enhancement and epidural extension (*arrows*) is easily seen with fat suppression.

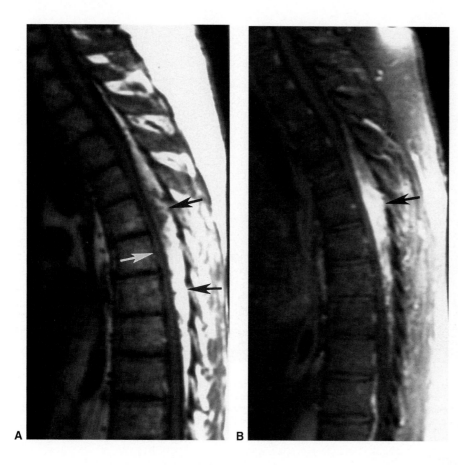

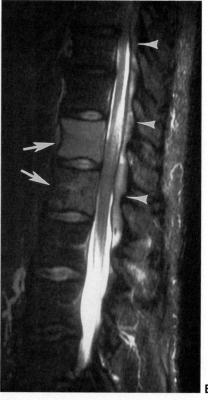

Figure 5-43 Thoracic epidural angiolipoma. **A:** Thoracic cord compression (*white arrow*), from a large posterior epidural mass (*black arrows*). **B:** The mass enhances heterogeneously with fat suppression (*arrow*). Angiolipoma was found at surgery.

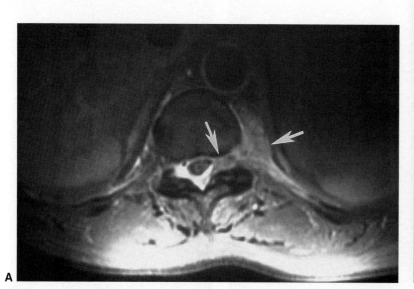

Figure 5-44 Lymphoma. **A:** Extension of paraspinal lymphoma through the neural foramen into the epidural space is best seen with contrast and fat suppression (*arrows*). **B:** Vertebral (*arrows*) and epidural (*arrowheads*) lymphoma (T2-weighted fast spin echo).

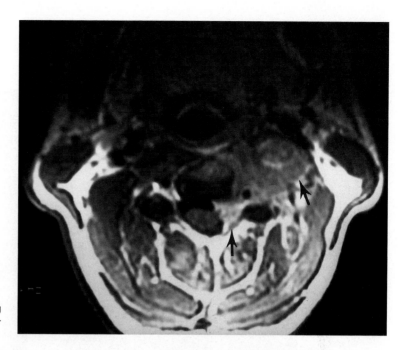

Figure 5-45 Cervical sarcoma. An enhancing paraspinal sarcoma extends through the neural foramen into the epidural space (*arrows*).

They are usually isointense to cord parenchyma on T1- and T2-weighted or gradient echo sequences. Areas of decreased signal relative to the cord parenchyma may also be observed depending on the presence or absence of calcium (see Fig. 5-46). Because these lesions lack a blood–brain barrier, they enhance homogeneously (105–107). A broad base of attachment to the dura or a dural tail may be present (see Fig. 5-47).

Neurogenic Tumor

In contrast to meningioma, neurogenic tumors (neurilemoma and neurofibroma) can occur anywhere in the spinal canal. There is no sex predilection, and they tend to occur in a slightly younger population. The presenting symptoms depend on their location (cervical, thoracic, lumbar) and may be similar to that seen in meningioma. They are more likely to be multiple. A neurilemoma (schwannoma) is a neoplasm of the nerve sheath that arises from the Schwann cells, whereas a neurofibroma is a neoplasm of the nerve itself. Neurofibromas may occur in patients without neurofibromatosis.

The typical appearance of a neurogenic tumor is a well-circumscribed, slightly lobulated, intradural extramedullary mass located lateral or posterolateral to the spinal cord. Sixteen percent have an extradural component that extends through the neural foramen into the paraspinal soft tissues (dumbbell tumor) (28). The extradural component may be quite prominent and often widens the neural foramen. Like meningiomas, neurogenic tumors tend to be isointense to the spinal cord parenchyma on T1- and T2-weighted or gradient echo sequences. However, their MR appearance is more variable, as neurogenic tumors have a propensity to undergo cystic degeneration and central necrosis that makes them hypointense on T1-weighted sequences and hyperintense on T2-weighted sequences, similar to CSF (108,109).

If large areas of cystic degeneration or necrosis are present, they may be difficult to identify on noncontrast studies, especially if a large FOV is used. Their appearance on post contrast T1-weighted sequences varies as they may

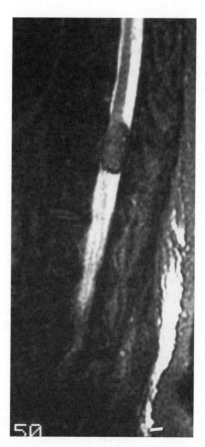

Figure 5-46 Meningioma. This well-circumscribed intradural extramedullary mass at T10 proved to be a calcified meningioma at surgery (TR 1,500 ms, TE 140 ms).

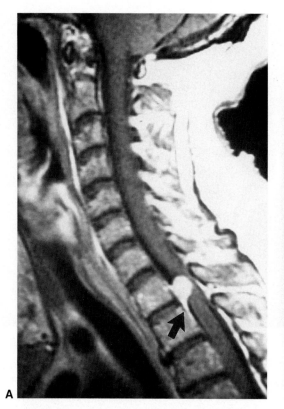

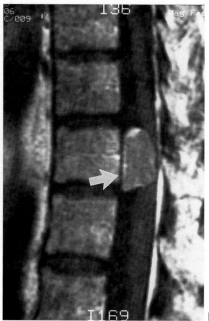

Figure 5-47 Meningioma. Two different patients with homogeneously enhancing intradural meningiomas. Note the dural tail in **(A)** (*arrow*) and the broad base of attachment to the dura in **(B)** (*arrow*).

enhance homogeneously, inhomogeneously, or peripherally, depending upon the degree of cystic degeneration (see Fig. 5-48).

Lipoma

Lipomas are congenital embryonal tumors (like dermoids and epidermoids) that arise from implantation of embryonic cutaneous ectoderm during neural tube closure. Intraspinal lipomas demonstrate signal changes similar to fat elsewhere and are hyperintense to the spinal cord parenchyma on T1-weighted and RARE T2-weighted sequences and hypointense on conventional T2-weighted or gradient echo sequences (see Fig. 5-49). The normal bright T1 signal can be confused with enhancement if contrast studies are obtained without fat suppression, which could lead to an erroneous diagnosis of meningioma or neurogenic tumor. These uncommon intraspinal lesions can occur anywhere in the spinal canal, but are often located at or near the conus medullaris in conjunction with spinal dysraphism. Tending to be well circumscribed, these slightly lobulated tumors usually do not deform the spinal cord. They often present in adolescence or early adulthood if they are associated with cord tethering. Some may cause symptoms if large (see Fig. 5-50); others are found incidentally in patients being evaluated for nonspinal indications.

Intradural Cyst

Spinal intradural cysts are a rare cause of symptomatic compressive myelopathy. Cysts in this location include meningeal, arachnoid, ependymal, enterogenous or neurenteric, teratogenous, and epithelial cysts (110). Most of these lesions are congenital and can have associated spinal anomalies. Ependymal cysts are thought to arise from ectopic ependymal fragments displaced from the central canal during development and can potentially occur anywhere along the spinal axis. Enterogenous cysts are derived from remnants of the primitive neurenteric canal and can be found in the thoracic spine or most commonly ventrally at the cervicothoracic junction. Meningeal cysts have been classified by Nabors et al. (111) Types I (without nerve roots) and II (with nerve roots) are usually asymptomatic but often result in adjacent bone remodeling. Type III or arachnoid cysts are the most common intradural cysts and have a peak incidence in the fifth decade, which is later than the other congenital cysts. They may also result from chronic inflammation or prior trauma and are then termed subarachnoid cysts. MR has been shown to be the most efficient preoperative study to diagnose and characterize the cysts and to evaluate for other associated spinal anomalies (see Fig 5-51) (112). Myelography may occasionally better define the cyst if MR findings are equivocal (see Fig. 5-52).

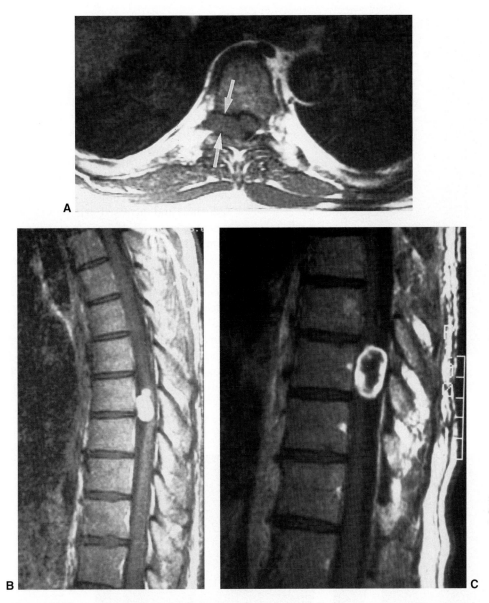

Figure 5-48 Neurilemoma. These three cases illustrate their varied appearances on T1-weighted imaging. **A:** This "dumbbell" neurilemoma expands the T8 neural foramen (*arrows*). **B:** Post-contrast image in another patient shows a slightly lobulated enhancing intradural mass at the T8 interspace. **C:** This necrotic enhancing neurilemoma was difficult to identify without contrast.

Intradural Metastasis

Intradural metastases may be dropped metastases from midline primary CNS neoplasms (pineal tumors, ependymoma, medulloblastoma, glioblastoma), local invasion from primary spinal cord neoplasms (ependymoma) or hematogenously disseminated to the CSF from aggressive nonneurologic primary neoplasms (breast, lung, melanoma). Unless large, these deposits of tumor are difficult to visualize on noncontrast sequences (113,114). On contrast sequences, nonspecific pial enhancement can be identified which may be focal or extensive, coating the pial surface of the cord and cauda equina (see Fig. 5-53). The accuracy of MR versus CT myelography in the detection

of meningeal tumor spread has not been determined although some researchers report increased detectability on contrast enhanced MR (see Fig. 5-54) (107). Certainly MRI is noninvasive and therefore the preferred imaging test. CSF cytology is more accurate than either imaging study and remains the gold standard for the diagnosis of meningeal metastases.

Intramedullary Lesions

Ependymoma

Ependymoma is the most common primary cord neoplasm, accounting for approximately 62% in some series (28). They commonly occur within the conus and filum

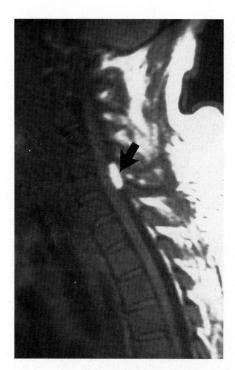

Figure 5-49 Intradural lipoma. The T1 signal of this incidental intradural mass is similar to the subcutaneous fat (*arrow*).

terminale but may be found anywhere in the spinal cord. There is no sex predilection and they most often occur in the third through the sixth decades of life. They are slow growing, benign, well-circumscribed lesions that may be focal or involve long segments of the cord. They often result in remodeling and expansion of the spinal canal. Ependymomas may contain areas of prior hemorrhage, cystic degeneration, calcium, or an associated spinal cord cyst that expands the cord above and/or below the neoplasm.

MR features include fusiform intramedullary expansion of the spinal cord parenchyma in conjunction with decreased signal relative to the cord on T1-weighted sequences and increased signal on T2-weighted or gradient echo sequences. If the ependymoma arises from the filum terminale, an intradural mass separate from the conus can be seen that cannot be differentiated from a neurogenic tumor (see Fig. 5-55). The signal changes are often complex depending on the presence or absence of hemorrhage, calcium, or necrosis. The presence of an associated spinal cord cyst often complicates the imaging appearance (115). The cyst usually contains a high protein fluid, may appear solid, and may be difficult to distinguish from the ependymoma or edema. The ependymoma may be disproportionately small relative to the length of the cord cyst and

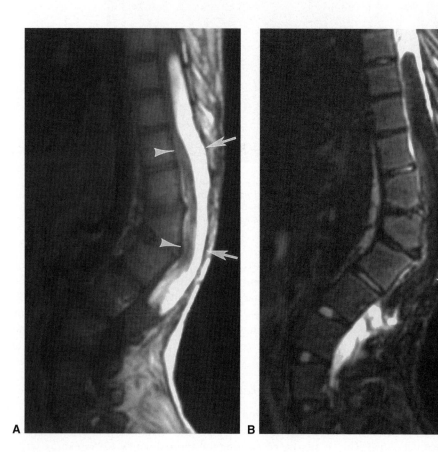

Figure 5-50 Large thoracic intradural lipoma. **A:** Thoracic cord compression (*arrow heads*) results from this large intradural lipoma, demonstrating typical bright T1 signal (*arrows*). **B:** STIR imaging results in expected fat suppression of the mass (*arrows*) (IR 150, TR 3,000, TE 100, echo train length 8).

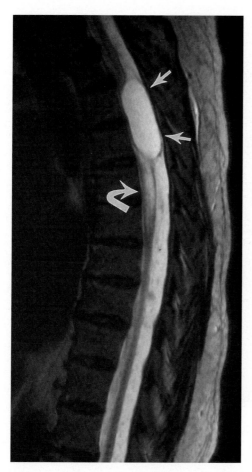

Figure 5-51 Thoracic intradural arachnoid cyst. Sagittal T2-weighted fast spin-echo image showing thoracic cord compression by a posterior intradural arachnoid cyst (*arrows*). Note signal changes in the cord below the cyst (*curved arrow*).

difficult to identify on noncontrast studies. Postcontrast T1-weighted sequences are essential in the evaluation of intramedullary neoplasms (96,105,106,109,116,117). The margins of the tumor enhance, allowing it to be separated from edema or a cord cyst. This better delineates the neoplasm within the cord, limiting the size of the laminectomy required (see Fig. 5-56).

Astrocytoma

Astrocytomas are the second most common spinal intramedullary glioma. However, they are more common than ependymomas if filum tumors are excluded. They present at a slightly earlier age than ependymomas (30s to 40s) and lack a sex predilection. They are the most common primary spinal cord neoplasms in children. The degree of malignancy varies, and higher grades of malignancy tend to afflict patients who present at the younger ages. The MR appearance is also variable and similar to that seen in ependymomas (106,109,117). In the young, these tumors tend to be more infiltrative, involve long segments

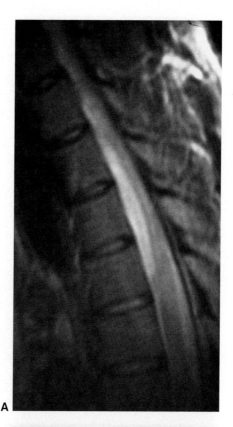

A

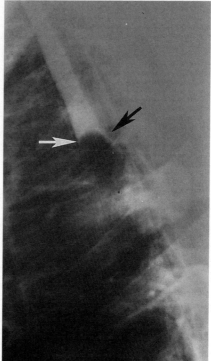

B

Figure 5-52 Thoracic intradural arachnoid cyst. **A:** T2-weighted fast spin-echo image shows posterior displacement of the thoracic cord, but no obvious mass. **B:** The anterior intradural mass is more evident on myelography with a meniscus sign (*white arrow*), compressing the thoracic cord (*black arrow*).

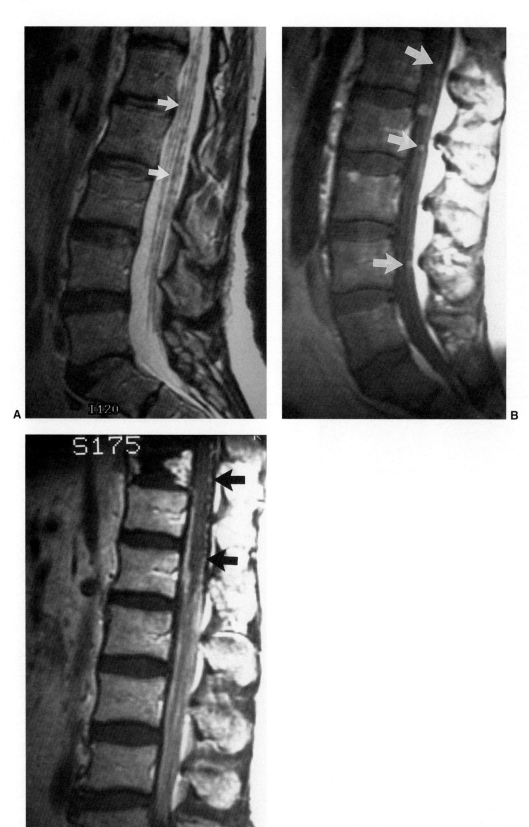

Figure 5-53 Intradural metastasis. **A:** Breast carcinoma metastasis. Sagittal T2-weighted fast spin-echo showing multiple tiny nodules adherent to the cauda equina (*arrows*). **B:** Metastatic melanoma. Note the larger enhancing deposits of neoplasm (*arrows*). **C:** Lymphoma. Diffuse "sheet-like" enhancement coats the cauda equina and spreads along the pial surface of the cord (*arrows*).

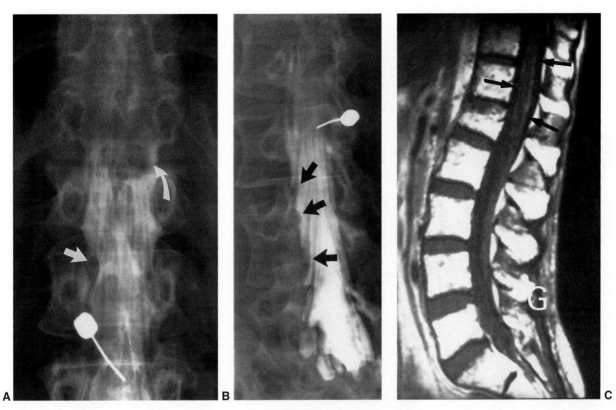

Figure 5-54 Intradural metastasis. **A:** AP and (**B**) oblique myelogram demonstrates metastatic deposits along multiple nerve roots of the cauda equina (*arrows*) and a larger deposit at the conus (*curved arrow*). **C:** This enhanced MR was obtained hours after the myelogram. Only equivocal pial enhancement of the cord surface is identified (*arrows*). Note the bright T1 vertebral body signal from radiation. (From Miller GM, Forbes GS, Onofrio BM. Magnetic resonance imaging of the spine. *Mayo Clin Proc* 1989;64:986–1004.)

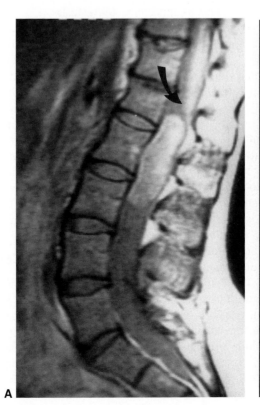

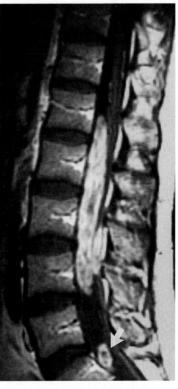

Figure 5-55 Ependymoma. **A:** A well-circumscribed intradural mass is seen that is separate from the conus (*curved arrow*) (TR 1,500 ms, TE 30 ms). **B:** This large enhancing ependymoma in another patient arose from the filum terminale and was easily removed at surgery. The second, smaller enhancing mass at S1 (*arrow*) was adherent to the dura and cauda equina and could not be removed, presumably a metastatic deposit.

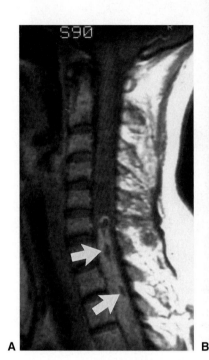

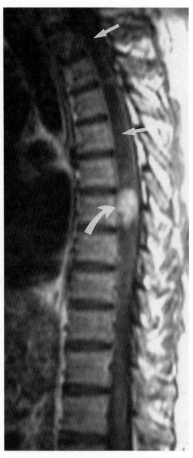

Figure 5-56 Ependymoma. **A:** Postcontrast image demonstrates a long enhancing intramedullary mass; the lower portion is not included on this image. Note the areas of necrosis (*arrows*) and mass effect. **B:** This T7 ependymoma (*curved arrow*) in another patient is small but results in a long syrinx cavity that extends well into the cervical region (*arrows*). (Fig. 5-46 B From Miller GM, Forbes GS, Onofrio BM. Magnetic resonance imaging of the spine. *Mayo Clinic Proc* 1989;64: 986–1004.)

of the spinal cord and have a more homogeneous appearance on MRI (see Fig. 5-57A). Astrocytomas that present in adults tend to be more heterogenous and may contain cysts, necrosis, or hemorrhage (see Fig 5-57 B to D). As in ependymoma, postcontrast T1-weighted sequences are necessary to define the extent of the neoplasm.

Hemangioblastoma

Hemangioblastoma is an uncommon, benign, primary spinal cord neoplasm often associated with von Hippel-Lindau disease. The neoplasm may be solitary or multiple, is pial based, and most often located in the cervical cord. Hemangioblastomas enhance intensely with contrast and may be associated with a tumor cyst (see Fig. 5-58) (105,106,117). These are intensely vascular neoplasms that drain into the posterior pial venous plexus. Associated findings include serpentine flow voids along the dorsal aspect of the cord (see Fig. 5-59). The combination of abnormal vasculature and a cystic intramedullary mass with an enhancing nodule suggests the diagnosis of hemangioblastoma, In the absence of a cystic intramedullary mass, the differential diagnosis would include a spinal vascular malformation.

Metastasis

Intramedullary metastases are uncommon, occurring in only 1% to 3% of tumor patients (118). They may be from primary CNS neoplasms spread via CSF pathways with secondary spinal cord invasion or hematogenously spread from non–CNS primary tumors. The metastatic deposits may be single or multiple and result in fusiform or irregular cord enlargement or no enlargement at all. The involved spinal cord often shows decreased signal on T1-weighted and increased signal on T2-weighted sequences predominately secondary to edema. The metastatic deposit itself is often small, asymmetrically involving only a portion of the cord parenchyma. It may only be identified on postcontrast images (see Fig. 5-60).

Inflammatory Conditions

Inflammatory processes may affect both the spinal column and the spinal cord. Inflammatory diseases of the spinal column include disc space infection, osteomyelitis of the vertebral bodies, paraspinal abscess, and epidural inflammation or abscess. These patients present with a wide variety of symptoms, including sepsis, localized pain and tenderness,

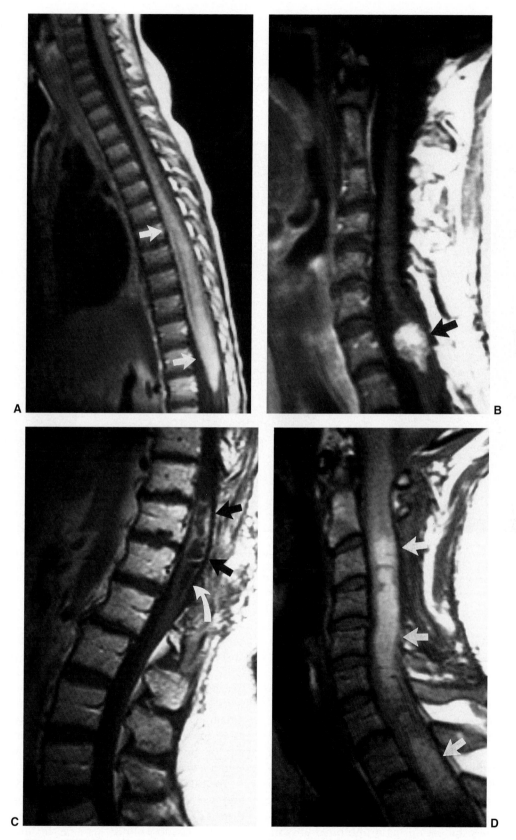

Figure 5-57 Astrocytoma. **A:** This child has an infiltrative enhancing mass within the distal spinal cord and conus (*arrows*). **B:** This C7 astrocytoma in an adult is well circumscribed and enhances homogeneously (*arrow*). **C:** Partially cystic or necrotic enhancing recurrent astrocytoma (*arrows*) results in a syrinx below the neoplasm (*curved arrow*). **D:** Noncontrast view shows high T1 signal changes (*arrows*) within an expanded cervical cord. At surgery, acute hemorrhage (hematomyelia) into an astrocytoma was found.

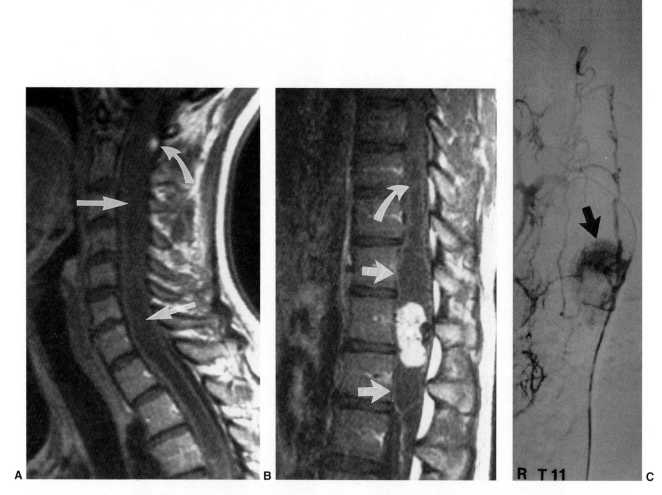

Figure 5-58   Hemangioblastoma. **A:** Postcontrast image demonstrates an expanded cord from a long syrinx cavity (*arrows*). The pial-based hemangioblastoma is located at C1 (*curved arrow*). **B:** This enhancing hemangioblastoma in another patient is much larger and is associated with a tumor cyst (*arrows*) and a syrinx (*curved arrow*). **C:** Spinal angiogram from the patient illustrated in **B** confirms the presence of a vascular neoplasm (*arrow*) fed by the right T11 intercostal artery.

and paraplegia. MRI is particularly suited for evaluation of suspected spinal infection as myelography risks iatrogenic meningitis.

Pyogenic Discitis

Disc space infection may be localized to one disc space or uncommonly may involve multiple intervertebral discs. Pyogenic organisms from remote septic foci spread hematogenously to the spinal column initially to the vertebral body endplates. From there, these organisms gain access to the intervertebral discs. The discs are relatively avascular and are unable to mount an inflammatory reaction which allows the organisms uninhibited growth. This together with the proteolytic enzymes released results in rapid destruction of the intervertebral disc. The adjacent endplate is then quickly invaded. Depending on the time course and the virulence of the organism, the

entire vertebral body can be involved with osteomyelitis. There may be an associated paraspinal or epidural abscess. Once the infection has spread to the epidural space, it is free to extend above and below the involved interspace for several segments. The epidural component may consist of inflammatory reaction (pannus) or abscess. If large, it may cause spinal cord compromise, resulting in a compressive myelopathy or cord infarction from thrombophlebitis of epidural spinal veins.

The MR findings in pyogenic disc space infection have been well described (119,120). On T1-weighted sequences there is decreased signal intensity within the involved intervertebral disc, loss of disc space height, and loss of normal marrow signal within the adjacent vertebral body endplates. The vertebral body changes may be minimal or extensive, depending on the degree of associated osteomyelitis. The intervertebral disc demonstrates high signal on T2-weighted

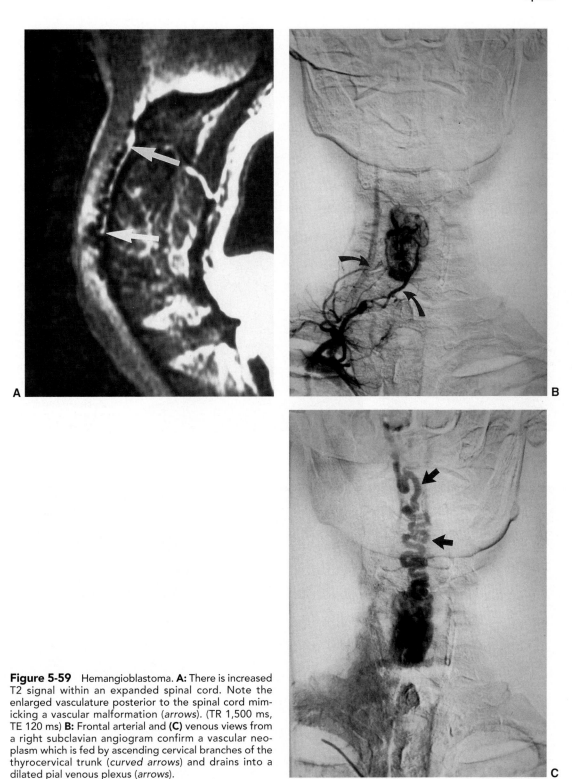

Figure 5-59 Hemangioblastoma. **A:** There is increased T2 signal within an expanded spinal cord. Note the enlarged vasculature posterior to the spinal cord mimicking a vascular malformation (*arrows*). (TR 1,500 ms, TE 120 ms) **B:** Frontal arterial and **(C)** venous views from a right subclavian angiogram confirm a vascular neoplasm which is fed by ascending cervical branches of the thyrocervical trunk (*curved arrows*) and drains into a dilated pial venous plexus (*arrows*).

images and enhances following contrast administration. The adjacent endplates may also demonstrate increased T2-weighted signal, but this is not a consistent finding (see Fig. 5-61) (121). These findings are thought to be fairly specific for pyogenic infection because metastasis rarely involves the intervertebral discs and adjacent vertebral bodies.

Paraspinal or Epidural Abscess

Paraspinal abscesses are best identified on axial T1- or T2-weighted sequences as soft tissue masses or fluid collections that may be loculated or enhance (see Fig. 5-62). Hematogenously disseminated pyogenic organisms may primarily infect the epidural space. MRI is ideal to evaluate

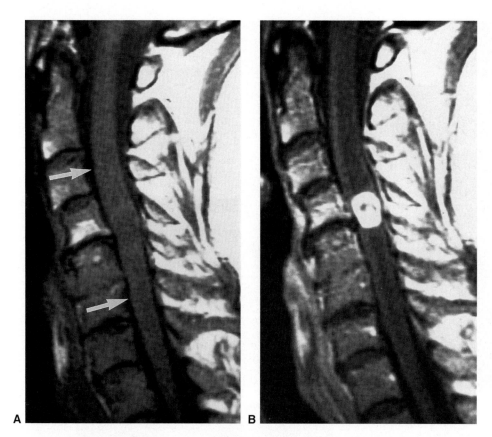

A

B

Figure 5-60 Intramedullary metastasis. **A:** Sagittal T1-weighted image showing nonspecific mass effect within a long segment of the spinal cord (*arrows*). **B:** On the postcontrast image, an enhancing mass, which proved to be a metastasis at surgery, is identified.

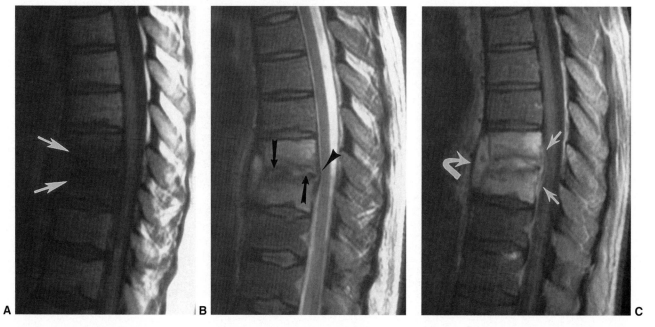

A   B   C

Figure 5-61 Pyogenic disc space infection. **A:** There is abnormal T1 vertebral body marrow signal (*arrows*) and the intervertebral disc is difficult to discern in this intravenous drug abuser. **B:** On a T2-weighted fast spin-echo image, the disc and adjacent vertebral bodies have high signal (*arrows*). Epidural inflammation partially compresses the spinal cord (*arrowhead*). **C:** Diffuse enhancement, including prevertebral (*curved arrow*) and epidural (*arrows*) extension, is best seen with fat suppression.

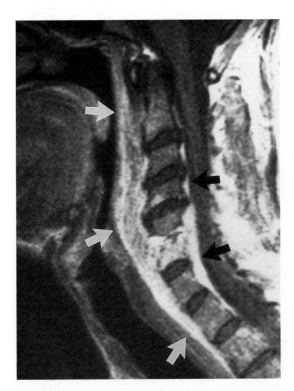

Figure 5-62 Pyogenic disc space infection. This postcontrast image in a patient with a C5 disc space infection has enhancing prevertebral (*white arrows*) and epidural (*black arrows*) spread of inflammation.

epidural spread of inflammation, which is best identified on the T2-weighted sequences (see Fig. 5-63) (122,123). An epidural abscess may be difficult to distinguish from adjacent CSF signal changes in the presence of spinal meningitis (123). Contrast is particularly useful for diagnosis in these cases. It is also helpful in determining the extent and location of the abscess and monitoring the response to treatment (124). Although MRI should be the initial screening procedure in patients with spinal infection, occasionally myelography with CT may be needed as a supplemental study in patients with a nondiagnostic study.

Spinal neuropathic arthropathy (Charcot spine) is an uncommon destructive process that affects the intervertebral disc space, adjoining vertebral bodies, and facet joints. Differentiation from pyogenic discitis, both clinically and radiographically, can be difficult. Vacuum disc, facet involvement, vertebral body spondylolisthesis, intervertebral joint disorganization and debris (osseous fragments), diffuse vertebral body signal abnormality, and rim enhancement of the disc have been shown by Wagner et al. (125) to indicate spinal neuropathic arthropathy.

Tuberculous Spondylitis

Tuberculous spondylitis is uncommon and differs from pyogenic discitis and osteomyelitis clinically and on MRI (126–128). Its onset is insidious, with symptoms ranging from months to years as opposed to days to months in patients with pyogenic infections. The MR findings, which resemble neoplasm, include widespread destruction of the vertebral bodies and relative preservation of the disc spaces. The anterior inferior aspect of the vertebral body is classically affected first, resulting in a gibbous deformity. The entire vertebral body may be involved, including the posterior elements. The infection tends to spread subligamentously, often affecting multiple vertebral bodies (126–128). Extension into the paraspinal soft tissues with abscess formation is common. Differentiation from neoplasm may be impossible on the basis of MR images alone. Other uncommon infections that may have a similar imaging appearance include brucellosis and blastomycosis (see Fig. 5-64).

Spinal Cord Infection or Inflammation

Inflammatory diseases of the spinal cord parenchyma are rare. Cord infections and inflammation from pyogenic organisms, fungi, tuberculosis, cysticercosis, and sarcoidosis have been reported (129–132). The MR appearance of these lesions is limited to individual case reports. In general, these lesions show nonspecific intramedullary mass effect with decreased signal on T1-weighted and increased signal on T2-weighted sequences within the cord parenchyma. Postcontrast studies help localize areas of active inflammation, granuloma, or abscess formation, differentiating them from the surrounding edema. We have observed patchy intramedullary enhancement and linear leptomeningeal enhancement in both tuberculosis (see Fig. 5-65) and sarcoid myelitis (see Fig. 5-66). Although it is difficult, or impossible, to distinguish cord infections from neoplasm, their extensive nature, patchy enhancement following contrast administration, and propensity for leptomeningeal involvement may suggest an inflammatory or infectious etiology.

Transverse Myelitis

Idiopathic acute transverse myelitis is an inflammatory condition of the spinal cord of indeterminate etiology. Suggested etiologies have focused on an autoimmune process with a possible contribution from small vessel vasculopathy (133).

It may present in a variety of clinical settings, including acquired immunodeficiency syndrome, and may be related to an allergic, viral, or paraneoplastic process. Patients usually present clinically with a rapid onset of bilateral motor, sensory, and autonomic dysfunction in the spinal cord. The midthoracic cord is commonly involved. The study may be normal initially. Long segmental intramedullary expansion can be seen with decreased signal on T1-weighted and increased signal on T2-weighted sequences (see Fig. 5-67) (130,134,135). Holocord involvement of both gray and white matter is usually seen. The enhancement pattern is variable but tends to be patchy and peripheral. The findings may be indistinguishable from neoplasm or multiple sclerosis (MS), although MS plaques tend to be located more peripherally in the cord (i.e., white

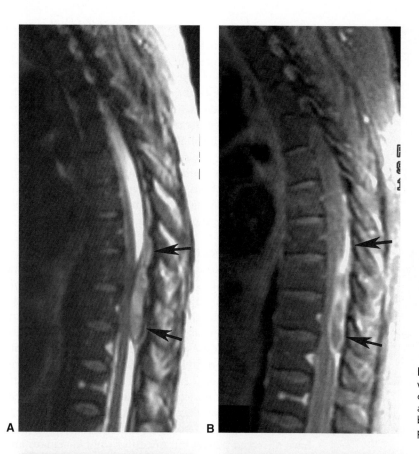

A   B

Figure 5-63 Epidural abscess. **A:** Sagittal T2-weighted fast spin-echo image shows thoracic cord compression from a posterior epidural abscess (*arrows*). **B:** Epidural enhancement is best seen with fat suppression (*arrows*). The patient had a recent liver transplant.

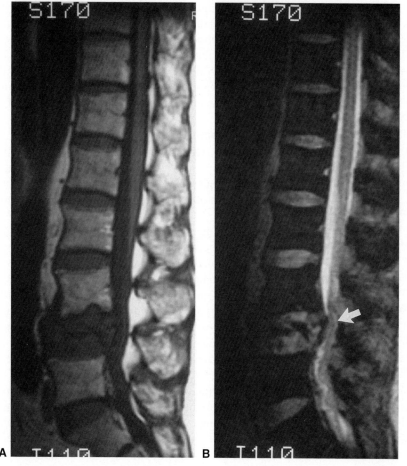

A   B

Figure 5-64 Blastomycosis. **A:** T1-weighted image showing destruction and near complete collapse of L4 vertebra with relative sparing of the intervertebral discs and adjacent vertebral bodies. **B:** Retropulsion of the posterior aspect of the L4 body into the spinal canal results in central canal stenosis (*arrow*) (TR 400 ms, TE 20 ms, 12° flip angle).

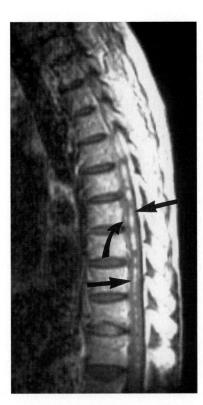

Figure 5-65 Tuberculous myelitis. Contrast enhanced image demonstrates unusual nodular parenchymal enhancement (*arrows*) and subtle pial enhancement (*curved arrow*). An open biopsy performed for diagnosis demonstrated acid fast bacilli.

matter) and have a length less than two vertebral segments. The MR abnormalities are often more extensive than predicted clinically. This disparity, as well as the relative acute onset of symptoms, helps distinguish this condition from neoplasm.

Radiation Myelitis

Radiation-induced damage to the spinal cord is a known serious complication of radiation treatment for head and neck neoplasms, lung carcinoma, Hodgkin disease, and thymoma. The spectrum of conditions associated with prior radiation range from acute transient radiation myelopathy to chronic progressive radiation myelitis. The incidence of radiation damage is related to a number of factors including the total radiation dose [>5,500 rads (cGy)], dose fraction size, treatment time, length of cord irradiated, and technical errors (136). The latent period of chronic progressive radiation myelitis is typically 2 to 19 months, after which patients present with a subacute onset of a progressive myelopathy. The diagnosis is one of exclusion, and the role of imaging is to exclude other causes of myelopathy such as extradural compression or intramedullary metastasis/primary neoplasm.

The MR appearance of radiation myelitis has been described (137–139). The findings have been found to be related more to the timing of the MR after the onset of symptoms than to the radiation dose (137,138). Mass

Figure 5-66 Sarcoid myelitis. **A:** This enhanced view demonstrates intramedullary cord expansion, patchy parenchymal enhancement, which is broad based to the pial surface (*straight arrow*) and subtle linear pial enhancement (*curved arrow*). The diagnosis was made by an open biopsy. Note the decompressive laminectomy performed elsewhere for presumed compressive myelopathy. **B:** Follow-up contrast enhanced study shows resolution of abnormal enhancement and mass effect (TR 500 ms, TE 20 ms). (From Nesbit GM, Miller GM, Baker HL Jr, et. al. Spinal cord sarcoidosis: a new finding at MR imaging with Gd-DTPA enhancement. *Radiology* 1989; 173:839–843.)

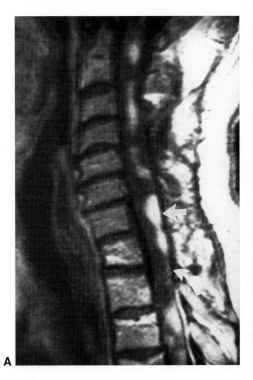

A

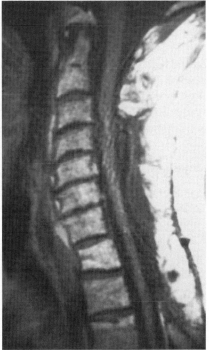

B

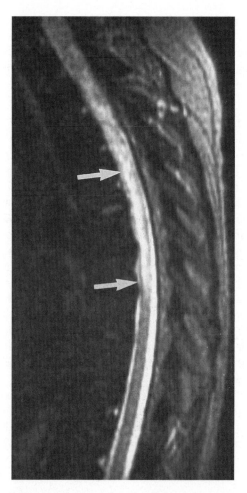

Figure 5-67 Transverse myelitis. Subtle intramedullary mass effect and abnormal T2 signal in a long segment of the upper and mid thoracic spinal cord. An open biopsy performed to exclude neoplasm demonstrated only inflammation. (TR 1,500 ms, TE 140 ms).

(141) and fast STIR sequences have been found to improve detection of spinal plaques (see Fig. 5-69) (142,143). Spinal cord plaques present as asymmetric areas of increased T2 signal within the cord parenchyma and most often involve the posterior (41%) and lateral (25%) columns (144,145). The plaques can be seen anywhere along the entire length of the spinal cord (see Fig. 5-70), but most tend to occur in the cervical region (see Fig. 5-71). They range in length from 2 to 64 mm, with 84% of the lesions measuring less than 15 mm. About two thirds of the time they are solitary, with 13% of patients showing three or more lesions. Mass effect is uncommon, being seen in up to 14% (145).

In our series, approximately half of the plaques enhanced with gadolinium on the initial examination (see Fig. 5-72) (145). Other series have also shown variable plaque enhancement (117,146). The findings from these series imply that the enhancement characteristics of cord plaques may parallel those seen in the head where enhancement indicates active lesions. The lack of enhancement does not necessarily imply inactivity, however. Interestingly, Larsson et al. (146) noted that the enhancement was maximal on delayed images obtained 45 to 60 minutes after contrast infusion. This characteristic is different from intraspinal neoplasms where enhancement is usually, but not always, maximal immediately following injection (147).

In patients in whom the spinal images suggest a demyelinating lesion, a head MRI may be of value in that up to 76% of patients may have additional lesions on the head MRI at the time of presentation (see Fig. 5-73) (145). Occasionally, a biopsy may be necessary to exclude the possibility of neoplasm.

Congenital Spinal Abnormalities

Congenital spinal abnormalities encompass a wide variety of conditions, including spinal dysraphism, sacral anomalies and caudal regression, vertebral body abnormalities and congenital scoliosis, and the Arnold-Chiari malformation. There is considerable overlap among these conditions that may occur by themselves or in association with the others. MR is the imaging modality of choice for the noninvasive evaluation of patients with known or suspected congenital abnormalities.

Spinal Dysraphism

Spinal dysraphism is a general term that denotes incomplete midline fusion of mesenchymal, bone, and neural elements. Spina bifida refers to failure of fusion of the vertebral column that may be occult or obvious with a prominent skin defect and exposure of neural elements. The latter condition is referred to as spina bifida aperta and encompasses a variety of conditions including meningocele, myelocele, meningomyelocele, and myelocystocele. In meningocele, only the meninges and subarachnoid spaces protrude through the skin defect. A myelocele is a condition where the distal spinal cord terminates in a neural placode with

effect and high T2 signal within the cord parenchyma can be seen within 8 months after the onset of symptoms. The T2 changes extend over multiple levels within the boundary of the radiation field. Focal patchy enhancement can also be present. Spinal cord atrophy is a late finding (see Fig. 5-68).

Demyelinating Disease

MRI is the modality of choice in evaluating patients for the presence of spinal cord demyelinating plaques and is the only modality that allows direct visualization of these lesions. Although the clinical diagnosis of MS is well-established in many patients at the time of imaging, a spinal cord plaque may be the initial presenting symptom in 10% of patients.

The evolution of MR technology brings with it controversy concerning the optimal pulse sequence or combination of sequences for detecting spinal cord plaques. Fast fluid attenuated inversion recovery (FLAIR) sequences have not been found to be as useful in the spine as in the brain (140), while magnetization transfer-prepared gradient echo

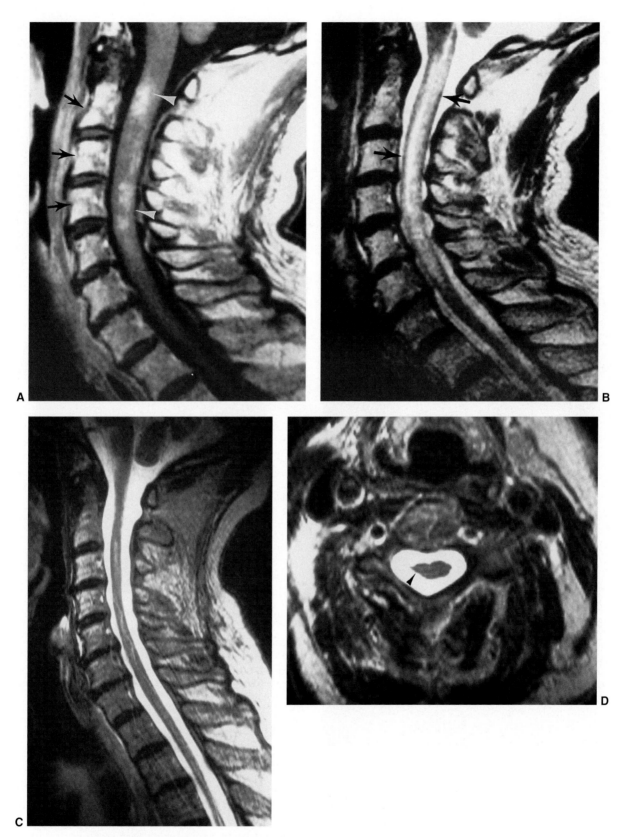

Figure 5-68   Radiation myelitis. This patient presented with myelopathy months following radiation for a right facial cancer. **A:** Patchy enhancement of the cord (*white arrowheads*) is within the radiation field as shown by the marrow changes in the vertebral bodies (*black arrows*). **B:** T2-weighted fast spin-echo shows cord swelling with T2 signal (*arrows*). Sagittal **(C)** and axial **(D)** images from a later study show predominantly right-sided cord atrophy (*arrowhead*). An extensive workup to exclude other causes of parenchymal enhancement was negative.

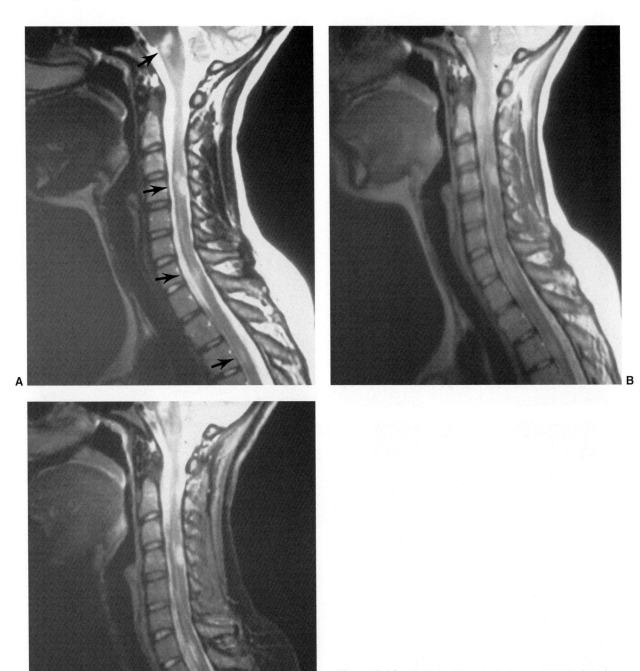

Figure 5-69 Multiple sclerosis. Brain stem, cervical, and upper thoracic demyelinating plaques (*arrows*) are demonstrated on multiple pulse sequences. **A:** T2-weighted (TR 4,000 ms, TE 120 ms, echo train length 16). **B:** Proton density weighted (TR 3,000 ms, TE 20 ms, echo train length 4). **C:** Short TI inversion recovery (IR 150 ms; TR 2,500 ms, TE 20 ms, echo train length 8).

neural tissues being exposed at the skin surface. The protruding myelocele may be surrounded by the meninges and subarachnoid space forming a meningomyelocele. In myelocystocele, cystic dilatation of the distal spinal cord central canal protrudes through the defect. This condition may be difficult to distinguish from meningomyelocele. However, in myelocystocele, the cystic cavity is lined by ependymal cells rather than arachnoid.

Spina bifida occulta or occult spinal dysraphism denotes a group of skin-covered abnormalities that may be minimal with isolated failure of fusion of the posterior elements of a vertebral body. More severe forms of occult spinal dysraphism include tethered cord, thickened filum terminale, dorsal dermal sinus, diastematomyelia, and spinal lipomas. An abnormal skin patch, nevus, or dimple may signify the presence of the more severe intraspinal abnormalities.

MRI is particularly useful for the noninvasive evaluation of patients with known or suspected spinal dysraphism (see Fig. 5-74) (148–151). In addition to the risk of ionizing radiation and contrast reaction, the presence of a congenital abnormality increases the morbidity of the myelogram, because a spinal tap from the lumbar route risks puncture of a low-lying spinal cord and a cervical puncture risks quadriparesis or death from intraspinal hematoma or inadvertent cerebellar tonsillar puncture. In spinal dysraphism, the level of the neural placode or conus medullaris as well the presence and nature of an associated intraspinal mass can be easily identified. MRI is particularly well-suited for the screening of patients with suspected occult spinal dysraphism as the location of the conus medullaris can usually be determined on sagittal or coronal images (see Fig. 5-75). In questionable cases, axial sequences can be performed for precise localization. The conus medullaris usually reaches the adult level sometime during the first few months of life with a normal level of termination above the second lumbar interspace. A conus termination at or below the third lumbar interspace is abnormal at any age. A termination at L3 is abnormal in adults but indeterminate in the pediatric population (152). A thickness of the filum terminale greater than 2 mm is abnormal. The presence or absence of a tethering mass, as well as its composition (fatty or fibrous), can easily be determined.

Congenital Scoliosis and Segmentation Anomalies

Segmentation abnormalities of the vertebral bodies such as hemivertebrae, butterfly vertebrae, and block vertebrae

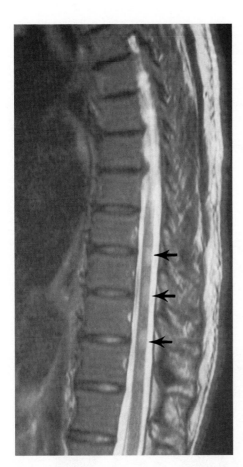

Figure 5-70   Thoracic multiple sclerosis. Sagittal T2-weighted fast spin-echo in a patient who presented with plaques only in the thoracic cord (*arrows*).

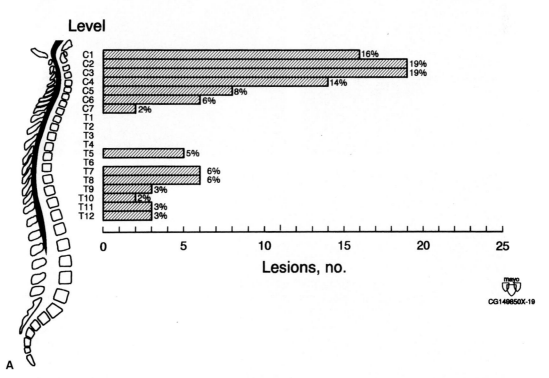

A

Figure 5-71   Multiple sclerosis. These bar graphs show the location of demyelinating plaques by **(A)** spinal cord level and **(B)** location in the transverse plane.

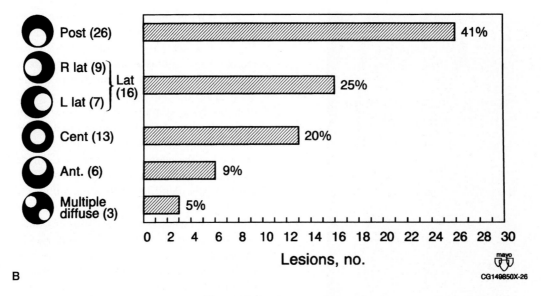

B

Figure 5-71 *(continued)*

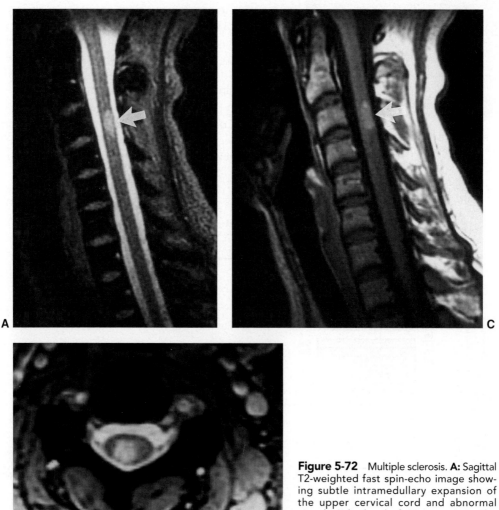

Figure 5-72 Multiple sclerosis. **A:** Sagittal T2-weighted fast spin-echo image showing subtle intramedullary expansion of the upper cervical cord and abnormal signal at the level of C3 (*arrow*). **B:** The cord plaque is located within the posterior column on the right (TR 300 ms, TE 20 ms, 10° flip angle). **C:** Note the subtle enhancement on this sagittal postcontrast image (*arrow*).

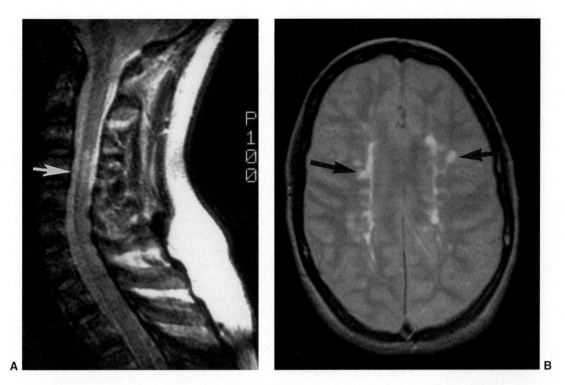

Figure 5-73   Multiple sclerosis. **A:** Sagittal T2-weighted fast spin-echo image shows abnormal signal within the cord parenchyma at C4 without mass effect (*arrow*). **B:** This axial image of the head confirms the diagnosis because multiple intracranial demyelinating plaques are also seen (*arrows*) (TR 2,000 ms, TE 40 ms).

Figure 5-74   Meningocele/meningomyelocele. **A:** The meninges and subarachnoid space extend through a bone defect in the upper sacrum (*arrows*) (TR 2,000 ms, TE 70 ms). **B:** T1-weighted image in another patient with spina bifida aperta. In addition to the meninges, neural elements extend through the defect in this child (*arrow*).

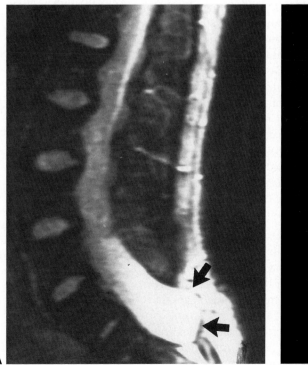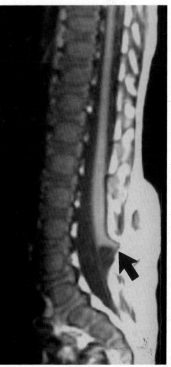

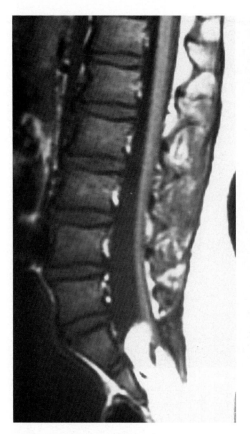

Figure 5-75 Tethered cord. The spinal cord ends at S1, tethered by a fibro-fatty mass with characteristic bright T1 signal.

result in congenital scoliosis. Intraspinal abnormalities seen in patients with congenital scoliosis include Chiari I and II malformations, syrinx, spinal cord tumor, tethered cord, myelomeningocele, and diastematomyelia (see Figs. 5-76 and 5-77) (153). Plain films best evaluate the vertebral body anomalies, whereas MRI best evaluates the presence or absence of associated intraspinal disorders. As previously discussed, patients with scoliosis are difficult to image by MRI because only small portions of spinal cord and canal are included on any one section. Curved reformatting or multiple oblique sagittal and coronal planes are needed for complete evaluation (see Fig. 5-78). Contrast agents may have a role in the evaluation of congenital scoliosis by increasing the conspicuity of an associated intraspinal mass.

Caudal Regression Syndrome

Sacral anomalies in the caudal regression syndrome cover a wide spectrum, ranging from minimal with absence of the coccyx to severe with absence of the distal spinal column, anal atresia, and malformation of the external genitalia. Associated conditions include tethered cord, meningocele, myelocele, and meningomyelocele (154).

When caudal regression is suspected, imaging the lower lumbar and sacral regions should be performed to verify the diagnosis. The level of vertebral regression, the presence of central spinal stenosis, and vertebral dysraphic anomalies

can be determined. A characteristic wedge-shaped (longer dorsally) cord terminus has been described (154).

Chiari Malformation

Arnold-Chiari malformations are complex hindbrain developmental abnormalities that are divided into three types depending on the degree of deformity present. Type I, the adult type, is characterized by inferior displacement of the cerebellar tonsils and medulla through the foramen magnum into the upper spinal canal. The cerebellar tonsils have an abnormal configuration, being pointed or beak shaped, indicating compression. There may be associated brain stem kinking or angulation present at the junction between the spinal cord medulla, or a spinal cord syrinx that may be septated. The fourth ventricle is near its normal position (see Fig. 5-79). Normally, the cerebellar tonsils project at or slightly below the posterior margin of the foramen magnum. However, in these instances the normal rounded configuration of the tonsils is preserved, which helps differentiate this condition from a mild type I malformation. Syringomyelia is likely caused by CSF flow obstruction due to the tonsillar ectopia, resulting in noncommunicating dilatation of the central canal. This often resolves following posterior fossa decompression (see Fig. 5-80) (155,156).

More severe hindbrain abnormalities are present in the type II malformation that presents in childhood. The posterior fossa is small, with caudal displacement of the medulla, cerebellar tonsils, and vermis through an enlarged foramen magnum. The fourth ventricle is inferiorly displaced. Because the cervical cord is firmly anchored by the dentate ligaments, downward descent of the medulla may result in a buckled or kinked appearance at the cervicomedullary junction. The inferior tip of the medulla forms a "spur" posterior to the cervical cord. Descent of the cerebellar tonsils can result in another tongue of tissue, or "peg," posterior to the medullary spur (see Fig. 5-81). Spinal dysraphism, such as meningocele or meningomyelocele, and hydrocephalus nearly always coexist. Other associated spinal abnormalities include syrinx and diastematomyelia. The type III malformation is the most severe, with caudal displacement of nearly the entire cerebellar hemisphere into an upper cervical or occipital encephalocele.

Abnormalities of the craniovertebral junction, such as the Chiari malformations, are best imaged on MR using sagittal or coronal sequences that allow accurate determination of the location of the cerebellar tonsils. The presence or absence of associated conditions, such as syringohydromyelia and spinal dysraphism, can also be determined (157–160).

Trauma

MR has been successfully used in the evaluation of both acute and chronic trauma (161–164). However, significant logistical hurdles exist that limit the usefulness of MRI in

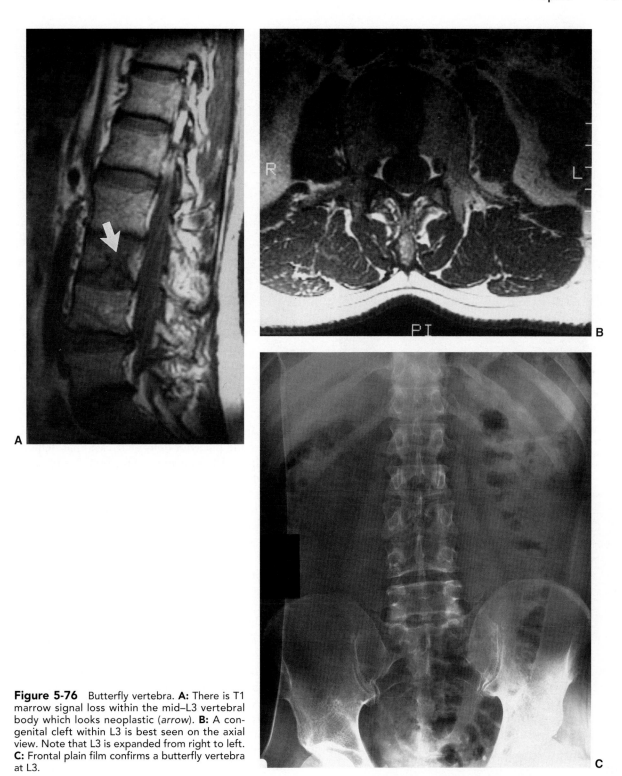

Figure 5-76 Butterfly vertebra. **A:** There is T1 marrow signal loss within the mid–L3 vertebral body which looks neoplastic (*arrow*). **B:** A congenital cleft within L3 is best seen on the axial view. Note that L3 is expanded from right to left. **C:** Frontal plain film confirms a butterfly vertebra at L3.

the acute spinal cord injury patient. These include limited availability of MR-compatible life support systems, limited access to the patient by support staff while in the scanner, and lack of MR-compatible immobilization or traction devices. Many vendors have developed MR-compatible systems that increase the utilization of MR in the acute setting.

MR can best identify ligamentous injury in acute spinal injury. These structures have been classified by Denis (165) into three columns: the anterior (consisting of the anterior longitudinal ligament, anterior anulus, and anterior vertebral body); the middle (consisting of the posterior longitudinal ligament, posterior anulus, and posterior vertebral

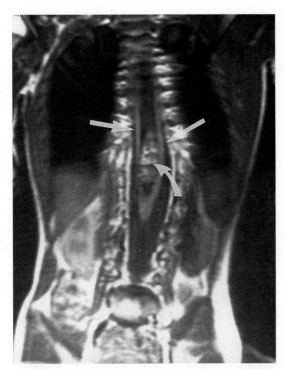

Figure 5-77 Diastematomyelia. Coronal image in an infant with congenital scoliosis demonstrates diastematomyelia with diplomyelia. The two spinal cords (*arrows*) are separated by a bone spur which contains marrow fat (*curved arrow*). The hemicords unite inferior to the bone spur. (TI 900 ms, TR 2,000 ms, TE 40 ms). (Reprinted with permission from Miller GM, Forbes GS, Onofrio BM. Magnetic resonance imaging of the spine. *Mayo Clin Proc* 1989;64: 986–1004.)

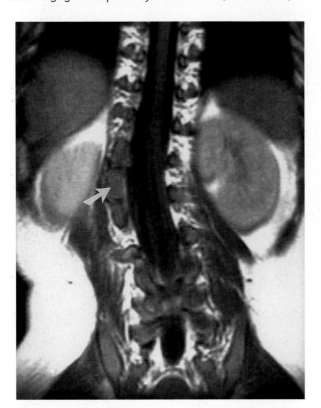

Figure 5-78 Congenital scoliosis. The coronal plane can be useful in the evaluation of these patients. Note the hemivertebra at L1 (*arrow*) (TR 500 ms, TE 20 ms).

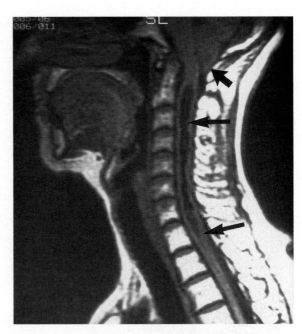

Figure 5-79 Type I Arnold-Chiari malformation. T1-weighted image showing the low position of the cerebellar tonsils (*short arrow*) and the associated intramedullary cord syrinx that extends from C2 to T2 (*long arrows*).

body); and posterior (consisting of the posterior ligament complex and posterior bony arch). MRI has demonstrated reliability in detecting injury to the posterior ligament complex, which consists of the supraspinous ligament, interspinous ligament, flaval ligaments, and capsules of the facets (166). Identification of ligamentous injury has important surgical implications, since stability is dependent on both middle and posterior column integrity (see Fig. 5-82).

MRI can directly visualize traumatic cord avulsions or cord compression from bone fragments or traumatic disc protrusions (see Fig. 5-83) (163). MRI can provide valuable information about the cord parenchyma that is not available on the myelogram. Intraparenchymal hematoma can be reliably distinguished from spinal cord edema on the basis of signal characteristics on T2-weighted sequences (161,167,168). Hours after the traumatic event, acute hematomas demonstrate decreased signal on T2-weighted sequences, presumably due to deoxyhemoglobin and intracellular methemoglobin. These changes are best seen on gradient-echo sequences (essential in the trauma patient) with a 1.5-T system (see Fig. 5-84). Cord edema and contusion, on the other hand, demonstrate increased T2-weighted signal. No corresponding signal changes are usually seen in either condition on T1-weighted sequences. The distinction between acute hematomas and cord contusion has important prognostic significance. Patients with cord hemorrhage usually have severe or complete lesions and are unlikely to recover neurologic function in most cases (151). Patients with edema or cord contusion usually have incomplete or less severe neurologic deficits and may recover significant neurologic function.

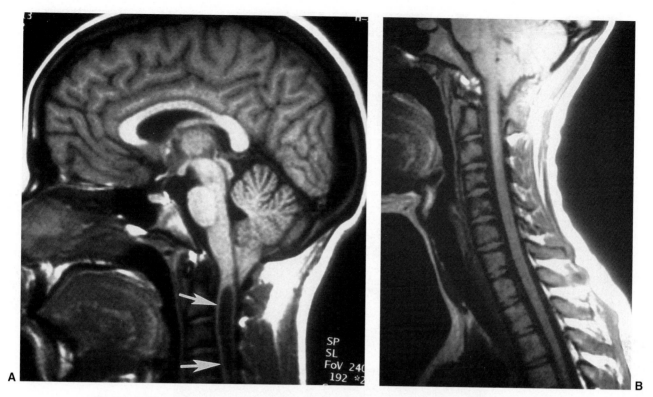

Figure 5-80 Type I Arnold-Chiari malformation. **A:** Chiari I malformation with syrinx (*arrows*). **B:** Near complete resolution of the syrinx following suboccipital craniectomy and C1 laminectomy.

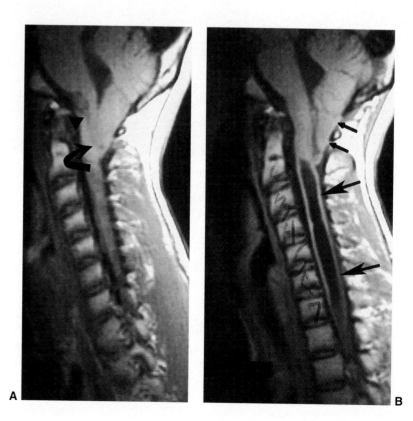

Figure 5-81 Type II Arnold-Chiari malformation. **A:** There is a "kink" (*arrowhead*) at the cervicomedullary junction, a medullary "spur" (*curved arrow*), and **(B)** a tonsillar "peg" (*small arrows*). Note the cord syrinx (*large arrows*).

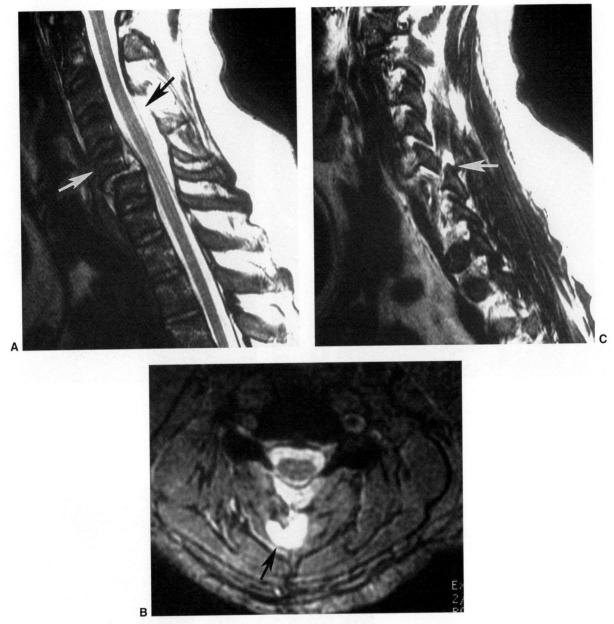

Figure 5-82 Ligamentous injury with locked facets. **A:** Sagittal T2-weighted fast spin-echo image showing acute traumatic anterior subluxation of C5 (*white arrow*) with posterior epidural fluid/hemorrhage (*black arrow*). **B:** Fluid from interspinous ligament injury (*arrow*). (TR 500 ms, TE 20 ms, 20° flip angle). **C:** Locked C5 and C6 facets (*arrow*).

MRI has been particularly useful in the evaluation of the chronically injured spine (162,164). Patients with a spinal cord injury and a new or progressive neurologic deficit months to years after the initial injury are best assessed by this technique. Etiologies of posttraumatic progressive myelopathy include spinal cord cysts, which may extend cephalad or caudad from the level of the injury, and arachnoiditis with subsequent adhesions and cord tethering. MRI more accurately distinguishes myelomalacia from spinal cord cysts than myelography with delayed CT (162,164). Lesions that parallel the intensity of CSF on T1-weighted, proton density, and T2-weighted sagittal sequences most likely represent a cord cyst (see Fig. 5-85). This distinction has important neurosurgical implications, as a patient with an ascending myelopathy and a spinal cord cyst above the level of the initial injury is likely to benefit from a shunt procedure, particularly if the cyst is large. Similarly, a patient with incomplete neurologic deficits, a descending myelopathy, and a spinal cord cyst extending below the level of the injury may also benefit. Patients with myelomalacia tend to have a poor response to therapy of any kind, although the surrounding myelomalacia signal changes in the cord may

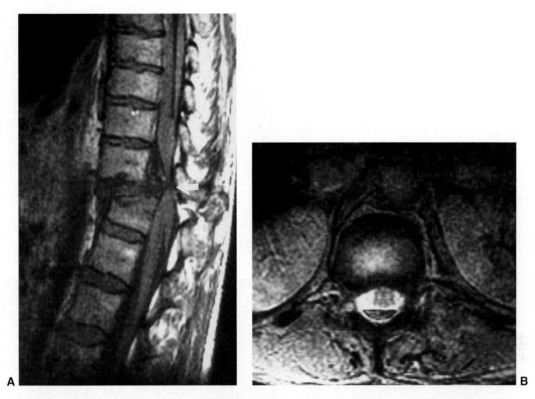

Figure 5-83 Acute trauma. **A:** T1-weighted image in a patient with a Chance fracture with dislocation of T11 posteriorly that results in compression of the spinal cord (*arrow*). **B:** Note the cerebrospinal fluid/blood level posteriorly in the spinal canal on the axial image (TR 400 ms, TE 20 ms, 12° flip angle).

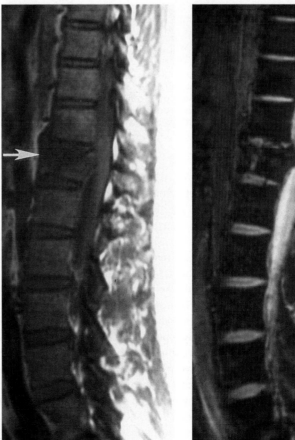

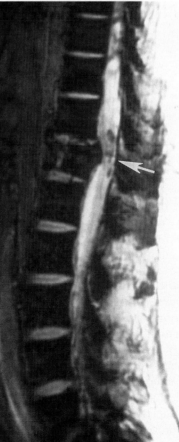

Figure 5-84 Traumatic cord hematoma. **A:** An acute hematoma within the thoracic cord associated with a T12 compression fracture (*arrow*) is difficult to detect on a T1-weighted image. **B:** The hematoma (*arrow*) is easier to see with gradient echo (TR 500 ms, TE 20 ms, 20° flip angle).

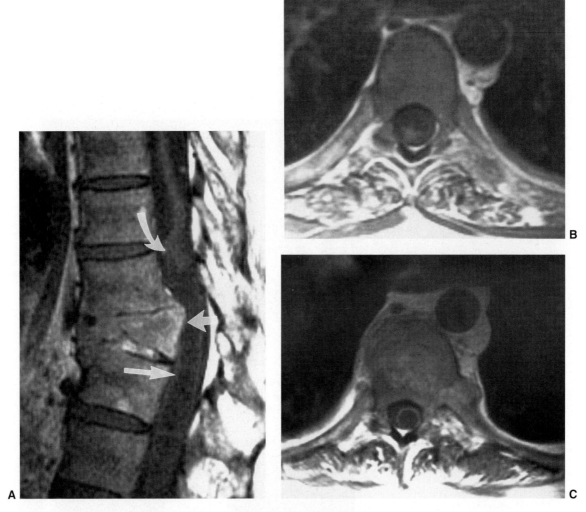

Figure 5-85 Chronic trauma. **A:** Sagittal T1-weighted image of the thoracic spine shows a burst fracture of T8 with a retropulsed fragment (*short arrow*). Note the deformity of the spinal cord above the injury (*curved arrow*) and the posttraumatic cord cyst (*long arrow*) below. **B:** Axial T1-weighted image at T7. **C:** Axial T1-weighted image at T9.

resolve after cyst shunting (162,164,169). Alteration in CSF flow due to arachnoiditis and cord tethering at the level of the trauma may also play a role in the development of myelomalacia in some cases. Cord signal changes may resolve following untethering (170).

Trauma can result in brachial plexus nerve root injury. The location of the injury has surgical and prognostic relevance. Nerve rootlet avulsion from the spinal cord is termed preganglionic and presently is incompatible with spontaneous or surgical recovery. Postganglionic nerve rupture can theoretically be surgically repaired (171) (see Fig. 5-86A). MRI can noninvasively detect brachial plexus nerve root injury. While nerve root avulsion can be inferred on MRI by the presence of a pseudomeningocele, high-resolution CT myelography has been shown to be superior for detecting these injuries (67,172). However, improvements in MR hardware and software are enabling

more consistent and reliable identification of avulsion injuries (see Fig. 5-86B and C).

VASCULAR

Spinal vascular malformations are divided into three types depending on the location of the nidus. The nidus may be located within the cord parenchyma [intramedullary arterial venous malformation (AVM)], within the pia/arachnoid (intradural AVM or fistula), or within the dura [dural arterial venous fistula (AVF)] (173). The intramedullary AVM and the dural AVF present with different clinical syndromes. The intradural AVM/AVF has clinical features that overlap the other two groups. MRI has been particularly useful as the screening examination for intramedullary AVM but may fail to diagnose the dural and intradural

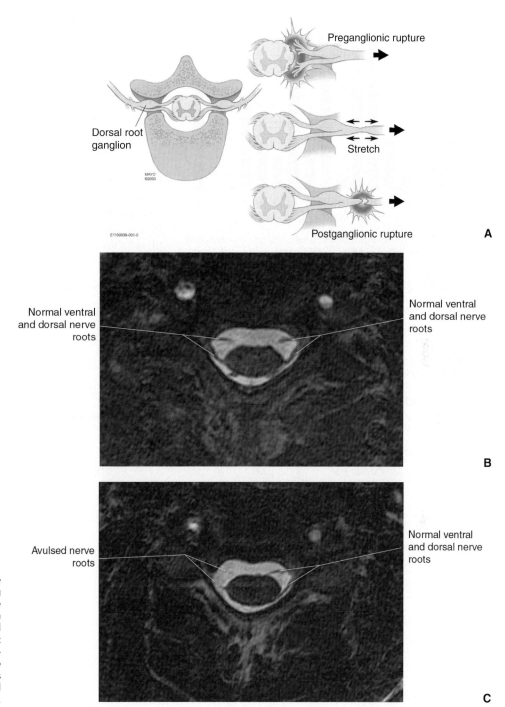

Figure 5-86 Cervical nerve root avulsion. **A:** Drawing depicting the types of nerve root injuries. High-resolution and enhanced cerebrospinal fluid and nerve root contrast provided by axial three-dimensional constructive interference in steady state imaging allows optimal delineation of normal **(B)** and avulsed **(C)** nerve roots.

malformations. The MR findings may be so subtle that clinically important lesions are missed.

Dural Arterial Venous Fistula

Dural AVF (DAVF) is the most common spinal vascular malformation. It typically occurs in older individuals, with an average age of 61 years (range, 45 to 82 years). The most common signs and symptoms include lower extremity weakness (55%), myelopathy or a mixed upper motor neuron/lower motor neuron pattern on physical exam (84%), and a chronic progressive clinical course (68%) (174). Bowel and bladder dysfunction occurs in the late stages. The symptoms are chronic, confusing, and may lead to ill-advised lumbar laminectomy unless the patient is carefully evaluated.

These lesions are most likely acquired. The nidus of the fistula is located within the dural sleeve of an exiting lower

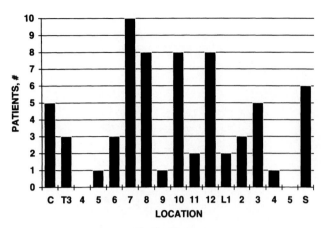

Figure 5-87 Dural arterial venous fistula. Bar graph illustrating the location of the fistula in 66 patients. C, cranial; S, sacral.

thoracic or upper lumbar nerve root. Approximately 8% of fistulas arise from an intracranial nidus and about 9% arise from a sacral nidus (see Fig. 5-87). The blood supply to the nidus is via a meningeal branch of the dorsal ramus of an aortic intercostal artery. The arteriovenous fistula subsequently drains retrograde into a radicular vein communicating with the posterior pial plexus that dilates due to the elevated pressure and increased flow (see Fig. 5-88). Clinical symptoms are thought to result from ischemia induced by venous hypertension and prolonged arteriovenous transit time (174–176).

The MR findings of DAVF include direct signs such as visualization of the dilated posterior pial venous plexus or indirect signs of cord ischemia. The dilated posterior pial plexus may produce serpentine flow voids posterior to the

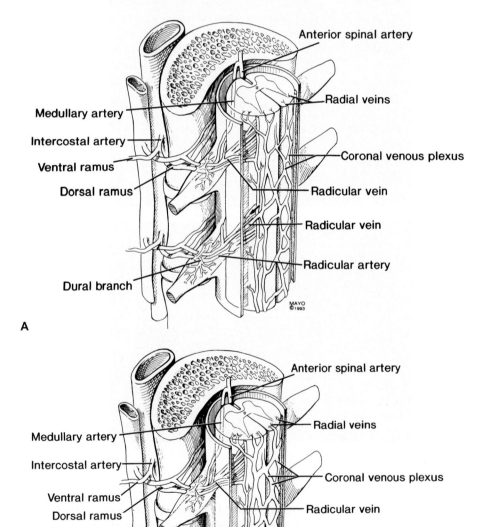

Figure 5-88 Dural arterial venous fistula. Artist drawing depicting **(A)** the normal vascular supply to the spinal cord and meninges and **(B)** the changes that occur with a dural arterial venous fistula. Note that the flow within the radicular vein is antegrade in **A** and retrograde in **B**.

thoracic spinal cord and conus on sagittal T1- and T2-weighted sequences (176,177). However, cerebrospinal fluid pulsation artifacts can both obscure or simulate this (3). Subtle scalloping of the posterior cord margin has been described on T1-weighted sequences because the dilated vessels lie immediately adjacent to the cord surface (178). Sequences obtained in the coronal plane may show the vessels to better advantage. Intravenous contrast administration is useful because subtle enhancement of the pial plexus along the posterior cord surface has been described (105,174).

In our series of 31 patients, the most common MR finding was increased T2 signal in the spinal cord (174). The signal changes extended over an average length of seven vertebral body segments and involved the tip of the conus 87% of the time. Flow voids from pial vessels were seen in only 45% of the patients on T2-weighted and 35% on T1-weighted sequences and were often difficult to distinguish from flow artifact. Mass effect was present in about half of the patients and pial or parenchymal enhancement was relatively common, observed in 88% of patients who received contrast (see Fig. 5-89).

A supine myelogram may be more sensitive than MRI in detecting DAVF. There are anecdotal reports of patients with proven dural fistulas and a normal MRI, although this has not been our experience. On the supine myelogram, serpentine defects, which represent the dilated pial venous plexus, can be identified within the contrast column along the dorsal aspect of the cord. Spinal angiography is necessary for definitive diagnosis and to determine the location of the nidus for surgical excision or endovascular embolization. Treatment results in the complete or partial resolution of MR findings (see Fig. 5-90) (179).

Spinal MRA has recently been advocated as a noninvasive method to detect abnormal medullary veins associated with DAVF (180–185). The MRA diagnosis of spinal DAVF is made on the basis of the radiologist's perception of the size, number, and tortuosity of the intradural vessels rather than on the direct visualization of the fistula (see Figs. 5-91 and 5-92). The study can obviate the need for myelography to determine the presence of abnormal vessels, and can aid the angiographer in targeting the spinal level most likely to harbor the fistula. This can significantly reduce catheter time and contrast load (185).

Intramedullary Arterial Venous Malformation

Intramedullary AVM is less common than DAVF and is believed to be a congenital lesion. Most patients present with symptoms of either acute intraparenchymal spinal cord hemorrhage or spinal subarachnoid hemorrhage before 30 years of age (186). The nidus is located within the cord parenchyma and may be large or small in size, superficial or deep in location, or involve only one side of the cord. These lesions are always fed by the anterior spinal (artery of Adamkiewicz) and/or one or both posterior spinal arteries (173). If the nidus of the AVM is small, there

may only be one medullary arterial feeder. If the nidus is large and extensive, several aortic intercostal arteries may contribute blood supply. If the nidus has been obliterated by the hemorrhage, the spinal angiogram may be normal.

MRI is the screening modality of choice for clinically suspected intramedullary AVM. Localized intramedullary enlargement of the spinal cord at the site of the nidus has been described. Serpentine flow voids may or may not be identified (175,177,178,187). The degree of pial plexus enlargement may be more prominent than that seen with the DAVF if the nidus is large (see Fig. 5-93). An intraparenchymal hematoma may be present, particularly if the patient presents with acute symptoms of paraplegia or quadriplegia. The signal changes seen depend on the age of the hematoma, with acute hematomas demonstrating no signal change on T1-weighted and decreased signal on T2-weighted sequences, subacute hematomas changing to increased signal on T1- and T2-weighted sequences, and chronic hematomas showing a well-defined ring of decreased signal on T2-weighted or gradient-echo sequences from hemosiderin deposition. Associated edema may be present in the acute phase as an area of decreased signal on T1-weighted and increased signal on T2-weighted sequences. Acute hemorrhage into the nidus may partially or completely obliterate it, particularly if the nidus is small. In these instances, the differential diagnosis would include hemorrhage into a neoplasm or a cavernous angioma (see Fig. 5-94). Ultimately, the diagnosis of intramedullary AVM is made on spinal angiography or at surgery.

Perimedullary Arterial Venous Fistula/Arterial Venous Malformation

Perimedullary AVF/AVM are the rarest and most complex spinal vascular malformations. The fistula or nidus is usually located within the posterior pia mater, although the nidus may be located anteriorly or extend intramedullary. The imaging appearance, age at presentation, and clinical symptoms vary and overlap considerably with the intramedullary AVM and DAVF (173). These patients may present at a young age with acute symptoms from hemorrhage, or later in life with symptoms of progressive thoracic myelopathy from chronic venous spinal cord ischemia. They are always supplied by spinal arteries similar to the intramedullary AVM. The blood supply may come from one or multiple aortic intercostal arteries.

Spinal Hemorrhage

Spinal hemorrhage can occur in the same compartments as typically described with spinal neoplasms, and can be posttraumatic or spontaneous.

Intramedullary Hemorrhage

As previously described, a spinal cord hemorrhage can occur following trauma. Other causes include hemorrhage within a vascular malformation or tumor.

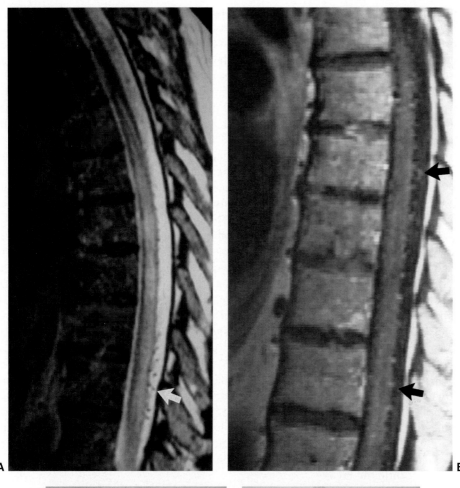

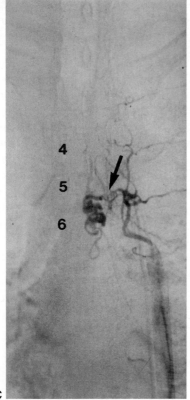

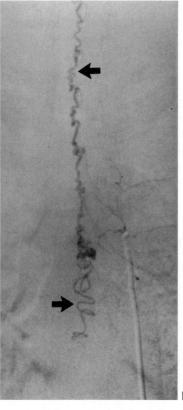

Figure 5-89 Dural arterial venous fistula. **A:** Sagittal T2-weighted fast spin-echo image showing bright signal in the thoracic spinal cord, mild mass effect, and flow voids from a dilated venous plexus (*arrow*). **B:** Subtle punctate pial enhancement of the venous plexus (*arrows*) is identified in another patient. **C:** The diagnosis is made on the spinal angiogram. The nidus in this patient is located inferior to the left T5 pedicle (*long arrow*). **D:** The enlarged pial veins are identified on this slightly later image from the angiogram (*arrows*). (Fig. 5–89 C and D From Miller GM, Forbes GS, Onofrio BM. Magnetic resonance imaging of the spine. *Mayo Clin Proc* 1989;64:986–1004.)

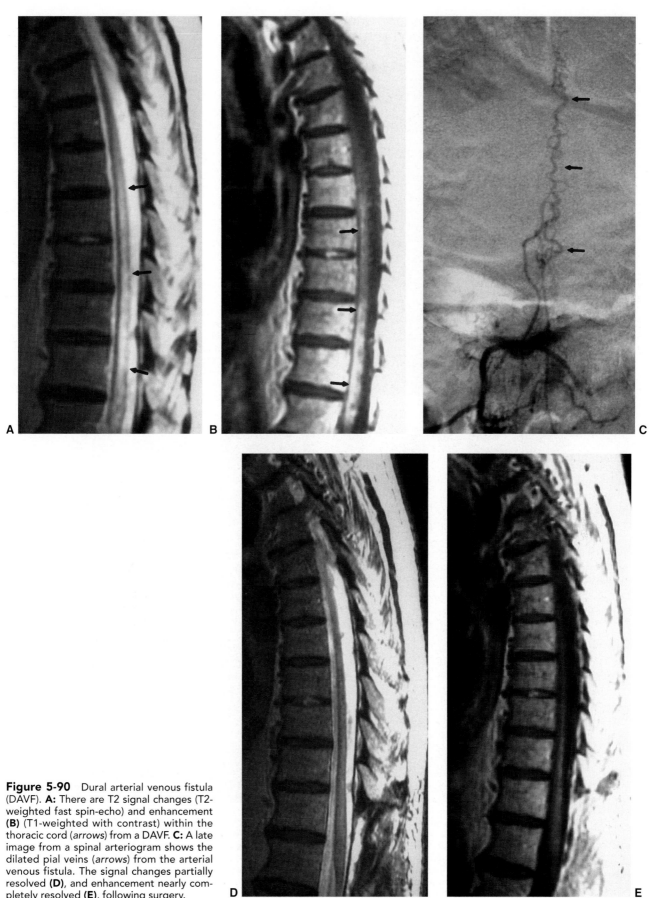

Figure 5-90 Dural arterial venous fistula (DAVF). **A:** There are T2 signal changes (T2-weighted fast spin-echo) and enhancement **(B)** (T1-weighted with contrast) within the thoracic cord (*arrows*) from a DAVF. **C:** A late image from a spinal arteriogram shows the dilated pial veins (*arrows*) from the arterial venous fistula. The signal changes partially resolved **(D)**, and enhancement nearly completely resolved **(E)**, following surgery.

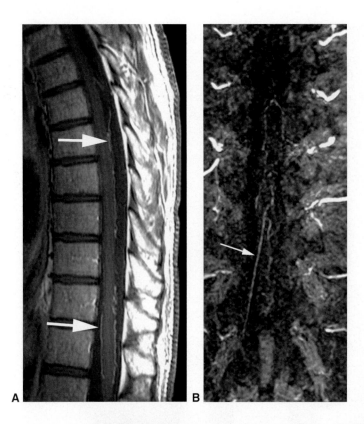

Figure 5-91 Normal spinal cord venous anatomy. **A:** T1-weighted sagittal image with contrast shows normal curvilinear enhancement along the dorsal and ventral surfaces of the spinal cord (*arrows*). **B:** Bolus gadolinium MRA of the spine with compressed coronal MIP images (from a sagittal slab acquisition) through the spinal canal demonstrate superimposition of the dorsal and ventral medullary venous plexus (*arrow*) in a patient with no vascular pathology.

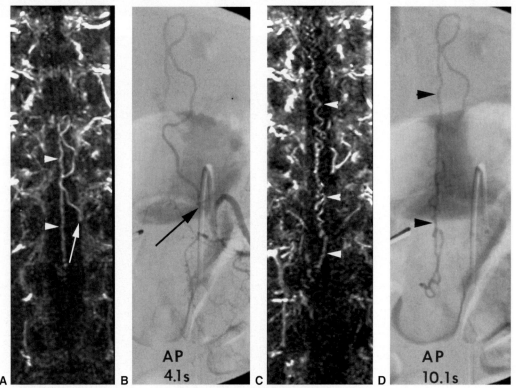

Figure 5-92 Spinal dural arterial venous fistula. **A:** Coronal maximum intensity projection (MIP) image from a bolus gadolinium MRA (sagittal slab acquisition) shows a large arteriolized radiculomedullary vein (*arrow*) on the left at the T12 level that drains into the dilated ventral medullary vein (*arrowheads*). **B:** Corresponding early image from a catheter (*arrow*) angiogram. **C:** 6 mm coronal MIP posterior to **A** demonstrates tortuous dilated dorsal medullary veins (*arrowheads*). **D:** The dilated veins are demonstrated on a later image from the catheter angiogram (*arrowheads*). [From Luetmer PH, Lane JI, Gilbertson JR, Bernstein et al. Preangiographic evaluation of spinal dural arteriovenous fistulae (AVFs) with elliptic centric contrast-enhanced MRA and impact on radiation and iodinated contrast dose. *Am J Neuroradiol*: In press, with permission.]

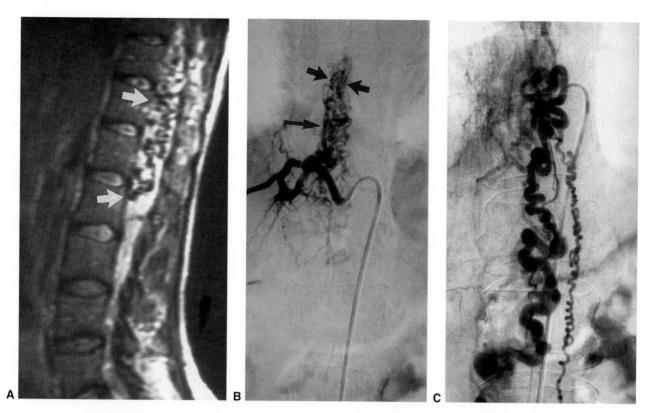

Figure 5-93 Intramedullary AVM. **A:** There are large abnormal vessels in the spinal canal on the sagittal T2-weighted image *(arrows)* (TR 1,500 ms, TE 80 ms). **B:** Selective right T11 intercostal artery angiogram confirms the presence of a vascular malformation *(short arrows)* that is fed by an enlarged left posterior spinal artery *(long arrow)*. **C:** The massively dilated pial venous plexus fills on a slightly later film from the angiogram.

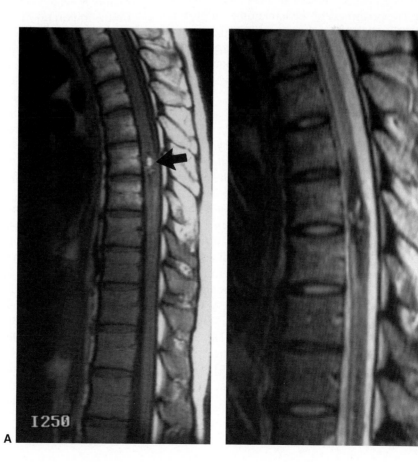

Figure 5-94 Intramedullary cavernous angioma. **A:** A chronic hematoma with bright T1 signal (extracellular methemoglobin) is identified within the spinal cord *(arrow)*. **B:** Note the hemosiderin deposition and mild intra-medullary mass effect on the sagittal T2-weighted fast spin echo. This was resected because of the risk of rehemorrhage in this patient, who has a partial deficit.

Spinal Subarachnoid Hemorrhage

Spontaneous spinal subarachnoid hemorrhage is uncommon, accounting for less than 1% of all cases of subarachnoid hemorrhage (188). The cause is often an AVM of the cord. Spinal tumors, particularly of the conus and cauda equina, are rare causes of spinal subarachnoid hemorrhage. Superficial siderosis is a rare condition that can result from repeated or continuous subarachnoid hemorrhage. The disease is characterized by subpial and leptomeningeal hemosiderin deposition in the brain (particularly cerebellum), brainstem and cranial nerves (particularly CN VIII), and spinal cord (189). These patients typically present with ataxia, hearing loss, and myelopathy. Prior to MRI, the diagnosis was usually made at autopsy. MRI can often demonstrate the hypointense hemosiderin deposits on T2-weighted images, which are accentuated on gradient echo. These can be seen coating the cerebellum, brainstem, and spinal cord (see Fig. 5-95) (190,191).

Spinal Epidural Hematoma

Spinal epidural hematomas are also uncommon and can be either posttraumatic or spontaneous. Patients with spontaneous hematomas may present with symptoms similar to an acutely herniated disc. CT findings in the lumbar spine are similar to a large, extruded, free-fragment disc herniation (192). The MR appearance of spontaneous lumbar epidural hematomas varies. It is often associated with adjacent degenerated discs, small anular tears, or disc herniations. The brightness of the hematoma on proton density and T2-weighted images varies, but is brighter and easily separated from the adjacent disc. Unlike typical free-fragment disc herniations, the hematomas are largest at the midvertebral body level (see Fig. 5-96) (192).

Infarct

Spinal cord infarcts are difficult to document by imaging and difficult to confirm histologically. Only isolated case reports are found in the literature (105,130). The diagnosis is made clinically. Spinal cord infarcts occur in association with abdominal aortic aneurysm repair procedures from inadvertent occlusion of an intercostal artery supplying a spinal artery, in patients with severe atherosclerotic disease from stenosis of an intercostal artery supplying a spinal artery, in patients with a vasculitis, or from thrombosis of an intraspinal vascular malformation (Foix-Alajouanine syndrome) (105). The MRI may be normal, or there may be intramedullary expansion and edema within the segment of infarct (see Fig. 5-97). Acute infarcts may show enhancement following contrast administration mimicking a neoplasm (105). In the chronic stage of infarction, the spinal cord may become atrophic.

Osteoporotic Compression Fractures and Percutaneous Intervention

Vertebral compression fractures secondary to osteoporosis are estimated to account for 700,000 hospital admissions per year, with a lifetime risk in women approximating 15%. These numbers are expected to increase with an aging population. Treatment options have expanded with the recent development of percutaneous vertebroplasty and kyphoplasty (193–195). Both of these procedures are used to primarily treat back pain related to unhealed compression fractures by injection of bone cement into the region of the fracture. Both are felt to produce fracture fragment stabilization, reducing the stimulation of pain generators in the periosteal layer of the vertebral cortex. Kyphoplasty achieves vertebral height restoration by inflating high-pressure balloons within the fractured vertebra to create trabecular bone cavities prior to cement injection.

In both procedures, polymethylmethacrylate (PMMA) is injected into the vertebral body, usually through a transpedicular approach in the thoracic and lumbar spine, and an anterolateral approach in the cervical spine (see Fig. 5-98). The PMMA appears dark on T1-weighted and T2-weighted images (see Fig. 5-99). These areas have a characteristic globular appearance and should not be misinterpreted as sclerotic metastases. The procedure has been used to treat back pain from vertebral angiomas, osteoporotic and malignant vertebral compression. The procedure is detailed elsewhere (196–198).

MRI is important in the evaluation of a patient with a compression fracture prior to vertebroplasty. Particular attention should be given to certain imaging findings in these patients. Often, more than one compression fracture is seen on plain film. Recent fractures with edematous changes on MRI will benefit from PMMA stabilization versus a healed fracture with normal marrow signal. The level (or levels) of the fracture(s) need to be accurately identified, allowing optimal correlation with pain localization on the physical examination. The degree of vertebral collapse should be quantified, since the procedure is difficult if the vertebral height is reduced by greater than one half. It is often helpful to employ fat-saturation to highlight edematous changes. Any degree of retropulsion should be mentioned, since significant canal compromise could be a relative contraindication to the procedure.

Approximately 30% of fractures will have evidence of a fluid-filled cleft beneath the compressed endplate on MRI or an air-filled cleft on plain film (see Fig. 5-100) (199). They are most commonly encountered at the thoracolumbar junction. Depending on the age of the fracture, they may represent sites of fracture nonunion secondary to flexion–extension forces along the plane of the fracture. These should be described, since most operators will attempt to fill the cleft with cement in order to

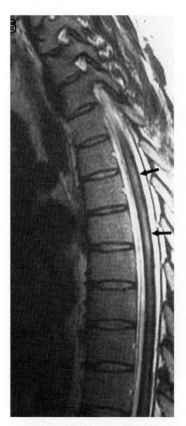

Figure 5-95 Superficial siderosis. Hypointense hemosiderin coats the thoracic cord (*arrows*) (T2-weighted fast spin echo).

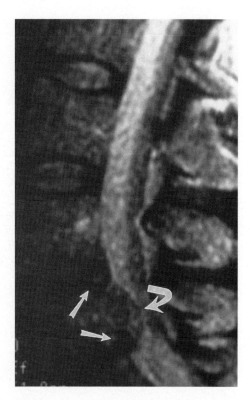

Figure 5-96 Epidural hematoma. An anterior epidural hematoma (*curved arrow*) is widest at the L5 midvertebral level. The signal intensity is greater than the adjacent discs (*arrows*) (TR 2,400 ms, TE 96 ms).

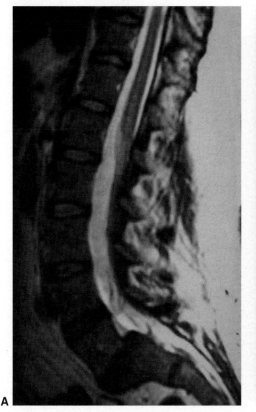
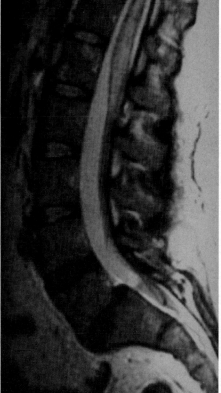

Figure 5-97 Recent infarct. **A:** This study was obtained within 24 hours of an acute neurologic deficit. The conus is normal (TR 2,800 ms, TE 96 ms). **B:** A repeat study three days later shows T2 signal and mass effect in the conus (TR 2,800 ms, TE 96 ms).

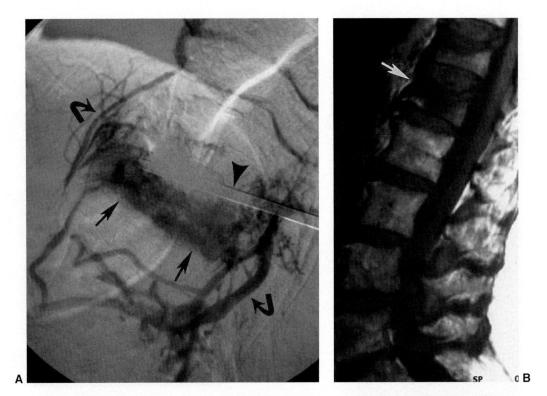

Figure 5-98 Percutaneous vertebroplasty. **A:** An 11-gauge needle (*arrowhead*) is positioned transpedicularly into the L1 vertebral body. Opacification of the compressed vertebral body (*arrows*) and draining veins (*curved arrows*) during the venogram portion of the study prior to PMMA instillation. **B:** Multiple compressed vertebral bodies are present on a T1-weighted sagittal image. The L1 fracture (*arrow*) was felt to be the source of the patient's pain on physical exam.

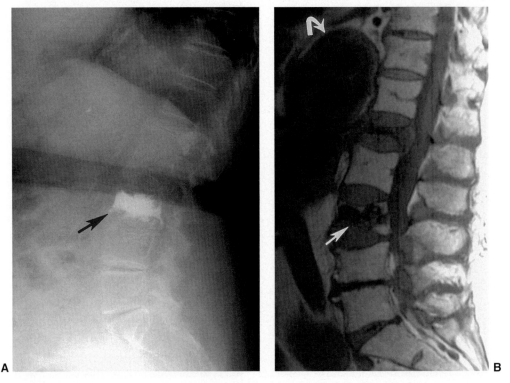

Figure 5-99 Magnetic resonance appearance of vertebroplasty. **A:** Lateral radiograph following L-3 vertebroplasty (*arrow*). The PMMA (*arrow*) appears dark on both T1-weighted fast spin-echo **(B)** and T2-weighted fast spin-echo **(C).** Known large aortic aneurysm (*curved arrow*).

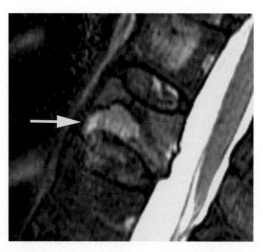

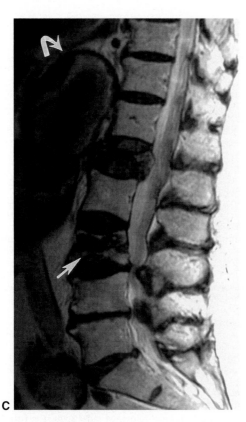

Figure 5-99 *(continued)*

Figure 5-100 Intravertebral cleft. Fat-saturated sagittal T2-weighted fast spin-echo image showing a fluid-filled thoracic vertebral body cleft *(arrow)*. (From Lane JI, Maus TP, Wald JT, et al. Intravertebral clefts opacified during vertebroplasty: Pathogenesis, technical implications, and prognostic significance. *Am J Neuroradiol* 2002;23(10):1642–1646.)

achieve better stabilization and height restoration. Finally, imaging features suspicious for a pathologic fracture must be clearly stated, since a biopsy could be performed before PMMA injection.

Approximately 20% of patients may return with recurrent pain secondary to a new compression within a year of the procedure. Marrow edema at the treated level can persist for months even after successful treatment (see Fig. 5-101) (200). Mild asymptomatic progressive collapse of the treated vertebra can also occur after successful vertebroplasty (200). These imaging findings should not be assumed to be the cause of a persistent source of pain in treated patients on follow-up studies.

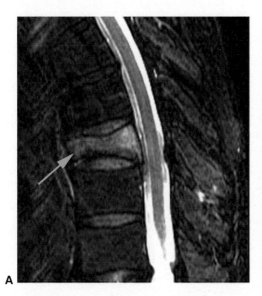

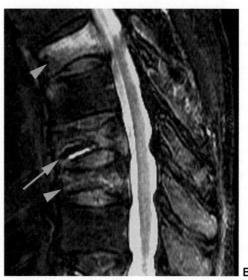

Figure 5-101 Residual marrow edema in a previously treated compression fracture. **A:** Fat-saturated sagittal T2-weighted fast spin echo obtained prior to T8 vertebroplasty, demonstrates an acute or subacute compression fracture associated with marrow edema *(arrow)*. **B:** Mild asymptomatic edema persists at T8 on a study obtained 13 months after T8 vertebroplasty *(arrow)*. Recurrent pain was from new T6 and T9 fractures *(arrowheads)*.

ACKNOWLEDGMENT

The authors wish to thank Dr. Daniel F. Broderick for Figs. 5-53A and 5-74 B, and Sharon Schouweiler for assistance in the preparation of the manuscript.

REFERENCES

1. Bellon EM, Haacke EM, Coleman PE, et al. MR artifacts: a review. *AJR Am J Roentgenol* 1986;147:1271–1281.
2. Rubin JB, Enzmann DR, Wright A. CSF-gated MR imaging of the spine: theory and clinical implementation. *Radiology* 1987; 163:784–792.
3. Rubin JB, Enzmann DR. Optimizing conventional MR imaging of the spine. *Radiology* 1987;163:777–783.
4. Enzmann DR, Rubin JB, Wright A. Use of cerebrospinal fluid gating to improve T2-weighted images. Part I. The spinal cord. *Radiology* 1987;162:763–767.
5. Rubin JB, Enzmann DR. Imaging of spinal CSF pulsation by 2DFT MR: significance during clinical imaging. *AJR Am J Roentgenol* 1987;148:973–982.
6. Rubin JB, Enzmann DR. Harmonic modulation of proton MR precessional phase by pulsatile motion: origin of spinal CSF flow phenomena. *AJR Am J Roentgenol* 1987;148:983–994.
7. Rubin JB, Wright A, Enzmann DR. Lumbar spine: motion compensation for cerebrospinal fluid on MR imaging. *Radiology* 1988;166:225–231.
8. Bronskill MJ, McVeigh ER, Kucharczyk W, et al. Syrinx-like artifacts on MR images of the spinal cord. *Radiology* 1988;166:485–488.
9. Czervionke LF, Czervionke JM, Daniels DL, et al. Characteristic features of MR truncation artifacts. *AJNR Am J Neuroradiol* 1988; 9:815–824.
10. Levy LM, Di Chiro G, Brooks RA, et al. Spinal cord artifacts from truncation errors during MR imaging. *Radiology* 1988; 166:479–483.
11. Petersilge CA, Lewin JS, Duerk JL, et al. Optimizing imaging parameters for MR evaluation of the spine with titanium pedicle screws. *AJR Am J Roentgenol* 1996;166:1213–1218.
12. Rudisch A, Kremser C, Peer S, et al. Metallic artifacts in magnetic resonance imaging of patients with spinal fusion. A comparison of implant materials and imaging sequences. *Spine* 1998; 23:692–699.
13. Bergman RA, Thompson SA, Afifi AK, et al. Compendium of human anatomic variation: text atlas, and world literature. Baltimore: Urban & Schwarzenberg, 1988.
14. Ralston MD, Dykes TA, Applebaum BI. Verification of lumbar vertebral bodies (letter). *Radiology* 1992;185:615–616.
15. Hahn PY, Strobel JJ, Hahn FJ. Verification of lumbosacral segments on MR images: identification of transitional vertebrae. *Radiology* 1992;182:580–581.
16. Netter FH. Nervous System. Part I. Anatomy and physiology. In: Brass A, ed. *Volume 1: The CIBA collection of medical illustrations.* West Caldwell, NJ: CIBA Pharmaceutical Company, 1986.
17. Czervionke LF, Daniels DL, Ho PSP, et al. Cervical neural foramina: correlative anatomic and MR imaging study. *Radiology* 1988; 169:753–759.
18. Pech P, Daniels DL, Williams AL, et al. The cervical neural foramina: correlation of microtomy and CT anatomy. *Radiology* 1985;155:143–146.
19. Pech P, Haughton VM. Lumbar intervertebral disk: correlative MR and anatomic study. *Radiology* 1985;156:699–701.
20. Grenier N, Kressel HY, Schiebler ML, et al. Normal and degenerative posterior spinal structures: MR imaging. *Radiology* 1987; 165:517–525.
21. Modic MT, Masaryk TJ, Ross JS, et al. Imaging of degenerative disk disease. *Radiology* 1988;168:177–186.
22. Modic MT, Pavlicek W, Weinstein MA, et al. Magnetic resonance imaging of intervertebral disk disease. *Radiology* 1984;152:103–111.
23. Aguila LA, Piraino DW, Modic MT, et al. The intranuclear cleft of the intervertebral disk: magnetic resonance imaging. *Radiology* 1985;155:155–158.
24. Yu S, Haughton VM, Lynch LK, et al. Fibrous structure in the intervertebral disk: correlation of MR appearance with anatomic sections. *AJNR Am J Neuroradiol* 1989;10:1105–1110.
25. Schellinger D. Patterns of anterior spinal canal involvement by neoplasms and infections. *AJNR Am J Neuroradiol* 1996;17: 953–959.
26. Grenier N, Greselle JF, Vital JM, et al. Normal and disrupted lumbar longitudinal ligaments: correlative MR and anatomic study. *Radiology* 1989;71:197–205.
27. Ho PSP, Yu S, Sether LA, et al. Ligamentum flavum: appearance on sagittal and coronal MR images. *Radiology* 1988;168: 469–472.
28. Sloof JL, Kernohan JW, McCarty CS. *Primary intramedullary tumors of the spinal cord and filum terminale.* Philadelphia, PA: WB Saunders, 1964.
29. Czervionke LF, Daniels DL, Ho PSP, et al. The MR appearance of gray and white matter in the cervical spinal cord. *AJNR Am J Neuroradiol* 1988;9:557–562.
30. Flannigan BD, Lufkin RB, McGlade C, et al. MR imaging of the cervical spine: neurovascular anatomy. *AJNR Am J Neuroradiol* 1987;8:27–32.
31. Miller GM, Rasmusson JJ, Onofrio BM. Clinical evaluation of phased array multicoil for spine MR imaging. Presented at the Radiological Society of North America Annual Meeting, Chicago, IL, Nov. 25-30, 1990.
32. Yousem DM, Schnall MD. MR examination for spinal cord compression: impact of a multicoil system on length of study. *J Comp Assist Tomogr* 1991;15(4):598–604.
33. Enzmann DR, Rubin JB. Cervical spine: MR imaging with a partial flip angle, gradient-refocused pulse sequence. Part I. General considerations and disk disease. *Radiology* 1988;166: 467–472.
34. Enzmann DR, Rubin JB. Cervical spine: MR imaging with a partial flip angle, gradient-refocused pulse sequence. Part II. Spinal cord disease. *Radiology* 1988;166:473–478.
35. VanDyke C, Ross JS, Tkach J, et al. Gradient-echo MR imaging of the cervical spine: evaluation of extradural disease. *AJNR Am J Neuroradiol* 1989;10:627–632.
36. Katz BH, Quencer RM, Hinks RS. Comparison of gradient-recalled-echo and T2-weighted spin-echo pulse sequences in intramedullary spinal lesions. *AJNR Am J Neuroradiol* 1989;10: 815–822.
37. Runge VM, Clanton JA, Lukehart CM, et al. Paramagnetic agents for contrast-enhanced NMR imaging: a review. *AJR Am J Roentgenol* 1983;141:1209–1215.
38. Weinmann HJ, Brasch RC, Press WR, et al. Characteristics of gadolinium-DTPA complex: a potential NMR contrast agent. *AJR Am J Roentgenol* 1984;142:619–624.
39. Brasch RC. Safety profile of gadopentetate dimeglumine. *MRI Decisions* 1989;3(6):13–17.
40. Goldstein HA, Kashanian FK, Blumetti RF, et al. Safety assessment of gadopentetate dimeglumine in U.S. clinical trials. *Radiology* 1990;174:17–23.
41. Runge VM, Carollo BR, Wolf CR, et al. Gd DTPA: a review of clinical indications in central nervous system magnetic resonance imaging. *Radiographics* 1989;9:929–958.
42. Fardon DF, Millette PC. Nomenclature and classification of lumbar disc pathology. Recommendations of the Combined Task Forces of the North American Spine Society, American Society of Spine Radiology, and American Society of Neuroradiology. *Spine* 2001;26(5):E93–E113.
43. Jarvik JG. Imaging of adults with low back pain in the primary care setting. *Neuroimaging Clin N Am* 2003;13(2):293–305.
44. Teresi LM, Lufkin RB, Reicher MA, et al. Asymptomatic degenerative disk disease and spondylosis of the cervical spine: MR imaging. *Radiology* 1987;64:83–88.
45. Daffner RH, Dalinka MK. Chronic neck pain. American College of Radiology. ACR Appropriateness Criteria. *Radiology* 2000;215: 345–356.
46. Anderson RE, Drayer BP. Acute low back pain-radiculopathy. American College of Radiology. ACR Appropriateness Criteria. *Radiology* 2000;479–785.
47. Yu S, Haughton VM, Sether LA, et al. Anulus fibrosis in bulging intervertebral disks. *Radiology* 1988;169:761–763.

48. Yu S, Sether LA, Ho PSP, et al. Tears of the anulus fibrosis: correlation between MR and pathologic findings in cadavers. *AJNR Am J Neuroradiol* 1988;9:367–370.
49. Ross JS, Modic MT, Masaryk TJ. Tears of the anulus fibrosis: assessment with Gd-DTPA-enhanced MR imaging. *AJNR Am J Neuroradiol* 1989;10:1251–1254.
50. Modic MT, Steinberg PM, Ross JS, et al. Degenerative disk disease: assessment of changes in vertebral body marrow with MR imaging. *Radiology* 1988;166:193–199.
51. Weishaupt D, Zanetti M, Hodler J, et al. MR imaging of the lumbar spine: prevalence of intervertebral disk extrusion and sequestration, nerve root compression, endplate abnormalities and osteoarthritis of the facet joints in asymptomatic volunteers. *Radiology* 1998;209:661–666.
52. Jinkins JR, Whittemore AR, Bradley WG. The anatomic basis of vertebrogenic pain and the autonomic syndrome associated with lumbar disk extrusion. *AJNR Am J Neuroradiol* 1989;10:219–231.
53. Osborn AG, Hood RS, Sherry RG, et al. CT/MR spectrum of far lateral and anterior lumbosacral disk herniations. *AJNR Am J Neuroradiol* 1988;9:775–778.
54. Weinreb JC, Wolbarsht LB, Cohen JM, et al. Prevalence of lumbosacral intervertebral disk abnormalities on MR images in pregnant and asymptomatic nonpregnant women. *Radiology* 1989;170:125–128.
55. Jenson MC, Brant-Zawadzki MN, Obuchowski N, et al. Magnetic resonance imaging of the lumbar spine in people without low back pain. *N Engl J M* 1994;331:69–73.
56. Stadnik TW, Lee RR, Coen HL, et al. Annular tears and disk herniation: prevalence and contrast enhancement on MR images in the absence of low back pain or sciatica. *Radiology* 1998;206:49–55.
57. Masaryk TJ, Ross JS, Modic MT, et al. High-resolution MR imaging of sequestered lumbar intervertebral disks. *AJNR Am J Neuroradiol* 1988;9:351–358.
58. Ross JS, Modic MT, Masaryk TJ, et al. Assessment of extradural degenerative disease with Gd-DTPA-enhanced MR imaging: correlation with surgical and pathologic findings. *AJNR Am J Neuroradiol* 1989;10:1243–1249.
59. Modic MT, Masaryk TJ, Boumphrey F, et al. Lumbar herniated disk disease and canal stenosis: prospective evaluation of surface coil MR, CT, and myelography. *AJR Am J Roentgenol* 1986;147:757–765.
60. Miller GM. Controversies, communication, and diagnosis in lumbar disc disease. Presented at the Radiological Society of North America, Chicago, IL, Dec. 1–6, 1991.
61. Brown BM, Schwartz RH, Frank E, et al. Preoperative evaluation of cervical radiculopathy and myelopathy by surface-coil MR imaging. *AJNR Am J Neuroradiol* 1988;9:859–866.
62. Hedberg MC, Drayer BP, Flom RA, et al. Gradient echo (GRASS) MR imaging in cervical radiculopathy. *AJNR Am J Neuroradiol* 1988;9:145–151.
63. Modic MT, Masaryk TJ, Mulopulos GP, et al. Cervical radiculopathy: prospective evaluation with surface coil MR imaging, CT with metrizamide, and metrizamide myelography. *Radiology* 1986;161:753–759.
64. Ryan RW, Lally JF, Kozic Z. Asymptomatic calcified herniated thoracic disks: CT recognition. *AJNR Am J Neuroradiol* 1988;9:363–366.
65. Ross JS, Perez-Reyes N, Masaryk TJ, et al. Thoracic disk herniation: MR imaging. *Radiology* 1987;165:511–515.
66. Houser OW, Onofrio BM, Miller GM, et al. Cervical spondylotic stenosis and myelopathy: evaluation with computed tomographic myelography. *Mayo Clin Proc* 1994;69:557–563.
67. Ramanauskas WL, Wilner HI, Metes JJ, et al. MR imaging of compressive myelomalacia. *J Comp Assist Tomogr* 1989;3:399–404.
68. Takahashi M, Yamashita Y, Sakamoto Y, et al. Chronic cervical cord compression: clinical significance of increased signal intensity on MR images. *Radiology* 1989;3:219–224.
69. Awwad E, Martin D, Smith K Jr, et al. MR imaging of lumbar juxta-articular cysts. *J Comp Assist Tomogr* 1990;14(3):415–417.
70. Jackson D Jr, Atlas S, Mani J, et al. Intraspinal synovial cysts: MR imaging. *Radiology* 1989;70:527–530.
71. Silbergleit R, Geborski S, Brunberg J, et al. Lumbar synovial cysts: correlation of myelographic CT, MR, and pathologic findings. *AJNR Am J Neuroradiol* 1990;11:777–779.
72. Krauss WE, Atkinson JLD, Miller GM. Juxtafacet cysts of the cervical spine. *Neurosurgery* 1998;43:1363–1368.
73. Bundschuh CV, Modic MT, Ross JS, et al. Epidural fibrosis and recurrent disk herniation in the lumbar spine: MR imaging assessment. *AJNR Am J Neuroradiol* 1988;9:169–178.
74. Frocrain L, Duvauferrier R, Husson J-L, et al. Recurrent postoperative sciatica: evaluation with MR imaging and enhanced CT. *Radiology* 1989;170:531–533.
75. Hochhauser L, Kieffer SA, Cacayorin ED, et al. Recurrent post-diskectomy low back pain: MR-surgical correlation. *AJNR Am J Neuroradiol* 1988;9:769–774.
76. Hueftle MG, Modic MT, Ross JS, et al. Lumbar spine: postoperative MR imaging with Gd-DTPA. *Radiology* 1988;167:817–824.
77. Ross JS, Blaser S, Masaryk TJ, et al. Gd-DTPA enhancement of posterior epidural scar: an experimental model. *AJNR Am J Neuroradiol* 1989;10:1083–1088.
78. Ross JS, Delamarter R, Hueftle MG, et al. Gadolinium-DTPA-enhanced MR imaging of the postoperative lumbar spine: time course and mechanism of enhancement. *AJNR Am J Neuroradiol* 1989;10:37–46.
79. Ross JS, Masaryk TJ, Modic MT, et al. Lumbar spine: postoperative assessment with surface-coil MR imaging. *Radiology* 1987;164:851–860.
80. Sotiropoulos S, Chafetz NI, Lang P, et al. Differentiation between postoperative scar and recurrent disk herniation: prospective comparison of MR, CT, and contrast-enhanced CT. *AJNR Am J Neuroradiol* 1989;10:639–643.
81. Ross JS, Masaryk TJ, Modic MT, et al. MR imaging of lumbar arachnoiditis. *AJNR Am J Neuroradiol* 1987;8:885–892.
82. Braun IF, Hoffman JC Jr, Davis PC, et al. Contrast enhancement in CT differentiation between recurrent disk herniation and postoperative scar: prospective study. *AJR Am J Roentgenol* 1985;145:785–790.
83. Firooznia H, Kricheff II, Rafii M, et al. Lumbar spine after surgery: examination with intravenous contrast-enhanced CT. *Radiology* 1987;163:221–226.
84. Teplick JG, Haskin ME. Intravenous contrast-enhanced CT of the postoperative lumbar spine: improved identification of recurrent disk herniation, scar, arachnoiditis, and diskitis. *AJR Am J Roentgenol* 1984;143:845–855.
85. Akansel G, Haughton VM, Papke RA, et al. Diffusion into human intervertebral disks studied with MR and gadoteridol. *AJNR Am J Neuroradiol* 1997;18:443–445.
86. Avrahami E, Tadmor R, Dally O, et al. Early MR demonstration of spinal metastases in patients with normal radiographs and CT and radionuclide bone scans. *J Comp Assist Tomogr* 1989;13:598–602.
87. Daffner RH, Lupetin AR, Dash N, et al. MRI in the detection of malignant infiltration of bone marrow. *AJR Am J Roentgenol* 1986;146:353–358.
88. Mehta RC, Wilson MA, Perlman SB. False-negative bone scan in extensive metastatic disease: CT and MR findings (case report). *J Comp Assist Tomogr* 1989;13:717–719.
89. Smoker WRK, Godersky JC, Knutzon RK, et al. The role of MR imaging in evaluating metastatic spinal disease. *AJNR Am J Neuroradiol* 1987;8:901–908.
90. Jones KM, Schwartz RB, Mantello MT, et al. Fast spin-echo MR in the detection of vertebral metastases: comparison of three sequences. *AJNR Am J Neuroradiol* 1994;15:401–407.
91. Mehta RC, Marks MP, Hinks RS, et al. MR evaluation of vertebral metastases: T1-weighted, short-inversion-time inversion recovery, fast spin-echo, and inversion-recover fast spin-echo sequences. *AJNR Am J Neuroradiol* 1995;16:281–288.
92. Lecouvet FE, VandeBerg BC, Maldague BE, et al. Vertebral compression fractures in multiple myeloma. Part I. Distribution and appearance at MR imaging. *Radiology* 1997;204:195–199.
93. Lecouvet FE, Malghem J, Michaux L, et al. Vertebral compression fractures in multiple myeloma Part II. Assessment of fracture risk with MR imaging of spinal bone marrow. *Radiology* 1997;204:201–205.
94. Carmody RF, Yang PJ, Seeley GW, et al. Spinal cord compression due to metastatic disease: diagnosis with MR imaging versus myelography. *Radiology* 1989;173:225–229.

95. Quint DJ, Patel SC, Sanders WP, et al. Importance of absence of CSF pulsation artifacts in the MR detection of significant myelographic block at 1.5 T. *AJNR Am J Neuroradiol* 1989;10: 1089–1095.

96. Breger RK, Williams AL, Daniels DL, et al. Contrast enhancement in spinal MR imaging. *AJNR Am J Neuroradiol* 1989;10: 633–637.

97. Sze G, Krol G, Zimmerman RD, et al. Malignant extradural spinal tumors: MR imaging with Gd-DTPA. *Radiology* 1988;167: 217–223.

98. Moulopoulos LA, Yoshimitsu K, Johnston DA, et al. MR prediction of benign and malignant vertebral compression fractures. *J Magn Reson Imaging* 1996;6:667–674.

99. Cuénad CA, Laredo JD, Chevret S, et al. Acute vertebral collapse due to osteoporosis or malignancy: appearance on unenhanced and gadolinium-enhanced MR images. *Radiology* 1996;199: 541–549.

100. Baur A, Stabler A, Arbogast S, et al. Diffusion-weighted MR imaging of bone marrow: differentiation of benign versus pathologic compression fractures. *Radiology* 1998;207:349–356.

101. Baker LL, Goodman SB, Perkash I, et al. Benign versus pathologic compression fractures of vertebral bodies: assessment with conventional spin-echo, chemical shift, and STIR MR imaging. *Radiology* 1990;174:495–502.

102. Pagni CA, Canavero S. Spinal epidural angiolipoma: rare or unreported? *Neurosurgery* 1992;31:758–764.

103. Provenjale JM, McLendon RE. Spinal Angiolipomas: MR features. *AJNR Am J Neuroradiol* 1996;17:713–719.

104. Holtas MHLIS, Larsson EM. MR imaging of spinal lymphomas. *Acta Radiol* 1992;33:338–342.

105. Dillon WP, Norman D, Newton TH, et al. Intradural spinal cord lesions: Gd-DTPA-enhanced MR imaging. *Radiology* 1989;170: 229–237.

106. Parizel PM, Baleriaux D, Rodesch G, et al. Gd-DTPA-enhanced MR imaging of spinal tumors. *AJNR Am J Neuroradiol* 1989;10: 249–258.

107. Sze G, Abramson A, Krol G, et al. Gadolinium-DTPA in the evaluation of intradural extramedullary spinal disease. *AJNR Am J Neuroradiol* 1988;9:153–163.

108. Burk DL Jr, Brunberg JA, Kanal E, et al. Spinal and paraspinal neurofibromatosis: surface coil MR imaging at 1.5 T. *Radiology* 1987;162:797–801.

109. Valk J. Gd-DTPA in MR of spinal lesions. *AJNR Am J Neuroradiol* 1988;9:345–350.

110. Osenbach RK, Godersky JC, Traynelis VC, et al. Intradural extramedullary cysts of the spinal canal: clinical presentation, radiographic diagnosis, and surgical management. *Neurosurgery* 1992;30:35–42.

111. Nabors MW, Pait TG, Byrd EB, et al. Updated assessment and current classification of spinal meningeal cysts. *J Neurosurg* 1988; 68:366–377.

112. Sklar E, Quencer RM, Greeen BA, et al. Acquired spinal subarachnoid cysts: evaluation with MR, CT myelography, and intraoperative sonography. *AJNR Am J Neuroradiol* 1989;10:1097–1104.

113. Barloon TJ, Yuh WTC, Yang CJC, et al. Spinal subarachnoid tumor seeding from intracranial metastasis: MR findings. *J Comp Assist Tomogr* 1987;11:242–244.

114. Krol G, Sze G, Malkin M, et al. MR of cranial and spinal meningeal carcinomatosis: comparison with CT and myelography. *AJNR Am J Neuroradiol* 1988;9:709–714.

115. Goy AMC, Pinto RS, Raghavendra BN, et al. Intramedullary spinal cord tumors: MR imaging, with emphasis on associated cysts. *Radiology* 1986;161:381–386.

116. Stimac GK, Porter BA, Olson DO, et al. Gadolinium-DTPA-enhanced MR imaging of spinal neoplasms: preliminary investigation and comparison with unenhanced spin-echo and STIR sequences. *AJNR Am J Neuroradiol* 1988;9:839–846.

117. Sze G, Krol G, Zimmerman RD, et al. Intramedullary disease of the spine: diagnosis using gadolinium-DTPA-enhanced MR imaging. *AJNR Am J Neuroradiol* 1988;9:847–858.

118. Donovan Post MJ, Quencer RM, Green BA, et al. Intramedullary spinal cord metastases, mainly of nonneurogenic origin. *AJNR Am J Neuroradiol* 1987;8:339–346.

119. Deeb ZL, Schimel S, Daffner RH, et al. Intervertebral disk-space infection after chymopapain injection. *AJR Am J Roentgenol* 1985;144:671–674.

120. Modic MT, Feiglin DH, Piraino DW, et al. Vertebral osteomyelitis: assessment using MR. *Radiology* 1985;57:157–166.

121. Dagirmanjian A, Schils J, McHenry M, et al. MR imaging of vertebral osteomyelitis revisited. *AJR Am J Roentgenol* 1996;167: 1539–1543.

122. Angtuaco EJC, McConnell JR, Chadduck WM, et al. MR imaging of spinal epidural sepsis. *AJNR Am J Neuroradiol* 1987;8: 879–883.

123. Donovan Post MJ, Quencer RM, Montalvo BM, et al. Spinal infection: evaluation with MR imaging and intraoperative US. *Radiology* 1988;169:765–771.

124. Donovan Post MJ, Sze G, Quencer RM, et al. Gadolinium enhanced MR in spinal infection. *J Comput Assist Tomogr* 1990; 14:721–729.

125. Wagner SC, Schweitzer ME, Morrison WB, et al. Can imaging findings help differentiate spinal neuropathic arthropathy from disk space infection? Initial experience. *Radiology* 2000; 214:693–699.

126. de Roos A, van Persijn V Meerten E, Bloem JL, et al. MRI of tuberculous spondylitis. *AJR Am J Roentgenol* 1986;147:79–82.

127. Sharif HS, Aideyan OA, Clark DC, et al. Brucellar and tuberculous spondylitis: comparative imaging features. *Radiology* 1989; 171:419–425.

128. Smith AS, Weinstein MA, Mizushima A, et al. MR imaging characteristics of tuberculous spondylitis vs vertebral osteomyelitis. *AJNR Am J Neuroradiol* 1989;10:619–625.

129. Castillo M, Quencer RM, Donovan Post MJ. MR of intramedullary spinal cysticercosis. *AJNR Am J Neuroradiol* 1988;9:393–395.

130. Enzmann DR, DeLaPaz RL, Rubin JB. *Magnetic resonance of the spine*. St. Louis, MO: The C.V. Mosby Company, 1990.

131. Kelly RB, Mahoney PD, Cawley KM. MR demonstration of spinal cord sarcoidosis: report of a case. *AJNR Am J Neuroradiol* 1988;9:197–199.

132. Nesbit GM, Miller GM, Baker HL Jr, et al. Spinal cord sarcoidosis: a new finding at MR imaging with Gd-DTPA enhancement. *Radiology* 1989;173:839–843.

133. Tartaglino LM, Croul SE, Flanders AE, et al. Idiopathic acute transverse myelitis. MR imaging finding. *Radiology* 1996;201:661–669.

134. Barakos JA, Mark AS, Dillion WP, et al. MR imaging of acute transverse myelitis and AIDS myelopathy. *J Comp Assist Tomogr* 1990;14(1):45–50.

135. Jeffery DR, Mandler RN, Davis LE. Transverse myelitis. Retrospective analysis of 33 cases, with differentiation of cases associated with multiple sclerosis and parainfectious events. *Arch Neurol (US)* 1993;59(5):532–535.

136. Ang KK, Stevens LC. Prevention and management of radiation myelopathy. *Oncology* 1994;8:71–81.

137. Melki PS, Halimi P, Wibault P, et al. MRI in chronic progressive radiation myelopathy. *J Comp Assist Tomogr* 1994;18(1):1–6.

138. Wang P-Y, Shen W-C, Jan J-S. MR imaging in radiation myelopathy. *AJNR Am J Neuroradiol* 1992;13:1049–1055.

139. Zweig G, Russell EJ. Radiation myelopathy of the cervical spinal cord: MR findings. *AJNR Am J Neuroradiol* 1990;11:1188–1190.

140. Keiper MD, Grossman RI, Brunson JC, et al. The low sensitivity of fluid-attenuated inversion-recovery MR in the detection of multiple sclerosis of the spinal cord. *AJNR Am J Neuroradiol* 1997;18:1035–1039.

141. Nijeholt GJ, Lycklama A, Barkhof F, et al. Comparison of two MR sequences for the detection of multiple sclerosis lesions in the spinal cord. *AJNR Am J Neuroradiol* 1996;17:1533–1538.

142. Hittmair K, Mallek R, Prayer D, et al. Spinal cord lesions in patients with multiple sclerosis: comparison of MR pulse sequences. *AJNR Am J Neuroradiol* 1996;17:1555–1565.

143. Rocca MA, Mastronardo G, Horsfield MA, et al. Comparison of three MR sequences for the detection of cervical cord lesions in patients with multiple sclerosis. *AJNR Am J Neuroradiol* 1999; 20:1710–1716.

144. Maravilla KR, Weinreb JC, Suss R, et al. Magnetic resonance demonstration of multiple sclerosis plaques in the cervical cord. *AJR Am J Roentgenol* 1985;144:381–385.

145. Thielen KR, Miller GM, Noseworthy JH. *Multiple sclerosis of the spinal cord: the MR appearance.* Presented at the American Society of Neuroradiology Annual Meeting, Vancouver, BC May 16–20 1993.

146. Larsson EM, Holtas S, Nilsson O. Gd-DTPA-enhanced MR of suspected spinal multiple sclerosis. *AJNR Am J Neuroradiol* 1989;10:1071–1076.

147. Sze G, Bravo S, Krol G. Spinal lesions: quantitative and qualitative temporal evolution of gadopentetate dimeglumine enhancement in MR imaging. *Radiology* 1989;170:849–856.

148. Altman NR, Altman DH. MR imaging of spinal dysraphism. *AJNR Am J Neuroradiol* 1987;8:533–538.

149. Barnes PD, Lester PD, Yamanashi WS, et al. MRI in infants and children with spinal dysraphism. *AJR Am J Roentgenol* 1986; 147:339–346.

150. Davis PC, Hoffman JC Jr, Ball TI, et al. Spinal abnormalities in pediatric patients: MR imaging findings compared with clinical, myelographic, and surgical findings. *Radiology* 1988;166:679–685.

151. Raghavan N, Barkovich AJ, Edwards M, et al. MR imaging in the tethered spinal cord syndrome. *AJR Am J Roentgenol* 1989; 152:843-852.

152. Wilson DA, Prince JR. MR imaging determination of the location of the normal conus medullaris throughout childhood. *AJNR Am J Neuroradiol* 1989;10:59–262.

153. Nokes SR, Murtagh FR, Jones JD III, et al. Childhood scoliosis: MR imaging. *Radiology* 1987;164:791–797.

154. Barkovich AJ, Raghavan N, Chuang S, et al. The wedge-shaped cord terminus: a radiographic sign of caudal regression. *AJNR Am J Neuroradiol* 1989;10:1223–1231.

155. Fischbein NJ, Dillon WP, Cobbs C, et al. The "Presynrinx" state: a reversible myelopathic condition that may precede syringomyelia. *AJNR Am J Neuroradiol* 1999;20:7–20.

156. Milhorat TH, Johnson RW, Milhorat RH, et al. Clinicopathological correlations in syringomyelia using axial magnetic resonance imaging. *Neurosurgery* 1995;37:205–213.

157. El Gammal T, Mark EK, Brooks BS. MR imaging of Chiari II malformation. *AJNR Am J Neuroradiol* 1987;8:1037–1044.

158. Samuelsson L, Bergstrom K, Thuomas K-A, et al. MR imaging of syringohydromyelia and Chiari malformations in myelomeningocele patients with scoliosis. *AJNR Am J Neuroradiol* 1987;8: 539–546.

159. Smoker WRK, Keyes WD, Dunn VD, et al. MRI versus conventional radiologic examinations in the evaluation of the craniovertebral and cervicomedullary junction. *Radiographics* 1986;6: 953–994.

160. Wolpert SM, Anderson M, Scott RM, et al. Chiari II malformation: MR imaging evaluation. *AJNR Am J Neuroradiol* 1987;8: 783–792.

161. Flanders AE, Spettell CM, Tartaglino LM, et al. Forecasting motor recovery after cervical spinal cord injury: value of MR imaging. *Radiology* 1996;201:649–655.

162. Gebarski SS, Maynard FW, Gabrielsen TO, et al. Posttraumatic progressive myelopathy: clinical and radiologic correlation employing MR imaging, delayed CT metrizamide myelography, and intraoperative sonography. *Radiology* 1985;157:379–385.

163. Mirvis SE, Geisler FH, Jelinek JJ, et al. Acute cervical spine trauma: evaluation with 1.5-T MR imaging. *Radiology* 1988;166:807–816.

164. Quencer RM, Sheldon JJ, Donovan Post MJ, et al. MRI of the chronically injured cervical spinal cord. *AJR Am J Roentgenol* 1986;147:125–132.

165. Denis F. The three-column spine and its significance in the classification of acute thoracolumbar spinal injuries. *Spine* 1983;8: 817–831.

166. Terk MR, Hume-Neal M, Fraipont M, et al. Injury of the posterior ligament complex in patients with acute spinal trauma: evaluation by MR imaging. *AJR Am J Roentgenol* 1997;168:1481–1486.

167. Chakeres DW, Flickinger F, Bresnahan JC, et al. MR imaging of acute spinal cord trauma. *AJNR Am J Neuroradiol* 1987;8:5–10.

168. Hackney DB, Asato R, Joseph PM, et al. Hemorrhage and edema in acute spinal cord compression: demonstration by MR imaging. *Radiology* 1986;61:387–390.

169. Jenkins JR, Reddy S, Leite CC, et al. MR of parenchymal spinal cord signal change as a sign of active advancement in clinically

170. Lee TT, Arias J, Andrus HL, et al. Progressive post-traumatic myelomalacic myelopathy: treatment with untethering and expansive duraplasty. *J Neurosurg* 1997;86:624–628.

171. McGillicuddy JE. Surgical anatomy and management of brachial plexus injury. In: Tindall GT, Cooper PR, Barrow DL, eds. *The practice of neurosurgery,* Baltimore: Williams & Wilkins, 1996:2859–2877.

172. Walker AT, Chaloupka JC, De Lotbiniere ACJ, et al. Detection of nerve rootlet avulsion on CT myelography in patients with birth palsy and brachial plexus injury after trauma. *AJR Am J Roentgenol* 1996;167:1283–1287.

173. Riche MC, Reizine D, Melki JP, et al. Classification of spinal cord vascular malformations. *Radiat Med* 1985;3(1):17–24.

174. Gilbertson JR, Miller GM, Goldman MS, et al. Spinal dural arteriovenous fistulas: MR and myelographic findings. *AJNR Am J Neuroradiol* 1995;16:2049–2057.

175. Dormont D, Gelbert F, Assouline E, et al. MR imaging of spinal cord arteriovenous malformations at 0.5 T: study of 34 cases. *AJNR Am J Neuroradiol* 1988;9:833–838.

176. Masaryk TJ, Ross JS, Modic MT, et al. Radiculomeningeal vascular malformations of the spine: MR imaging. *Radiology* 1987; 164:845–849.

177. Doppman JL, Di Chiro G, Dwyer AJ, et al. Magnetic resonance imaging of spinal arteriovenous malformations. *J Neurosurg* 1987;66:830–834.

178. Minami S, Sagoh T, Nishimura K, et al. Spinal arteriovenous malformation: MR imaging. *Radiology* 1988;169:109–115.

179. Willinsky RA, terBrugge K, Montanera W, et al. Post-treatment MR findings in spinal dural arteriovenous malformations. *AJNR Am J Neuroradiol* 1995;16:2063–2071.

180. Gelbert F, Guichard JP, Kourier KL, et al. Phase-contrast MR angiography of vascular malformations of the spinal cord at 0.5 T^1. *J Magn Reson Imaging* 1992;2:631–636.

181. Mascalchi M, Bianchi MC, Quilici N, et al. MR angiography of spinal vascular malformations. *AJNR Am J Neuroradiol* 1995; 16:289–297.

182. Mascalchi M, Quilici N, Ferrito G, et al. Identification of the feeding arteries of spinal vascular lesions via phase-contrast MR angiography with three-dimensional acquisition and phase display. *AJNR Am J Neuroradiol* 1997;18:351–358.

183. Provenzale JM, Tien RD, Felsbert GJ, et al. Spinal dural arteriovenous fistula: demonstration using phase contrast MRA. *J Comput Assist Tomogr* 1994;18:811–814.

184. Bowen BC, Kraser K, Kochan JP, et al. Spinal dural arteriovenous fistulas: evaluation with MR angiography. *AJNR Am J Neuroradiol* 1995; 16:2029–2043.

185. Luetmer PH, Lane JI, Gilbertson JR, et al. Pre-angiographic evaluation of spinal dural arteriovenous fistulae (AVFs) with elliptic centric contrast-enhanced MRA and impact on radiation and iodinated contrast dose. *AJNR Am J Neuroradiol* 2005 *(in press).*

186. Tobin WD, Layton DD Jr. The diagnosis and natural history of spinal cord arteriovenous malformations. *Mayo Clin Proc* 1976; 51:637–646.

187. Di Chiro G, Doppman JL, Dwyer AJ, et al. Tumors and arteriovenous malformations of the spinal cord: assessment using MR. *Radiology* 1985;156:689–697.

188. Walton JN. Subarachnoid hemorrhage of unusual etiology. *Neurology* 1953;3:517–543.

189. Hughes JT, Oppenheimer DR. Superficial siderosis of the central nervous system; a report on nine cases with autopsy. *Acta Neuropathol* 1969;13:556–574.

190. Bourgouin PM, Tampieri D, Melancon D, et al. Superficial siderosis of the brain following unexplained subarachnoid hemorrhage: MRI diagnosis and clinical significance. *Neuroradiology* 1992;34:407–410.

191. Gomori JM, Grossman RI, Bilaniuk LT, et al. High-field MR imaging of superficial siderosis of the central nervous system. *J Comp Assist Tomogr* 1985;9:972–975.

192. Gundry CR, Heithoff KB. Epidural hematoma of the lumbar spine: 18 surgically confirmed cases. *Radiology* 1993;187:427–431.

193. Kallmes D, Jensen M. Percutaneous vertebroplasty. *Radiology* 2003;229:27–36.

194. Mathis J, Ortiz A, Zoarski G, et al. Vertebroplasty versus Kyphoplasty: a comparison and contrast. *AJNR Am J Neuroradiol* 2004;25:840–845.

195. Rhyne AI, Banit D. Kyphoplasty: report of eighty-two thoracolumbar osteoporotic vertebral fractures. *J Orhtop Trauma* 2005;18(5):294–299.

196. Cotton A, Boutry N, Cortet B, et al. Percutaneous vertebroplasty: state of the art. *Radiographics* 1998;18:311–320.

197. Cyteval CM, Baron Sarrabere MP, et al. Acute osteoporotic vertebral collapse: open study on percutaneous injection of acrylic surgical cement in 20 patients. *AJR Am J Roentgenol* 1999; 173:1685–1690.

198. Deramond H, Depriester C, Galibert P, et al. Percutaneous vertebroplasty with polymethylmethacrylate. *Radiol Clin North Am* 1998;36:533–546.

199. Lane J, Maus T, Shalabh Bobra, et al. Intravertebral clefts opacified during vertebroplasty: pathogenesis, technical implications, and prognostic significance. *AJNR Am J Neuroradiol* 2002; 23(10):1642–1646.

200. Dansie D, Luetmer P. MR findings after successful vertebroplasty. *AJNR Am J Neuroradiol* 2005 *(in press)*

Pelvis, Hips, and Thigh

6

Thomas H. Berquist

Magnetic resonance imaging (MRI) of the pelvis and hips has achieved wide acceptance as an imaging technique. This was initially due to the sensitivity and specificity of MRI for early detection of avascular necrosis (AVN) (1–6). However, as with other musculoskeletal regions, the applications for MRI of the pelvis, hips, and thighs continue to expand. New pulse sequences, intravenous and intraarticular contrast enhancement, and other technological improvements have contributed significantly to the growth of MRI.

TECHNIQUE

The image planes and pulse sequences chosen for evaluation of the pelvis, hips, and thighs depend upon the clinical indication. The patient's age and clinical status is also important. Sedation may be required for certain adults (pain, claustrophobia, etc.) and is commonly required in young children (see Chapter 3) (1,7,8). Specific techniques will be discussed later, however, there are certain standard techniques that can be used for screening examinations.

Pelvis and Sacroiliac Joints

Examinations for suspected pathology of the pelvis and/or sacroiliac joints can be accomplished using the torso coil. Smaller coils may be used for infants and children (7,8). Scout images are obtained in three planes with the patient in the supine position (see Fig. 6-1). Every effort should be made to be certain the patient is properly positioned (see Fig. 6-2) with the hips at the same level. The legs should be internally rotated (toes touching) to assure a symmetric appearance of the trochanters and soft tissues to allow easy comparison. A bolster can be positioned under the knees for patient comfort. This results in flexion of the

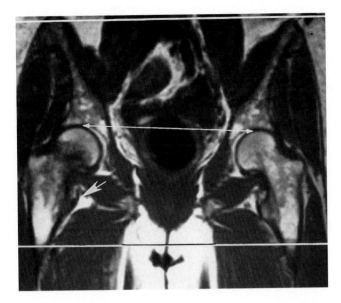

Figure 6-1 Coronal SE 400/20 scout image of the pelvis [128 × 256, 1 NEX, 42 cm field of view (FOV)] with axial images selected from the iliac crests to below the lesser trochanter (*white lines*). The number of axial images can be reduced or expanded depending upon the indication. Thin sections are used when smaller regions are examined. There is slight malpositioning of the right femur (*arrow*) as the lesser trochanters are not seen in the same profile on this section. The femoral heads are also slightly tilted indicating asymmetric patient position (*white line with arrows on femoral heads*).

hips (~15°). Therefore, we try to avoid using this approach when hip pathology is suspected. If a soft tissue abnormality is suspected posteriorly, the patient should be placed in the prone position. This reduces compression of the soft tissues and anatomic distortion (9,10). After the initial scout images, axial images are obtained using spin-echo T1-weighted and turbo spin-echo T2-weighted sequences (Table 6-1) (10). The same sections are selected for both sequences. This allows more accurate comparison of T1- and T2-weighted sections. In the same fashion, coronal images are obtained using short TI inversion recovery (STIR) and T1-weighted sequences (Table 6-1) (see Fig. 6-3). Some

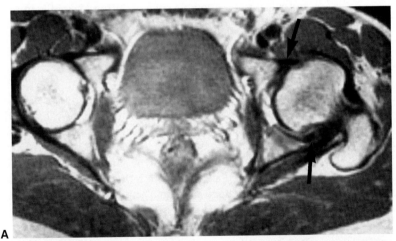

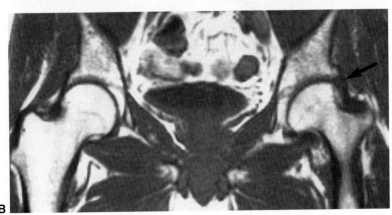

Figure 6-2 Axial images of the pelvis with the patient improperly positioned. **A:** Axial SE 450/12 image with the patient improperly positioned. The femoral heads are at different levels. Note the deformity of the left femoral head due to old developmental dysplasia. *Arrows* mark the labra on the *left*. The patient is also slightly off center in the gantry. **B:** Coronal SE 500/15 image of the pelvis with the patient slightly rotated and tilted. The greater trochanter is identified on the *right*. The femoral heads are clearly not comparable. *Arrow* on the *left* marks the labrum.

TABLE 6-1
MR EXAMINATIONS OF THE PELVIS, HIPS, AND THIGHS

	Pulse Sequence	Slice Thickness	Matrix	Field of View (FOV) cm	Acquisitions (NEX)	Image Time
Pelvis–SI joints						
Scout-axial	15/5 FA 40°	3-5 1 cm slices	256	40	1	26 s
Coronal sagittal axial	SE 410/17	6 mm	512	34–40[a]	2	5 min 20 s
Axial	TSE 4,000/102	6 mm	512	34–40[a]	2	4 min 36 s
Coronal	SE 580/13	5 mm	512	34–40[a]	1	5 min 2 s
Coronal	STIR 5,600/109/165	5 mm	256	34–40[a]	2	4 min 34 s
Hips						
Coronal	SE 536/15	4 mm	320	20–24	1	4 min 38 s
Axial	TSE 4,000/102	6 mm	512	20–24	2	4 min 36 s
Sagittal	SE 536/15	4 mm	320	20–24	1	4 min 38 s
Thighs						
Coronal scout	SE 400/15–20	3 1-cm slices	128 × 256	42	1	51 s
Axial	TSE 4,000/102	6 mm	512	30–42[a]	2	4 min 36 s
Coronal or sagittal	SE 536/15	4 mm	320	30–42[a]	1	4 min 38 s
Arthrography						
Axial	SE 568/15	4 mm	256	18	1	4 min 55 s
Sagittal	SE 568/15	4 mm	256	18	1	4 min 55 s
Coronal	SE 420/15	4 mm	256	18	1	3 min 36 s
Coronal	TSE 4,000/92 (fat suppressed)	4 mm	256	18	1	3 min 39 s
Oblique coronal	SE 420/15	4 mm	256	18	1	3 min 39 s
Oblique sagittal	SE 420/15	4 mm	256	18	1	3 min 39 s

TSE, turbo spin echo; FA, flip angle; SI, sacroiliac; SE, spin echo; STIR, short inversion time recovery.
[a] Varies with patient size and area of interest

institutions advocate a single coronal STIR sequence for a limited screening examination in patients with hip pain (11). When the coronal or sagittal plane is used, the slice thickness varies depending on the tissue volume of the area to be studied. These sequences and image planes generally provide an adequate screening examination for the pelvis (Table 6-1). In certain circumstances, which will be discussed later, further pulse sequences and image planes may be indicated (10,12). The field of view (FOV) selected varies with patient size, but generally 34 to 40 cm is adequate for adults. A matrix of 256 × 256 or 512 × 512 with 1 or 2 acquisitions (NEX) is obtained. Respiratory compensation techniques should be used to reduce motion artifact in the upper pelvis. Thinner slices can be used if a more defined area of the anatomy is to be studied.

When pathology of the sacrum or sacroiliac joints is suspected, a different approach may provide additional information (13,14). This is especially true in patients with suspected sacroiliac arthropathy. Additional oblique coronal images in the plane of the sacrum (see Fig. 6-4) and sacroiliac joints are performed using T1-, T2-weighted, and STIR sequences (10,15). Fat suppression techniques are useful, especially when intravenous gadolinium is injected. Gadolinium is useful for identification of early or acute inflammatory changes in patients with sacroiliitis (8).

Hips

Evaluation of patients with symptoms more defined to the hip region is performed with a slightly different technique. Using a three-plane scout sequence as a guide, a T1-weighted coronal sequence (SE 540/15) is performed using 4-mm-thick sections with no interslice gap. This technique will usually define AVN and other obvious marrow abnormalities in the hips. When there is no evidence of AVN or if other abnormalities are suspected, a second turbo spin-echo or fat suppressed T2-weighted axial sequence is performed similar to above (pelvis and sacroiliac joints) (Table 6-1). In certain situations such as AVN or subtle osteochondral abnormalities of the femoral heads, it may be of benefit to use a surface coil or dual coupled coils to improve image quality (10,16,17). Sagittal images are useful to quantify surface area involvement of the femoral head (see Fig. 6-5). In this setting, a small FOV (12 to 16 cm) should be used (4,17,18).

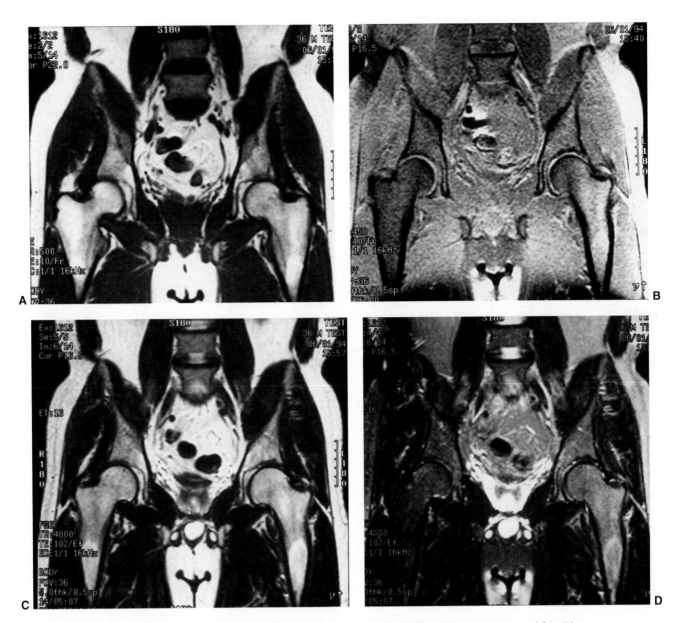

Figure 6-3 Coronal SE 500/10 **(A)** and fat-suppressed SE 450/10 **(B)** images. Coronal fast T2 (4800/102) **(C)** and fat-suppressed fast spin-echo T2 (4800/102) **(D)** sequences. There are contrast differences and there is less fat suppression with fast spin-echo T2-weighted sequences compared to conventional spin-echo T2-weighted sequences. Note the uneven suppression of fat signal and signal intensity loss on the *left* compared to *right* on these images. Uniform fat suppression is important to prevent errors in image interpretation.

Evaluation of subtle femoral head changes, articular cartilage, synovial or labral pathology may require additional sequences and intravenous or intraarticular gadolinium (4,19,20). In these clinical settings, a surface coil, or coupled coils and smaller FOV (12 to 16 cm) is also required (4,10,17). Early changes in articular cartilage may be more evident with fat-suppressed T2-weighted fast spin-echo sequences. Three-dimensional spoiled gradient-echo sequences have also been advocated, with accuracy reported at over 90% for detection of cartilage lesions (TR 60, TE 5, flip angle 40°) (21). Axial and coronal or sagittal T1-weighted spin-echo and T2-weighted turbo spin-echo sequences provide initial screening of the thighs (Table 6-1).

Intravenous gadolinium is useful for detection of subtle ischemic disease in adults (AVN) and children, and changes in articular cartilage and synovium (19,22,23). Conventional sequences are usually performed followed by fat-suppressed T1-weighted sequences after contrast injection (see Fig. 6-6).

Magnetic Resonance Arthrography

Intraarticular contrast has become more popular in recent years to better define specific hip disorders (see Fig. 6-7) (20,24–27). MR arthrograms can more readily identify intraarticular abnormalities such as cartilage defects, loose

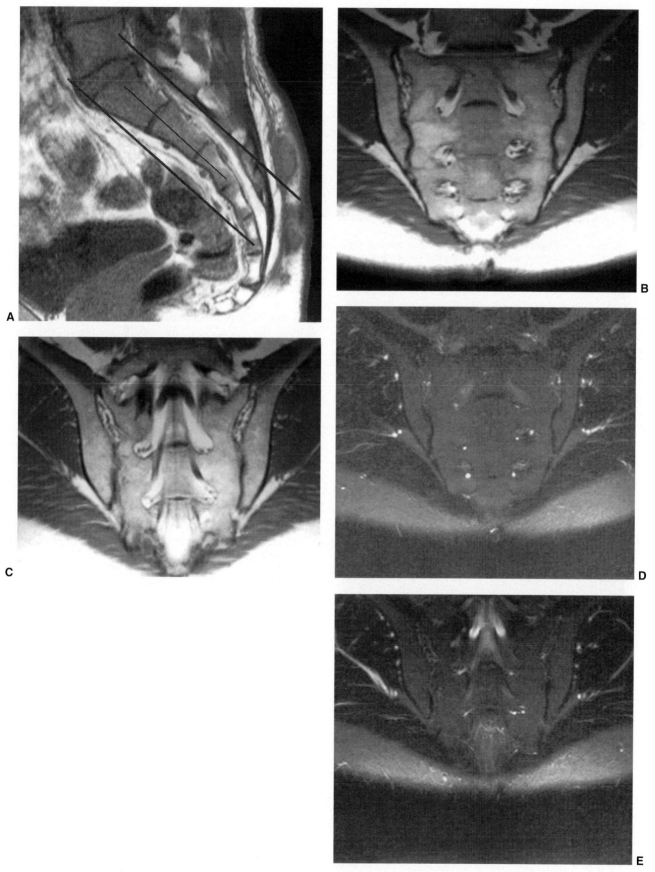

Figure 6-4 Scout sagittal image **(A)** to select image planes and sections for evaluation of the sacrum and sacroiliac joints. Oblique coronal images of the sacrum and sacroiliac joints using T1-weighted **(B, C)** images and fat-suppressed, T2-weighted **(D, E)** images at similar levels.

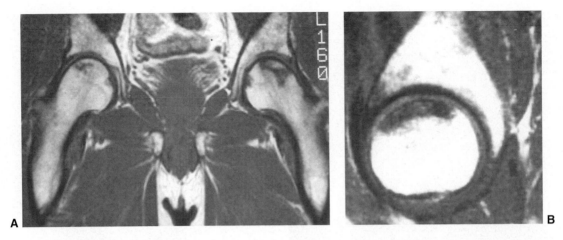

Figure 6-5 Coronal **(A)** torso coil and sagittal **(B)** surface coil images of the femoral head in a patient with AVN. The extent of involvement is more accurately assessed when both coronal and sagittal sections are obtained.

bodies, and labral tears compared to conventional MRI (20,27). Though an arthrographic effect can also be achieved by delayed imaging (>15 minutes after injection) after intravenous contrast, there is no control of contrast volumes and joint fluid cannot be obtained for study. Therefore, direct MR arthrography (Fig. 6-7) is preferred in most cases. Contrast (8 to 20 mL of 1 mmol solution of gadolinium) is injected using fluoroscopic

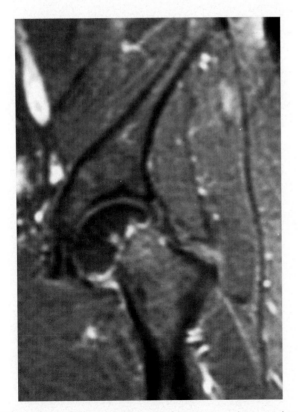

Figure 6-6 Coronal postcontrast fat-suppressed T1-weighted image demonstrates a femoral neck fracture with no enhancement of the femoral head due to vascular injury.

guidance. We mix 50% iodinated contrast and 50% Marcaine to dilute the gadolinium. This assists in confirming the hip is the source of symptoms, specifically pain. The patient is exercised and transferred to the MR gantry. MR arthrography requires a surface coil with a small field of view (12 to 18 cm). Axial, coronal, sagittal, oblique, or radial images can be obtained depending upon the suspected pathology (Table 6-1) (28–30). T1-weighted fat-suppressed spin-echo and turbo spin-echo T2-weighted sequences are most commonly used with MR arthrography (20,27). Three-dimensional gradient-echo sequences (30/9, 45° flip angle) can also be utilized (24,31).

MR arthrograms of the hip are invasive and carry the same minimal risks associated with conventional arthrography. Examination time and cost also exceed conventional MRI studies (10,24,31).

Thighs

Generally, both T1- and T2-weighted sequences are required to fully evaluate the soft tissues of the thighs and the upper femurs. Again, a coronal scout through the hip and thigh region is generally obtained, from which conventional or fat-suppressed T2-weighted axial images are selected. Depending upon the findings noted with the T2-weighted images, a second series of T1-weighted images is performed in either the coronal or sagittal plane. The second sequence is important in characterizing the nature of the lesion. Two different planes are essential if the extent of a lesion is important to define, such as for a neoplasm, abscess, or hematoma. Short TI inversion recovery (STIR) or gadolinium enhanced T1-weighted images are useful for evaluating subtle changes (2,10).

New angiographic sequences (see Chapters 1 and 3) are useful when vascular abnormalities are suspected in the pelvis or thighs (32). Variations in techniques will be discussed more fully later with specific clinical applications.

ANATOMY

It is essential that the anatomy of the bone and soft tissue structures be clearly understood in all image planes typically used with MRI (see Figs. 6-8 to 6-10) (2,10,33–35).

Osseous Anatomy

The pelvis is formed by the two innominate bones that articulate posteriorly with the sacrum at the sacroiliac joints and anteriorly at the pubic symphysis. Each innominate bone is composed of an ilium, ischium, and pubis. The

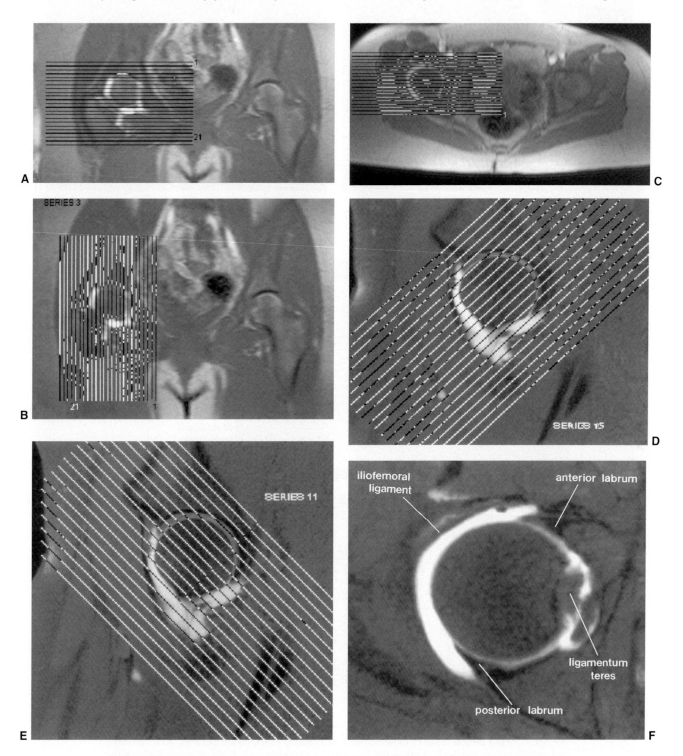

Figure 6-7   Normal MR arthrogram. Scout axial **(A)**, sagittal **(B)**, coronal **(C)**, and oblique coronal **(D)**, and oblique sagittal **(E)** images. Normal axial **(F)**, coronal **(G)**, and sagittal **(H)** arthrogram images. The joint capsule attaches several millimeters proximal to the superior labrum (*arrow* in **G**) creating the superior acetabular recess.

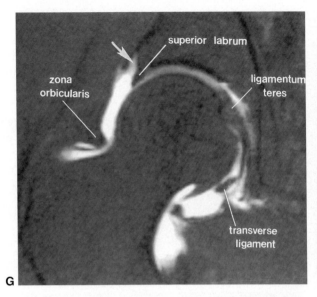

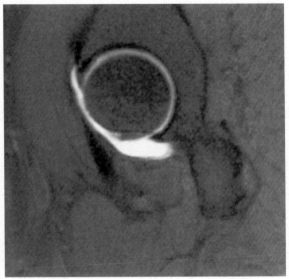

Figure 6-7 *(continued)*

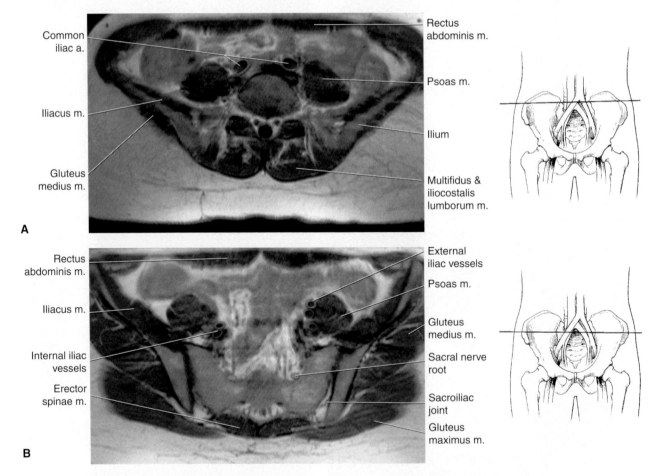

Figure 6-8 Axial MR images (SE 405/16) of the pelvis, hips, and upper thighs with accompanying illustration of the section levels to demonstrate MRI anatomy of the pelvis and hips. **A:** Axial image through the upper pelvis. **B:** Axial image through the upper sacrum. **C:** Axial image through the lower sacroiliac joint. **D:** Axial image through the sciatic notch. **E:** Axial image through the anterior inferior iliac spine. **F:** Axial image through the upper femoral head. **G:** Axial image through the femoral head and greater trochanter. **H:** Axial image through the femoral neck. **I:** Axial image through the lesser trochanter. **J:** Axial image through the upper femur. **K:** Axial image through the upper thigh.

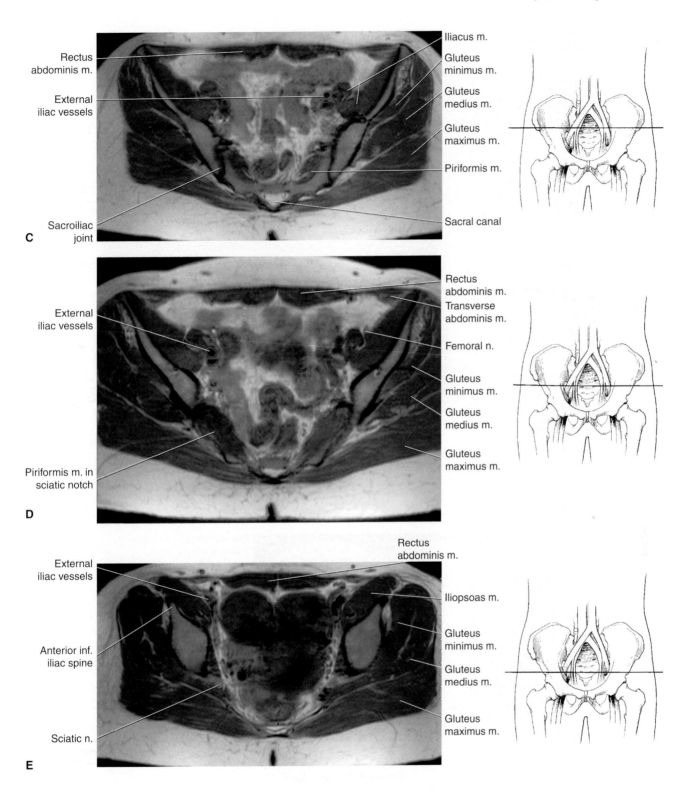

Rectus
abdominis m.

External
iliac vessels

Sacroiliac
joint

C

Iliacus m.

Gluteus
minimus m.

Gluteus
medius m.

Gluteus
maximus m.

Piriformis m.

Sacral canal

External
iliac vessels

Piriformis m. in
sciatic notch

D

Rectus
abdominis m.

Transverse
abdominis m.

Femoral n.

Gluteus
minimus m.

Gluteus
medius m.

Gluteus
maximus m.

External
iliac vessels

Anterior inf.
iliac spine

Sciatic n.

E

Rectus
abdominis m.

Iliopsoas m.

Gluteus
minimus m.

Gluteus
medius m.

Gluteus
maximus m.

Figure 6-8 (*continued*)

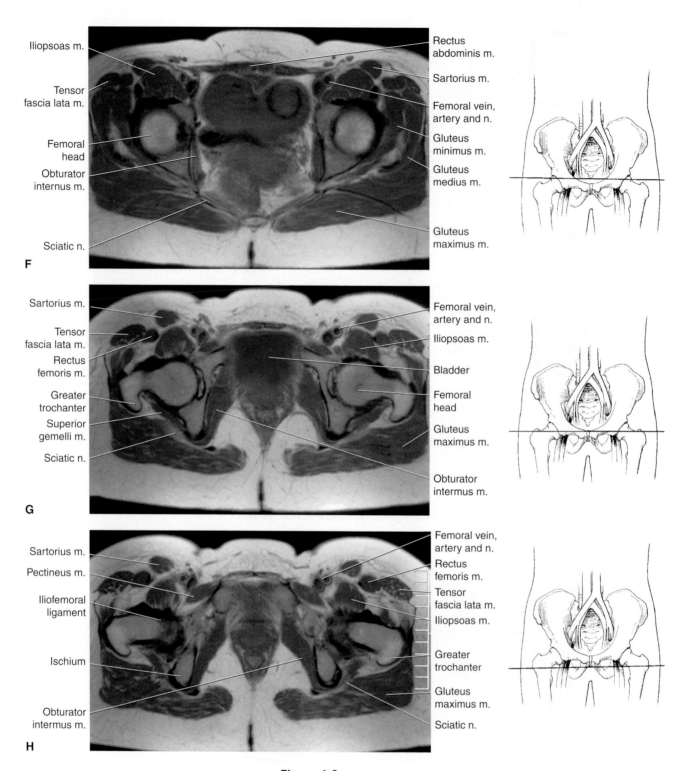

Iliopsoas m.
Tensor fascia lata m.
Femoral head
Obturator internus m.
Sciatic n.

Rectus abdominis m.
Sartorius m.
Femoral vein, artery and n.
Gluteus minimus m.
Gluteus medius m.
Gluteus maximus m.

F

Sartorius m.
Tensor fascia lata m.
Rectus femoris m.
Greater trochanter
Superior gemelli m.
Sciatic n.

Femoral vein, artery and n.
Iliopsoas m.
Bladder
Femoral head
Gluteus maximus m.
Obturator intermus m.

G

Sartorius m.
Pectineus m.
Iliofemoral ligament
Ischium
Obturator intermus m.

Femoral vein, artery and n.
Rectus femoris m.
Tensor fascia lata m.
Iliopsoas m.
Greater trochanter
Gluteus maximus m.
Sciatic n.

H

Figure 6-8 (continued)

acetabulum is formed by the junction of these osseous structures. The posterior acetabulum is stronger and along with the dome comprises the weight-bearing portion of the acetabulum (10,34). The margin of the acetabulum is surrounded by a fibrocartilaginous labrum (Fig. 6-7). Identification of the shape of this labrum, its relationship to the femoral head, and whether the structure is intact is important in infants, children, and adults (10,26,27,36). Special image planes and intraarticular gadolinium may be required to demonstrate the entire labrum. These techniques will be discussed later in this chapter.

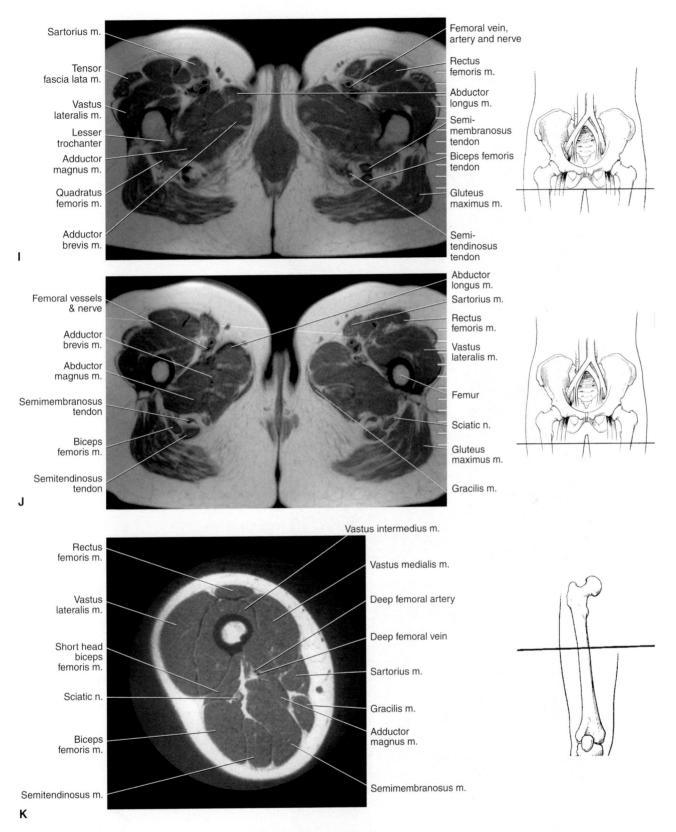

Sartorius m.

Tensor fascia lata m.

Vastus lateralis m.

Lesser trochanter

Adductor magnus m.

Quadratus femoris m.

Adductor brevis m.

Femoral vein, artery and nerve

Rectus femoris m.

Abductor longus m.

Semi-membranosus tendon

Biceps femoris tendon

Gluteus maximus m.

Semi-tendinosus tendon

I

Femoral vessels & nerve

Adductor brevis m.

Abductor magnus m.

Semimembranosus tendon

Biceps femoris m.

Semitendinosus tendon

Abductor longus m.

Sartorius m.

Rectus femoris m.

Vastus lateralis m.

Femur

Sciatic n.

Gluteus maximus m.

Gracilis m.

J

Vastus intermedius m.

Rectus femoris m.

Vastus lateralis m.

Short head biceps femoris m.

Sciatic n.

Biceps femoris m.

Semitendinosus m.

Vastus medialis m.

Deep femoral artery

Deep femoral vein

Sartorius m.

Gracilis m.

Adductor magnus m.

Semimembranosus m.

K

Figure 6-8   (*continued*)

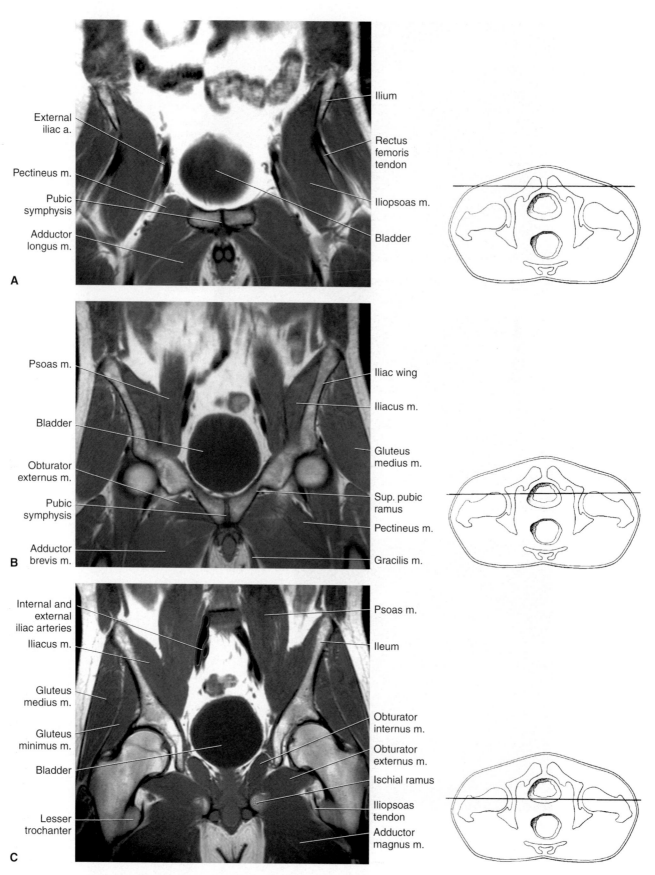

Figure 6-9 Coronal MR images (SE 450/15) and accompanying illustrations of section levels of the pelvis, hips, and thighs. **A:** Coronal image through the pubic symphysis. **B:** Coronal image through the anterior aspect of the hips. **C:** Coronal image through the midjoint space of the hip. **D:** Coronal image through the greater trochanteric level of the hips. **E:** Coronal image through the ischium.

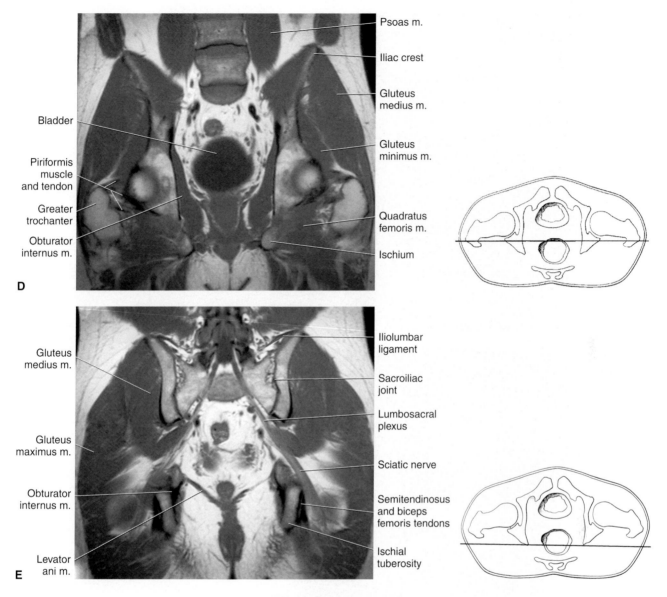

Figure labels (top image, D):
Psoas m.
Iliac crest
Gluteus medius m.
Gluteus minimus m.
Quadratus femoris m.
Ischium
Bladder
Piriformis muscle and tendon
Greater trochanter
Obturator internus m.

Figure labels (bottom image, E):
Iliolumbar ligament
Sacroiliac joint
Lumbosacral plexus
Sciatic nerve
Semitendinosus and biceps femoris tendons
Ischial tuberosity
Gluteus medius m.
Gluteus maximus m.
Obturator internus m.
Levator ani m.

Figure 6-9 (continued)

Further discussion of the articulations in the pelvis is important, as these areas are easily assessed with MRI. Anteriorly, the pubic symphysis is formed by the two pubic bones. The joint is supported by the superior pubic and arcuate ligaments that encase a fibrocartilaginous disc. The disc lies between the two pubic bones (see Figs. 6-9 and 6-11) (37,38). The sacroiliac joint is a synovial joint with posterior and anterior ligamentous support (Fig. 6-11). The posterior ligaments are stronger than the anterior ligaments, which allow some anterior motion. In addition, there are several accessory ligaments that assist in the support of the sacroiliac joint. These include the sacrotuberous ligament, which extends from the inferolateral margin of the sacrum to the ischial tuberosity; the sacrospinous ligament, which extends from the lower margin of the sacrum to the ischial spine; and the iliolumbar ligament, which extends from the anterior

inferior transverse process of L5 and passes inferiorly to blend with the anterior sacroiliac ligament along the base of the sacrum. These ligamentous structures appear dark or have no signal intensity on MR images. The synovial cavity of the sacroiliac joint contains only a small amount of fluid. Joint fliud is most easily identified on axial T2-weighted or contrast-enhanced MR images (Fig. 6-6) (37,38).

The hip is a ball and socket joint. The fibrous capsule of the hip joint is lined with synovial membrane and hyaline cartilage covers the articular surfaces of the acetabulum and femoral head (see Figs. 6-7 and 6-12). There are several important intraarticular structures that should be identified on MR images. Ligamentum teres is a firm ligament extending from the fovea of the femoral head to the acetabulum. The ligament enters a small notch in the medial acetabular

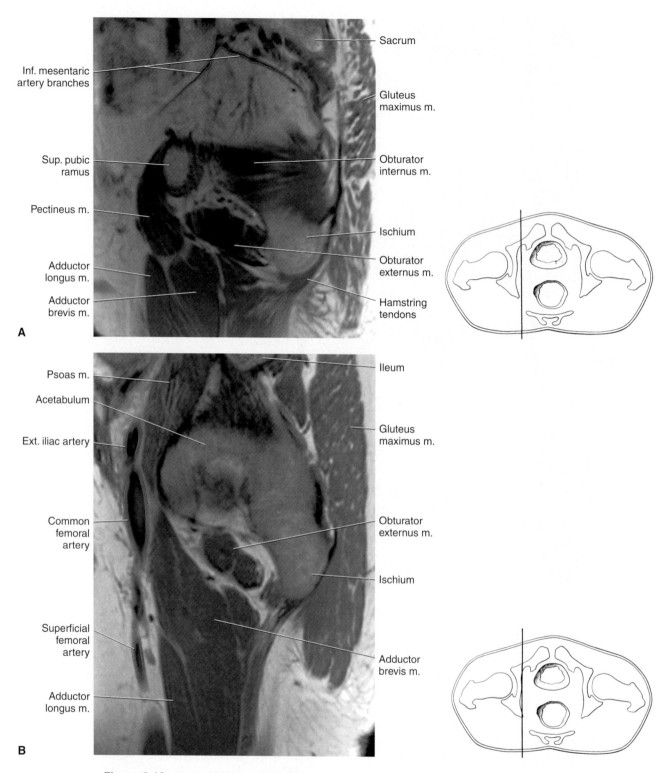

Figure 6-10   Sagittal MR images (SE 450/15) and accompanying anatomic illustrations section levels of the pelvis, hips, and thighs progressing from medial to lateral. **A:** Sagittal image through the medial ilium near the sciatic notch. **B:** Sagittal image through the level of the iliopectineal imminence. **C:** Sagittal image through the medial joint space. **D:** Sagittal image through the medial femoral head. **E:** Sagittal image through the femur. **F:** Sagittal image through the level of the greater trochanter.

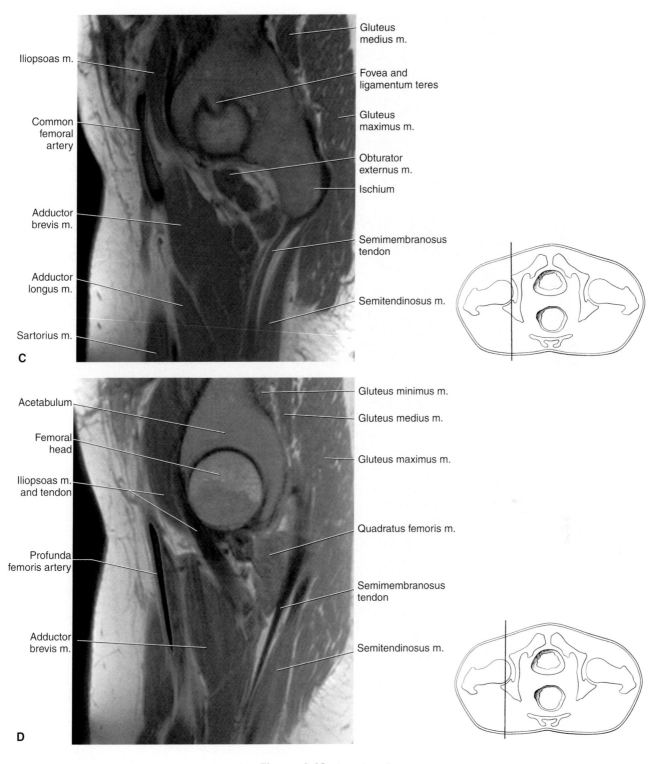

Figure 6-10 *(continued)*

wall where it is surrounded by fat (Figs. 6-9 E and 6-12). A fibrocartilaginous acetabular labrum surrounds the acetabular rim. This structure is more clearly defined on MR arthrograms than conventional MR images (Figs. 6-7 and 6-9) (20,39,40). Axial, coronal, oblique (Fig. 6-7) or radial images

(see Fig. 6-13) may be necessary to completely define this structure (10,26). Inferiorly the labrum is incomplete but connected by the transverse ligament (Figs. 6-7G and 6-12). This ligament has an elliptical configuration and should not be confused with an acetabular labral tear. The ligaments that

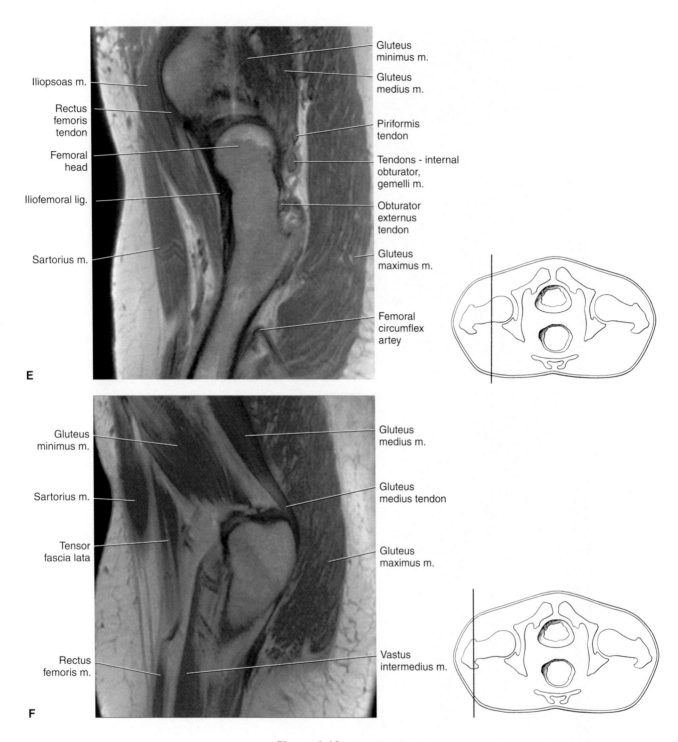

Figure 6-10 (continued)

surround the capsule of the hip blend with the capsule and are not easily defined by MRI. Major ligaments (see Fig. 6-14) include the pubofemoral ligament that arises from the body of the pubis close to the acetabulum and passes anterior to the lower part of the femoral head, blending with the lower limb of the iliofemoral ligament as it attaches to the lower margin of the femoral neck. The iliofemoral ligament is thicker and probably the strongest

of the supporting ligaments of the hip. It is more triangular with its apex attached to the lower part of the anterior inferior iliac spine and body of the ilium. The base of this triangular ligament attaches to the intertrochanteric lines (Fig. 6-14). The ischiofemoral ligament, the thinnest of the three major ligaments, arises from the ischium behind and below the acetabulum. Its upper fibers are horizontal; its lower fibers extend upward and laterally and attach to the

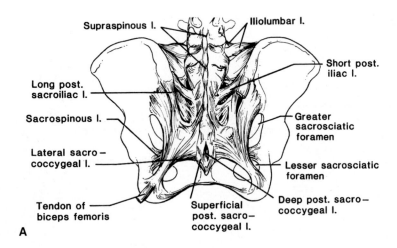

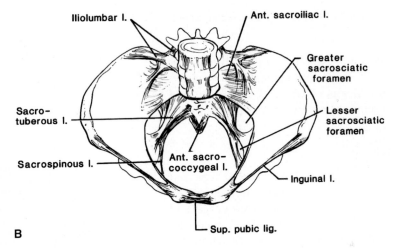

Figure 6-11 Illustration of the ligaments of the posterior sacroiliac region (**A**) and anterior sacroiliac region (**B**) and symphysis. (From Berquist TH. *Imaging of orthopedic trauma.* New York: Raven Press, 1992.)

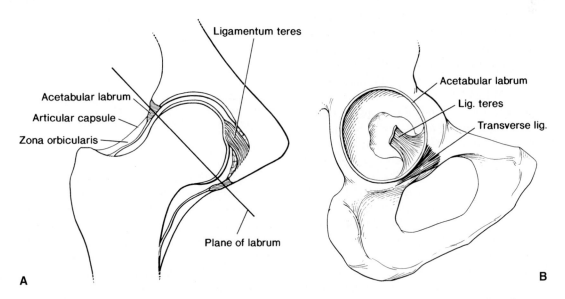

Figure 6-12 **A:** Coronal illustration of the hip demonstrating the major articular components and capsule and the plane (*line*) of the labrum. **B:** Enface illustration of the acetabular fossa and labrum.

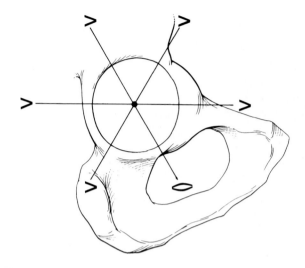

Figure 6-13 Illustration of radial planes and labral configurations.

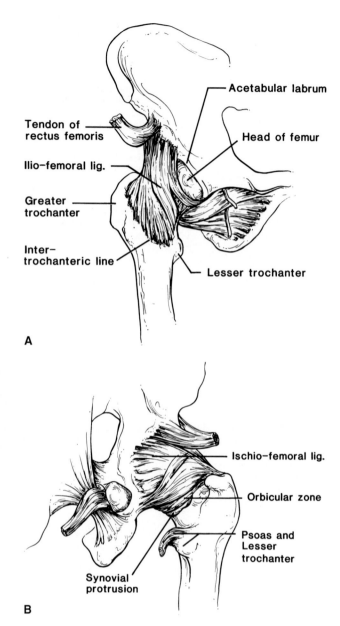

Figure 6-14 Illustration of the supporting ligaments of the hip from anterior **(A)** and posterior **(B)**. (From Berquist TH. *Imaging of orthopedic trauma.* New York: Raven Press, 1992.)

upper posterior neck at the junction of the greater trochanter. The vascular supply of the hip and femoral head is important, especially in the etiology of AVN. This will be discussed more thoroughly later in the section on AVN (34,38,41,42).

Muscular Anatomy

The anatomy of the muscles acting on the pelvis, hips, and thighs in axial, coronal, sagittal, and even oblique planes must be thoroughly understood to interpret MR images and evaluate symptoms related to these structures. The muscles acting on the hip joint *per se* are numerous. Therefore, it is simplest to discuss them based upon their function (2,10,33,34,36–38).

The chief extensors of the hip include the gluteus maximus and posterior portion of the adductor magnus (see Fig. 6-15). Extension is also accomplished to some degree by assistance from the semimembranosus, semitendinosus, biceps femoris, gluteus medius, and gluteus minimus (Table 6-2) (34,43).

The primary flexor of the hip is the iliopsoas muscle (see Fig. 6-16). However, the pectineus, tensor fasciae latae, adductor brevis and sartorius also function in this regard. Accessory flexors include the adductor longus, adductor magnus, gracilis, and gluteus minimus (34,38).

Adduction of the femur is primarily accomplished by the adductor muscle group and gracilis (Figs. 6-8, 6-10, and 6-16). Adductor group includes the adductor brevis, adductor longus, and adductor magnus. Accessory adductors include the gluteus maximus, pectineus, and obturator externus. The hamstring muscles also assist slightly in this regard. Medial or internal rotation of the hip is primarily accomplished by the gluteus medius and minimus and the tensor fasciae latae. Semitendinosus, semimembranosus, and to some degree the gracilis also participate in internal rotation. External rotation of the hip is accomplished by the gluteus maximus and the short rotators of the gluteal

region including the piriformis, obturator internus, and the gemelli muscles (see Fig 6-17) (34,38).

Table 6-2 summarizes the muscles of the pelvis and hips along with their origins, insertions and functions. Identification of these muscles in all planes is essential in properly evaluating the pelvis, hips, and thighs with MRI. It is also important to know the relationships of these muscles to the various neurovascular structures.

The gluteus maximus (Table 6-2) is a large oblique muscle that largely contributes to the shape of the buttock (Figs. 6-8, 6-10, 6-15, and 6-17). This muscle arises from the posterior ilium and dorsal surface of the sacrum and coccyx. The gluteus maximus has both superficial and

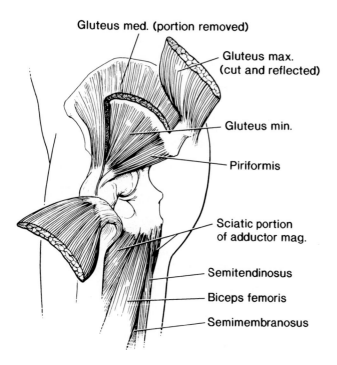

Gluteus med. (portion removed)

Gluteus max. (cut and reflected)

Gluteus min.

Piriformis

Sciatic portion of adductor mag.

Semitendinosus

Biceps femoris

Semimembranosus

Figure 6-15   Illustration of the extensors of the thigh.

deep insertions. Portions of the insertion blend with the tendinous fibers of the fasciae latae and form a portion of the iliotibial tract. The deeper part of the muscle inserts into the gluteal tuberosity of the femur. This lies below the level of the trochanters along the posterior margin of the femur. A subcutaneous bursa frequently lies over the superficial portion of the tendon at the level of the greater trochanter. There is a larger bursa (see Fig. 6-18) that typically lies between the tendon and the greater trochanter (10,34,44). When inflamed, these bursae are seen as well defined, high intensity lesions near the insertions (T2-weighted sequences) (10,45).

The gluteus medius (Figs. 6-8 through 6-10, and 6-17) arises from a large area on the posterior wing of the ilium, below the iliac crest. It extends inferiorly and laterally to insert on the greater trochanter along its posterolateral surface. An additional bursa typically lies between the anterior fibers and the adjacent trochanter (Fig. 6-18). Major fibers of the superior gluteal nerve and vessels lie between the gluteus medius and minimus (Fig. 6-8). The gluteus minimus is also a fan-shaped muscle arising from a more inferior aspect of the posterior ilium and extending along a similar course to insert in the upper anterior surface of the greater trochanter. There is also a bursa between this muscle and the trochanter. These two muscles combine to form the major abductors of the hip. The gluteus medius and minimus muscles are innervated by the superior gluteal nerve (10,34,38).

The tensor fasciae latae (Fig. 6-16) arises from the anterior-most aspect of the iliac crest and passes posteriorly

and inferiorly, inserting in the anterior part of the iliotibial tract. It is innervated by the superior gluteal nerve and serves primarily as a flexor, internal rotator, and abductor of the thigh (38).

The piriformis (Figs. 6-8 and 6-17) is the most superior of the small muscles in the gluteal region and plays a significant role in vascular disorders in the gluteal region. This muscle largely fills the greater sciatic notch (Fig. 6-8), through which the sacral plexus and associated neurovascular structures pass. The superior gluteal nerve and vessels typically lie along the upper border of this muscle, while the pudendal nerve and vessels and inferior gluteal nerve and vessels along with the sciatic nerve typically lie along its lower margin (see Fig. 6-26). In up to 10% of patients, the piriformis is actually perforated by the sciatic nerve or its branches. The muscle arises from the lateral aspect of the sacrum at the level of the second through fourth sacral segments and extends laterally and posterior to the hip joint to insert on the posterior aspect of the greater trochanter (37,38).

The obturator internus takes its origin from the internal pelvic wall of the bones forming the obturator foramen (Figs. 6-8 and 6-10). The muscle passes laterally through the lesser sciatic foramen, posterior to the lesser sciatic notch of the ischium, running posterior to the hip joint to insert on the medial surface of the greater trochanter just above the trochanteric fossa. Again, a bursa typically separates the tendon from the bone in this region (34,37,38). This bursa is typically not identified on MR images unless inflamed and distended with fluid (10).

The superior and inferior gemelli muscles (Figs. 6-8 and 6-17) lie above and below the obturator internus respectively. The superior gemellus originates from the posterior ischial spine and the inferior gemellus from the upper part of the ischial tuberosity. Both muscle bundles converge to insert with the obturator internus tendon and assist this muscle in external rotation of the hip (34,38).

The final muscle in the external rotator group is the quadratus femoris (Fig. 6-17). This muscle takes its origin from the lateral aspect of the ischial tuberosity and inserts on the posterior aspect of the femur just below the intertrochanteric line (Figs. 6-9 and 6-17).

The anterior muscles of the thigh (see Fig. 6-19), with which the iliopsoas are included, are the sartorius and the four segments of the quadriceps muscle. The pectineus muscle is also included in this muscle group (34,38).

The iliopsoas as it appears in the thigh is a combination of two muscles, the iliacus and the psoas major (Figs. 6-8 and 6-19). The psoas major arises in the retroperitoneum at the lateral margin of the T12 through L5 lumbar vertebrae. This muscle passes inferiorly and slightly laterally where it joins the iliacus to insert on the lesser trochanter (34). The psoas minor is an inconsistent muscle that typically arises from the adjacent borders of the last thoracic and first lumbar vertebrae and extends along the anterolateral margin of the psoas major to insert on the iliopectineal eminence of the innominate bone. The

TABLE 6-2

MUSCLES OF THE PELVIS, HIPS, AND THIGH

Muscle	Origin	Insertion	Function	Innervation
Gluteus maximus	Posterior ilium Dorsolateral sacrum and coccyx	Gluteal tuberosity of femur Iliotibial tract	Hip extensor External rotator	Inferior gluteal nerve (L5–S1)
Gluteus medius	Posterior ilium below crest	Posterolateral greater trochanter	Hip abductor	Superior gluteal nerve (L4–S1)
Gluteus minimus	Posterior mid ilium	Anterior greater trochanter	Hip abductor	Superior gluteal nerve (L4–S1)
Tensor fasciae latae	Anterior iliac crest	Iliotibial tract	Flexor Internal rotator Abductor	Superior gluteal nerve (L4–S1)
Piriformis	Anterolateral sacrum S2–S4	Superior border greater trochanter	External rotator Abductor	S1, S2
Obturator internus	Pubic and ischial margins	Medial greater trochanter	External rotator	L5–S2
Superior gemelli	Posterior ischial spine	Obturator internus tendon	External rotator	L5–S2
Inferior gemelli	Ischial tuberosity	Obturator internus tendon	External rotator	L5–S2
Quadratus femoris	Lateral ischial tuberosity	Posterior femur below intertrochanteric line	External rotator Abductor	L4–S1
Iliopsoas				
Psoas major	Lateral margin T12–L5	Lesser trochanter	Thigh flexor Accessory adductor	L2–L4
Psoas minor	Lateral margin T12–L5	Iliopectineal eminence	Tilt pelvis upward	T12–L2
Iliacus	Inner iliac surface below crest	Lesser trochanter	Thigh flexor	L2–L4
Sartorius	Anterior superior iliac spine	Proximal anteromedial tibia	Thigh flexor Accessory external rotator	Femoral nerve (L2–L3)
Quadriceps femoris				
Rectus femoris	Anterior inferior iliac spine	Upper patella	Extensor of knee Accessory thigh flexor	Femoral nerve (L3–L4)
Vastus lateralis	Upper lateral and posterolateral femur	Upper lateral patella	Extensor of knee	L3–L4

(continued)

TABLE 6-2
(Continued)

Muscle	Origin	Insertion	Function	Innervation
Vastus medialis	Medial posterior femur	Medial tendon of rectus femoris	Extensor of knee	L3–L4
Vastus intermedius	Anterior mid femur	Upper posterior patella	Extensor of knee	L3–L4
Pectineus	Superior pubic ramus	Pectineal line femur	Thigh flexor	Femoral nerve (L2, L3)
Adductor longus	Anterior pubic bone	Medial linea aspera	Thigh adductor	Obturator nerve (L2–L3)
Adductor brevis	Pubic bone and inferior ramus	Upper linea aspera	Thigh adductor	Obturator nerve (L2–L3)
Adductor magnus	Ischium and inferior pubic ramus	Linea aspera Adductor tubercle	Thigh adductor	Obturator and tibial nerve (L3–L5)
Gracilis	Inferior pubic ramus near symphysis	Upper anterior tibia	Thigh adductor Medial rotator thigh	Obturator nerve (L3–L4)
Obturator externus	Outer margins obturator foramen	Intertrochanteric fossa	Lateral rotator	Obturator nerve (L3–L4)
Semitendinosus	Posteromedial ischial tuberosity	Upper anterior tibia	Thigh extensor Knee flexor	Tibial side of sciatic (L5–S1)
Biceps femoris	Long head: posteromedial ischial tuberosity	Fibular head	Extend thigh	Long head: tibial side of sciatic nerve (L5–S1)
	Short head: lateral lip linea aspera	Fibular head	Flex knee	Short head: peroneal side of sciatic nerve (L5–S2)
Semimembranosus	Posterolateral ischial tuberosity	Posteromedial upper tibia	Thigh extensor Accessory medial rotator and thigh adductor	Tibial side of sciatic nerve (L5–S2)

From Baum PA, Matsumoto AH, Teitelbaum GP, et al. Anatomic relationship between the common femoral artery and vein. CT evaluation and clinical significance. *Radiology* 1989;173:775–777 and Rosse C, Rosse PC. *Hollinshead's textbook of anatomy.* Philadelphia, PA: Lippincott–Raven, 1997.

iliacus takes its origin from the internal surface of the ilium below the iliac crest and passes slightly obliquely anterior to the hip joint, inserting with the psoas muscle in the lesser trochanter (Fig. 6-19). An important bursa (can cause clinical symptoms and local hip pain) is the iliopsoas bursa, which lies beneath the iliopsoas muscle just as it crosses the anterior surface of the hip joint. This bursa may approach 3 to 7 cm in length and 2 to 4 cm in width. The bursa communicates with the hip joint in up to 15% of patients (see Fig. 6-20) (34,38,44).

The sartorius is a long, straplike muscle that originates from the anterior superior iliac spine and passes obliquely and medially to run along the inner thigh. Below the level of the knee joint it inserts on the anteromedial aspect of the upper tibia (Fig. 6-19). At its insertion it lies largely above the gracilis and semitendinosus. The combination of these three tendons forms the pes anserinus tendon. A bursa typically lies deep to the insertion of the sartorius. This bursa tends to separate it from the insertions of the gracilis and semitendinosus (34,38).

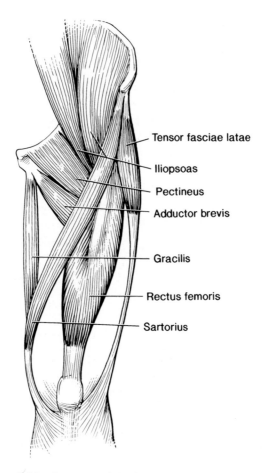

Figure 6-16 Illustration of the flexors of the thigh.

The quadriceps femoris is composed of four muscles. These include the rectus femoris, vastus lateralis, vastus intermedius, and vastus medialis, all of which blend at their patellar insertions (Figs. 6-8, 6-9, and 6-19). The most anterior muscle of the group is the rectus femoris that arises from the anterior inferior iliac spine. This muscle has the distinction of being the only member of the quadriceps group that crosses the hip joint as it passes along its anterior superficial course to insert with the other muscles in the quadriceps tendon, which inserts in the upper border of the patella. A second, more inconsistent origin is also noted from the upper margin of the acetabulum. This is important in that a bursa typically lies deep to this reflected tendon of the rectus femoris. The quadriceps tendon, with the patella, continues to form the patellar ligament that inserts on the tibial tuberosity (34).

The vastus lateralis is a large member of the quadriceps group that is covered anteriorly by the rectus femoris and tensor fasciae latae (Figs. 6-8 and 6-19). The muscle itself lies anterior and lateral to the vastus intermedius. Its origin is from the femur just below the greater trochanter and posterolaterally along the margin of the linea aspera and intermuscular septum. The vastus intermedius inserts along the upper lateral margin of the patella forming a portion of the quadriceps tendon. The vastus medialis makes its origin from just below the lesser trochanter anteriorly and the medial and posterior aspect of the femur. It extends inferiorly and inserts into the medial aspect of the rectus femoris tendon. The vastus intermedius covers a major portion of the front and medial and lateral aspects of the femur (Fig. 6-19) (34,37,46). It is completely covered superficially by the vastus lateralis and medialis on its sides and the rectus femoris anteriorly. Distally, its fibers fuse with the vastus medialis and lateralis to insert in the posterior upper surface of the patella (33,34,37,38).

The pectineus arises from the superior anterior aspect of the superior pubic ramus and extends obliquely in an inferolateral direction to insert along the pectineal line of the femur that extends inferiorly from the lesser trochanter to the linea aspera (Fig. 6-19) (37,38). Anatomists often include the adductor brevis, adductor longus, adductor magnus, gracilis, and obturator externus in the anterior medial muscle group, as all of these muscles are innervated

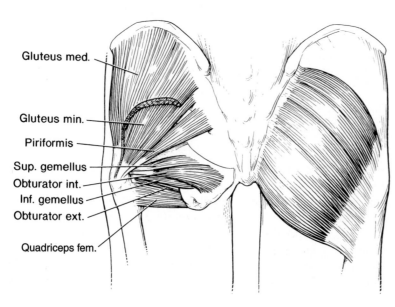

Figure 6-17 Illustration of the external rotators of the hip.

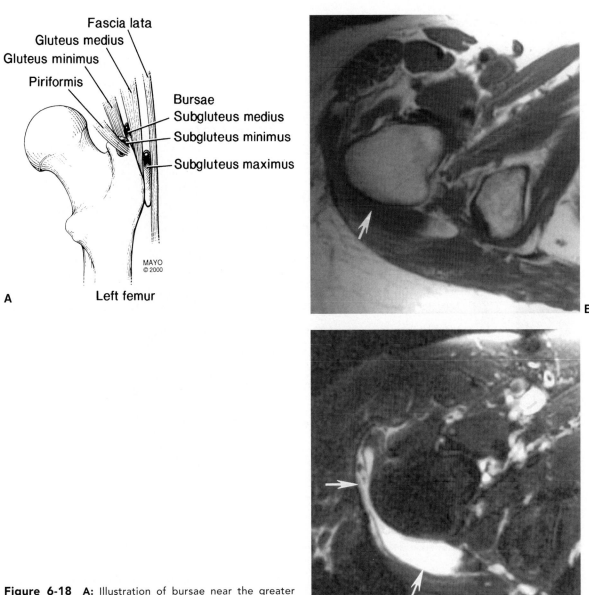

Fascia lata
Gluteus medius
Gluteus minimus
Piriformis

Bursae
Subgluteus medius
Subgluteus minimus
Subgluteus maximus

MAYO
© 2000

A   Left femur

B

C

Figure 6-18 A: Illustration of bursae near the greater trochanter. Axial T1- **(B)** and T2-weighted **(C)** images demonstrating trochanteric bursitis (*arrows*).

by the obturator nerve (Table 6-2) (38). In the axial plane, the adductor longus is the most anterior of the adductor muscles in the upper thigh (Fig. 6-8). The adductor longus takes its origin from the pubic bone superiorly near the pubic symphysis and extends in a triangular fashion inferiorly and laterally to insert along the medial aspect of the linea aspera at the level of the mid femur. This muscle forms the floor of the femoral triangle along with the pectineus and iliopsoas muscle. The adductor brevis arises from a broad tendon from the body and inferior ramus of the pubis and expands in a triangular fashion to insert in the upper half of the linea aspera. It is typically seen between the adductor longus and magnus on the axial views with the gracilis running along its medial aspect (Figs. 6-8 and 6-19) (10,33,34,37,38).

The adductor magnus, like the other adductor muscles, is triangular but much larger (Fig. 6-19). It arises from the lower part of the inferior pubic ramus and the entire length of the ramus of the ischium. It courses inferiorly and laterally with the upper portion, inserting on the linea aspera with lower fibers inserting in the adductor tubercle just above the medial femoral condyle (34,38).

The gracilis is a long, thin muscle that arises from the inferior aspect of the pubic bone close to the symphysis (Figs. 6-8, 6-9, and 6-19). It passes medially along the thigh, superficial to the adductor muscles (Fig. 6-9). Near the knee, it lies first between the sartorius and semimembranosus and then between the sartorius and semitendinosus. Below the knee, the tendon curves anteriorly and inserts in the upper medial anterior tibia with a bursa termed the anserine

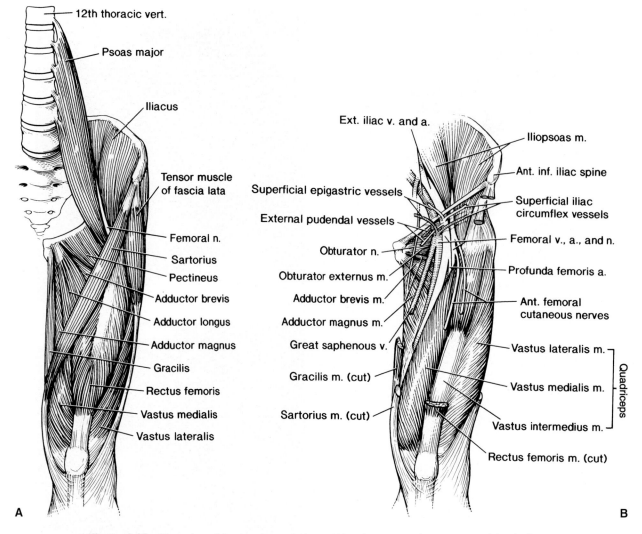

Figure 6-19 illustrations with labels:

A (left):
- 12th thoracic vert.
- Psoas major
- Iliacus
- Tensor muscle of fascia lata
- Femoral n.
- Sartorius
- Pectineus
- Adductor brevis
- Adductor longus
- Adductor magnus
- Gracilis
- Rectus femoris
- Vastus medialis
- Vastus lateralis

B (right):
- Ext. iliac v. and a.
- Superficial epigastric vessels
- External pudendal vessels
- Obturator n.
- Obturator externus m.
- Adductor brevis m.
- Adductor magnus m.
- Great saphenous v.
- Gracilis m. (cut)
- Sartorius m. (cut)
- Iliopsoas m.
- Ant. inf. iliac spine
- Superficial iliac circumflex vessels
- Femoral v., a., and n.
- Profunda femoris a.
- Ant. femoral cutaneous nerves
- Vastus lateralis m.
- Vastus medialis m.
- Vastus intermedius m.
- Rectus femoris m. (cut)
- Quadriceps

Figure 6-19 Illustration of the anterior musculature (**A**) and neurovascular structures of the thigh (**B**).

bursa intervening between gracilis, sartorius, and semitendinosus tendons and the tibia (10,34).

The obturator externus (Figs. 6-8, 6-9, and 6-19) is the most deeply placed muscle in the adductor group. This

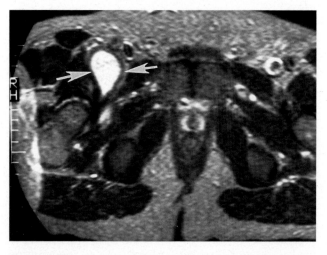

Figure 6-20 Axial T2-weighted image of the pelvis demonstrating an enlarged iliopsoas bursa (*arrows*).

muscle arises from the external margins of the obturator foramen, namely the superior pubic ramus, inferior pubic ramus, and upper margin of the ischium, and extends laterally and posterior to the hip capsule it may be separated from the capsule proper by a bursa (38,47). The obturator internus functions primarily as a lateral rotator (38).

The posterior muscles of the thigh, commonly referred to as the hamstring muscles, include the semitendinosus, the biceps femoris, the semimembranosus, and a portion of the adductor magnus that arises from the ischial tuberosity (see Fig. 6-21). All of the hamstring muscles take their origin from the ischial tuberosity except for the short head of the biceps femoris. The semitendinosus arises from the posteromedial aspect of the ischial tuberosity. Its origin is fused with the long head of the biceps. Just above the medial condyle the tendinous portion of the muscle continues posterior to the knee and forward along the medial aspect to insert in the upper anterior tibia, just posterior to the insertions of the gracilis and sartorius. As noted previously, this is, along with the above tendons, a part of the pes anserinus complex (34,38).

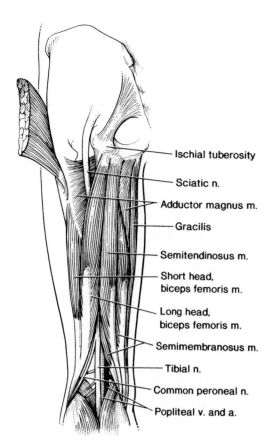

- Ischial tuberosity
- Sciatic n.
- Adductor magnus m.
- Gracilis
- Semitendinosus m.
- Short head, biceps femoris m.
- Long head, biceps femoris m.
- Semimembranosus m.
- Tibial n.
- Common peroneal n.
- Popliteal v. and a.

Figure 6-21 Illustration of the hamstring muscle group.

The biceps femoris has two heads, a short and long head (Fig. 6-21). The long head of the biceps arises from the posteromedial aspect of the inferior aspect of the ischial tuberosity in common with the semitendinosus tendon. The short head of the biceps originates from the lower lateral aspect of the linea aspera. This muscle lies lateral to the belly of the long head as it extends inferiorly, and at the level of the knee joint, a common tendon forms that crosses the knee and inserts into the head of the fibula (34,38).

The semimembranosus arises from a long, flat tendon at the posterolateral aspect of the ischial tuberosity that is lateral to the common origin of the biceps femoris and semitendinosus (Fig. 6-21). The muscle becomes tendinous posterior to the medial meniscus as it crosses the knee. At the level of the joint, it gives off an oblique expansion that also attaches to the medial collateral ligament. Its insertion is the posterior medial aspect of the upper tibia just below the knee (33,34,37,43).

NEUROVASCULAR STRUCTURES

The neurovascular anatomy of the pelvis, hips, and thigh is complex and the relationships of these structures to the sacrum and the above muscles is important in evaluating pathology along the course of the neurovascular bundles

(see Figs. 6-22 and 6-23) (2,32,34,38,48). Demonstration of these structures can be accomplished using axial planes (Fig. 6-8) but may be difficult with coronal and sagittal planes because of the difficulty in following the changes in the course of the neurovascular structures (Figs. 6-9 and 6-10). The lumbosacral plexus can be identified on coronal (see Fig. 6-24), sagittal, and oblique coronal planes. The last is preferred for evaluating neural structures in the sacral foramina (see Fig. 6-25) (48).

The abdominal aorta usually bifurcates at the L-4 level, forming the iliac arteries. The iliac arteries divide at the level of the sacroiliac joints to form the internal and external iliac vessels (Fig. 6-22). The internal iliac artery gives off the superior and inferior gluteal arteries that supply the posterior or buttock muscles (see Fig. 6-26). These vessels and their branches are difficult to define on conventional orthogonal MR images. The common femoral artery is a continuation of the external iliac below the inguinal ligament. The circumflex arteries and branches of the obturator artery (via ligamentum teres) supply the hip. The superficial femoral and deep femoral (profunda) arteries form slightly distal to this level (Fig. 6-22) (2,38,41); they branch at about the same level as the superficial femoral and saphenous veins (Fig. 6-22). The course of the major arteries and companion veins is easily followed on contiguous axial MR images (Fig. 6-8). In the upper thigh (Fig. 6-22), the superficial femoral artery lies anterior to the adductor longus and deep to the sartorius. The profunda femoris artery and vein lie more laterally between the adductor longus and magnus near the linea aspera of the femur (Fig. 6-8). Perforating branches are usually identifiable between the adductor magnus and hamstring muscles just posterior and slightly lateral to the linea aspera of the femur (34,38). Today, MR angiography is capable of demonstrating all major vessels (see Fig. 6-27).

The major neural structures are derived from the lumbosacral plexus (L1 through S2) (Fig. 6-23) (2,48). Portions of the T12 and S3 ventral rami also contribute to this plexus. The sacral branches exit the ventral foramina along with the L4 through L5 segments for the sciatic nerve (L4 through S3) (Figs. 6-24 and 6-25). The sciatic nerve exits the pelvis posteriorly and lies just posterior to the hip (Fig. 6-24). This is best seen on axial MR images (Figs. 6-8 and 6-23) (2,34,38).

The sciatic nerve enters the buttock below the piriformis (Fig. 6-26) in about 85% of patients. In some cases, the sciatic nerve may pass through the piriformis. Alternatively, the peroneal and tibial segments of the sciatic nerve may be separated by the piriformis (38). The nerve lies posterior to the obturator externus, gemelli, and quadriceps femoris, and it passes distally (Figs. 6-8 and 6-26). The posterior femoral cutaneous branch also exits below the piriformis but is less easily identified on MR images. The superior gluteal nerve lies between the gluteus minimus and medius above the level of the piriformis (Fig. 6-26). In the posterior thigh, the sciatic nerve lies posterior to the adductor magnus and deep to the

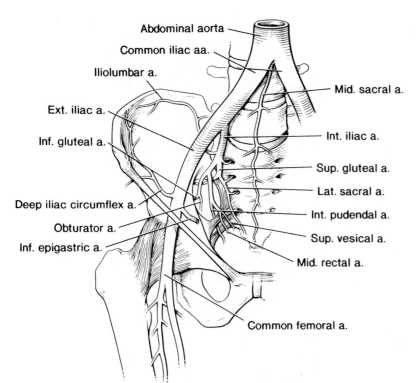

Figure 6-22 Illustration of the major vessels to the pelvis and thighs.

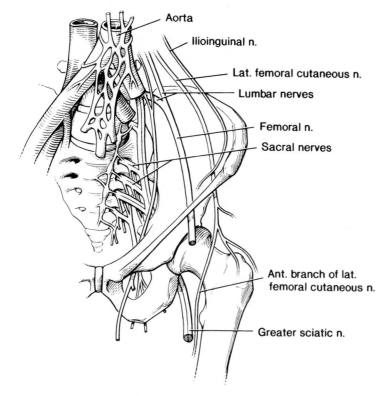

Figure 6-23 Illustration of the major neural structures of the pelvis and hips.

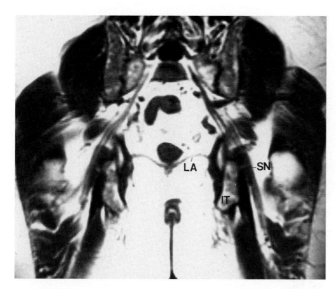

Figure 6-24 Coronal SE 450/15 image of the pelvis demonstrating the course of the sacral plexus and sciatic nerve. Note the relationship of the sciatic nerve to the ischium. *SN*, sciatic nerve; *IT*, ischial tuberosity; *LA*, levator ani.

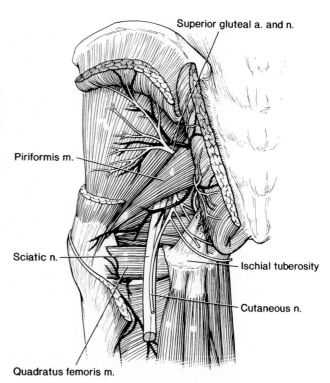

Figure 6-26 Neurovascular anatomy of the gluteal region.

biceps femoris (Fig. 6-8). The nerve branches innervate the hamstring group. Just above the knee, the sciatic nerve generally divides into common peroneal and tibial branches (Fig. 6-21) (34,38).

The anterior musculature of the pelvis and thighs are innervated by the obturator and femoral nerve (Table 6-2). Both are derived from the L2 through L4 segments. The femoral nerve lies just lateral to the artery and vein in the femoral triangle (Fig. 6-19). In the upper portion of the femoral triangle it divides into muscular and cutaneous branches (38). The largest branches may be identified on MR images. These branches (saphenous nerve and nerve to

the vastus medialis) lie anterior to the adductor group and deep to the sartorius (Fig. 6-8) (34,37,38). The obturator nerve enters the thigh through the obturator canal, deep to the pectineus (Fig. 6-19). Its anterior branch lies between the adductor longus and brevis and the posterior branch posterior to the adductor brevis (34,38).

PITFALLS

Certain errors in interpreting MR images can be reduced by reviewing radiographic findings. Pitfalls in MR imaging of the pelvis, hips, and thighs do not differ significantly from other areas in regard to hardware and software artifacts (see Figs. 6-28 to 6-30). Metal artifact from orthopedic implants is common in the pelvis and hips due to the increasing number of patients with arthroplasty or fracture fixation devices. (Fig. 6-30) The role of MRI in this patient group will be discussed later in this chapter. However, artifact from orthopedic implants can be reduced by orienting implants parallel to the magnetic field and modifying pulse sequences to reduce frequency shift. Titanium implants cause less artifact than cobalt-chromium alloys due to reduced ferromagnetic content (49,50). This section will focus on bone and soft tissue variants, which require further discussion (51,52).

Soft tissue variants are important when evaluating patients with suspected soft tissue masses (see Fig. 6-31) or sciatic nerve pathology (10,38,52–54). Knowledge of

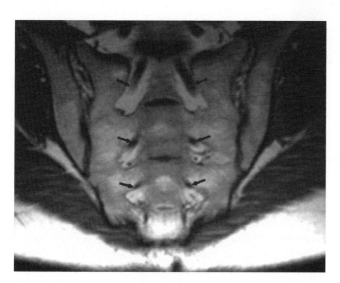

Figure 6-25 Oblique T1-weighted coronal images demonstrating the sacral nerve roots (*arrows*) surrounded by fat as they exit the ventral foramina. The sacroiliac joints are also well demonstrated.

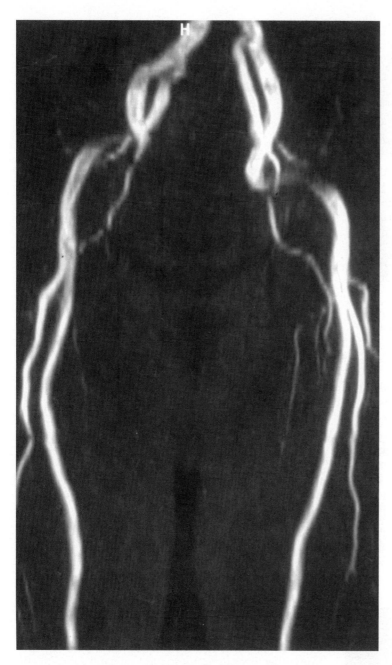

Figure 6-27 Normal MR angiogram of the lower abdomen, pelvis, and thighs.

the normal variants in the sciatic–piriformis muscle anatomy is important in patients with suspected piriformis syndrome. As noted above, the sciatic nerve typically passes deep to the piriformis muscle, but it may pass through the muscle or separate the tibial and peroneal tracts (34,38).

The psoas minor is absent in up to 51% of patients. Other muscle anomalies in the pelvis and thighs typically result in fusion of muscles (i.e., quadratus femoris and adductor magnus) or separate muscle bellies. The smaller muscles such as the gemelli and quadratus femoris may be absent, resulting in muscle mass asymmetry (34,38). In young, active patients, one can identify changes in muscle signal intensity related to exercise. These changes vary with the extent, eccentric nature, and time since the activity

occurred (55). Typically, the entire muscle is involved and changes usually are not similar to neoplasms or other soft tissue pathology.

Inflamed bursae (Figs. 6-18 and 6-20) should not be confused with neoplasms. Most of these bursae were described in the anatomy section of this chapter. The obturator externus bursa is seen less frequently than iliopsoas or trochanteric bursae (45,47). This bursa communicates with the posterior inferior hip joint and, when enlarged, displaces the obturator externus inferiorly (see Fig. 6-32) (47). Infrequently, bursae may develop between the piriformis and the femur, between the gluteal muscles, and over the ischial tuberosities. When present, these bursae appear as well-marginated, high-intensity lesions on T2-weighted sequences

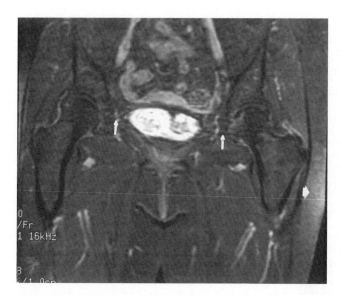

Figure 6-28 Coronal T2-weighted, fat-suppressed MR image of the pelvis demonstrating motion artifact (*upper arrows*) and asymmetric fat suppression (*large white arrow*).

and are low intensity on T1-weighted sequences (see Fig. 6-33). Size of the bursae may vary significantly (44,54,56).

Variations in marrow patterns in the pelvis, hips, and femurs and focal areas of abnormality in the femoral head can be very confusing (2,10,57,58). A more thorough discussion of marrow imaging is presented in Chapter 14. However, certain common problems and variants deserve mention here.

The transition from hemopoietic to fatty marrow occurs normally with aging. This may be partially related to decreased medullary blood flow (58–60). In younger patients, the capital epiphysis and greater trochanter are typically composed of fatty marrow, resulting in high signal intensity on T1-weighted sequences (see Fig. 6-34). Also, partial volume effects can cause confusion on axial images (Fig. 6-34) in the physeal region. Changes should not be confused with pathology and can usually be clarified on coronal or sagittal images. With age, the hemopoietic marrow in the intertrochanteric region becomes replaced with fatty marrow so that after age 50 most of the

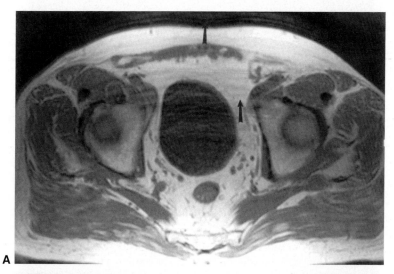

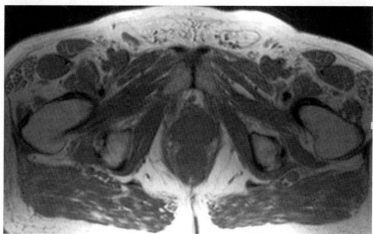

Figure 6-29 Respiratory motion artifact in the phase encoding direction. Axial T1-weighted images of the upper pelvis **(A)** and more inferiorly at the level of the ischial tuberosities **(B).** There is considerable artifact in **A** (*arrows*) due to respiratory and bowel motion.

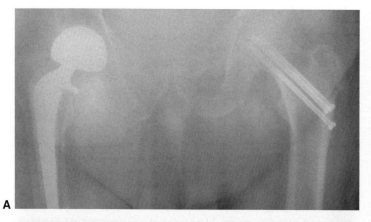

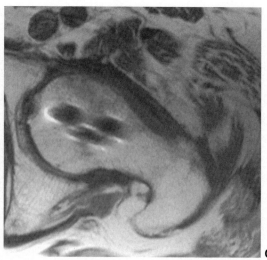

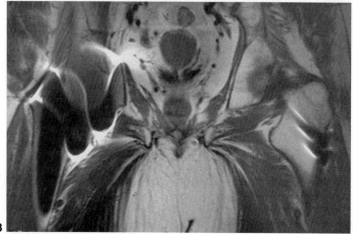

Figure 6-30 A: Anteroposterior view of the pelvis in a patient with a bipolar implant on the right and three cannulated screws on the left. Coronal **(B)** T1-weighted image shows artifact bilaterally, greater on the right. Axial T1-weighted image of the left hip **(C)** shows minimal artifact around the hip pins. The marrow is clearly demonstrated.

marrow in this region is fatty (see Fig. 6-35) (59). The compressive and tensile trabeculae in the femoral head and neck are seen as linear areas of low signal intensity on both T1- and T2-weighted sequences (Fig. 6-35B) (2,58). Lack of familiarity with the changes normally seen in the marrow of the acetabulum and femur can lead to a false-positive diagnosis such as AVN or metastasis (see Fig. 6-36) (61).

Well-defined areas of abnormal signal intensity may be noted in the femoral neck. These herniation pits are due to mechanical effects of the anterior capsule. The result is a focal cortical defect that allows soft tissue erosion into the femoral neck. These defects are noted in about 5% of the adult population (30,51,62). Radiographically, these defects are nearly always in the anterior outer quadrant of the femoral neck (see Fig. 6-37). They are generally 1 cm in diameter with sclerotic, well-defined margins. Multilobulated herniation pits have also been described (30,51,58). Herniation pits may enlarge over time but maintain their characteristic appearance on imaging studies. In this setting, fractures may occur (62). On MR images the appearance is also typical. The location and typical low intensity on T1-weighted images and high intensity with a low intensity margin on T2-weighted images should not be confused with AVN, metastasis, or interosseous ganglia (57). Comparison with radiographs will confirm the diagnosis when MR features seem atypical.

A simple but common mistake is failure to compare other studies, especially routine radiographs, with MR images (10,63,64). This is especially important in the pelvis and hips, where marrow patterns can be confusing (see Fig. 6-38) (10). Also, areas of heterotopic ossification and periarticular calcification, common about the hips, may be confused with other pathology if radiographs or computed tomography (CT) are not available for review (see Fig. 6-39) (65).

APPLICATIONS

Most patients referred for musculoskeletal MRI examinations of the pelvis, hips, and thighs present with pain, a history of trauma, or suspected soft tissue or skeletal neoplasms (66–69). There are numerous causes of hip pain (70). Applications for MR imaging of the pelvis and hips have evolved in adults and children. The following sections will review current applications for MR imaging of the pelvis and hips. Pediatric disorders will be discussed separately in the last section of this chapter.

Osteonecrosis: Marrow Edema Patterns

Avascular necrosis of the femoral head is usually easily diagnosed with MRI in the later stages. However, confusion

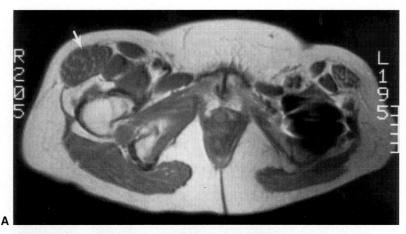

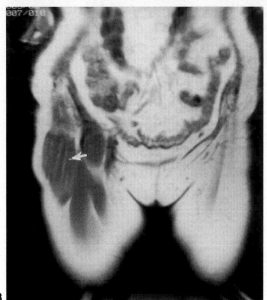

Figure 6-31 Hypertrophy of the tensor fascia lata. Axial **(A)** and coronal **(B)** T1-weighted images demonstrate marked enlargement of the muscle that was felt to be a soft tissue mass clinically.

can occur in the early phases prior to development of the typical geographic abnormality, double-line sign, and other features commonly noted on MR images (71–77). Diffuse marrow edema may be the initial feature, presenting with low signal intensity changes in the femoral head and neck on T1-weighted images, and high signal intensity on T2-weighted images (72,78,79). Iida et al. (74) reported high-risk patients with bone marrow edema (steroids, renal transplants, etc.) progressed to advanced AVN in 85% of cases. However, marrow edema can be identified with numerous conditions including transient bone marrow edema, migratory osteoporosis, transient osteoporosis, infection, trauma, neoplasms, and altered weight bearing (72,76,80–82). The MR features of transient bone marrow edema, transient osteoporosis, and early osteonecrosis, though controversial, have been clarified in recent years (76,83–85). Though not always clear-cut, the data from radiographs, radionuclide scans, MR images, and clinical data, specifically risk factors, are useful in differentiating these conditions and selecting conservative

treatment or surgical intervention (i.e., core decompression) (72,86–90).

Osteonecrosis

Osteonecrosis is a general term applied to conditions resulting in cellular necrosis of bone and marrow elements (85,91,92). The term AVN is most commonly applied when the epiphysis or subchondral bone is involved. Osteonecrosis of the metaphyseal or diaphyseal bone is commonly referred to as a bone infarct (93).

Bone necrosis occurs when flow is disrupted by thrombosis, external compression, vessel wall disease, or traumatic disruption of vessels. Jiang and Shih (94) evaluated physeal scars and their association with AVN (Fig. 6-35A). Many physeal scars (seen as a linear low signal intensity structure) are incomplete. Complete physeal scars that extend from cortex to cortex were associated with AVN in 32 of 72 (44%) femoral heads (94). The numerous causes of osteonecrosis are summarized in Table 6-3. Though

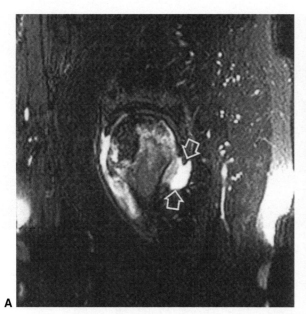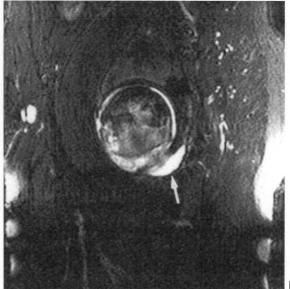

Figure 6-32 Sagittal T2-weighted fat-suppressed fast spin-echo images **(A,B)** in a patient with AVN demonstrate a joint effusion with an obturator externus bursa. **A:** Posterior communication with the joint (*open arrows*). **B:** The bursa extending medially. (From Robinson P, White LM, Agur A, et al. Obturator externus bursa: Anatomic origin and MR imaging features of pathologic involvement. *Radiology* 2003;228:230–234.)

osteonecrosis can occur in any area of the skeleton, it is a frequent and significant problem in the femoral head. Therefore, the major discussion of pathophysiology and MR features will be discussed here.

Susceptibility to AVN in the hip is due in part to the vascular anatomy. The foveal artery supplies only the area of the femoral head immediately adjacent to the fovea (see Fig. 6-40). Distally, the medial and lateral femoral circumflex arteries supply the remainder of the femoral head and neck (Fig. 6-40). Their location makes them particularly susceptible to damage with femoral neck fractures and dislocations (35,91,92,95,98).

Nontraumatic cell death may occur from direct effects (chemotherapy, radiation therapy, or thermal injury) or

intraosseous extravascular changes such as edema or marrow infiltration diseases such as Gaucher disease (90,91,99).

Fat embolism and/or disorders in fat metabolism are frequently implicated in nontraumatic osteonecrosis. Jones (91) described three potential mechanisms and four phases that evolve due to lipid disorders. Fat embolism may develop due to fatty liver, destabilization and coalescence of plasma lipoproteins, or disruption of fatty marrow or fatty tissues in nonosseous regions. Fat embolism (stage 0) leads to interosseous vascular occlusion (phase I) that increases lipase, which in turn increases free fatty acids and prostaglandins (phase II). These changes can lead to focal intravascular coagulation, platelet aggregation, and thrombosis, which result in osteonecrosis (91).

Early diagnosis and selection of the most appropriate therapy has been particularly challenging for patients with AVN of the hips (28,90,100–105). Early detection permits more conservative therapy such as non-weight bearing with crutches, core decompression, and vascularized grafts (5,103,106).

Early detection of AVN with imaging techniques has been challenging (2,83,107,108). Radiographs are often normal in early stages of AVN. Changes may be subtle even during stage II disease. Detection at this time (Table 6-4) may require more sophisticated studies than anteroposterior and oblique radiographs. Isotope studies have been very useful at this stage (2,104). However, early changes can be difficult to evaluate with radionuclide scans, as well. Comparison with the opposite hip may not be useful since the disease is bilateral in up to 81% of patients (2,81,83,107).

TABLE 6-3

ETIOLOGY OF OSTEONECROSIS

Trauma
Corticosteroids
Sickle cell disease
Alcoholism
Gaucher disease
Nitrogen narcosis
Radiation
Collagen disease
Pancreatitis
Idiopathic

From references 91, 92, and 95–97.

TABLE 6-4

STAGING OF AVASCULAR NECROSIS OF THE HIP

Stage	Clinical	Radiograph	MRI	Pathology
0	No symptoms	Normal	Normal to uniform edema ($\downarrow$ signal T1WI, $\uparrow$ signal T2WI) (Fig. 6-45)	Hematopoietic cell necrosis followed by fat cell necrosis and osteocytes
			Subchondral zone of nonenhancement or $\uparrow$ enhancement due to edema with Gd. (Fig. 6-48)	
I	May have symptoms	Normal or may have patchy osteoporosis (Fig. 6-41A)	Normal to uniform edema ($\downarrow$ signal T1WI, $\uparrow$ signal T2WI) or low intensity zone on T1WI (Fig. 6-42)	Sinus congestion, fibroblastic, hypoplastic marrow, empty lacunae
			Subchondral zone of nonenhancement or $\uparrow$ enhancement due to edema with Gd. (Fig. 6-45)	
II	Pain, stiffness	Osteopenia mixed, osteopenia and sclerosis, cystic changes (Figs. 6-41C and 6-52)	Wedge-shaped crescent sign (x-ray stage III)	Necrotic central tissue, margin fibrous with revascularization and new bone on dead trabeculae
III	Stiffness, groin and knee pain	Crescent sign, sequestra, cortical collapse, joint preserved (Fig. 6-41, D through F)	Crescent sign sequestra cortical collapse joint preserved (Fig. 6-53)	Necrosis surrounded by granulation tissue
IV	Pain and limp, may be severe	III plus degenerative changes with narrowed joint space (Fig. 6-41 E and F)	III plus degenerative changes with narrowed joint space (Fig. 6-54)	Changes of stage III exaggerated

T1WI, T1-weighted image; T2WI, T2-weighted image; Gd, Gadolinium.
From references 10, 96 and 109–111.

Ficat (112) and Ficat and Arlet (113) described the stages of AVN of the femoral head based on radiographic and clinical features (see Fig. 6-41). This staging is also useful in evaluating MR images (Table 6-4). Stages 0 and I have no radiographic findings and clinical symptoms are subtle. Stage II changes are often overlooked on routine radiographs but consist of focal areas of subchondral lucency or sclerosis. Stages III and IV are usually easily detected on radiographs due to the crescent sign and progressive subchondral collapse and degenerative joint disease (Table 6-4) (112,113).

Due to the increased use of core decompression and vascularized grafts, the Ficat and Arlet classification has been modified by Steinberg et al. (114) (Table 6-5). The most recent classification system, the University of Pennsylvania classification and staging system, incorporates imaging features which will become important later in this section when we discuss management approaches for femoral head osteonecrosis (96,115,116). Stage 0 is normal imaging studies, including MRI. Stage I disease has normal radiographs with abnormal radionuclide scans and MRI. Stage II AVN demonstrates lytic and/or sclerotic changes in the femoral head and

stage III subchondral collapse (crescent sign). Stage III disease progresses to flattening of the femoral head, stage V joint space narrowing and acetabular changes, and stage VI advanced degenerative joint disease. There are subcategories based on image features for stages I–V (Table 6-5).

MR imaging approaches should be selected to fit the classification system and provide the surgeon with the extent of femoral head involvement, acetabular involvement, and the accurate stage of AVN (103,114,115,117).

Before discussing the corresponding MR features, we will review specific aspects of technique that were not fully discussed in the introductory technique section of this chapter. When positive, coronal T1-weighted (SE 500/10) images are adequate for diagnosis of AVN (Fig. 6-42A) (10,21,59,118–120). This sequence can be performed quickly (2 to 4 minutes) using a 30- to 42-cm FOV, 4-mm-thick sections, 1 NEX, and a 256 $\times$ 256 or 192 $\times$ 256 matrix. This approach may provide a simple screening technique for high risk patients (10). Tervonen et al. (121) detected occult AVN in 6% of asymptomatic high-risk patients. More recently, Iida et al. (74) demonstrated 85%

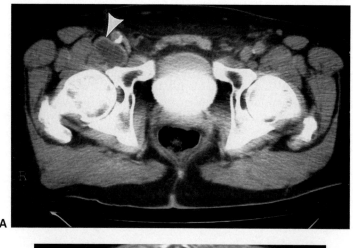

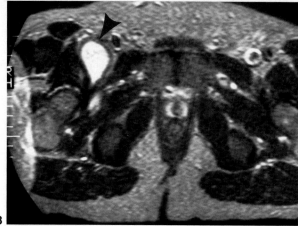

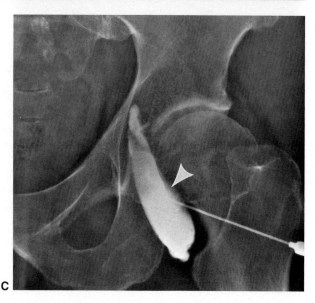

Figure 6-33 Enlarged iliopsoas bursa (*arrowhead*) mistaken for a mass. CT (**A**) and SE 2000/80 (**B**) MR images demonstrate a characteristic enlarged bursa (*arrowhead*). The bursa was injected with contrast medial (**C**) and aspirated for diagnosis and treatment. Aspiration is usually not successful for long-term treatment.

of high-risk patients (steroid, transplant, etc.) progressed from marrow edema to advanced osteonecrosis.

We also perform sagittal images of both hips in abnormal cases to define the extent of articular involvement and improve mapping of the femoral head for treatment planning (see Fig. 6-42B). T2-weighted or fat-suppressed, fast

spin-echo T2-weighted sequences in the sagittal and/or coronal planes are important to define joint anatomy and articular cartilage changes. Surface coils and a small FOV are useful for evaluation of subtle articular changes (10,81,115,122).

It is also important to assess the acetabular side of the joint for cartilage loss, geode formation, and ischemic

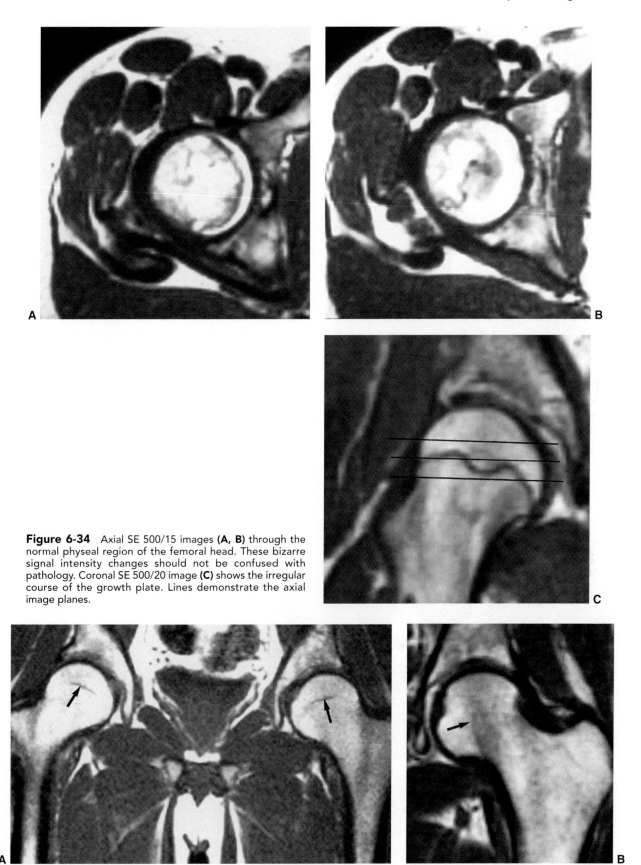

Figure 6-34 Axial SE 500/15 images **(A, B)** through the normal physeal region of the femoral head. These bizarre signal intensity changes should not be confused with pathology. Coronal SE 500/20 image **(C)** shows the irregular course of the growth plate. Lines demonstrate the axial image planes.

Figure 6-35 Adult hips. **A:** SE 500/30 image of the pelvis and hips demonstrating predominantly fatty marrow in the femoral heads and necks. The physeal scars (*arrows*) should not be confused with AVN. **B:** Coronal SE 500/20 image of the left hip. The low intensity region (*arrow*) created by the trabecular pattern in the femoral neck is normal.

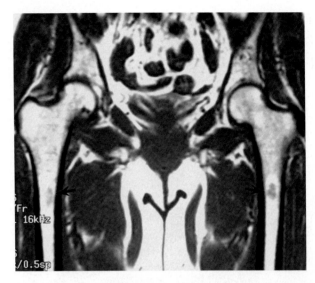

Figure 6-36 Coronal SE 500/15 images of the hips and femurs show targetlike areas in the marrow (*arrows*) of the femurs in the subtrochanteric regions. This is normal.

changes (see Fig. 6-43) (96,115). These findings may lead to a different surgical approach. In most cases a bipolar implant is used for AVN of the femoral head. However, when there are acetabular abnormalities (Fig. 6-43), a total hip arthroplasty may provide more optimal results (96,112). Fink et al. (123) detected AVN of the acetabulum in 9.5% of patients with femoral head necrosis.

In high-risk patients (systemic disease, steroids, renal transplant, etc.), more aggressive studies using fat suppressed T1-weighted images after gadolinium injection may detect ischemic changes earlier (see Fig. 6-44) (10,89).

During the earliest phases of AVN, conventional sequences can appear normal (124–126). Early findings are more easily appreciated using gadolinium (Fig. 6-44) and fat-suppressed T1-weighted sequences (124). Red marrow enhances more than yellow marrow. Gadolinium is freely distributed into the extracellular space, so enhancement may be related to flow, increased capillary permeability, or both (127,128). Normal marrow enhances rapidly, with increase in signal intensity of more than 80% typically within 36 seconds of injection. There is no enhancement in regions of ischemia (Fig. 6-44). In later phases (7 days), an enhancing zone is usually identified around the ischemic zone (see Fig. 6-45). Li et al. (128) described three patterns using gadolinium-enhanced fat-suppression MR techniques. Stage I changes demonstrate focal low intensity in the femoral head surrounded with a high-intensity margin or hyperemic zone. Stage II changes are typical of bone marrow edema with diffuse enhancement in the femoral head and neck (Fig. 6-43B). Combined features of stages I and II were considered stage III. Though marrow edema may not progress to AVN, many believe that this is the earliest phase (76,83,85,127–129). Differentiation of marrow edema from AVN will be discussed further later; however, follow-up imaging is the

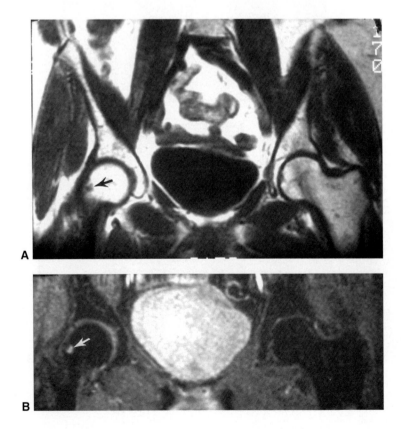

Figure 6-37 Coronal SE 500/20 **(A)** and axial SE 2000/60 **(B)** images of the pelvis demonstrating a typical herniation pit (*arrow*).

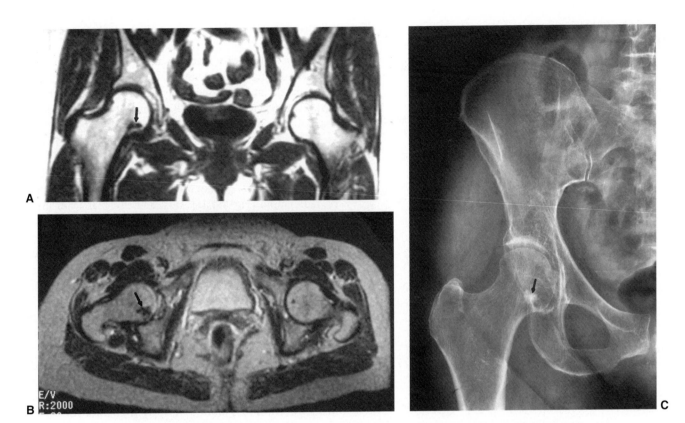

Figure 6-38   Benign bone island. Coronal T1- **(A)** and axial T2-weighted **(B)** images demonstrate an area of low signal intensity in the right femoral neck (*arrow*). Anteroposterior **(C)** radiograph demonstrates faint chondrocalcinosis, degenerative arthritis, and a sclerotic bone island (*arrow*), which created the signal abnormality on the MR images.

only way to be sure the transient bone marrow edema has resolved (72,76,130).

Regardless of the technique used, the MR features can be correlated to some degree with histologic changes. Though not required for diagnosis in later stages, gadolinium clearly helps understand the ischemic and reactive changes that occur around the necrotic bone (Figs. 6-44 and 6-45) (76,82,127).

The MR signal intensity in the femoral head and neck depends upon the presence of fat cells, hemopoietic cells, and trabecular bone (see Fig. 6-46) (2,3,131). Marrow patterns are age-related. These variations must be considered when interpreting MR images. During fetal development, bone marrow in the hip is entirely hemopoietic in nature (59). After birth and during early childhood, the marrow in the epiphysis and trochanters is fatty (see Fig. 6-47 A and B) (120,132). Fatty marrow in the epiphysis is normally evident by age 2 (59,133). In children, red marrow predominates in the metaphysis, intertrochanteric regions, and pelvis (see Fig. 6-47C). In young adults (ages 20 to 40 years), hemopoietic or red marrow is present in the femoral neck and intertrochanteric region, and proximal shaft is evident in 94% of patients. Fatty marrow is present in the femoral head and trochanters (59). These regions are composed of fatty marrow in 88% of adults over 50 years of age. (see Fig. 6-47D) (59).

Femoral AVN can result from numerous conditions (Table 6-3) (59,74). All osseous elements become necrotic at different times after an ischemic event. Hemopoietic cells are most sensitive and become necrotic prior to fat cell necrosis (91,92). Osteocytes show necrotic changes shortly after hemopoietic cells (85). It is not unusual to demonstrate mixed necrosis and survival if changes are early. Early animal studies show MR images remain normal until about the seventh day. Beginning on the seventh day an inhomogeneous loss of signal intensity can be demonstrated on T1-weighted images. These changes correspond histologically to lymphocytic infiltration (96,109). This inhomogeneity progresses over the first 16 days until day 20, when a more homogeneous loss of signal intensity in the femoral head becomes evident (see Fig. 6-48). This correlates with increased lymphocyte infiltration and early fibrosis. As expected, radiographs remain normal during this time period (Table 6-4) (10,112,113). Early uniform loss of signal intensity in the femoral head and neck on T1-weighted images that is similar to transient bone marrow edema has also been reported (Fig. 6-48) (10,73,117, 119,129,134). Conservative management is employed with

TABLE 6-5

CLASSIFICATION OF FEMORAL HEAD AVN

Stage	Criteria
Stage 0	Normal or nondiagnostic radiograph, bone scan, and magnetic resonance imaging
Stage 1	Normal radiograph; abnormal bone scan, and/or magnetic resonance imaging
A	Mild (<15% of head affected)
B	Moderate (15%–30% of head affected)
C	Severe (>30% of head affected)
Stage II	Lucent and sclerotic changes in femoral head
A	Mild (<15% of head affected)
B	Moderate (15%–30% of head affected)
C	Severe (>15% of head affected)
Stage III	Subchondral collapse (crescent sign) without flattening
A	Mild (<15% of articular surface)
B	Moderate (15%–30% of articular surface)
C	Severe (>30% of articular surface)
Stage IV	Flattening of femoral head
A	Mild (<15% of surface and <2-mm depression)
B	Moderate (15%–30% of surface or 2- to 4-mm depression)
C	Severe (>30% of surface or >4-mm depression)
Stage V	Joint narrowing and/or acetabular changes
A	Mild
B	Moderate
C	Severe
Stage VI	Advanced degenerative changes

From Lieberman JR, Berry DB, Mont MA, et al. Osteonecrosis of the hip: Management in the twenty-first century. *J Bone Joint Surg Am* 2002; 84A:834-853; Cherian SF, Laorr A, Saleh KJ, et al. Quantifying the extent of femoral head involvement in osteonecrosis. *J Bone Joint Surg Am* 2003;85A:309–314; and Steinberg ME, Hayken GD, Steinberg DR. A quantitative system for staging avascular necrosis. *J Bone Joint Surg Am* 1995;77B:34–41.

either condition. However, follow-up studies are important in clarifying which disorder is present and to exclude other inflammatory diseases, specifically infection (73,126,129).

Also during the early phase, a low intensity line of demarcation may be evident at the margin of the necrotic zone. This is easily appreciated on T1-weighted coronal images (see Fig. 6-49). The signal intensity of the necrotic zone may be indistinguishable from normal fatty marrow (10,115,117). This low intensity zone surrounding the necrotic bone is most likely due to hyperemia. During this phase of AVN the radiographs are typically normal, though slight sclerosis or lucency may be evident with early stage II AVN (Tables 6-4 and 6-5) (1,2,118). Photopenia (cold spots) may be evident on radionuclide scans at this point (119).

Gradually (>2 weeks), the cells around the necrotic zone modulate into fibroblasts that have low signal intensity on T1-weighted sequences. Hyperemia causes mixed low and high signal intensity margins on T2-weighted images (10, 59,119,120). Hyperemic changes may be more clearly defined on contrast-enhanced images (see Fig. 6-50). Little

progression is evident on radiographs or isotope scans at this point (72).

Reinforcement of trabeculae and persistent hyperemia lead to widening of the low-intensity margin on T1-weighted, T2-weighted, and postcontrast sequences (see Figs.6-50 and 6-51). The hyperemia remains high intensity on T2-weighted sequences. At this stage, a clear stage II radiographic picture (see Fig. 6-52) is usually evident, namely a lucent or sclerotic area surrounded by a geographic pattern (10,59,120).

With progression, the subchondral bone collapses resulting in stage III AVN (Tables 6-4 and 6-5) or the crescent sign on radiographs (Fig. 6-41D). This can be seen as a subchondral low intensity line on T1-weighted sequences or a high intensity area on T2-weighted sequences with deformity of the femoral contour (see Fig. 6-53 and 6-54). The latter may be more easily appreciated due to the high contrast between the dark cortical bone and high signal seen with T2-weighted sequences (91,92,95,96). Early subchondral collapse may only be seen with coronal and sagittal surface coil images. In fact, subchondral fracture may be most easily appreciated on coronal reformatted CT images (135).

Once stage IV AVN (Tables 6-4 and 6-6) has been reached, the appearance of the MR images and radiographs are similar. However, effusions are more obvious on MR images at this stage (136,137). Subtle joint space changes are definitely more easily assessed with radiographs (Fig. 6-41E and F) than with conventional large FOV (8,37,103,109,138–146) body coil MR images of the hip (Fig. 6-53).

Several reports have correlated extent of effusion and marrow edema with symptoms and the stage of AVN (117,129,134,147). Huang et al. (117) evaluated the stage for maximal bone marrow edema and the extent of joint effusion in correlation with the stage of AVN. Effusions were graded 0, no fluid; grade 1, minimal fluid; grade 2, sufficient fluid to extend along the femoral neck; and grade 3, large effusion with joint distention (see Fig. 6-55) (117). Both edema and effusions (grade 2) were most common at stage III (Tables 6-4 and 6-5) osteonecrosis. Bone marrow

TABLE 6-6

MR SIGNAL INTENSITY IN AVASCULAR NECROSIS OF THE FEMORAL HEAD

Signal Intensity		Signal Intensity Analogous to	Radiologic Stage
Short TR/TE	Long TE/TR		
High	Intermediate	Fat	I–II
High	High	Blood	I–II
Low	High	Fluid	III–IV
Low	Low	Fibrous tissue bone	III–IV

From Beltran J, Burk JM, Herman LJ, et al. Avascular necrosis of the femoral head: early MRI detection and radiological correlation. *Magn Reson Imaging* 1987;5:431–442; and Mitchell DG, Rao VM, Dalinka MK, et al. Femoral head avascular necrosis: correlation of MR imaging, radiographic staging, radionuclide imaging, and clinical findings. *Radiology* 1987;162:709–715.

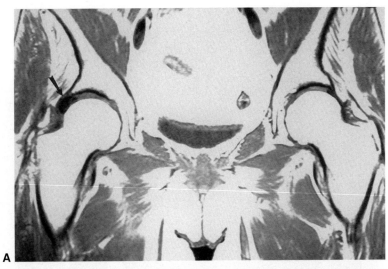

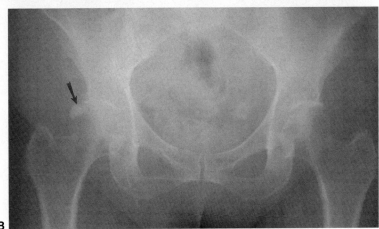

Figure 6-39 Coronal T1-weighted image **(A)** demonstrates a low signal intensity area in the peri-labral region. Anteroposterior radiograph **(B)** shows obvious dense calcification (*arrow*).

edema was a more consistent feature in patients with pain than joint effusion (117,134).

The MR patterns of AVN, though imperfect, are useful in understanding the histologic phases of AVN (59,120,148).

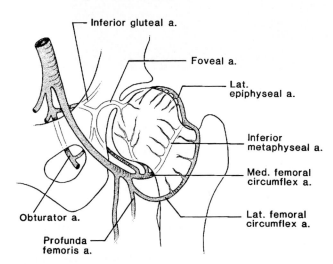

Figure 6-40 Illustration of the vascular anatomy of the hip. (From Berquist TH, Coventry MB. The Pelvis and Hips. In: Berquist TH, ed. *Imaging of Orthopedic Trauma and Surgery*. Philadelphia; W.B. Saunders, 1986:181–279.)

Mitchell et al. (120) correlated the MR signal intensity with radiographic features. Signal intensity was evaluated on both T1- and T2-weighted spin-echo sequences (Table 6-6). When signal intensity was similar to fat or marrow, the symptoms and radiographic features were generally early (stage I or II). Signal intensity that corresponded to fluid or fibrous tissue (Table 6-6) was nearly always associated with more advanced (stage III or IV) disease. Beltran et al. (101) also described MR imaging patterns and divided stages into early, intermediate, and late. We prefer comparing MRI and histologic changes (Table 6-4) and staging with the imaging features (Table 6-5) to assist with treatment selection (96,112–114). A thorough understanding of these histologic changes and the morphologic patterns of AVN improves the sensitivity and specificity of MRI. When compared with radiography, CT, and isotope scans, MRI is clearly the technique of choice for diagnosis and follow-up evaluation (1,10,120,124). Glickenstein et al. (149) reported specificity of 98% and sensitivity of 97% in differentiating AVN from normal hips. MRI was 91% sensitive in differentiating AVN from other types of hip pathology. The sensitivity of MRI was 96% compared to 86% for radionuclide scans. Also, false-negative isotope studies have been reported in up to 18% of patients with biopsy-proven AVN (3).

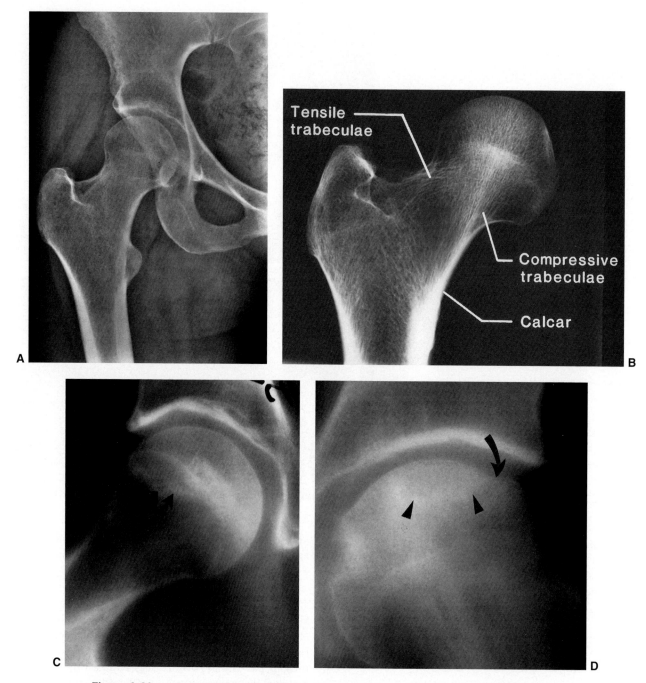

Figure 6-41 Radiographic features of AVN. **A:** Normal anteroposterior view of the hip. **B:** Specimen demonstrating normal femoral head contour and trabecular pattern. Stage 0 to I. **C:** Oblique tomogram demonstrates a normal joint space and the articular surface of the femoral head is normal. There is a lucent area with marginal sclerosis (*curved arrow*) due to AVN. Stage II. **D:** Anteroposterior tomogram demonstrating lucent area (*arrowheads*) with articular collapse (*curved arrow*). Stage III AVN. Anteroposterior of the pelvis (**E**) and oblique view of the right hip (**F**) show advanced articular collapse with osteoarthritis. Ficat stage IV or modified stage V AVN.

Morphologic changes on T1- and T2-weighted images play an important role in detection and treatment planning (10,120,127,150,151). Conventional spin echo, fast spin echo with fat suppression, spoiled gradient-recalled steady state (GRASS), and contrast-enhanced images are useful to evaluate articular cartilage and acetabular involvement (Figs. 6-43B and 6-50).

Axial, coronal, sagittal, and three-dimensional image data have been used to quantify the extent of femoral head involvement and the extent of weight-bearing surface

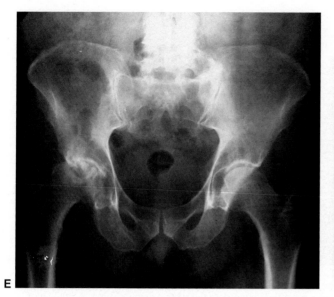

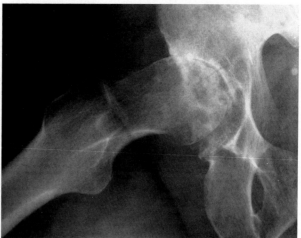

Figure 6-41 (continued)

included in the area of necrosis (96,101,114,115,127,150). Several methods have been suggested to help stage the extent of involvement for prognosis and treatment planning.

Lafforgue et al. (152) measured three parameters to evaluate the extent and location of lesions. Measurements can be obtained from the coronal T1-weighted image, which makes the technique simple, reproducible, and therefore easy to repeat on follow-up studies. The alpha angle was measured on the coronal image selecting the largest area of necrosis and determining the angle formed at the center of the femoral head (see Fig. 6-56). Patients with angles at least 75° had a

poor prognosis and patients with angles less than or equal to 45° had a more satisfactory clinical response and the lesions were less likely to progress if treated. This method was further modified by Koo and Kim (18) and later by Cheng (115).

Koo and Kim (18), (see Fig. 6-57) measured the angle formed from the center of the femoral head on midcoronal and midsagittal images to quantify the extent of femoral head involvement. Cheng modified this to measure the section with maximal involvement on the coronal and sagittal images (115). The combined angles coronal/180 × sagittal/180 × 100 resulted in the necrotic index (18,114,115).

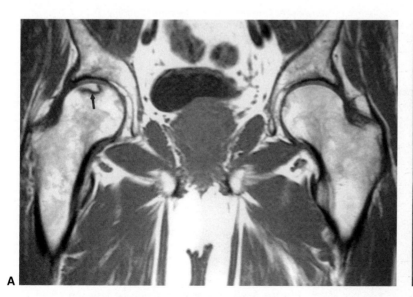

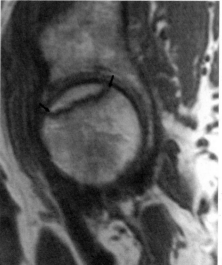

Figure 6-42   SE 500/10 images of the hips in a patient with early AVN on the right. Radiographs were normal. **A:** Coronal image demonstrating a small linear subchondral defect (arrow). **B:** Sagittal image of the right hip more clearly defines the extent of involvement (arrows).

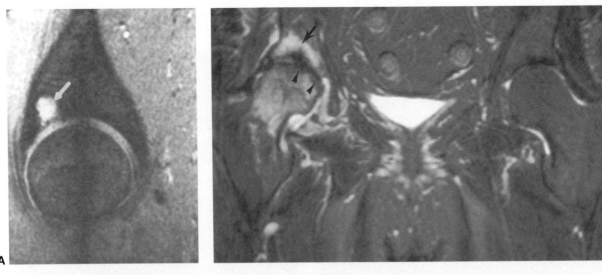

Figure 6-43 A: Sagittal gradient echo T2*-weighted image demonstrating an acetabular geode (*arrow*). **B:** Coronal fat suppressed fast spin-echo T2-weighted image demonstrates marrow edema, osteonecrosis (*arrowheads*) and an acetabular insufficiency fracture (*arrow*).

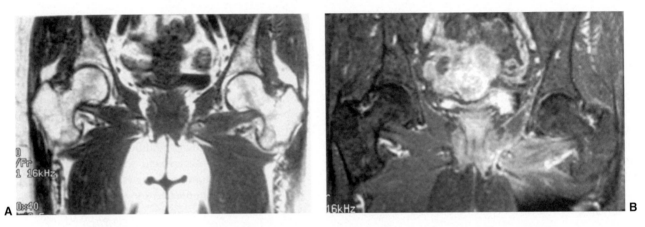

Figure 6-44 Patient with systemic disease on steroids. **A:** Coronal SE 500/11 image is normal. **B:** Postgadolinium fat-suppressed SE 500/10 image shows no increased signal in the femoral heads bilaterally, suggesting decreased flow. Compare to the signal intensity of the intertrochanteric and acetabular regions.

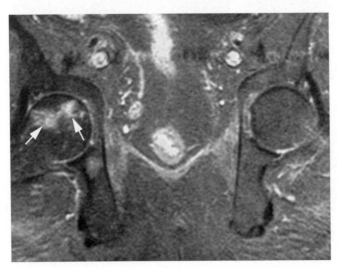

Figure 6-45 Coronal postcontrast fat-suppressed T1-weighted image demonstrates a focal area of necroses in the femoral head with surrounding enhancement or hyperemia (*arrows*).

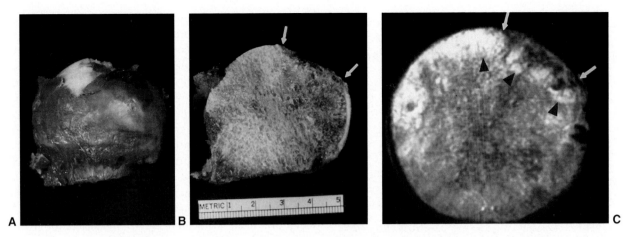

Figure 6-46 Gross **(A)** and coronal cut section **(B)** in a patient with AVN and articular collapse (*white arrows*). Axial section **(C)** shows the articular defect (*white arrows*) with reactive changes (*arrowheads*) at the necrotic interface and in the adjacent subchondral bone.

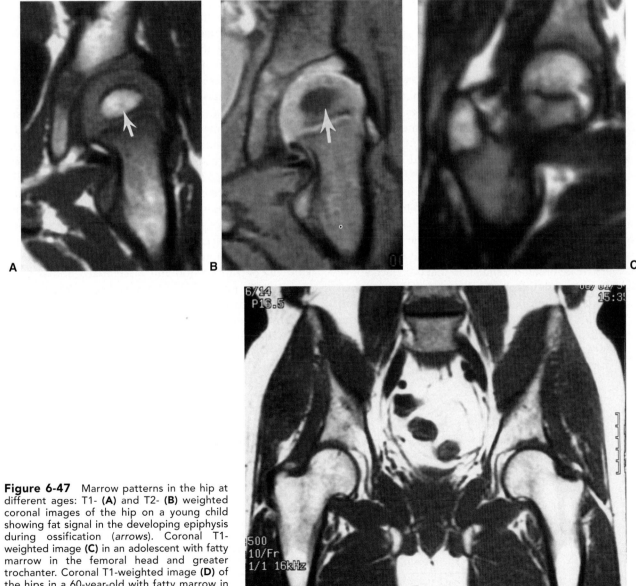

Figure 6-47 Marrow patterns in the hip at different ages: T1- **(A)** and T2- **(B)** weighted coronal images of the hip on a young child showing fat signal in the developing epiphysis during ossification (*arrows*). Coronal T1-weighted image **(C)** in an adolescent with fatty marrow in the femoral head and greater trochanter. Coronal T1-weighted image **(D)** of the hips in a 60-year-old with fatty marrow in both upper femurs.

TABLE 6-7

TREATMENT OPTIONS, AVASCULAR NECROSIS OF THE FEMORAL HEAD

Nonweight bearing
Core decompression
Core decompression/vascularized fibular graft
Core decompression/non-vascularized fibular graft
Osteotomy
Resurfacing arthroplasty
Bipolar hip arthroplasty
Total hip arthroplasty

From Cherian SF, Laorr A, Saleh KJ, et al. Quantifying the extent of femoral head involvement in osteonecrosis. *J Bone Joint Surg Am* 2003;85A:309–314; Lieberman JR, Berry DJ, Mont MA, et al. Osteonecrosis of the hip: management in the twenty-first century. *J Bone Joint Surg Am* 2002;84A:834–853; and Scully SP, Aaron RK, Wibaniak JR. Survival analysis of hips treated with core decompression or vascularized fibular grafting because of avascular necrosis. *J Bone Joint Surg Am* 1998;80A:1270–1275.

Another accepted method (Table 6-5) is estimating the percentage of the area of head involved and dividing the result into three categories: <15%, 15% to 30%, and >30%.

The percentage of necrosis of the femoral articular surface can be evaluated using several techniques. Lafforgue et al. (152) configured a circle about the femoral head by extending the articular surface (see Fig. 6-58). The surface area (A × B) divided by the diameter squared × 100 equals the percentage of head involvement (Fig. 6-58).

Shimizu et al. (150) used a similar technique to predict femoral head collapse. This system combines weight-bearing and femoral head involvement. T1-weighted coronal images are used with this technique that permits easy reproducibility and decreased cost and examination time. A circle is configured similar to that described above (Fig. 6-58). Necrosis was classified as grade A if its maximal distance from the articular margin was less than one fourth the diameter. Grade B necrosis (see Fig. 6-59) is between one fourth and one half, and grade C necrosis is greater than one half the diameter. In addition to weight-bearing described above, Shimizu also evaluated signal intensity of the necrotic zone on T1-weighted images. Intensity was categorized as high, mixed, or lower than the normal marrow. Following these changes, a predictable outcome could be established. When less than one fourth of the femoral head was involved, collapse did not occur. Thirty-five percent of grade B lesions collapsed and 62% of grade C lesions collapsed within 32 months. If less than 33% of the femoral head weight-bearing surface was involved, collapse did not occur. When at least two thirds of the weight-bearing surface of the femoral head was involved, the survival rate was only 29% (153). Femoral heads with high signal intensity (similar to fat) survived in 79% (32 months) of cases, mixed-intensity cases had only 15% survival at 11 months, and none of the femoral heads considered low intensity (Fig. 6-55) collapsed (150).

More recently, Malizos et al. (154) used three-dimensional, reformatted, 4-mm-thick sections to quantify femoral head involvement. Of these multiple techniques, we prefer the modified method used by Cheng (115) to measure maximal involvement on coronal and sagittal images. However, it is best to use the method preferred by the referring orthopedic surgeon.

Prior to MRI, the radiographic stage (Table 6-4) was used to determine treatment of AVN. Patients with stages I and II disease were considered as potential candidates for core decompression. Treatment of stages III and IV changes usually requires arthroplasty (10,114,120). As noted above, the MR features can be correlated with histologic change and are evident earlier than radiographic features. Previous studies using radiography have demonstrated progression of AVN after core decompression in the majority of patients (109). However, more recently MRI features and experience with core decompression and vascularized fibular grafts in early AVN (stages I and II) have been more positive (10,35,80,96,115,150).

Core decompression has regained popularity with the increased ability to detect subtle marrow edema and early

TABLE 6-8

TREATMENT APPROACHES TO AVASCULAR NECROSIS OF THE FEMORAL HEAD

Imaging Stage[a]	Symptoms	Treatment
I, II	None	Observation ± core decompression ± bone grafting
I, II	Present	Core decompression ± bone grafting
IC, IIC, III, IVA	Present	Bone grafting, resurfacing or total hip arthroplasty
IIIB, IVC	Present	Resurfacing or total hip arthroplasty
V, VI	Present	Total hip arthroplasty

[a] Indicates sub-stages A,B,C included (Table 6-5).
From Lieberman JR, Berry DJ, Mont MA, et al. Osteonecrosis of the hip: Management in the 21st century. *J Bone Joint Surg Am* 2002; 84A:834–853.

TABLE 6-9

TRANSIENT OSTEOPOROSIS, BONE MARROW EDEMA AND AVASCULAR NECROSIS: CLINICAL AND IMAGE FEATURES

	Transient Osteoporosis	Bone Marrow Edema	Avascular Necrosis
Onset	Acute	Usually insidious	Gradual or insidious
Symptoms	Pain with weight bearing, limp	Pain at rest, limp later in course	Pain at rest, limp later in course
Etiology	Unknown	Unknown	Circulation interrupted
Male:Female ratio	3:1	~Equal	Equal
Incidence	Rare	Uncommon	Common
Risk factors for AVN	Absent	May be present	Present
Bilateral	No	No	50–80%
Radiographic features	Osteopenia 4–6 weeks after onset	± Osteopenia	Sclerosis, lucency, subchondral collapse
Bone scan	Diffusely increased tracer in head, neck and trochanteric region	Diffusely increased tracer in head and neck	Localized increased tracer or photopenia
MRI	↑ signal T2WI	↑ signal T2WI	Focal subchondral defect ± marrow edema
	↓ signal T1WI in head, neck and trochanteric regions	↓ signal T1WI, head and neck	
Prognosis	Resolves 2–6 months	Resolves 2–6 months	70–80% progress
Treatment	Conservative, non-weight bearing	Conservative vs. core decompression	Core decompression, vascularized graft, arthroplasty

T2WI, T2-weighted image; T1WI, T1-weighted image.
From references 72, 73, 85, 116, 155, 172, and 173.

AVN. Appropriate use of core decompression and vascularized bone grafts can reduce or delay the need for hip arthroplasty (77,90,105,106,155,156). Scully et al. (90) compared results of core decompression with vascularized grafts in patients with stage I to stage III AVN. Both techniques were effective for stage I disease. However, with more advanced stage II and III AVN the results with core decompression were less satisfactory. Satisfactory results at four years for core decompression were 65% for stage II and 21% for stage III disease compared with 89% and 81% respectively for vascularized grafts (90). Similar results have been reported by Camp (109) and Hopson et al. (28).

Lieberman et al. (96) reviewed treatment options based upon the classification system described in Table 6-5, which incorporates radiographic and MRI features. Multiple procedures were included in their report (Table 6-7). Core decompression is the most common approach for early (stage I and stage II) disease (90,96,103,115). Results demonstrate success rates (no symptoms, no progression) of up to 95% for stage I and stage IIA (sclerotic radiographic features without cystic changes) (103). Others report success rates of over 80% for stages I and II (Table 6-5) disease (96).

Core decompression with vascularized fibular grafts provides the benefit of decompression plus strut support and revascularization (96). Success rates of 91% were achieved for stages I and II AVN (96,157). Non-vascularized grafts were 90% successful for stage I and stage II disease (96). Resurfacing arthroplasty (Fig. 6-56) has a success rate of 91% at 5 years and 61% at 10 years (96,158). Total hip arthroplasty has the highest likelihood of providing a long term successful result (96).

Based upon their review using the classification in Table 6-5, Lieberman et al. (96) suggested treatment approaches summarized in Table 6-8.

Bone infarcts in the pelvis and upper femurs (see Fig. 6-60) also have a very typical MR appearance (10,93). Radiographic, CT, and radionuclide features of bone infarcts may be nonspecific, appear more aggressive than bone infarction (i.e., malignancy or infection) or be totally unremarkable (10,93). T1-weighted MR images show an area of low intensity in the diaphysis or metaphysis. This may have a well-defined serpiginous margin and multiple foci of involvement are common. On T2-weighted sequences, the margins are more clearly defined and form a "double line" of low and high signal intensity (122,159). This appearance may be due to chemical shift artifact, in which case the high

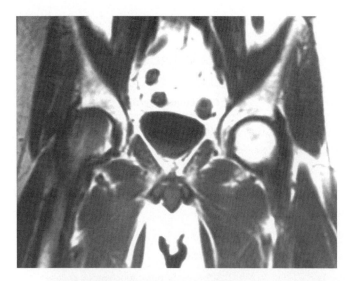

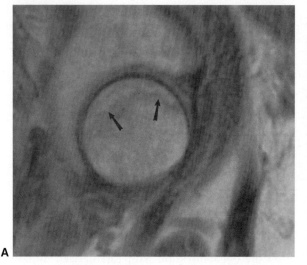

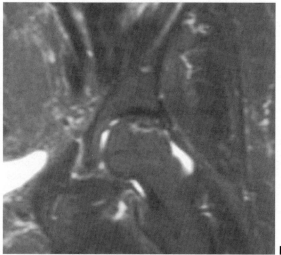

A

B

Figure 6-48 Axial SE 456/15 image demonstrating diffuse low signal intensity in the right femoral head due to early AVN.

Figure 6-49 Sagittal spin-echo 456/15 image of the hip **(A)** in early AVN. There is a low intensity margin around the necrotic area (*arrows*). The necrotic area maintains fat signal intensity. Fat-suppressed T2-weighted coronal image **(B)** shows high signal intensity at the margin with the necrotic zone. The necrotic zone maintains the same fat-suppressed signal intensity as the remainder of the femoral head and neck.

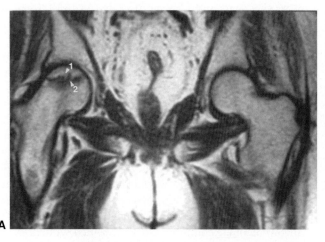

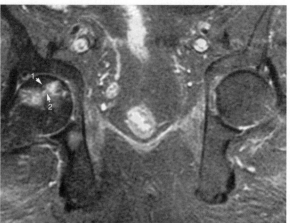

A

B

Figure 6-50 Coronal T1-weighted **(A)** and contrast enhanced fat-suppressed T1-weighted images **(B)** demonstrate the necrotic zone (*1*) and hyperemic response zone (*2*). Contrast enhancement more clearly differentiates hyperemia from fibrous tissue.

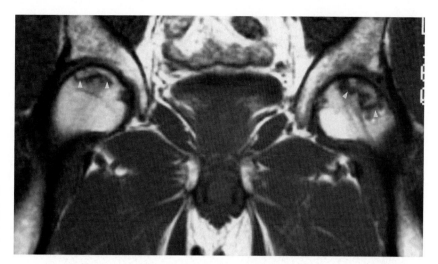

Figure 6-51 Coronal spin-echo T1-weighted image with early AVN on the right and a thin, low-intensity zone (*arrowheads*). The changes on the left have progressed to trabecular reinforcement, leading to a widening of the reactive zone (*arrowheads*).

intensity will be on opposite sides of the dark line, or due to hyperemia and new bone formation or calcification, in which case the high intensity zone remains along the same margin of the lesion throughout (87,136,151). Bone sclerosis and calcification appear as areas of low intensity on both T1- and T2-weighted sequences and are usually seen in chronic infarcts (132).

Rapidly Destructive Hip Disease

Ryu et al. (160) described a more aggressive destructive process of the femoral head termed rapidly destructive hip disease (RDHD). This unusual condition was noted in 20 hips over a 5-year period. Unlike typical AVN, this condition results in rapid destruction of the femoral head over 2 to 12 months (160). Most cases presented with radiographs suggesting stage III or IV AVN. Bone fragmentation and loss of

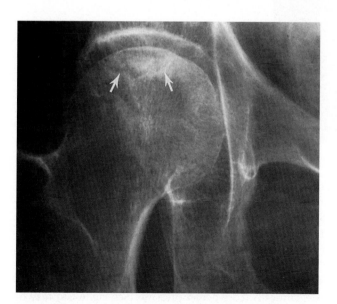

Figure 6-52 Anteroposterior radiograph of the hip demonstrating stage II avascular necroses with a clearly defined area of mixed sclerosis and lucency (*arrows*).

the femoral articular surface with large joint effusions were common (see Fig. 6-61). Acetabular erosions were noted in 55% of cases (60). More recently, Watanabe et al. (161) and Yamamota et al. (162) described subchondral insufficiency fractures in elderly females and renal transplant patients which also lead to rapid hip destruction (rapidly destructive coxathrosis). Differential diagnosis of these disorders would include rheumatoid arthritis, infection, and neurotrophic arthropathy. These conditions are usually excluded based on clinical features or joint fluid studies. Though etiology is uncertain, ischemic bone necrosis was evident in all surgical specimens (68,135).

Bone Marrow Edema

Bone marrow edema or transient marrow edema is a controversial entity that may represent early AVN, or represent a transient condition with no sequelae (Table 6-9) (70,77,83,163). Radiographs demonstrate transient osteopenia and scintigrams increased uptake in the femoral head and intertrochanteric region (10,163). This is a diagnosis of exclusion and must be differentiated from early osteonecrosis, transient osteoporosis of the hip and other causes of edema such as infection, trauma, and neoplasm (72,87,108,164–168). Marrow edema has low signal intensity on T1-weighted images, high signal intensity on T2-weighted and STIR sequences, and enhances with gadolinium in the presence of patent vessels or flow to the femoral head (72,164). The extent of involvement is more diffuse than characteristic osteonecrosis and generally involves the femoral head and neck (see Fig. 6-62) (15,87,169–171). Follow-up MR examinations in 6 to 12 weeks usually show improvement or no progression to typical osteonecrosis (108,166). Routine radiographs in patients with transient osteoporosis are usually positive within 8 weeks after the onset of symptoms. Therefore, comparison of MR features with radiographs is important. If there are no features of transient osteoporosis (osteopenia of femoral head

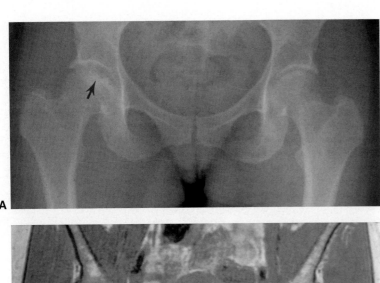

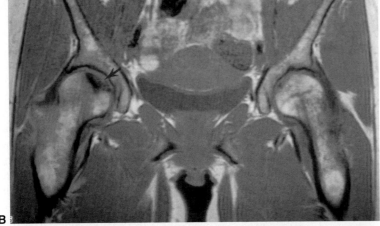

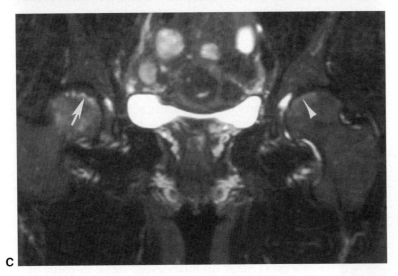

Figure 6-53 A: Anteroposterior radiograph demonstrates sclerosis (*arrow*) and collapse of the right femoral head. Coronal T1-weighted image **(B)** shows mixed signal intensity in the necrotic zone with deformity (*arrow*) of the femoral head. Coronal T2-weighted image **(C)** shows marrow edema with increased signal intensity in the area of subchondral collapse (*arrow*). There are also early subchondral changes on the left (*arrowhead*).

and upper femur) by 8 weeks, the diagnosis is in question and further follow-up with MRI is indicated to assure that osteonecrosis or some other process is not the cause (72).

Recently, Lecouet et al. (116) and VandeBerg et al. (77) described subchondral features on MR images that assist in predicting lesions that may be transient rather than irreversible. All lesions that did not demonstrate any subchondral changes on T2-weighted or contrast enhanced T1-weighted images were transient. Patients with bone marrow edema and subchondral lesions (see Fig. 6-63)

measuring 12.5 mm in length or with thickness ≥4 mm had positive predictive values of 85% and 73% on T2-weighted images for AVN. Positive predictive values for these features were 87% and 86% respectively on contrast enhanced T1-weighted images (77).

Patients with bone marrow edema may be treated conservatively. However, with subchondral changes or risk factors clinically, core decompression (see Fig. 6-64) may be indicated (72,166). Histology obtained in patients with marrow edema during core decompression shows edema

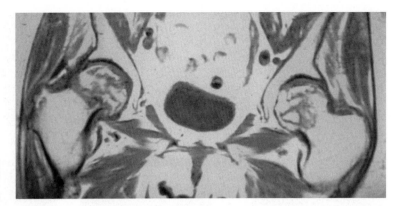

Figure 6-54 Coronal SE 456/15 image of the pelvis and hips (field of view, 42 cm) with bilateral advanced AVN. There is joint space narrowing and osteophyte formation indicating stage IV disease (*Tables 6-4 and 6-5*).

and necrosis, which supports the theory that this condition is the earliest phase of AVN (174).

Transient Osteoporosis

Transient osteoporosis of the hip is one of several conditions that presents with pain and bone marrow edema pattern. The etiology is unknown (72,73,105). The condition was commonly described in the third trimester of pregnancy. Calcium demand during this phase of pregnancy may cause bone loss. Also, genetic disorders have been considered as a possible etiology (96,128,172,175–177). It is now clear that the condition is seen in men and women. The condition is more common in males than females (M:F = 3:1) and most commonly presents in young or middle-age males (Table 6-9).

Guerra and Steinberg (172) described three clinical stages. The initial phase presents with acute pain, limp, and reduced functional capacity in the involved hip. This phase lasts about one month. The second phase lasts about two months during which the symptoms plateau and radiographs demonstrate osteopenia involving the femoral head, neck and often the upper femur (see Fig. 6-65) (96,172). Symptoms regress during the third phase, which typically lasts about 4 months (172). After symptoms resolve, other joints may be affected resulting in migratory osteoporosis (72,73).

Image features are useful (Table 6-9) with osteopenia occurring 4 to 6 weeks after the onset of symptoms (Fig. 6-65). Bone scan and MR image features occur early. Scintigrams demonstrate diffusely increased tracer in the femoral head and neck (see Fig. 6-66) (72,73,96). MR images

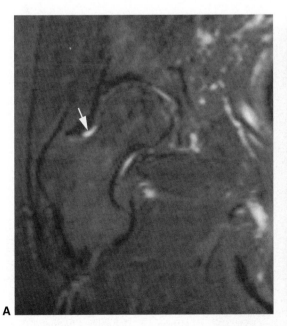

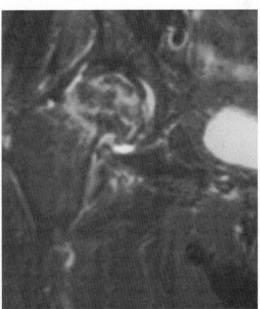

Figure 6-55 Coronal T2-weighted images on patients with early AVN treated with core decompression (**A**) and advanced AVN (**B**). There is sufficient fluid to extend along the femoral neck (grade 2) (*arrow* in **A**) and a larger effusion (grade 3) in **B**.

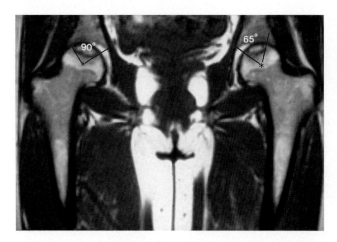

Figure 6-56 Coronal MR image demonstrating the alpha α angle of necrosis in the femoral head. Lines are drawn from the necrotic margins to the center (*) of the head. The angle formed (α angle) is a useful prognostic indicator. Angles ≥75° have a more guarded prognosis. Angles ≤45° have a better prognosis. The angle on the *right* measures 90° and on the *left* 65°. (From Lafforgue P, Dahan E, Chagnaud C, et al. Early stage avascular necrosis of the femoral head: MR imaging of prognosis in 31 cases with at least two years follow-up. *Radiology* 1993;187:199–204.)

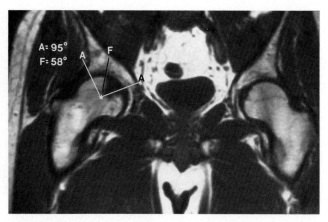

Figure 6-57 Coronal image of the pelvis and hips demonstrating the weight-bearing surface calculation. The acetabular weight bearing angle **A** is formed by lines (*white lines, A*) from the weight bearing area to the center (*) of the femoral head. In this case A = 95°. The angle **F** of femoral head involvement is formed by the margin of necrosis within the acetabular weight-bearing lines. In this case, F = 58°. F/A × 100 = % weight-bearing involvement. In this case, 58/95 × 100 = 61%. Weight-bearing involvement >45% has a poor prognosis and <45% a favorable prognosis. (From Koo K-H, Kim R. Quantifying the extent of osteonecrosis of the femoral head. A method using MRI. *J Bone Joint Surg Am* 1995;77B: 825–880.)

demonstrate increased signal intensity on T2-weighted images. Signal intensity is decreased on T1-weighted images. The abnormality is seen in the head and neck. There is no subchondral defect to suggest AVN. Effusions are common (see Fig. 6-67) (10,72,73,178).

The differential diagnosis includes other causes of marrow edema including reflex sympathetic dystrophy (70,73,133,172). Radiographic features of transient osteoporosis and reflex sympathetic dystrophy are similar. Reflex sympathetic dystrophy more commonly involves the upper extremities, is more debilitating than transient osteoporosis, and skin changes and vasomotor dysfunction are more often seen with reflex sympathetic dystrophy (72).

Symptoms spontaneously resolve in patients with transient osteoporosis (Table 6-9). Therefore, conservative therapy is selected once the diagnosis is established.

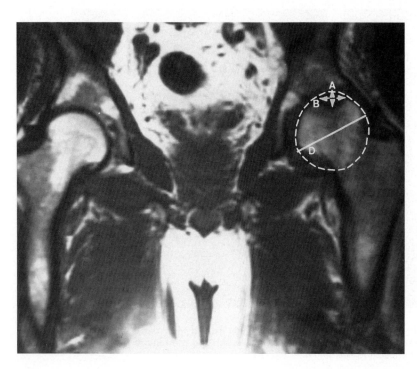

Figure 6-58 Percentage of femoral head involved with AVN. The articular surface of the head is extended to create a circle. The area of necrosis (A × B) divided by the diameter (D) (*white line*) squared × 100 yields the percentage of femoral head involved. In our experience, this technique is more difficult to use than those demonstrated in Figs. 6-56 and 6-57. (After Lafforgue P, Dahan E, Chagnaud C, et al. Early stage avascular necrosis of the femoral head: MR imaging of prognosis in 31 cases with at least two years follow-up. *Radiology* 1993;187:199–204.)

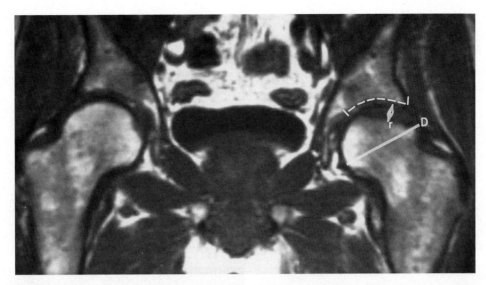

Figure 6-59 Femoral head involvement described by Shimizu et al. Coronal T1-weighted image of the hips with an area of necrosis on the *left* that has lower signal intensity than normal marrow. *Line D* is the diameter of the femoral head circle. The radial distance (*r*) is less than one fourth the diameter (*D*) or grade A. The area of necrosis involves over two thirds of the weight-bearing surface (*broken line*), which increases the likelihood of femoral head collapse. (After Shimizu K, Moriya H, Akita T, et al. Prediction of collapse with magnetic resonance imaging of avascular necrosis of the femoral head. *J Bone Joint Surg Am* 1994;76A:215–223.)

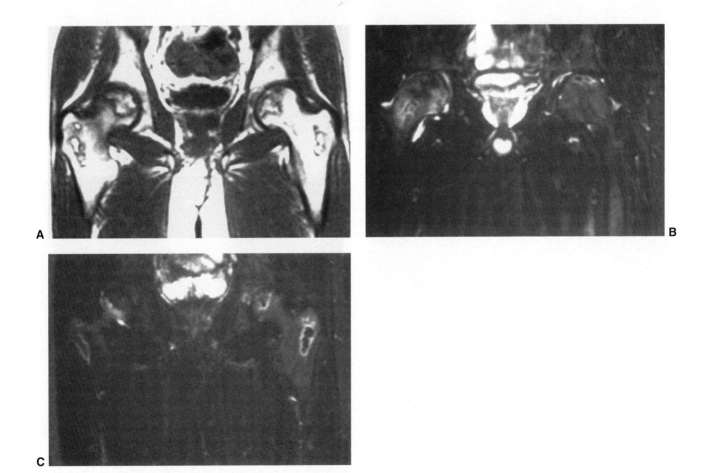

Figure 6-60 Patient on steroids for Crohn disease. Coronal T1-weighted image **(A)** demonstrates bilateral AVN of the femoral heads and trochanteric bone infarcts. Fat-suppressed postcontrast images **(B, C)** show marginal enhancement around the necrotic bone due to hyperemia.

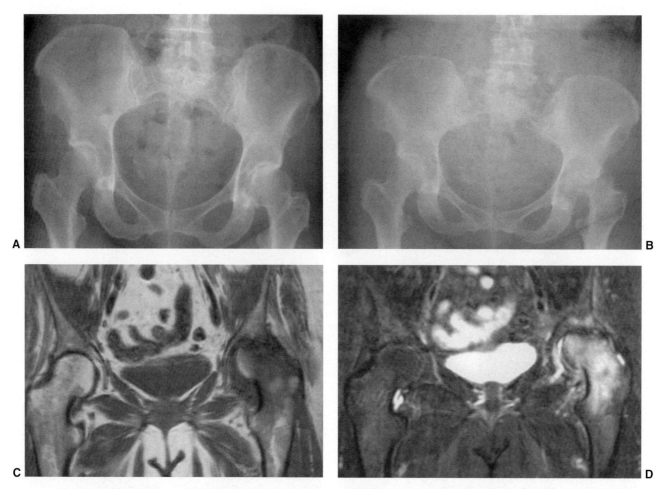

Figure 6-61 Radiographs **(A,B)** 3 months apart demonstrate rapid destruction of the left femoral head. T1- **(C)** and T2-weighted **(D)** MR images demonstrate marked deformity of the femoral head and extensive marrow edema.

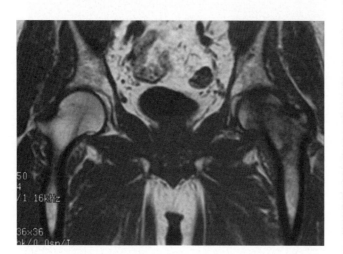

Figure 6-62 Transient bone marrow edema. T1-weighted coronal image shows reduced signal intensity in the left femoral head and neck. Acetabular signal intensity is normal.

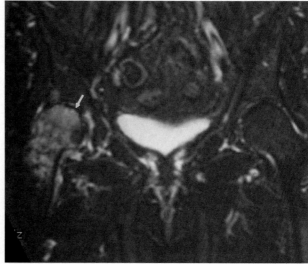

Figure 6-63 Bone marrow edema seen on a T2-weighted image with high signal intensity in the right femoral head and neck. There is a low intensity subchondral linear area (*arrow*) that indicates an irreversible lesion or early AVN.

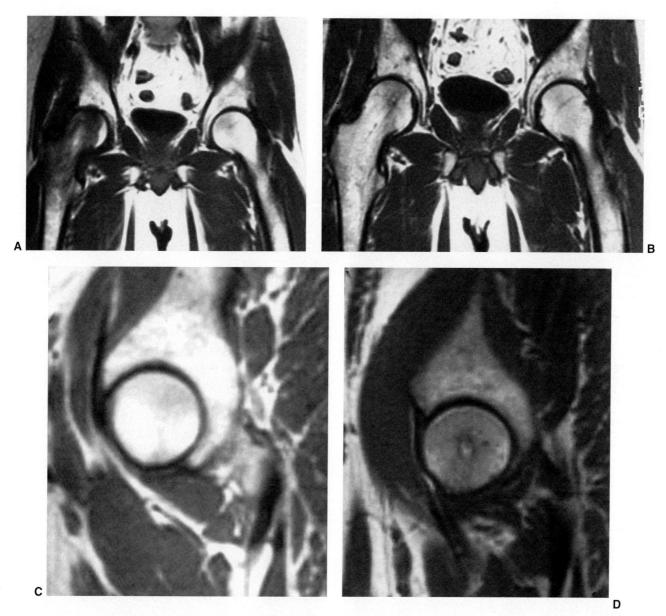

Figure 6-64   Bone marrow edema treated with core decompression in a patient with risk factors for osteonecrosis. **A:** Coronal T1-weighted image demonstrating edema in the right femoral head and proximal femur. Coronal T1-weighted image **(B)** and sagittal images **(C,D)** one year after core decompression are normal.

Trauma

Osseous Trauma

MRI has become an effective tool for detection of osseous, articular, and soft tissue trauma in the pelvis, hips, and thighs (10,143,179–188) (Table 6-10). Generally, MRI is not requested for most acute skeletal injuries because routine radiography, CT, and isotope studies are usually diagnostic (10,189,190). However, subtle fractures, such as stress fractures (see Fig. 6-68), femoral neck fractures, avulsion fractures, and unsuspected fractures can be defined early using MRI (see Fig. 6-69) (9,97,165–167,182,188,191–195). Deutsch et al. (182) reported detection of hip fractures by

MRI in all nine patients with normal radiographs. Also, up to 74% of patients with trauma have soft tissue injuries that were detected by MRI but not suspected clinically (180).

In recent years, MRI has replaced radionuclide scans as a more cost-effective technique to exclude subtle hip and pelvic fractures in children and adults (Fig. 6-65) (23,98,130,180,186,196–198). Bogost et al. (180) reported detection of unsuspected pelvic and hip fracture in 23% and 375 of patients, respectively. Conventional T1-weighted coronal images provide an effective screening tool for osseous injury (see Figs. 6-68B and 6-70) (98,186). Examinations can be performed quickly and treatment decisions made early, which reduces delays

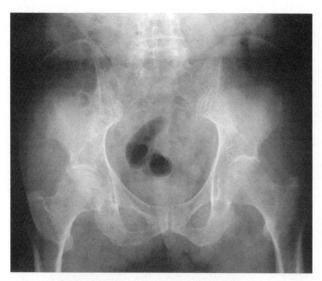

Figure 6-65 Transient osteoporosis of the hip. There is osteopenia involving the upper left femur. The joint space and acetabular bone density is normal.

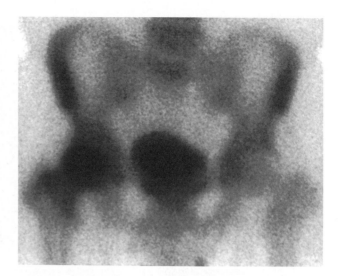

Figure 6-66 Bone scan [Tc-99m methylene diphosphonate (MDP)] shows diffusely increased traces in the right femoral head and neck.

TABLE 6-10

INJURIES IN THE PELVIS AND HIPS

Osseous	Soft Tissue
Avulsion fractures	Muscle, tendon tears
Stress/Insufficiency fractures	Muscle strain
Osteochondral fractures	Muscle contusion
Bone bruises	Bursitis
	Ligament tears
	Acetabular labral tears
	Trochanteric pain syndrome

From references 98, 180, 182, 183, and 195.

and hospital costs. Diagnosis based upon radionuclide scans can result in delays of 2 to 3 days prior to instituting appropriate therapy (Fig. 6-70) (186,199). MRI may also more clearly define the extent of bone and soft tissue injury in the acute setting (23,180,186,199).

The role of MRI for evaluating osseous trauma in the pelvis and hips continues to expand as more experience is gained with different categories of injury (Table 6-10).

Avulsion fractures are common in children and adolescents and uncommon in adults. Injury results from strong muscle contractions causing fracture of the physis. Common avulsion injuries include the anterior superior iliac spine (sartoseus), inferior iliac spine (rectus femoris), greater trochanter (gluteus), lesser trochanter (iliopsoas), and

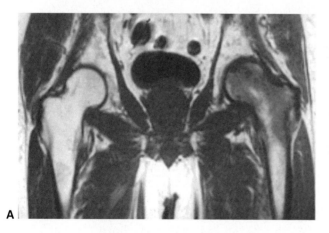
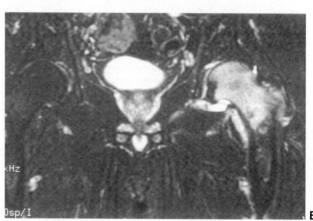

Figure 6-67 Transient osteoporosis of the hip. **A:** T1-weighted coronal image demonstrating decreased signal intensity in the femoral head and neck. There are no geographic subchondral changes to suggest AVN. **B:** Coronal T2-weighted image shows increased signal intensity in the left femoral head and neck with a joint effusion.

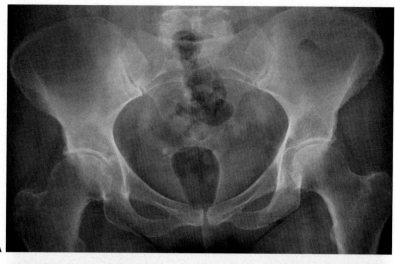

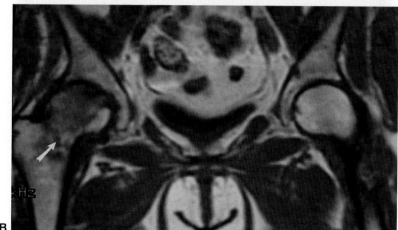

Figure 6-68   Patient with right hip pain and normal radiograph **(A)**. Coronal T1-weighted image **(B)** demonstrates decreased signal intensity due to edema and a fracture at the base of the femoral neck (*arrow*).

ischial tuberosity (hamstrings) (see Fig. 6-71) (6,10). In younger patients, injuries are often related to sports such as soccer, gymnastics, cheerleading, and track. In adults, these injuries are uncommon. In fact, if an avulsion fracture of the lesser trochanter is identified, with no significant trauma history, the finding is indicative of underlying malignancy or metastasis. Avulsion fractures in this setting have been reported in the anterior superior iliac spine, anterior inferior iliac spine, and ischial tuberosity (144).

Most displaced fractures are easily identified radiographically. However, subtle fractures may be overlooked. MR examinations can be planned based on radiographic features. T1-weighted and fat-suppressed T2-weighted fast spin-echo sequences may be adequate. Contrast enhanced, fat-suppressed T1-weighted images may be useful in subtle cases (see Figs. 6-72 and 6-73) (166,167,193,200,201).

Stress fractures are due to repetitive trauma of insufficient magnitude to cause an acute fracture (2). Imbalance in bone resorption and formation lead to weakening, with microtrabecular fracture leading to eventual cortical fracture if activity is continued (200). Stress fractures account for 10% of cases in sports medicine practices and occur in up to 30% of military recruits (195,202). Several studies have documented the incidence and location of stress fracture in the pelvis and proximal femurs (165–167,193, 202,203). Stress fractures in this region account for 1% to 10% of all stress fractures (44,161,204). Kiuru et al. (166) reviewed stress fractures in 340 military recruits. Sixty percent involved the femur, and 40% involved the pelvis. The majority of femoral fractures involved the neck (67%), the proximal femur was involved in 32%, and 1% involved the femoral head (166). Stress fractures in the femoral neck may be compressive or distractive. Compressive fractures occur along the lower medial femoral neck (see Fig. 6-74). They appear sclerotic on radiographs and less likely to displace. Distractive fractures appear as lucent areas in the superior lateral femoral neck and tend to displace (Fig. 6-69) (205,206).

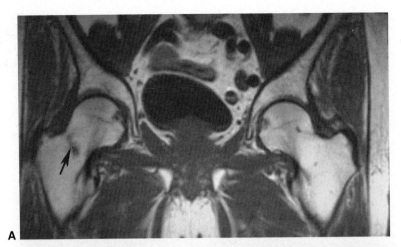

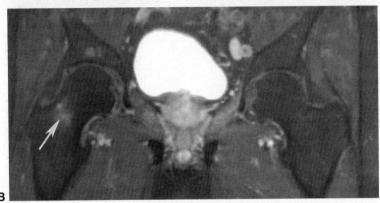

Figure 6-69 Lateral femoral neck insufficiency fracture. Radiograph was normal. T1- **(A)** and T2-weighted fast spin-echo **(B)** coronal images clearly demonstrate the fracture (*arrow*).

Forty percent of fractures involved the pelvis (166). The inferior pubic ramus was involved in 49%, the sacrum 41%, the superior pubic ramus 4%, iliam 4%. and acetabulum 1% (see Fig. 6-75). Multiple fractures were evident in 24% of patients (166). Williams et al. (207) reported a

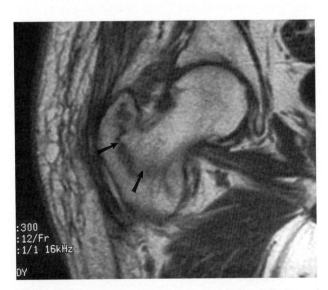

Figure 6-70 Undisplaced intertrochanteric fracture. Radiograph was normal. T1-weighted coronal image clearly demonstrates the fracture (*arrows*).

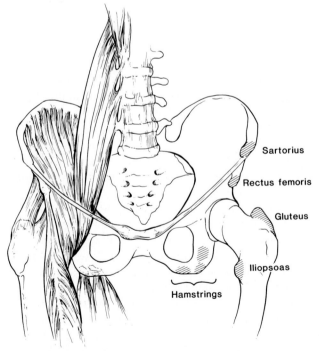

Figure 6-71 Illustration of locations of muscle-related avulsion fractures. (From Berquist TH. *Imaging of Orthopedic Trauma*. 2nd ed. New York: Raven Press, 1992.)

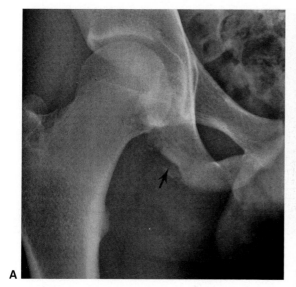

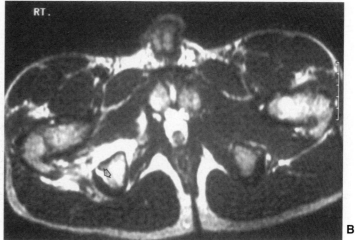

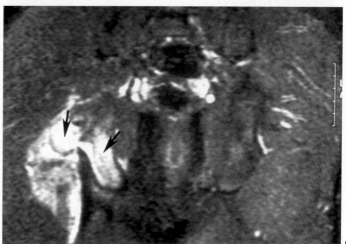

Figure 6-72   Ischial tuberosity physis avulsion in young athlete. **A:** Routine radiograph demonstrates a defect in the ischium (*arrow*). Axial **(B)** and coronal **(C)** T2-weighted images show fluid in the physis (*open arrow*) not evident on the opposite side and increased signal intensity in the bone and soft tissue (*arrows*).

higher incidence of acebabular fractures (6.7%) in a similar patient population. Seventy percent of acetabular fractures involve the roof, and 30% the anterior column (207).

Radiographs have a sensitivity of 37%, specificity of 79%, and accuracy of 60% for detection or early stress fractures. MRI has a sensitivity of 100%, specificity of 86%, and accuracy of 95% (166,193). Kiuru et al. (193) graded MR image features of stress fractures. Grade I is marrow edema, with grade V representing marrow edema, periosteal changes, a fracture line, and callus formation (Table 6-11). MR features can be identified on T1-weighted, T2-weighted, and STIR sequences. Dynamic contrast studies may be useful, especially for evaluating the fracture line, callus, and muscle edema (165). We have not used this dynamic technique routinely. However, as described by Kiura et al. (165), 0.1 mmol per Kg of gadolinium is injected as a bolus followed by a 20-mL saline flush. A short T1-fast spoiled gradient-echo multiphase sequence (8/2, flip angle 45°, 60 axial and 60 coronal sections) is used. Contrast studies are also useful to assess flow in patients with femoral neck fractures (208).

Marrow edema or bone bruise has also been described in the pubic bones in 77% of Australian rules football players by Verrrall et al. (202) Inflammation in the pubic symphisis is also common and may respond well to injection (209).

Insufficiency fractures are common in the sacrum, pubic rami, supra acetabular region, and femoral neck

TABLE 6-11

STRESS FRACTURES: KIURU CLASSIFICATION

Grade	MR Image Feature
I	Marrow edema
II	Marrow and periosteal edema
III	Marrow, periosteal, and muscle edema
IV	Fracture line
V	Endosteal or periosteal callus

From Kiuri MJ, Pihlajamaki HK, Hietanen HJ, et al. MR imaging, bone scintigraphy and radiography in bone stress injuries of the pelvis and lower extremities. *Acta Radiol* 2002;43(2):207–212.

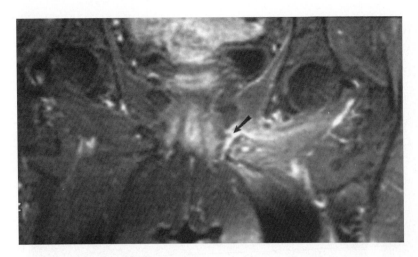

Figure 6-73 Adult with groin pain. T2-weighted, fat-suppressed fast spin-echo image demonstrates a partial avulsion of the adductor muscle (*arrow*).

(see Figs. 6-76 through 6-80) (184,206,210). These fractures are a common cause of low back and groin pain in the elderly, specifically osteoporotic females (206). In many cases, there is a history of previous malignancy or radiation therapy. Therefore, metastatic disease must be differentiated from an insufficiency fracture or fractures (107,203,206,211).

Until recently, radionuclide scans and CT were used to diagnose insufficiency fractures (10,211). CT may still be more specific (Fig. 6-76) (2,10,212). MRI features of insufficiency fractures are now more clearly defined. Bone marrow edema (↑ signal on T2-weighted, ↓ signal on T1-weighted images) may be evident as early as 18 days after insufficiency fracture (107,184). The linear fracture line is usually low intensity and therefore more easily appreciated on T2-weighted or STIR sequences (see Figs. 6-78D and 6-79B) (10,78). In more chronic fractures there may be fluid in the fracture line (35,153,198). Contrast-enhanced, fat-suppressed T1-weighted images are usually not indicated. However, in some cases it makes the fracture line more evident (107). If present, a linear edema pattern and fracture line is very helpful when excluding metastatic disease. In difficult cases, CT may be required to confirm the diagnosis (Fig. 6-76).

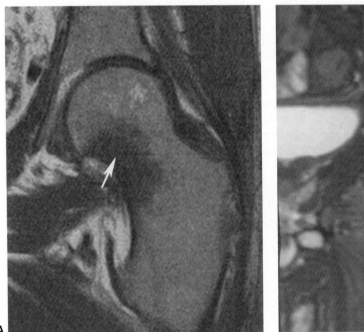
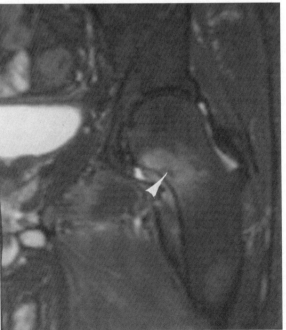

Figure 6-74 Medial femoral (compressive) neck stress fracture. Coronal T1-weighted image **(A)** shows a large area of edema medially (*arrow*). Fast spin-echo T2-weighted image **(B)** demonstrates edema and a low intensity fracture line (*arrowhead*).

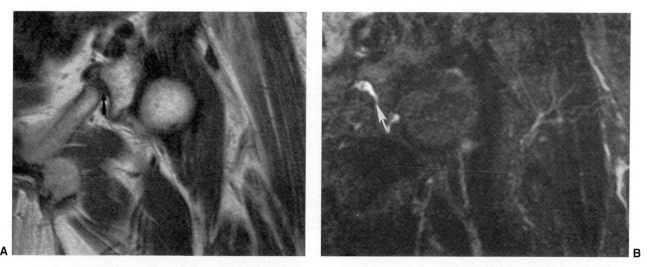

Figure 6-75 Chronic ununited superior pubic ramus fracture. Coronal T1-weighted image **(A)** demonstrates well-marginated fracture fragments with low intensity between the fragments (*arrow*). T2-weighted image **(B)** demonstrates high signal intensity fluid (*arrow*) due to nonunion.

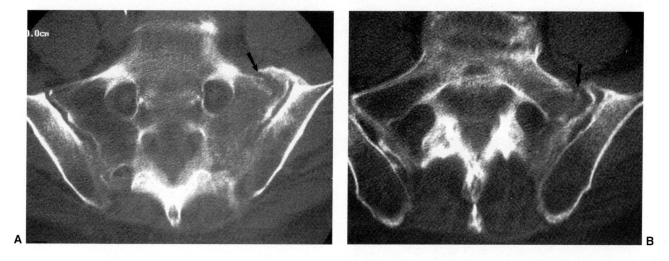

Figure 6-76 Axial CT images **(A,B)** of a sacral insufficiency fracture (*arrow*).

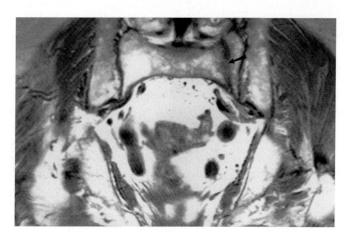

Figure 6-77 Coronal T1-weighted image demonstrating a sacral insufficiency fracture on the left (*arrow*).

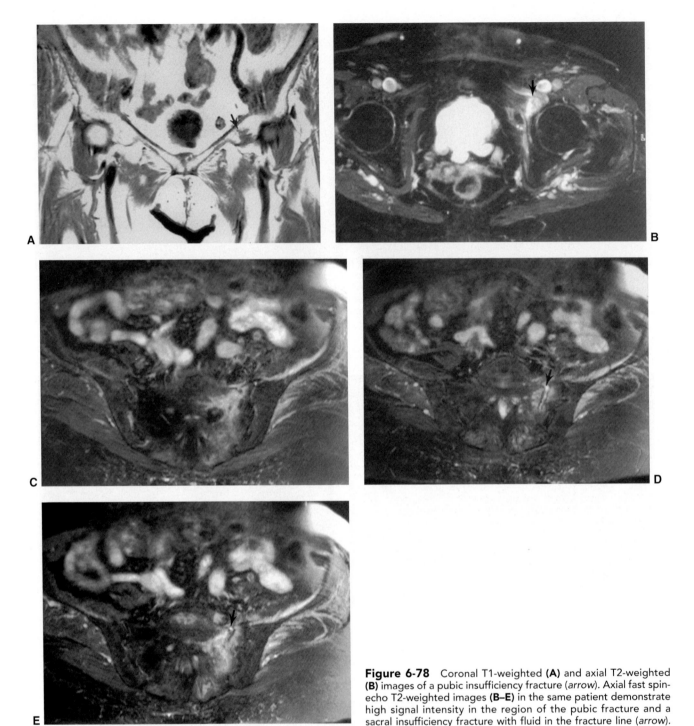

Figure 6-78 Coronal T1-weighted **(A)** and axial T2-weighted **(B)** images of a pubic insufficiency fracture (*arrow*). Axial fast spin-echo T2-weighted images **(B–E)** in the same patient demonstrate high signal intensity in the region of the pubic fracture and a sacral insufficiency fracture with fluid in the fracture line (*arrow*).

Osteochondral injuries can also occur. Acute osteochondral injuries may occur with subluxation or dislocation of the femoral head (14,58,77,118,143,186,197,213). Impaction injuries may also result in cartilage and subchondral bone microfractures (200).

Osteochondritis dissecans may have a similar MR appearance. Lesions are uncommon in the hip. However, when present, the lesion is usually near the fovea. Most patients are adolescents and present with pain on ambulation and decreased rotation. Patients may have prior developmental hip dysplasia, Legg-Calvé-Perthes disease, or trauma (190).

Cartilage lesions have been graded based upon MR image features. Grade 1 lesions have intact cartilage with signal abnormality in subchondral bone. Grade 2 injuries show partial detachment of the osteochondral fragment, grade 3 lesions are completely detached (fluid signal intensity surrounds the fragment), and grade 4 lesions are displaced (10,200).

MR imaging can accurately locate the lesions and determine the extent of involvement. T2-weighted or dual echo steady state (DESS) images define the articular cartilage, but accuracy of grading is suboptimal. MR

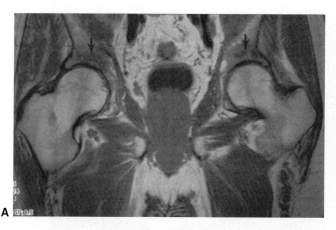
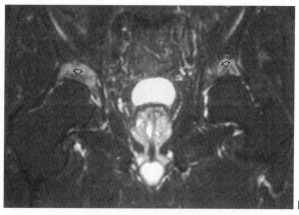

Figure 6-79 Bilateral acetabular insufficiency fractures. Coronal T1-weighted image **(A)** demonstrates low signal intensity in both acetabular regions (*arrows*). T2-weighted image **(B)** shows high signal intensity edema with fracture lines easily appreciated (*open arrows*).

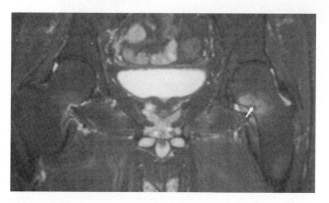

Figure 6-80 Fat-suppressed fast spin-echo T2-weighted coronal image demonstrates a medial insufficiency fracture with a fracture line (*arrow*) centrally.

arthrography is over 90% accurate for grading osteochondral lesions (23,58,200).

Soft Tissue Trauma

MRI is ideally suited for detection, classification, and therapy monitoring of acute and chronic soft tissue injuries (muscle, tendon, ligament, neurovascular structures) (56,180,196,204,214–221).

Muscle/Tendon Injuries

Muscle and tendon injuries in the pelvis and thighs are common in athletes and patients engaged in strenuous exercise programs. Injuries may also result from underlying disorders (renal failure, diabetes mellitus, connective tissue diseases, etc.) or patients on steroids (10,177,222). Differentiating muscle and tendon injury from an avulsion is important, as surgical intervention, especially for hamstring avulsions, may be indicated (200,223,224).

Classification of the type and extent of injury is useful for treatment planning and predicting rehabilitation time (10,225). A muscle contusion generally is due to a direct blow with a blunt object. The quadriceps and gluteal muscles

are most commonly involved (200). MR images demonstrate a poorly defined, feathery area of increased signal intensity on T2-weighted or STIR sequences (10,200). Grade 1 strains result in tearing of a few muscle/tendon fibers. Grade 2 strains involve about 50% of the fibers, and grade 3 strains are complete tears (10,200,225–227). T2-weighted sequences in two image planes (axial and coronal or sagittal) permit classification of the injury (10,225).

Hematomas are fluid collections that vary, though not entirely predictably, depending upon whether the injury is acute, subacute, or chronic. Acute hematomas are typically hypo- or isointense to muscle on T1- and T2-weighted sequences due to the presence of deoxyhemoglobin in intact red blood cells (10,200). Subacute hematomas have high intensity on T1-weighted sequences and inhomogeneous signal intensity on T2-weighted sequences due to methhemoglobin. Chronic hematomas develop a low intensity wall due to fibrous tissue and hemosiderin. Unfortunately, most hematomas have mixed signal intensity on both T1- and T2-weighted sequences by the time the injury is imaged (10,180,200).

Myositis ossificans is more accurately diagnosed with CT. Peripheral calcification or ossification is more easily appreciated compared to MR images. MRI may reveal an inhomogeneous central region with fluid–fluid levels in some cases. A low-intensity peripheral capsule can be seen with fibrous tissue or calcification on T2-weighted sequences (10).

Myotendenous injuries may involve the abdominal, gluteal, iliopsoas, adductor, or hamstring muscles (85,190,200,216,228).

The hamstring muscles (biceps femoris, semimembranosus, and semitendonosus) are most frequently injured in athletes (see Fig. 6-81) (203). The biceps femoris is most commonly involved. The semimembranosus may also be affected, but involvement of the semitendonosus is uncommon (223). Most injuries occur at the musculotendenous junction proximally. Koulouris and Connell (223) reported 16 avulsion injuries and five partial tears in 21 patients. Multiple muscles were involved in 33% of patients. Distal injuries occur in up to 40% of athletes (see Fig. 6-82).

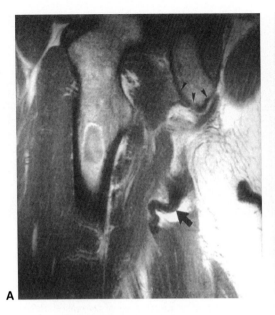
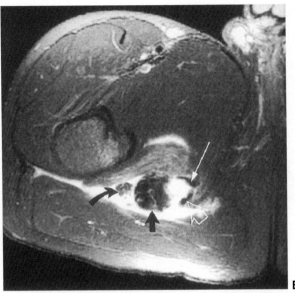

Figure 6-81 A 32-year-old football player developed severe pain in the ischial region while kicking. **A:** Oblique coronal MR image shows a ligamentous avulsion of the conjoined tendon (*black arrow*). The amount of retraction is evident. **B:** Axial image shows abnormal signal intensity due to edema and hemorrhage. The adjacent adductor magnus (*white arrow*) and semimembranosus tendons (*open arrow*) with the relationship of the muscles (*black arrow*) to the sciatic nerve (*curved arrow*) is demonstrated. (From Koulouris G, Connell D. Evaluation of the hamstring complex following acute injury. *Skeletal Radiol* 2003;32:582–589.)

Axial and sagittal or coronal MR images using T2-weighted or STIR sequences permit grading of the injury that is useful for treatment planning and predicting rehabilitation time (225).

Injuries to the adductor muscle group and gracilis (Table 6-2) are not uncommon in athletes, especially soccer players (see Fig. 6-83). Injuries may be acute or due to repetitive microtrauma (overuse). Most injuries occur near the anterior pubic attachment. Myotendonous or avulsion injury may occur. Osteitis pubis with bone marrow edema may also be evident (200,202). Patients typically present with acute or recurring groin pain (10,229).

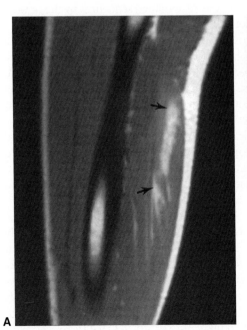
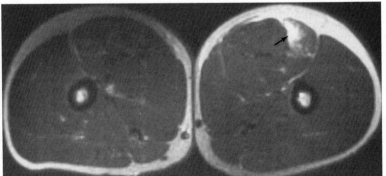

Figure 6-82 Sagittal **(A)** and axial **(B)** T2-weighted images of the thigh in a football player with hamstring hemorrhage (*arrows*) in the biceps femoris. There is no hematoma. The athlete returned to active participation in 6 weeks.

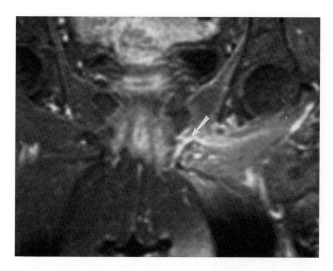

Figure 6-83 Fat–suppressed, T1-weighted, postcontrast coronal image of an adductor avulsion injury (*arrow*).

The disc of the pubic symphysis may extrude with disruption of the adductor attachment, gracilis, and rectus abdominus aponeurosis. Changes with region of the symphysis are most easily appreciated on coronal and axial T2-weighted or STIR images (10,200,202) (see Fig. 6-84).

Tears of the external oblique muscle may result in groin pain. An associated hernia (sportsman's hernia) is a common cause of chronic groin pain in athletes. The condition is more common in males than females (2.5:1) (200). MR images demonstrate muscle disruption with fat and/or bowel extruding through the defect. Axial T1- and T2-weighted images are most useful to confirm this diagnosis.

Gluteus medius and minimus tears are becoming recognized more frequently. These injuries may be difficult to diagnose clinically. Gluteal tears will be discussed

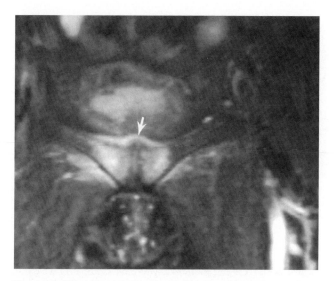

Figure 6-84 Coronal fast spin-echo T2-weighted image with fat-suppression demonstrates edema adjacent to the pubic symphysis with ligament swelling and edema (*arrow*) superiorly.

more completely later in this chapter along with greater trochanteric pain syndrome (200,222,228,230).

Increased signal intensity in muscles may also be evident after exercise or in patients with delayed onset muscle soreness (DOMS) (55,218,231). DOMS presents with pain in the involved muscles about 24 hours after exercise. Symptoms peak in 1 to 3 days and usually resolve in a week. MR image changes may persist several weeks after symptoms clear (218,231).

Compartment syndromes are more common in the lower leg (see Chapter 8). However, they have been reported in the thigh (232–234). Persistent pain and circulatory compromise occur due to increased intracompartmental pressure. If not properly diagnosed and treated, the changes may progress to myonecrosis and fibrous replacement (205,233,234). Exercise-induced rhabdomyolysis may also occur due to overuse (see Fig. 6-85). This process results from loss of cell membrane integrity that allows fluids to escape into the extracellular space. Enzyme levels (CK, IDH, GOT) are elevated (235). Early diagnosis and evaluation of the extent of involvement is important. This can be accomplished with radionuclide scans (236). However, T2-weighted or STIR images in the axial and sagittal or coronal planes more clearly defines the extent of muscle involvement (237). Sequelae of myonecrosis include renal failure, hyperkalemia, and hypocalcemia (235,236).

Piriformis Syndrome

Piriformis syndrome is a rare condition that may be due to entrapment of the sciatic nerve by an abnormal piriformis muscle or trauma (238,239). The piriformis arises from the anterior sacrum, the gluteal surface of the ilium, and extends to the superior border of the greater trochanter through the sciatic notch (38,238). The sciatic nerve most commonly passes adjacent to the muscle (90%), but in 10% of patients the nerve passes through the muscle (238).

An anomalous muscle or posttraumatic inflammation of the muscle and fascia may both result in compressive neuropathy of the sciatic nerve. Up to 6% of patients with low back pain or sciatica may actually have piriformis syndrome. The patient's symptoms are reproduced by digital pressure on the piriformis or lateral rectal wall on rectal or pelvic examination (238,239).

Antiinflammatory medication, physical therapy, steroid injection, and surgical release may be required for patients who do not respond to conservative treatment (238).

MRI is useful to exclude lumbar disc disease and may demonstrate signal abnormality in the muscle and nerve. T2-weighted or STIR sequences in the axial plane are most useful for detection of piriformis syndrome (see Fig. 6-86). We also add contrast-enhanced, fat-suppressed T1-weighted images in the axial and oblique coronal planes.

Greater Trochanteric Pain Syndrome

Greater trochanteric pain syndrome is a common disorder seen by rheumatologists, orthopedic surgeons, and sports

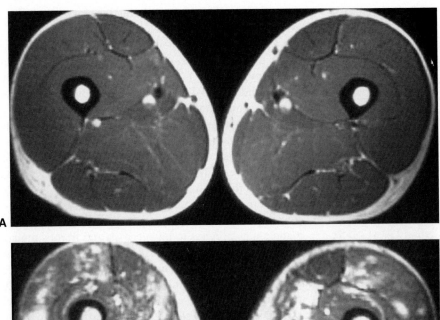

A

B

Figure 6-85 Rhabdomyolysis due to overuse in a bicycle racer. **A:** Axial T1-weighted image is normal. Axial T2-weighted image **(B)** at the same level shows diffuse edema and hemorrhage in both thighs, especially in the adductors and quadriceps muscle groups.

medicine and primary care physicians (228,240). The condition is common in middle-aged to elderly women, as well as runners and individuals engaged in step aerobics (204). Patients present with lateral hip pain and local tenderness over the greater trochanteric region (228,204). Pain is exacerbated by lying on the affected side and by climbing stairs (228). Differential diagnostic considerations include lumbar spine disorders, fibromyalgia, bursitis, arthritis, iliotibial band syndrome, and abductor tendonitis.

A brief review of the anatomy in the greater trochanteric region is useful to understand the pathology and imaging features of greater trochanteric pain syndrome. The greater

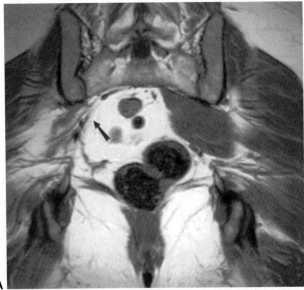

A

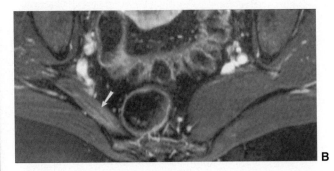

B

Figure 6-86 Chronic piriformis syndrome. Coronal T1-weighted image **(A)** demonstrates piriformis atrophy (*arrow*) on the right. Fat-suppressed fast spin-echo image **(B)** shows atrophy and inflammation (*arrow*).

trochanter has four facets: anterior, lateral, posterior, and superoposterior (228,38). The anterior facet (see Fig. 6-87) serves as the insertion site for the gluteus minimus tendon. This facet is most easily identified on axial MR images but also can be seen on sagittal and coronal images (45). The lateral facet serves as the attachment point for the gluteus medius tendon and is most easily identified on coronal MR images (Fig. 6-87D and E).

The posterior facet is covered by the trochanteric bursa. This facet is best seen on sagittal images (Fig. 6-87 A–C) (45,38). The superoposterior facet serves for insertion of the main tendon of the gluteus medius. This facet (Fig. 6-87 A–C) is most easily identified on sagittal MR images (45).

There are three bursae associated with the greater trochanter. The subgluteus maximus bursa is lateral to the greater trochanter and closely related to the gluteus medius insertion (Fig. 6-18A). The subgluteus medius bursa lies beneath the gluteus medius, posterior and superior to the

greater trochanter. The subgluteus minimus bursa is less frequently identified (minor bursa), and lies anteriorly deep to the gluteus minimus tendon and adjacent to the hip capsule. Communication with the joint can occur (38,45,228).

Pain may be related to bursal inflammation (see Fig. 6-88) or degeneration or tearing of the gluteus medius and/or minimus (see Figs. 6-89 and 6-90). This tendon complex is analogous to the rotator cuff, as much pathology is age-related. There is also a vascular watershed region in the tendon complex similar to the rotator cuff (222). Osteophytes may be visible on the greater trochanter in up to 50% of patients (222). Calcifications in the tendon or bursae may also be evident radiographically (228). Osteophytes may result in impingement. Bursitis is also frequently evident with gluteal tendon tears (204,222,228). MR images should be performed using a small FOV (18cm) and T2-weighted images in axial, coronal, and sagittal planes.

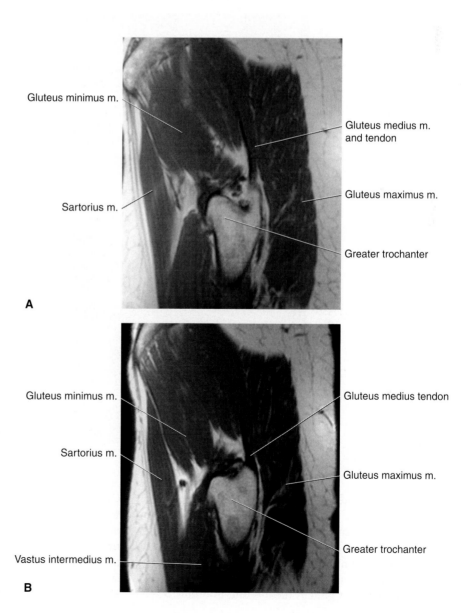

Figure 6-87 Greater trochanteric anatomy. Sagittal images **(A-C)** of the greater trochanter from medial to lateral and coronal images **(D,E)** demonstrating myotendinous anatomy.

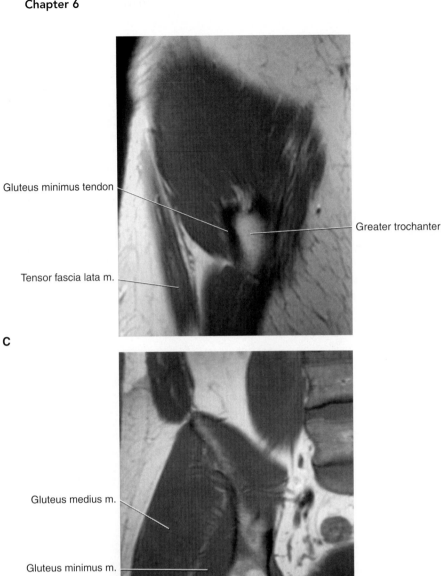

Gluteus minimus tendon

Greater trochanter

Tensor fascia lata m.

C

Gluteus medius m.

Gluteus minimus m.

Greater trochanter

Piriformis m. and tendon

D

Figure 6-87 (continued)

Contrast enhancement may be useful for subtle tendon pathology and to confirm synovial inflammation (45,200,228). Bursal distention is evident in 85% of patients with greater trochanteric pain syndrome compared to 30% of asymptomatic patients (228).

A recent article evaluated the features and accuracy of MRI for detection of gluteus medius and minimus tears.

Cvtanic et al. (240) described increased signal intensity superior to the greater trochanter, tendon elongation, tendon discontinuity, and increased signal lateral to the greater trochanter or T2-weighted sequences (Figs. 6-89 and 6-90). MR accuracy was 91%. A region of increased signal intensity superior to the greater trochanter had the highest sensitivity (73%) and specificity (95%) for muscle tears.

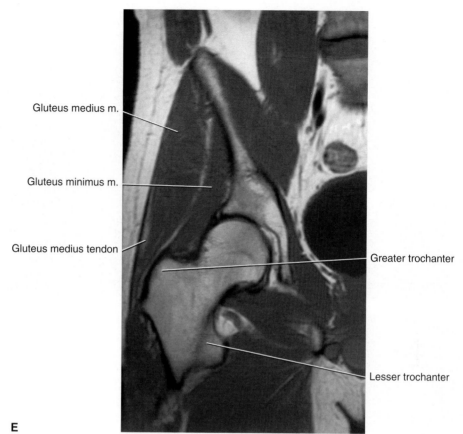

Gluteus medius m.

Gluteus minimus m.

Gluteus medius tendon

Greater trochanter

Lesser trochanter

Figure 6-87   *(continued)*   **E**

Atrophy of the gluteal muscles may also be evident. This can easily be evaluated by comparison with the unaffected hip (240).

Treatment of greater trochanteric pain syndrome consists of steroid injections, physical therapy, and ultrasound therapy (222,228,230).

Morel-Lavallée Lesions

Morel-Lavallée lesions result from abrupt separation of skin and subcutaneous tissues from the underlying fascia. Lesions are particularly common in the greater trochanteric region and the thigh (241).

The vascular plexus passes through the fascia in these regions. When disrupted, blood, lymphatic fluid, and debris form. Mellado et al. (241) described MR features of this condition. Lesions were oval to fusiform and located adjacent to the fascia of the greater trochanter or upper thigh. Fluid signal intensity varied, but was typically low on T1-weighted signals and high on T2-weighted sequences. A thin, fibrous or hemosiderin-laden capsule was identified (see Fig. 6-91). Differential diagnosis should include fat necrosis and hematoma. Lesions may enlarge and become painful. Surgical resection may be required in this setting (241).

Bursitis

There are 20 bursae located about the hip. Bursae are lined with synovial membrane and typically form in areas with tendon friction (47). The trochanteric bursae were discussed in the prior section. The other two significant bursae are the iliopsoas and ischiogluteal bursae (45,200,228). Ischiogluteal bursitis is often related to direct trauma to the ischial region. Iliopsoas bursitis may occur with chronic friction of the iliopsoas tendon (200). However, iliopsoas bursitis is commonly associated with osteoarthritis (56%), rheumatoid arthritis, pigmented villonodular synovitis, AVN, gout, infection, and following total hip arthroplasty (242,56).

The iliopsoas bursa lies between the hip capsule and the musculotendinous junction of the iliopsoas. The bursa extends from the marginal ligament inferiorly to the level of the lesser trochanter. It is bordered medially by the femoral vessels and laterally by the femoral nerve (Fig. 6-33) (56,242). The bursa communicates with the hip joint in 15% to 20% of symptomatic patients (242). The iliopsoas bursa can be imaged using bursography, ultrasound, CT, and MRI (41). However, T2-weighted axial and sagittal or coronal MR images are most useful to identify the communication and extent of the bursa (56). Contrast enhancement is generally not required to exclude other pathology.

Robinson et al. (47) recently described MR image features of the obturator externus bursa. Though described as a bursa, some may consider it a recess. The bursa is located contiguous to the joint capsule along the obiturator externus (Fig. 6-32). Ten patients demonstrated communication

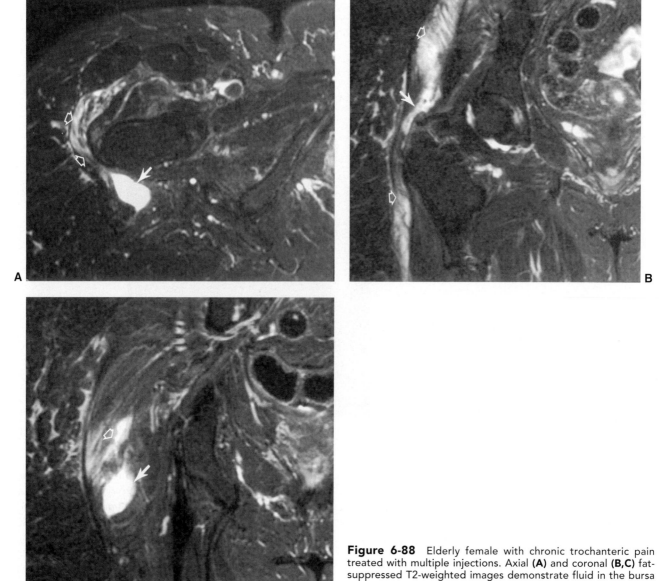

Figure 6-88 Elderly female with chronic trochanteric pain treated with multiple injections. Axial **(A)** and coronal **(B,C)** fat-suppressed T2-weighted images demonstrate fluid in the bursa (*arrow*) and increased signal intensity about the bursa (*open arrows*) due to multiple recent injections.

with the hip joint in all cases. All patients had underlying conditions similar to those with iliopsoas bursitis (47). Axial and sagittal T2-weighted images define the extent of the bursa.

Snapping Hip

Snapping hip is an audible click or snap that occurs with flexion and extension. Extraarticular snapping may be due to the iliotibial band, the anterior gluteus maximus as it moves over the greater trochanter, or the iliopsoas tendon as it crosses the iliopectineal eminence or lateral femoral head (see Fig. 6-92) (243). Intraarticular causes such as loose bodies, lateral tears, and osteochondral fractures may also cause snapping (10,45).

Confirming iliopsoas snapping may be accomplished with tenography and motion studies as ultrasound (146,244).

Sufficient motion cannot be achieved with MR in most cases. Therefore, MRI is most useful to identify inflammation of the tendons or iliotibial band and to exclude intraarticular pathology (see Fig. 6-93).

Articular injuries can also be defined with MRI. However, a small FOV and surface coil techniques are essential to define subtle labral and osteochondral lesions. In most cases intraarticular contrast is required to clearly define the capsule, cartilage, and labral anatomy (24,167,245–247). Conventional MR images may be useful in some cases (see Fig. 6-94). However, MR arthrography is usually preferred (23,24,31).

MR arthrographic techniques have been described by several authors (20,24,26,27,31,172,248,249). When articular lesions are suspected, a closely coupled coil, small FOV (Fig. 6-79), and intraarticular contrast provide optimal image quality (Table 6-1) (24,27,31,247).

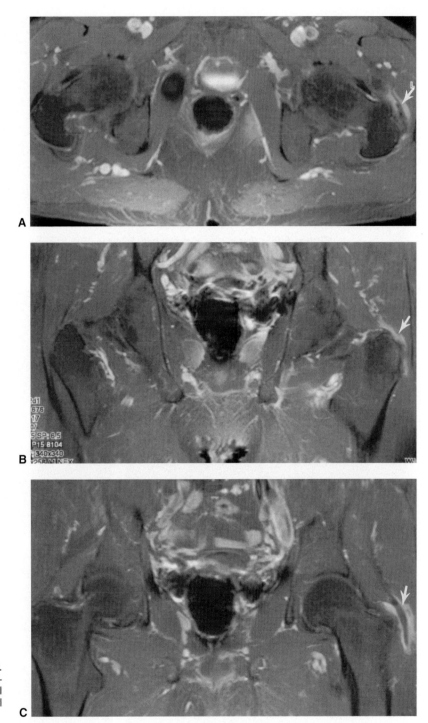

Figure 6-89 Gluteus medius tendon tear. Axial **(A)** and coronal **(B,C)** fast spin-echo T2-weighted images demonstrate increased signal about the tendon (*arrows*) due to a partial attachment tear.

MR arthrographic technique for the hip was discussed briefly in the introductory technique section, but it deserves more in-depth review. The patient is supine on the fluoroscopic table, and the area over the involved hip is prepared using sterile techniques. Prior to injection of superficial local anesthetic, the femoral vessels are palpated. An area over the lateral aspect of the femoral neck is typically selected for approaching the joint. A small (5 cc) syringe with local anesthetic is used to determine the injection site fluoroscopically. The superficial soft tissues are injected with local anesthetic.

A 20-gauge spinal needle is used to enter the hip with a direct vertical or slightly oblique approach so that the joint is entered near the lateral junction of the femoral head and neck. Most institutions confirm the intraarticular needle placement by fluid aspiration or injection of a small amount of iodinated contrast medium (20,25,27). After needle position is confirmed, 8 to 12 mL of contrast [0.1 mL gadopentetate dimeglumine (Magnevist, Berlex Laboratories, Wayne, NJ) diluted in 25 mL of normal saline] is injected. We use a slightly different approach, as a solution of 50% iodinated

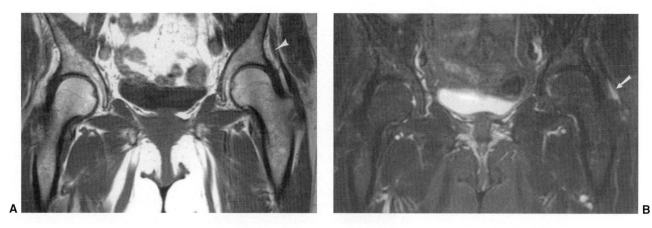

Figure 6-90 Partial tear of the gluteus minimus with atrophy. Coronal T1-weighted **(A)** and fast spin-echo T2-weighted **(B)** images demonstrate increased signal intensity in the distal minimus tendon (*arrow*) with muscle atrophy (*arrowhead*).

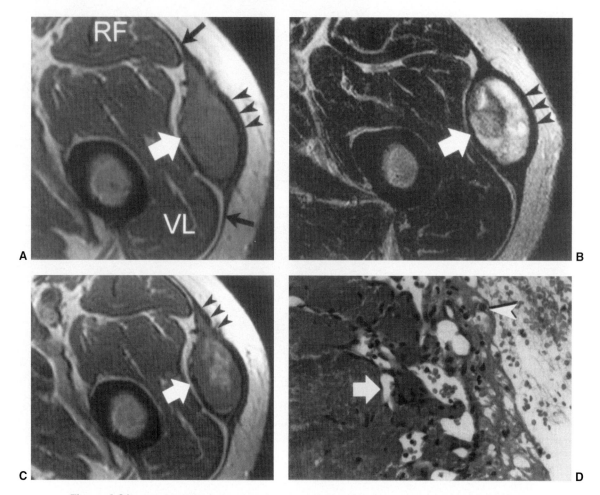

Figure 6-91 Morel-Lavallée lesion. Sixty-five-year-old male with history of a motorcycle accident 34 years earlier. **A:** Axial T1-weighted image shows a longstanding Morel-Lavallée lesion (*white arrow*) in deep subcutaneous tissues adjacent to the fascia lata (*black arrows*) and vastus lateralis (VL) and rectus femoris (RF) muscles in the proximal thigh. The lesion is mildly hyperintense related to muscle and surrounded by a thick hypointense capsule. **B:** Axial T2-weighted images show heterogeneous hyperintensity in the lession (*arrow*) and a thick hypointense capsule (*arrowheads*). Axial contrast enhanced image **(C)** reveals patchy internal enhancement (*arrow*). The anterior aspect of the capsule (*arrowheads*) also shows mild enhancement. **D:** Photomicrograph of the specimen shows abundant fibrin, areas of recent hemorrhage, aggregates of organizing thrombus, newly formed capillaries (*arrow*), and inflammatory infiltrate with hemosiderin laden histiocytes (*arrowhead*). (From Mellado JM, Perez del Palomar L, Diaz L, et al. Long-standing Morel-Lavallée lesions in the trochanteric region and proximal thigh. MRI features in five patients. *AJR Am J Roentgenol* 2004;182:1289–1294.)

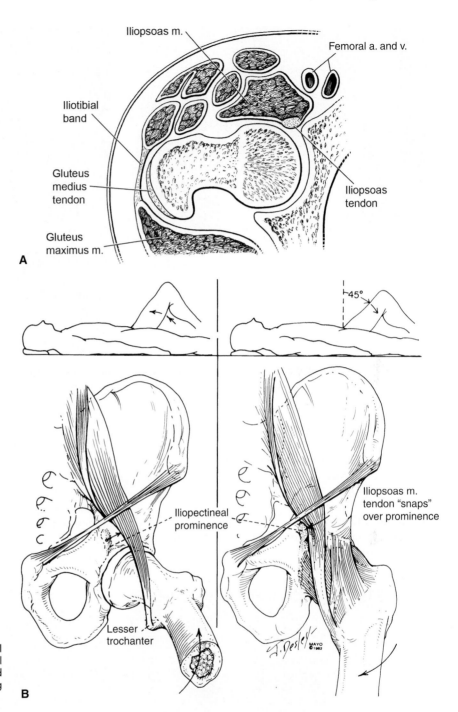

Figure 6-92 A: Illustration of the normal relationships of the iliopsoas and iliotibial band to the neurovascular structures and greater trochanter. **B:** Illustration of snapping iliopsoas tendon in flexion and extension.

contrast medium and 50% Marcaine is used to dilute the 0.1 mL of gadolinium. The exact amount injected is monitored by pressure and patient tolerance and will vary with capsule size (10,27). The patient is moved to the MR gantry and placed supine with a phased-array coil (i.e., shoulder or other closely coupled coil) positioned on the involved hip. Patient comfort may be improved by placing a bolster under the knees. Some prefer internal rotation of the hips and others have used leg traction to optimize labral visualization (178,250). The latter may result in motion artifact, so we do not use this approach.

Images are obtained using an 18-cm FOV and 256 × 256 matrix (Table 6-1). Several image sequences and planes have been suggested for optimal evaluation of the labrum. The oblique orientation of the labrum would suggest that oblique coronal, oblique sagittal or three-dimensional imaging would be optimal. Some authors simply perform sagittal, axial, and coronal images with fat-suppressed, T1-weighted images (20,24,25,26,27,31,249).

Plötz et al. (247) compared radial images taken at 10° increments to conventional image planes including axial and coronal obliques. Sensitivity improved from 60% with

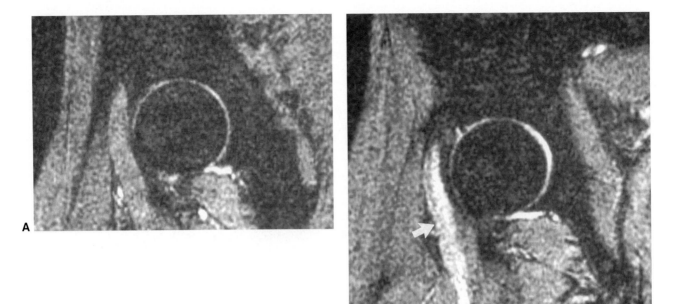

Figure 6-93 Iliopsoas inflammation due to snapping tendon syndrome. Sagittal gradient-echo images of the normal **(A)** and abnormal **(B)** high signal intensity inflammed iliopsoas (*arrow*).

conventional planes to 80% with radial images. Specificity was 100% for both, while accuracy improved from 70% to 85% with radial images.

Acetabular Labral Tears

The normal acetabular labrum is of low signal intensity and is triangular in configuration (see Figs. 6-94 and 6-95)

(35,251). The labrum attaches to the acetabular margin anteriorly, superiorly, and posteriorly. Its inferior position merges into the transverse ligament. Inferiorly, the labrum may be separated from the transverse ligament, which should not be confused with a labral tear (20,26). The labrum is generally thinner anteriorly and thicker posteriorly (Fig. 6-95) (20).

The labrum has minimal vascularity. The most vascular regions (anterior, inferior, posterior) are also the most

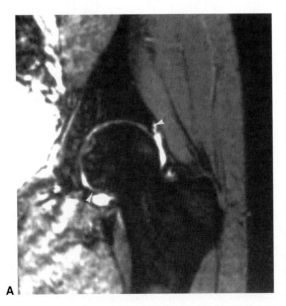

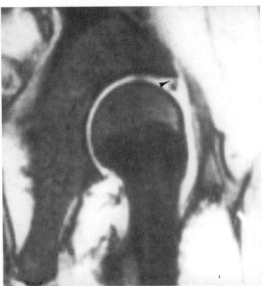

Figure 6-94 Acetabular labral tear. Radial GRIL [gradient-recalled steady state (GRASS), interleaved] images show normal **(A)** superior and inferior labrum (*arrowheads*) with high signal intensity joint fluid. The labrum in side **(B)** is partially separated superiorly (*arrowhead*).

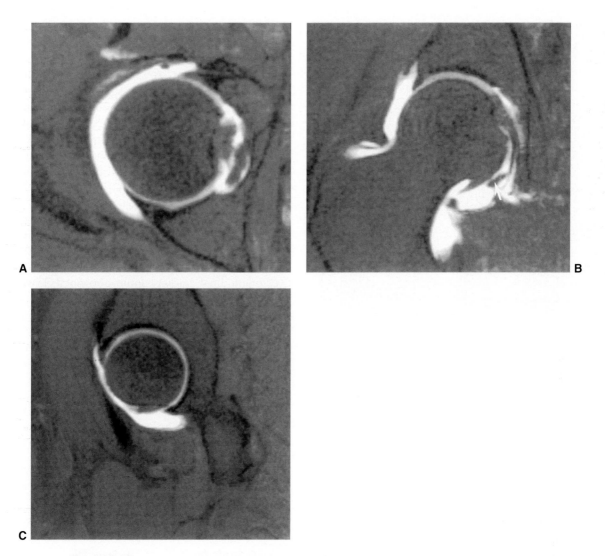

Figure 6-95 Axial **(A)**, coronal **(B)**, and sagittal **(C)** MR arthrographic images demonstrating the normal triangular appearance of the acetabular labrum. The transverse ligament (*arrow*) is seen on coronal image **B.**

common sites for injury and subjected to the greatest mechanical stress (23,40,252).

There have been multiple studies evaluating labral variations in children and asymptomatic adults (24,39,164,253). In children younger than 11 years of age, the anterior superior labrum is triangular with linear intersubstance increased signal intensity. The midsuperior labrum is triangular and low intensity. The posterosuperior labrum is flat. In children 12 to 13 years of age, the appearance is similar but the area of increased signal intensity in the anterior superior labrum is less frequently identified (164). The size of the labrum is larger though acetabular coverage is less in children as compared to adults (164,253).

Aydürgöz and Ózürk (39) evaluated 360 labra in 180 asymptomatic patients. The patients were evaluated in five different age groups (10 to 19, 20 to 29, 30 to 39, 40 to 49, 50+ years). There were differences in labral appearance between hips in 15% of patients. Size differences were evident in 25%. As expected, changes in shape and internal

signal intensity varied with age. The incidence of increased signal intensity in the labrum was 18% for women and 32% for men age 10 to 19 years. This increased slightly in the 20-to-29-year age group. Over age 30, increased signal intensity was evident in 37% of women and 50% of men, and in volunteers over 50 years of age, increased signal intensity was evident in 55% of women and 90% of men (Fig. 6-95) (39).

The labrum was triangular in 69%, round in 16%, flat in 12.5%, and absent in 2.5% (39). Though most consider absence abnormal, others have reported absence in 10% to 14% (5,6,20,26,27,45,245,248).

As with the menisci in the knee, appearance of the acetabular labrum has been defined and classified based upon changes in shape and signal intensity (24–26,31,172). Czerny et al. (31) classified labral lesions based upon MR arthrographic features including shape and acetabular attachment (see Fig. 6-96). Normal labra (Fig. 6-94A) are triangular with low signal intensity, and the labral recess is clearly visible. Stage IA labra have increased signal intensity

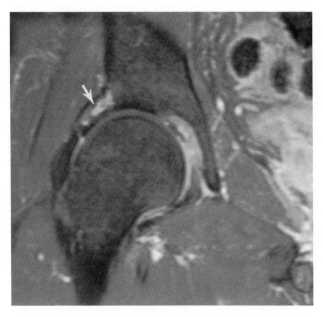

Figure 6-96 Coronal fat-suppressed, fast spin-echo, T2-weighted image in an elderly man demonstrating increased signal intensity and superior labral degeneration.

that does not communicate with the articular surface, and the recess is visible (see Fig. 6-97B). Stage IB labra are thickened (Fig. 6-97B) and the recess is not seen. Stage IIA labral lesions show contrast extending into the articular surface, but the recess is visible. Stage IIB lesions are similar, but the recess is no longer evident (see Fig. 6-97C). Stage IIIA lesions demonstrate labral detachment, but the normal triangular shape is maintained (see Fig. 6-97D). Stage IIIB lesions show

detachment with thickened labra with abnormal signal intensity, and the recess is no longer evident (Fig. 6-97D) (31,25). Using these criteria, the sensitivity of MR arthrography was 91%, specificity 71%, and accuracy 88% (31).

Most labral tears occur in the superior and anterior quadrants (25,27,31,249). Findings should be correlated with clinical symptoms (pain, snapping or clicking, and locking). Certain features such as thickening, central degeneration (Fig. 6-96), marginal irregularity, and absent labra may also be seen in asymptomatic patients. Up to 28% of asymptomatic patients may have abnormalities in labral morphology (20,26,27).

Labral pathology may include detachment or substance tears similar to the menisci of the knee (see Fig. 6-98). Detachment is more common than a labral tear (27). Tears have configurations not unlike the knee (radial, degenerative, longitudinal, bucket handle, horizontal cleavage, etc). Tears are identified by intersubstance contrast on MR arthrograms. Contrast passes between the acetabulum and labrum in case of labral detachment. Displacement may be evident, as well (27). Degeneration may result in labral enlargement and/or increased labral size (Figs. 6-96 and 6-98A). An absent anterosuperior labrum with a small superior remnant may be a normal variant. Absence of the labrum in any other region is considered abnormal (27). It is not unusual to note associated cartilage abnormalities in the femoral head, again similar to findings with meniscal tears in the knee (see Fig. 6-99) (20,26,27,40).

Articular Cartilage Lesions

Cartilage lesions involving the femoral head and acetabulum should be carefully evaluated on MR arthrograms. Acetabular

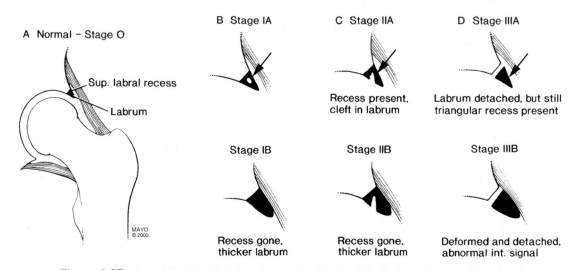

Figure 6-97 Acetabular labral injuries. Czerny classification (31). **A:** Stage 0: normal low signal intensity triangular labrum with normal superior labral recess. **B:** Stage IA: increased signal that does not communicate with the articular surface. The recess (*arrow*) is preserved. Stage IB: Labrum thickened and superior recess no longer visible. **C:** Stage IIA: There is a cleft in labrum communicating with articular surface. The recess (*arrow*) is preserved. Stage IIB: Thickened labrum with cleft and recess not visible. **D:** Stage IIIA: Labrum detached but still triangular. Recess (*arrow*) is preserved. Stage IIIB: Labrum detached and thickened with abnormal internal signal intensity. Recess not visible. (From Czerny C, Hofmann S, Neuhold A, et al. Lesions of the acetabular labrum: accuracy of MR imaging and MR arthrography in detection and staging. *Radiology* 1999;220:225–230.)

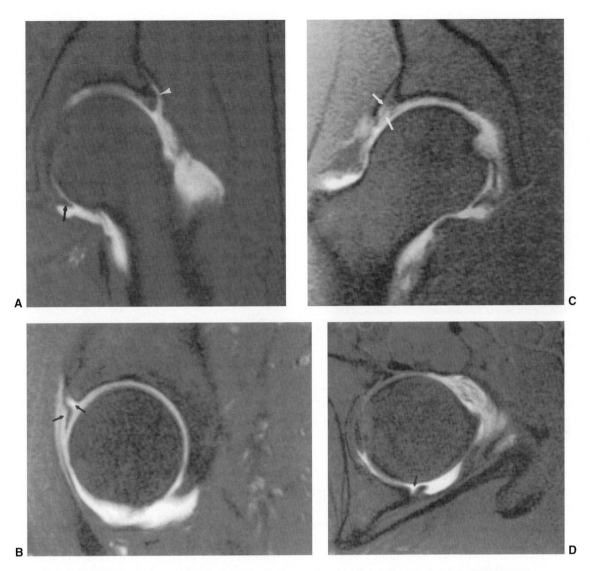

Figure 6-98 Acetabular labral tears. MR arthrogram images demonstrating **(A)** a thickened superior labrum with recess (*arrowhead*) still visible. The inferior labrum (*arrow*) is normal. **B:** Deformed partially detached superior labrum (*arrows*). **C:** Advanced degenerative tear (*arrows*). **D:** Tear and partial detachment posteriorly (*arrow*).

cartilage lesions are most common in the anterior superior acetabulum. Changes are usually related to labral pathology or femoroacetabular impingement (see Fig. 6-99) (23,254). Lesions are often associated with and likely follow labral tears. Impingement is related to anatomic variation in the femoral head and neck, including decreased femoral anteversion, head–neck offset, and shallower tape between the femoral head and neck (254).

Paralabral Cysts

Labral tears and, more commonly detachments, are also associated with labral cysts (see Figs. 6-100 and 6-101) (24,26,27). Labral cysts are usually located in the superior region anteriorly or posteriorly (252). There is an increased incidence of labral cysts in patients with developmental hip

dysplasia. Cysts may cause acetabular bone erosion. This radiographic finding should suggest labral pathology as the possible etiology for hip pain (20,27). Sciatic nerve compression by paralabral cysts has also been reported (251). Cysts are well-defined (see Fig. 6-102) but may be septated or lobulated (Figs. 6-100 and 6-101). Signal intensity is low on T1-weighted and high on T2-weighted sequences (10,27,251,255). Rim enhancement occurs on postcontrast fat-suppressed, T1-weighted images (251).

Neoplasms

MRI examinations of the pelvic region are frequently requested to evaluate patients with suspected musculoskeletal neoplasms. Metastatic disease is common in this location (256,257). Chapter 12 discusses musculoskeletal neoplasms

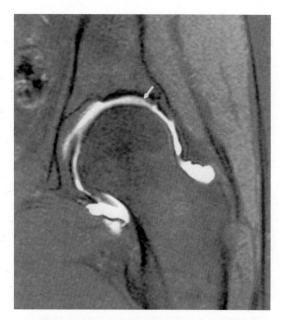

Figure 6-99 Coronal MR arthrogram shows cartilage loss beginning at the labral base (*arrow*).

more fully; however, certain neoplasms and imaging considerations in the pelvis deserve mention. Table 6-12 summarizes common skeletal and soft tissue neoplasms in the pelvic region (256–258).

Soft Tissue Masses

The appearance of soft tissue lesions does not differ significantly according to location. Benign lesions tend to be homogeneous and well-marginated and do not cause neurovascular encasement (see Chapter 12). Exceptions are hemangiomas and desmoids that have more inhomogeneous signal intensity and irregular margins (10,260). Lesions

TABLE 6-12

BONE AND SOFT TISSUE NEOPLASMS ABOUT THE PELVIS, HIPS, AND UPPER THIGH

Bone Tumors

Metastasis	
Malignant primary	#/11,087 cases
Chondrosarcoma	293
Osteosarcoma	251
Lymphoma	146
Chordoma	133
Ewings	131
Myeloma	114
Fibrosarcoma	54
Postradiation sarcoma	25
Benign	
Osteochondroma	115
Osteoid osteoma	80
Giant cell tumor	67
Chondroma	23
Chondroblastoma	19
Soft Tissue Tumors	
Liposarcoma	130
Desmoids	67
Alveolar sarcoma	42
Synovial sarcoma	22
Epithelioid sarcoma	22

From Berquist TH. *MRI of the musculoskeletal system*, 4th ed. New York: Lippincott Williams & Wilkins, 2001; Unni KK. *Dahlin's bone tumors. General aspects and data on 11,087 cases*, 5th ed. Philadelphia, PA: Lippincott–Raven, 1996; and Weiss SW, Goldblum JR. *Enzinger and Weiss soft tissue tumors*, 4th ed. St. Louis, MO: Mosby, 2001.

that become necrotic can also cause confusion. Synovial sarcomas may also appear well-defined and cystic and may be confused with a more benign process. This is an important factor to consider due to their significant incidence about the

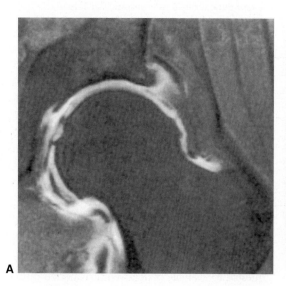

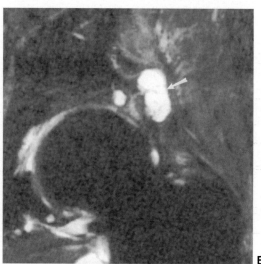

Figure 6-100 Coronal images from MR arthrogram images demonstrating a degenerative labral tear (**A**) and and associated ganglion cyst (**B**) (*arrow*).

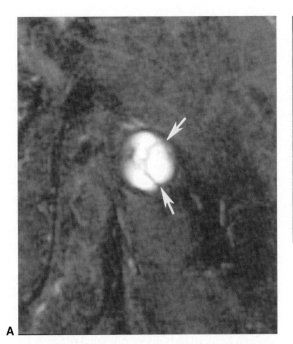

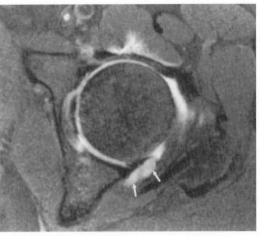

Figure 6-101   Coronal **(A)** and axial **(B)** arthrogram images demonstrating a large septated para-labral cyst (*arrows*).

pelvis (42,157,260). As a rule, malignant soft tissue masses are inhomogeneous, have irregular margins, and more often encase neurovascular structures (10).

An enlarged iliopsoas bursa (Fig. 6-33) can be confused with neoplasm clinically. These lesions are often palpable and can be symptomatic. CT and arthrography can be used for diagnosis. Communication with the hip joint is common. T2-weighted MR images clearly demonstrate the nature of the lesion as communication with the joint can be demonstrated. This is most easily evaluated in the axial plane. Lesions also have homogeneous high signal intensity with well-defined margins, which is typical of a periarticular cyst.

There are numerous bursae about the hip. Therefore, this diagnosis is more common than ganglion cysts. Ganglion cysts are typically small, deep, and nonpalpable.

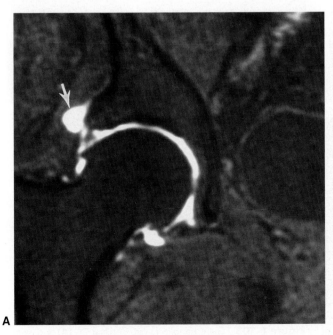

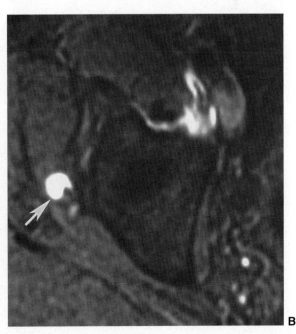

Figure 6-102   Coronal **(A)** and axial **(B)** MR arthrogram images demonstrating a smooth septated paralabral cyst (*arrow*) in a patient with a labral tear.

However, ganglia may be large, septated, and palpable or intrapelvic (145,261). As noted earlier, paralabral cysts are commonly associated with labral tears and hip dysplasia (177). Ganglia in the hip, though considered less common, are not unlike those described in the hand, wrist, knee, and foot (261). The etiology is unclear, but ganglia may develop due to an outpouching of the capsule, a developmental synovial remnant, or connective tissue weakness (145). Synovial cysts have a similar appearance and are related to joint pathology leading to synovial outpouching. This finding is typically seen in patients with rheumatoid arthritis, gout, infection, and degenerative arthritis (145).

MR features are similar to those of bursae in that they are well-defined with or without septations. Lesions are low intensity on T1-weighted images, high intensity on T2-weighted images, and rim enhancement occurs on contrast-enhanced images (see Fig. 6-103) (10,145,261).

Lipomas are not uncommon in the pelvis, hips, and thighs. Lipoma arborescens is a rare condition with extensive proliferation of synovium and subsynovial fat. This lesion is typically seen in the knee, but can occur in the hip (262). Characteristic fat signal intensity makes the diagnosis obvious.

Liposarcomas have areas of signal irregularity when low grade (see Fig. 6-104). High-grade lipomas may have very little fat signal (10). These lesions are common in the pelvis and thighs (Table 6-12) (257).

Osseous Neoplasms

Soft tissue neoplasms are more easily characterized than skeletal tumors. The marrow pattern in the pelvis and upper femurs is often inhomogeneous due to the trabecular pattern and variations in fatty and hemopoietic marrow (see Chapter 14) (52,58,61,99,256,263). Metastasis (see Fig. 6-105) and myeloma (see Fig. 6-106) are common in the pelvis and hips (259).

When evaluating skeletal neoplasms it is imperative to have routine radiographs for comparison. Radiographs are useful for characterizing the lesions. Blastic lesions (Fig. 6-38) may be confused with other conditions such as benign bone islands. Paget disease (see Fig. 6-107) can also

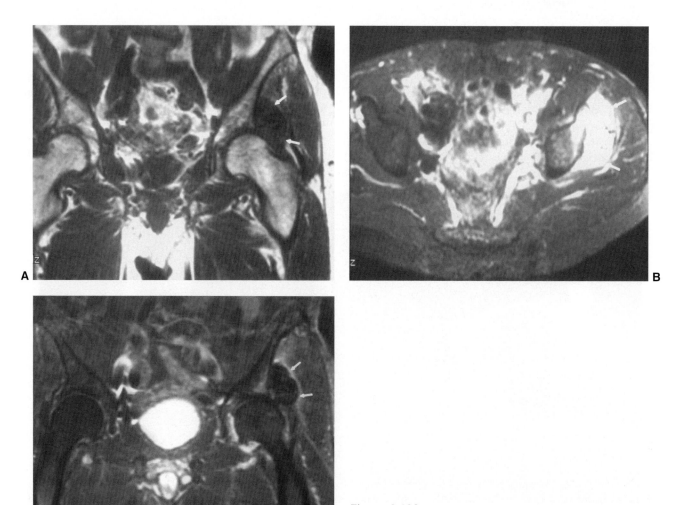

Figure 6-103 Giant ganglion cyst. Coronal T1- **(A)** and axial T2-weighted **(B)** images demonstrate a large ganglion cyst. Postcontrast image **(C)** shows peripheral enhancement (*arrows*).

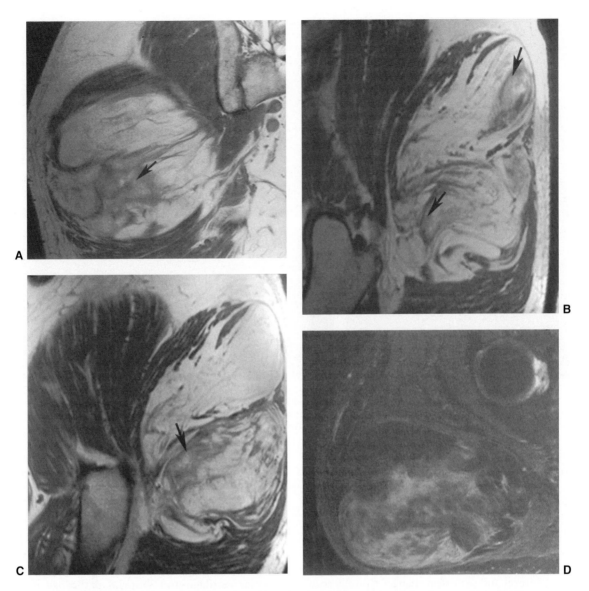

Figure 6-104 Low-grade liposarcoma. There is a large fatty mass with focal areas of low signal intensity (*arrows*) seen on T1-weighted coronal **(A)** and sagittal **(B,C)** images. Axial T2-weighted image **(D)** shows areas of high signal intensity with fat suppressed.

cause confusion if radiographs are not available to compare with MR images (10). MRI is generally reserved for staging suspected malignancy and evaluating the extent of lymphoma or other infiltrative processes (Fig. 6-106) (10,259,264). Generally, T1- and T2-weighted sequences are used to define the extent and nature of lesions in marrow and cortical bone. However, especially in the pelvis, STIR images may be very useful to evaluate subtle changes in bone marrow, cortical bone, and soft tissues (9,201,260). We also routinely add contrast-enhanced, fat-suppressed T1-weighted sequences.

Sundarum et al. (265) described the utility of T1-weighted images alone in detecting malignant degeneration of Paget disease (see Chapter 15). Malignant degeneration occurs in about 1% of patients with Paget disease. Radiographic comparison is imperative. Lytic areas or osteolysis is common in

early Paget disease, but less frequently seen with advanced disease. If a lytic area on radiographs shows fatty marrow on T1-weighted images, biopsy is not indicated. Low signal intensity in lytic regions on radiographs is a good indicator of malignant degeneration (265).

Because of the difficulty in diagnosis and often-confusing MR features, it is important to discuss osteoid osteoma in this section as well as Chapter 12.

Osteoid osteomas account for 11% of benign bone tumors (259,266,267). The lesion is more common in males (M:F, 2:1 to 3:1) and 90% occur in patients younger than 30 years of age (266,267). Though lesions can be medullary, cortical, or periosteal, in the femoral neck they are more often medullary or parosteal (266). The clinical features can be as confusing as the imaging findings, especially with intracapsular osteoid osteomas. Pain is not

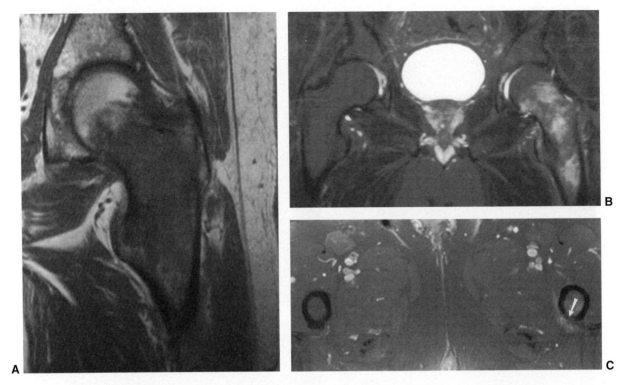

Figure 6-105 Lung metastasis. Coronal T1- **(A)** and T2-weighted **(B)** images demonstrate a large area of abnormal signal intensity in the proximal left femur. Axial T2-weighted image **(C)** demonstrates cortical destruction (*arrow*) and soft tissue extension.

always typical and response to aspirin or naprosin is not as clear-cut compared to extracapsular osteoid osteomas. Also, pain may be referred to the knee, adding to the confusing clinical picture (266,267).

Image features can also be difficult to interpret. Osteopenia and joint space widening may be evident on routine radiographs, suggesting infection. Joint space widening is due to the effusion and reactive synovitis created by the lesion (268). Cortical and periosteal changes typically seen with extracapsular lesions are not usually seen with intracapsular lesions (266).

MR image features may cause confusion. The frequent dramatic bone (see Fig. 6-108) and soft tissue changes may be easily mistaken for a more aggressive lesion. The typical nidus seen with osteoid osteoma can be evident with extracapsular lesions (see Fig. 6-109) in the pelvis and hips; however, the nidus may be overlooked because of the narrow edema or soft tissue changes. Though MR image features are more readily appreciated today, we find thin-section CT guided by radiographic or radionuclide image findings to be still effective (13,48). CT sections of 2 mm or less should be performed to avoid missing subtle intracapsular lesions (see Fig. 6-110).

Arthropathies

A more complex discussion of the role of MRI in evaluating arthropathies can be found in Chapter 15. However, there are several conditions including osteoarthritis and synovial chondromatosis that deserve mention in this chapter. Osteoarthritis is most often evaluated with routine radiography. Occasionally, CT or arthrography is required to evaluate subtle articular changes and exclude other causes of hip pain (2,10,139). The role of MRI for evaluation of articular cartilage and synovial changes has increased with new pulse sequences, radial imaging, and MR arthrography (10,110,134,142,159,190,269–271). The ability to evaluate articular cartilage and synovial pathology is useful in patients with early rheumatoid arthritis and osteoarthritis (10,20,26,27,271). Intravenous and intraarticular contrast have provide effective evaluation of subtle changes in the synovium and articular cartilage (25).

Li et al. (272) correlated MRI, radiographic, and functional factors in ten patients with osteoarthritis. The correlations are useful in understanding the role of MRI in evaluating patients with osteoarthritis. Table 6-13 demonstrates that MRI features compare favorably with patients' symptoms in the early stages of disease but do not provide much utility in more advanced stages (see Fig. 6-111). Bone marrow edema may correlate with symptoms and radiographic staging (272).

Anterior impingement of the femoral head–neck junction on the anterior acetabulum is recognized as an early cause of osteoarthritis in active young patients. Patients have a "pistol grip" appearance of the femoral head–neck junction on radiographs. MR images have also demonstrated reduced femoral anteversion and head–neck offset (57).

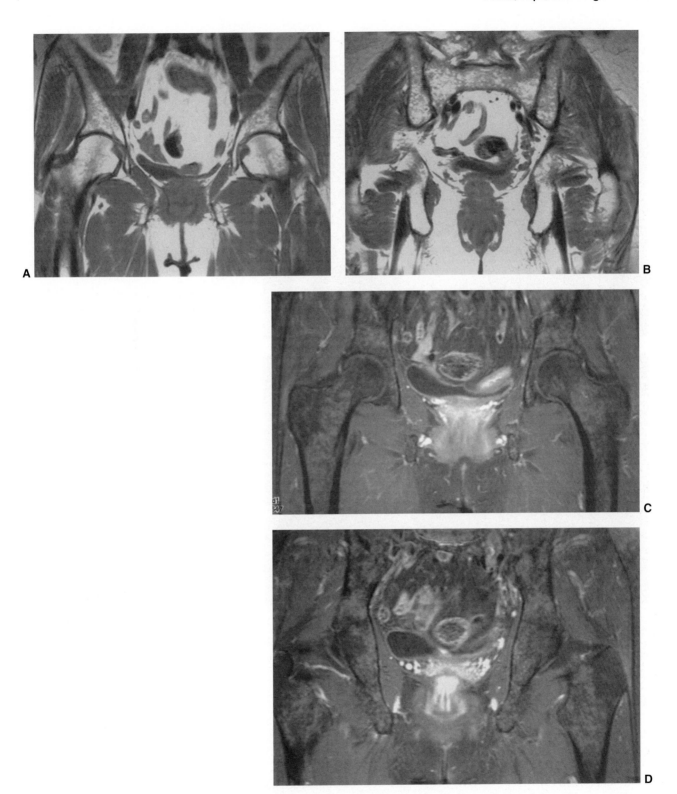

Figure 6-106 Multiple myeloma. Coronal T1-weighted images **(A,B)** demonstrate diffuse small areas of low signal intensity. Coronal T2-weighted images **(C,D)** show high signal intensity in these regions.

Symptoms are reproduced on physical examination by internal rotation and 90° of hip flexion. MR images demonstrate changes described above on conventional images with loss of articular cartilage in the anterior acetabulum on MR arthrograms (10,57).

Synovial chondromatosis or osteochondromatosis results from metaplasia of the synovium (43,70). The condition is uncommon but frequently involves the hip. Patients present with hip pain and reduced motion. Patients may present over a wide range of ages, but most

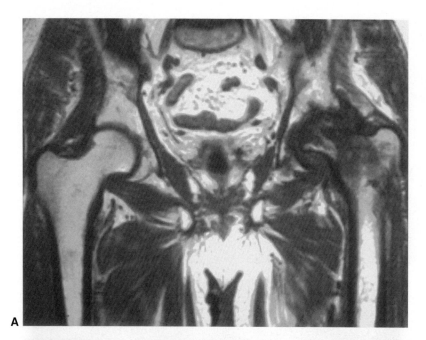

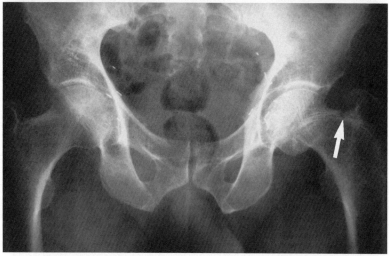

Figure 6-107 Coronal T2-weighted image **(A)** demonstrates abnormal signal intensity in the left femoral head and neck. Could this be neoplasm? AP radiograph **(B)** demonstrates Paget disease with a fracture superiorly (*arrow*).

often the diagnosis is made in the 40s and 50s. Men are affected two to four times more frequently than females (273). Radiographs may be normal initially. However, as the condition progresses, osteopenia, bone erosion, and calcified or ossified densities may be detected (see Fig. 6-112). The appearance differs from advanced degenerative arthritis with large osteochondral fragments, though over time, degenerative changes do occur (70,273). Extracapsular extension may occur along the iliopsoas and obturator externus fat planes (43).

MR features of synovial chondromatosis are now more clearly defined. In the earliest stages, small irregularities in the synovium may be the only finding (see Fig. 6-113). This finding may be evident on T2-weighted images in the presence of significant joint effusion. MR arthrography is more accurate at this stage.

In later phases, intraarticular loose bodies become more obvious. In addition, synovial thickening (87%),

bone erosion (73%), and extracapsular cysts (40%) may be evident (273).

Infection

MRI is a sensitive technique for early detection of osteomyelitis (see Fig. 6-114), joint space infection, and for differentiating osseous from soft tissue infection (274–277). MRI is particularly useful in detecting early infection in children. Recent studies also indicate MRI may be useful for differentiating infection from transient synovitis of the hip (275). Lee et al. (275) evaluated joint effusions, synovial changes, and marrow signal intensity in patients with infection and transient synovitis. Significant joint effusions and pericapsular signal intensity changes may be seen in both conditions. The most useful MR feature is marrow abnormalities (low signal intensity on T1-weighted, and increased intensity on T2-weighted or contrast-enhanced

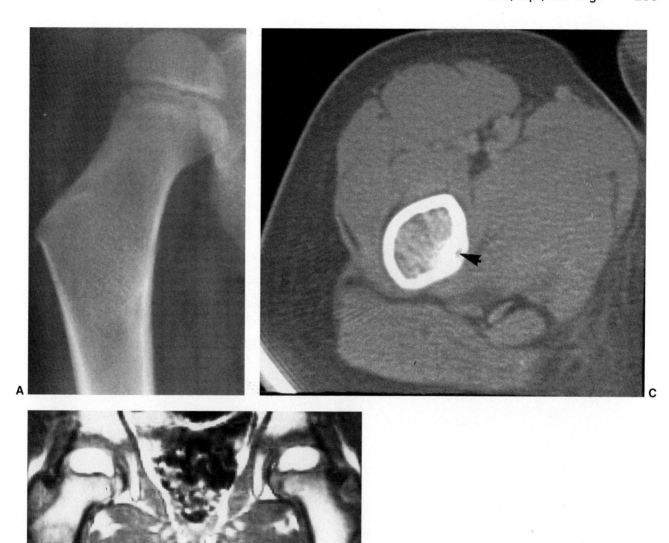

Figure 6-108 **A:** Anteroposterior radiograph of the upper femur is normal. No lytic or blastic lesions are identified. **B:** Coronal SE 500/20 image shows a large area of low signal intensity (*arrow*) in the upper right femur. This is nonspecific and could be edema secondary to infection, tumor, or a stress fracture. **C:** CT scan demonstrates cortical thickening with a lucent nidus (*arrowhead*) typical of osteoid osteoma.

images) in the femoral head. This finding was present on patients with infection, but in none of the patients with transient synovitis of the hip (275) (see Chapter 13).

Hip Arthroplasty

Evaluation of potential complications such as infection, loosening, and osteolysis has been accomplished using serial radiographs, arthrography and radionuclide studies including PET imaging. CT has also proved to be useful for evaluating periprosthetic bone and soft tissue changes (50).

To date, MRI has only been used in selected situations due to problems with metal artifact and cost. However, modification of MR parameters can reduce artifact, specifically about the femoral component, adding to the value of MR imaging for evaluating complications of hip arthroplasty (49,50,278). Early studies demonstrated that artifact was reduced with low field (<0.2 T) images. Also, T1-weighted (SE 500/10) and intermediate (SE 1,000/60) sequences minimize metal artifact about the femoral component. Artifact is more significant about the acetabular component or when wires or screws are in place (9,10,279).

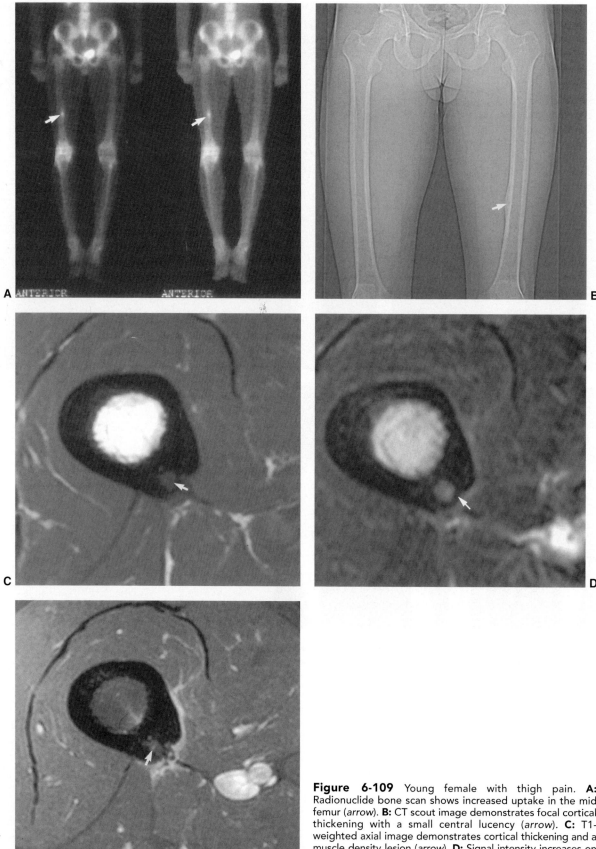

Figure 6-109 Young female with thigh pain. **A:** Radionuclide bone scan shows increased uptake in the mid femur (*arrow*). **B:** CT scout image demonstrates focal cortical thickening with a small central lucency (*arrow*). **C:** T1-weighted axial image demonstrates cortical thickening and a muscle density lesion (*arrow*). **D:** Signal intensity increases on the T2-weighted image (*arrow*). **E:** Contrast enhanced image shows a small central vessel (*arrow*) and periosteal enhancement.

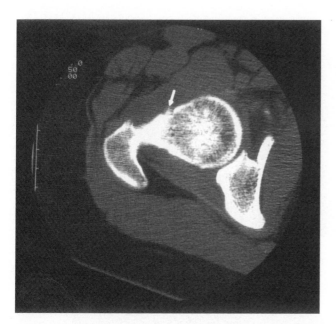

Figure 6-110 Thin-section CT demonstrating an intracapsular osteoid osteoma (*arrow*).

Recent experience with modification of multiple MR parameters has resulted in increased utility of MRI for evaluating patients with hip arthroplasty regardless of the suspected abnormality in the adjacent tissues (278,279).

Artifacts associated with metal implants (see Chapter 3) include geometric distortion of signal intensity in the frequency encoding direction (misregistration), section thickness variation, increased signal intensity loss, and increased dephasing with gradient echo-imaging (279).

MR imaging parameters can be modified (Table 6-14) to minimize artifact and signal voids and increase tissue resolution. Thus far, imaging in the coronal plane along the femoral component is useful for evaluating loosening and areas of osteolysis (279). Soft tissue abnormalities such as enlarged bursae and soft tissue abscesses, and abductor muscle avulsions and heterotopic ossification can also be demonstrated by MRI (65,278).

Pulse sequences should include fast STIR (3,000/40/100, echo train 6, 5-mm sections, 32 kHz bandwidth, 256 × 160 matrix and 4 acquisitions, frequency encoding parallel to femoral component), T1-weighted (340/15, 5-mm sections, 16 kHz bandwidth, 256 × 224 matrix and 3 acquisitions) and postcontrast T1-weighted images. Coronal and axial image planes are most useful (see Fig. 6-115) (278,279).

PEDIATRIC DISORDERS

Routine radiographs, computed tomography, radionuclide scans, arthrography, ultrasound and magnetic resonance imaging all play a role in evaluation of disorders of the pelvis and hips in children (10,35,84,167,280–282). This section will review common applications for magnetic resonance

TABLE 6-13
OSTEOARTHRITIS RADIOGRAPHIC AND MRI STAGES

Grade	Radiographic Staging	MRI Staging (Coronal Images)
0	Normal	Normal
1	? joint space narrowing and subtle osteophytes	Inhomogeneous high signal intensity in cartilage (T2WI)
2	Definite joint space narrowing, osteophytes and sclerosis, especially in acetabular region	Inhomogeneity with areas of high signal intensity in articular cartilage (T2WI); indistinct trabeculae or signal intensity loss in femoral head and neck (T1WI)
3	Marked joint space narrowing, osteophytes, cyst formation, and deformity of femoral head	Criteria of stage 1 and 2 plus indistinct zone between femoral head and acetabulum; subchondral signal loss (both T1WI and T2WI) due to bone sclerosis
4	Gross loss of joint space with above features plus large osteophytes and increased deformity of the femoral head and acetabulum	Above criteria plus deformity of femoral head

T2WI, T2-weighted image; T1WI, T1-weighted image.
From Li KCP, Higgs J, Aisen AM, et al. MRI in osteoarthritis of the hip: gradation of severity. *Mag Res Imag* 1988;6:229–236.

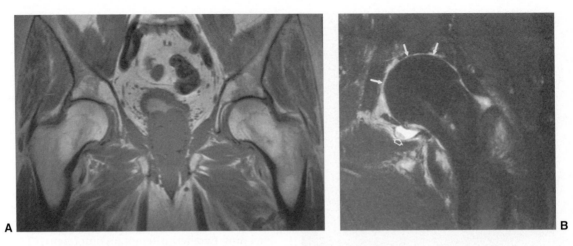

Figure 6-111   Osteoarthritis. **A:** Coronal T1-weighted image demonstrates uniform joint space narrowing in both hips with no subchondral cysts or marrow edema. **B:** Small field of view, fat-suppressed, T2-weighted image shows marked loss of cartilage (*arrows*) and a loose body (*open arrow*).

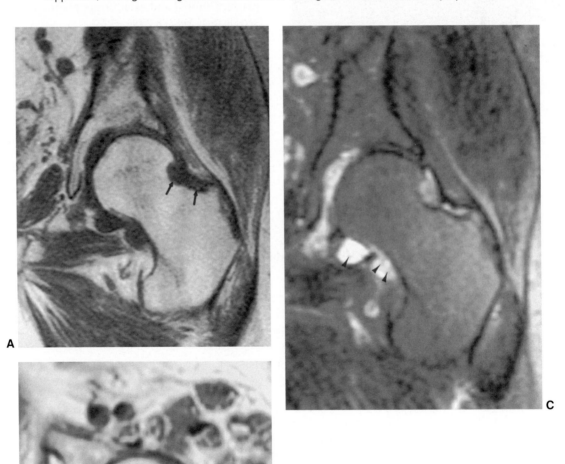

Figure 6-112   Synovial chondromatosis. Coronal **(A)** and axial **(B)** T1-weighted images demonstrate a joint effusion with bone erosions (*arrows*). Coronal T2-weighted image **(C)** demonstrates the effusion and faint low signal intensity chondromas (*arrowheads*).

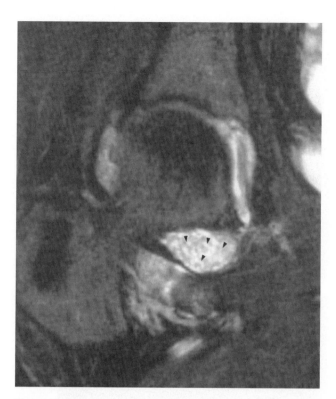

Figure 6-113 Coronal T2-weighted image shows multiple low signal intensity bodies in the joint fluid.

imaging studies in children. Though anatomy and technique were discussed in the earlier sections of this chapter, certain specific features deserve review as they relate to infants and children.

Technique

Sedation and patient monitoring may be required in infants and young children. These methods were reviewed in Chapter 3 and will not be repeated here. Additional approaches to the examination include the type of MR unit desired, whether motion or positioning studies will be required and whether intravenous or intraarticular contrast are indicated (19,283,284). The initial decision must also include whether a screening examination of both hips is needed or higher detail images of one hip would be preferred. A routine screening examination may be accomplished with coronal T1- and axial T2-weighted spin-echo or fast spin-echo sequences. The field of view should be selected based upon patient size but should include the pelvis and femurs to just below the lesser trochanters. The head coil may be used for infants and smaller children (35).

When higher detail is required, the hip should be studied with a surface coil and smaller FOV (8 to 16 cm) should be used (10,16). T1-weighted and T2-weighted images may once again provide adequate information for detection of bone, joint, and soft tissue abnormalities. Fast scan techniques may be preferred in children depending upon their level of cooperation. Three-dimensional

TABLE 6-14	
METAL ARTIFACT REDUCTION TECHNIQUES	
Technique	**Comments**
↑ frequency encoding	↓ misregistration
Gradient strength	Artifact
Selective orientation of frequency and phase encoding direction	Improves tissue resolution near implant
Implant oriented longitudinally in magnetic field	↓ misregistration artifact
Fast spin-echo sequences	↑ signal intensity in tissue near implant
↓ Voxel size	↓ signal voids
High bandwidth/pixel	↓ artifact
Frequency encoding along axis of prosthesis	↓ artifact
Lower field strength	↓ artifact

From Twair A, Ryan M, O'Connell M, et al. MRI of failed total hip replacement caused by abductor muscle avulsion. *AJR Am J Roentgenol* 2003;181:1547–1550; and White LM, Kim JD, Mehta M, et al. Complications of total hip arthroplasty: MR imaging—initial experience. *Radiology* 2000;215:254–262.

gradient-echo techniques are useful for fine detail or when reformatting may be indicated (10,35). T2-weighted fat-suppressed fast spin-echo techniques are useful for evaluation of articular cartilage. Intravenous contrast may be useful to evaluate early ischemic or synovial changes (10,283). However, in children we attempt to minimize the invasiveness of studies when possible.

Anatomy

The ossified and developing skeleton is clearly demonstrated with MRI. Changes in signal intensity due to fat, cartilage, and red marrow are readily apparent. Soft tissue anatomy and the ligaments, labrum, and supporting structures of the hip are also easily identified (see Fig. 6-116). Radiographs demonstrate only the ossified portions of the immature skeleton (285).

Bone formation on the pelvis and hips results in signal intensities quite different from the adult hip. The metaphysis and diaphyses are composed of red marrow during the early years. This has low signal intensity on T1-weighted MR images (Fig. 6-116A). The cartilage model of the epiphyses is intermediate signal intensity. As ossification evolves the epiphyseal marrow, which is fatty and has high signal intensity on T1-weighted images (Fig 6-116C). The signal is low on T2-weighted or fat-suppressed images (10).

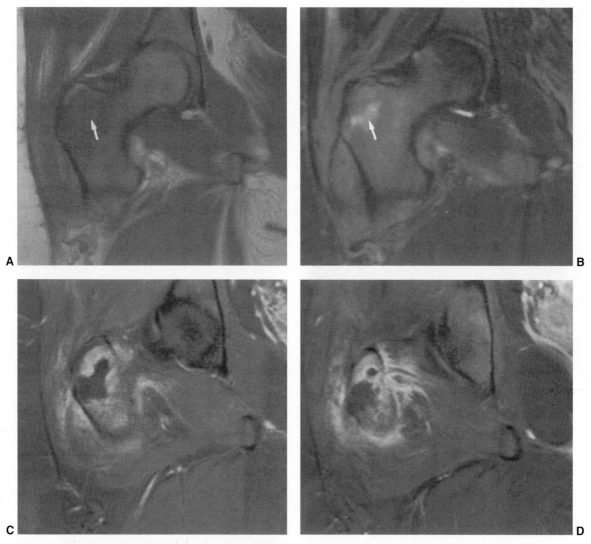

A

B

C

D

Figure 6-114 Greater trochanteric abcess. Coronal T1- **(A)** and T2-weighted **(B)** images demonstrate abnormal signal intensity in the greater trochanter (*arrow*). Contrast-enhanced images **(C,D)** show peripheral enhancement and soft tissue inflammation due to a bone abscess.

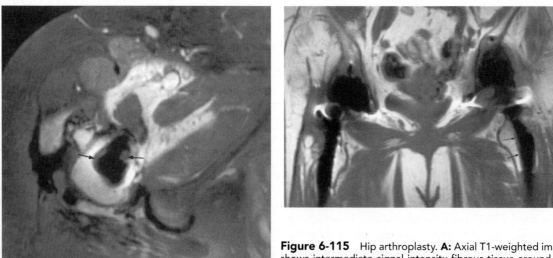

A

B

Figure 6-115 Hip arthroplasty. **A:** Axial T1-weighted image shows intermediate signal intensity fibrous tissue around the component (*arrows*). Similar findings (*arrows*) are noted on the coronal image **(B)** in a different patient.

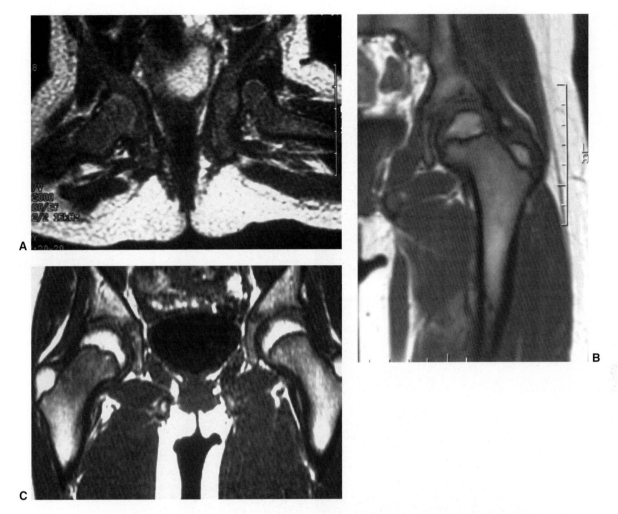

Figure 6-116 Pelvis and hips in infant and child. **A:** Infant with developmental hip dysplasia on the *left*. The low signal intensity is due to red marrow. **B:** T1-weighted image in a young child with developing ossification centers with fat signal intensity in the epiphyses. **C:** Adolescent with fatty marrow in the femoral leads and greater trochanter.

Legg-Calvé-Perthes Disease

Legg-Calvé-Perthes disease is an ischemic disease of the femoral head seen most commonly in males between the ages of 3 and 12 years. Patients present most commonly between 5 and 8 years of age. The condition can be bilateral (15%), though findings are generally asymmetrical in this setting (35,42,129,286,287). Patients typically present with pain and a Trendelenberg gait, though pain symptoms may be confusing or referred to the knee.

Unlike adult avascular necrosis, the femoral head generally remodels with variable deformity and secondary joint incongruency (see Fig. 6-117) (129). Early diagnosis is essential to minimize deformity, reduce degenerative hip disease, and maintain normal articular relationships (19,288). Routine radiographs are normal for 6 to 8 weeks. Radiographic features vary depending upon the stage of the disease (devascularization, subchondral collapse, fragmentation, reossification). Sclerosis of the epiphysis, join space incongruency, fragmentation, and flattening of

the femoral head may be evident (289,290). Radionuclide scans and MR images are positive earlier than when seen in radiographs. MRI also provides significant advantages over bone scans in demonstrating the osseous and articular anatomy (5,133,140,284,291,292).

Several classification systems have been developed to assist in evaluating prognoses and management of Legg-Calvé-Perthes disease. Catterall (293) classified the extent of disease based upon the extent of femoral head involvement on routine anteroposterior radiographs (see Fig. 6-118). Group I patients have ≤25% of the femoral head involved, group II 25% to 50%, group III 50% to 75%, and group IV 100% (293,294). Herring classified Legg-Calvé-Perthes disease based on the radiographic height of the femoral head or epiphysis. Group A patients maintained normal height (100%), group B 50% of normal height, and group C less than 50% of the normal height (294,295).

MR features may appear more advanced compared to radiographs. Hochbergs et al. (174,294,296) devised an MR system based upon two central and two peripheral

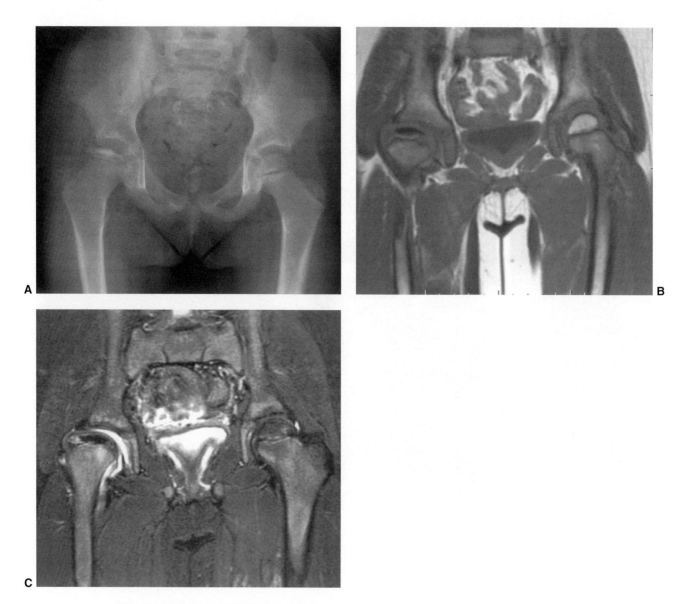

Figure 6-117   Legg-Calve-Perthes disease. **A:** Anteroposterior radiograph demonstrates sclerosis and deformity of the right femoral epiphysis. Coronal T1- **(B),** and T2-weighted **(C)** images show marked deformity of the femoral head with an effusion, lateral subluxation, and areas of necrosis and deformity in the epiphysis.

zones in the femoral head (see Fig. 6-119). These features correlate with radiographic extend. With more severe disease, the peripheral zones are involved. The peripheral regions are also the sites of initial revascularization, which can be evaluated with contrast enhanced T1-weighted images (174,283,294,296).

Conservative therapy is preferred when possible. However, surgical intervention may be required. Conventional arthrography is useful to evaluate seating of the femoral head in the acetabulum, joint congruency, and the extent of femoral head deformity. These factors are important when surgery is a consideration. Static MR images are effective for evaluating deformity of the femoral head (19). However, different positions (external rotation, abduction,

etc.) are important to evaluate more accurately congruency and containment of the femoral head within the acetabulum. Jaramello et al. (283) used an open magnetic to compare positioned MR images to arthrography. Results were equal when trying to define these three parameters (femoral head, congruency, and joint containment). MR arthrography has not been used frequently in young children.

MR imaging may also be useful to follow the healing and remodeling process. Contrast-enhanced T1-weighted images provide information regarding revascularization and femoral head deformity. Because of cost, most cases can be followed with radiographs and clinical correlation. Therefore, MRI is used selectively.

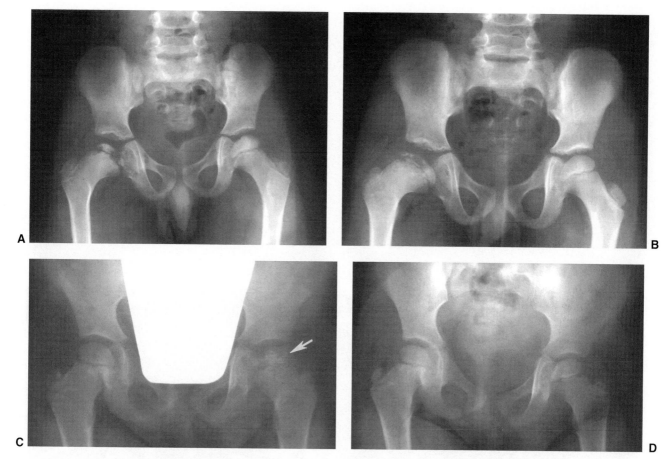

Figure 6-118   Radiographs at different stages of Legg-Calvé-Perthes disease. **A,B:** Flattening and fragmentation of the femoral head with widening of the femoral neck **A** with reossification 1 year later **B. C,D:** Fragmentation and sclerosis of the epiphysis on the left (*arrow* in **C**). Reossification is seen six months later **D.**

Developmental Hip Dysplasia

Developmental hip dysplasia (DHD) classically affects first-born white males. Though etiology is controversial,

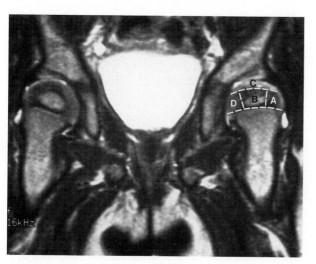

Figure 6-119   MR in a patient with Legg-Calvé-Perthes disease demonstrating the four zone classification of Hochbergs. Zones *C* and *B* are central, and *A* and *D* peripheral.

the condition is related to joint laxity that may be anatomic, hormonal, or due to intrauterine position (129,141,285,292,297,298). Ninety-eight percent result from *in utero* alterations during the last 4 weeks of pregnancy (132). Most subluxations become evident in the first 2 to 4 weeks after birth (170,192,280). Early detection and reduction by 4 years of age can result in normal development in up to 95% of cases (170,192,299).

Radiographic localization of the femoral head is difficult in early stages, as ossification may not be evident until 6 months after birth (see Fig. 6-120). Acetabular changes in developmental hip dysplasia occur late (129). Ultrasound is available and can be more easily performed on infants than MRI (132,250). MRI is expensive, infants must be sedated, and positioning can be difficult unless an open-bore system is used (see Fig. 6-121).

MRI or MR arthrography can identify the unossified femoral head and acetabular structures including the labrum. Complications such as ischemic necrosis can also be readily identified (see Fig. 6-122) (300,297). However, in most cases, clinical, radiographic, and ultrasound features are most commonly used for diagnoses and follow-up (129).

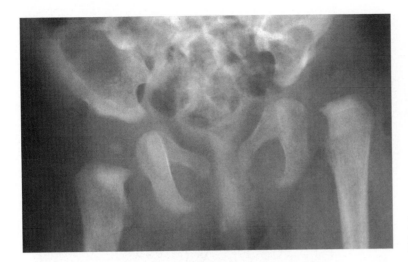

Figure 6-120 Developmental hip dysplasia on the *left*. There is minimal ossification of the right femoral head.

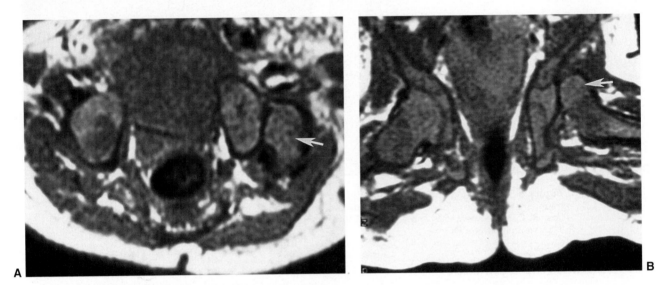

Figure 6-121 Developmental hip dysplasia (DHD) in an infant. MR images with the legs abducted and externally rotated in the axial **(A)** and coronal **(B)** planes demonstrate DHD on the *left* with the femoral head dislocated superiorly (*arrow*).

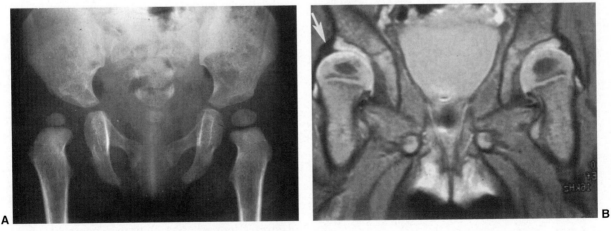

Figure 6-122 Developmental hip dysplasia. **A:** Anteroposterior radiograph demonstrates a dysplastic right hip. After treatment, the coronal proton density MR image **(B)** clearly demonstrates the position of the femoral head and labral coverage. There is still slight medial joint space widening.

Slipped Capital Femoral Epiphysis

Slipped capital femoral epiphysis is the most common hip disorder in adolescence. It is also a frequent cause of early osteoarthritis (138). Men are affected more commonly than women. Ages for men range from 10 to 17 years (most common at 13 to 14 years of age), and women 8 to 15 years (most common at 11 to 12 years of age) (138). The condition is bilateral in 23% to 81% of patients. If one hip is involved, the contralateral hip most often is affected within the first 2 years of diagnosis (12,138,301).

Patients present with pain and a limp. Hip pain is evident in 50%; however, symptoms may be referred to the knee in a significant number of cases resulting in missed or delayed diagnosis in 26% (12,138).

Slipped capital femoral epiphysis can be staged based upon clinical and radiographic criteria. Clinically, patients may be considered pre-slip, acute, or chronic. During the pre-slip phase, clinical symptoms (weakness, thigh or knee pain) may obscure the diagnosis. There is generally mild widening of the physis on radiographs, but an actual slip is not apparent (see Fig. 6-123) (138). Once the slip occurs, it can be categorized as mild, moderate, or severe, depending upon the degree of displacement (138).

MRI is useful to detect early physeal changes and to evaluate changes in the contralateral hip. Coronal and oblique sagittal T1- and T2-weighted images should be

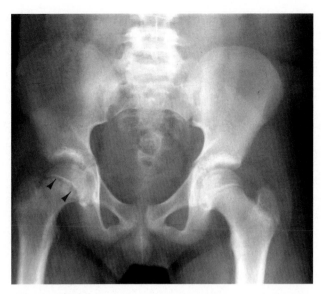

Figure 6-123 Anteroposterior radiograph of the pelvis shows physeal irregularity on the *right* (*arrowheads*) without slip.

obtained (see Fig. 6-124) (12). Fast spin-echo T2-weighted sequences have replaced conventional spin-echo techniques. Physeal changes on T1-weighted sequences demonstrate low signal irregularity and widening of the physis. Signal intensity is increased on T2-weighted images, and joint effusions

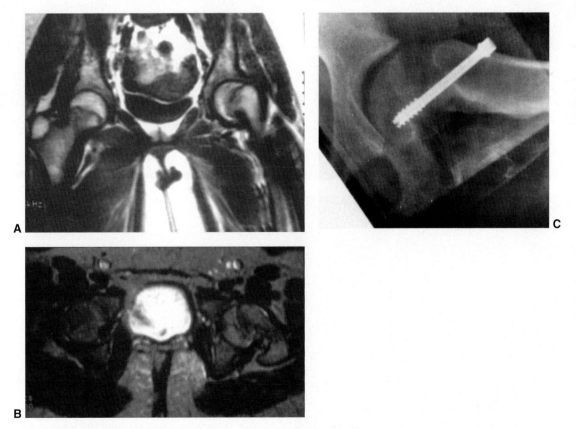

Figure 6-124 Coronal T1- **(A)** and axial T2-weighted **(B)** MR images of a slipped capital femoral epiphysis on the left. There is significant displacement and irregularity of the physis. **C:** Oblique radiograph after pinning.

are commonly demonstrated. The degree of slippage can be easily assessed. Both hips should be evaluated, as bilateral changes are common even if only one hip is symptomatic (12,94,138).

The involved hip is treated with pinning. Postoperatively, MRI is useful to evaluate physeal closure and complications such as AVN (12).

Rotational Deformities

Rotational deformities are due to torsion of the distal femur relative to the proximal femur. These deformities are seen in patients with neuromuscular disorders, Legg-Calvé-Perthes disease, developmental hip dysplasia, and idiopathic excessive antetorsion (111,129,157,302,303). Treatment of rotational deformities includes femoral neck osteotomy, which requires accurate measurements of the degree of

deformity prior to planning the surgical approach and degree of correction required (302).

Radiographic measurements have been performed using multiple modalities including routine radiographs, CT, ultrasound, and MRI (171,302–304). To date, CT has been the gold standard. However, MRI can also be used and offers several advantages over CT (171,302). Axial images can be obtained in the true plane of the femoral neck (see Fig. 6-125) and in infants and young children, the unossified cartilage is easily demonstrated, so measurements can be accurately obtained (302).

MR measurements can be easily obtained using T1-weighted images. A coronal scout serves to select oblique and axial images to measure the α angle (Fig. 6-125B). This angle is the angle formed by a line through the central axis of the femoral neck and the horizontal. A second angle, the β angle is measured on axial images through the distal femoral

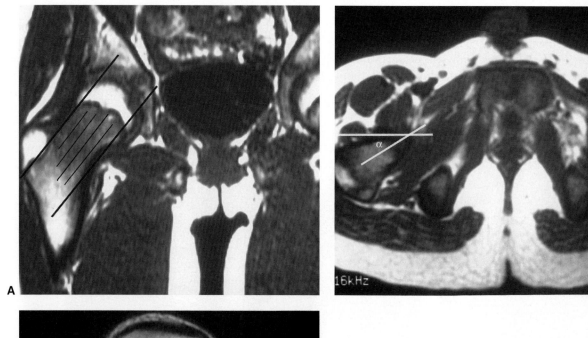

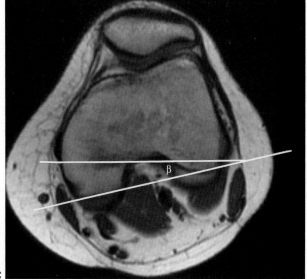

Figure 6-125 MR images demonstrating methods for measuring femoral anteversion. **A:** Coronal image with oblique planes selected to optimize visualization of the femoral neck (lines). **B:** Axial image demonstrating the alpha (α) angle (horizontal line and femoral neck). **C:** Axial image of the knee demonstrating the beta angle (β) formed by the orientation of the condyles to the horizontal reference.

condyles (Fig. 6-125C). The degree of rotational deformity is the difference between the β and α angles. Both legs are measured for comparison (171,302).

REFERENCES

1. Beltran J, Herman LJ, Burk JM, et al. Femoral head avascular necrosis: MR imaging and clinical-pathologic and radionuclide correlation. *Radiology* 1988;166:215–220.
2. Berquist TH, Coventry MB. The pelvis and hips. In: Berquist TH, ed. *Imaging of orthopedic trauma*, 2nd ed. New York: Raven Press, 1992:207–310.
3. Bieber E, Hungerford D, Leunox DW. Factors in the diagnosis of avascular necrosis of the femoral head. *Adv Orthop Surg* 1985; 147:221–226.
4. Hayes CB, Balbissoon AA. Magnetic resonance imaging of the musculoskeletal system: II. The hip. *Clin Orthop* 1996;322:297–309.
5. Pinto MR, Peterson HA, Berquist TH. Magnetic resonance imaging in early diagnosis of Legg-Calvé-Perthes disease. *J Pediatr Orthop* 1989;9:19–22.
6. Pisacano RM, Miller TT. Comparing sonography with MR imaging of apophyseal injuries of the pelvis in four boys. *AJR Am J Roentgenol* 2003;181:223–230.
7. Boechat MI. MR imaging of the pediatric pelvis. *MRI Clin North Am* 1996;4(4):679–696.
8. Bollow M, Braun J, Biedermann T, et al. Use of contrast enhanced MR imaging to detect sacroiliitis in children. *Skeletal Radiol* 1998;27:606–616.
9. Berquist TH. Magnetic resonance techniques in musculoskeletal diseases. *Rheum Clin North Am* 1991;17:599–615.
10. Berquist TH. *MRI of the musculoskeletal system*, 4th ed. New York: Lippincott Williams & Wilkins, 2001.
11. Kent JA, Bolinger L, Strear CM, et al. Proton image T1 measurements in human calf muscle during exercise. Presented at the Society of Magnetic Resonance in Medicine. Amsterdam, Netherlands, 1989.
12. Futami T, Suzuki S, Seto Y, et al. Sequential magnetic resonance imaging in slipped capital femoral physis: assessment of preslip in the contralateral hip. *J Pediatr Orthop* 2001;10(4):298–303.
13. Gierada DS, Erickson SJ. MR imaging of the sacral plexus: abnormal findings. *AJR Am J Roentgenol* 1993;160:1067–1071.
14. Puhakka KB, Melsen F, Jurik AG, et al. MR imaging of the sacroiliac joint with correlation to histology. *Skeletal Radiol* 2004;33:15–28.
15. Sturzenbecher A, Braun J, Paris F, et al. MR imaging of septic sacroiliitis. *Skeletal Radiol* 2000;29:439–446.
16. Do-Dai DD, Youngberg RA. MRI of the hip with a shoulder surface coil in off-coronal plane. *J Comput Assist Tomogr* 1995;19(2): 336–338.
17. Niitsu M, Mishima H, Miyakawa S, et al. High resolution MR imaging of the bilateral hips with dual phased-array coil. *J Magn Reson Imaging* 1996;6:950–953.
18. Koo K-H, Kim R. Quantifying the extent of osteonecrosis of the femoral head. A method using MRI. *J Bone Joint Surg Br* 1995;77B:825–880.
19. Jaramillo D, Villegas-Medina OL, Laor T, et al. Gadolinium-enhanced MR imaging of pediatric patients after reduction of hip dysplasia: assessment of femoral head position and factors impeding reduction and femoral head ischemia. *AJR Am J Roentgenol* 1998;170:1633–1637.
20. Petersilge CA. Current concepts of MR arthrography of the hip. *Semin Ultrasound CT MR* 1997;18(4):291–301.
21. McCauley TR, Disler DG. MR imaging of articular cartilage. *Radiology* 1998;209:629–640.
22. Jaramillo D, Villegas-Medina OL, Doty DK, et al. Gadolinium enhanced MR imaging demonstrates abduction-caused hip ischemia and its reversal in piglets. *AJR Am J Roentgenol* 1996;166:879–887.
23. Schmid MR, Nötzli HP, Zanetti M, et al. Cartilage lesions of the hip: diagnostic effectiveness of MR arthrography. *Radiography* 2003;226:382–386.
24. Czerny C, Hofmann S, Urban M, et al. MR arthrography of the adult acetabular capsular-labral complex: correlation with surgery and anatomy. *AJR Am J Roentgenol* 1999;173:345–349.
25. Haims A, Katz LD, Busconi B. MR arthrography of the hip. *Radiol Clin North Am* 1998;36(4):691–702.
26. Petersilge CA, Hague MA, Petersilge WJ, et al. Acetabular labral tears: evaluation with MR arthrography. *Radiology* 1996;200: 231–235.
27. Petersilge CA. MR arthrography for evaluation of the acetabular labrum. *Skeletal Radiol* 2001;30:423–430.
28. Hopson CN, Siverhus SW. Ischemic necrosis of the femoral head. Treatment by core decompression. *J Bone Joint Surg Am* 1988;70: 1048–1051.
29. May DA, Purins JL, Smith DK. MR imaging of occult traumatic fractures and muscular injuries of the hip and pelvis in elderly patients. *AJR Am J Roentgenol* 1999;166:1075–1078.
30. Pitt MJ, Graham AR, Shipman JH, et al. Herniation pits of the femoral neck. *AJR Am J Roentgenol* 1982;138:1115–1121.
31. Czerny C, Hofmann S, Neuhold A, et al. Lesions of the acetabular labrum: accuracy of MR imaging and MR arthrography in detection and staging. *Radiology* 1999;220:225–230.
32. Yucel EK, Silver MS, Carter AP. MR angiography of normal pelvic arteries: comparison of signal intensity and contrast-to-noise ratio of three different in flow techniques. *AJR Am J Roentgenol* 1994;163:197–201.
33. El-Khoury G, Bergman RA, Montgomery WJ. *Sectional anatomy by MRI*, 2nd ed. New York: Churchill-Livingstone, 1995.
34. Gray H, Williams PL. *Anatomy of the human body*, 38th ed. New York: Churchill Livingstone, 1995.
35. Sebag GH. Disorders of the hip. *MRI Clin North Am* 1998;6(3): 627–641.
36. Johnson ND, Wood BP, Noh KS, et al. MR imaging anatomy of the infant hip. *AJR Am J Roentgenol* 1989;153:127–133.
37. Carter BL, Morehead J, Walpert SM, et al. *Cross-sectional anatomy: computed tomography and ultrasound correlation*. New York: Appleton-Century-Crofts, 1977.
38. Rosse C, Rosse PC. *Hollinshead's textbook of anatomy*. Philadelphia, PA: Lippincott–Raven, 1997.
39. Aydingoz U, Ozturk MH. MR imaging of the acetabular labrum: a comparative study of both hips in 180 asymptomatic volunteers. *Eur Radiol* 2001;11(4):567–574.
40. Binningsley D. Tear of the acetabular labrum in an elite athlete. *Br J Sports Med* 2003;37(1):84–88.
41. Baum PA, Matsumoto AH, Teitelbaum GP, et al. Anatomic relationship between the common femoral artery and vein. CT evaluation and clinical significance. *Radiology* 1989;173: 775–777.
42. Egund N, Wingstrand H. Legg-Calvé-Perthes disease: imaging with MR. *Radiology* 1991;179:89–92.
43. Robinson P, White LM, Kandel R, et al. Primary synovial oseochondromatosis of the hip: extracapsular patterns of spread. *Skeletal Radiol* 2004;33:210–215.
44. Varma DGK, Parihar A, Richli WR. CT appearance of the distended trochanteric bursa. *J Comput Assist Tomogr* 1993;17(1):141–143.
45. Pfirrmann CWA, Chang CB, Theumann WH, et al. Greater trochanter of the hip: attachment of the abductor mechanism and a complex of three bursae—MR imaging and MR bursography in cadavers and MR imaging in asymptomatic volunteers. *Radiology* 2001;221:469–477.
46. McMaster PE. Tendon and muscle ruptures. *J Bone Joint Surg* 1933;15A:705–722.
47. Robinson P, White LM, Agur A, et al. Obturator externus bursa: anatomic origin and MR imaging features of pathologic involvement. *Radiology* 2003;228:230–234.
48. Gierada DS, Erickson SJ, Haughton VM, et al. MR imaging of the sacral plexus: normal findings. *AJR Am J Roentgenol* 1993;160: 1059–1065.
49. Cook SM, Pellicci PM, Potter HG. Use of magnetic resonance imaging in the diagnosis of occult fracture of the femoral component after total hip arthroplasty. *J Bone Joint Surg Am* 2004;86A:149–153.
50. Cyteval C, Hamm V, Sarrabere MP, et al. Painful infection at the site of hip prosthesis CT imaging. *Radiology* 2002;224:477–483.
51. Nokes SR, Vogler JB, Spritzer CE, et al. Herniation pits of the femoral neck: appearance at MR imaging. *Radiology* 1989;172: 231–234.
52. Ricci C, Cova M, Kang YS, et al. Normal age related patterns of cellular and fatty bone marrow distribution in the axial skeleton: MR imaging study. *Radiology* 1990;177:83–88.

53. Ilaslan H, Wenger DE, Shives TC, et al. Unilateral hypertrophy of tensor fascia lata: a soft tissue simulator. *Skeletal Radiol* 2003;32: 628–632.

54. Weinreb JC, Cohen JM, Maravilla KR. Iliopsoas muscles: MR study of normal anatomy and disease. *Radiology* 1985;156:435–440.

55. Takahashi H, Kuno S-Y, Miyamoto T, et al. Changes in magnetic resonance images in human skeletal muscle after eccentric exercise. *Eur J Appl Physiol* 1994;69:408–413.

56. Wunderhaldinger P, Bremer C, Schellenberger E, et al. Imaging features of iliopsoas bursitis. *Eur Radiol* 2002;12(2):409–415.

57. Notzli HP, Wyss TF, Stoeklin CH, et al. The contour of the femoral head-neck junction as a predictor of the risk for anterior impingement. *J Bone Joint Surg Br* 2002;84B:556–560.

58. Vogler JB, Murphy WA. Bone marrow imaging. *Radiology* 1988; 168:679–693.

59. Mitchell DG, Rao VM, Dalinka M, et al. Hematopoietic and fatty bone marrow distribution in the normal and ischemic hip: new observations with 1.5-T MR imaging. *Radiology* 1986;161:199–202.

60. Potter H, Moran M, Schneider R, et al. Magnetic resonance imaging in diagnosis of transient osteoporosis of the hip. *Clin Orthop* 1992;280:223–229.

61. Levine CD, Schweitzer MR, Ehrlich SM. Pelvic marrow in adults. *Skeletal Radiol* 1994;23:343–347.

62. Daenen B, Preidler KW, Padmanabhan S, et al. Symptomatic herniation pits of the femoral neck. *AJR Am J Roentgenol* 1997;168: 149–153.

63. . Major NM, Helms CA. Absence or interruption of the supraacetabular line: a subtle film indicator of hip pathology. *Skeletal Radiol* 1996;25:525–529.

64. Yu W, Fent F, Dion E, et al. Comparison of radiography, computed tomography and magnetic resonance imaging in the detection of sacroiliitis accompanying ankylosing spondylitis. *Skeletal Radiol* 1998;27:311–320.

65. Ledermann HP, Schweitzer ME, Morrison WB. Pelvic heterotopic ossification: MR imaging characteristics. *Radiology* 2002;222: 189–195.

66. Edwards DJ, Lomas D, Villar RN. Diagnosis of the painful hip by magnetic resonance imaging and arthroscopy. *J Bone Joint Surg Br* 1995;77B:374–376.

67. Gibbon WW, Hession PR. Diseases of the pelvis and pubic symphysis: MR imaging appearances. *AJR Am J Roentgenol* 1997;169:849–853.

68. Lang P, Jergesen HE, Moseley ME, et al. Avascular necrosis of the femoral head: high-field-strength MR imaging with histologic correlation. *Radiology* 1988;169:517–524.

69. Stover MD, Morgan SJ, Bosse MJ, et al. Prospective comparison of contrast-enhanced computed tomography versus magnetic resonance venography in detection of occult deep pelvic vein thrombosis in patients with pelvic and acetabular fractures. *J Orthop Trauma* 2002;16(9):613–621.

70. Newberg AH, Newman JS. Imaging of the painful hip. *Clin Orthop Relat Res* 2003;406:19–28.

71. Chin CS, Ooi C, Ma SK, et al. Bone marrow necrosis in bone marrow transplantation: the role of MR imaging. *Bone Marrow Transplant* 1998;22:1125–1128.

72. Conway WF, Hayes CW, Daniel WW. Bone marrow edema pattern on MR imaging: transient osteoporosis or early osteonecrosis of bone? *RSNA categorical course in musculoskeletal radiology* 1993;141–154.

73. Hayes CW, Conway WF, Daniel WW. MR imaging of bone marrow edema pattern: transient osteoporosis, transient bone marrow edema or osteonecrosis. *Radiographics* 1993;13:1001–1011.

74. Iida S, Harada Y, Shimizu K, et al. Correlation between bone marrow edema and collapse of the femoral head in steroid-induced osteonecrosis. *AJR Am J Roentgenol* 2000;174:735–743.

75. Takatori Y, Kokulo T, Ninomiya S, et al. Transient osteoporosis of the hip: magnetic resonance imaging. *Clin Orthop* 1991;271: 190–194.

76. VandeBerg B, Malghem JJ, Labaisse MA, et al. MR imaging of avascular necrosis and transient marrow edema of the femoral head. *Radiographics* 1993;13:501–520.

77. VandeBerg BC, Malghen JJ, Lecouvet FE, et al. Idiopathic bone marrow edema lesions of the femoral head. Predictive value of MR imaging findings. *Radiology* 1999;212:527–535.

78. Hosono M, Kobayashi H, Fujimoto R, et al. MR appearance of parasymphyseal insufficiency fractures of the os pubis. *Skeletal Radiol* 1997;26:525–528.

79. Wilson AJ, Murphy WA, Hardy DC, et al. Transient osteoporosis: transient bone marrow edema? *Radiology* 1988;167:757–760.

80. Schweitzer ME, White LM. Does altered biomechanics cause bone marrow edema. *Radiology* 1996;198:851–853.

81. Sissons HA, Nuovo MA, Steiner GC. Pathology of osteonecrosis of the femoral head. *Skeletal Radiol* 1992;21:229–238.

82. VandeBerg B, Malghem J, Labaisse MA, et al. Apparent focal bone marrow ischemia with marrow disorders: MR studies. *J Comput Assist Tomogr* 1993;17:792–797.

83. Koo K-H, Ahn I-O, Kim R, et al. Bone marrow edema and associated pain in early stage osteonecrosis of the femoral head. Prospective study with serial MR images. *Radiology* 1999;213: 715–722.

84. Krany R, Casser HR, Reguardt H, et al. A new holder and surface MRI coil for the examination of the newborn infant hip. *Pediatr Radiol* 1993;23:538–540.

85. MacDougall L, Conway WF. Controversies in magnetic resonance imaging of the hip. *Top Magn Reson Imaging* 1996;8(1):44–50.

86. Bluemke DA, Petri M, Zerhouni EA. Femoral head perfusion and composition: MR imaging and spectroscopic evaluation of patients with systemic lupus erythematosus and at risk for avascular necrosis. *Radiology* 1995;197:453–438.

87. Chan TW, Dalinka MK, Steinberg ME, et al. MRI appearance of femoral head osteonecrosis following core decompression and bone grafting. *Skeletal Radiol* 1991;20:103–107.

88. Daniel WW, Sanders PC, Alarcon GS. The early diagnosis of transient osteoporosis by magnetic resonance imaging. *J Bone Joint Surg Am* 1992;74A:1262–1264.

89. Fujisawa K, Hirata H, Inada H, et al. Value of dynamic MR scan in predicting vascular in growth from full vascularized scapular transplant used for treatment of avascular femoral head necrosis. *Microsurgery* 1995;16(10):673–678.

90. Scully SP, Aaron RK, Urbaniak JR. Survival analysis of hips treated with core decompression or vascularized fibular grafting because of avascular necrosis. *J Bone Joint Surg* 1998;80A:1270–1275.

91. Jones JP Jr. Osteonecrosis. In: McCarty DJ ed. *Arthritis and allied conditions: a textbook of rheumatology*, 11th ed. Philadelphia, PA: Lea & Febiger, 1989: 1545–1562.

92. Jones JP Jr. Etiology and pathogenesis of osteonecrosis. *Semin Arthroplasty* 1991;2:160–168.

93. Munk PL, Helms CA, Holt RG. Immature bone infarcts: findings of plain radiographs and MR scans. *AJR Am J Roentgenol* 1989; 152:547–549.

94. Jiang C-C, Shih TTF. Epiphyseal scar of the femoral head: risk factor for osteonecrosis. *Radiology* 1994;191:409–412.

95. Jones JP Jr. Intravascular coagulation and osteonecrosis. *Clin Orthop* 1992;277:41–53.

96. Lieberman JR, Berry DJ, Mont MA, et al. Osteonecrosis of the hip: management in the twenty-first century. *J Bone Joint Surg Am* 2002;84A:834–853.

97. Poggi JJ, Callaghan JJ, Spritzer CE, et al. Changes on magnetic resonance images after traumatic hip dislocation. *Clin Orthop* 1995;319:249–259.

98. Quinn SF, McCarthy JL. Prospective evaluation of patients with suspected hip fracture and indeterminate radiographs: use of T1-weighted MR images. *Radiology* 1993;187:469–471.

99. Blocklet D, Abramowicz M, Schoutens A. Bone, bone marrow and MIBI scintigraphic findings in Gaucher's disease "bone crisis." *Clin Nucl Med* 2001;26(9):765–769.

100. Bassett LW, Gold RH, Reicher M, et al. Magnetic resonance imaging in the early diagnosis of ischemic necrosis in the femoral head. *Clin Orthop* 1987;214:237–248.

101. Beltran J, Burk JM, Herman LJ, et al. Avascular necrosis of the femoral head: early MRI detection and radiological correlation. *Magn Reson Imaging* 1987;5:431–442.

102. Beltran J, Caudill JL, Herman LA. Rheumatoid arthritis: MR imaging manifestations. *Radiology* 1987;165:153–157.

103. Bozic KJ, Zurakowski D, Thornhill TS. Survivorship analysis of hips treated with care decompression for nontraumatic osteonecrosis of the femoral head. *J Bone Joint Surg* 1999;81A: 200–208.

104. Greiff J, Lang S, Hoilund-Carlsen PF, et al. Early detection of 99Tc-SN-pyrophosphate scintigraphy of femoral head necrosis following femoral neck fractures. *Acta Orthop Scand* 1980;51:119–125.

105. Hofmann S, Engel A, Neuhold A, et al. Bone marrow edema and transient osteoporosis of the hip. An MR controlled study of treatment by core decompression. *J Bone Joint Surg* 1993;75B:210–216.

106. Wang GJ, Dughman SS, Reger SI, et al. The affect of core decompression on the femoral head blood flow in steroid-induced avascular necrosis of the femoral head. *J Bone Joint Surg* 1985;67A:121–124.

107. Grangier C, Garcia J, Howarth NR, et al. Role of MRI in diagnosis of insufficiency fractures of the sacrum and acetabular roof. *Skeletal Radiol* 1997;26:517–524.

108. Koch E, Hofer HO, Sialer G, et al. Failure of MR imaging to detect reflex sympathetic dystrophy of the extremities. *AJR Am J Roentgenol* 1991;156:113–115.

109. Camp JF, Colwell CW. Core decompression of the femoral head for osteonecrosis. *J Bone Joint Surg Am* 1986;68A:1313–1319.

110. Esobedo EM, Hunter JC, Zink-Brody GC, et al. Magnetic resonance imaging of dialysis-related amyloidosis of the shoulder and hip. *Skeletal Radiol* 1996;25:41–48.

111. Falliner A, Muble C, Brossmann J. Acetabular inclination and anteversion in infants using 3D MR imaging. *Acta Radiol* 2002;43(2):221–224.

112. Ficat RF. Treatment of avascular necrosis of the femoral head. *Hip* 1983;2:279–295.

113. Ficat RF, Arlet J. Bone necrosis of known etiology. In: Hungerford P ed. *Ischemia and necrosis of bone*, Baltimore, MD: Williams & Wilkins, 1980.

114. Steinberg ME, Hayken GD, Steinberg DR. A quantitative system for staging avascular necrosis. *J Bone Joint Surg Br* 1995;77B:34–41.

115. Cherian SF, Laorr A, Saleh KJ, et al. Quantifying the extent of femoral head involvement in osteonecrosis. *J Bone Joint Surg Am* 2003;85A:309–314.

116. Lecouvet FE, VandeBerg BC, Maldaque BE, et al. Early irreversible osteonecrosis versus transient lesions of the femoral condyles: prognostic value of subchondral bone and marrow changes on MR imaging. *AJR Am J Roentgenol* 1998;170:71–72.

117. Huang GS, Chan WP, Chang YC, et al. MR imaging of bone marrow edema and joint effusion in patients with osteonecrosis of the femoral head: relationship to pain. *AJR Am J Roentgenol* 203;181(2):545–549.

118. Mitchell B, McCory P, Brukner P, et al. Hip joint pathology: clinical presentation and correlation between magnetic resonance arthrography, ultrasound and arthroscopic findings in 25 patients. *Clin J Sport Med* 2003;13(3):152–156.

119. Mitchell DG, Using MR. imaging to probe the pathophysiology of osteonecrosis. *Radiology* 1989;171:25–26.

120. Mitchell DG, Rao VM, Dalinka MK, et al. Femoral head avascular necrosis: correlation of MR imaging, radiographic staging, radionuclide imaging, and clinical findings. *Radiology* 1987;162:709–715.

121. Tervonen O, Mueller DM, Matteson EL, et al. Clinically occult avascular necrosis of the hip: prevalence in an asymptomatic population at risk. *Radiology* 1992;182:845–847.

122. Steinberg ME, Corces A, Fallon M. Acetabular involvement with osteonecrosis of the femoral head. *J Bone Joint Surg Am* 1999;81A:60–65.

123. Fink B, Assheuer J, Enderle A, et al. Avascular necrosis of the acetabulum. *Skeletal Radiol* 1997;26:509–516.

124. Mitchell MD, Kunkel HL, Steinberg ME, et al. Avascular necrosis of the hip: comparison of MR, CT and scintigraphy. *AJR Am J Roentgenol* 1986;147:67–71.

125. Turner DA, Templeton AC, Selzer PM, et al. Femoral capital osteonecrosis: MR finding of diffuse marrow abnormalities without focal lesions. *Radiology* 1989;171:135–140.

126. VandeBerg B, Malghem J, Labaisse MA, et al. Avascular necrosis of the hip: comparison of contrast-enhanced and nonenhanced MR imaging with histologic correlation. *Radiology* 1992;182:445–450.

127. Kramer J, Hoffman S Jr, Engel A Jr, et al. Bone marrow edema in transient osteoporosis: initial stage of avascular necrosis of the hip [abstract]. *Radiology* 1991;181(P):136.

128. Li KCP, Hiette P. Contrast enhanced fat saturation magnetic resonance imaging for studying the pathophysiology of osteonecrosis of the hips. *Skeletal Radiol* 1992;21:375–379.

129. Hubbard AM, Dormans JP. Evaluation of developmental dysplasia, Perthes disease, and neuromuscular dysplasia of the hip in children before and after surgery: an imaging update. *AJR Am J Roentgenol* 1995;164:1062–1073.

130. Laorr A, Greenspan A, Anderson MW, et al. Traumatic hip dislocation—early MRI findings. *Skeletal Radiol* 1995;24:239–245.

131. Genez BM, Wilson MR, Houk RW, et al. Early osteonecrosis of the femoral head: detection in high-risk patients with MR imaging. *Radiology* 1988;168:521–524.

132. Murray KA, Crim JP. Radiographic imaging for treatment and follow-up of developmental dysplasia of the hip. *Semin Ultrasound CT MR* 2001;22(4):306–340.

133. Nadel SN, Debatin JF, Richardson WJ, et al. Detection of acute avascular necrosis of the femoral head in dogs: dynamic contrast enhanced MR imaging vs. spin-echo and STIR sequences. *AJR Am J Roentgenol* 1992;159:1255–1261.

134. Yoshida T, Kanayama Y, Okamura M, et al. Long term observation of avascular necrosis of the femoral head in systemic lupus erythematosis: an MRI study. *Clin Exp Rheumatol* 2002;20(4):525–530.

135. Stevens K, Tao C, Lee S-U, et al. Subchondral fractures in osteonecrosis of the femoral head: comparison of radiography, CT and MR imaging. *AJR Am J Roentgenol* 2003;180:363–368.

136. Cohen JM, Hodges SC, Weinreb JC, et al. MR imaging of iliopsoas bursitis and concurrent avascular necrosis of the femoral head. *J Comput Assist Tomogr* 1985;9:969–971.

137. Mitchell DG, Rao V, Dalinka M, et al. MRI of joint fluid in the normal and ischemic hip. *AJR Am J Roentgenol* 1986;146:1215–1218.

138. Boles CA, El-Khoury GY. Slipped capital femoral epiphysis. *Radiographics* 1997;17:809–823.

139. Bongartz G, Bock E, Horback T, et al. Degenerative cartilage lesions in the hip—magnetic resonance evaluation. *Magn Reson Imaging* 1989;7:179–186.

140. Bos CFA, Bloem JL, Bloem RM. Sequential magnetic resonance imaging in Perthes disease. *J Bone Joint Surg Br* 1991;73B:219–224.

141. Bos CFA, Bloem JL. Treatment of dislocation of the hip, detected in early childhood, based on magnetic resonance imaging. *J Bone Joint Surg Am* 1989;71A:1523–1529.

142. Boutry N, Paul C, Leroy X, et al. Rapidly destructive osteoarthritis of the hip: MR image findings. *AJR Am J Roentgenol* 2002;179(3):657–663.

143. Bruce W, Higgs RJ, Manidasa D, et al. Acute osteochondral injuries of the hip. *Clin Nucl Med* 2002;27(8):547–549.

144. Bui-Monsfield LT, Chen FS, Lenchik L, et al. Nontraumatic avulsions of the pelvis. *AJR Am J Roentgenol* 2002;178:423–427.

145. Campeas S, Rafic M. Pelvic presentation of a hip joint ganglion: a case report. *Bull Hosp Joint Dis* 2002-2003;61(1-2):89–92.

146. Cardinal E, Buckwalter KA, Capello WN, et al. US of the snapping iliopsoas tendon. *Radiology* 1996;198:521–522.

147. Chan WP, Liu YJ, Huang GS, et al. MRI of joint fluid in femoral head avascular necrosis. *Skeletal Radiol* 2002;31:624–630.

148. Plenk H, Gstettner M, Grosschmidt K, et al. Magnetic resonance imaging and histology of repair in femoral head osteonecrosis. *Clin Orthop Relat Res* 2001;386:42–53.

149. Glickstein MF, Burk DL Jr, Schiebler ML, et al. Avascular necrosis versus other diseases of the hip: sensitivity of MR imaging. *Radiology* 1988;169:213–215.

150. Shimizu K, Moriya H, Akita T, et al. Prediction of collapse with magnetic resonance imaging of avascular necrosis of the femoral head. *J Bone Joint Surg* 1994;76A:215–223.

151. Sugimoto H, Okubo RS, Ohsawa T. Chemical shift and the double-line sign in MRI of early femoral avascular necrosis. *J Comput Assist Tomogr* 1992;16:727–730.

152. Lafforgue P, Dahan E, Chagnaud C, et al. Early stage avascular necrosis of the femoral head: MR imaging of prognosis in 31 cases with at least two years follow-up. *Radiology* 1993;187:199–204.

153. Seo GS, Aoki J, Karakida O, et al. Ischiopubic insufficiency fractures: MRI appearances. *Skeletal Radiol* 1997;26:705–710.

154. Malizos KN, Siafakas MS, Fotiadis DI, et al. An MRI-based semi-anatomical volumetric quantification of hip osteonecrosis. *Skeletal Radiol* 2001;30:686–693.

155. Kopecky KK, Braunstein EM, Brandt KD, et al. Apparent avascular necrosis of the hip: appearance and spontaneous resolution of MR findings in renal allograft recipients. *Radiology* 1991;179: 523–527.

156. Springfield DS, Enneking WJ. Surgery of aseptic necrosis of the femoral head. *Clin Orthop Relat Res* 1978;130:175–178.

157. Urbaniak JR, Coogan PG, Gurnalson EB, et al. Treatment of osteonecrosis of the femoral head with free vascularized fibular grafting. A long- term study of one hundred and three hips. *J Bone Joint Surg* 1995;77A:681–694.

158. Krachow KA, Mont MA, Maar DC. Limited femoral endoprosthesis for avascular necrosis of the femoral head. *Orthop Radiol* 1993;22:457–463.

159. Summers RM, Brune AM, Choyke PL, et al. Juvenile idiopathic inflammatory myopathy: exercise induced changes in muscle at short inversion time inversion-recovery MR imaging. *Radiology* 1998;209:191–196.

160. Ryu KN, Kim EJ, Yoo MC, et al. Ischemic necrosis of the entire femoral head and rapidly destructive hip disease: potential causative relationship. *Skeletal Radiol* 1997;26:143–149.

161. Watanabe W, Itoi E, Yamada S. Early MRI findings of rapidly destructive coxarthrosis. *Skeletal Radiol* 2002;31:35–38.

162. Yamamoto T, Takabataki K, Iwamoto Y. Subchondral insufficiency fracture of the femoral head resulting in rapid destruction of the hip joint. A sequential radiographic study. *AJR Am J Roentgenol* 2002;178:435–437.

163. Hodler J, Yu JS, Goodwin D, et al. MR arthrography of the hip: improved imaging of the acetabular labrum with histologic correlation in cadavers. *AJR Am J Roentgenol* 1995;165:887–891.

164. Hachiya Y, Kubo T, Morii M, et al. Characteristic features of the acetabular labrum in healthy children. *J Ped Ortho* 2001;10(3): 169–172.

165. Kiuru MJ, Pihlajamaki HK, Perkio JP, et al. Dynamic contrast enhanced MR imaging in symptomatic bone stress of the pelvis and lower extremity. *Acta Radiol* 2001;47(3):277–285.

166. Kiuru MJ, Pihlajamaki HK, Ahovuo JA. Fatigue stress injuries of the pelvic bone and proximal femur: evaluation with MR imaging. *Eur Radiol* 2003;13(3):605–611.

167. Kneeland JB. MR imaging of sports related injuries of the hip. *Magn Reson Imaging Clin N Am* 1999;7(1):105–115.

168. Lambiase RE, Levine SM, Froehlick JA. Rapid osteolysis of the femoral neck after fracture. *AJR Am J Roentgenol* 1999;172: 489–491.

169. Theodorou DJ, Theodorou SJ, Haghighi P, et al. Distinct focal lesions of the femoral head: imaging features suggesting atypical and minimal form of bone necrosis. *Skeletal Radiol* 2002;31: 435–444.

170. Toby EB, Koman LA, Bechtold RE. Magnetic resonance imaging of pediatric hip disease. *J Pediatr Orthop* 1985;5:665–671.

171. Tomczak RJ, Guenther KP, Rieber A, et al. MR imaging measurement of the femoral anteversion angle as a new technique: comparison with CT in children and adults. *AJR Am J Roentgenol* 1997;168:791–794.

172. Guerra JJ, Steinberg MR. Distinguishing transient osteoporosis from avascular necrosis of the hip. *J Bone Joint Surg* 1995;77A: 616–624.

173. LeParc J-M, Andre T, Helenon O, et al. Osteonecrosis of the hip in renal transplant recipients. Changes in functional status and magnetic resonance imaging findings over three years in three hundred five patients. *Rev Rhum Engl Ed* 1996;63(6):413–420.

174. Hockbergs P, Echenwall G, Wingstrand H, et al. Epiphyseal bone marrow abnormalities and restitution in Legg-Calvé-Perthes disease. Valuation by MR imaging in 86 cases. *Acta Radiol* 1997;38:855–862.

175. Bloem JL. Transient osteoporosis of the hip: MR imaging. *Radiology* 1988;167:753–755.

176. Boissonnault WG, Boissonnault JS. Transient osteoporosis of the hip associated with pregnancy. *J Orthop Sports Phys Ther* 2001; 31(7):359–365.

177. Lim IG, Berger M, Bertouch J. An unusual cause of pain in both hips. *Ann Rheum Dis* 2003;62(6):510–511.

178. Moss SG, Schweitzer ME, Jacobson JA, et al. Hip joint fluid: detection and distribution at MR imaging and US with cadaveric correlation. *Radiology* 1998;208:43–48.

179. Asnis SE, Gould ES, Bansal M, et al. Magnetic resonance imaging of the hip after displaced femoral neck fractures. *Clin Orthop* 1994;298:191–198.

180. Bogost GA, Lizerbram EK, Crues JV III. MR imaging in evaluation of suspected hip fracture: frequency of unsuspected bone and soft-tissue injury. *Radiology* 1995;197:263–267.

181. DeSmet AA, Best TM. MR imaging of the distribution and location of acute hamstring injuries in athletes. *AJR Am J Roentgenol* 2000;174:393–399.

182. Deutsch AL, Mink JH, Waxman AD. Occult fractures of the proximal femur: MR imaging. *Radiology* 1989;170:113–116.

183. Haramati N, Staron RB, Barox C, et al. Magnetic resonance imaging of occult fractures of the proximal femur. *Skeletal Radiol* 1994;23:19–22.

184. Mammone JF, Schweitzer ME. MRI of occult sacral insufficiency fractures following radiotherapy. *Skeletal Radiol* 1995;24:101–104.

185. Peh WCG, Cheng KC, Ho WY, et al. Transient-bone marrow edema: a variant pattern of sacral insufficiency fractures. *Austral Radiol* 1998;42:102–105.

186. Rizzo PF, Gould ES, Lyden JP, et al. Diagnosis of occult fractures about the hip. *J Bone Joint Surg Am* 1993;75A:395–401.

187. Rubel IF, Kloen P, Potter HG, et al. MRI assessment of the posterior acetabular wall fracture in traumatic dislocation of the hip in children. *Pediatr Radiol* 2002;32(6):435–439.

188. Weaver CT, Major NM, Garrett WE, et al. Femoral head osteochondral lesions in painful hips of athletes: MR image findings. *AJR Am J Roentgenol* 2002;178:973–977.

189. Lewis SL, Rees JIS, Thomas GV, et al. Pitfalls of bone scintigraphy in suspected hip fractures. *Br J Radiol* 1991;64:403–408.

190. Linden B, Jonsson K, Redland-Johnell I. Osteochondritis dissecans of the hip. *Acta Radiol* 2003;44(1):67–71.

191. Ahovuo JA, Kiuru MJ, Kinnunen JJ, et al. MR imaging of fatigue stress injuries to bones: intra- and inter observer agreement. *Magn Reson Imaging* 2002;20(5):401–406.

192. Jaramillo D, Shapiro F. Musculoskeletal trauma in children. *Magn Reson Imaging Clin N Am.* 1998;6:521–536.

193. Kiuri MJ, Pihlajamaki HK, Hietanen HJ, et al. MR imaging, bone scintigraphy and radiography in bone stress injuries of the pelvis and lower extremities. *Acta Radiol* 2002;43(2):207–212.

194. Slocum KA, Gorman JD, Puckett ML, et al. Resolution of abnormal MR signal intensity in patients with stress fractures of the femoral neck. *AJR Am J Roentgenol* 1997;168:1295–1299.

195. Warwick B, Higgs RJED, Munidasa D, et al. Acute osteochondral injuries of the hip. *Clin Nucl Med* 2002;27(8):547–549.

196. Gabriel H, Fitzgerald SW, Myers MT, et al. MR imaging of hip disorders. *Radiographics* 1994;14:763–781.

197. Moorman CT, Warren RF, Hershman EB, et al. Traumatic posterior hip subluxation in American football. *J Bone Joint Surg Am* 2003;85A:1190–1196.

198. Schultz E, Miller TT, Boruchov SD, et al. Incomplete intertrochanteric fractures: imaging features and clinical management. *Radiology* 1999;211:237–240.

199. Rubin SJ, Marquardt JD, Gottlieb RH, et al. Magnetic resonance imaging: a cost-effective alternative to bone scintigraphy in evaluation of patients with suspected hip fractures. *Skeletal Radiol* 1998;27:199–204.

200. Bencardino JT, Palmer WE. Imaging of hip disorders in athletes. *Radiol Clin North Am* 2002;40(2):267–287.

201. Khoury NJ, Birnjawi GA, Chaaya M, et al. Use of limited MR protocol (coronal STIR) in evaluation of patients with hip pain. *Skeletal Radiol* 2003;32:567–574.

202. Verrall GM, Slavotinek JP, Fon GT. Incidence of pubic bone marrow edema in Australian rules football players: related to groin pain. *Br J Sports Med* 2001;35(1):28–33.

203. Major NM, Helms CA. Sacral stress fractures in long-distance runners. *AJR Am J Roentgenol* 2000;174:727–729.

204. Walsh G, Archibald CG. MRI in greater trochanteric pain syndrome. *Australian Radiol* 2003;47(1):85–87.

205. O'Donoghue DH. *Treatment of injuries to athletes,* 4th ed. Philadelphia, PA: WB Saunders, 1984.

206. Peh WCG, Khong P-L, Yur Y, et al. Imaging of pelvic insufficiency fractures. *Radiographics* 1996;16:335–348.

207. Williams TR, Puckett ML, Denison G, et al. Acetabular stress fractures in military endurance athletes and recruits: incidence and

MRI and scintigraphic findings. *Skeletal Radiol* 2002;31(5): 277–281.

208. Lang P, Mauz M, Schörner W, et al. Acute fracture of the femoral neck: assessment of femoral head perfusion with gadopentetate dimeglumine-enhanced MR imaging. *AJR Am J Roentgenol* 1993;160:335–441.

209. O'Connell MJ, Powell T, McCaffray NM, et al. Symphyseal cleft injection in the diagnosis and treatment of osteitis pubis in athletes. *AJR Am J Roentgenol* 2002;179:955–959.

210. Otte M, Helms CA, Fritz RC. MR imaging of supra-acetabular insufficiency fractures. *Skeletal Radiol* 1997;26:279–283.

211. Blomlie V, Rofstad EK, Talle K, et al. Incidence of radiation induced insufficiency fractures of the female pelvis: evaluation with MR imaging. *AJR Am J Roentgenol* 1996;167:1205–1210.

212. Blomlie V, Lien HH, Iversen T, et al. Radiation-induced insufficiency fractures of the sacrum: evaluation with MR imaging. *Radiology* 1993;188:241–244.

213. Remström P. Swedish research on traumatology. *Clin Orthop* 1984;191:144–158.

214. Bartlett ML, Ginn L, Beitz L, et al. Quantitative assessment of myositis in the thigh using magnetic resonance imaging. *Magn Reson Imag* 1999;17(2):183–191.

215. Chung CB, Robertson JE, Cho GJ, et al. Gluteus medius tendon tears and avulsive injuries in elderly women. Imaging findings in six patients. *AJR Am J Roentgenol* 1999;173:351–353.

216. DeSmet AA, Fisher DR, Heiner JP, et al. Magnetic resonance imaging of muscle tears. *Skeletal Radiol* 1990;19:283–286.

217. Ekberg O, Sjoberg S, Westlin N. Sports-related groin pain: evaluation with MR imaging. *Eur Radiol* 1996;6:52–55.

218. Fleckenstein JL, Canby RC, Parkey RW, et al. Acute effects of exercise on MR imaging of skeletal muscles in normal volunteers. *AJR Am J Roentgenol* 1988;151:231–237.

219. Fleckenstein JL, Weatherall PT, Parkey RW, et al. Sports-related muscle injuries: evaluation with MR imaging. *Radiology* 1989;172: 793–798.

220. Khoury NJ, El-Khoury GY, Kathol MH. MRI diagnosis of diabetic muscle infarction: report of 2 cases. *Skeletal Radiol* 1997;26: 122–127.

221. McKeag DB. The concept of overuse: the primary care aspects of overuse syndromes in sports. *Prim Care* 1984;11:43–59.

222. Lonner JH, Van Kleunen JP. Spontaneous rupture of the gluteus medius and minimus tendons. *Am J Orthop* 2002;31(10): 579–581.

223. Koulouris G, Connell D. Evaluation of the hamstring muscle complex following acute injury. *Skeletal Radiol* 2003;32:582–589.

224. Oakes BW. Hamstring muscle injuries. *Aust Fam Physician* 1984; 13:587–591.

225. Slavotinek JP, Verrall GM, Fon GT. Hamstring injury in athletes: using MR imaging measurements to compare the extent of muscle injury with the amount of time lost for competition. *AJR Am J Roentgenol* 2002;179:1621–1628.

226. Dooms GC, Fisher MR, Hricak H, et al. MR imaging of intramuscular hemorrhage. *J Comput Assist Tomogr* 1985;9:908–913.

227. Pomeranz SJ, Heidt RS. MR imaging in the prognostication of hamstring injuries. *Radiology* 1993;189:897–900.

228. Bird PA, Oakley SP, Shnier R, et al. Prospective evaluation of magnetic resonance imaging and physical examination findings in patients with greater trochanteric pain syndrome. *Arthritis Rheum* 2001;44(9):2138–2145.

229. Baker BE. Current concepts in diagnosis and treatment of musculotendinous injuries. *Med Sci Sports Exerc* 1984;16:323–327.

230. Kingzett-Taylor A, Tiroran PFJ, Feller J, et al. Tendinosis and tears of the gluteus medius and minimum muscles as a cause of hip pain: MR image findings. *AJR Am J Roentgenol* 1999;173:1123–1226.

231. Asinger DA, El-Khoury GY. Tensor fascia lata muscle tear: evaluation by MRI. *Iowa Orthop J* 1998;18:146–149.

232. An HS, Simpson JM, Gale S, et al. Acute anterior compartment syndrome in the thigh: a case report and review of the literature. *J Orthop Trauma* 1987;1(2):180–182.

233. Kahan JS, McClellan RT, Burton DS. Acute bilateral compartment syndrome of the thigh induced by exercise. *J Bone Joint Surg Am* 1994;76A:1068–1071.

234. Raether PM, Lather LD. Recurrent compartment syndrome in the posterior thigh. A report of a case. *Am J Sports Med* 1982;10:40–43.

235. Siegel AJ, Silverman LM, Holman BL. Elevated creatinine kinase MG isoenzyme levels in marathon runners. *JAMA* 1981;246: 2049–2051.

236. Matin P, Lange G, Caretta R, et al. Scintigraphic evaluation of muscle damage following extreme exercise. Concise communication. *J Nucl Med* 1983;24:308–311.

237. Zagoria RJ, Karstaedt N, Koubek TD. MR imaging of rhabdomyosis. *J Comput Assist Tomogr* 1986;10:268–270.

238. Benson ER, Schutzer SF. Post traumatic piriformis syndrome. Diagnosis and results of operative treatment. *J Bone Joint Surg Am* 1999;81A:941–949.

239. Lee EY, Margherita AJ, Gierada DS, et al. MRI of piriformis syndrome. *AJR Am J Roentgenol* 2004;183:63–64.

240. Cvtanic O, Henzie G, Skezas N, et al. MRI diagnosis of tears of the abductor tendons (gluteus medius and gluteus minimus). *AJR Am J Roentgenol* 2004;182:137–143.

241. Mellado JM, Perez del Palomar L, Diaz L, et al. Long standing Morel-Lavallee lesions of the trochanteric region and proximal thigh. *AJR Am J Roentgenol* 2004;182:1289–1294.

242. Coulier B, Cloots V. Atypical retroperitoneal extension of iliopsoas bursitis. *Skeletal Radiol* 2003;32:298–301.

243. Dobbs MB, Gordon JE, Luhmann SJ, et al. Surgical correction of the snapping iliopsoas tendon in adolescents. *J Bone Joint Surg Am* 2002;84A(3):420–424.

244. Pelsser V, Cardinal E, Hobden R, et al. Extraarticular snapping hip: sonographic findings. *AJR Am J Roentgenol* 2001;176:67–73.

245. Cotton A, Boutry N, Demondion X, et al. Acetabular labrum: MRI in asymptomatic volunteers. *J Comput Assist Tomogr* 1998; 22(1):1–7.

246. Konrath GA, Hamel AJ, Olson SA, et al. The role of the acetabular labrum and the transverse acetabular ligament in load transmission in the hip. *J Bone Joint Surg Am* 1998;80A:1781–1788.

247. Plotz GM, Brossmann J, Von Kusch M, et al. Magnetic resonance arthrography of the acetabular labrum: value of radial reconstructions. *Arch Orthop Trauma Surg* 2001;121(8):450–457.

248. Lecouvet FE, VandeBerg BC, Malghem BE, et al. MR imaging of the acetabular labrum: variations in 200 asymptomatic hips. *AJR Am J Roentgenol* 1996;167:1025–1028.

249. Leunig M, Werlen S, Undersbock A, et al. Evaluation of the acetabular labrum by MR arthrography. *J Bone Joint Surg Br* 1997;79B:230–234.

250. Nishii T, Makanishi K, Sugano N, et al. Acetabular labral tears: contrast-enhanced MR imaging under contiguous leg traction. *Skeletal Radiol* 1996;25:349–356.

251. Sherman PM, Matchette MW, Sanders TG, et al. Acetabular paralabral cyst: an uncommon cause of sciatica. *Skeletal Radiol* 2003;32:90–94.

252. Schnaskowski P, Steinbach LS, Tirman PFJ, et al. Magnetic resonance imaging of labral cysts of the hip. *Skeletal Radiol* 1996;25:733–737.

253. Horii M, Kubo T, Hachiya Y, et al. Development of the acetabulum and acetabular labrum in the normal child: analysis with radial sequence magnetic resonance imaging. *J Pediatr Ortho* 2002;22(2):222–227.

254. Ito K, Minka MA, Leunig M, et al. Femora acetabular impingement and the cam-effect: a MRI based quantitative anatomical study of the femoral head-neck offset. *J Bone Joint Surg* 2001; 83B:171–176.

255. Magee T, Hinson G. Association of paralabral cysts with acetabular disorders. *AJR Am J Roentgenol* 2000;174:1381–1384.

256. Daffner RH, Lupetin AR, Dash N, et al. MRI in the detection of malignant infiltration of bone marrow. *AJR Am J Roentgenol* 1986;146:353–358.

257. Weiss SW, Goldblum JR. *Enzinger and Weiss soft tissue tumors*, 4th ed. St. Louis, MO: Mosby, 2001.

258. Finnelli A, Babyn P, Melorie GA, et al. The use of magnetic resonance imaging in diagnosis and follow-up of pediatric rhabdomyosarcoma. *J Urol* 2000;163:1952–1953.

259. Unni KK. *Dahlin's bone tumors. General aspects and data on 11,087 cases*, 5th ed. Philadelphia, PA: Lippincott–Raven, 1996.

260. Berquist TH. MRI of musculoskeletal neoplasms. *Clin Orthop* 1989;244:101–118.

261. Mahrlein R, Weiand G, Schmelzeisen H. Ganglion of the hip: report of 5 cases. *J South Orthop Assoc* 2001;10(1):1–5.

262. Wolf RS, Zoys GN, Saldivar JA, et al. Lipoma arborescens of the hip. *Am J Orthop* 2002;31(5):276–279.

263. Smith SR, Williams CE, Davies JM, et al. Bone marrow disorders: characterization with quantitative MR imaging. *Radiology* 1989;172:805–810.

264. Sundarum M, McDonald DJ. The solitary tumor or tumor like lesion of bone. *Top Magn Reson Imaging* 1989;1(4):17–29.

265. Sundarum M, Khanna G, El-Khoury GY. T1-weighted imaging for distinguishing large osteolysis of Paget's disease from sarcomatous degeneration. *Skeletal Radiol* 2001;30(7):278–383.

266. Goldman AB, Schneider R, Pavlov H. Osteoid osteomas of the femoral neck: report of four cases evaluated with isotope bone scanning, CT and MR imaging. *Radiology* 1993;186:227–232.

267. Goldstein HA, Treves S. Bone scintigraphy of osteoid osteoma: a clinical review. *Clin Nucl Med* 1978;3:359–363.

268. Woods ER, Martel W, Mandell SH, et al. Reactive soft tissue mass associated with osteoid osteoma: correlation of MR imaging features with pathologic findings. *Radiology* 1993;186:221–225.

269. Otake S, Tsuruta Y, Yamana D, et al. Amyloid arthropathy of the hip joint: MR demonstration of presumed amyloid lesions in 152 patients with long-term hemodialysis. *Eur Radiol* 1998;8:1352–1356.

270. Rayner CK, Burnet SP, McNeil JD. Osseous sarcoidosis–a magnetic resonance imaging diagnosis. *Clin Exp Rheumatol* 2002;20(4):546–548.

271. Yulish BS, Lieberman JM, Newman AJ, et al. Juvenile rheumatoid arthritis: assessment with MR imaging. *Radiology* 1987;165:149–152.

272. Li KC, Higgs J, Aisen AM, et al. MRI in osteoarthritis of the hip: gradation of severity. *Magn Reson Imaging* 1988;6:229–236.

273. Kim SH, Hong SJ, Park JS, et al. Idiopathic osteochondromatosis of the hip: radiographic and MR appearances in 15 patients. *Korean J Radiol* 2002;3(4):254–259.

274. Fletcher BD, Scoles PV, Nelson AD. Osteomyelitis in children: detection by magnetic resonance. *Radiology* 1984;150:57–60.

275. Lee SK, Suh KJ, Kim YW, et al. Septic arthritis versus transient synovitis at MR imaging: preliminary assessment with signal intensity alterations in bone marrow. *Radiology* 1999;211:459–465.

276. Mason MD, Zlatkin MB, Esterhai JL, et al. Chronic complicated osteomyelitis of the lower extremity: evaluation with MR imaging. *Radiology* 1989;173:355–359.

277. O'Connor DA, Ridha H, Roche CJ, et al. SAPHO syndrome presenting as septic arthritis in the hip. *Ir Med J* 2003;96(2):41–42.

278. Twair A, Ryan M, O'Connell M, et al. MRI of failed total hip replacement caused by abductor muscle avulsion. *AJR Am J Roentgenol* 2003;181:1547–1550.

279. White LM, Kim JD, Mehta M, et al. Complications of total hip arthroplasty: MR imaging—initial experience. *Radiology* 2000;215:254–262.

280. Cohen MD. Magnetic resonance imaging of the pediatric musculoskeletal system. *Semin Ultrasound CT MRI* 1991;12:506–523.

281. Dietrich RB. *Pediatric MRI*, 2nd ed. Philadelphia, PA: Lippincott Williams & Wilkins, 2002.

282. Siegel MJ. Magnetic resonance imaging of the pediatric pelvis. *Semin Ultrasound CT MR* 1991;12:475–505.

283. Jaramillo D, Galen TA, Winalski CS, et al. Legg-Calvé-Perthes disease: MR imaging evaluation during manual positioning of the hip—comparison with conventional arthrography. *Radiology* 1999;212:519–525.

284. Kaniblideo C, Lonnerholm T, Moberg A, et al. Legg-Calvé-Perthes disease: comparison of conventional radiography, MR imaging, bone scintigraphy and arthrography. *Acta Radiol* 1995;36:434–439.

285. Keller MS, Weltin GG, Rattner Z, et al. Normal instability of the hip in the neonate: US standards. *Radiology* 1988;169:733–736.

286. Eckerwall G, Hochbergs P, Simesen K, et al. Metaphyseal histology and magnetic resonance imaging in Legg-Calvé-Perthes disease. *J Pediatr Orthop* 1997;17:659–662.

287. Wenger DR, Ward WT, Herring JA. Current concepts review: Legg-Calvé-Perthes disease. *J Bone Joint Surg Am* 1991;73A:778–788.

288. Uno A, Hattori T, Noritaki K, et al. Legg-Calvé-Perthes disease in the evolutionary period: comparison of magnetic resonance imaging with bone scintigraphy. *J Pediatr Orthop* 1995;15:362–367.

289. Rush BH, Bramson RT, Ogden JA. Legg-Calvé-Perthes disease: detection of cartilaginous and synovial changes with MR imaging. *Radiology* 1988;167:473–476.

290. Salter RB, Thompson GH. Legg-Calvé-Perthes disease. The prognostic significance of subchondral fractures and a two-group classification of femoral head involvement. *J Bone Joint Surg Am* 1984;66A:479–489.

291. Henderson RC, Renner JB, Stardivant MC, et al. Evaluation of magnetic resonance imaging of Legg-Perthes disease. A prospective blinded study. *J Pediatr Orthop* 1990;10:289–297.

292. Johnson ND, Wood BP, Jackman KV. Complex infantile and congenital hip dislocation: assessment with MR imaging. *Radiology* 1988;168:151–156.

293. Catterall A. Legg-Calvé Perthes disease. *RSNA Instr Course Lect* 1989;9:19–22.

294. Hochbergs P, Echenwall G, Egund N, et al. Synovitis in Legg-Calvé-Perthes disease: evaluation with MR imaging in 84 hips. *Acta Radiol* 1998;39:532–537.

295. Herring JA, Neustadt JB, Williams JJ, et al. The lateral pillar classification of Legg-Calvé-Perthes disease. *J Pediatr Orthop* 1992;12:143–150.

296. Hochbergs P, Echewall G, Egund N, et al. Femoral head shape in Legg-Calvé-Perthes disease. Correlation between conventional radiography, arthrography and MR imaging. *Acta Radiol* 1994;35:545–548.

297. Guidera KJ, Einbecker ME, Berman CG, et al. Magnetic resonance imaging evaluation of congenital dislocation of the hips. *Clin Orthop* 1990;261:96–101.

298. Horii M, Kubo T, Inoue S, et al. Coverage of the femoral head by the acetabular labrum in dysplastic hips: quantitative analysis with radial MR imaging. *Acta Ortho Scand* 2003;74(3):287–292.

299. Weinstein SL, Mubarak SJ, Wenger DR. Developmental hip dysplasia and dislocation. *J Bone Joint Surg* 2003;85A:2024–2035.

300. Duffy CM, Taylor FN, Coleman L, et al. Magnetic resonance imaging evaluation of surgical management of developmental dysplasia of the hip in childhood. *J Pediatr Ortho* 2002;22(1):92–100.

301. Umans H, Liebling MS, Moy L, et al. Slipped capital femoral epiphyses: a physeal lesion diagnosed by MRI with radiographic and CT correlation. *Skeletal Radiol* 1998;27:139–144.

302. Guenther KP, Tomczak R, Kessler S, et al. Measurement of femoral anteversion by magnetic resonance imaging-evaluation of a new technique in children and adolescents. *Eur J Radiol* 1995;21:47–52.

303. Prasad SS, Bruce C, Crawford S, et al. Femoral anteversion in infants: a method using ultrasound. *Skeletal Radiol* 2003;32:462–467.

304. Iwasada S, Hasegawa Y, Iwasi T, et al. Bone scintigraphy and magnetic resonance imaging after transtrochanteric rotational osteotomy. *Skeletal Radiol* 1999;28:251–259.

Knee

Elizabeth Ann Kelley   Thomas H. Berquist

The value of magnetic resonance imaging (MRI) for imaging the knee was apparent almost immediately after the introduction of this modality in the early 1980s (1–7).

With the introduction of special closely coupled extremity coils, high field systems, open systems, extremity units (see Chapter 3), and other technical advances, the utility of MRI in the knee has expanded dramatically (3,8–17). These capabilities have made knee imaging one of the most widely accepted applications of MRI. MRI has replaced arthrography in the evaluation of knee pathology (18–21). Studies have demonstrated MRI is equally effective when requested by orthopedic surgeons and primary care physicians (22). MRI has also been demonstrated as a cost-effective technique by reducing unnecessary surgical or arthroscopic interventions (23,24). Improved diagnostic accuracy has been clearly demonstrated and MRI resulted in changes in patient management in 41% of patients (25). MR examinations obtained prior to more expensive arthroscopic studies can reduce the need for arthroscopy in up to 42% of patients (26,27).

More recent literature by Alioto et al. (28) revealed that MR examinations beneficially altered the treatment plans of the orthopedic surgeon in 18% of patients. Furthermore, they found MRI to be more useful in the decision-making process when pathology involved the meniscus or chondral surfaces. MRI was not as useful for evaluating anterior cruciate ligament (ACL) insufficiency (28).

TECHNIQUES

The techniques used for evaluating the knee should be tailored to the clinical indication and the imaging system that is employed. Although many techniques and image planes may be used, the following discussion is oriented toward the routine screening examination that is commonly used to evaluate most articular and periarticular disorders of the knee. More specific techniques are discussed later in the applications section as they apply to specific clinical disorders.

Positioning and Coil Selection

Typically, the patient is placed in the supine position with the knee placed in a closely coupled extremity coil (see Fig. 7-1). The knee may be externally rotated 15° to 20° to facilitate visualization of the ACL on sagittal images (14,21,29,30). This practice is not routinely performed at all MR imaging centers. The knee should be flexed slightly (5° to 10°) to increase the accuracy of assessing the patellofemoral compartment and patellar alignment (31). Excessive flexion or hyperextension does not permit accurate evaluation of patellar alignment (31). Different coil systems and positions may be required if motion studies are required for patellofemoral evaluation. Recently, Antonio et al. (32) added targeted imaging using a 4-cm loop receive coil to obtain more detail in the area of interest. A 10-cm field of view (normal 14-cm in our practice) with 256 × 512 (displayed at 512 × 512) matrix was utilized.

Most high field imagers allow more limited motion than the open gantries of lower field units. New extremity units also limit positioning options. Positioning techniques will be discussed more completely later with patellofemoral disorders.

Pulse Sequences/Image Planes

When selecting pulse sequences, physicians have many options, ranging from spin-echo sequences, fast spin-echo (FSE) sequences, various gradient-echo (GRE) sequences, and three-dimensional imaging (Table 7-1) (33–50). The contrast requirements in knee imaging demand some variation in sequences. Meniscal tears are best imaged with MR sequences that are neither purely T1- or

T2-weighted. Other structures such as ligaments are best evaluated with T2-weighted images (1,2).

A technical requirement that should not be underestimated is the need to use adequate image geometry. The menisci and the cruciate ligaments are complex structures, and it is unreasonable to expect to be able to evaluate them reliably using a single slice orientation.

The pulse sequences that are now widely available for knee imaging include spin-echo and FSE techniques, GRE techniques, both slice-selective and three-dimensional Fourier transform (3DFT) versions. Short inversion time recovery (STIR) and FSE STIR sequences may also be selected (51).

In the spin-echo category, we can consider short repetition time/echo time (TR/TE) sequences and long TR multi-echo sequences. At this time, there seems to be little to recommend the sole use of short TR/TE spin-echo sequences for knee imaging. Although they are technically undemanding, rapidly acquired, and sensitive for medullary bone lesions, they only provide low contrast for meniscal lesions, they are not well-suited for demonstrating acute ligamentous injuries or the interface between joint fluid and articular cartilage, and they require special windowing during photography (see Fig. 7-2).

Long TR, multiecho spin-echo sequences are very effective for knee imaging. A short first echo provides intermediate contrast that is excellent for identifying meniscal lesions, and a second, long echo provides T2-weighted contrast that is critical for evaluation of the cruciate ligaments and other structures (5–7,52).

A commonly used approach for knee imaging is to perform sagittal and coronal spin-echo acquisitions (see Fig. 7-3) (53,54). The exact technical approach will depend on the imaging hardware utilized. We have found the parameters summarized in Table 7-1 to be efficient and reliable using a 1.5 T imager.

Long TR multiecho sequences have the advantages of high slice throughput (in terms of images per unit time) and favorable contrast characteristics. They have the disadvantage of requiring longer acquisition times, and the long TE T2-weighted images are technically demanding in terms of imager performance.

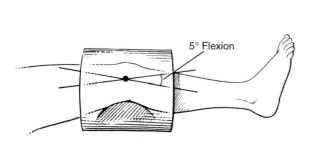

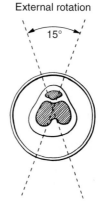

Figure 7-1 Knee positioned in a volume coil. The knee is flexed 5° to 10° and externally rotated 15°.

TABLE 7-1

MR SCREENING EXAMINATION OF THE KNEE

Image Plane Author's	Pulse Sequence	Slice Thickness	Field of View (cm)	Matrix	Acquisitions (NEX)	Image Time
Axial scout localizer	FLASH 15/5	8 mm/skip 8 mm	14	256 × 128	1	11 s
Coronal/sagittal scout localizer	FLASH 15/5	8 mm/skip 8 mm	14	256 × 128	1	21 s
Coronal						
T1WI	SE 689/14	4 mm/skip 0.5 mm	14	512 × 256	2	4 min
DESS	DE 23.87/6.73	1 mm/ 20%	14	256 × 192 with interpolation	2	6 min 54 s
Sagittal						
PD FSE	TSE 2,500/26, echo train 7	4 mm/skip 0.5 mm	14	512 × 256	2	3 min 47 s
T2WI FSE	TSE 4,000/83, echo train 7	4 mm/skip 0.5 mm	14	512 × 256	2	3 min 54 s
Axial						
PD FSE with fat sat	TSE 4,000/26, echo train 7	4 mm/ skip 0.5 mm	14	256 × 192	2	4 min 22 s
				Image time scouts		32 s
				Image time coronals		10 min 54 s
				Image time sagittals and axials		12 min 5 s
				Total imaging time		24 min 1 s
Additional Sequences:						
Fat-suppressed fast spin-echo T2WI (Axial, coronal, or sagittal)	3,500/20–30 (echo train 2–8)	4 mm/skip 0.5	14	512 × 256	2	3 min 58 s
STIR FSE (axial, coronal, or sagittal)	4,230/86, TI160	5 mm/skip 1 mm	14	256 × 192	2	4 min 58 s
Conventional T2 (axial)	2,230/20	6 mm/skip 1.5	14	256 × 192	1	9 min 52 s

T1WI, T1-weighted image; T2WI, T2-weighted image; FSE, fast spin echo; TSE, turbo spin echo; PD, proton density; DESS, dual echo steady state; STIR, short inversion time recovery; DE, dual echo; SE, spin echo; FLASH, fast low-angle single-shot; SAT, saturation.

In recent years, new FSE sequences have essentially replaced conventional spin-echo sequences (24,45,52,55). These sequences permit, in theory, faster data acquisition with repeated spin echoes following a 180° pulse. The echoes have different degrees of phase encoding and all contribute to a single image. We have used this technique sparingly in the knee as both short- and long-effect TE FSE sequences appear to have less contrast and fat suppression than conventional spin-echo sequences even though the sequences can be performed in half the time (see Fig. 7-4). When we select FSE sequences, we generally add fat suppression. Rubin et al. (45) reported that FSE sequences were less useful than conventional spin-echo sequences for detection of meniscal tears. More recently, Escobedo et al. (52) reported that FSE sequences with a short echo train were comparable to proton density (SE 2,000/20) images and could be performed in 5 minutes and 20 seconds compared to 7 minutes and 38 seconds for spin-echo sequences.

GRE techniques (Fig. 7-4) have seen increasing use for musculoskeletal imaging in the last several years. They provide interesting capabilities in terms of contrast and speed. These techniques can be broadly divided into "steady state" sequences such as gradient-recalled steady state (GRASS) and fast imaging with steady-state free precession (FISP), and "spoiled" sequences such as fast low-angle single-shot (FLASH) and spoiled GRASS (see Chapter 2) (44,56,57).

Multislice GRE acquisitions can be performed in two ways: Sequentially acquiring each slice individually, or acquiring the slices in an interleaved fashion similar to multislice spin-echo imaging. In the first alternative, the TR must be very short so that the total imaging time to acquire the entire set of slices will not be excessively long. It turns out that for knee imaging with GREs, the short-TR, sequential, single-slice approach is less favorable than a long TR, multislice approach. In the specific application of knee

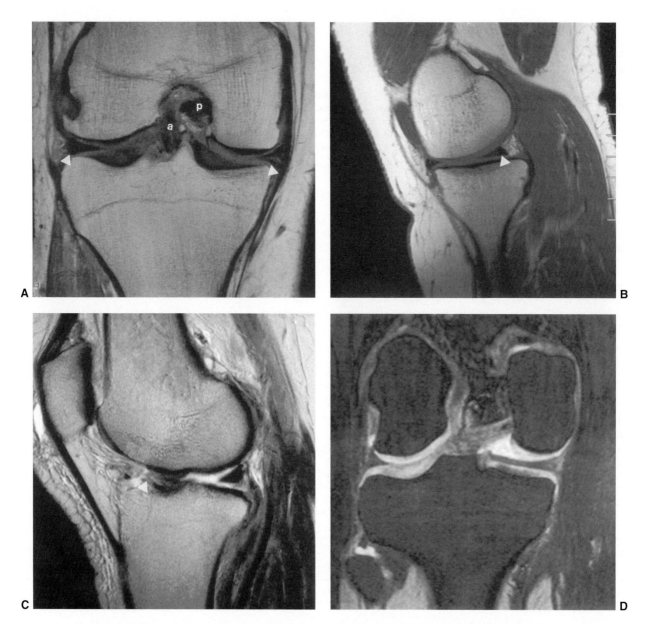

Figure 7-2   A: Coronal SE 450/15 image of the knee demonstrates normal signal intensity in the marrow. The menisci are low signal intensity and the articular cartilage is intermediate signal intensity. The cruciate ligaments (*a*, anterior; *p*, posterior) are seen in the intercondylar notch. The collateral ligaments (*arrowheads*) are also low signal intensity. **B:** Sagittal proton density (2,300/26) image of the posterior medial knee demonstrates the posterior horn of the medial meniscus with intrasubstance increased signal intensity (*arrowhead*), but not communication with the articular surface. **C:** Sagittal fast spin-echo T2-weighted sequence (3,300/80) image of the knee demonstrates abnormal signal and truncation of the anterior horn and body of the lateral meniscus (*arrowhead*). **D:** Coronal dual echo steady state image (three-dimensional, 23.87/6.73) demonstrates normal meniscal signal intensity and excellent cartilage detail.

imaging, the longer TR of the interleaved approach has the effect of improving the contrast and signal-to-noise characteristics of the images, compared with short TR gradient echoes (Table 7-1).

These long-TR, medium-TE GREs provide excellent contrast for delineating meniscal tears. An advantage of this technique is that special windowing of the images is not required at photography. Long-TR GRE sequences can provide very pronounced T2-weighted contrast for depicting

ligamentous lesions. Long-TR GRE images seem to have special capabilities for depicting chondral and osteochondral lesions as shown in these images, but these have not been fully explored as yet.

Most authors now advocate 3DFT acquisition for knee imaging (36,38–41,43,58). The great attraction of this technique is that a high-resolution volume data set can be processed retrospectively to generate any arbitrarily oriented plane of section (Table 7-1). Three-dimensional

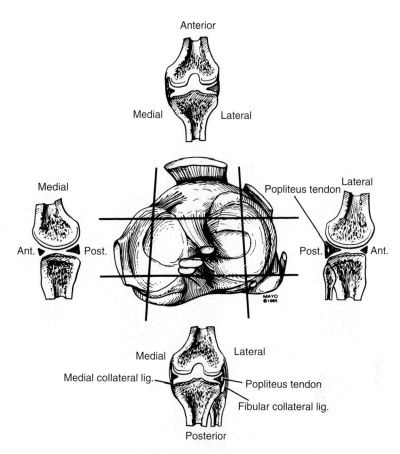

Anterior

Medial   Lateral

Medial

Ant.   Post.

Popliteus tendon   Lateral

Post.   Ant.

MAYO ©1985

Medial   Lateral

Medial collateral lig.

Popliteus tendon

Fibular collateral lig.

Posterior

Figure 7-3 Axial anatomy of the knee and selected coronal and sagittal sections.

imaging may be particularly useful for evaluating articular cartilage (see Fig. 7-5) (10,11,17,38–40,44,49,56,59).

The advantages of three-dimensional imaging are: The ability to acquire thin sections without gaps and the potential for three-dimensional rendering and reformatting. The disadvantage of 3DFT imaging is that the costs include a significantly larger requirement for resources such as computing power, memory, display, and storage. Other, less well-established concerns are that the examinations may take longer to interpret, given that more sections must be viewed, and that there may be a penalty in signal-to-noise and contrast, which accompanies the requirement for isotropic resolution in three-dimensional imaging. This is imposed by the short repetition time that must be used (57,60,61).

Additional sequences commonly employed or used as alternatives include FSE STIR sequences, FSE T2-weighted imaging, as well as occasionally performing conventional T2-weighted axial images for evaluation of mass lesions. Fast STIR sequences are useful for detection of subtle soft tissue and marrow abnormalities (34,62,63) (Table 7-1).

Gadolinium-diethylenetriamine pentaacetic acid (Gd-DTPA) has also been used to evaluate the knee. However, the need for intraarticular contrast medium for examinations of the knee has not been clearly established (18,19,50,64–67). Intravenous gadolinium may be useful in certain arthropathies for enhancing synovium and joint fluid (68–70).

There are many good approaches for imaging the knee. Techniques should be tailored to the specific clinical situation. Our current screening examinations (Table 7-1) include axial proton density FSE, sagittal FSE proton density and T2-weighted images with fat suppression and coronal T1-weighted and DESS (three-dimensional gradient echo) sequences. Additional technical considerations will be discussed in more detail with specific knee disorders.

ANATOMY

The multiple image planes that are used to evaluate the knee increase the need to completely understand the articular and periarticular anatomy of the knee in all commonly used image planes (see Figs. 7-6 to 7-8) (55,71,72). In addition, a thorough knowledge of this anatomy is essential to properly select special image planes to demonstrate properly certain anatomic structures (73–76).

Bone and Articular Anatomy

The knee is formed by the femoral and tibial condylar articulations. The tibiofibular articulation (Fig. 7-7B), though often considered a part of the knee, is in fact not a portion of the true knee joint (77,78). The knee is primarily a hinge joint that is protected anteriorly and posteriorly by muscles

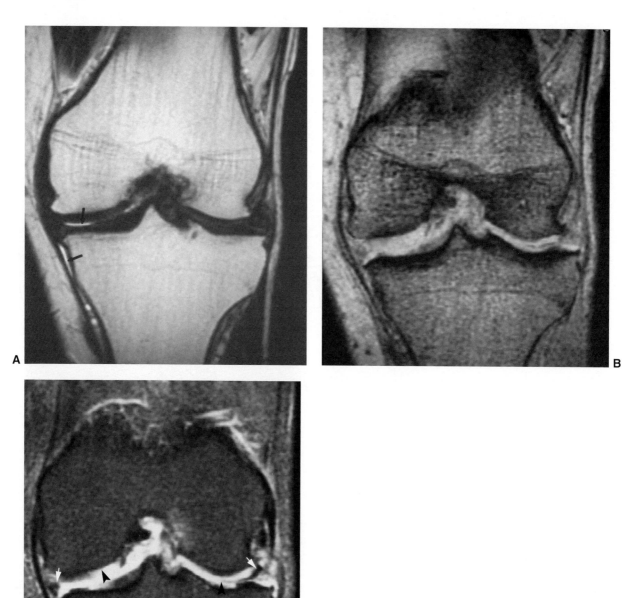

Figure 7-4 Coronal images of the knee with the same plane of section in a patient with meniscal tears and articular cartilage loss. **A:** Fast spin-echo (4,000/108) is similar in appearance to a T1-weighted spin-echo sequence (marrow and fat have high signal intensity) except for high signal intensity of joint fluid and vessels (*arrows*). Other intraarticular structures are not clearly defined. **B:** Gradient echo (700/31, flip angle 25°) and **(C)** fat-suppressed spin-echo (SE 2,000/80) images demonstrate the meniscal tears (*arrows*) and loss of articular cartilage (*arrowheads*) more clearly.

with special ligamentous attachments to the capsule. The articular surfaces of both the femoral condyles and tibial condyles are covered with hyaline cartilage. Hyaline cartilage has four zones with variations in chondrocytes, collagen fiber orientation, and proteoglycans. MR image features described in normal and abnormal articular cartilage are due to variation in normal content of hyaline cartilage. Normal cartilage is 60% to 80% water. Collagen makes up 50% of the weight of cartilage and proteoglycans contribute 30% to 35% (65,79).

The femoral condyles are oval anteriorly and rounded posteriorly to provide increased stability in extension and increased motion and rotation in flexion (Fig. 7-6) (77). The medial femoral condyle is larger and important in load transmission across the knee. Medial and lateral tibial condyles form the expanded articular portion of the tibia. The condyles are separated by the intracondylar eminence that serves for cruciate attachment. The intercondylar eminence has medial and lateral tubercles (Fig. 7-8). The weight-bearing surfaces of the tibial and femoral condyles

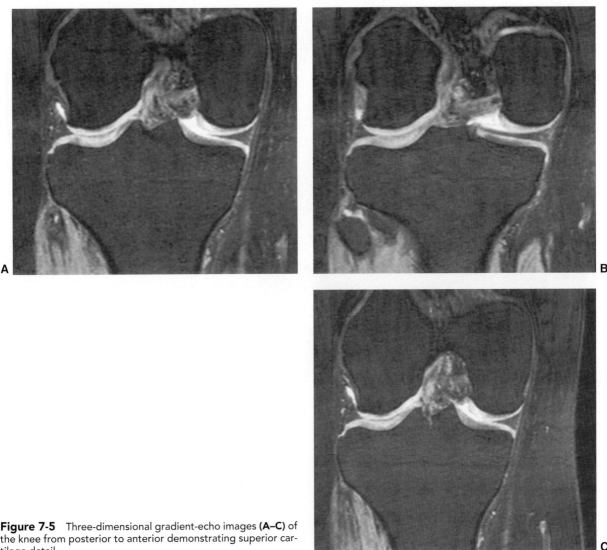

Figure 7-5 Three-dimensional gradient-echo images **(A–C)** of the knee from posterior to anterior demonstrating superior cartilage detail.

are separated by fibrocartilaginous menisci. The menisci are triangular when viewed tangentially and thicker laterally than medially (see Fig. 7-9) (33,77,78,80,81).

The patella is the largest sesamoid bone in the body and develops in the tendon of the quadriceps (extensor mechanism) (Figs. 7-6 and 7-7) (78,82). The patellar retinacula are formed by expansions in the quadriceps tendon and fascia that extend from the sides of the patella to the femoral and tibial condyles (Fig. 7-6). The patella is divided into several Wiberg types. The medial and lateral facets are of equal size in type I. Type II, the most common configuration, has a smaller medial than lateral facet (Fig. 7-6). Type III has a very small medial facet that is convex and a large, concave lateral facet. Both facets are covered with hyaline cartilage and most easily seen on axial MR images (Fig. 7-6) (77,83,84).

The capsule of the knee is lined by synovial membrane that is subdivided into several communicating compartments (78). Anteriorly, the synovial membrane is attached to the articular margins of the patella (see Fig. 7-10A).

From the medial and lateral sides, the synovium extends circumferentially (Fig. 7-10C), in contact with the retinacula (Fig. 7-6). From the inferior aspect of the patella, the synovial membrane extends downward and backward and is separated from the patellar ligament by the infrapatellar fat pad (Fig. 7-10A and B). At the lower margin of the patella there is a central fold, the intrapatellar synovial fold that is also sometimes referred to as the ligamentum mucosum (Fig. 7-10B). This structure is joined by two lesser alar folds or plicae that extend down from the sides of the patella. As the synovial fold extends into the femoral notch, it attaches to the intracondylar fossa of the femur anteriorly (Fig. 7-10A and B). The membrane fans out at its sides medially and laterally so that it covers the front and sides of the femoral attachment of the posterior cruciate ligament (PCL) (Fig. 7-10D and E). Inferiorly, the synovial membrane continues down to the intracondylar area of the tibia covering the attachment of the ACL (Fig. 7-10B and E). Due to the fact that the fold attaches to both the femur and the tibia, it in fact divides

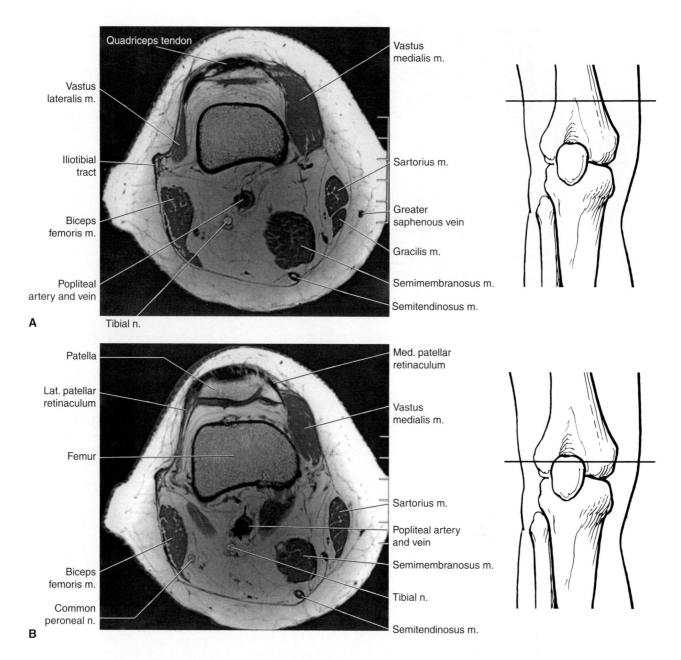

Figure 7-6 Axial SE 500/15 MR images through the knee with level of section demonstrated. **A:** Axial image through the distal femoral shaft above the patella. **B:** Axial image through the upper patella. **C:** Axial image through the upper femoral condyles and patella. **D:** Axial image through the femoral condyles and lower patella. **E:** Axial image through the lower femoral condyles below the patella. **F:** Axial image and illustration through the upper tibia. **G:** Axial image and illustration through the tibia and fibular head. **H:** Axial image through the upper tibia and fibula.

the knee into medial and lateral synovial cavities separated by the extrasynovial space that houses the cruciate ligaments (Fig. 7-10E) (28,77,78,85).

The synovial membrane extends superiorly from the upper margin of the patella for a variable distance and is closely applied to the quadriceps muscle (Fig. 7-10A and B). It then reflects onto the anterior aspect of the femur. This forms the suprapatellar bursa that lies between the quadriceps and the front of the femur (Fig. 7-10A and B). Along

the medial, lateral, and posterior aspects of the capsule, the synovial membrane attaches to the femur at the edges of the articular surfaces posteriorly. Medially and laterally it passes from the articular margins inferiorly to attach to the articular margins of the tibial condyles (Fig. 7-10D). The intrasynovial space that extends from the intracondylar fossa superiorly to the intracondylar area of the tibia inferiorly houses the cruciate ligaments. The cruciate ligaments are, therefore, covered superiorly, medially, laterally, and anteriorly by synovial

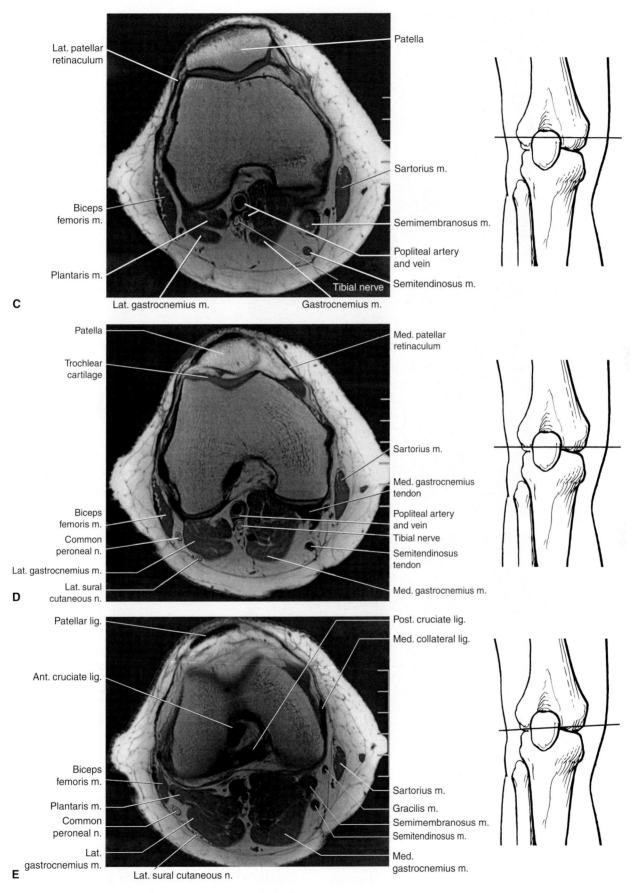

Lat. patellar retinaculum

Patella

Sartorius m.

Semimembranosus m.

Biceps femoris m.

Popliteal artery and vein

Plantaris m.

Semitendinosus m.

Tibial nerve

C   Lat. gastrocnemius m.   Gastrocnemius m.

Patella

Med. patellar retinaculum

Trochlear cartilage

Sartorius m.

Med. gastrocnemius tendon

Biceps femoris m.

Popliteal artery and vein

Common peroneal n.

Tibial nerve

Lat. gastrocnemius m.

Semitendinosus tendon

Lat. sural cutaneous n.

Med. gastrocnemius m.

D

Patellar lig.

Post. cruciate lig.

Med. collateral lig.

Ant. cruciate lig.

Biceps femoris m.

Plantaris m.

Sartorius m.

Common peroneal n.

Gracilis m.

Semimembranosus m.

Semitendinosus m.

Lat. gastrocnemius m.

Med. gastrocnemius m.

E   Lat. sural cutaneous n.

Figure 7-6   (*continued*)

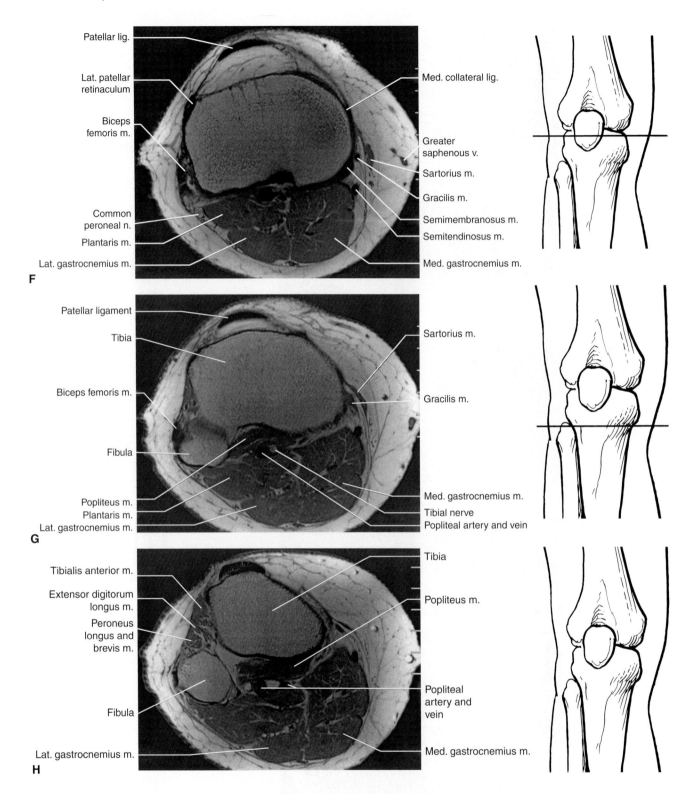

Patellar lig.

Lat. patellar retinaculum

Biceps femoris m.

Common peroneal n.

Plantaris m.

Lat. gastrocnemius m.

Med. collateral lig.

Greater saphenous v.

Sartorius m.

Gracilis m.

Semimembranosus m.

Semitendinosus m.

Med. gastrocnemius m.

F

Patellar ligament

Tibia

Biceps femoris m.

Fibula

Popliteus m.
Plantaris m.
Lat. gastrocnemius m.

Sartorius m.

Gracilis m.

Med. gastrocnemius m.
Tibial nerve
Popliteal artery and vein

G

Tibialis anterior m.

Extensor digitorum longus m.

Peroneus longus and brevis m.

Fibula

Lat. gastrocnemius m.

Tibia

Popliteus m.

Popliteal artery and vein

Med. gastrocnemius m.

H

Figure 7-6 (*continued*)

membrane but not posteriorly (Fig. 7-10A, B, and E). Posterolaterally, the synovial membrane is separated from the fibrous capsule by the popliteus tendon. It is not unusual to identify a bursa along the popliteus tendon that communicates with the joint space posterolaterally. The other common bursae about the knee are listed in Table 7-2 (see Fig. 7-11) (28,78). There is also a lateral synovial extension that may be implicated in iliotibial band syndrome (86).

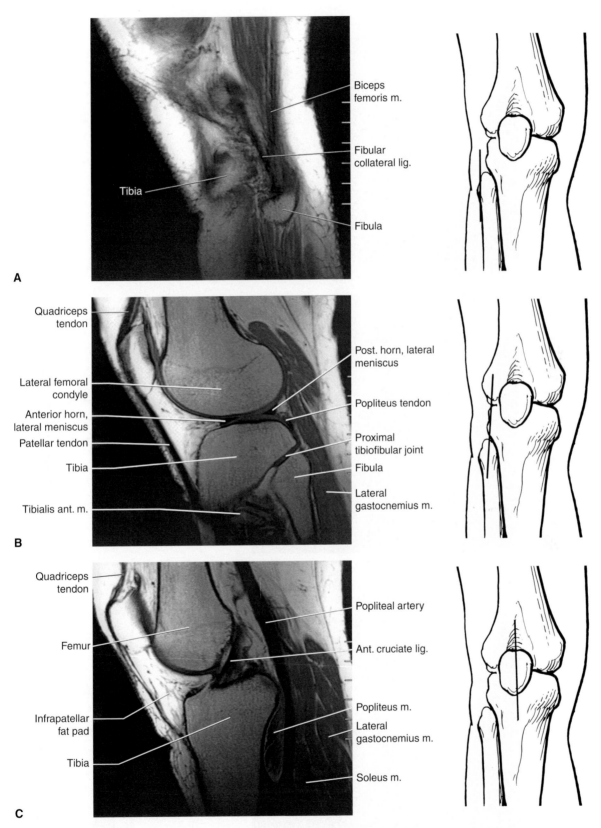

Figure 7-7 Sagittal SE 500/15 images of the knee from lateral to medial with plane of section demonstrated. **A:** Sagittal image through the lateral margin of the fibular head. **B:** Sagittal image through the fibular head. **C:** Sagittal image through the anterior cruciate ligament. **D:** Sagittal image through the posterior cruciate ligament. **E:** Sagittal image through the medial compartment. **F:** Sagittal image through the medial soft tissues and margin of the femoral condyle.

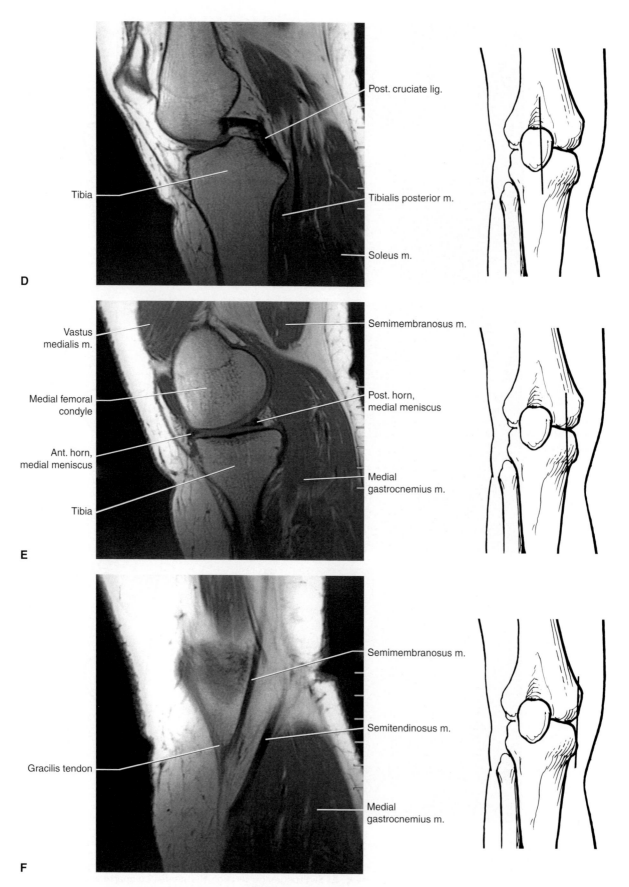

D

Post. cruciate lig.

Tibialis posterior m.

Soleus m.

Tibia

E

Vastus
medialis m.

Medial femoral
condyle

Ant. horn,
medial meniscus

Tibia

Semimembranosus m.

Post. horn,
medial meniscus

Medial
gastrocnemius m.

F

Gracilis tendon

Semimembranosus m.

Semitendinosus m.

Medial
gastrocnemius m.

Figure 7-7   (continued)

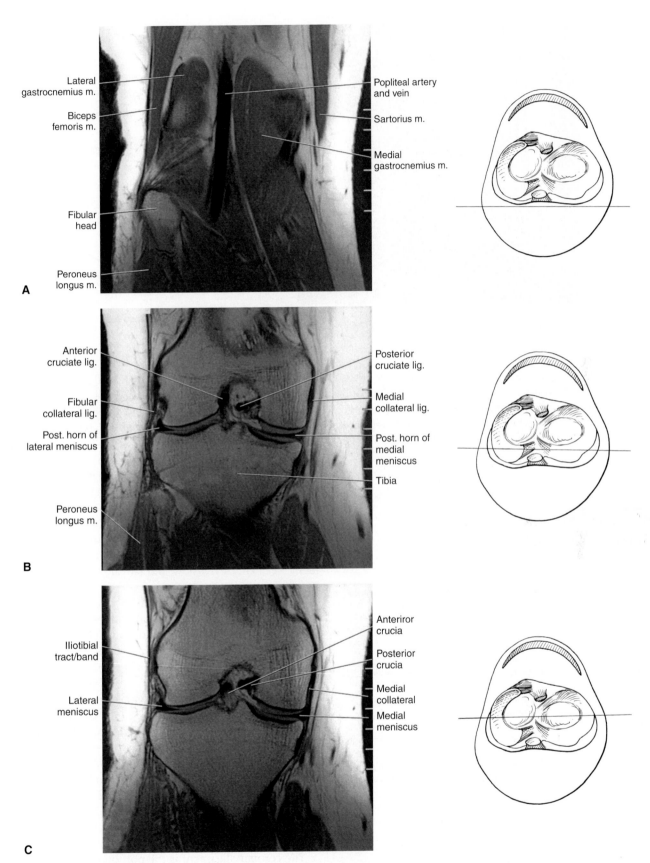

Lateral gastrocnemius m.

Biceps femoris m.

Fibular head

Peroneus longus m.

Popliteal artery and vein

Sartorius m.

Medial gastrocnemius m.

A

Anterior cruciate lig.

Fibular collateral lig.

Post. horn of lateral meniscus

Peroneus longus m.

Posterior cruciate lig.

Medial collateral lig.

Post. horn of medial meniscus

Tibia

B

Iliotibial tract/band

Lateral meniscus

Anteriror crucia

Posterior crucia

Medial collateral

Medial meniscus

C

Figure 7-8 Coronal SE 500/15 images of the knee from posterior to anterior with level of section demonstrated. **A:** Coronal image through the soft tissues and fibular head. **B:** Coronal image through the posterior tibia and femoral condyles. **C:** Coronal image through the mid joint. **D:** Coronal image through the anterior joint.

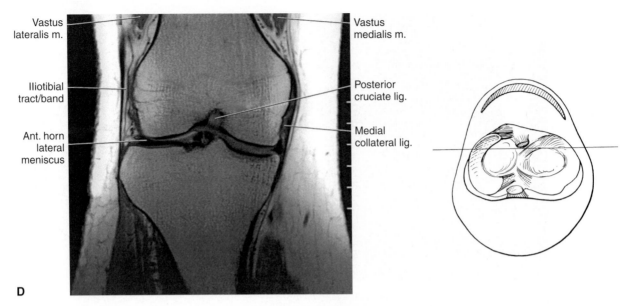

Vastus lateralis m.

Vastus medialis m.

Iliotibial tract/band

Posterior cruciate lig.

Ant. horn lateral meniscus

Medial collateral lig.

D

Figure 7-8 *(continued)*

The fibrous capsule and periarticular ligaments of the knee are important for support and must be understood if one is to completely evaluate MR images of the knee (90–95). Anteriorly, the knee capsule is essentially replaced by the quadriceps and its tendon, the patella, and the patellar

ligament and retinacula (Figs. 7-6 and 7-11) (78,96). Medially and laterally the capsule is attached to the femur just outside the synovial membrane and extends from the articular margin of the femoral condyles to the articular margin of the tibial condyles (Figs. 7-10 and 7-11). Laterally, the primary ligamentous support is provided by the lateral or fibular collateral ligament. The lateral collateral ligament is clearly separated from the capsule (Fig. 7-11). The posterolateral support structures are restraints to prevent varus angulation and external rotation of the tibia (91,97). The main restraints are the fabellofibular and arcuate ligaments and the popliteal muscle and tendon (98). The coronary ligament, ligament of Winslow, and lateral collateral ligament are secondary restraints (78).

The medial capsule is supported by the medial or tibial collateral ligament. Unique medial features include the fact that the medial collateral ligament (MCL) blends with the capsule and the medial meniscus is attached to the capsule (Fig. 7-11A). The posteromedial supporting structures are classically divided into three layers (77,90). The first or superficial layer is composed of fascial extensions from the sartorius and vastus medialis (77,78,90). The intermediate layer consists of the MCL and posterior oblique ligament. The MCL (Figs. 7-8D and 7-11A and B) extends from the femoral condyle to attach to the tibia 5 to 7 cm below the joint line and deep to the gracilis and semitendinosis tendons. The posterior oblique ligament lies posterior to the MCL and extends from the adductor tubercle to the posteromedial meniscus (90). The third or deep layer is the joint capsule (77,90,99).

The coronary ligament is the portion of the capsule to which the meniscus is attached to the tibia (Fig. 7-11A). This ligament has some laxity that allows slight motion of the menisci on the tibia (77,78).

TABLE 7-2

BURSAE ABOUT THE KNEE

Anterior

Prepatellar	Between patella and skin
Retropatellar	Between patellar ligament and upper tibia
Pretibial	Between tibial tuberosity and skin
Suprapatellar[a]	Between quadriceps and femur (communicates with joint)

Lateral

Gastrocnemius	Between large gastrocnemius and capsule
Fibular	Between fibular collateral ligament and biceps tendon
Fibulopopliteal	Between fibular collateral ligament and popliteus tendon
Popliteal[a]	Between popliteus tendon and lateral femoral condyle (communicates with joint)

Medial

Gastrocnemius[a]	Between medial head of gastrocnemius and capsule (often communicates with joint)
Pes anserine	Between tibial collateral ligament and gracilis, sartorius, and semitendinosus tendons
Semimembranous-tibial collateral ligament	Between semimembranosus tendon and medial collateral ligament

[a] Communicating bursae.
From references 78, 80, and 87–89.

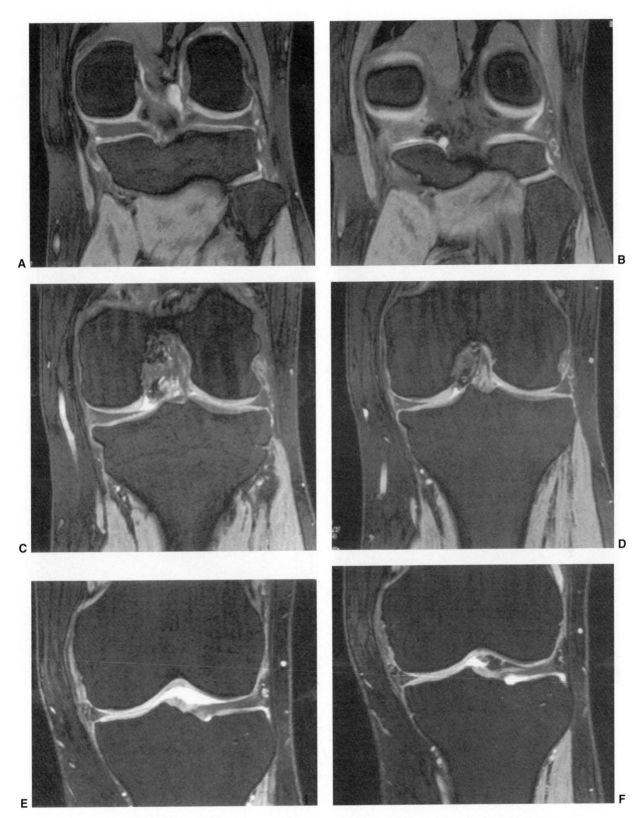

Figure 7-9 Coronal DESS three-dimensional (23.87/6.73, field of view 14 cm, matrix 256 × 192, two acquisitions) images **(A–F)** of the knee demonstrating both medial and lateral menisci and superior cartilage detail.

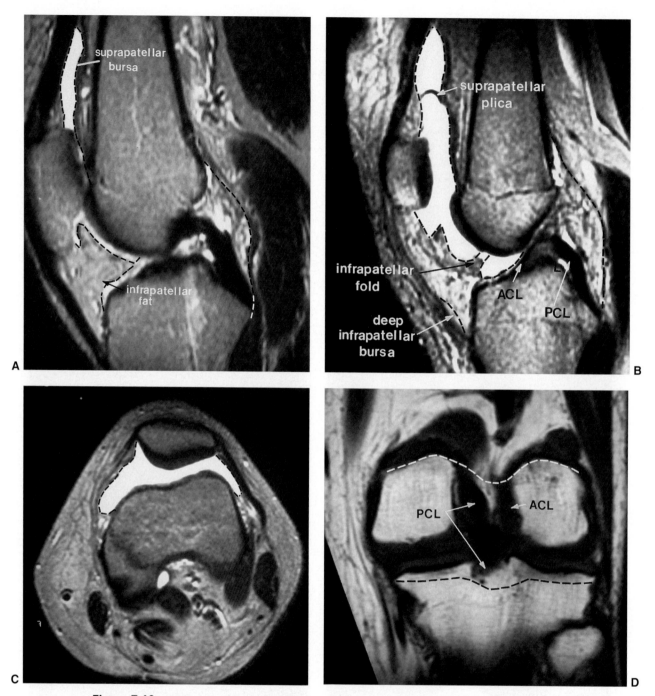

Figure 7-10 MR images of the knee demonstrating the synovial and capsular attachments (*dotted lines*) of the knee. **A:** Sagittal image in the plane of the posterior cruciate ligament. **B:** Sagittal image in the plane of the anterior cruciate ligament (ACL, anterior cruciate ligament; PCL, posterior cruciate ligament). **C:** Axial image at the patellar level demonstrating the synovial reflection (*broken lines*). **D:** Posterior coronal image demonstrating the posterior synovial and capsular margins (*broken lines*) (ACL, anterior cruciate ligament; PCL, posterior cruciate ligament). **E:** Axial image of the tibial articular surface demonstrating meniscal and cruciate attachments and synovial reflections.

The cruciate ligaments are intraarticular but lie outside the synovial compartment of the knee (Fig. 7-10E) and are covered by synovial membrane anteriorly, medially and laterally, but not posteriorly. The ACL arises from the anterior nonarticular surface of the intracondylar area of the tibia adjacent to the medial condyle. It extends obliquely, superiorly, and posteriorly to attach the medial side of the lateral femoral condyle. The ACL has significant variability in its appearance and is typically more slender and longer than the posterior cruciate. This and its oblique course account for some of the difficulty encountered in evaluating this structure with MRI (Fig. 7-11A) (1,77,78).

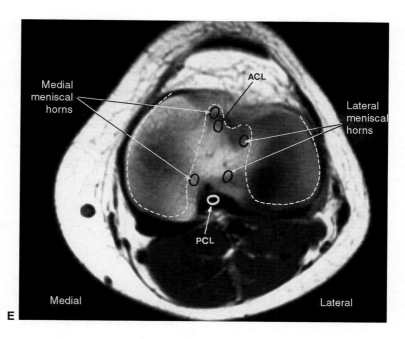

Figure 7-10 (*continued*) **E**

The PCL arises from the posterior intercondylar area and passes obliquely upward and forward in a nearly sagittal plane to attach to the anterior intercondylar fossa of the lateral surface of the medial femoral condyle (Figs. 7-8 and 7-11). The posterior cruciate, because of its larger transverse diameter and straight sagittal course, is consistently identified on sagittal MR images (Fig. 7-8) (1).

The fibrocartilaginous menisci have a differing shape, with the medial meniscus being larger and thicker in transverse diameter posteriorly than anteriorly (Figs. 7-7, 7-9, and 7-11A). The lateral meniscus is more C-shaped and uniform in width (Fig. 7-11A). There are several ligamentous attachments that may cause confusion on MR images. For example, the posterior horn of the lateral meniscus is closely applied to the PCL and may give off a band of fibers, termed the meniscofemoral ligament, that follows the PCL to its attachment on the femur. Between the anterior horns of the medial and lateral meniscus there is a transverse band of fibers termed the transverse ligament of the knee. This can easily be confused with an anterior meniscal tear, especially on the medial side (see Fig. 7-12) (77,78). Another variant, the meniscomeniscal ligament, may also be confused with meniscal pathology. The medial meniscomeniscal ligament extends from the anterior horn of the medial meniscus to the posterior horn of the lateral meniscus. The lateral meniscomeniscal ligament extends from the anterolateral to posteromedial meniscus (100).

Muscles About the Knee

The muscles of the thigh, calf, and foot and ankle are discussed in Chapters 6 and 8. Therefore, a thorough review of their origins and insertions would be redundant. However, it is important to review the muscles about the

knee and their neurovascular and biomechanical function. Chief movements at the knee are those of flexion and extension. Mild rotation, however, can occur. If one starts from the flexed position (see Fig. 7-13), the posterior condyles of the femur are in contact with the posterior horns of both menisci. The medial and lateral collateral ligaments are also relaxed in this position. In full flexion, both anterior and PCLs are taut. In this flexed position more rotary motion is allowed. As one goes from the flexed to the extended position, the femoral condyles shift such that the more anterior parts of the menisci and tibial condyles are now in contact (Fig. 7-13) (77,78).

The primary flexors of the knee are the hamstring muscle group (semimembranosus, semitendinosus, and biceps femoris) along with the gracilis and sartorius (Figs. 7-6 to 7-8). The popliteus muscle has some significance in the early phases of flexion due to its rotary action upon the femur or tibia (Table 7-3) (98). In the nonweight-bearing state, the gastrocnemius muscle is also utilized in flexion of the knee. The quadriceps group is the chief extensor of the knee (Figs. 7-6 to 7-8) (Table 7-3) (77,78).

Neurovascular Supply of the Knee

The arterial supply about the knee is primarily via branch vessels of the distal superficial femoral and popliteal arteries (see Fig. 7-14). Superiorly there are medial and lateral genicular arteries as well as muscular branches at the level of the knee joint. Inferiorly, medial and lateral inferior genicular arteries supply the knee. There are numerous anastomoses that interconnect this vascular supply (78).

Innervation of the knee (Table 7-3) is primarily by branches of the femoral, obturator, and sciatic nerves.

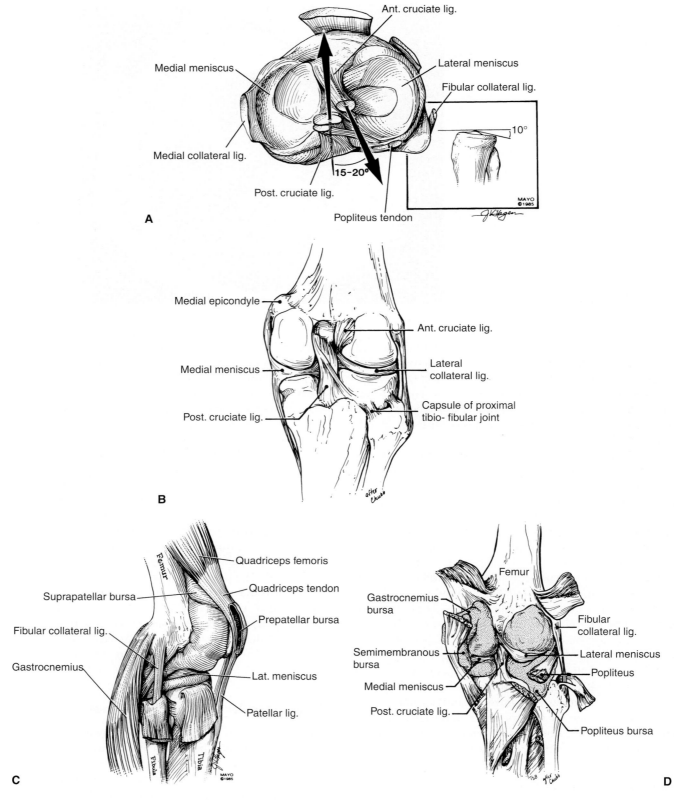

Figure 7-11 Axial (**A**), coronal (**B**), sagittal (**C**), and posterior (**D**) illustrations of the ligaments, menisci, and bursae of the knee.

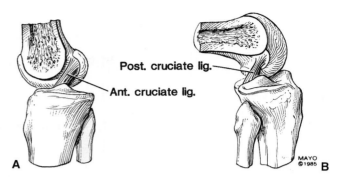

Figure 7-13 Sagittal illustrations of the knee and cruciate ligaments in the extended **(A)** and flexed **(B)** positions.

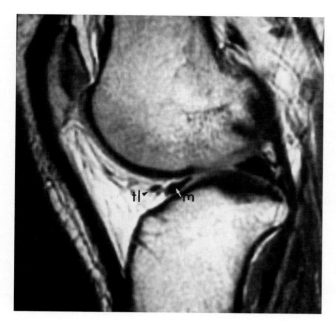

Figure 7-12 Sagittal SE 500/20 image of the knee demonstrating a normal anterior horn of the medial meniscus (*m*) and the transverse ligament (*tl*). This should not be confused with a meniscal tear.

Posterolaterally, recurrent branches of the peroneal nerve also supply the knee (77,78).

PITFALLS

The majority of the pitfalls in evaluating the knee are related to normal anatomy or variants and artifacts created

by flow, motion, and software problems (101–105). Partial volume effects must also be considered when evaluating the knee. As with any anatomic region, failure to compare MR images with routine radiographs or other available imaging studies can result in significant errors in interpretation.

Problems with flow artifacts occur less frequently during examination of the knee than in the more peripheral extremities, where the number of vascular structures per unit area is more numerous (see Chapters 3 and 11). The largest problem with flow artifact occurs in the sagittal plane, where the midline anatomy can be distorted by flow artifact from the popliteal artery (see Fig. 7-15). This can be corrected by swapping the phase to the superior inferior direction instead of the anteroposterior (AP) direction (3,106). The artifact can also be reduced to some degree by placing the patient prone. In the latter situation, the pulsatile effect of the

TABLE 7-3
KNEE FLEXORS AND EXTENSORS

Muscle	Origin	Insertion	Innervation
Flexors			
Semitendinosus	Posteromedial ischial tuberosity	Medial tibia posterior to gracilis and sartorius	Tibial nerve (L5–S1)
Biceps femoris	2 head: long head with semitendinosus, short head — midlinea aspera	Fibular head	Peroneal (L5–S1)
Semimembranosus	Posterolateral ischial tuberosity, medial meniscus	Proximal medial tibia	Tibial (L5–S1)
Gracilis	Inferior pubic ramus near symphysis	Medial upper tibia between sartorius and semitendinosus	Obturator (L3–L4)
Sartorius	Anterior superior iliac spine	Upper medial tibia above gradilis and semitendinosus	Femoral (L3–L4)
Extensors			
Rectus femoris	Anterior inferior iliac spine	Quadriceps tendon to patella	Femoral (L3–L4)
Vastus lateralis	Below greater trochanter	Quadriceps tendon to patella	Femoral (L3–L4)
Vastus medialis	Below lesser trochanter	Quadriceps tendon to patella	Femoral (L3–L4)
Vastus intermedius	Midfemur	Quadriceps tendon to patella	Femoral (L3–L4)

From Rosse C, Rosse PG. *Hollinshead's textbook of anatomy*. Philadelphia, PA: Lippincott–Raven, 1997.

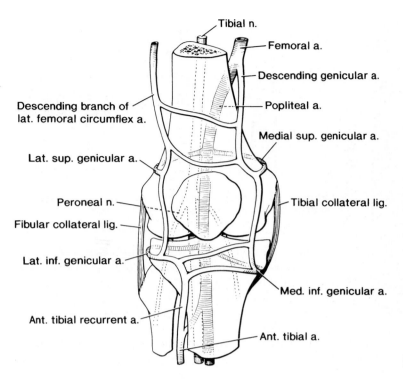

Figure 7-14   Neurovascular anatomy of the knee.

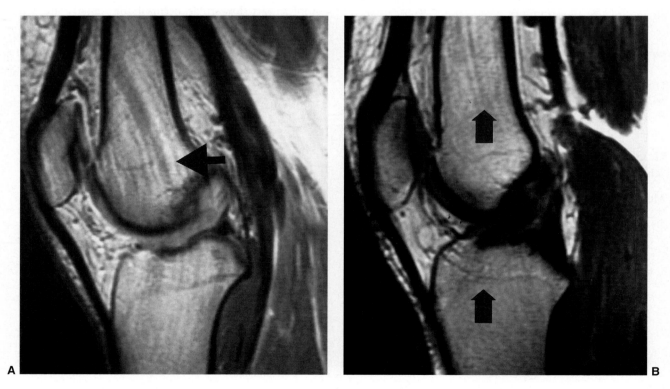

Figure 7-15   **A:** Sagittal proton density image of the knee demonstrating pulsatile motion artifact from the popliteal artery. The phase encoding is in the anteroposterior direction (*arrow*). Artifact is decreased **(B)** by switching the phase encoding to the superior-inferior (*arrows*) direction.

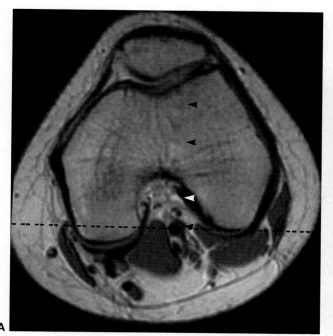
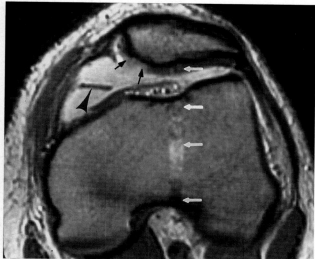

Figure 7-16 **A:** Axial proton density image in a patient referred for patellofemoral pain. The focal defect in the lateral femoral condyle (*large arrowhead*) is due to flow artifact (*small arrows*). This should not be confused with an articular defect. This problem can be avoided by swapping phase direction to the transverse (*dotted line*) plane. **B:** Axial T2-weighted image through the patellofemoral compartment. There is an effusion, a medial plica (*arrowhead*) and grade IV chondro-malacia on the medial patellar facet (*small arrows*). Flow artifact (*white arrows*) with phase encoding in the anteroposterior direction creates a false lesion (increased signal) in the lateral facet.

popliteal artery does not create as much motion artifact as when the patient is supine (1,3).

Flow artifact can create false positive interpretations if the phase direction is not considered. For example, when patellofemoral disease is being evaluated in the axial plane, phase encoding should be in the "X" or transverse direction (see Fig. 7-16). This prevents the artifact from entering the area of interest.

Marrow changes have also been reported in highly trained athletes and marathon runners (see Fig. 7-17). Shellock et al. (107), reported an increase in hematopoietic marrow in 43% of marathon runners, compared to only 15% of patients with knee disorders and 3% of normal healthy patients. This marrow conversion pattern may be due to "sports anemia," which has been attributed to numerous problems such as hemolysis, hematuria, increased plasma volume, and gastrointestinal blood loss (107).

A significant number of interpretation errors are related to lack of familiarity with normal anatomy and anatomic variants (Table 7-4) (31,73,101,104,108–110). The majority of these pitfalls are related to normal variations in the appearance of the menisci and/or variation in lesser known ligaments associated with the menisci (73,111). There is vascular tissue and variable amounts of fat and synovial tissue near the attachment of the menisci, especially the

TABLE 7-4

COMMON VARIANTS AND ARTIFACTS IN MR IMAGING OF THE KNEE

Popliteal tendon sheath near posterior horn of lateral meniscus
Accessory popliteus muscle
Meniscofemoral ligament variations
Transverse ligament
Meniscomeniscal ligaments
Increased signal near central attachment in anterior horns of lateral meniscus
Truncation artifact
Magic angle effect

From references 114–118.

posterior medial meniscus (112,113). Signal intensity created by this tissue is a more difficult problem on nontangential sagittal and coronal images as tissue is projected between the meniscus and the margin of the capsule. This should not be confused with a peripheral tear in the meniscus (see Fig. 7-18). Typically this tissue has the appearance of fat or similar signal intensity to fat on T1- and T2-weighted

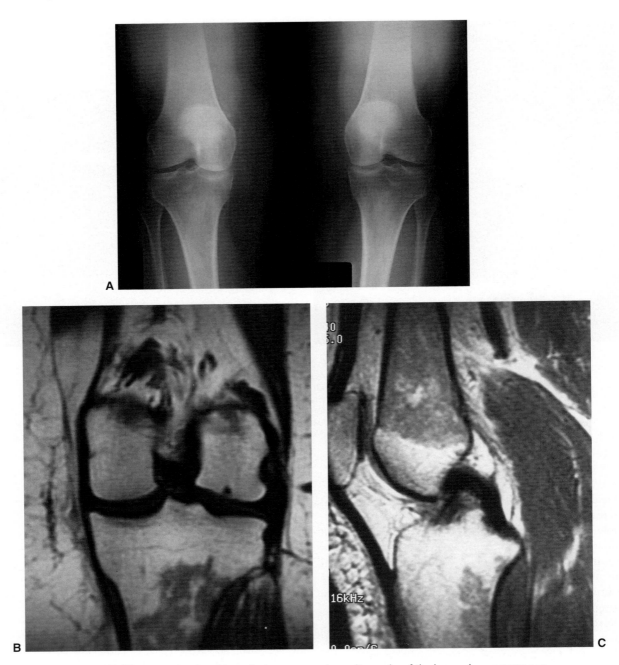

Figure 7-17 Normal male athlete. **A:** Anteroposterior radiographs of the knees demonstrate normal marrow and medial compartment narrowing. T1-weighted coronal **(B)** and sagittal **(C)** images show decreased signal intensity in the femoral metaphysis and diaphysis and upper tibia due to red marrow reconversion.

images. Meniscal tears are seen as an area of high signal intensity, similar to fluid. Fat-suppression techniques can reduce confusion in this region.

As with arthrography, evaluation of the posterior lateral meniscus can be difficult due to the popliteus tendon and its sheath (Table 7-4) that pass between the capsule and meniscus posteriorly. This should not be mistaken for a meniscal tear (see Fig. 7-19) (119–121). Additional anatomic structures that can cause confusion are the inferior lateral geniculate vessels that course along the margin of the lateral meniscus anteriorly. The signal intensity of these vessels can give the appearance of a peripheral detachment (Figs. 7-14 and 7-20) (112). Irregular increased signal intensity may also be seen in normal anterior lateral menisci near the central attachment. The transverse meniscal ligament is seen anteriorly and can be confused with a horizontal tear in the anterior horn of the meniscus (Fig. 7-12) (73,109,122).

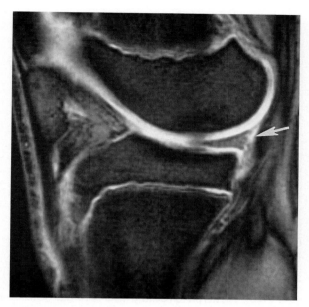

Figure 7-18 Sagittal gradient-echo image of the posterior medial meniscus demonstrating increased signal intensity at the meniscosynovial junction (*arrow*), which can be confused with a tear.

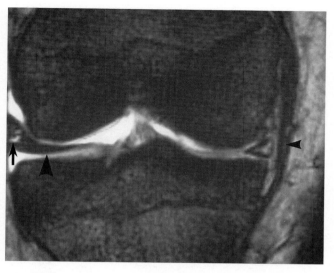

Figure 7-20 Coronal gradient-echo image of the knee demonstrating a discoid lateral meniscus (*large arrowhead*). Note the inferior genicular vessels (*black arrow*), which should not be confused with a tear. Medially (*arrowhead*) there is fat between the fibers of the medial collateral ligament that is normal.

Discoid menisci can cause significant problems if one does not consider this variant. Discoid menisci are more common laterally and occur in 1% to 2% of arthrographic and 2% to 5% of surgical series. The meniscus has a wafer-like appearance on the coronal T1-weighted and DESS images (see Fig. 7-20) and projects farther into the joint space on sagittal images. Discoid menisci are more prone to tears and are important to recognize (62,73,123).

Other meniscal or perimeniscal features have also been described that can be confused with pathology. These include vacuum phenomena, truncation artifacts, the "magic angle" effect, and artifacts created by recent orthopedic interventions (62,73,124–126).

Turner et al. (126) described truncation artifacts in the meniscus on sagittal images when using 128 × 256 matrix and phase encoding in the superior-inferior (SI) direction. This subtle linear area of high signal intensity (see Fig. 7-21) is commonly identified two pixels from the meniscal joint fluid interface. This defect can be seen extending beyond the meniscal margins when images are optimally windowed.

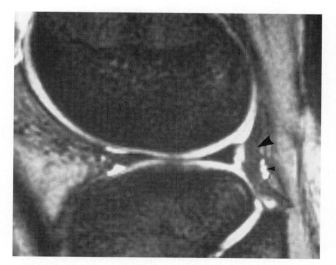

Figure 7-19 Sagittal gradient-echo image of the knee. The popliteus tendon (*large arrowhead*) and tendon sheath pass between the lateral meniscus and capsule. This should not be mistaken for a meniscal tear. The small areas of high signal intensity (*small arrowhead*) are due to the inferior genicular vessels.

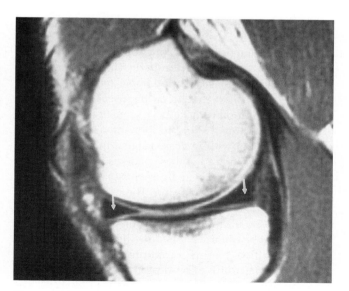

Figure 7-21 Sagittal proton density image of the knee using a 128 × 256 matrix and 16-cm field of view. The phase encoding is in the superior-inferior (SI) direction. The truncation artifact creates a faint linear area of increased signal intensity approximately 2 pixels from the meniscal margin (*arrows*).

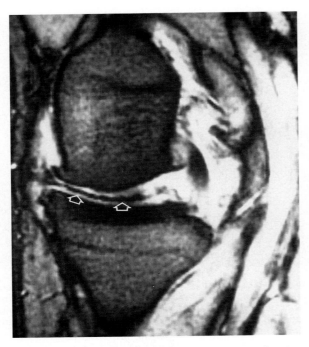

Figure 7-22 Oblique radial gradient-echo image showing an irregular low intensity structure (*open arrows*) extending into the joint from the meniscal margin due to vacuum phenomenon.

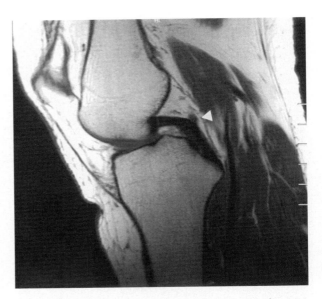

Figure 7-23 Sagittal proton density-weighted image demonstrating a normal posterior cruciate ligament. The ligament of Wrisberg (*arrowhead*) should not be confused with a posterior cruciate defect.

This artifact can be removed using 256 × 256 or 192 × 256 matrix and/or by switching the phase direction to the AP direction (126).

The vacuum phenomenon (see Fig. 7-22) can simulate discoid menisci or articular abnormalities in the joint (125). Careful review of multiple image planes should prevent interpretation errors in this setting.

The magic angle phenomenon has been described with tendons and menisci when collagen fibers are oriented approximately 55° to the static magnetic field. At this angle, the interactions that contribute to T2 relaxation among water protons are nulled. This can result in increased signal intensity on the upper medial portion of the posterior horn of the lateral meniscus (124). This is particularly common with short TE sequences. Peterfy et al. (124) reported this finding in 74% of 42 patients. The meniscal segment with increased signal intensity was oriented 55° to 60° in 80% of these patients (124).

Variations in the cruciate ligaments and collateral ligaments may also cause confusion. The main problem with the ACL is its oblique course (Fig. 7-11A). This can result in incomplete visualization of the ligament. Further oblique views should be obtained when the ligament is not completely identified. Normal variations in the posterior ligaments can be confused with partial tears in the PCL, a meniscal tear, or osteochondral fragment (127–129). The meniscal femoral ligament extends from near the posterior capsular attachment of the lateral meniscus to the medial femoral condyle and may have two branches. The most common segment is the ligament of Wrisberg that is seen just posterior to the PCL (see Fig. 7-23). This is evident in 23% to 32.5% of sagittal MR images and should not be confused with a partial tear (101,104,110,112,129). The anterior bundle of this ligament or the ligament of Humphrey is seen in 34% of patients (see Fig. 7-24) (104,110). This lies just anterior to the PCL.

Cho et al. (101) described several variations in the meniscofemoral ligaments. Familiarity with these variants

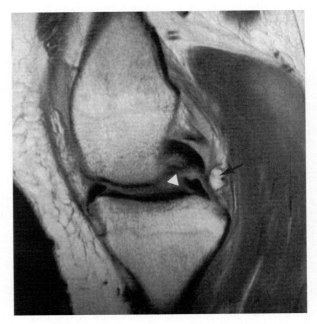

Figure 7-24 Sagittal proton density-weighted image of the posterior cruciate ligament. Note the ligament of Humphrey (*arrowhead*) anteriorly that should not be confused with a posterior cruciate abnormality. There is also a loose body (*arrow*) posteriorly.

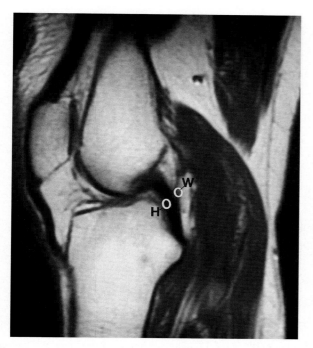

Figure 7-25 Sagittal proton density-weighted MR image demonstrating the usual locations of the meniscofemoral ligaments of Humphrey (*H*) and Wrisberg (*W*).

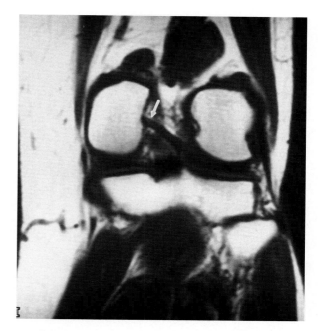

Figure 7-26 Coronal T1-weighted image demonstrating a type I meniscofemoral ligament inserting on the medial femoral condyle (*arrow*).

will assist in proper interpretation of coronal and sagittal MR images. Previous reports describe how meniscofemoral ligaments can be identified in 33% to 59% of patients. This report noted an incidence of 93% (101). The ligament of Wrisberg was identified in 90% and Humphrey in 17% of cases (see Fig. 7-25) (101). The meniscofemoral ligament can be classified into three types based on the proximal insertion. Type I ligaments (see Fig. 7-26) insert on the medial femoral condyle and were completely separated from the PCL. Type II ligaments blend with the PCL and are less vertically oriented (see Fig. 7-27). Type III ligaments blend with the inferior PCL forming a distal thickening on the sagittal images. Type I ligaments are most common (45%, Fig. 7-26). Type II ligaments were noted in 31% and type III in 21% of 90 cases (101).

There is frequently a linear collection of fat (Fig. 7-20) between the fibers of the MCL and between the lateral collateral ligament and capsule (104,110). These areas can be confused with tears. However, the fat signal is suppressed on T2-weighted sequences. Fluid and blood from a tear should have high signal intensity. Using double-echo or fat-suppressed sequences is useful, as fat signal is suppressed on the second echo and the signal intensity of fluid increases (1,62).

Deformity or buckling of the patellar tendon is usually due to position and should not be confused with pathology, especially if signal intensity is normal (see Fig. 7-28) (62). Subtle increase in signal intensity at the junction of the lower pole of the patella and tibial insertion is noted in 74% and 32% of normal patients. Increased signal intensity

that does not increase on the second echo using T2- or T2*-sequences should be insignificant (62).

Familiarity with the anatomic variations and normal ligamentous attachments in the knee is critical in evaluating MR images so that false positive interpretations do not occur. Recently, Duc et al. (103) described an accessory popliteal muscle. Other accessory muscles about the knee include the accessory semimembranosus and tensor fasciae suralis muscle (78,103). The accessory popliteus muscle merges with the popliteal muscle at the posteromedial

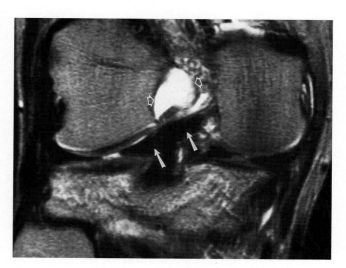

Figure 7-27 Coronal T2-weighted image demonstrating a type II meniscofemoral ligament (*arrows*) that is less vertically oriented than the type I in Fig. 7-26. There is high signal (*open arrows*) due to an ACL tear.

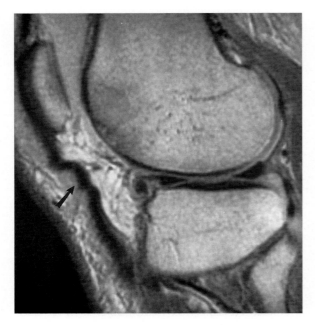

Figure 7-28 Sagittal proton density-weighted image demonstrating buckling of the patellar tendon (*arrow*) due to the extended position of the knee.

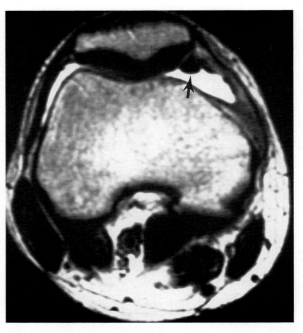

Figure 7-30 Axial T2-weighted image of the knee in a patient with knee pain. There is an effusion with a low signal intensity structure (*arrow*) medially. This could be mistaken for a loose body, medial patellar fragment, or thickened soft tissue structure. The signal abnormality was created by an air collection from arthroscopy two days previously.

aspect of the tibia. The muscle lies deep in the posterior compartment and may pass ventral or dorsal to the popliteal vessels (see Fig. 7-29) (103).

Artifacts can also be created by previous percutaneous (arthroscopy, injection) or open orthopedic procedures (see Figs. 7-30 to 7-32). The patient's history should be carefully reviewed or the case reviewed with the referring physician so errors in interpretation related to these procedures can be avoided. Technique can also be varied to

minimize metal artifact. Titanium causes less artifact than stainless steel implants (62). Suh et al. (130) found that metal oriented perpendicular to the magnet bore caused more significant artifact compared to metal parallel to the magnet bore. Therefore, modifying the patient position to change the orientation of the metal should

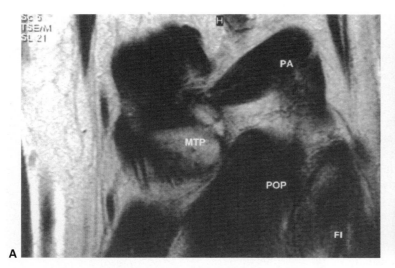

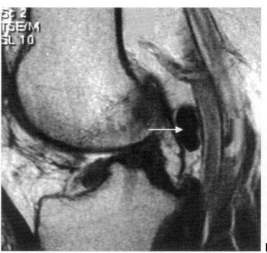

Figure 7-29 Accessory popliteal muscle. Coronal **(A)** and sagittal **(B)** T1-weighted images of the accessory popliteal muscle (*arrow* in **B**, *PA* in **A**). (From Duc SR, Wentz KU, Kach KP, et al. First report of an accessory popliteal muscle: detection with MRI. *Skeletal Radiol* 2004;33:429–431.)

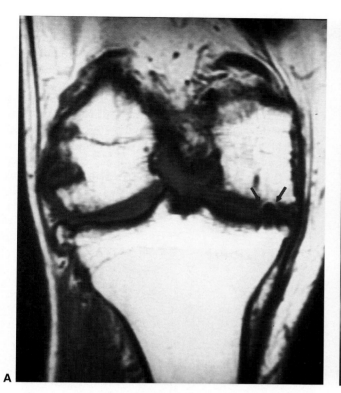

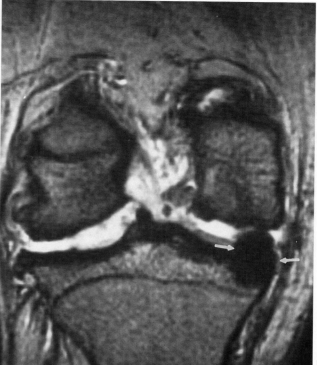

Figure 7-31 Patient with advanced osteoarthritis and a low signal intensity defect medially (*arrows*). The artifact is subtle on the coronal T1-weighted image **(A)** and more obvious on the gradient-echo image **(B)**. This artifact was created by a small metal remnant from previous arthroscopy.

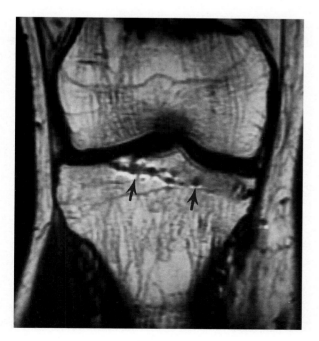

Figure 7-32 Coronal T1-weighted image demonstrating artifacts from a previous screw tract (*arrows*) created by residual microscopic metal fragments.

be considered prior to imaging. Variations in pulse sequence parameters and decreasing voxel size may also reduce metal artifacts (130).

APPLICATIONS

MRI provides excellent soft tissue contrast and is capable of evaluating the soft tissue and bony structures of the knee in multiple image planes, which provides significant advantages over conventional arthrography, computed tomography (CT), and other imaging techniques. The major application for MRI of the knee has been evaluation of patients with trauma or suspected internal derangement of the knee (4,30,131–136).

Most patients are referred for MRI of the knee to exclude tears in the menisci or ligamentous structures. Prior to the acceptance of MRI, arthrography was the imaging technique of choice for evaluation of the menisci. Accuracy of arthrography, especially using double contrast technique, approaches 95% for medial meniscal tears and approximately 90% for the lateral meniscus (74,77,117,137). However, this technique does have shortcomings in evaluating the collateral and cruciate ligaments, and the accuracy is reduced when large effusions or hemarthrosis are present (77). Arthroscopy usually is considered the gold standard for evaluating the accuracy of imaging techniques. However, keep in mind the accuracy of arthroscopy varies from 69% to 98% depending on the experience of the examiner (9,19).

MENISCAL LESIONS

Meniscal Tears

The most common causes of knee pain and disability are tears in the medial and/or lateral menisci. Pain due to meniscal tears can be mediated via the neurovascular bundle that is in the outer third of the meniscus or can occur when innervated synovium invaginates into a tear. Patients may also present with locking, which is usually related to a bucket-handle tear, or giving way, which is more often related to pain (7,77,135,138,139).

Prior to discussing the MR features of meniscal tears, it is essential to review certain anatomic and pathophysiology aspects of meniscal injury. The lateral meniscus is C-shaped and thicker than the medial meniscus. The transverse diameter is similar in the body, posterior, and anterior horns (see Fig. 7-33). The lateral meniscus is also less firmly attached to the capsule and is in fact separated posteriorly by the popliteus tendon and tendon sheath (Figs. 7-19, 7-21, and 7-33).

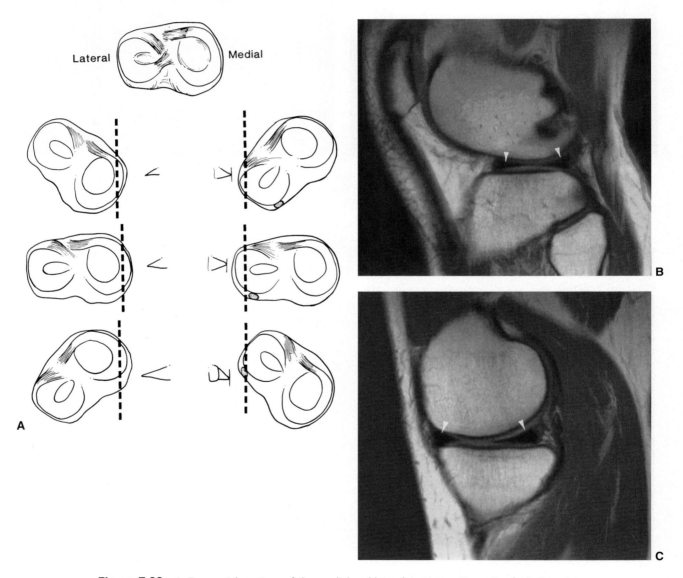

Figure 7-33   A: Tangential sections of the medial and lateral meniscus. (From Rand JA, Berquist TH. The knee. In: Berquist TH, ed. *Imaging of orthopedic trauma*, 2nd ed. New York: Raven Press, 1992:333–432.) **B:** Sagittal proton density-weighted image of the knee through the lateral meniscus demonstrating the similar size of the anterior and posterior horns (*small arrowheads*). **C:** Sagittal proton density-weighted image through the medial meniscus demonstrating the posterior horn is significantly larger than the anterior horn (*white arrowheads*).

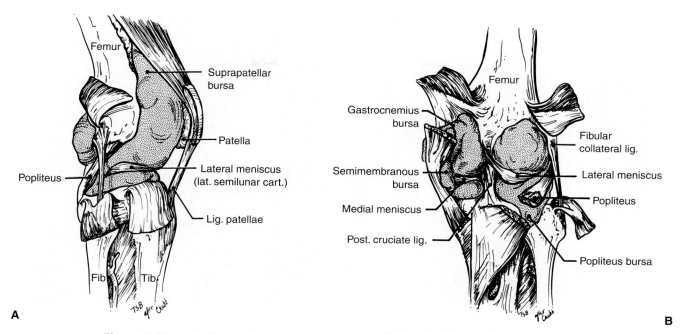

Figure 7-34 Lateral **(A)** and posterior **(B)** illustrations of the knee demonstrating the joint space and associated ligament and meniscal anatomy. (From Rand JA, Berquist TH. The knee. In: Berquist TH, ed. *Imaging of orthopedic trauma*, 2nd ed. New York: Raven Press, 1992:333–432.)

The horns of the meniscus attach to the tibia in the intercondylar region (Figs. 7-10E and 7-11). The medial meniscus is more firmly attached to the capsule. The anterior horn attaches to the intercondylar eminence anterior to the ACL (Figs. 7-10E and 7-11). The transverse diameter of the anterior horn is smaller (see Figs. 7-34 to 7-36) than the posterior horn. The posterior horn attaches to the intercondylar eminence anterior to the PCL (28,51,77,78).

The menisci perform an important function in load bearing and knee function. Up to 50% of load bearing is transmitted through the menisci when the knee is in extension and 85% in flexion (138). The contact area can be reduced significantly after partial menisectomy that can increase contact pressures by 350% (138).

Tears in the menisci may result from acute trauma or repetitive trauma and progressive degeneration (48,74,77, 140–145). Acute tears are usually due to athletic injuries, with crushing of the meniscus between the tibia and femoral condyles. Most tears extend from posterior to anterior (74). Chronic repetitive trauma is common both in athletes and nonathletes with aging (89,146–148). Chrondrocyte necrosis and increase in mucoid ground substance can lead to meniscal tears (149–151).

Examination techniques for meniscal pathology (see Technique section) vary depending on the software and preferences of the examiner (1,144,148,152,153). Throughput and ease of lesion detection are both important (Table 7-1). We prefer proton density and three-dimensional gradient-echo sequences for meniscal imaging (Fig. 7-36). The contrast of lesions (high signal intensity) compared to the normal low signal intensity (black) of the menisci allows defects to be more easily appreciated. Lesions are often less conspicuous on the second echo of spin-echo sequences. Some authors prefer T1-weighted sequences (36,41,154–157). T1-weighted sequences with short TE (<10ms) and TR of 700 show increased signal on meniscal tears consistently (148).

Figure 7-35 Menisci and their attachments and associated ligament and tendon anatomy. (From Rand JA, Berquist TH. The knee. In: Berquist TH, ed. *Imaging of orthopedic trauma*, 2nd ed. New York: Raven Press, 1992:333–432.)

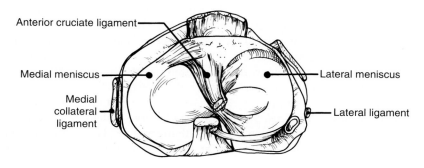

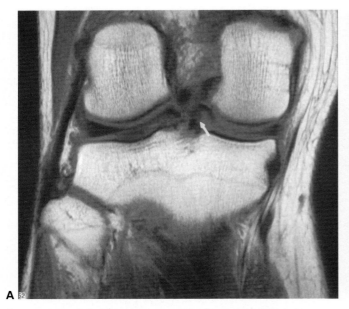

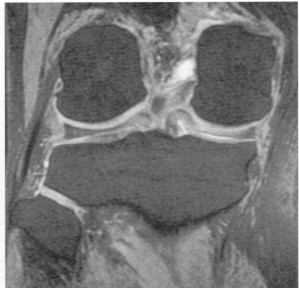

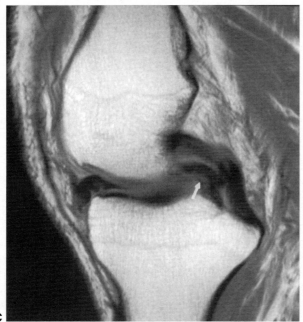

Figure 7-36 Coronal T1-weighted **(A)**, coronal three-dimensional DESS **(B)**, and sagittal proton density-weighted **(C)** images demonstrating a bucket-handle tear of the medial meniscus with a truncated meniscus and a medial fragment (*white arrows*) that creates a "double posterior cruciate ligament" sign. The lateral meniscus is normal. The abnormality is more clearly seen on both the coronal DESS **B** and sagittal proton density-weighted **C** images.

Some authors use 0.7-mm thick sections (28 contiguous), a 50/15 TR/TE, 20° flip angle, and 128 × 256 matrix with 3DFT to evaluate meniscal lesions. This technique yielded a sensitivity of 97% and specificity of 96% (1,62). Disler et al. (36), found three-dimensional techniques especially useful for posterior horn lesions (see Fig. 7-37).

The use of intraarticular contrast medium has also been investigated. Hajek et al. (64) reviewed the effects of air, blood, saline, Renografin 60, and Gd-DTPA as contrast agents for MRI. T1-weighted sequences can be used which affords excellent anatomy in less time than long-TE, TR, T2-weighted sequences. Applegate et al. (51) found that

injecting 40 to 50 mL of 1:100 gadopentetate dimeglumine in saline enhanced accuracy when evaluating patients with partial meniscectomy. However, the examination becomes invasive and more expensive. The time required for injection would likely negate or increase examination time gained by using T1- compared to T2-weighted sequences. Also, newer gradient-echo sequences achieve the same degree of contrast compared to T2-weighted sequences and they can be performed in about the same amount of time as a T1-weighted spin-echo sequence. Early studies with intravenous gadolinium have been encouraging (69). However, to date, contrast media are not frequently used

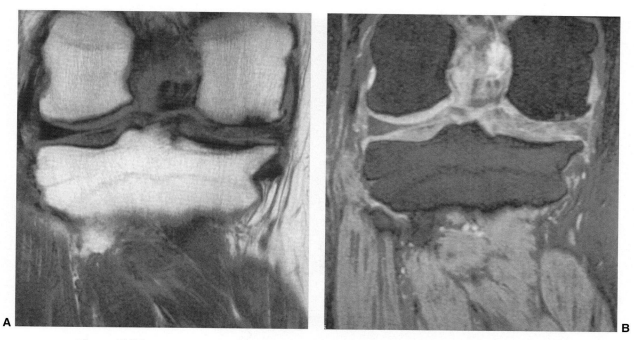

Figure 7-37 Coronal T1-weighted **(A)** and DESS **(B)** images demonstrate tearing of the medial meniscus posteriorly. The meniscal tear is more clearly defined on the DESS sequence.

for MR examinations of the menisci. Regardless of the imaging approach, the menisci should be evaluated in all planes prior to classifying the type of tear (120,158).

The appearance of normal menisci and meniscal tears has been well documented in MRI literature (see Fig. 7-38). Increased signal intensity has been noted on T1-, T2-, and

GRE sequences (5–7,31,149,159,160). These changes can be seen with mucoid degeneration as well as meniscal tears. Grading systems for meniscal tears have been described by Stoller (94), Crues (4–7), and Mesgarzadeh et al. (73) based on pathologic findings in cadaver specimens and operative features (see Figs. 7-38 and 7-39). A grade 1

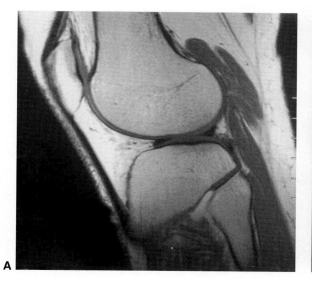

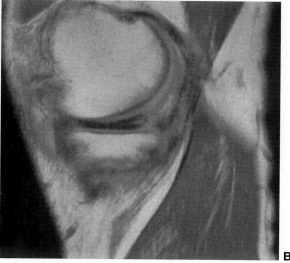

Figure 7-38 Normal and abnormal menisci. **A:** Normal sagittal proton density-weighted image of the lateral meniscus. There is no signal in the meniscus. **B:** Grade 2 globular increased signal intensity in the medial meniscus on a sagittal proton density-weighted image. **C:** Grade 3 increased signal intensity in the posterior horn of the medial meniscus communicating with the inferior articular surface (*small arrowhead*). **D:** Sagittal gradient-echo image demonstrating a grade 3A tear (*small arrowhead*) with an associated meniscal cyst (*large arrowhead*). **E:** Sagittal gradient-echo image demonstrating a more complex linear tear in the posterior horn of the medial meniscus. **F:** Grade 3B meniscal tear with a broad area of articular involvement (*arrowheads*).

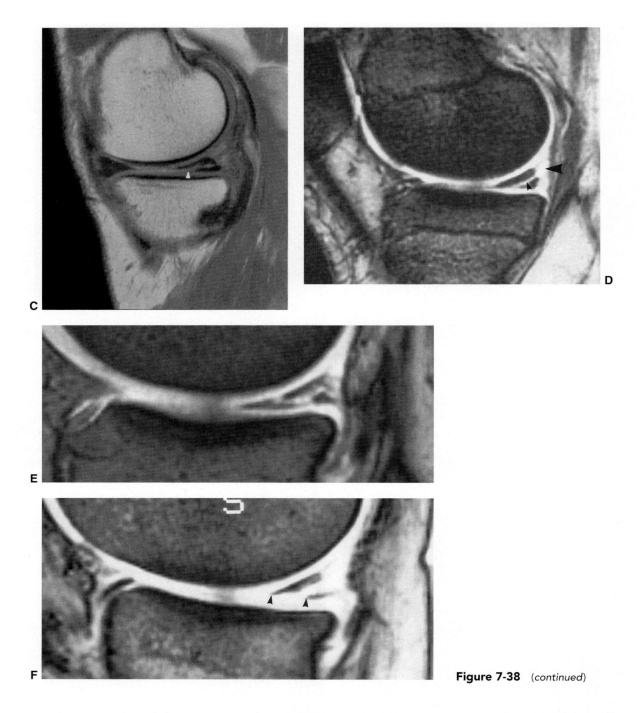

Figure 7-38 (continued)

meniscal lesion is globular in nature and does not communicate articular surface. Histologically, this stage correlates with early mucoid degeneration. It is felt that these changes are not symptomatic but represent a response to mechanical stress and loading that result in increased production of mucoid polysaccharide ground substance (94).

Grade 2 signal intensity is linear (Fig. 7-39) in nature and remains within the substance of the meniscus. Once again, there is no evidence of communication with the articular surface of the meniscus. Histologically, grade 2 menisci are characterized by more extensive bands of

mucoid degeneration. Most feel that grade 2 changes represent progression of grade 1. Some authors feel that grade 2 lesions are precursors to complete tears (51,94,161). However, Dillon et al. (162) found most were stable when followed for three years. Reinig et al. (151) found progression when evaluating football players over a period of one season.

With grade 3 tears (Fig. 7-39) there is increased signal intensity within the meniscus that extends to the articular surface (Fig. 7-38C). Demonstrating communication with the articular surface is important or the tear is not

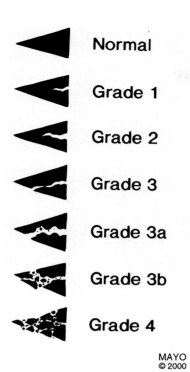

Normal

Grade 1

Grade 2

Grade 3

Grade 3a

Grade 3b

Grade 4

MAYO
© 2000

Figure 7-39 Meniscal tear grading system.

likely to be confirmed arthroscopically. Some authors have used narrow "meniscal windows" to assist in confirming communication with the articular surface. In our experience and that of Buckwalter et al. (156), there is little value in this technique. In fact, if done routinely without conventional windows, bone lesions and other abnormalities can be overlooked (see Fig. 7-40). Grade 3 tears

can be further divided into subcategories. Grade 3A signal intensity is a linear intrameniscal signal that abuts the articular margin (Fig. 7-38D). Grade 3B is a more irregular area of signal intensity that abuts the articular margin (Fig. 7-38F). The grade 3B lesions are most often associated with more extensive degenerative change in the adjacent areas of the meniscus associated with the tear. It is not unusual to have difficulty in differentiating grade 2 from grade 3 tears. Careful windowing and evaluating adjacent sections is useful in these cases. When still in doubt, we describe but do not specifically call linear abnormal signal that *may* communicate with the articular surface a tear.

Grade 4 menisci (Fig. 7-39) are distorted (see Fig. 7-37 and 7-41) in addition to changes described with grade 3 (149). With more severe meniscal tears, meniscal extrusion and associated articular cartilage loss are common (163).

These categories do not include all possible meniscal injuries such as truncated menisci, bucket-handle tears, etc. (73,74). The grading system is most useful in describing significant signal-intensity changes that communicate with the articular surface.

The MR appearance of different types of meniscal tears is similar to those that have been described with arthrography (see Fig. 7-42). Vertical tears are usually traumatic compared with horizontal cleavage tears that are more often degenerative. Degenerative fraying of the surface of the meniscus may also be evident on MR images and is demonstrated as areas of irregular increased signal intensity on the meniscal surface compared to the normal dark or low intensity of the body of the meniscus (see Fig. 7-43). Radial tears may be somewhat difficult to diagnose but are typically seen as areas of increased signal in the inner

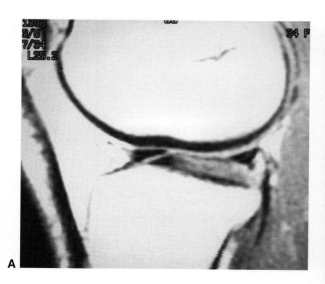

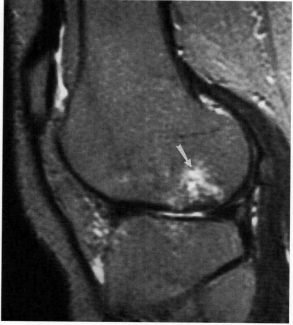

Figure 7-40 Sagittal MR images with meniscal windows **(A)** and conventional windowing **(B).** There is no meniscal tear, however, the "bone bruise" (*arrow*) is only visible on the conventionally windowed image **B.**

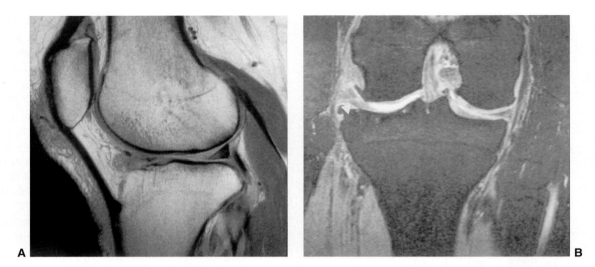

Figure 7-41 Sagittal proton density-weighted **(A)** and coronal three-dimensional DESS **(B)** images demonstrate complex degenerative tearing of the anterior horn and body of the lateral meniscus. Additionally, the coronal image **B** shows displacement of the fragments (*white arrowhead*).

margin of the menisci (see Figs. 7-42 and 7-44). Full-thickness radial tears are demonstrated on coronal and sagittal (Fig. 7-44) images as areas of increased signal involving the entire meniscus with normal meniscal signal on adjacent coronal sections (164).

A bucket-handle tear is a tear with displacement of an attached inner fragment for variable distances (see Figs. 7-42 and 7-45) (18,67). Up to 82% of bucket-handle tears involve the medial meniscus (67). When truncated menisci are identified, one must search carefully for the displaced (bucket-handle) fragment (Fig. 7-45). Loose bodies or fragments of menisci in the intercondylar regions are not uncommon (77,149). These lesions may be very subtle, such that reduction in the size of the meniscus may be the

only finding (Figs. 7-42 and 7-45) (18,67). Bucket-handle tears may involve only a small portion or the entire meniscus. When the entire meniscus is involved (Fig. 7-42), 84% of displaced fragments can be identified on MR images (67). MRI has overall sensitivity for detection of the displaced fragment of about 64%. Several signs (Table 7-5) have been described to assist in detection of bucket-handle tears. The double-PCL sign (see Fig. 7-46) is seen on coronal and sagittal images when the displaced fragment lies below the PCL, giving the appearance of two ligaments. This feature is more common with medial tears (53%) than lateral (14%) bucket-handle tears (Table 7-5) (18,67). The flipped-fragment sign (see Fig. 7-47) is seen with 44% of medial and 29% of lateral meniscal

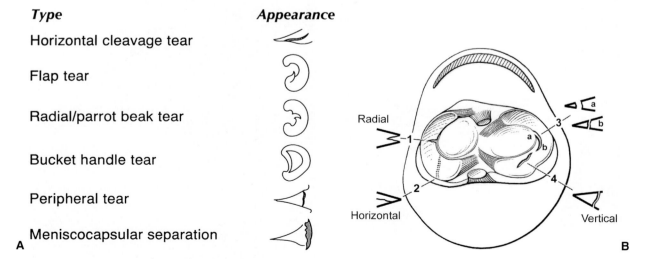

Figure 7-42 Types of meniscal tears. **A:** (*1*) Radial tear with cross sectional appearance. (*2*) Horizontal tear that is only seen on tangential view. (*3*) Flap tear, oriented oblique to the long axis of the meniscus. Note the distance from the apex increases (*a to b*) as the tear extends into the meniscus. (*4*) Vertical tear. **B:** Meniscal tears seen tangentially.

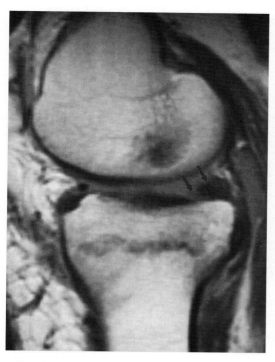

Figure 7-43 Proton density-weighted image demonstrating degeneration of the inner margin and dorsal articular surface of the posteromedial meniscus (*arrows*). There is also a proximal tibial stress fracture.

bucket-handle tears (Table 7-5) (67). Defining a fragment in the notch may be difficult, especially when they are small and the configuration of the meniscus is not significantly truncated (Fig. 7-45, Table 7-5). Larger fragments are identified with 66% of medial and 43% of lateral meniscal tears (67). Detection may be improved by using coronal STIR images. Magee and Hinson (18) reported

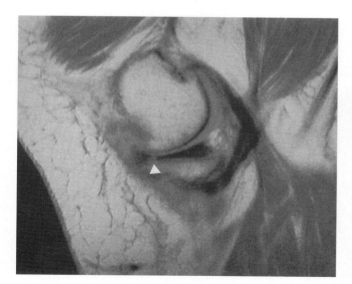

Figure 7-44 Sagittal proton density-weighted image of the medial meniscus demonstrating a small radial tear in the margin of the body of the meniscus (*arrowhead*).

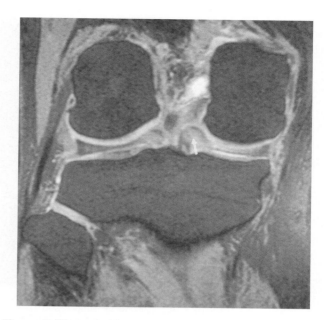

Figure 7-45 Bucket-handle tear with shortening of the medial meniscus and marked displacement of the inner fragment (*small arrow*).

detection of 93% of fragments using STIR sequences. Defining the fragments is important, as they need to be removed arthroscopically (18).

Parrot-beak tears (Fig. 7-42) are horizontal tears with vertical or radial components at the meniscal margin. These lesions are most common at the junction of the body and posterior horn of the lateral meniscus (149). These lesions are frequently asymptomatic (4). Peripheral tears or separations in the meniscus can also be identified. These are usually easily diagnosed with arthrography but can be subtle on MR images due to vascular tissue and the normally increased signal intensity at synoviomeniscal junction along the margins of the meniscus (Figs. 7-18, 7-20, 7-48). It is important to clearly define the location (see Fig. 7-48) (medial, lateral, inner margin, peripheral),

TABLE 7-5

BUCKET HANDLE TEARS: MRI FEATURES

Feature	Incidence	
	Medial Meniscus	Lateral Meniscus
Double posterior cruciate ligament sign (Fig. 7-46)	53%	14%
Flipped-fragment sign (Fig. 7-47)	44%	29%
Fragment in notch (Fig. 7-45)	66%	43%

From references 6, 18, 67, 139, and 165.

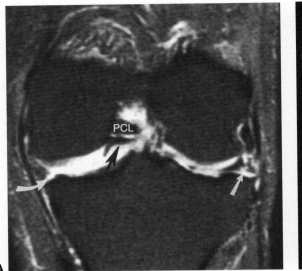
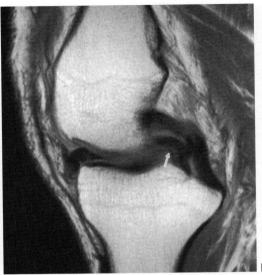

Figure 7-46 Coronal fat-suppressed T2-weighted image **(A)** demonstrating a medial tear (*curved arrow*) with a large displaced fragment (*black arrow*) that gives the appearance of two posterior cruciate ligaments (PCLs). There is also a complex tear of the lateral meniscus (*white arrow*) and loss of articular cartilage. Sagittal proton density-weighted image **(B)** demonstrating a medial meniscal tear with a large displaced fragment (*small arrow*), resulting in a double-PCL sign.

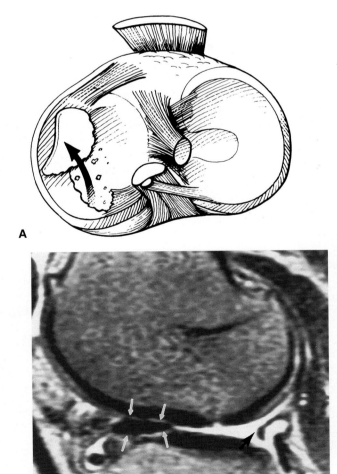
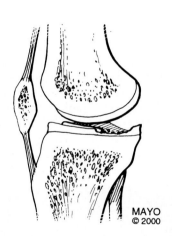

Figure 7-47 Flipped-fragment sign. **A:** Flipped fragment seen on the axial and sagittal planes. **B:** Sagittal gradient-echo image with posterior fragment flipped anteriorly (*white arrows*) creating a "large anterior meniscus." There is only a small remnant left posteriorly (*black arrow*).

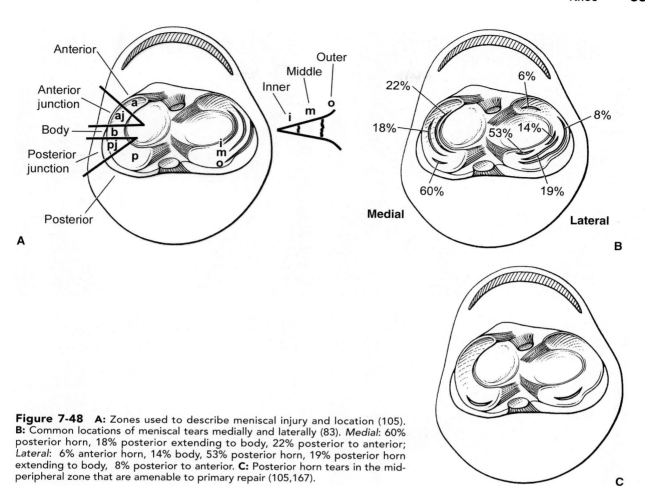

Figure 7-48 **A:** Zones used to describe meniscal injury and location (105). **B:** Common locations of meniscal tears medially and laterally (83). *Medial*: 60% posterior horn, 18% posterior extending to body, 22% posterior to anterior; *Lateral*: 6% anterior horn, 14% body, 53% posterior horn, 19% posterior horn extending to body, 8% posterior to anterior. **C:** Posterior horn tears in the mid-peripheral zone that are amenable to primary repair (105,167).

type of tear, and associated bone and/or ligament injury (4,159). Grade 1 and 2 lesions will not be identified arthroscopically (6,7,166). Certain lesions are stable and can heal with conservative therapy, so arthroscopy may be

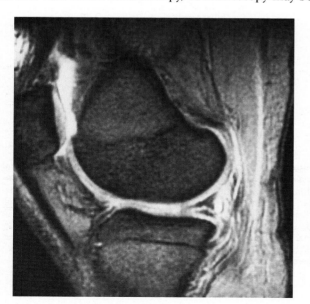

Figure 7-49 Sagittal gradient-echo image demonstrating a horizontal cleavage tear in the posterior horn.

avoided (22,25). Peripheral lesions are particularly suited for meniscal repair (Fig. 7-48) (4,51,105,167).

The type and location of meniscal tear are important in determining if the lesion is responsible for the symptoms so the appropriate therapy can be selected (4,25,149,168). Crues (4) summarized the typical meniscal lesions and correlated the type of lesion with symptoms. Horizontal cleavage tears (see Figs. 7-38 and 7-49) are grade 3 tears (linear extending to the articular surface) that are frequently asymptomatic, especially in patients over 50 years of age. Radial or parrot-beak tears (Fig. 7-42) are also often asymptomatic (167,169). Flap tears (horizontal or vertical tear with one end of the fragment displaced) (see Figs. 7-42 and 7-50) are more often symptomatic and respond to partial meniscectomy (4,159,167). Bucket-handle tears (see Figs. 7-42 and 7-51) are most often symptomatic, acute, and usually an indication for meniscal repair (3,4). Peripheral tears and meniscocapsular separations are also frequently symptomatic, but may heal with conservative therapy due to the peripheral vascular supply (see Fig. 7-52). Primary meniscal repair may also be successful (167). Certain repairs may be performed arthroscopically; however, open repairs may be preferred for peripheral tears or meniscocapsular separations involving the posterior one-third of the medial or lateral meniscus (138).

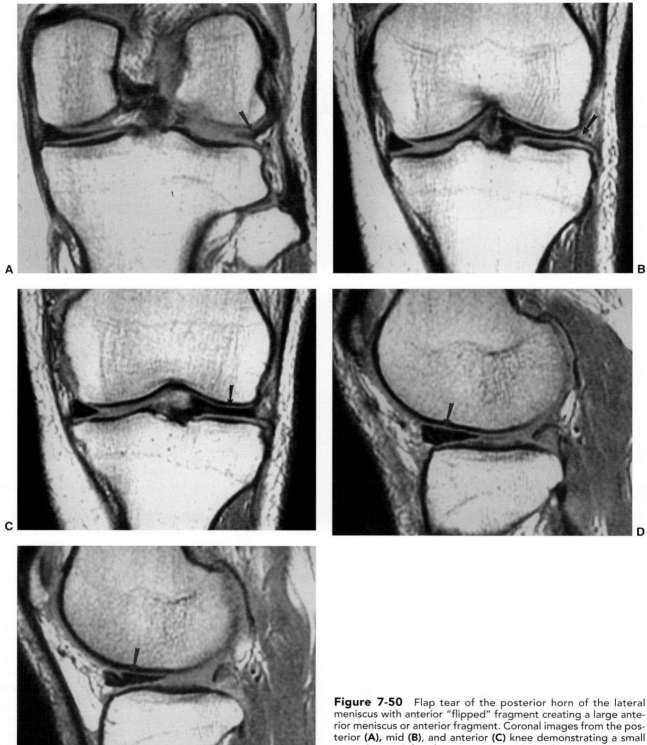

Figure 7-50 Flap tear of the posterior horn of the lateral meniscus with anterior "flipped" fragment creating a large anterior meniscus or anterior fragment. Coronal images from the posterior **(A)**, mid **(B)**, and anterior **(C)** knee demonstrating a small posterior peripheral remnant (*arrow*) **C,** absent meniscus in **B,** and a large, thick meniscal structure anteriorly. Note the normal medial meniscus. Sagittal proton density-weighted images **(D,E)** demonstrate the flipped fragment anteriorly (*arrow*) that gives the appearance of a very large anterior horn.

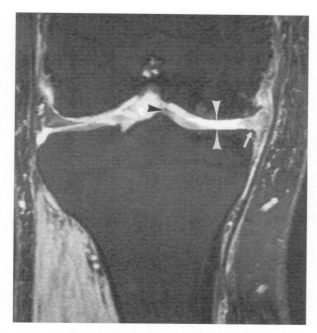

Figure 7-51 Coronal three-dimensional DESS image with truncation of the medial meniscus (*arrow*) and the medial fragment (*black arrowhead*) in the central joint space. There is also extensive articular cartilage loss (*white arrowheads*).

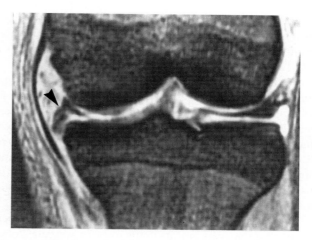

Figure 7-52 Coronal gradient-echo image demonstrates a discoid lateral meniscus and a complex medial meniscal separation and tear (*arrowhead*).

Several reports in the MR literature have described the accuracy of MRI for identification of meniscal tears (Table 7-6) (18,170–172). Sensitivity for MRI in detecting meniscal tears seen at arthroscopy ranges from 75% to 100%. Review of our data demonstrated a sensitivity of 99%, specificity of 90%, accuracy of 90%, positive predicted value of 96%, and negative predicted value of 98% for the medial meniscus. MRI of the lateral meniscus showed 97% sensitivity, 97% specificity, and 91% accuracy.

One could consider arthrography as an equally effective tool in evaluating meniscal lesions (accuracy 91% medial

meniscus, 81% lateral meniscus), though it is clearly not as valuable in evaluating the other structures in the knee (18,77). However, even in this setting there are two situations in which MRI is clearly superior and a more effective technique. This would include children with knee pain and patients with acute trauma and hemarthrosis (25,133).

Postoperative Meniscus

Detection and characterization of meniscal tears can establish the need for surgery and the type of procedure. Other injuries, such as occult bone injury or injury to the capsule or supporting structures, must be evaluated along with meniscal tears as explanations of patients' symptoms. Conservative therapy or watchful waiting has little downside risk in patients without locking of the knee (174).

The meniscus serves multiple important functions. It is a shock absorber and assists in joint lubrication and

TABLE 7-6

MRI OF MENISCAL TEARS

| | Mayo Series | | Glashow et al. (173) | Crues et al. (4–6) | | Munk et al. (21) | | Dorsay et al. (139)[a] | |
	MM	LM	Both menisci	MM	LM	MM	LM	MM	LM
No. of cases	129	129	50	144	144	242	242	43	43
Accuracy	90%	91%	—	89%	94%	94%	92%	—	—
Sensitivity	99%	97%	83%	87%	88%	97%	92%	86–96%	86–96%
Specificity	90%	97%	84%	91%	98%	89%	91%	89–98%	89–98%
Positive predictive value	96%	76%	75%	93%	96%	—	—	—	—
Negative predictive value	98%	99%	90%	84%	92%	—	—	—	—

MM, medial meniscus; LM, lateral meniscus.
[a]Multiple signs used.

chondrocyte nutrition. Stress to the articular cartilage is also reduced. The meniscus also restricts anterior displacement of the tibia on the femur, reducing stress on the ACL (77,175,176).

Decisions regarding surgical repair depend upon the type and location (peripheral or central) of the tear as well as what other injuries may be associated with the meniscal tear. Partial meniscectomy, complete removal, or replacement with cadaver allograft or prosthesis may be considered (175,177). Replacement procedures are relatively new and suggested for patients with previous total meniscectomy or partial meniscectomy with continued symptoms but good joint alignment (175).

As noted above, partial meniscectomy is usually performed for flap tears or tears in the inner or avascular zones of the meniscus (Fig. 7-48) (138,167,174). Peripheral tears are frequently repaired (sutured) so the normal meniscal configuration is maintained but with potentially confusing signal intensity changes on MR images (1,62,159).

MRI is also of value, though potentially more difficult to interpret, for studying patients who have had either partial or complete meniscectomy or primary arthroscopic repairs of the meniscus. Postoperatively, patients are generally referred to exclude residual fragments, remnants of a tear that was not completely resected, or new tears (1,159,176–178).

MR features noted following meniscal repair are similar to preoperative findings. Increased signal intensity that communicates with the articular surface (primary repair) or a truncated margin (partial meniscectomy) (see Fig. 7-53) are common findings (175,177). Though meniscal tears may

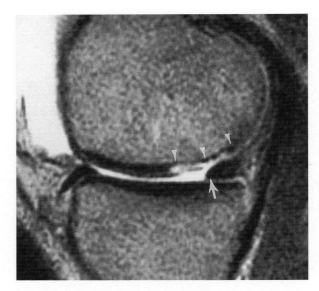

Figure 7-53 Sagittal T2-weighted image after partial resection of the inner margin of the posterior medial meniscus. There is new articular deformity (*white arrowheads*) involving the adjacent femoral condyle with erosion of the cartilage and uncovered bone. Note the rounded appearance (*arrow*) of the meniscal margin.

fill in with fibrous tissue (dark on MR images), the tear can also fill in with chondrocytes that will have increased intensity similar to a tear. Though the MR features at the operative site may be confusing, additional causes of pain such as bone (see Fig. 7-54) or ligament lesions and residual or new meniscal fragments (see Figs. 7-54 and 7-55) can be identified (1,4,159,177).

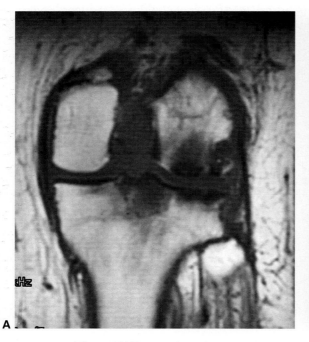

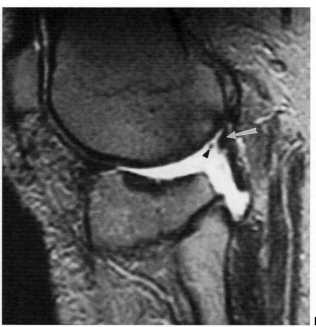

Figure 7-54 **A:** Coronal T1-weighted image after lateral meniscectomy demonstrating osteonecrosis of the femur and tibia. **B:** Sagittal T2-weighted image shows a residual peripheral remnant (*arrow*) and a small free fragment (*arrowhead*).

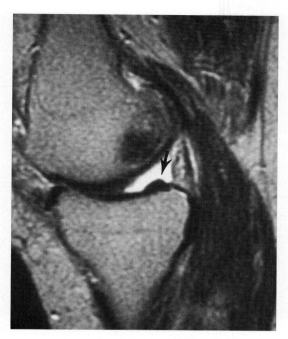

Figure 7-55 Sagittal T2-weighted image after medial menisectomy demonstrating a large retained fragment (*arrow*).

Accuracy can be improved when intraarticular gadolinium is used (51,179). Some authors also suggest conventional arthrography after meniscal repair (180). Sciulli et al. (178) compared conventional arthrography with MR arthrography using iodinated contrast and gadolinium. Intraarticular gadolinium studies were most accurate (92%) and conventional arthrograms least accurate (58%) for evaluating menisci after surgical procedures (178). In our experience, equivocal cases are most often reexamined arthroscopically.

Meniscal Cysts

Meniscal cysts have been reported in up to 1% of patients undergoing meniscectomy. Most cysts are located in the anterolateral meniscus, but they may occur along the margin of either meniscus (Fig. 7-38D) (13,181–184). Lateral meniscal cysts are two to four times more common than medial cysts (184,185). The patients typically present with localized tenderness and, occasionally, swelling along the joint line. Cysts may be palpable, especially when they involve the lateral joint line (184). Similar presentations can be noted in patients with periarticular ganglion cysts. Ganglion cysts may or may not have a clearly defined connection with the joint (182,186). Ganglion cysts may also occur along the periarticular tendon sheaths and tibiofibular joint (181). Popliteal cysts are typically located posteromedially near the medial head of the gastrocnemius (181,184). Distinction between these conditions is important since operative management of meniscal cysts is more commonly required. Popliteal cysts, however, if persistently symptomatic, may also require resection. Medial cysts, though less common, frequently tend to be asymptomatic

even though they may be larger than cysts in the lateral meniscus (181,183). Treatment of meniscal cysts requires decompression and treatment of meniscal pathology (184). Therefore, differentiation of intra- and parameniscal cysts from other fluid collections, including bursitis, is important (see Figs. 7-56 and 7-57) (181,184).

The etiology of meniscal cysts is controversial. Various theories have been proposed including chronic infection, hemorrhage, and mucoid degeneration. Since the fluid is similar to synovial fluid, most feel that a tear in the meniscus leads to fluid accumulation in the adjacent soft tissues resulting in cyst formation (Fig. 7-37D). It is likely that the etiology is multifactorial; however, most authors exclude hemorrhage and infection as causes (159,181,182,185).

MR features of meniscal cysts and ganglia are easily appreciated on T2-weighted and gradient-echo sequences. Both are well-marginated, high intensity lesions. Meniscal cysts tend to be within or at the margin of the meniscus, while ganglion cysts may extend from the capsule or be located in the periarticular soft tissues (see Fig. 7-58) (181,183,185,186). Atypical signal intensity can occur with hemorrhage (low T2-, high T1-weighted sequence) or when fluid is thick and proteinaceous. Meniscal cysts may be small (<1cm) (Fig. 7-58) or as large as 5 cm (Fig. 7-56) (184). Up to 47% may be septated, as noted in Fig. 7-56. Associated abnormalities may include ACL tears (11%) and bone injury (13%) (184).

Certain cysts may cause confusion due to their location. Lektrakul et al. (187) described cysts arising in the posteromedial meniscus that resemble a cruciate ligament ganglion cyst (see Fig. 7-59).

Discoid Menisci

Discoid menisci (Fig. 7-52) are uncommon and are reported in 1.5% to 15.5% of lateral menisci and 0.1% to 0.3% of medial menisci (137,188,189). Both the etiology and classification of discoid menisci are controversial. Hall (137) has described an arthrographic classification for discoid menisci that may also be applied to MR features.

Discoid menisci are typically broad and disk-shaped. This configuration and the extension into the joint make this meniscus more susceptible to tearing (see Fig. 7-60). Type 1 discoid menisci are thick, slablike menisci with parallel superior and inferior surfaces. Type 2 menisci are more slablike with a thin central portion. Type 3 discoid menisci are only slightly larger than normal menisci (Fig. 7-20). Type 4 menisci are asymmetric, with the anterior horn extending farther into the joint than the posterior horn. Type 5 is between normal and slab type, and type 6 is any of the above with an associated tear (Fig. 7-60) (77,137).

A commonly used orthopedic classification defines discoid menisci as complete, incomplete, or Wrisberg ligament types. Complete and incomplete vary depending upon the extent of coverage of the lateral tibial plateau. The Wrisberg ligament type has an abnormal posterior attachment with abnormal meniscal morbidity (190).

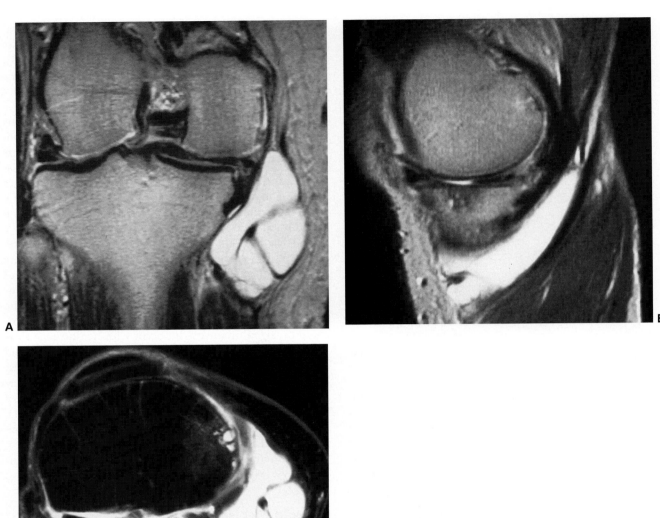

Figure 7-56 Large, septated meniscal cyst. Coronal **(A)** and sagittal **(B)** T2-weighted and fat-suppressed axial fast spin-echo **(C)** images demonstrate a large, septated meniscal cyst with degeneration of the medial meniscus. Features on the sagittal image in **B** could be confused with pes anserine bursitis.

Clinically, patients with discoid meniscus present with symptoms of snapping and occasionally pain, as these menisci are more prone to degeneration and tears. Until recently, there were no large series of MR findings in discoid menisci. Hartzman et al. did report a series describing the MR findings (152). The transverse diameter of the normal meniscus is approximately 10 to 11 mm and, therefore, the increased transverse diameter of a discoid meniscus can result in typical findings on both coronal and sagittal MR images. For example, on sagittal 4 to 5 mm slices, only two slices should demonstrate the meniscus (Fig. 7-60). Visualization of the meniscus in more than two slices is indicative of a discoid meniscus (Fig. 7-60) (159). Coronal and radial images of the meniscus are perhaps more useful in that the true extension into the joint can be better

demonstrated (Figs. 7-20 and 7-60) (124,137). Care should be taken not to mistake the thin, low-intensity line of the vacuum phenomenon for a discoid meniscus (see Fig. 7-61). MR features used for diagnosis of tears in nondiscoid menisci can also be applied to discoid menisci (191). However, accuracy is reduced due to factors such as degeneration and a high incidence of multiple tears (48%). Ryu et al. (189) reported a positive predictive value of only 57% for tears in discoid menisci.

Meniscal Ossicles

Meniscal ossicles are very uncommon (192,193). The etiology of these intrameniscal ossicles is uncertain. Lesions may mimic loose bodies on routine radiographs. The common

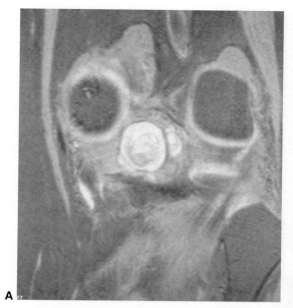

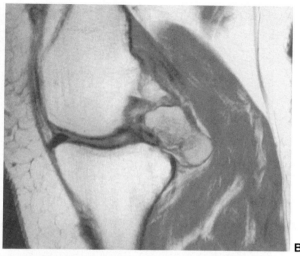

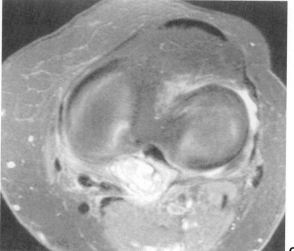

Figure 7-57 Large, complex medial meniscal cyst. Coronal three-dimensional DESS **(A)**, sagittal proton density **(B)**, and axial proton density, fat-suppressed **(C)** images show a complex cyst with associated meniscal tear.

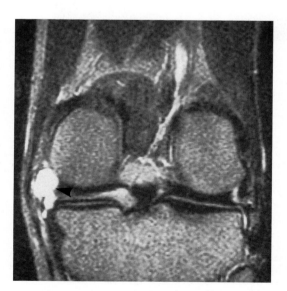

Figure 7-58 Coronal gradient-echo image demonstrating a medial meniscal cyst (*arrowhead*).

location in the posterior horn of the medial meniscus should raise the question of meniscal ossicle when seen on routine radiographs. Histology may demonstrate fatty marrow or lamellar bone (194).

Meniscal ossicles are usually asymptomatic. Radiographs demonstrate the abnormality, which is often confused with a loose body (195). MR images typically demonstrate a small marrow containing ossicle in the meniscus near the tibial attachment (194).

Ligament and Tendon Injuries

Complete evaluation of the capsule, medial, and lateral collateral ligaments, cruciate ligaments, and tendons about the knee has been difficult with conventional arthrography and CT arthrography. Multiplanar MR images provide significant improvement in our ability to assess these structures. The anatomy of the ligaments of the knee was discussed in the initial section of this chapter; however, some review is necessary for discussing the technical aspects for evaluating these

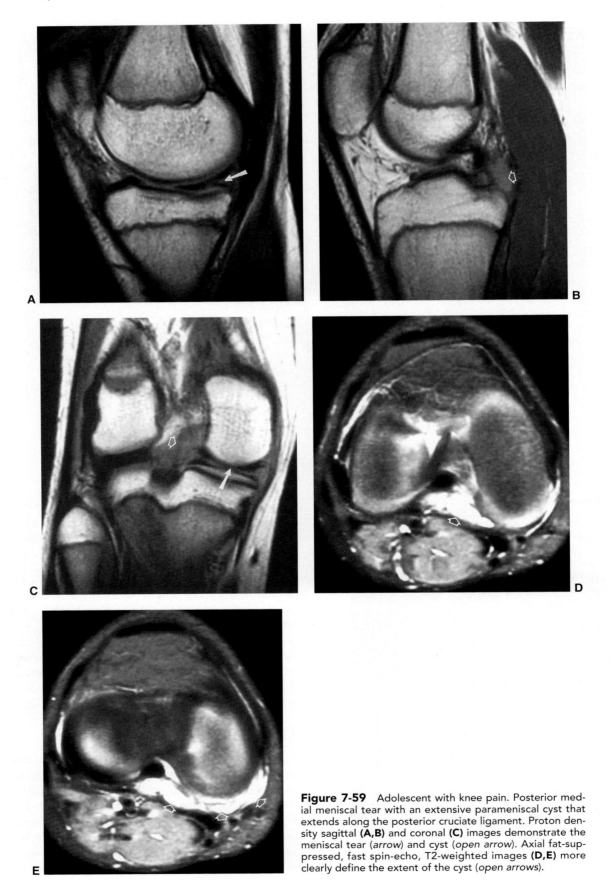

Figure 7-59 Adolescent with knee pain. Posterior medial meniscal tear with an extensive parameniscal cyst that extends along the posterior cruciate ligament. Proton density sagittal **(A,B)** and coronal **(C)** images demonstrate the meniscal tear (*arrow*) and cyst (*open arrow*). Axial fat-suppressed, fast spin-echo, T2-weighted images **(D,E)** more clearly define the extent of the cyst (*open arrows*).

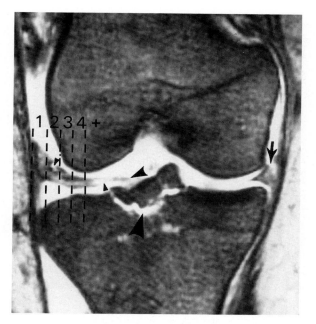

Figure 7-60 Gradient-echo image demonstrating a large discoid lateral meniscus extending into the midjoint *space* (*large arrowhead*). There are multiple tears (*small arrowheads*) and a tibial spine fracture (*lower arrowhead*). There is also a peripheral separation (*arrow*) of the medial meniscus. Dotted lines demonstrated the number of sagittal sections that include the meniscus (four or more 4-mm sections).

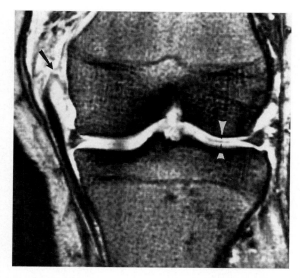

Figure 7-61 Coronal gradient-echo image demonstrating a low-intensity line (vacuum phenomenon) laterally (*arrowheads*). This is thinner than a discoid meniscus and confusion can be avoided by comparing coronal images with findings on sagittal or radial images. Note the medial collateral ligament tear (*arrow*).

structures. The ACL, because of its oblique course (Fig. 7-11A), can be more difficult to identify and in early studies, prior to oblique off-axis imaging, the ability to demonstrate the ACL in a given slice completely was significantly hindered. Our initial review demonstrated that incomplete evaluation of the ACL occurred in up to 30% of cases. Improved positioning (15% to 20% external rotation) and software developments have greatly improved our ability to demonstrate the ligaments of the knee (see Fig. 7-62) (99,175,186,196–198).

The anterior cruciate, through its oblique course, is intraarticular but extrasynovial (Fig. 7-10E) (78,199). This ligament is one of the main stabilizers of the knee preventing excessive anterior displacement of the femur on the tibia

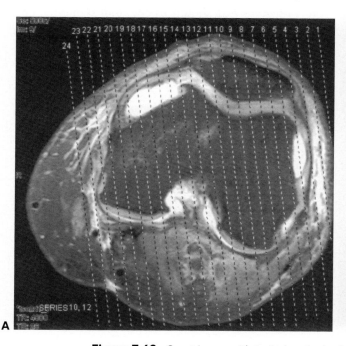

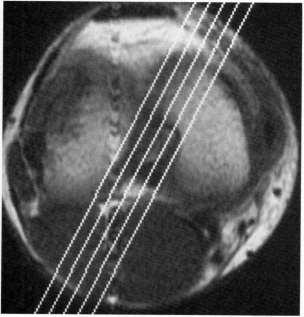

Figure 7-62 Scout image with typical sagittal selections **(A)** and oblique sagittal plane selection **(B)** to demonstrate the cruciate ligament.

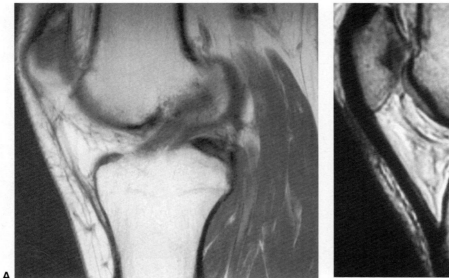
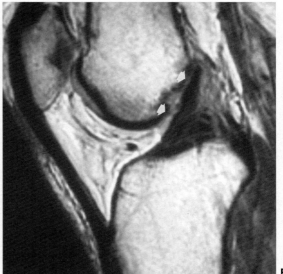

Figure 7-63 Variations in appearance of the normal ACL. **A:** T1-weighted sagittal image demonstrating the normal course of the cruciate ligament even though the femoral attachment is not completely seen. Note the thin low intensity fibers with interspersed bands of intermediate signal intensity. **B:** Sagittal T1-weighted image demonstrates a thicker low signal intensity normal anterior cruciate ligament. The entire structure is visualized. The normal course parallels the intercondylar roof (*arrows*).

(77,200). The ligament is broader at the tibial attachment with an average width of 11 mm and length of 4 cm (201,202). There are two distinct anatomic fiber bundles (anteromedial and posterolateral) that are not usually distinguishable on MR images. The anteromedial band is taut during flexion and the larger posterolateral band is taut with the knee extended (203,204). The anteromedial band is thinner and longer and contributes to stability in internal and external rotation in addition to limiting tibiofemoral translation during flexion. The thicker posterolateral band contributes to rotational stability (204). Typically, the anatomic appearance on MR images varies with the anterior cruciate having multiple fibers which are seen as linear areas of low signal intensity compared to the thicker and more uniform low signal intensity of the PCL (see Fig. 7-63). Though oblique sagittal or externally rotated (20° to 30°) true sagittal images are most often used, the ACL should also be studied in other image planes (see Figs. 7-64 and 7-65) (62).

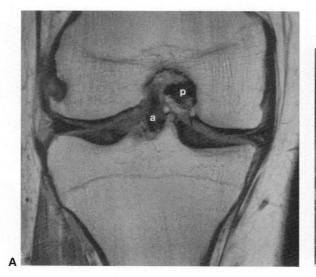
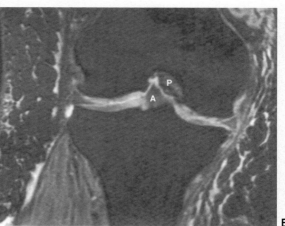

Figure 7-64 **A:** Coronal T1-weighted image demonstrating normal posterior (*p*) and anterior (*a*) cruciate ligaments. **B:** Coronal DESS image demonstrating the normal posterior (*P*) and anterior (*A*) cruciate ligaments.

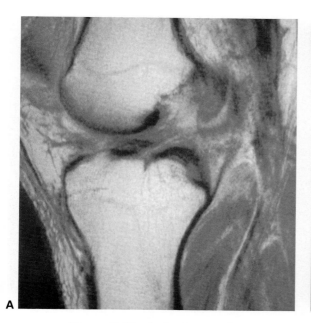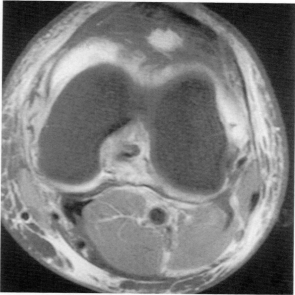

A   B

Figure 7-65 Sagittal proton density-weighted **(A)** and axial proton density fat-suppressed **(B)** images demonstrate no visualization of the anterior cruciate ligament.

Tears in the ACL can occur due to multiple mechanisms of injury. Injuries most often occur with forced valgus and external rotation, but anterior cruciate tears can also follow external rotation with hyperextension, internal rotation with extension and forward displacement of the tibia (see Fig. 7-66) (205). Up to 70% of patients have other intraarticular injuries, most often the MCL and/or the postero-medial meniscus (O'Donoghue's triad — ACL tear, MCL tear, medial meniscal tear) (Fig. 7-66) (77,206–211). The PCL is thicker and has a midline sagittal course and is, therefore, not difficult to visualize on MR sagittal images (1,77). This ligament serves as a stabilizer of the knee in flexion, extension, and internal rotation (77). Tears of the PCL occur with posterior force to the flexed knee or forced hypertension (203).

Technique for routine examination of the knee as described above is generally adequate for evaluation of the cruciate ligaments and medial and lateral collateral ligaments. In certain cases the ACL may be incompletely seen, in which case repeat oblique images can easily be obtained. One should strive to demonstrate both cruciate ligaments completely on a single slice to more easily assess abnormalities (Fig. 7-62). Review of axial and coronal images should also be performed to increase the accuracy of diagnosis (173,212–215). Axial images may be particularly useful for detection of partial tears (214).

Conventional spin-echo or FSE sequences may be equally effective for detection of ACL injuries (63). However, we still use conventional spin-echo sequences in the sagittal plane to evaluate the cruciate ligaments and menisci (3).

MR findings with acute disruption of either the anterior or PCL are similar (Table 7-7). The appearance or signal

intensity will, of course, vary with the age of the lesion. We prefer T2-weighted images for assessment of the cruciate ligaments as the high signal intensity seen with acute lesions provides excellent contrast compared to the normally low signal intensity (black) ligaments (Figs. 7-66). In recent years, FSE sequences have been found to be equally effective. Ha et al. (63) reported 98% accuracy, a positive

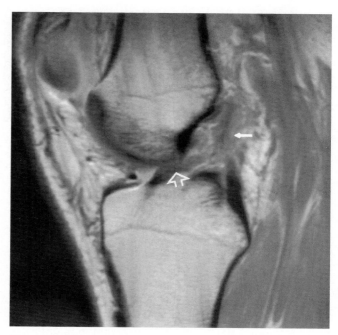

Figure 7-66 Sagittal proton density-weighted image demonstrates an anterior cruciate ligament tear at the femoral attachment (*arrow*) with a horizontal distal remnant (*open arrow*).

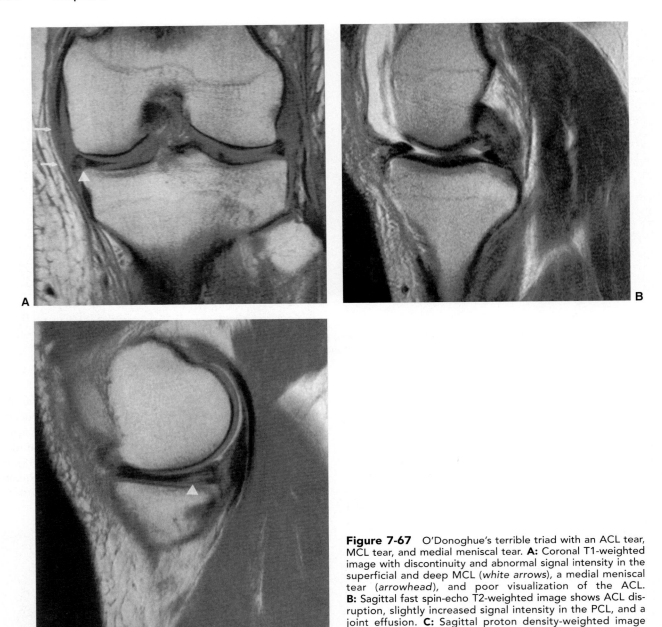

Figure 7-67 O'Donoghue's terrible triad with an ACL tear, MCL tear, and medial meniscal tear. **A:** Coronal T1-weighted image with discontinuity and abnormal signal intensity in the superficial and deep MCL (*white arrows*), a medial meniscal tear (*arrowhead*), and poor visualization of the ACL. **B:** Sagittal fast spin-echo T2-weighted image shows ACL disruption, slightly increased signal intensity in the PCL, and a joint effusion. **C:** Sagittal proton density-weighted image shows a posterior medial meniscal tear (*arrowhead*).

predictive value of 95%, and negative predictive value of 99% for detection of ACL injuries using FSE sequences.

Both primary and secondary signs for ligament tears have been described. Primary features can be applied to most ligament and tendon injuries. ACL tears are more common (posterior cruciate tears account for 2% to 23% of injuries) and can be difficult to evaluate (46,62,220,221). Acute tears are seen as areas of high signal intensity on T2-weighted sequences. Tears can occur in the midsubstance (90%) or at the femoral (7%) or tibial (3%) attachments. Disruption near the femoral attachment is more common in our practice (Fig. 7-66) (62,149). With complete tears, the signal intensity extends throughout the width of the ligament

and there is usually separation of the ligament ends at the site of the tear with laxity or loss of the normal course of the ACL (see Figs. 7-66 to 7-68). Barry et al. (206) described five features of ACL tears. Forty-eight percent presented with increased signal intensity and thickening on T2-weighted sequences, 21% demonstrated a horizontal ligament, in 18% the ligament could not be identified, and discontinuity of the ACL was seen in only 11% of cases. Features of ACL tears can be applied to MR images in adults and children (85,222). It is useful to evaluate all image planes (coronal, sagittal, and axial) to most accurately classify ACL injuries (see Fig. 7-69) (3,46). Chronic tears are seen as areas of intermediate signal intensity, typically with ligament thickening

TABLE 7-7

CRITERIA FOR ANTERIOR CRUCIATE LIGAMENT TEARS

Primary Features

Acute—complete
1. Discontinuity with increased signal intensity between segments or at the femoral or tibial attachments (T2-weighted sequence)
2. Flat or horizontal distal tibial segment with high signal intensity near the femoral attachment
3. Complete absence of the ligament with effusion and high signal intensity in the midjoint space (T2-weighted sequence)
4. Wavy ligament

Acute—incomplete
    Increased signal intensity (T2-weighted sequence) with thickening and normal course.

Chronic tears
1. Laxity with normal or intermediate signal intensity and thickening or poorly defined ligament (No signal intensity increase between first and second echo.)
2. Ligament atrophy

Secondary Signs
    Effusion
    Angulation of the posterior cruciate ligament
    Anterior tibial subluxation
    Bone bruise
    Segond fracture
    Uncovered lateral meniscus
    Deep femoral notch
    Medial collateral ligament tear
    Meniscal tear

From references 41, 60, 91, 92, 133, 143, and 216–219.

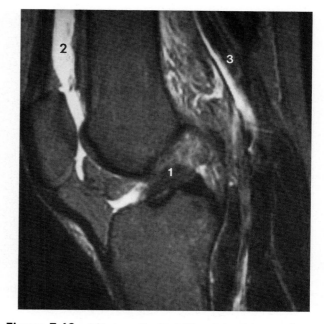

Figure 7-68 ACL tear. Sagittal T2-weighted image demonstrates a horizontal distal segment (*1*), joint effusion (*2*), and increased signal posteriorly (*3*) due to capsular tear.

and associated ligament laxity (see Fig. 7-71) Ligament atrophy or scar formation can make diagnosis difficult (see Figs. 7-70 to 7-72) (196,223–225).

Detection of partial ACL tears is more difficult with MR imaging (204,214). Detection of these injuries is important, as they frequently lead to ligament deficiency and instability (38% to 56%) (204). Tears of less than 25% of the ligament thickness have a more favorable prognosis. On MR images, one can expect to see high signal intensity that does not involve the entire thickness of the ligament

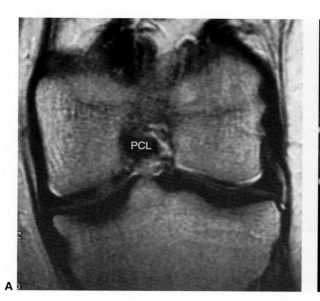
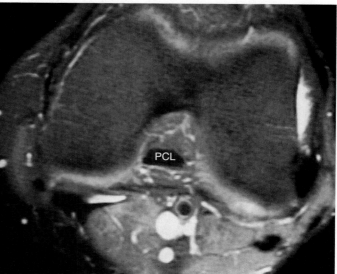

Figure 7-69 Chronic ACL injury. Coronal proton density-weighted (**A**) and axial fat-suppressed, T2-weighted, fast spin-echo (**B**) images clearly demonstrate the PCL. The ACL is attretic.

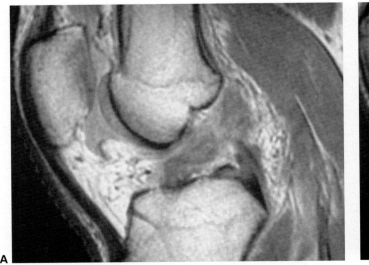
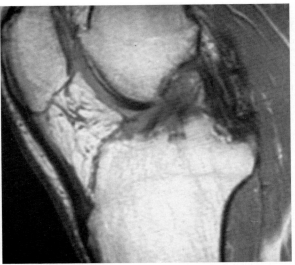

Figure 7-70   Chronic ACL injuries. Sagittal proton density-weighted images **(A,B)** show thickening of the ACL and involvement of the PCL in **B.**

(see Fig. 7-73). However, this finding may also be identified with a ligament contusion (204). Secondary signs may be helpful. When the posterior horn of the lateral meniscus and popliteal muscle injury are present, a complete tear is indicated (221).

Sonin et al. (16) reviewed PCL tears. Forty-five percent were complete, 47% partial (see Fig. 7-74), and bone avulsions were associated with 9% of PCL injuries. Twenty-eight percent of tears were isolated, and 72% were associated

with meniscal or ligament injuries or bone bruises. Most PCL tears (68%) involve the midsubstance, while 19% are proximal and the remainder distal segment injuries (16). The MR image findings in posterior cruciate tears are similar to anterior cruciate tears except that the course of the ligament is not as useful. The PCL typically has a more curved appearance, with convexity of its upper surface (see Fig. 7-75).

Numerous secondary signs have been described for evaluating ACL tears (Table 7-7) (101,127,215,216,

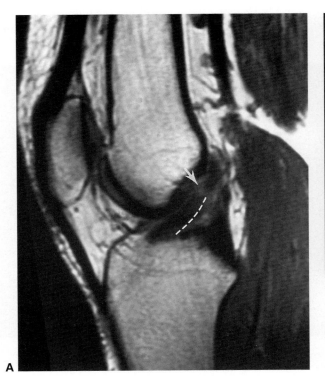
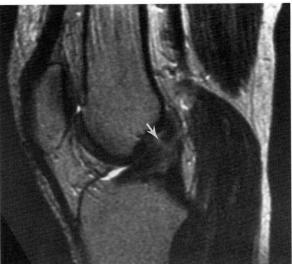

Figure 7-71   Sagittal proton density **(A)** and T2-weighted **(B)** images demonstrate an old tear (*arrow*) in the anterior cruciate ligament. The ligament is bowed (*white broken line*) and signal intensity does not increase on the second echo.

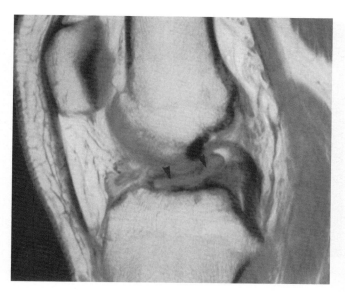

Figure 7-72 Chronic ACL tear. Sagittal proton density-weighted image demonstrates an old tear with a horizontal remnant (*arrowheads*). Note there is no joint effusion.

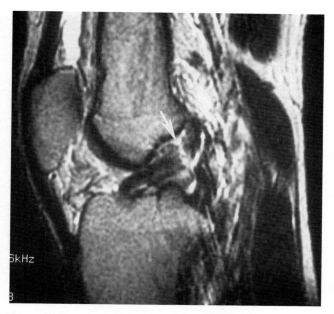

Figure 7-73 Sagittal T2-weighted image demonstrates a linear area of increased signal intensity (*arrow*). The ligament is lax; there is an effusion and high signal intensity posteriorly due to capsular tear. High-grade to complete tear.

221–227). Changes in the configuration of the PCL are useful as a secondary sign of ACL disruption (see Figs. 7-76 and 7-77). An acute angle in the upper portion of the PCL forming a "question mark" configuration suggests a positive drawer sign due to ACL tear (Fig. 7-77) (54,62,205,223). Tung et al. (215) described two measurements to quantify the PCL curve. A line *(y)* is drawn from the anterior femoral to the anterior tibial insertions (Fig. 7-76). A second line *(x)* is drawn perpendicular to *(y)* at the point of maximal curve or distance to line *(y)*. The curve value is calculated by dividing the length of *(x)* by *(y)* (Fig. 7-76). The mean value is

0.45 ± 0.12 in documented ACL tears compared to 0.27 ± 0.06 for normal patients.

The angle of the PCL can also be used to evaluate ACL tears. McCauley et al. (226) reported a PCL angle of $<105°$ (see Fig. 7-78) was 72% to 74% sensitive and up to 86% specific for predicting ACL tears. The mean normal PCL angle is $113°$ to $114°$ (226).

Anterior tibial subluxation can be inferred from PCL changes or measured on sagittal MR images (215,224).

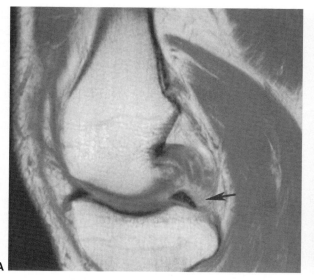
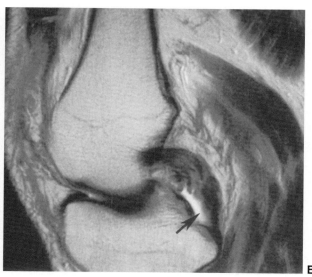

Figure 7-74 Sagittal proton density **(A)** and T2-weighted, **(B)** fast spin-echo images demonstrate thickening and increased signal intensity of the PCL with fluid at the tibial attachment (*arrow*) consistent with a high-grade partial tear.

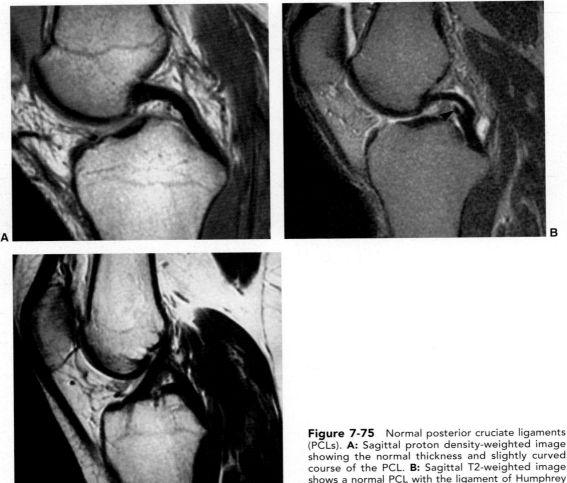

Figure 7-75 Normal posterior cruciate ligaments (PCLs). **A:** Sagittal proton density-weighted image showing the normal thickness and slightly curved course of the PCL. **B:** Sagittal T2-weighted image shows a normal PCL with the ligament of Humphrey anteriorly (*arrowhead*). **C:** Sagittal proton density-weighted image demonstrating normal anterior and posterior cruciate ligaments.

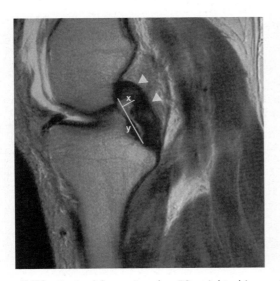

Figure 7-76 Sagittal fast spin-echo, T2-weighted image in a patient with an ACL tear and buckling of the PCL (*white arrowheads*). Line *y* is extended from the femoral to tibial attachments. Line *x* is perpendicular to *y* at the point of maximum curve. Curve value = x/y.

Subluxation was graded using 5-mm increments by Chan et al. (127). Patients with no subluxation were considered grade 0; those with 0- to 5-mm displacement, grade 1; and greater than 5 mm, grade 2, etc. Measurements were made through the midlateral femoral condyle (Fig. 7-78). Subluxation of more than 5 mm resulted in a sensitivity of 86% and specificity of 99% for ACL tears. Vahey et al. (225) reported 58% sensitivity, 93% specificity, and 69% accuracy using this technique for ACL tears.

Posterior displacement of the lateral meniscus with relation to the tibia on sagittal images is also a sign of tibial shift ("uncovered meniscus sign") (215). A vertical line constructed through the posterior cortical margin of the tibia should not intersect the lateral meniscus (see Fig. 7-79) (215,226). McCauley et al. (226) reported sensitivity of 56% and specificity of 97% using this technique.

Bone bruises, specifically involving the lateral femoral condyle and tibial plateau (see Fig. 7-80) have also been reported with ACL tears (306). McCauley et al. (226) reported a sensitivity of 50% and specificity of 97% for bone bruise in diagnosing ACL tears. Tung et al. (215) noted bone

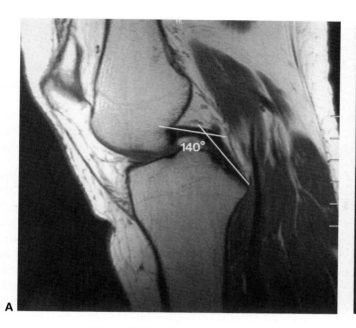

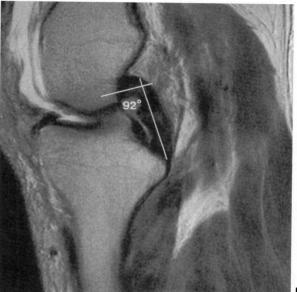

Figure 7-77   The PCL angle is formed by lines through the tibial and femoral segments of the ligament. Normal mean is 113° to 114°. **A:** Sagittal MR image demonstrating a normal patient with a PCL angle of 140°. **B:** Anterior cruciate ligament tear with a PCL angle of 92°. Angles of <105° have near 86% specificity for ACL tear (226).

bruises in 73% of patients with ACL tears studied within 9 weeks of injury. Therefore, it is important to know when the injury occurred to make this secondary sign meaningful (215,223). In children, ligament laxity may allow a bone bruise to occur while the ACL is still intact (220).

Articular abnormalities in the lateral femoral articular surface have also been described with ACL tears (129,203).

Cobby et al. (129) measured the depth of the lateral condylopatellar sulcus (see Fig. 7-81). In normal patients, the mean depth was 0.45 mm, compared to 0.89 mm in patients with ACL tears. In patients with a normal ACL, the sulcus was never deeper than 1.2 mm. A sulcus depth of 1.5 mm was three standard deviations above the mean and a reliable sign of ACL disruption (129).

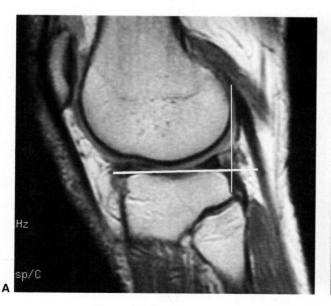

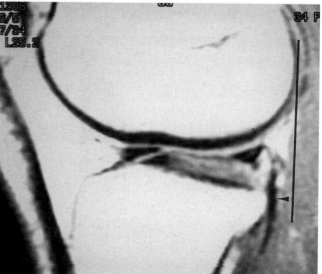

Figure 7-78   Tibial subluxation measured through the midlateral femoral condyle. Lines can be drawn vertically at the tibial and femoral margin or using the tibial surface **(A)** and drawing lines perpendicular to it (224). **A:** Normal sagittal proton density-weighted image with no subluxation. Note the normal position of the lateral meniscus. **B:** Sagittal image with meniscal windows demonstrating 6-mm subluxation (*arrowhead*).

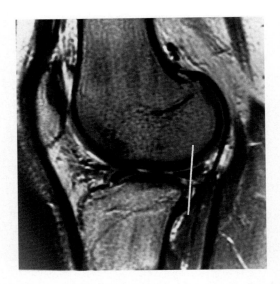

Figure 7-79 Sagittal MR image in a patient with an ACL tear and tibial subluxation with an "uncovered meniscus" sign. A line along the posterior tibial cortex passes through the meniscus.

Other signs and injuries associated with ACL tears (Table 7-7) include joint effusion, angle between tibia and ACL <45°, MCL tears (18%), meniscal tears (65% to 78% of ACL tears have an associated meniscal tear, but the normal ACL is with 63% of meniscal injuries), and the Segond fracture (see Fig. 7-82) (74,149,213,226,228,229).

MRI data for cruciate ligament tears continues to improve. Our data demonstrated an accuracy of 95%, specificity of 98%, positive predictive value of 88%, and a negative predictive value of 96%.

Evaluation of the medial and lateral collateral ligaments is generally easily accomplished using the routine MR examination. However, in some cases additional axial and coronal sections may be necessary to more clearly define subtle lesions (1,62,97,210,230). In addition, the coronal and axial images need to include enough of the tibia to show the distal ligament at the insertion (see Fig. 7-83). Subtle tears can be overlooked if this is not accomplished. The MCL is typically divided into layers (see Figs. 7-8 and 7-84) (78,210,231). The first layer is composed of deep

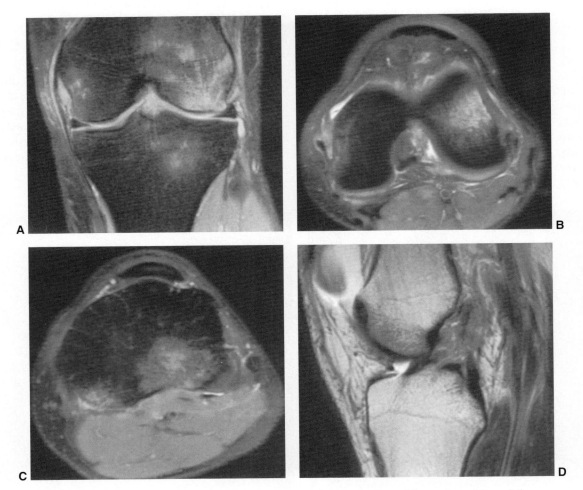

Figure 7-80 ACL tear with bone bruises involving the anterior lateral femoral condyle and the posterolateral tibia consistent with "kissing contusions." **A:** Coronal fat-suppressed, T2-weighted image demonstrating the femoral bone bruise as well as an MCL sprain. **B:** Axial T2-weighted, fat-suppressed image again shows the lateral femoral condylar bruise. **C:** Axial fat-suppressed, T2-weighted image showing the tibial bone bruise. **D:** Sagittal proton density-weighted image demonstrating complete disruption of the ACL as well as a joint effusion.

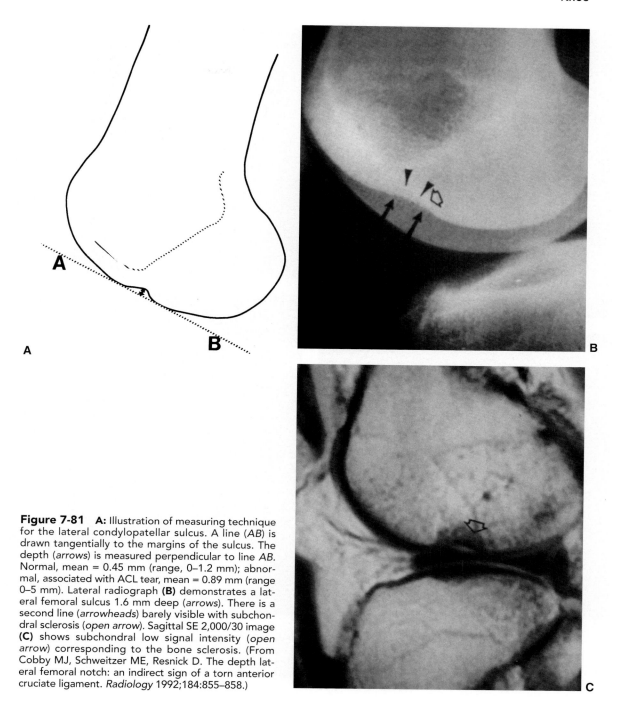

Figure 7-81 **A:** Illustration of measuring technique for the lateral condylopatellar sulcus. A line (*AB*) is drawn tangentially to the margins of the sulcus. The depth (*arrows*) is measured perpendicular to line *AB*. Normal, mean = 0.45 mm (range, 0–1.2 mm); abnormal, associated with ACL tear, mean = 0.89 mm (range 0–5 mm). Lateral radiograph **(B)** demonstrates a lateral femoral sulcus 1.6 mm deep (*arrows*). There is a second line (*arrowheads*) barely visible with subchondral sclerosis (*open arrow*). Sagittal SE 2,000/30 image **(C)** shows subchondral low signal intensity (*open arrow*) corresponding to the bone sclerosis. (From Cobby MJ, Schweitzer ME, Resnick D. The depth lateral femoral notch: an indirect sign of a torn anterior cruciate ligament. *Radiology* 1992;184:855–858.)

fascia that covers the quadriceps. The second layer includes the MCL and the third layer is the capsular ligament (38,228,231). Superficial portion of the ligament typically arises from the medial femoral condyle and passes distally to insert approximately 5 cm below the joint line and posterior to the pes anserinus (205,210,229,230). Superficial fibers are separated from the deep fibers by a bursa that may be inflamed and enlarged and should not be confused with a tear in the MCL (Figs. 7-20 and 7-84). The deep ligament is firmly attached to the capsule (Fig. 7-11) and midportion of

the medial meniscus and attaches to the femur and tibia more nearly adjacent to the joint. This anatomic association results in combination injuries of the ligament, capsule, and peripheral meniscocapsular separations (205,210,232). The MCL is a stabilizer that resists external rotation and anterior forces and is more often injured than its lateral counterpart. The MCL is typically injured during valgus stress with the knee in flexion (see Figs. 7-83, 7-85, and 7-86) (205,210,230,232). Associated injuries of the capsule and adjacent meniscus are common. Tears of the ACL are

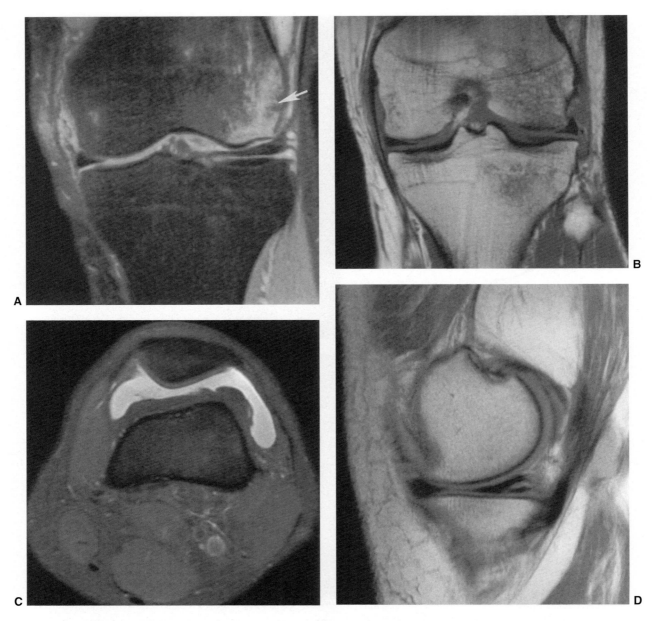

Figure 7-82 Athlete with an ACL tear, lateral condylar bone bruise, joint effusion, and medial meniscal tear. **A:** Coronal DESS image demonstrates the lateral bone bruise (*arrow*). **B:** Coronal T1-weighted image shows edema in the femur and tibia. **C:** Axial fat-suppressed, proton density-weighted image shows a large effusion. **D:** Sagittal proton density-weighted image demonstrating a tear in the posterior horn of the medial meniscus.

frequently noted in association with MCL tears (30%) (see Figs. 7-11, 7-85D, and 7-87) (192). O'Donahue's triad (medial meniscal tear, ACL tear, and MCL tear) is a frequently described injury pattern (77,210).

Acute incomplete tears result in areas of increased signal intensity in the soft tissues and within the normally dark-appearing ligaments (Fig. 7-85) on T2-weighted images. When an incomplete tear is present (Fig. 7-85A), the joint space is normal and the course of the ligament unchanged. Care should be taken not to misinterpret the MCL bursa or fat between its superficial and deep fibers as an incomplete

injury (Fig. 7-84). Complete tears in either ligament are identified by increased signal intensity at the site of the tear with lack of continuity of the ligament and typically retraction of the torn ends (see Figs. 7-85 and 7-88). Secondary findings, such as joint space widening, effusion, meniscal tears, cruciate tears, and bone bruises (Figs. 7-85, 7-87), are not unusual (3,77,149). Yao et al. (230) reported an 87% accuracy for MRI in classifying MCL injuries. Minor injuries are particularly easy to detect due to the high sensitivity of MRI. Partial or grade 2 tears are more difficult to correctly classify with MRI (230).

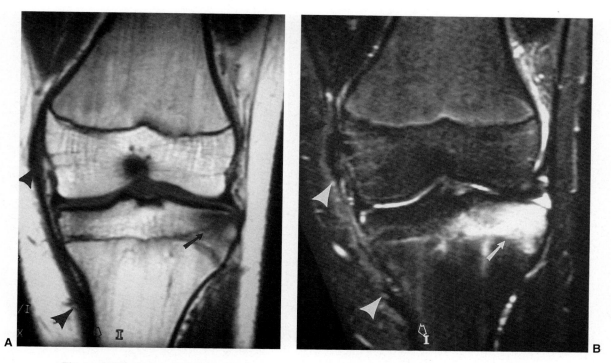

Figure 7-83   Football player with a valgus injury and bone bruise laterally. Coronal T1-weighted **(A)** and fat-suppressed, T2-weighted **(B)** images show the obvious bone bruise (*arrow*). There are multiple incomplete tears (*arrowheads*) in the MCL. The distal aspect (*open arrow*) is just included in the field of view.

The lateral support consists of three structures (54,77,97). The lateral capsular ligament is essentially a capsular thickening. The lateral collateral ligament is separated from the capsule (see Fig. 7-89). This well-defined cord (Figs. 7-11 and 7-89) extends from the lateral femoral condyle to the fibular head. This low intensity structure can be seen on coronal, sagittal, and axial MR images (54,232). The iliotibial band is a thinner structure that lies more anteriorly and can be identified on coronal images (Fig. 7-89C). The fibular collateral ligament is injured infrequently compared to the MCL. When the ligament is disrupted, it is not uncommon to identify associated tears in the PCL (3,77).

The anatomy of the extensor mechanism is easily assessed with MR images (3,78,233–236). The extensor

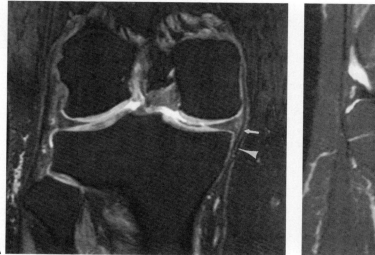

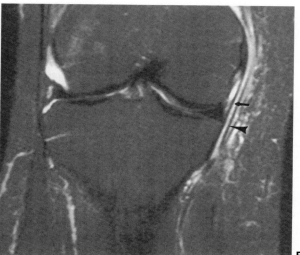

Figure 7-84   Coronal DESS images **(A,B)** of the knee demonstrating the superficial (*large arrowhead*), deep (*small arrow*) fibers of the MCL, with the bursa and fat between the superficial and deep fibers.

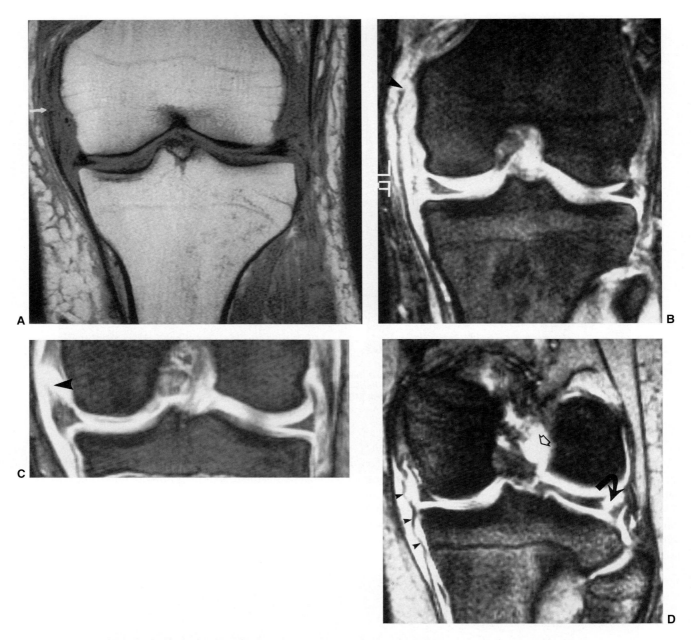

Figure 7-85 Medial collateral ligament (MCL) tears demonstrated on spin-echo and gradient-echo images. **A:** T1-weighted coronal image demonstrates a sprain (*arrow*) of the MCL at the femoral attachment. **B:** Coronal gradient-echo image with increased signal along the MCL and a complete tear (*arrowhead*) near the femoral origin. There is also a capsular tear and peripheral meniscal separation. **C:** Complete tear of the capsule and MCL (*arrowhead*) just above the meniscus. **D:** Wavy MCL (*arrowheads*) due to a complete tear proximally. There is also a torn (*curved arrow*) discoid meniscus laterally. The ACL (*open arrow*) is absent.

mechanism includes the quadriceps muscle group (vastus medialis, vastus lateralis, vastus intermedius, and rectus femoris), and tendon, patella, patellar tendon or ligament (these terms are often both applied), and the tibial tuberosity (78,234,236,237). The quadriceps tendon is formed by muscle slips resulting in layers that may be evident on axial and sagittal MR images (see Fig. 7-90). The superficial muscle layer is formed by the rectus femoris tendon, the intermediate layer by the vastus lateralis and medialis, and the deep layer by the vastus intermedius (Fig. 7-90) (236,238). The tendon attaches to the patella that typically has a larger lateral and smaller medial facet. Patellar anatomy and variants will be discussed more completely later. The patellar tendon extends from the inferior patella to the tibial tuberosity with

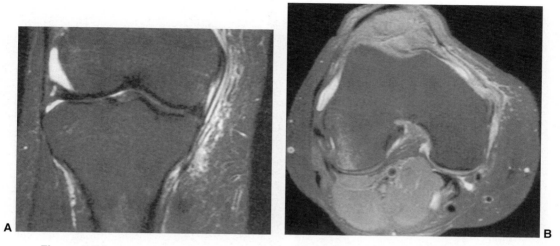

Figure 7-86 Coronal STIR **(A)** and axial fat-suppressed proton density **(B)** images demonstrate abnormal signal intensity along the MCL with fluid in the bursa consistent with a partial tear.

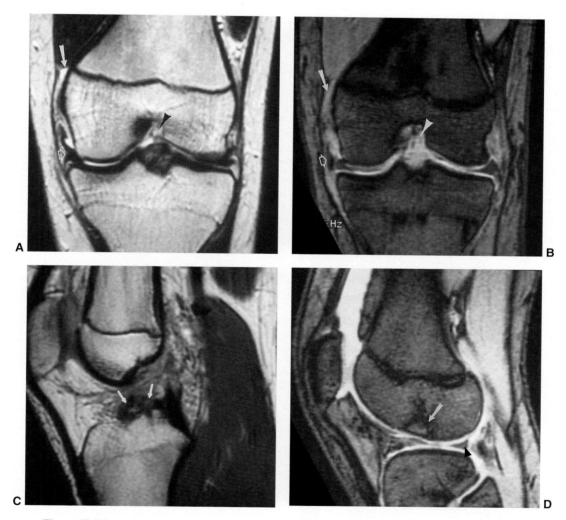

Figure 7-87 Soccer player with knee injury. Medial collateral ligament, anterior cruciate ligament, and meniscal tear. Coronal T1-weighted **(A)** and gradient-echo **(B)** images demonstrate a medial collateral ligament tear (*white arrow*), meniscocapsular separation (*open arrow*), and an absent ACL in the notch (*arrowhead*). Sagittal proton density-weighted image **(C)** demonstrates the distal ACL remnant (*arrows*). Sagittal gradient-echo image **(D)** shows an effusion, femoral condylar bruise (*arrow*), and posterior lateral meniscal tear (*arrowhead*).

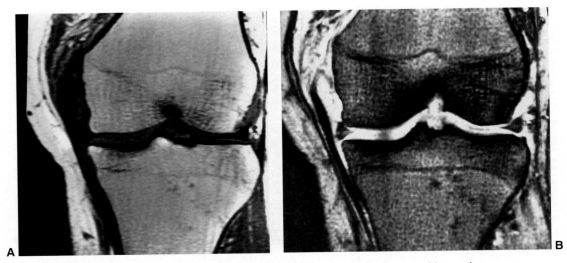

Figure 7-88 Complete tear of the medial collateral ligament with edema and hemorrhage near the femoral attachment seen on coronal T1-weighted **(A)** and gradient-echo **(B)** images. T2-weighted or T2* images are superior for injury detection and classification.

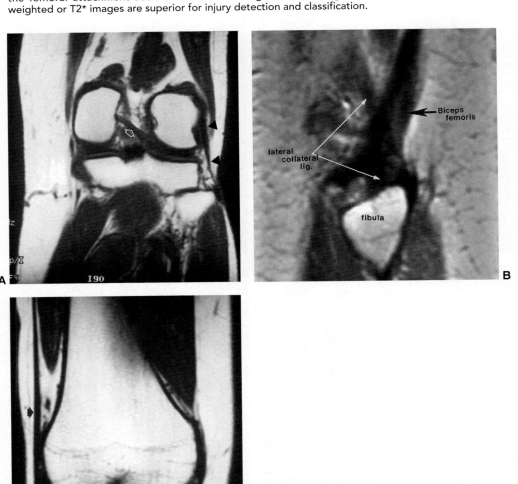

Figure 7-89 Lateral ligaments and support structures. **A:** Coronal image demonstrating the lateral collateral ligament extending from the fibular head to the lateral femoral condyle (*arrowheads*). Note also the ligament of Wrisberg (*open arrow*). **B:** Sagittal image at the level of the fibula demonstrating the biceps femoris tendon and lateral collateral ligament. **C:** Anterior coronal T1-weighted image demonstrating the iliotibial band (*arrows*).

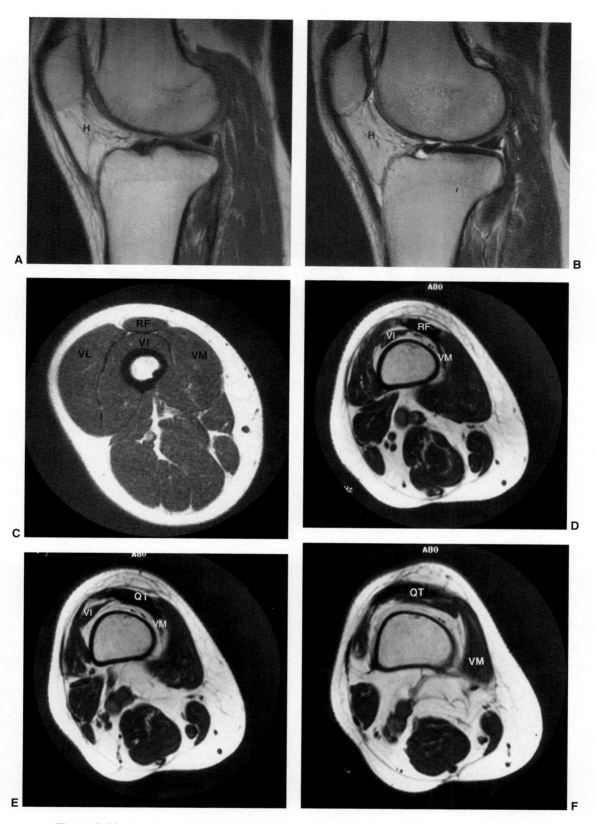

Figure 7-90 Quadriceps tendon anatomy. Sagittal MR images demonstrating uniformly low intensity in the quadriceps and patellar tendon on the proton density-weighted image **(A)** and a laminated appearance due to the superficial, intermediate and deep tendon fibers on the T2-weighted image **(B)**. Note Hoffa fat pad (*H*) posterior to the patellar ligament. Axial images demonstrating the quadriceps muscle group and tendons. **(C)** Axial image of the thigh demonstrating the rectus femoris (*RF*), vastus medialis (*VM*), vastus lateralis (*VL*), and vastus intermedius (*VI*). More distally **(D)** the tendon slips off the vastus intermedius (*VI*), vastus medialis (*VM*) and rectus femoris (*RF*) are clearly separated. The tendon slips blend as they progress inferiorly (**E–H**) to form the quadriceps tendon (*QT*).

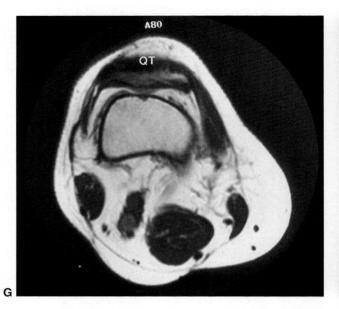

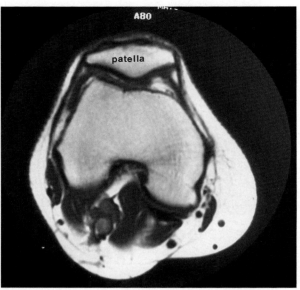

Figure 7-90 (continued)

distal expansions inserting into the anterior tibia (78,236). There is a thin layer of subcutaneous fat anterior to the tendon and a large fat pad (Hoffa fat pad) posterior to the patellar tendon (Fig. 7-90 A and B) (234,238). The prepatellar bursa is not usually seen on MR images (Fig. 7-90A) (3).

Injuries to the quadriceps and patellar tendons may be due to acute or repetitive trauma. Inflammation may result in thickening with increased signal intensity. Partial tears are seen as areas of increased signal intensity involving a portion of the tendon. Complete tears (see Fig. 7-91) are easily diagnosed by the high signal intensity in the region of the tear with separation of the involved tendon and patellar displacement (1,3,234,236,238–240).

Quadriceps tears are unusual except in elderly patients with predisposing conditions such as rheumatoid arthritis, systemic lupus erythematosus, metabolic disease, or degenerative disease (205,232,241,242). Tears, when they do occur, are usually located just above the patella (see Fig. 7-92) (241).

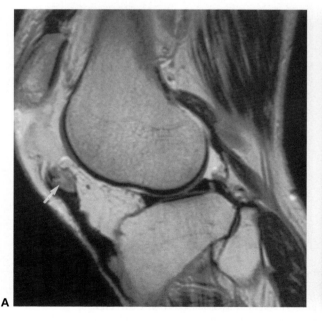

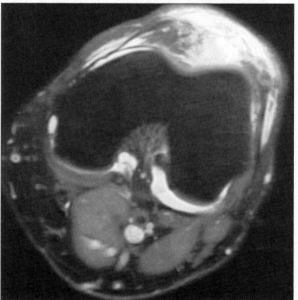

Figure 7-91 Acute patellar tendon avulsion from the lower pole of the patella. **A:** Sagittal proton density-weighted image shows the lax tendon with the avulsed bone fragment (*arrow*). **B:** Axial fat-suppressed, T2-weighted image demonstrates an absent tendon as well as a large fluid collection.

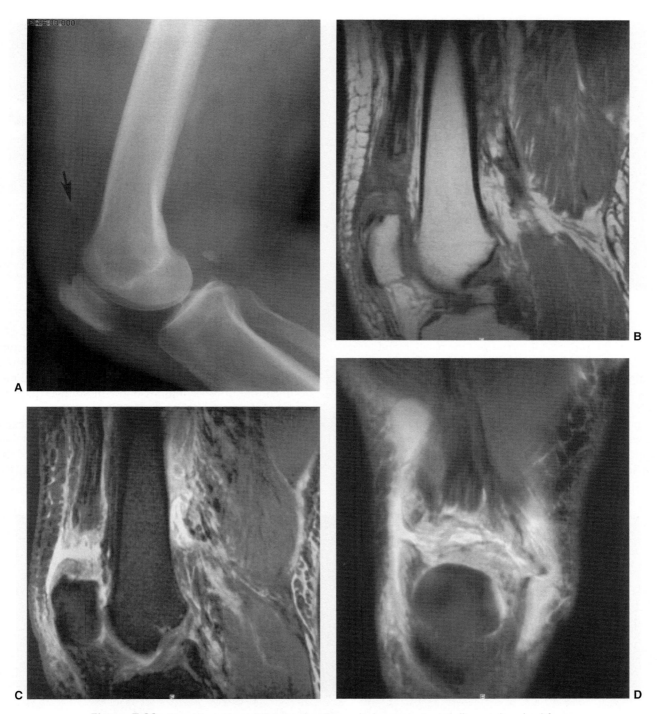

Figure 7-92 Quadriceps tear. **(A)** Lateral radiograph demonstrates swelling and avulsed fragments proximally (*arrow*). Sagittal T1- **(B)** sagittal fast spin-echo, T2-weighted **(C)** and coronal **(D)** images clearly demonstrate the tear near the patellar attachment.

Patellar tendon injuries are more frequently identified and include tendinitis, tendon tears and chronic overuse syndromes (149,233,234,236,238,239,243–246). Patellar tendinosus (jumper's knee) is a common problem in athletes involved in running and jumping sports. The etiology is most likely related to repetitive microtrauma, which leads to tendon degeneration and increased risk for tendon disruption (238,244,247). The differential diagnosis includes chondromalacia and infrapatellar plica syndrome (247). Patients usually present with point tenderness in the proximal patellar tendon. Imaging of this condition can be accomplished with ultrasound or MRI (247–249).

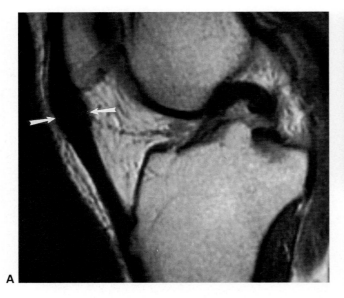

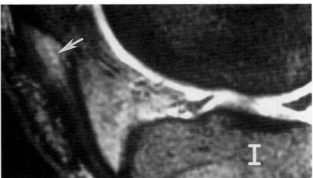

Figure 7-93 Jumper's knee. **A:** Sagittal T1-weighted image in a patient with jumper's knee demonstrating thickening of the proximal patellar tendon (*arrows*). **B:** Different patient with thickening and increased signal (*arrow*) on T2-weighted images.

MR features may be more specific. Almost all patients present with proximal thickening of the patellar tendon (see Fig. 7-93). Thickening is often greater medially, probably related to asymmetry in stress on the tendon (238). There may be variable increase in signal intensity near the inferior pole of the patella. Signal intensity is typically intermediate on proton density images and may or may not increase on T2-weighted sequences (3,247). Histologically, these areas demonstrate tenocyte hyperplasia, angiogenesis, and loss of collagen architecture with microtears (238). These areas

show enhancement after intravenous gadolinium (247). Tendinosus and degeneration may lead to complete disruption (238). Patellar tendon tears have an appearance similar to quadriceps tears (see Figs. 7-91 and 7-94). These injuries are uncommon. Most injuries occur in younger patients involved in athletic activities (1,238).

A similar presentation may be seen in adolescents (Sinding-Larsen-Johansson disease), but there is generally osseous fragmentation involving the lower pole of the patella (236,241). Osgood-Schlatter disease affects the

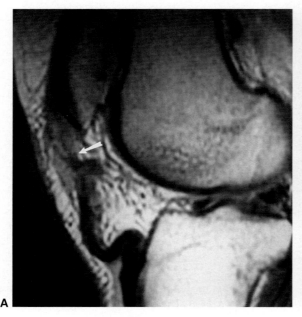

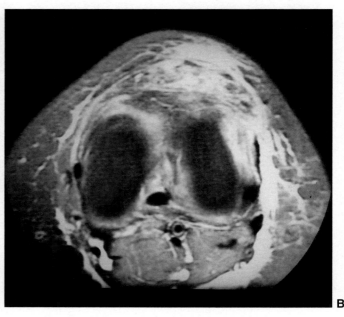

Figure 7-94 Complete tear of the patellar tendon in a weightlifter. Sagittal T1-weighted image **(A)** demonstrates a complete tear at the patellar attachment (*arrow*). Note the wavy appearance of the distal segment. Axial fat-suppressed, T2-weighted fast spin-echo image **(B)** shows high signal intensity with no remaining dark signal normally seen in the tendon.

distal tendon and tibial tuberosity. Clinical and radiographic features are usually characteristic, so MR imaging is not required (3,37,77).

Assessment of the quadriceps tendon and patellar ligament (tendon) is easily accomplished using sagittal and axial MR images (see Figs. 7-91 to 7-95) (3). Thus, routine knee screening examination is adequate (3,250,251). When a tear in either of these structures is identified, it is important to obtain axial images so that classification of the tear can be more accurately completed. Again, T2-weighted (SE or FSE) or GRE T2*sequences are preferred to identify and classify these injuries. Many extensor mechanism injuries can be detected clinically and complete tears can often be palpated. Therefore, MRI may not be necessary except to define the exact nature or the extent of the clinically suspected lesion (3,37,77).

Ligament–Tendon Reconstruction

Ligament and tendon injuries may require primary repair or reconstruction procedures using tendon grafts, allografts, or synthetic materials (119,197,252–254). Manaster and others have described radiographic and other imaging features of ligament repairs (111,119,255). Imaging studies are most frequently used to evaluate cruciate ligament reconstructions. Patellar tendon graft composed of the middle third of the tendon and a bone plug form the patella, and tibial tuberosity is frequently used (111,119,253,256).

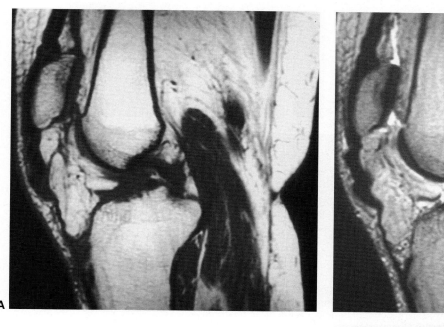

A

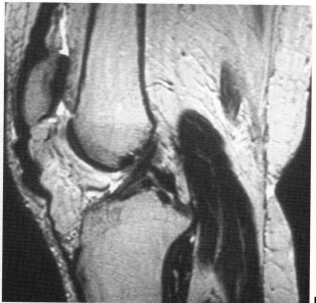

B

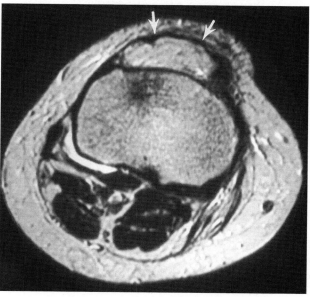

C

Figure 7-95 Old distal tear of the patellar tendon. Sagittal T1-weighted **(A)** and proton density **(B)** images show a wavy tendon with superior patellar displacement. There is marked thinning of the distal tendon. Axial proton density image **(C)** shows the marked distal thinning (*arrows*).

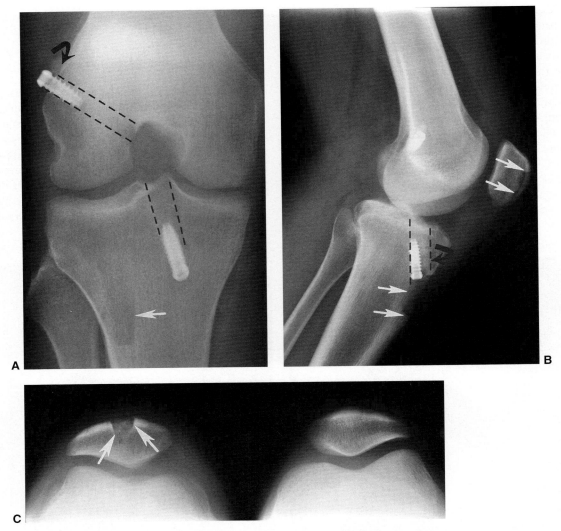

Figure 7-96 Notch **(A)**, lateral **(B)**, and merchant **(C)** radiographs after ACL reconstruction using patellar tendon graft and interference screws. The tunnels (*broken lines*), bone plug (*curved arrow*), and donor sites (*arrows*) are clearly defined. Bone plugs are often obscured, at least partially, on MR images due to metal artifact.

Gracilis, semitendinosus, and, less frequently, iliotibial band grafts may also be used (257). The graft is inserted through tibial and femoral tunnels (8- to 10-mm in diameter) and secured with interference screws in the tunnel, or bone staples and other soft tissue anchors outside the tunnel (see Fig. 7-96) (119). Most repairs can be evaluated with physical examination and routine radiography. Isometric positioning of the tunnels (see Fig. 7-97) is important for good results. Improper positioning is a common complication (Table 7-8). Grafts are usually incorporated 5 months after surgery (119,256).

Evaluation of complications and results is usually possible with physical examination and routine radiographs. Most complications (position, hardware, fracture, impingement, and instability) can be detected in this manner (Table 7-8) (119,121,259,260). A cross-table lateral view of the knee in extension is a simple method to evaluate graft impingement, which usually occurs in the terminal 5 degrees to 10 degrees of extension (see Fig. 7-98) (256).

MR imaging is also useful to evaluate the graft, tunnel position (see Fig. 7-99), and other bone and soft tissue abnormalities that may cause symptoms not directly related to the repair (119,128,149,259,260). Sagittal, coronal, and axial images are all useful. A bolster placed under the foot will hyperextend the knee, which enhances the value of sagittal images for evaluating graft impingement. T1-weighted spin-echo sequences are adequate for tunnel evaluation and metal artifact is less significant (3). Artifact is more significant with T2-weighted or GRE sequences. However, since orthopedic surgeons began using titanium screws, the artifact problem has been reduced (see Fig. 7-100). When indicated, T1-weighted images with intravenous

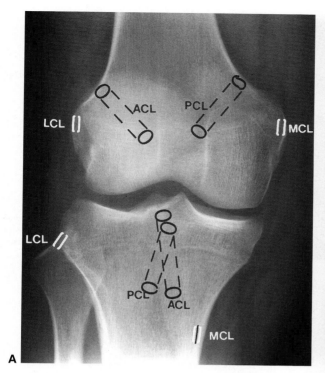

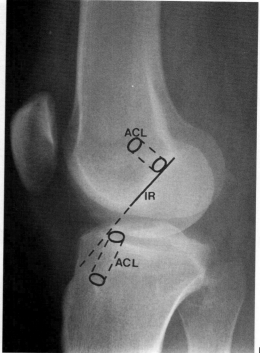

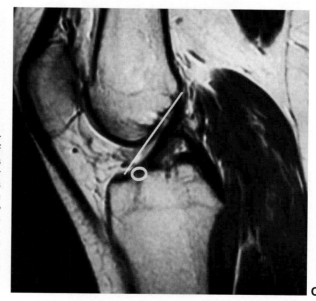

Figure 7-97 Positioning of tunnels and grafts for cruciate ligament repair. **A:** Anteroposterior view of the knee demonstrating the femoral and tibial tunnels for the *ACL* and *PCL* ligaments. The attachments for the medial (*MCL*) and lateral (*LCL*) collateral ligaments are also demonstrated. **B:** Lateral radiograph is an extension demonstrating the intercondylar roof (*line with broken extension*) and the normal position of the ACL tunnels. If the tibial opening is anterior to the intercondylar roof, ACL impingement can occur, limiting extension and reducing function (166,258). **C:** Sagittal proton density-weighted MR image demonstrating the intercondylar roof (*line*) and attachment site of the normal ACL (*circle*).

gadolinium can be useful. However, in our experience, this is rarely necessary. MR images should be evaluated to define tunnel position, bone plug integrity, signal intensity changes in the graft, and graft laxity (see Fig. 7-101). Signs similar to those described with conventional ligament tears can be used for graft rupture. Secondary signs, such as hooking of the PCL, can also be applied. Howell et al. (259) described increased signal intensity in the distal (tibial segment) graft in patients with impingement due to positioning the tibial tunnel anterior to the intercondylar roof. Four of 14 grafts failed in this setting, though function

may be acceptable. Extension is reduced up to 5°, depending on tunnel position (259,260).

Complications of Anterior Cruciate Ligament Reconstruction

ACL tears are one of the most common injuries of the knee in young adults and athletes (165,261–263). Reconstruction of the torn ACL has been described above. Long-term results are usually favorable; however, unsatisfactory results do occur, including graft failure, graft impingement,

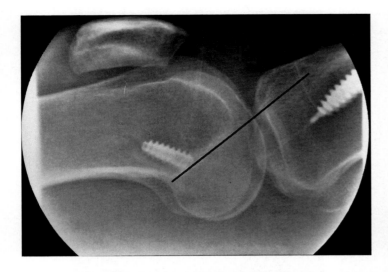

Figure 7-98 Fluoroscopically positioned lateral in full extension shows the tibial tunnel is completely posterior and parallel to the condylar roof (*black line*), which is the normal position.

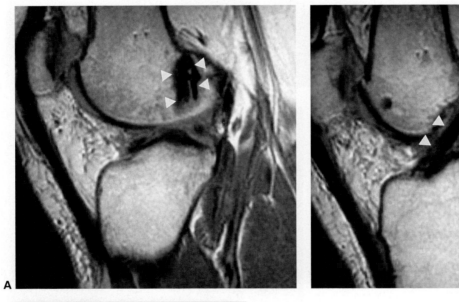

A

B

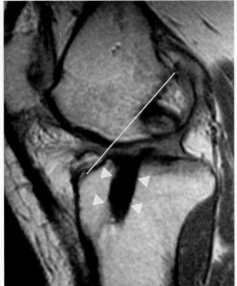

C

Figure 7-99 Sagittal proton density-weighted images after patellar tendon graft reconstruction of the ACL. **A:** Sagittal image demonstrating the femoral tunnel (*arrowheads*). **B:** Sagittal image showing the normal low intensity graft (*arrowheads*) with the normal straight course. **C:** Sagittal image demonstrating the tibial tunnel (*arrowheads*), normally positioned posterior to the intercondylar roof (*white line*).

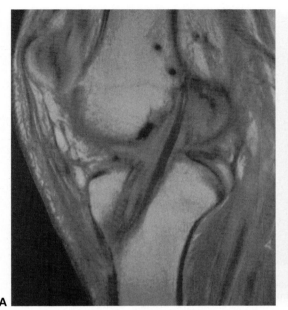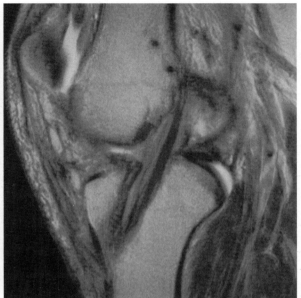

Figure 7-100   Sagittal proton density **(A)** and fast spin-echo T2-weighted **(B)** images demonstrate both the tibial and femoral graft tunnels. The graft is intact. Recent use of titanium screws has significantly decreased the metal artifact.

cystic degeneration in the graft, arthrofibrosis or cyclops lesions, and infection (263,264) (Table 7-8).

Graft Failure

The ACL graft is disrupted when no intact fibers can be identified, and partially disrupted when some of the fibers

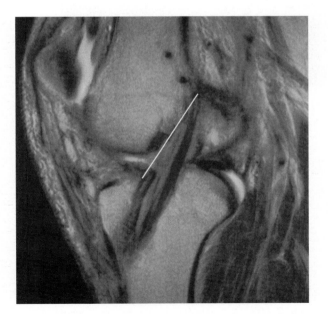

Figure 7-101   Sagittal fast spin-echo, T2-weighted image demonstrating a normal tibial tunnel. The graft is taut without ligamentous laxity. There is a small joint effusion that is not uncommon for 6 to 9 months following the surgery.

remain intact (3). Graft failure presents clinically as knee instability (see Fig. 7-102).

Arthrofibrosis and Cyclops Lesions

Cyclops lesion, or localized arthrofibrosis, refers to synovial hyperplasia with excessive production of fibrous tissue and inflammatory cells surrounding the ACL graft. This is the second most common cause of loss of extension of the knee. The most common cause is graft impingement (263). Arthroscopically, the cyclops lesion is identified as a headlike, fibrous lesion with purple-blue areas of discoloration resembling an eye (see Fig. 7-103).

MR imaging characteristics of the cyclops lesions demonstrate a well-circumscribed lesion or nodule with intermediate to low signal intensity on both T1- and T2-weighted images. The lesion lies anterior to the tibial insertion of the

TABLE 7-8

LIGAMENT RECONSTRUCTION COMPLICATIONS

Improper tunnel position
Hardware failure
Bone plug fracture
Patella fracture (stress riser from donor site)
Patellar tendon failure
Graft rupture
Graft impingement
Anterior arthrofibrosis (cyclops lesion)
Postoperative infection

From references 111, 121, 247, 256, 259, and 260.

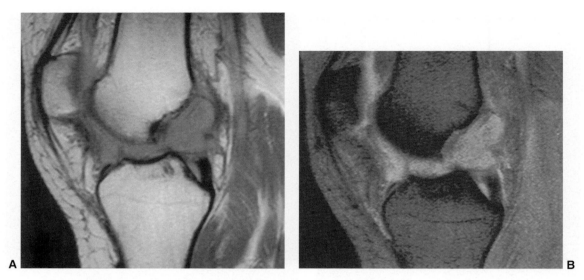

Figure 7-102 Graft rupture and failure shown as complete absence of any visualized graft fibers on sagittal proton density **(A)** and gradient-echo **(B)** images.

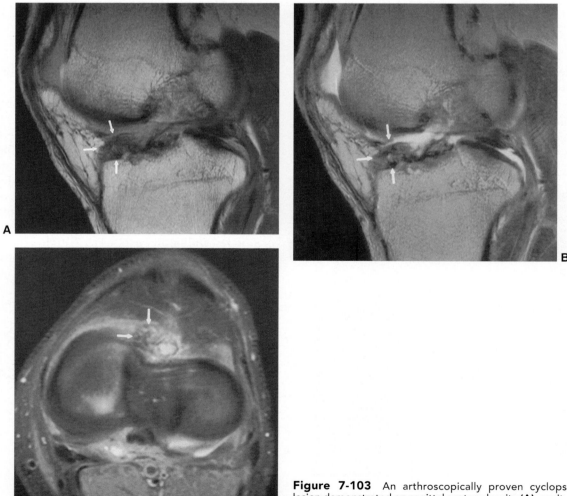

Figure 7-103 An arthroscopically proven cyclops lesion demonstrated on sagittal proton density **(A)**, sagittal fast spin-echo, T2- **(B)**, and axial proton density, fat-suppressed **(C)** images. The lesion (*small white arrows*) is located anterior to the ACL graft and posterior to the infrapatellar fat pad.

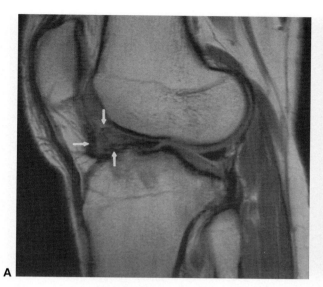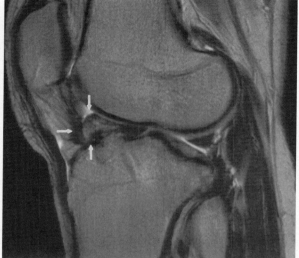

Figure 7-104 A cyclops lesion (*small white arrows*) is identified on sagittal proton density **(A)** and fast spin-echo, T2-weighted **(B)** images that demonstrate low signal intensity on both sequences.

ACL graft and posterior to the infrapatellar fat pad (see Figs. 7-103 and 7-104). There also exists a more diffuse form of cyclops lesion termed diffuse arthrofibrosis. This entity engulfs and surrounds the ACL graft both anteriorly and posteriorly, as well as abutting the joint capsule. The diffuse form demonstrates MR signal characteristics similar to the cyclops lesion with low to intermediate signal intensity on T1- and T2-weighted sequences (165,263).

Postoperative Infection

Postoperative infection of ACL reconstruction can occur. Septic arthritis is rare, affecting 0.5% of postoperative orthopedic patients (165,263). The most common pathogen is *Staphylococcus aureus*. Although aspiration is absolutely mandatory to establish a diagnosis and pathogen, MR can be extremely useful in assessing the extent of infection, including abscess formation, draining sinuses, and osteomyelitis. A sinus tract is seen as a linear tunnel with low signal intensity on T1-weighted images and increased signal intensity on T2-weighted images. Sinus tracts extend from the subcutaneous region to the underlying bone (see Fig. 7-105).

Plicae

The significance of synovial plicae was not fully recognized prior to the advent of arthroscopy (77,154,265,266). Plicae are embryonic synovial remnants that may be present in an asymptomatic knee. During fetal development, there are thin membranes that divide the knee into medial, lateral, and suprapatellar compartments. These membranes usually involute, resulting in a single cavity in the knee. When the membrane or a portion of it persists into adult life, it is termed a plica. These remnants are reported

in up to 20% of the population (267,268). The most common plicae (see Fig. 7-106) are classified as suprapatellar, mediopatellar, and infrapatellar (anterior) based on the location of the original fetal membrane (266,268,269).

The suprapatellar plica is the remnant that separated the suprapatellar bursa from the medial and lateral compartments (Fig. 7-106C). Several forms have been observed (266). A transverse septum may be complete (Fig. 7-106C), or partial medial, lateral, or central suprapatellar plicae may be present (266). The mediopatellar plica begins above the patella medially and progresses distally to insert on the synovium above the infrapatellar fat pad (154,267). The mediopatellar plica (Fig. 7-106B) is most often symptomatic (149,266). On sagittal MR or CT images, this can be seen as a fold of soft tissue extending through the suprapatellar bursa. On axial images this remnant extends into the suprapatellar bursa (see Fig. 7-107).

The infrapatellar plica is detected most frequently. This plica follows a course along the upper margin of the ACL (Fig. 7-106A). It is rarely symptomatic (154,266,267). However, the infrapatellar plica may be confused with an intact ACL, interfere with arthroscopy, or increase difficulty in removing loose bodies from the intercondylar region (269).

With chronic inflammation, these membranes can become thickened and cause clicking or snapping as they pass over the femoral condyles. When left untreated, synovitis and cartilage damage can occur (267,268). The exact etiology is unclear, but trauma and other associated conditions such as osteoarthritis, loose bodies, etc. may be evident (267,268). Most patients (90%) present with tenderness above the joint near the superior pole of the patella. A snap can be demonstrated in 71% of patients. Symptoms are generally due to thickening of the mediopatellar plica; however, the suprapatellar plica has

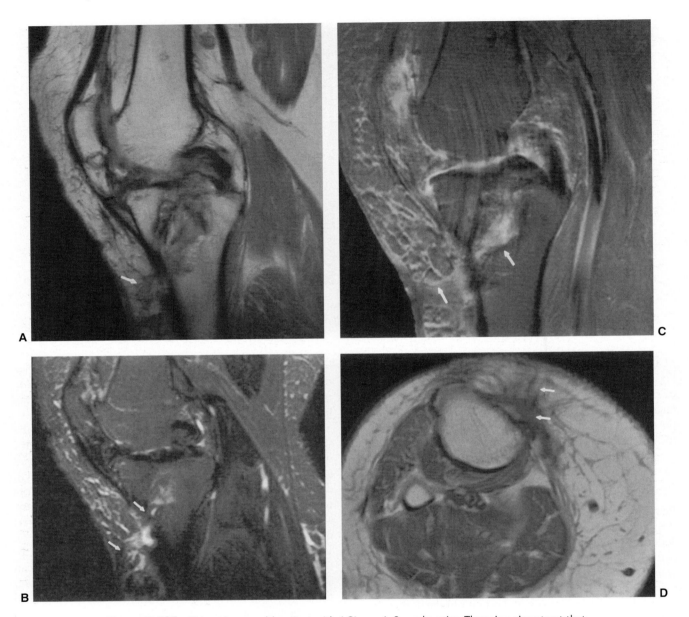

Figure 7-105 Thirty-six-year-old patient with ACL repair 3 weeks prior. There is a sinus tract that begins at the tibial insertion of the graft and extends to the subcutaneous tissues. Cultures were positive for *Staphylococcus aureus*. Sagittal T1-weighted **(A)**, STIR **(B)**, and postcontrast T1-weighted fat-suppressed **(C)** images demonstrate a linear sinus tract extending from the tibia (*white arrows*). Axial T1-weighted **(D)** and postcontrast, fat-suppressed T1-weighted **(E)** images demonstrate the sinus tract (*white arrows*). Blood pool **(F)** and delayed **(G)** images from a three-phase bone scan show no flow in **F** and increased uptake on all phases in the right knee in the distribution of the sinus tract and ACL graft. **H:** Radiograph of the right knee 2 months after intraoperative placement of antibiotic beads and cement.

been implicated in patellar tracking abnormalities (267). Symptoms are most common in children and young adults. The symptoms are not specific, making differentiation from other disorders difficult (Table 7-9) (266).

When patients present with symptoms suggesting plicae syndrome (snapping, peripatellar pain), the MR examination must be modified. The T2-weighted sagittal images are adequate for identification of the suprapatellar (see Fig. 7-108) and infrapatellar plicae. However, axial T2*- or T2-weighted images are indicated to identify the mediopatellar plica or more complex lesions (Fig. 7-109). The low signal intensity plicae is more easily seen contrasted to the high signal intensity synovial fluid (see Fig. 7-109) (3,149,266). Intraarticular or intravenous gadolinium is generally not indicated, as an effusion is invariably present when plicae become inflamed and symptomatic.

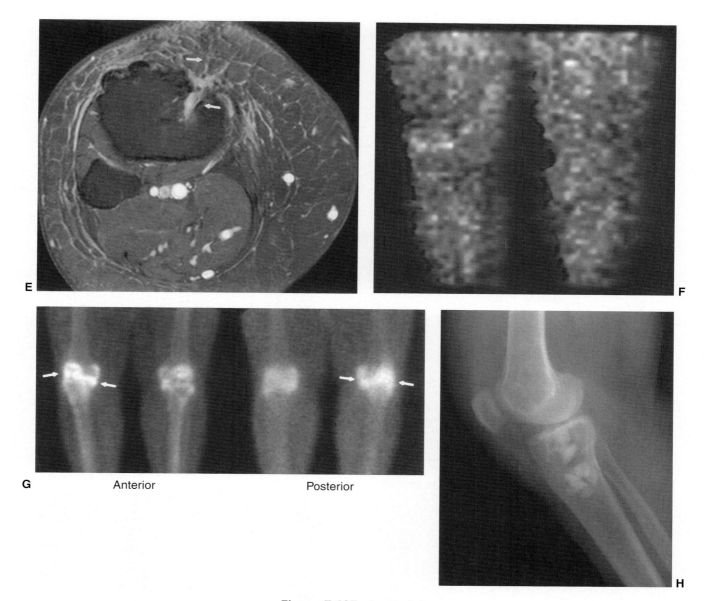

G   Anterior   Posterior

Figure 7-105 *(continued)*

Other conditions may mimic plica syndrome (Table 7-9). Most, except patellar tracking disorders, are easily detected using a standard MR knee examination (see Fig. 7-110). Thickened, symptomatic plicae can be treated conservatively, but arthroscopic division frequently yields much better results. Johnson et al. (266) reported 83% improved following division compared to only 29% of patients treated conservatively.

Patellar Disorders

Patellofemoral pain syndromes are commonly attributed to chondromalacia or instability due to abnormalities in the extensor mechanism (93,149,217,271–274). Imaging of patellofemoral disorders has been attempted with patellar views in 0° to 60° of flexion, arthrography, CT and arthrotomography, and MRI (4,5,23,29,275).

A review of patellar anatomy and normal relationships is important to assist in fully understanding symptoms related to the patellofemoral joint. The patella is a sesamoid bone contained in the quadriceps tendon. The patellar tendon (ligament) connects the patella to the tibial tuberosity (77,149,242). The articular surface of the patella has a medial and lateral facet that articulate with the companion femoral condyle (see Fig. 7-111) (77). The articular cartilage on the medial facet (4 to 5 mm thick) is somewhat thicker than the lateral facet (77,84). Various patellar configurations have been described. Wiberg (Fig. 7-111B)

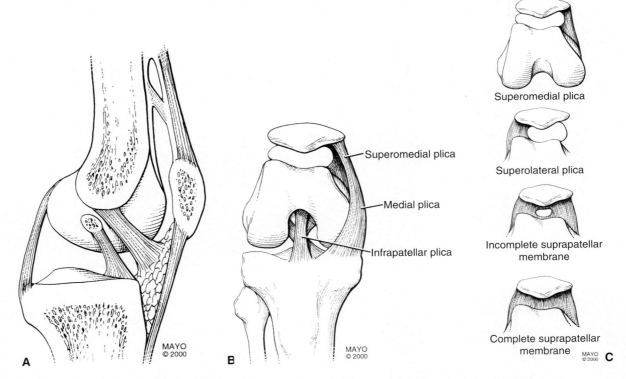

Figure 7-106   Illustrations of the plicae of the knee. **A:** Lateral illustration of anterior (infrapatellar) and suprapatellar plicae. **B:** Anterior illustration of the anterior and medial plicae with the knee flexed. **C:** Four suprapatellar plica variations.

(Labels in illustration B:) Superomedial plica, Medial plica, Infrapatellar plica

(Labels in illustration C:) Superomedial plica, Superolateral plica, Incomplete suprapatellar membrane, Complete suprapatellar membrane

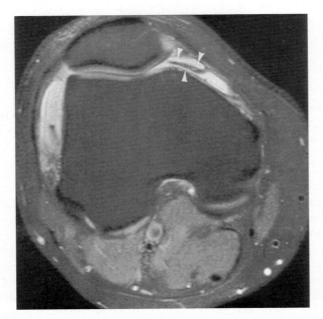

Figure 7-107   Axial fat-suppressed, proton density-weighted image in a patient with a small effusion and thickened mediopatellar plica (*arrowheads*).

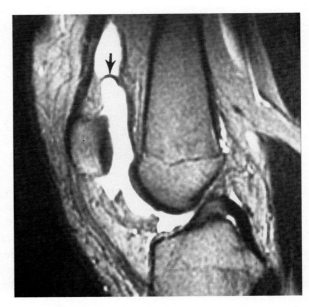

Figure 7-108   Sagittal T2-weighted image in a patient with an effusion and suprapatellar plica (*arrow*).

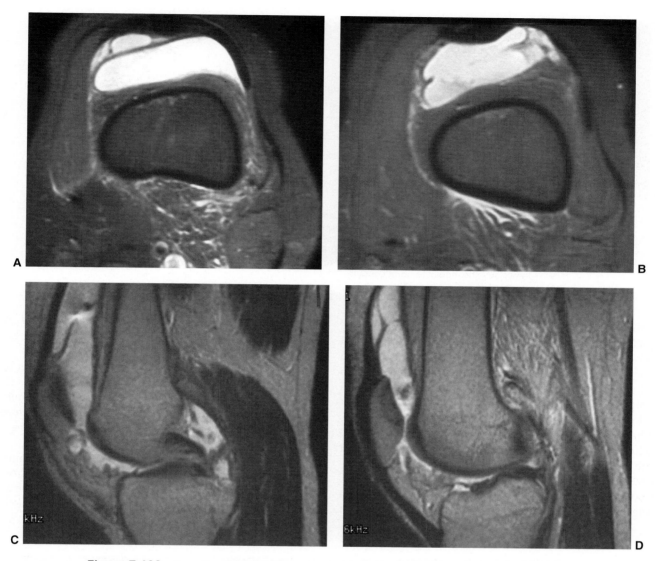

Figure 7-109 Complex plica. Axial fat-suppressed, T2-weighted, fast spin-echo images **(A,B)** demonstrate a complex plica. Sagittal T2-weighted images **(C,D)** demonstrate the configuration and thickening of the plica in the sagittal plane.

TABLE 7-9

CONDITIONS WITH SYMPTOMS THAT MIMIC PLICAE

Chondromalacia
Patellofemoral subluxation
Patellar compression syndrome
Meniscal tears
Loose bodies
Lateral retinacular injury

From references 101, 190, 241, and 270.

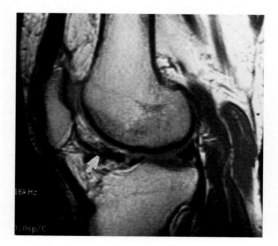

Figure 7-110 Sagittal SE 2,000/20 image of the knee in a patient with anterior pain and snapping due to a thick fibrous band in the fat anteriorly (*arrow*).

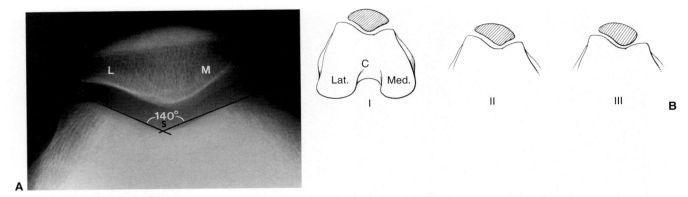

Figure 7-111 A: Merchant view of the knee demonstrating the patellofemoral relationships. The lateral facet (*L*) and medial facet (*M*) are nearly equal in size. The normal sulcus angle (*S*) formed by lines along the femoral condyles measures 138° to 142°. An increased angle indicates condylar dysplasia and a tendency for patellar subluxation. **B:** Patellar configurations. Type I, medial and lateral facets equal; type II, lateral facet larger than the medial facet (most common); type III, small medial facet with hypoplastic medial femoral condyle.

proposed a classification that includes the majority of patellar configurations (84). A type I patella has medial and lateral facets that are equal. This is the least common variation. The lateral facet is larger than the medial facet in Wiberg type II patellae. This configuration is the most common. Type III patellae have a very small medial facet and there is hypoplasia of the medial femoral facet (84). Other patellar configurations occur less commonly and include the Alpine hunter's cap (essentially a single facet with a 90 medial–lateral facet angle), flattened or hemi-patella, half-moon patella (flat posterior articular surface), hypoplastic (patella parva) and an enlarged patella (patella magna) (77,84,276). Bipartite patellae are reported in about

2% of the population. This variant usually is bilateral and typically involves the upper outer quadrant (see Fig. 7-112) (77,84,277).

The patella facilitates knee extension by increasing the distance between the extensor mechanism and the rotational axis of the femur. The patella also serves to centralize the quadriceps muscle, allowing transmission of its force around an angle during knee flexion with minimal loss of motion due to friction (77,277).

Lateral radiographs (see Fig. 7-113) are usually obtained in 30° of flexion to assist in patellar assessment. Routine MR images are usually obtained in 0° to 5° of flexion for most screening examinations. In this position the

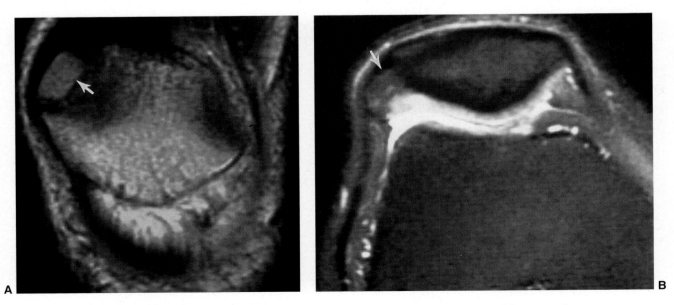

Figure 7-112 Bipartite patella. Coronal T1-weighted **(A)** and axial fat-suppressed fast spin-echo T2-weighted **(B)** images of the patellae demonstrating a bipartate patella (*arrow*).

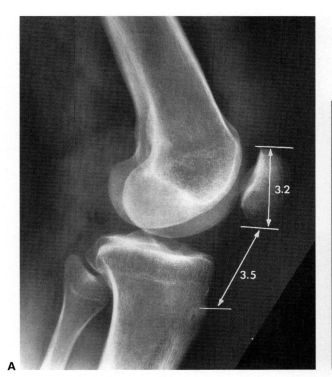
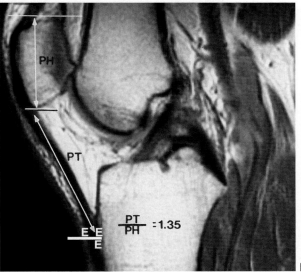

Figure 7-113   Lateral radiographic and sagittal MR patellar relationships. **A:** Lateral radiograph obtained with 35° of flexion. The patella is located over the trochlear surface of the femur. The normal relationship of the patella and patellar tendon is demonstrated. The Insall–Salvati Index (ratio of patellar tendon length to the patellar height). Normal 1.02 ±13. In this case, 3.5/3.2 = 1.09. A low-lying patella decreases the ratio (patella infra) and a high-riding patella increases the ratio (patella alta). Patella infra is usually postoperative, while patella alta is associated with subluxation, dislocation, and chondromalacia (94,240). **B:** Sagittal MR image demonstrating the patellar length and patellar tendon length. PT/PH = 1.35, where PT = patellar tendon, PH = patellar height. Normal 1.02 ±13, a difference of 20% is abnormal.

patella lies superior to the trochlear surface of the femur. The patella is also positioned somewhat laterally in 87% of patients with the knee extended. Contact with the trochlear articular surface typically begins in 10° to 20° of flexion. The patella becomes centered in the trochlea with increasing degrees of flexion (30° to 80°) (77,84).

Axial and sagittal images should be evaluated to measure patellofemoral relationships (33,278,279). Figs. 7-111A and 7-113 demonstrate the normal sulcus angle (138° to 142°) and the normal patellar tendon/patellar height ratio (1.02 ± 0. 13) (77,278).

There are several other important axial relationships. These patellofemoral indices and measurements are useful for evaluating instability and alignment disorders (77,273). The congruence angle is formed by a line (see Fig. 7-114A) bisecting the sulcus angle and a second line through the lowest point of the articular ridge of the patella. The lateral patellar angle (Fig. 7-114B) is formed by a line along the femoral condyles and a second line along the lateral patellar facet (77,84,273). The lines tend to be parallel in patients with chondromalacia and lateral patellar subluxation. Laurin (12) reported chondromalacia (10%), lateral subluxation (60%),

and lateral patellar tilt (4%) in patients with parallel lines (Fig. 7-114B).

The patellofemoral index (Fig. 7-114C) is the ratio of distance of the medial and lateral patellofemoral articulations measured at the narrowest distance. The normal ratio or index is 1.6 or less. In patients with chondromalacia (93%), lateral tilt, or subluxation (100% of patients), the index is increased (12).

Lateral patellar distance (Fig. 7-114C) is measured from the medial femoral articular margin. In normal patients, the patellar margin should be at or just medial to this margin (12). Patients with subluxation or chondromalacia have lateral patellar shift (+) (12).

Chondromalacia

Chondromalacia patella (cartilage softening) is a frequent topic in the radiology and orthopedic literature (33,55,65,116,149,217,276,280,281). The patellar articular changes may result from subluxation, fracture, or repetitive microtrauma with disruption of the vertical collagen fibers (84). Unfortunately, image features and

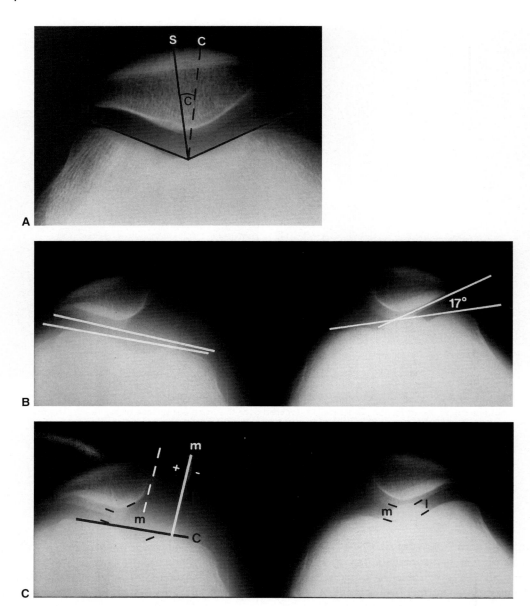

Figure 7-114   A: Merchant view of the knee demonstrating the congruence angle. This angle is formed by a line (*S*) bisecting the sulcus angle and a second line (*C, broken line*) through the lowest point in the articular surface of the patella. In this case, the congruence angle (*C*) measures −15°. If the apex of the patella is lateral to line *S* it is positive, and if medial it is negative. Normal is −8 ± 6°. A positive angle of >23° is seen on patients with recurrent dislocation. **B:** Merchant views of the knee with a lateral patellar angle of 17° on the right and lateral tilt and subluxation on the left. The lines used to form the angle do not cross within the condylar margins. **C:** Same patient as **B,** demonstrating the patellofemoral index (*m/l*). The narrowest distance in the medial joint space divided by the lateral is ≤1.6. An increase (left knee) is seen with subluxation, chondromalacia, and lateral patellar tilt. Right knee is 1.5 and the left 2.7. The lateral patellar displacement is measured using a line (*m*) perpendicular to the condylar line (*C*) at the medial margin of the medial femoral articular surface. In normal knees, the patella should be at or slightly medial to line *m*. Patients with chondromalacia and subluxation have positive measurements (12).

clinical symptoms do not always correlate with histologic changes. Chondromalacia affects men more often than women, involves the medial facet more frequently than the lateral facet, and more commonly involves the mid and lower patella (55,65,116,149,275).

Currently, arthroscopy is the technique of choice for evaluating the patellar surface (63,77). Outerbridge (282) described the appearance of cartilage in the various stages of chondromalacia (Table 7-10). During the earliest phases the normal bluish-white cartilage has a yellowish or dull

TABLE 7-10
ARTHROSCOPIC AND MR CLASSIFICATION OF CHONDROMALACIA PATELLAE

Arthroscopic Classification		MRI Classification & Image Features	
Grade 1	Softening of articular cartilage	Stage 1	Normal contour ± signal intensity change
Grade 2	Blister-like swelling	Stage 2	Focal areas of swelling with signal intensity changes on T1 and T2 weighted sequences
Stage 3	Surface irregularity and areas of thinning	Stage 3	Irregularity and focal thinning with fluid extending into cartilage
Stage 4	Ulceration and bone exposure	Stage 4	Focal bone exposure

From references 71, 119, 285, and 286.

appearance. Four stages of chondromalacia are typically described (149,282). These stages and corresponding MR features are summarized in Table 7-10. Changes progress from focal softening and blistering to ulceration and eventually exposure of the underlying bone (282). MRI is useful for detection of chondromalacia but is most accurate in stage III and IV disease (35,217,276,283,284). Correlation with arthroscopic findings (focal cartilage swelling, irregularity, thinning, and areas of base bone) has been achieved, especially in the more advanced stages (57).

MRI techniques in the axial (see Fig. 7-115) and sagittal (see Fig. 7-116) planes have been reported (37,55,65,149, 193,287,288). T1-, T2-, STIR, GRE, three-dimensional, fast spin-echo, and fat-suppression techniques have all been employed to evaluate chondromalacia (see Figs. 7-117 and 7-118) (15,276). T2-weighted sequences provide a high signal intensity interface between the femoral and patellar articular surfaces. This allows subtle changes to be easily detected. GRE and three-dimensional spoiled GRASS sequences provide similar information and excellent tissue

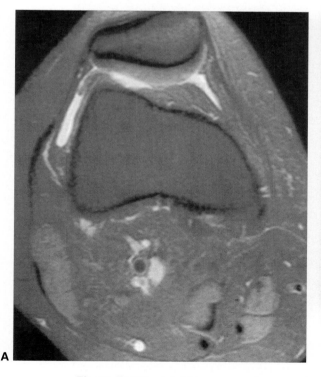

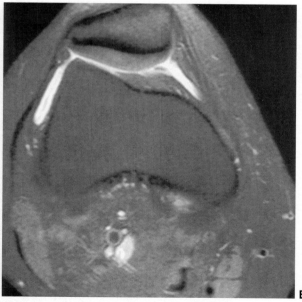

Figure 7-115 Axial fat-suppressed, proton density-weighted images **(A,B)** show normal patellar cartilage. The medial cartilage is usually thicker than the lateral.

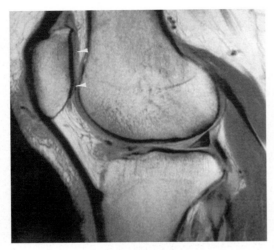

Figure 7-116 Sagittal proton density-weighted image shows diffuse thinning of the patellar cartilage (*arrowheads*). Note also the truncation and complex tearing of the anterior horn and body of the lateral meniscus.

contrast between the high signal intensity of the articular cartilage and low intensity of subchondral bone (15,37, 39,40,57,288). Recht et al. (15) reported sensitivity of 81%, specificity of 97%, and accuracies of 97% using three-dimensional fat-suppressed spoiled GRE sequences. MR features matched arthroscopy in 77% of patients. Intraarticular Gd-DTPA has also been advocated for more accurate delineation of articular cartilage (57,65,149,287). Intravenous gadolinium can also achieve intraarticular levels to provide an arthrographic effect approximately 15 minutes after injection (69,70).

We have attempted numerous pulse sequences and were initially impressed with fat-suppressed spoiled GRASS (Fig. 7-118) sequences. However, large effusions often created difficulty in detecting subtle changes in patellar cartilage. Recently, we have been more successful using axial proton density, fat-suppressed sequences (Table 7-1) (Fig. 7-117). Though late changes (grade III and IV) (see Fig. 7-119) can be detected with several techniques, early changes are more

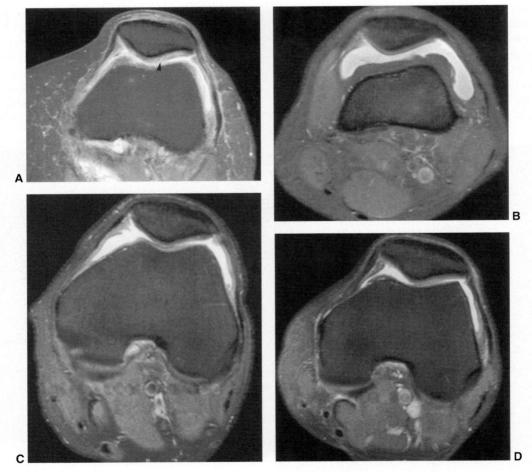

Figure 7-117 **A:** Axial fat-suppressed, proton density-weighted image demonstrating subtle flap tear of the lateral facet (*arrowhead*) and increased signal intensity in the medial and lateral cartilage. **B:** Axial fat-suppressed, proton density image demonstrating grade 2 chondromalacia in the medial and lateral facets. **C:** Axial fat-suppressed, proton density image with grade 3 chondromalacia in the medial and lateral facets. **D:** Axial fat-suppressed, proton density image showing grade 4 changes medially.

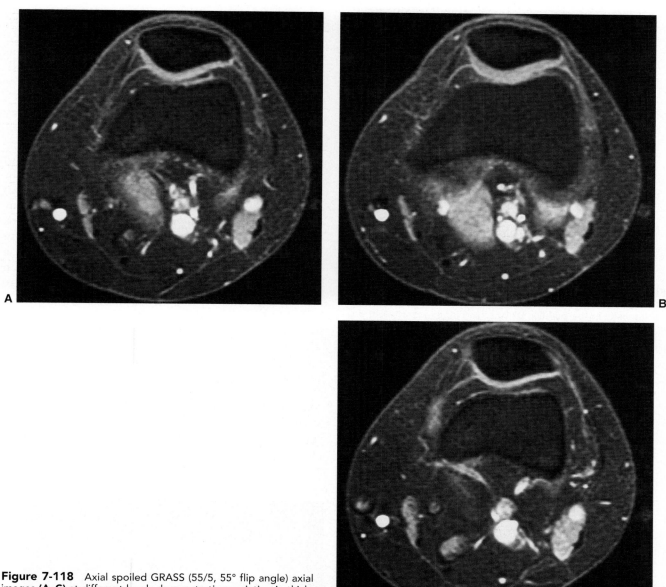

Figure 7-118 Axial spoiled GRASS (55/5, 55° flip angle) axial images **(A–C)** at different levels demonstrating variation in thickness of the cartilage. The high signal intensity of cartilage makes subtle change more apparent.

easily appreciated using this sequence even in the presence of an effusion.

Axial images are most useful. A volume coil and small field of view (14 to 16 cm) are also important. The phase encoding direction (see Fig. 7-120) should be left to right or flow artifact may cause confusion as it extends through the patella.

Patellar Tracking/Instability

Patellofemoral instability is potentially complex and can be difficult to image accurately with consistently reproducible results (77,248,249). Normally, the apex of the patella should be centered between the medial and lateral

femoral condyle (Figs. 7-111 through 7-114) (77,273). This position should be maintained when changing from the extended to the flexed (up to 30°) positions (77, 289–292). Translation and rotation or progressive asymmetry of the medial and lateral facets with relation to the femoral condyles needs to be assessed in the extended and flexed positions. Conditions that may be detected are (77,290,293) as follows:

- Lateral subluxation—lateral translation of the patella so the patellar facet extends beyond the articular margin of the femoral condyle.
- Excessive lateral pressure syndrome—lateral facet joint narrowed or patella tilted with no subluxation.

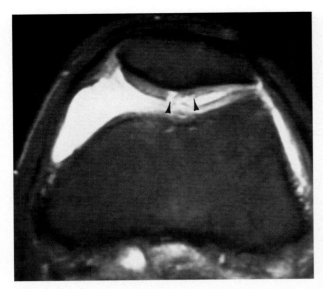

Figure 7-119 Axial fat-suppressed, fast spin-echo, proton density-weighted image demonstrating an effusion with increased signal intensity in the patellar articular cartilage (*arrowheads*) due areas of grade III and IV chondromalacia.

- Medial subluxation—medial translation of the patella so the patellar facet extends beyond the articular margin of the medial femoral condyle.
- Lateral-medial subluxation—the patella starts in lateral subluxation but shifts to medial subluxation during flexion.

- Dislocation—complete loss of articular interface with the femoral condyles (115).

The above syndromes may be due to congenital abnormalities (condylar dysplasia, patellar-shape variations), muscle imbalance, retinacular abnormalities (overly lax or taut), or previous surgery (see Fig. 7-121) (43,48,149,237). Hughston reported that 73% of patients with instability had at least one congenital deformity (294).

Imaging of instability usually requires motion or flexion of the knee. This can be accomplished with MRI or fast CT (87,149,217,271,290,292). Both knees should be examined simultaneously for comparison purposes, but static images (Figs. 7-111 through 7-114) provide many clues to problems of alignment or instability. Therefore, the body or head coil is used with the patient supine. For motion studies, the knees should be imaged in extension and up to 30° of flexion at 5° to 10° increments. This can be most effectively performed using GRE sequences to reduce image time (289–292).

MR features have also been described in patients with acute and chronic subluxation or dislocation (96,249, 279,295). Awareness of these findings can reduce the difficulty in detecting instability problems on motion and static images. Lance et al. (296) reported hemarthrosis, medial retinacular rupture, and lateral femoral contusion in 82% of acute dislocations (see Figs. 7-122 and 7-123). Osteochondral fractures (Fig. 7-123) have also been described. Patients with transient or recurrent subluxation/dislocation may have

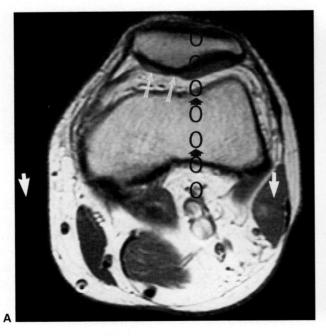
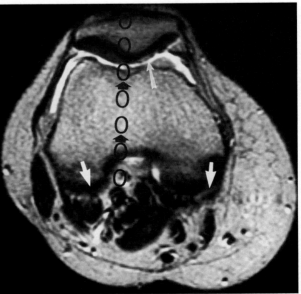

Figure 7-120 Axial proton density **(A)** and T2-weighted **(B)** images in two different patients with chondromalacia (*arrows*). The phase encoding is left to right so the flow artifact (*white arrows*) does not extend through the patella. If the phase encoding were in the anteroposterior direction (*black arrows and "O"s*), it would extend into the articular cartilage and could be mistaken for a focal defect.

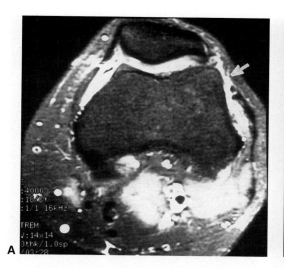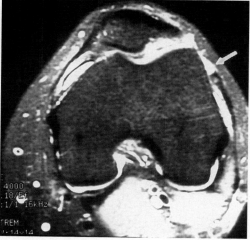

Figure 7-121 Axial fast spin-echo T2-weighted images **(A,B)** with fat-suppression in a patient with previous lateral release (*arrow*), resulting in medial patellar subluxation and impingement on the femoral condyle with chondromalacia.

similar findings (249). Kirsch et al. (249) described the features and incidence of findings:

- Effusion—100%
- Rupture or strain medial retinaculum—96%
- Lateral patellar subluxation—92%
- Lateral femoral contusion—81%
- Osteochondral fracture—58%
- Meniscal tear/ligament injuries—31%

Loose Bodies

Detection of osseous or cartilaginous fragments in the joint can be difficult. Loose bodies develop following fracture, meniscal tears, and in patients with osteochondromatosis, synovial chondromatosis, and osteochondritis dissecans (53,77,143,297). Loose bodies may be osseous, cartilaginous, fibrous, or a combination of tissues. Patients generally present with pain, recurrent effusions, and locking or restricted motion (77).

Identification of loose bodies has been accomplished using arthrography with or without CT and arthroscopy (53,77). Routine radiographs (see Fig. 7-124) can detect calcified or osseous bodies, but it is difficult to determine if the lesion is a loose body or calcification or ossification in the cruciate ligament or attached to the capsule. Technically a loose body should move in the joint and on arthrograms should be surrounded by contrast material (3,77).

Brossman et al. (53) described common locations for loose bodies. On coronal images, there are six common locations (see Fig. 7-125A) in the suprapatellar bursa and medial or lateral gutters. On sagittal images, loose bodies occur most frequently in the intercondylar area, near the

ACL attachment to the tibia, behind Hoffa fat pad and posteriorly above or below the joint line (Fig. 7-125B) (53).

MRI or MR arthrography can also identify loose bodies (see Fig. 7-126). Calcification or ossification has low signal intensity, though osseous loose bodies may actually contain marrow. Cartilage or chronic synovial proliferation may also have low signal intensity on both T1- and T2-weighted sequences. T2-weighted and GRE sequences

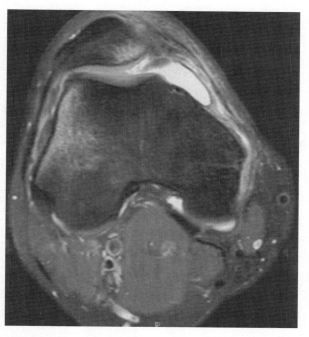

Figure 7-122 Classic lateral patellar subluxation with associated high-grade tearing of the medial retinaculum. Axial fat-suppressed, proton density-weighted image demonstrates an osseous contusion in the lateral femoral condyle and medial patella with a joint effusion.

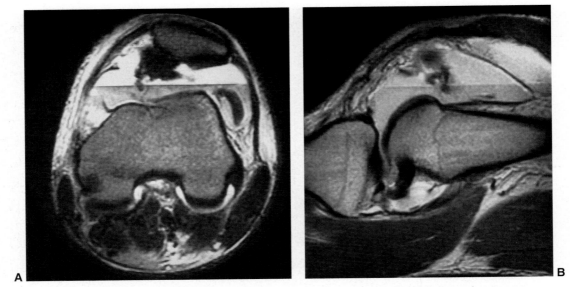

Figure 7-123   Axial **(A)** and sagittal **(B)** T2-weighted images after patellar dislocation demonstrating a lipohemarthrosis, retinacular tear, and lateral patellar displacement.

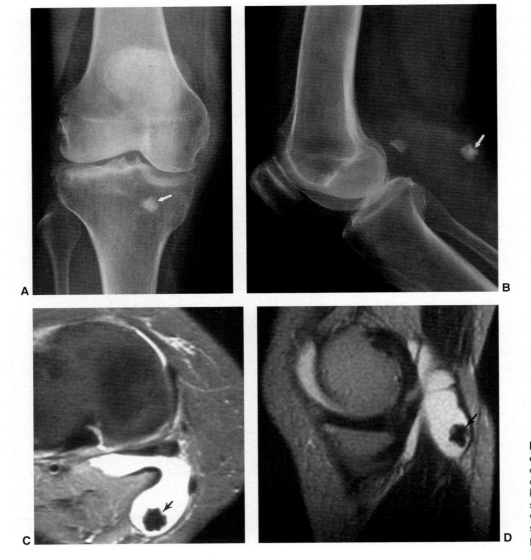

Figure 7-124 Anteroposterior **(A)** and lateral **(B)** radiographs demonstrate a bony density (*arrow*) posterior to the knee. Axial fat-suppressed, fast spin-echo **(C)**, and sagittal T2-weighted images **(D)** demonstrate a loose body (*arrow*) in a popliteal cyst.

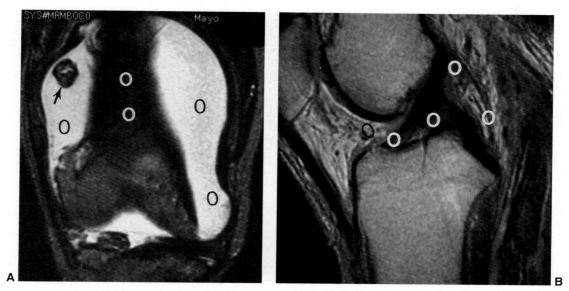

Figure 7-125 Coronal fat-suppressed T2-weighted image shows a distended suprapatellar bursa with a large loose body (*arrow*). Other common locations for loose bodies are noted with black and white *O's* on the coronal (**A**) and sagittal (**B**) images.

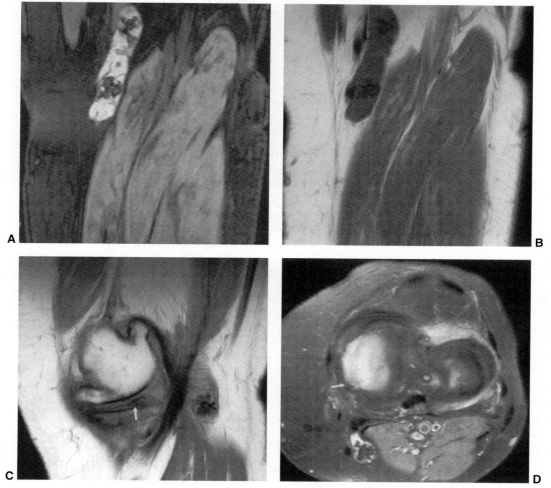

Figure 7-126 Multiple ossified loose bodies in a popliteal cyst. Coronal DESS (**A**) and T1-weighted (**B**) images clearly demonstrate the fluid surrounding the loose bodies in the popliteal cyst. Sagittal proton density (**C**) and axial fat-suppressed, proton density-weighted (**D**) images demonstrate the multiple ossified loose bodies. Note also the complex degenerative tear in the medial meniscus (*arrow*).

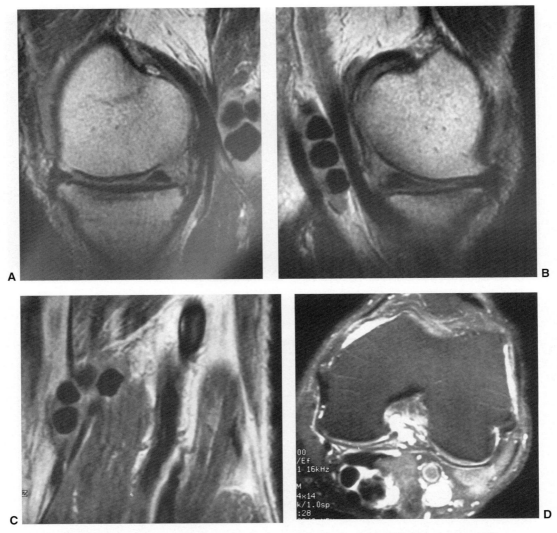

Figure 7-127 Multiple ossified loose bodies in a popliteal cyst. Sagittal **(A,B)** and coronal **(C)** proton density images demonstrate multiple large loose bodies. Fat-suppressed, T2-weighted fast spin-echo axial image **(D)** shows the fluid around the loose bodies in the popliteal cyst more clearly.

are generally used to identify loose bodies, as these lesions are more easily detected in the presence of high signal intensity synovial fluid (see Fig. 7-127). However, there are numerous structures that can cause confusion. These include the transverse ligament anteriorly, the ligament of Wrisberg and Humphrey posteriorly, and areas of synovial hypertrophy (3,104,110). Comparison with radiographs is very useful in evaluating loose bodies. Ossification near the tibia spines is common and should not be confused with a loose body (3). MR arthrography is superior to conventional MRI and CT arthrography for identification of loose bodies (see Fig. 7-128) (53). Defects in the articular cartilage may also be more easily evaluated.

Fractures

Routine radiography, CT, and isotope scans are typically used to identify fractures about the knee (3,77). During the early stages of development, MRI was considered primarily a soft tissue imaging technique. As use of MRI expanded, especially for evaluating patients with suspected internal derangement or other soft tissue injuries of the knee, it became apparent the complete fractures and subtle bone injuries could be identified that had not been demonstrated on routine radiographs (298). Multiple osseous injuries have been identified (198,299,300). Stress fractures, plateau fractures, bone bruises, osteochondral fractures, physeal injuries, and other fractures and associated soft tissue injuries have been identified and classified using MRI (1,29,31,82,285,301–308).

Stress fractures are not uncommon in the upper tibia. MR features of stress fractures are usually easily appreciated, even in the presence of normal radiographs (307, 309). T1-weighted images demonstrate linear or irregular areas of low signal intensity along the fracture line. Adjacent edema is seen as an area of high signal intensity

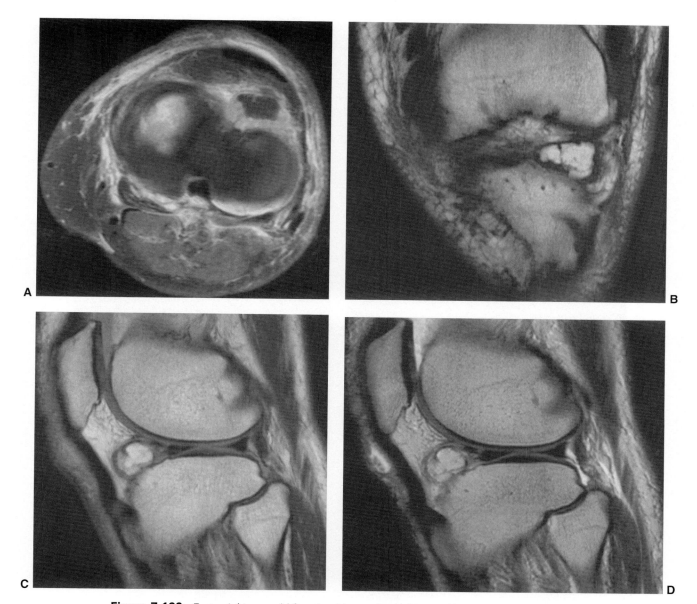

Figure 7-128 Forty-eight-year-old female with anterior locking and knee pain. Arthroscopy confirmed a 3.0 × 2.5 cm loose body anteriorly. **A:** Axial fat-suppressed proton density, **(B)** coronal T1-weighted, **(C)** sagittal proton density, and **(D)** sagittal fast spin-echo, T2-weighted images demonstrate the well-circumscribed loose body anterior to the transverse ligament. No donor site could be identified.

on T2-weighted sequences. Compressed trabeculae are low intensity on T1- and T2-weighted sequences (see Fig. 7-129) (1,3,198,308,310).

"Bone bruises" are subtle fractures that typically involve the tibial plateau or femoral condyles (see Fig. 7-130) (3,311). Radiographs are usually normal. These injuries may mimic meniscal tears or other soft tissue injuries. When isolated (no associated meniscal or ligament injury), bone bruises can explain the patient's symptoms and reduce the need for further imaging or arthroscopic procedures (34,302,305,311). The majority of these fractures occur in the lateral compartment secondary to valgus injuries. When both the tibial

plateau and lateral femoral condyle are involved, anterior subluxation with femoral–tibial impaction is suggested. The location of the injuries depends upon the degree of knee flexion during the injury. Femoral bruises tend to be located more posteriorly with increasing degrees of flexion at the time of injury (29,305). Three categories of injury have been described. Type 1 injuries involve the medullary bone in the metaphyseal and/or epiphyseal regions. Type 2 injuries are linear, similar to the stress fracture in (Fig. 7-129), and type 3 injuries are subchondral or juxtacortical.

When a bone bruise is identified, a careful search for ligament and meniscal injury is required. Kaplan et al. (223)

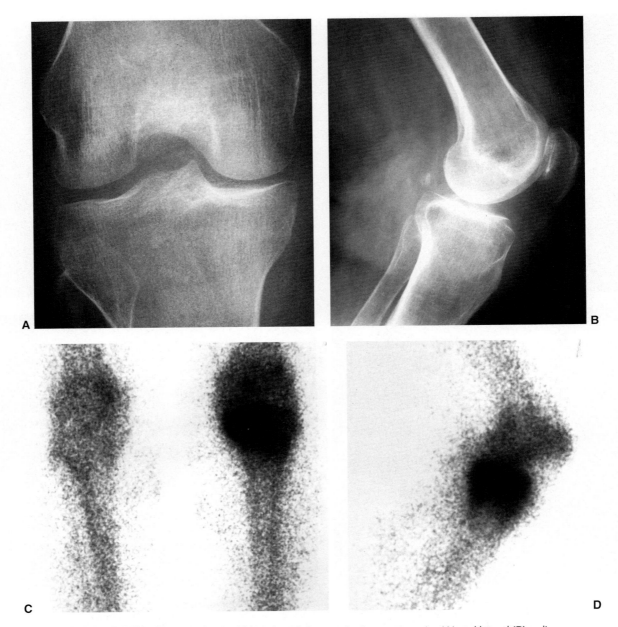

Figure 7-129 Fifty-three-year-old female with knee pain. Anteroposterior **(A)** and lateral **(B)** radiographs are normal. Radionuclide scans show increased uptake in the tibia on frontal **(C)** and lateral **(D)** views. Is this osteonecrosis or metastasis? **E:** T1-weighted coronal image demonstrates a stress fracture (*arrowheads*). There is also buckling of the lateral cortex (*arrow*).

reported that 89% of patients with ACL tears had bone bruises involving posterolateral tibial plateau (see Fig. 7-130). Associated femoral bruises were common.

Weber et al. (312) noted tibial bruises, frequently without an identifiable Segond fragment, near the posterior tibial capsular junction in patients with ACL tears and medial meniscal injuries. Segond fractures have associated ACL and meniscal tears in 75% to 100% and 67% of patients, respectively (196,223,312).

Murphy et al. (304) reported 94% of patients had posterior tibial bruises and 91% lateral femoral condyle bruises

when complete ACL tears were present. Only 17% of patients with partial ACL tears had associated bone bruises.

Complete fractures, such as femoral fractures or tibial plateau fractures, can be detected with routine radiographs. However, recent studies suggest MRI is superior to CT for defining articular separation and depression (see Fig. 7-131) (115). MRI provides the additional advantage of detecting associated soft tissue injury (115,301,313).

MRI is particularly useful for detection and follow-up evaluation of physeal injuries in children. These fractures can be subtle. Follow-up evaluation is important to evaluate

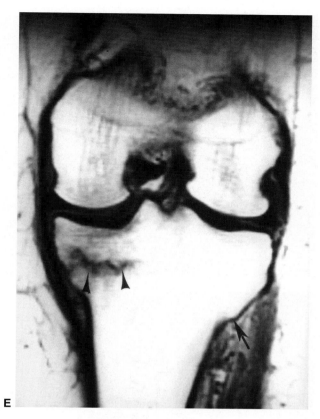

E

Figure 7-129 (continued)

potential physeal arrest, bone bars, and growth plate deformities (31,285,314).

The screening examination of the knee described in the early portion of this chapter is quite adequate for detection of fractures. T1- and T2- weighted sequences are generally sufficient for diagnosis. We prefer T2- or T2*- GRE sequences to identify fractures (see Fig. 7-132) and the frequently associated ligament and meniscal injuries. STIR and fat-suppressed FSE sequences are useful for subtle cases and increased throughput respectively (34,302,305,311). Gadolinium is not commonly used in our practice. However, it has been reported that gadolinium is useful in certain physeal injuries.

Though MRI is very sensitive for detection of most osseous injuries, there are certain injuries that may be overlooked. Impaction injuries result in marrow edema. However, distraction injuries may have little edema, which may reduce the likelihood of detection (315). In addition, small flake fractures (i.e., Segond fracture) may be overlooked due to reduced marrow edema and difficulty in detecting the small cortical fragment (1,3). Joint effusion and fluid–fluid levels are useful when osteochondral fractures are suspected (275,299).

Osteochondritis Dissecans

Osteochondritis dissecans is a disease of teenagers. The average age of onset is 15 years. Males outnumber females by a 3:1 ratio. The lesion most commonly involves the lateral aspect of the medial femoral condyle, but the lateral condyle, patella, and other areas in the knee can also be involved (77). The right knee is involved slightly more commonly than the left, but bilateral involvement is reported in up to 25% of cases. The etiology is unclear, but the lesion is probably related to repetitive trauma and/or ischemia (29,77).

Symptoms, such as pain or instability, and the radiographic appearance dictate whether a conservative approach (rest), arthroscopic surgery, or open surgery is required. Many lesions are asymptomatic and found incidentally

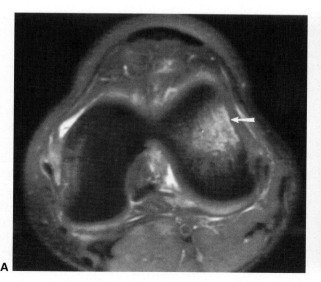

A

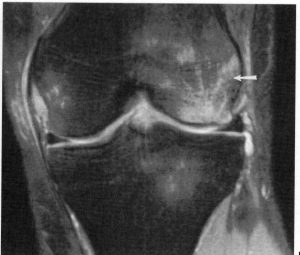

B

Figure 7-130 Axial proton density with fat-suppression **(A)** and coronal DESS **(B)** images demonstrating a lateral femoral condyle bone bruise (*arrow*).

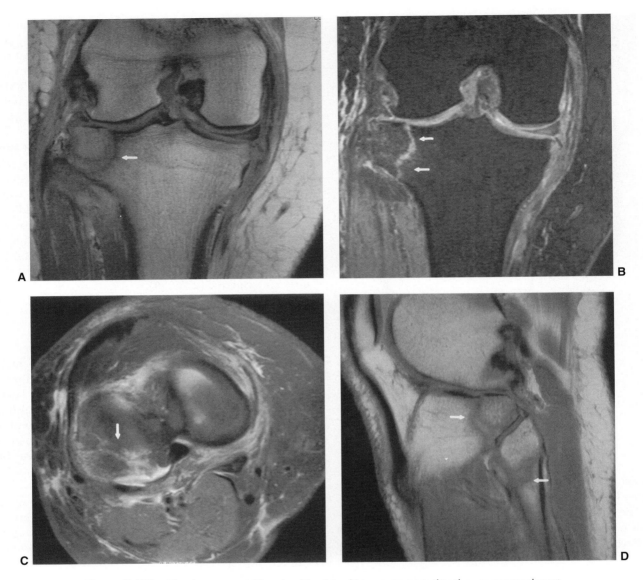

Figure 7-131 Fifty-three-year-old female with minimal trauma presented to the emergency department complaining of knee pain. Radiographs were normal. Coronal T1-weighted **(A)** and DESS **(B)**, axial fat-suppressed proton density **(C)** and sagittal proton density-weighted **(D)** images clearly demonstrate the lateral tibial plateau fracture (*arrows*). Coronal T1-weighted **(E)** and DESS **(F)** and axial fat-suppressed proton density-weighted **(G)** images also show a proximal fibular fracture (*arrow*).

(29). It is important to assess the size, location, position, and cartilaginous articular surface of the lesion (77,299).

Osteochondritis dissecans is classified by gross arthroscopic or surgical appearance and MR imaging features (Table 7-11) (299,316). Surgically normal cartilage is Grade 0. Grade 1 lesions demonstrate softening or fissuring without a definable fragment. Grade 2 lesions have a definable fragment without displacement. Grade 3 lesions are partially displaced but still attached, and grade 4 lesions are completely displaced (see Fig. 7-133).

MRI features compare to the surgical appearance and classification. Grade 0 is normal. Grade 1 lesions show signal intensity abnormality, but cartilage is intact with normal

thickness. Grade 2 lesions demonstrate a breach, usually linear, in the articular cartilage. Grade 3 lesions have a linear area of increased signal intensity on T2-weighted sequences that defines the size and location of the defect. Grade 4 lesions show mixed or low signal intensity lying in or displaced from its bed (Fig. 7-133).

Conventional or CT arthrography was used in the past. However, MRI or, less commonly, MR arthrography provide ideal techniques for evaluating these lesions. Both coronal and sagittal images (see Fig. 7-134) are needed to fully evaluate the size and position of the lesion. GRE, DESS, or T2-weighted sequences (see Fig. 7-135) are most useful (38,228,297). Loose fragments may be displaced

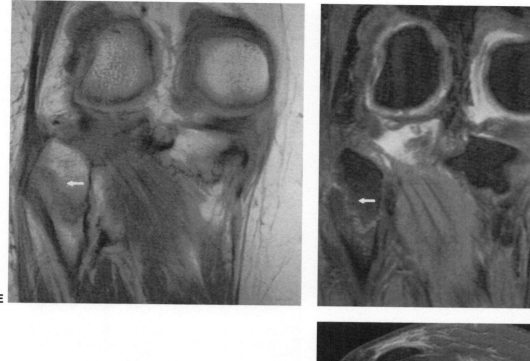

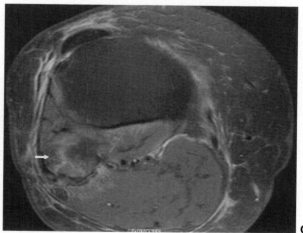

Figure 7-131 *(continued)*

From Bohndorf K. Imaging of acute injuries of the articular surfaces (chondral, osteochondral and sub-chondral fractures). *Skeletal Radiol* 1999;28:545–560; and Nelson DW, Pipaola J, Colville M, et al. Osteochondritis dissecans of the talus and knee: prospective comparison of MR and arthroscopic classifications. *J Comput Assist Tomogr* 1990;14:804–808.

TABLE 7-11

OSTEOCHONDRITIS DISSECANS HISTOLOGIC AND MR FEATURES

Grade	Arthroscopic Features	MR Features
Grade 0	Normal	Normal
Grade 1	Focal-softening, fibrillation or fissuring	Cartilage intact, signal intensity abnormal in bone and cartilage
Grade 2	Defect in cartilage	Breach in articular cartilage
Grade 3	Fragment partially detached around fragment	Thin rim of abnormal signal intensity
Grade 4	Displaced fragment or loose in joint	Mixed signal intensity with fragment in place or loose in joint

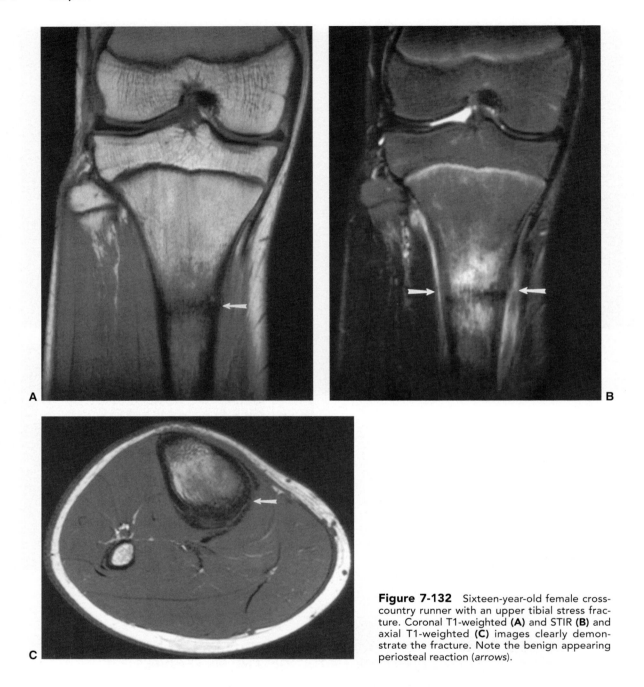

A

B

C

Figure 7-132 Sixteen-year-old female cross-country runner with an upper tibial stress fracture. Coronal T1-weighted **(A)** and STIR **(B)** and axial T1-weighted **(C)** images clearly demonstrate the fracture. Note the benign appearing periosteal reaction (*arrows*).

or simply have a linear fluid collection (high intensity on T2-weighted sequences) between the native bone and osteochondral fragments. MRI is also effective in assessing the cartilage to determine whether it is intact or incompletely covers the lesion (228,305). DeSmet et al. (297) described four signs used to evaluate osteochondritis dissecans. These are similar to those described in Table 7-11. Findings include an abnormal signal intensity line (Fig. 7-134) around the fragment, lytic changes proximal to the fragment, abnormal signal intensity in the cartilage, and subchondral bone or a linear cleft in the cartilage (297). Using T2-weighted images for evaluation, the sensitivity

and specificity for MR imaging was 97% and 100%, respectively. A high signal intensity line (T2-weighted images) or low intensity line on T1-weighted images is common in unstable lesions (see Fig. 7-136) (297).

Osteonecrosis and Osteochondrosis

Osteonecrosis, including the histologic changes and pathophysiology, are discussed in Chapter 6. However, though the etiology and MR appearance of avascular necrosis (AVN) in the knee are similar compared to the hip, there are certain differences that should be emphasized.

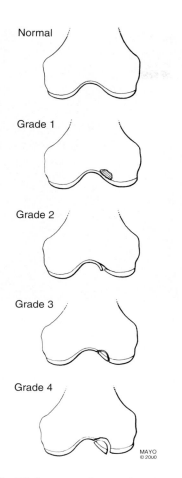

Normal

Grade 1

Grade 2

Grade 3

Grade 4

MAYO
© 2000

Figure 7-133 MR features of osteochondritis dissecans. **A:** Normal, grade 0. **B:** Grade 1, abnormal signal intensity, cartilage intact. **C:** Grade 2, linear break in articular cartilage. **D:** Grade 3, abnormal signal intensity (↑ *T2WI,* ↓ *T1WI*) around fragment. **E:** Grade 4, fragment has abnormal signal intensity and may be in normal position or loose in joint.

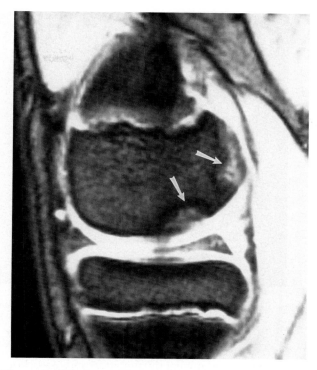

Figure 7-135 Sagittal gradient-echo image demonstrating two areas of osteochondritis in the posterior femoral condyle (*arrows*).

The incidence of AVN in the femoral condyles follows the hip and shoulder. MR image features are also similar and the stages described in Chapter 6, Table 6-4, can be applied to the knee as well as the hip (see Fig. 7-137). There are several variations peculiar to the knee. These include spontaneous osteonecrosis, which typically involves the medial femoral condyle but can also involve the lateral

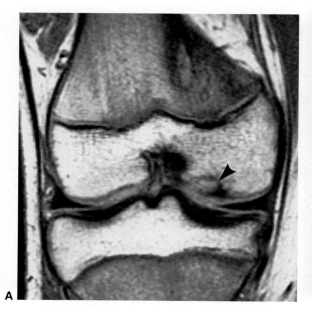

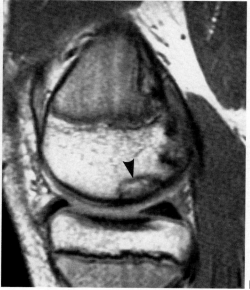

Figure 7-134 Osteochondritis dissecans. Coronal **(A)** and sagittal **(B)** proton density-weighted images define the linear defect (*arrowhead*) around the lesion with intact articular cartilage.

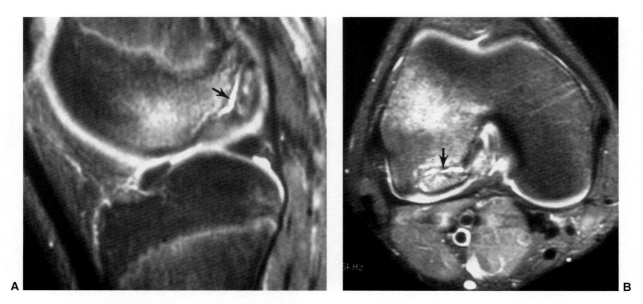

Figure 7-136 Osteochondritis dissecans. Sagittal **(A)** and axial **(B)** fat-suppressed, T2-weighted fast spin-echo images demonstrate fluid (*arrow*) between the fragment and femoral condyle.

femoral condyle and medial tibial plateau and osteochondrosis (152,286,317).

Osteonecrosis is a condition associated with females 50 years of age or older. Patients typically present with persistent knee pain, and tenderness over the affected area (29). The pain, often worse at night, progresses for 6 to 8 weeks before subsiding (29). The disorder is of unknown etiology but most likely is traumatic, with osteopenic or weakened bone predisposing to the condition. Patients on steroids (secondary) may develop changes in similar sites. The medial femoral condyle is most frequently involved. However, the lateral femoral condyle and tibial plateau can also be affected. The clinical history is similar regardless of the location involved.

Radiographs are normal in early stages of the disease (Table 7-12). Isotope scans will demonstrate increased uptake. However, this is nonspecific and often not useful in patients of this age group (318,319). MRI features are

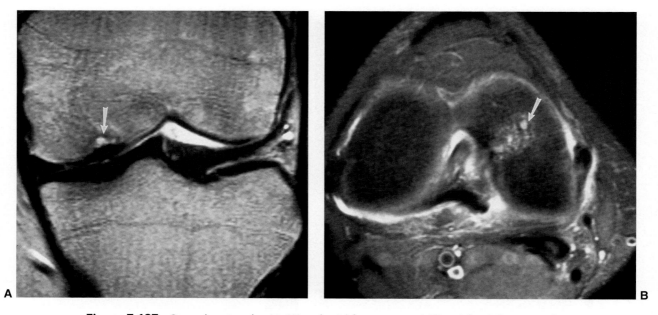

Figure 7-137 Coronal proton density **(A)** and axial fat-suppressed, T2-weighted, fast spin-echo **(B)** images demonstrate an area of osteonecrosis in the medial femoral condyle (*arrow*).

TABLE 7-12

SPONTANEOUS OSTEONECROSIS OF THE KNEE: RADIOGRAPHIC AND MRI FEATURES

	Routine Radiographs	MRI
Stage 1	Normal	Geographic area of ↑ intensity T2WI, ↓ intensity T1WI
Stage 2	Slight flattening of the femoral condyle, sclerosis of subchondral tibial bone	Geographic area with surrounding low intensity on T1WI
Stage 3	Subchondral lucency with surrounding sclerosis	Subchondral area of reduced to normal signal intensity surrounded by low intensity area on both T1 & T2WIs
Stage 4	Same but wider area of sclerosis	Same as stage 3 but wider area of low intensity
Stage 5	Above changes plus degenerative joint disease	Geographic area of low intensity with joint space narrowing

T2WI, T2-weighted image; T1WI, T1-weighted image.
From Lotke PA, Ecker ML. Current concepts review. Osteonecrosis of the knee. *J Bone Joint Surg Am* 1988;70:470–473.

more useful and appear earlier than radiographic changes (see Fig. 7-138) (Table 7-12) (318). As with AVN of the hip, the MRI and radiographic features are more easily correlated in the later stages of the disease. An additional advantage of MRI is the ability to differentiate osteonecrosis from other conditions that may have similar clinical presentations such as meniscal tears, pes anserine bursitis, and simple osteoarthritis (see Fig. 7-139) (3,318).

Osteochondroses involving the knee include Blount disease, Sinding-Larsen-Johansson disease, and Osgood-Schlatter disease (29,320). Blount disease presents in infantile and adolescent forms. The infantile variety is seen as a varus deformity of the knee with progressive bowing. The adolescent form presents from 8 to 15 years of age, and unlike the infantile type is often unilateral with pain in the involved knee (61,321).

Clinical features and radiographic changes have been sufficient for diagnosis of this disorder. Radiographic features were used by Lankenshiold to stage Blount disease. Stages I to VI show progressive deformity with bone bridge formation between the epiphysis and metaphysis (320). Experience with MR imaging indicates that early changes, especially in the unossified epiphysis and physis, are more easily evaluated. The coronal plane and T2-weighted, DESS or three-dimensional fat-suppressed spoiled GRASS sequences, are best suited for this purpose (see Fig. 7-140) (3,320).

Osgood-Schlatter disease is a common problem in adolescent males. The condition is frequently bilateral and occurs in active or athletic patients. Patients usually present with pain and swelling over the tibial tuberosity. The clinical presentation and demonstration of fragmentation

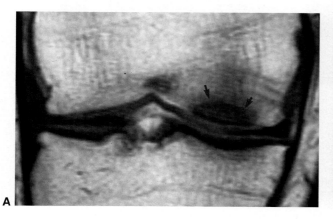
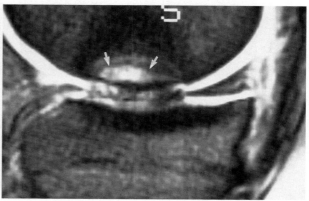

Figure 7-138 Coronal proton density **(A)** and sagittal gradient-echo **(B)** images demonstrate spontaneous osteonecrosis of the femoral condyle (*arrows*).

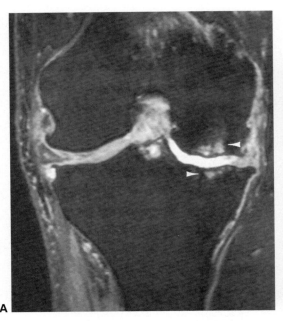

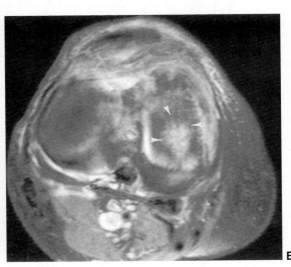

Figure 7-139 Coronal DESS (**A**) and axial fat-suppressed proton density-weighted (**B**) images demonstrate grade 4 chondromalacia of the medial compartment with extensive underlying reactive changes in the medial femoral condyle and tibia (*arrowheads*). Cartilage can be seen in the lateral compartment, where there is grade 2-3 chondromalacia. Note the marginal osteophytes.

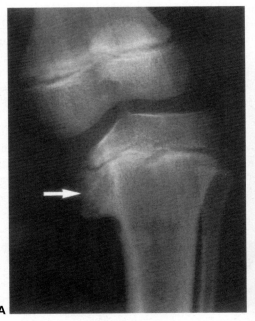

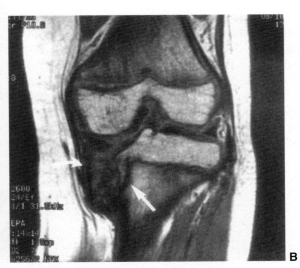

Figure 7-140 Seven-year-old female with increasing varus deformity in the left leg. **A:** Anteroposterior radiograph shows marked irregularity of the medial tibia consistent with Langenshiold type V changes (*arrow*). **B:** Coronal fast proton density image shows marked depression of the medial growth plate (*straight arrow*) and delayed ossification of the medial epiphysis (*curved arrow*). **C:** Coronal fat-suppressed, T2-weighted fast spin-echo image shows depression of the medial growth plate (*arrow*), delay in ossification of the medial epiphysis, and edema in the metaphysis (*curved arrow*). **D:** Sagittal fat-suppressed, three-dimensional spoiled GRASS image shows irregular depression of most of the medial growth plate (*large arrow*). In addition, there are small intrusions of cartilage into the metaphysis (*small arrows*). **E:** Coronal reformatted three-dimensional spoiled GRASS image shows depression and irregularity of the medial growth plate (*straight arrow*). The delayed ossification of the medial epiphysis (*curved arrow*) is clearly displayed, as is the depression of the medial tibial plateau. (From Craig JG, van Holsbeeck M, Zaltz I. The utility of MR in assessing Blount disease. *Skeletal Radiol* 2002;31:208–213.)

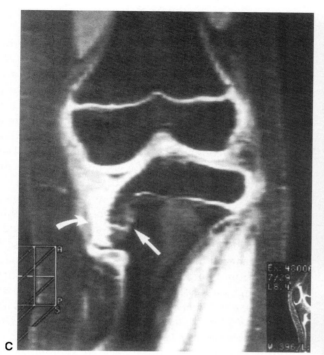

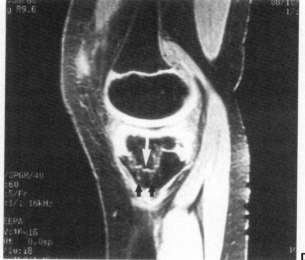

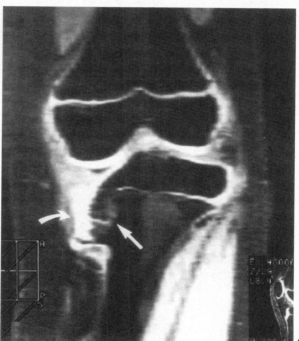

Figure 7-140 (continued)

of the tuberosity on radiographs usually are sufficient to confirm the diagnosis (321). Sagittal T2-weighted MR images are useful in evaluating the patellar tendon and associated soft tissue changes (see Fig. 7-141). Rosenberg et al. (322) noted increased signal intensity at the tendon insertion (Fig. 7-141) in all patients with symptomatic improvement, even in the presence of tuberosity fragmentation. Therefore, bone changes may be less important than soft tissue findings. This finding suggests MRI may be

an important imaging technique for diagnosis and follow-up of patients with Osgood-Schlatter disease (29). However, in our experience the diagnosis is usually obvious based on clinical features, and MRI is reserved for difficult or atypical cases.

Sinding-Larsen-Johansson disease is similar to Osgood-Schlatter disease but involves the lower pole of the patella or patellar tendon origin. Similar soft tissue changes may be seen on MR images (29).

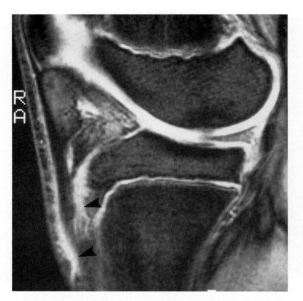

Figure 7-141 Sagittal T2-weighted image of the knee in a 14-year-old male. There is inflammation along the distal patellar tendon (*arrowheads*) due to Osgood-Schlatter disease.

Musculoskeletal Neoplasms and Soft Tissue Masses

A complete discussion of musculoskeletal neoplasms is included in Chapter 12. However, there are certain applications and technical aspects for evaluating the knee that are more appropriately discussed in this chapter.

Skeletal lesions are most easily characterized using routine radiography (2,62,3). Primary bone tumors in the knee are common (Table 7-13). About half of osteosarcomas occur in the knee. This excludes the subcategories [telangiectatic osteogenic sarcoma (OGS), perosteal OGS, etc.] that are also common in this location. Sixty percent of Ewing sarcomas involve the pelvis or knee. Certain benign tumors are also common about the knee (see Fig. 7-142) (166,323). Thirty-two percent of chondroblastomas and more than half of giant cell tumors are located in the knee (323,324). Patellar tumors are rare. Patellar tumors accounted for only 0.06% of 8,542 bone tumors of Dahlin and Unni's series (324). Kransdorf et al. (325) reported a series of 42 cases. Thirty-eight were benign (chondroblastoma 16, giant cell tumor 8, simple cyst 6, hemangioma 3, osteochondroma 2, lipoma 2, and osteoblastoma 1). Three of four malignant lesions were lymphomas and there was one hemangioendotheliosarcoma. At this time, MRI is primarily reserved for staging and therapy planning of skeletal neoplasms (see Chapter 12).

Soft tissue masses about the knee are summarized in Table 7-14 (326). The MR features of these lesions and techniques for examination are discussed in Chapter 12. Other soft tissue masses of the knee, which may mimic benign or malignant lesions, are more properly discussed here. These lesions include popliteal cysts, ganglia, and

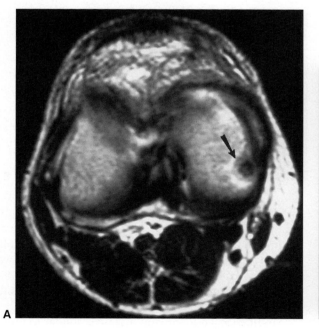

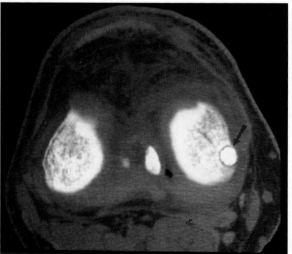

Figure 7-142 Osteoid osteoma. The knee is not the most common location, and symptoms may mimic more common knee pathology. **A:** Axial T1-weighted image demonstrates a well-defined circular area of the low signal intensity in femoral condyle (*arrow*). An axial CT image **(B)** demonstrates an osteoid osteoma that may be more easily characterized with the more familiar CT features. (Courtesy of Michael J. Collins, Hinsdale Orthopedic Associates, Hinsdale, IL.)

TABLE 7-13

PRIMARY SKELETAL NEOPLASMS OF THE KNEE (BASED ON 11,087 CASES)

	Knee / %Total Lesions
Malignant	
Osteosarcoma	795/48%
Chondrosarcoma	143/16%
Reticulum cell sarcoma	79/11%
Fibrosarcoma	80/31%
Ewings sarcoma	71/14%
Benign	
Osteochondroma	325/37%
Giant cell tumor	282/50%
Aneurysmal bone cysts	68/24%
Chondroma	44/15%
Osteoid osteoma	41/12%
Chondroblastoma	44/37%
Chondromyxoid fibroma	17/38%

From Dahlin DC, Unni KK. *Bone tumors: general aspects and data on 8,542 cases*, 4th ed. Springfield, IL: Charles C Thomas Publisher, 1986; and Unni KK. *Dahlin's bone tumors. General aspects and data on 11,087 cases*, 5th ed. Philadelphia, PA: Lippincott–Raven Publishers, 1996.

TABLE 7-14

SOFT TISSUE TUMORS OF THE KNEE AND LEG

Type of Lesion	No. of Cases
Liposarcoma	321
Fibrosarcoma	170
Synovial sarcoma	102
Alveolar sarcoma	63
Hemangioma	50
Rhabdomyosarcoma	40
Hemangiopericytoma	37
Epithelioid sarcoma	31
Desmoid tumor	27
Giant cell tumor of tendon sheath	15

From Weiss SW, Goldblum JR. *Enzinger and weiss soft tissue tumors*, 4th ed. St. Louis, MO: Mosby, 2001.

other soft tissue lesions commonly seen in the knee (106,118,183,327–330). Posterior soft tissue lesions are common. These include popliteal cysts, meniscal cysts, ganglion cysts, popliteal varices, popliteal artery aneurysm, and hemangiomas. Lipomas, lymphadenopathy, and malignant neoplasms may also be identified posteriorly (106,186,187,218,327,329–331). Popliteal or Baker's cysts were reported in 5% of 1,000 MR examinations by Fielding et al. (270) and in 10% to 41% of posterior masses by Butler et al. (327). These lesions typically communicated with the joint at the junction of the medial head of the gastrocnemius and insertion of the semimembranosus (see Fig. 7-143) (181,183). Popliteal (Baker's) cysts are commonly associated with joint effusion. Large joint effusions increase joint pressure, forcing fluid through the weak posterior capsule between the medial gastrocnemius and semimembranosus (see Fig. 7-144 and 7-145) (327,328). Popliteal cysts are also commonly associated with meniscal tears and degenerative joint disease. Cysts may be noted in up to 38% of knees with these associated abnormalities. ACL and MCL tears are not typically seen with popliteal cysts (328). Cysts or bursal enlargements can also occur along the popliteus tendon and biceps femoris. Popliteal cysts may vary in size and they can be large and multiloculated or contain septations. Patients usually present with knee pain, and a posterior mass may be palpable. Rupture of these cysts may result in dissection of fluid between the soleus and gastrocnemius (2,332). Symptoms may be difficult to differentiate

from deep venous thrombosis (see Fig. 7-146). Additionally, the popliteal cyst may become inflamed, leading to synovitis and significant pain (see Fig. 7-147).

MRI is ideally suited for diagnosis of either of these conditions. Popliteal cysts are homogeneous with high signal intensity on T2-weighted sequences and low intensity on T1-weighted sequences (Figs. 7-143 through 7-145). Sagittal and axial images are most useful for defining the joint communication (Fig. 7-143 through 7-146) and size. Other lesions such as distended bursae (Table 7-2) and ganglia have similar MR features (see Fig. 7-148). Ganglion cysts may be extraarticular or intraarticular (333,334). Ganglia are more common along tendon sheaths and near the tibiofibular joint (see Fig. 7-149) (333). Size and location are important to define. Lesions near the tibiofibular joint can cause compression of the common peroneal nerve (335–337). However, many are asymptomatic. Ilahi et al. (333) reported that over 50% of proximal tibiofibular ganglia were asymptomatic. Intraarticular ganglia make up 1.3% of lesions (113,331). Most present with pain. The majority of intraarticular ganglia (61%) are located in the intracondylar notch. Thirteen percent are located in Hoffa fat pad, 43% involve the ACL, and 35% the PCL (see Fig. 7-150) (331). However, any intraarticular structure may be involved.

Meniscal cysts may be intrameniscal or parameniscal due to extension into the soft tissues. The latter are more common. Meniscal cysts are located along the joint line adjacent to the menisci and are usually associated with an adjacent meniscal tear (183). Pericruciate meniscal cysts arise from tears in the posterior horn of the medial meniscus. These may be confused with PCL ganglia. Axial, sagittal, and coronal image planes should be carefully evaluated to differentiate meniscal cysts from PCL cysts, as treatment approaches may differ (187).

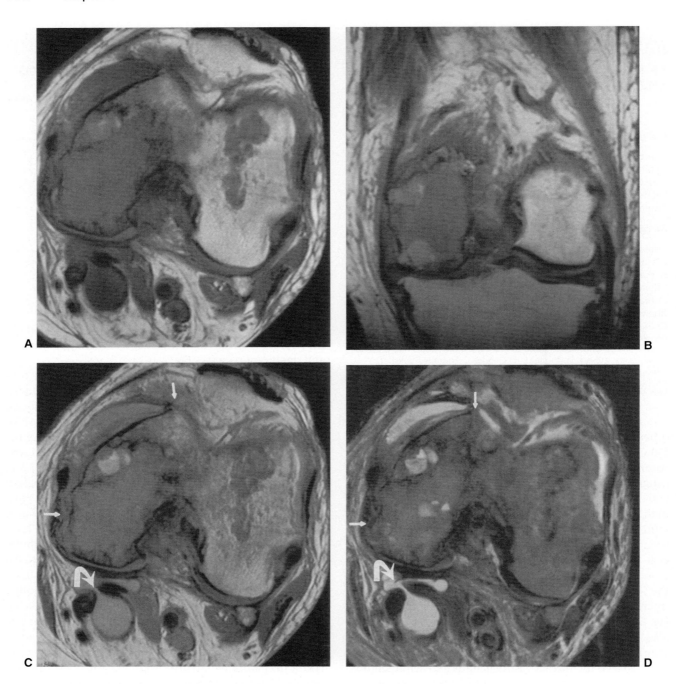

Figure 7-143 Eighty-two-year-old male seen for possible knee arthroplasty. MR images demonstrated a pathologic fracture with biopsy-confirmed metastatic lesion. Axial **(A)** and coronal **(B)** T1-weighted and axial proton density **(C)** and fast spin-echo T2-weighted **(D)** images demonstrate a hemorrhagic infiltrative lesion with a pathologic fracture (*arrows*). Axial images **C,D** demonstrate a popliteal cyst (*curved arrow*) extending between the tendons.

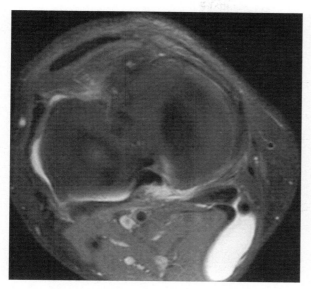

Figure 7-144 Axial fat-suppressed, proton density-weighted image demonstrates a popliteal cyst with the neck clearly demonstrated.

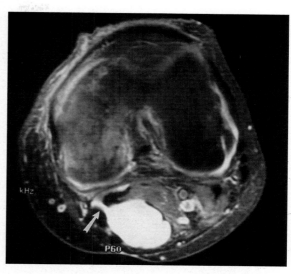

Figure 7-145 Fat-suppressed fast spin-echo axial image demonstrating a popliteal cyst with a well-defined neck (*arrow*) and a femoral bone bruise.

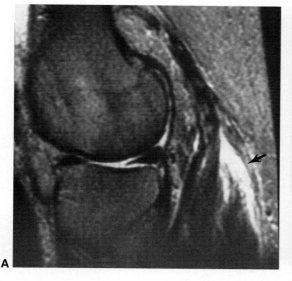

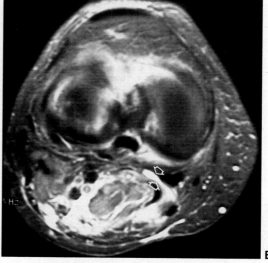

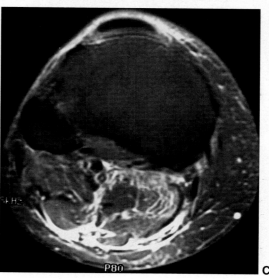

Figure 7-146 Dissecting popliteal cyst. Sagittal T2-weighted image **(A)** demonstrates fluid in the posterior soft tissues dissecting distally (*arrow*). Axial fat-suppressed T2-weighted fast spin-echo images **(B,C)** demonstrate the fluid dissection and neck of the cyst (*open arrows*).

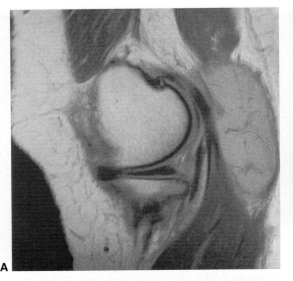

A

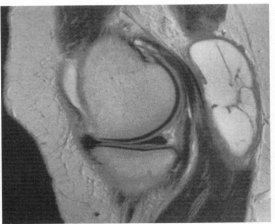

B

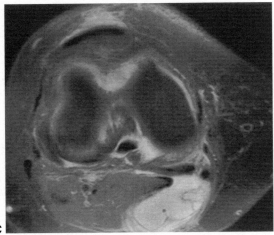

C

Figure 7-147 Large symptomatic popliteal cyst with synovitis demonstrated on sagittal proton density **(A)**, fast spin-echo T2-weighted **(B)**, and axial proton density fat-suppressed **(C)** images.

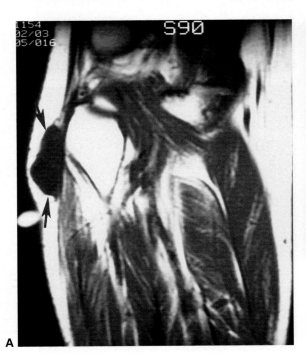

A

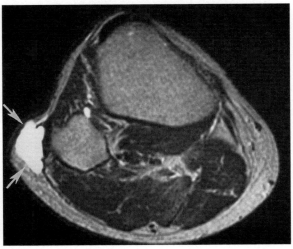

B

Figure 7-148 Coronal T1- **(A)** and axial T2-weighted **(B)** images demonstrating a ganglion cyst along the upper fibula (*arrows*).

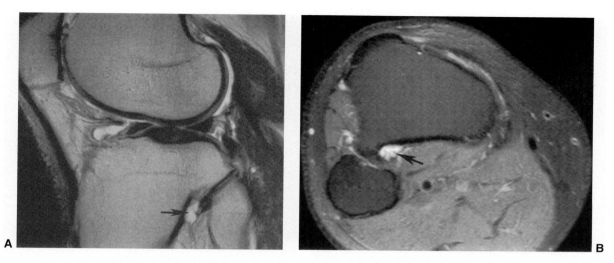

Figure 7-149 Sagittal fast spin-echo T2-weighted **(A)** and axial fat-suppressed T2-weighted **(B)** images show a tibiofibular ganglion cyst (*arrow*).

Another typically benign-appearing lesion is the giant cell tumor of the tendon sheath. These lesions can appear similar to other cysts. However, often there is hemosiderin deposition which results in reduced signal intensity on T2-weighted sequences. This is a useful finding for characterizing the lesion (see Fig. 7-151).

The routine screening examination used for knee trauma is typically not used in patients referred for suspected bone or soft tissue neoplasms of the knee. Typically both T1- and T2- weighted sequences are required to properly characterize the nature of the lesions, especially in the soft tissues (2,104,113,338). We prefer to obtain images

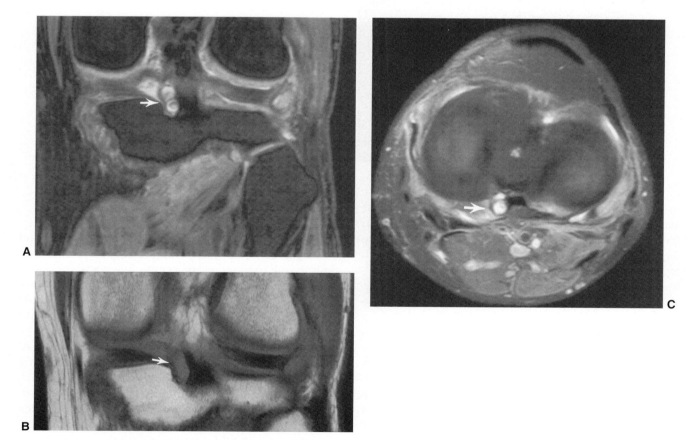

Figure 7-150 Patient with a previous partial posterior cruciate ligament tear and persistent pain. Coronal DESS **(A)**, T1-weighted **(B)** and axial fat-suppressed proton density-weighted **(C)** images demonstrate an intraarticular ganglion (*arrow*) in the region of the prior ligament tear.

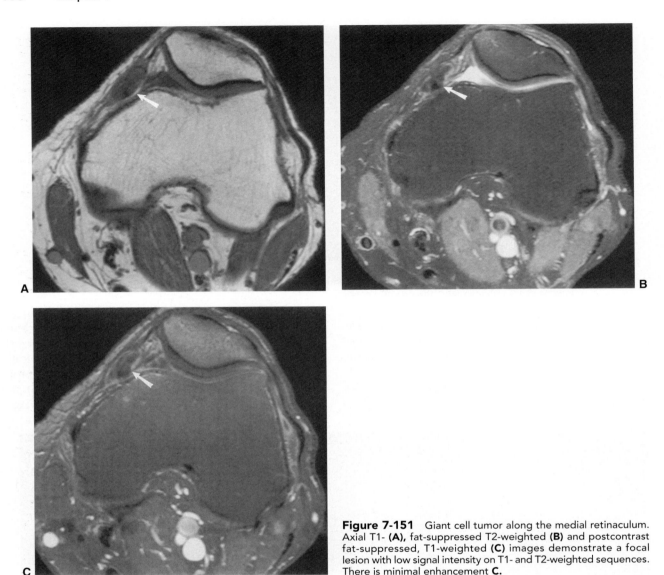

Figure 7-151 Giant cell tumor along the medial retinaculum. Axial T1- **(A)**, fat-suppressed T2-weighted **(B)** and postcontrast fat-suppressed, T1-weighted **(C)** images demonstrate a focal lesion with low signal intensity on T1- and T2-weighted sequences. There is minimal enhancement **C.**

in two planes to evaluate the extent of lesions fully. The axial and sagittal or coronal planes are utilized. Obvious lesions can be identified and classified using two sequences and two image planes. The axial image plane is typically performed using a T2-weighted sequence and followed by either a sagittal or coronal T1-weighted sequence. This minimizes examination time without hindering diagnosis (2,3).

More subtle lesions, especially in the marrow, may require a STIR sequence to assess the abnormalities in the marrow more easily (319). Subtle soft tissue changes may dictate that the T1- and T2-weighted sequences be performed in the same image plane to more easily characterize the lesion. Vascular lesions or lesions that may encase or displace vessels may be further studied using MR angiography to better define the vascular anatomy (3).

Arthropathies

Early detection and characterization of arthropathies and synovial inflammatory diseases (see Fig. 7-152) has been difficult with conventional imaging techniques (65). Routine radiographs may demonstrate soft tissue swelling, effusions, bony erosions, sclerosis, and osteophytes. Radionuclide scans can identify changes earlier, but findings are not specific (3).

Recently, MRI has provided a new method of evaluating early articular and synovial inflammatory disease (34,65,68,69,70,143,232,281,339–341). Articular cartilage is easily identified due to the contrast between cartilage and the low intensity cortical bone. T2-weighted spin-echo, fat-suppressed FSE, GRE, and coronal DESS sequences are useful for evaluating subtle changes in the

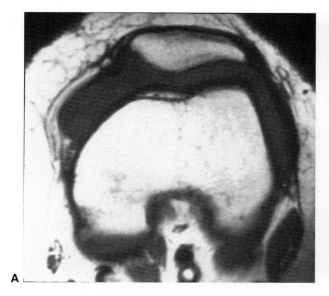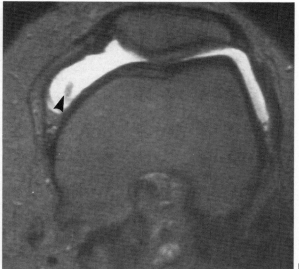

Figure 7-152 Axial T1- **(A)** and T2-weighted **(B)** images of the knee. The articular cartilage and synovial proliferation (*arrowhead* in **B**) are more easily evaluated on the T2-weighted image.

articular cartilage (see Fig. 7-153). Disler et al. (38) found fat-suppressed three-dimensional spoiled GRASS (60/5/40°, 16-cm FOV, 256 ×160 matrix, 1 acquisition, 60 contiguous 1.5-mm sections) superior to other conventional MR imaging sequences for evaluating articular cartilage. The ability to reformat images in multiple image planes is an added benefit of three-dimensional techniques (see Fig. 7-154). Also, T2 values of articular cartilage are higher with more severe osteoarthritis, especially in the medial compartment (342).

The routine screening examination is adequate for detecting cartilage erosions earlier than routine radiographs.

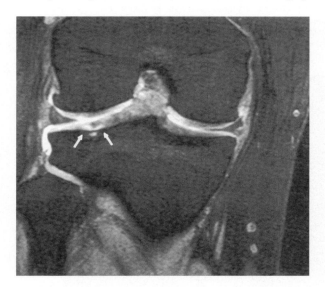

Figure 7-153 Coronal DESS image demonstrating cartilage loss (*arrows*) and osteophyte formation.

Also, changes in the growth plate and ossifying epiphysis can be easily assessed. Therefore, changes can be detected earlier in osteoarthritis, juvenile rheumatoid arthritis, rheumatoid arthritis, hemophilic arthropathy, and other cartilaginous disorders (202,232,343–347). The causes of synovial inflammation are numerous. Unfortunately, changes noted on MRI may not always indicate the etiology. Synovial proliferation can lead to irregular fronds that extend into the joint space (348,349). These appear as low signal intensity filling defects on T2-weighted sequences (Fig. 7-153) (3,349). These changes can be identified with any chronic synovial inflammatory process. Therefore, they are not useful in separating the types of arthropathy. Calcifications, such as those seen with chondrocalcinosis or calcium pyrophosphate deposition disease, may be difficult to detect (3,350). However, MR imaging is capable of identifying these findings, especially in the femoral condyles (351).

Certain specific features have been noted with pigmented villonodular synovitis. This condition is a monoarticular disease that involves the knee in 80% of cases. Hemorrhagic effusions lead to histologic changes including synovial proliferation and hemosiderin-laden macrophages (352–354). The latter result in focal areas of low signal intensity on T2-weighted images, presumably due to the paramagnetic effects of hemosiderin (see Fig. 7-155). The areas of low intensity tend to be larger and more globular than typical synovial fronds or synovial chondromatosis (see Figs. 7-153 and 7-156). Amyloid arthropathy also presents as an aggressive disorder with extensive erosions and synovial masses (see Fig. 7-157).

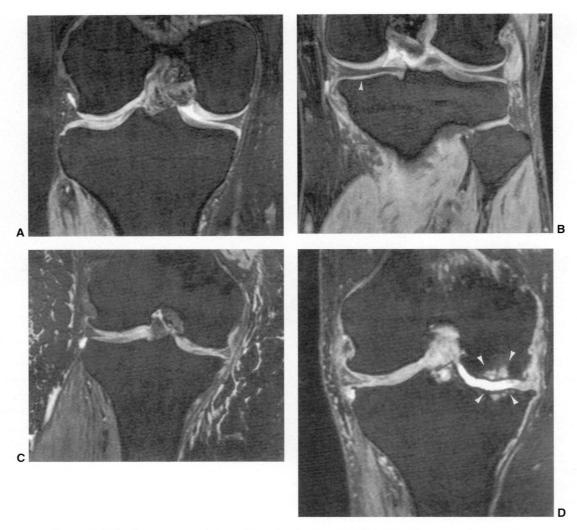

Figure 7-154 Fat-suppressed three-dimensional coronal DESS images demonstrating superior articular detail with different grades of chondromalacia. **A:** Normal articular cartilage. **B:** Grade 1–2 chondromalacia with thinning of the medial tibial cartilage (*arrowhead*). **C:** Grade 3 lateral and Grade 4 medial chondromalacia. **D:** Grade 4 medial compartment chondromalacia with extreme reactive marrow changes in the underlying tibia and femur (*arrowheads*).

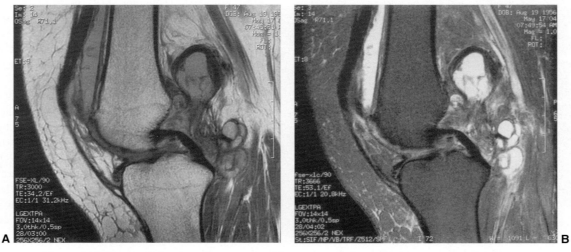

Figure 7-155 Sagittal proton density **(A)** and fast spin-echo T2-weighted **(B)** images of the knee in a patient with pigmented villonodular synovitis. Note the multiple large areas of decreased intensity in the distended joint on the T2-weighted sequence.

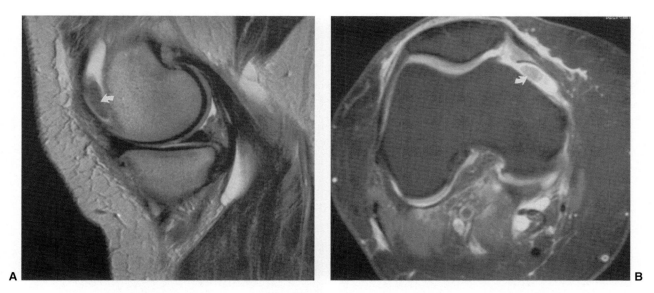

Figure 7-156 Seventeen-year-old female with focal pigmented villonodular synovitis (*arrow*) demonstrated on sagittal fast spin-echo, T2-weighted **(A)**, and axial fat-suppressed proton density-weighted **(B)** images.

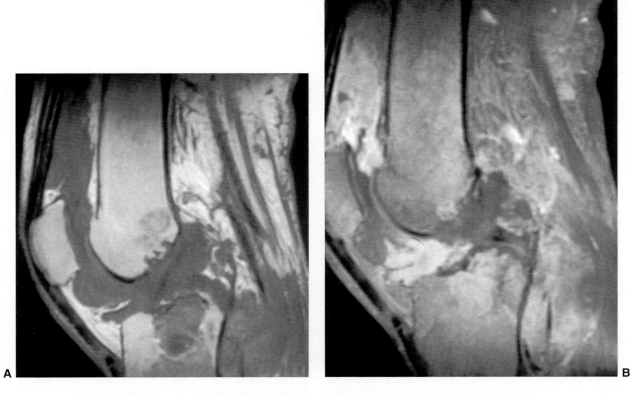

Figure 7-157 Amyloid arthropathy. Sagittal T1- **(A)** and postcontrast T1-weighted **(B)** images, and axial precontrast **(C,D)**, coronal postcontrast **(E)**, and sagittal fat-suppressed, T2-weighted **(F)** images demonstrate extensive synovial infiltration and proliferation with large osseous erosions.

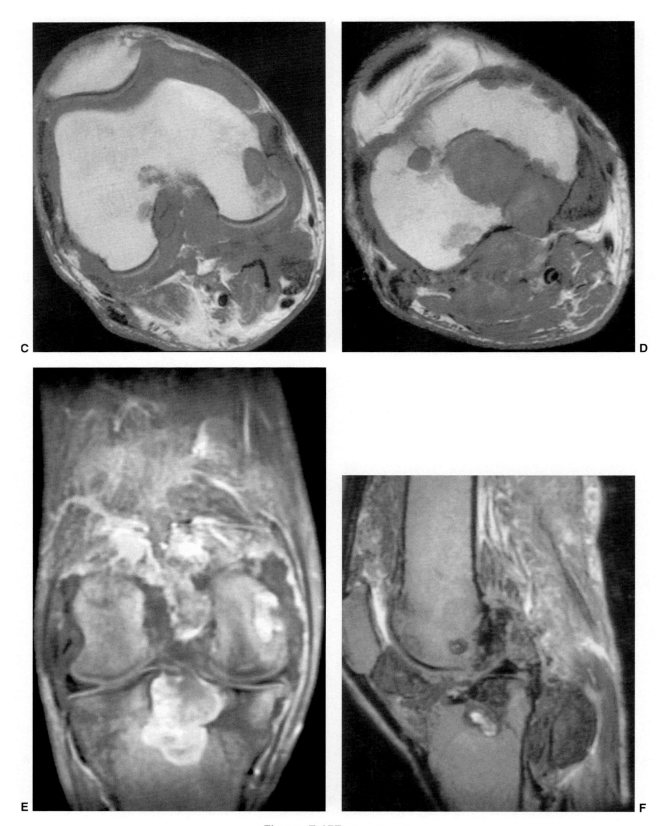

Figure 7-157 (continued)

Attempts to characterize changes in synovial fluid including T1 and T2 relaxation times, spectroscopy, and correlation of signal intensity with normal, infected, or inflamed synovial fluid have been unsuccessful (232,355).

The use of intravenous and intraarticular contrast material has progressed in recent years (64,68–70,341). Gadolinium can be injected (≈ 30 to 40 mL, diluted in normal saline 0.1:25) into the knee to improve visualization of subtle changes in articular cartilage. Intravenous injection results in synovial enhancement and later enhancement in joint fluid in 15 to 30 minutes (68,70). Joint fluid enhances more rapidly after exercise or when there is not an effusion already present. Large effusions increase joint pressure resulting in slower fluid enhancement (69,70). Fluid enhancement may also occur more rapidly, with actively inflamed synovium such as in patients with rheumatoid arthritis. Intravenous contrast with conventional or bolus injection and rapid sequence imaging provides valuable information regarding active synovitis, synovial volume, and response to therapy (341).

Chronic Overuse Syndromes/Miscellaneous Conditions

There are numerous inflammatory conditions in and about the knee that can result in pain and symptoms that reduce activity or effective participation in sports or exercise programs. Conditions such as osteochondroses have been discussed previously. Tendinitis, bursitis, muscle injuries, and other overuse syndromes can mimic more serious knee injuries or soft tissue masses (3,95,356). Awareness of these conditions can lead to proper conservative therapy or local injections while obviating the need for arthroscopy or more invasive procedures.

Bursitis

There are numerous bursae about the knee (Table 7-2) (see Fig. 7-158). Bursae may become inflamed and fluid-distended, which will produce well-defined, though occasionally lobulated or multifocal, cyst-like lesions about the tendons of the knee. These distended bursae are high signal intensity on T2-weighted and low intensity on T1-weighted MR images (see Fig. 7-159) (95,356). Pes anserine bursitis leads to medial knee pain (see Fig. 7-160) (89,357). This bursa lies deep to the pes anserine (gracilis, semitendinosus, and sartorius) tendons. Pain or a palpable mass may be the presenting complaint. It is not uncommon for patients to have underlying osteoarthritis or rheumatoid arthritis (357). Other fluid collections or bursae may also present with medial joint line pain. The MCL and semimembranosus–tibial collateral ligament bursae may also become inflamed. Location and appearance (see Figs. 7-161 and 7-162) are important for differentiating these anatomic structures (89,99).

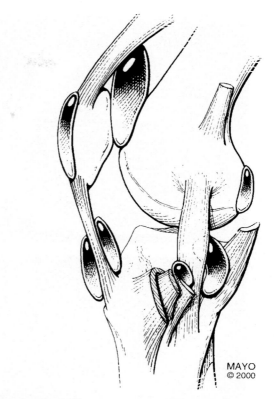

Figure 7-158 The bursae about the knee.

Differential diagnosis in these patients should include meniscal cysts, ganglion cysts, and other soft tissue masses.

Acute trauma to bursae can lead to hemorrhage and chronic problems (see Figs. 7-163 and 7-164) if not properly treated. Aspiration and/or resection may be required.

Tendinitis

Tendon inflammation can occur alone or with bursitis and other chronic overuse injuries. Tendon snapping can occur in either setting. The semitendinosus tendon can snap over a bony prominence or inflamed bursa (Fig. 7-164). Tendinitis involving the extensor mechanism was discussed previously. Inflammation in the juxtapatellar regions, especially the patellar tendon, is easily detected as areas of high signal intensity on axial and sagittal T2-weighted or STIR sequences.

Iliotibial Band Syndrome

This overuse syndrome is common in long distance runners, cyclists, and football players (114,20,219). There is usually a history of increasing distance or running on hills.

The iliotibial band extends from the greater trochanter to insert distally on the supracondylar tubercle of the femur, the intermuscular septum, and distally on the anterolateral aspect of the tibia (Gerdy's tubercle) (114,201,258).

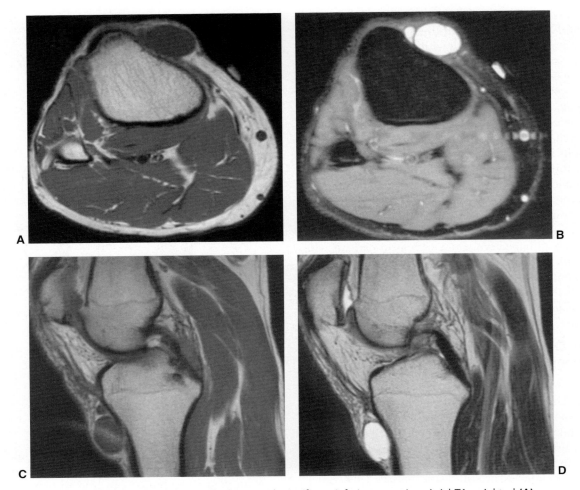

Figure 7-159 Deep infrapatellar bursa with significant inferior extension. Axial T1-weighted **(A)** and fat-suppressed fast spin-echo T2-weighted **(B)**, and sagittal T1-weighted **(C)** and T2-weighted **(D)** images demonstrate a well-circumscribed, fluid-filled bursa.

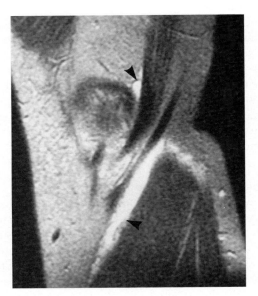

Figure 7-160 Sagittal T2-weighted image demonstrating an inflamed pes anserine bursa (*arrowheads*) along the medial tendons.

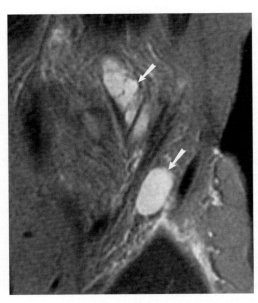

Figure 7-161 Sagittal T2-weighted image demonstrating multiple small areas of bursal distention (*arrows*). The lower collection is a distended semimembranous–tibial collateral ligament bursa.

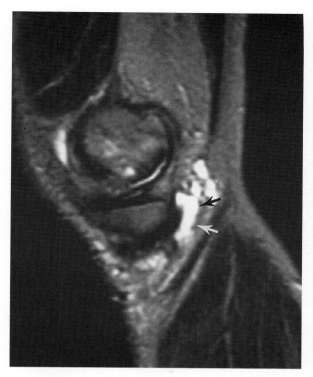

Figure 7-162 Middle-aged jogger with multiple areas of bursal distention (*arrows*) medially.

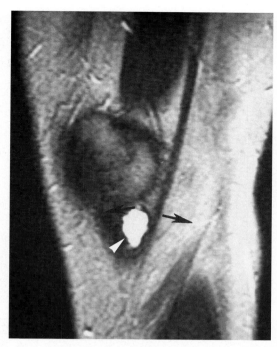

Figure 7-164 Sagittal T2-weighted image demonstrates a focal bursal enlargement (*arrowhead*) which caused snapping of the adjacent tendon with flexion and extension (*arrows*).

The syndrome is due to friction of the iliotibial band over the supracondylar femur and underlying tissues. This results in lateral joint line pain that is reproducible during flexion and extension of the knee (20). Differential diagnosis includes lateral meniscal tears, lateral collateral ligament injuries, popliteal tendon, and lateral hamstring strains (20).

Imaging can be accomplished with ultrasound. However, MRI is more definitive for confirming the diagnosis and excluding other bone or soft tissue injuries. MR features may vary with the extent and chronicity of the injury. Poorly defined or localized fluid collections with or without thickening of the iliotibial band are most commonly identified (see Figs. 7-165 and 7-166) (201,258,358).

Coronal and axial T2 or T2* images are most useful for detection of changes in thickness of the iliotibial band and the adjacent inflammation or fluid collections (20).

Muscle Tears

Muscle tears occur more commonly in the thigh and calf than the region of the knee joint where ligament and tendon injuries predominate (359). Tears in the extensor mechanism may involve the quadriceps (Figs. 7-91 and 7-92). Injuries to the plantaris and popliteus deserve mention in this section.

The plantaris is a small muscle arising from the lateral femoral condyle where it descends deep to the lateral head of the gastrocnemius. The long tendon courses between the gastrocnemius and soleus to join the Achilles tendon as it attaches to the calcaneus (78). Tears on the plantaris are common in athletes, especially tennis players (146). Injuries are sometimes misdiagnosed as gastrocnemius tears or deep vein thrombosis. A plantaris tear is usually

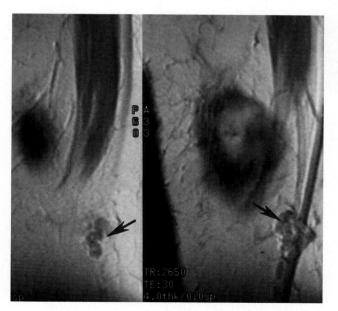

Figure 7-163 Superficial sagittal images in a patient with chronic bursitis treated with multiple injections leading to multiple small granulomas (*arrows*).

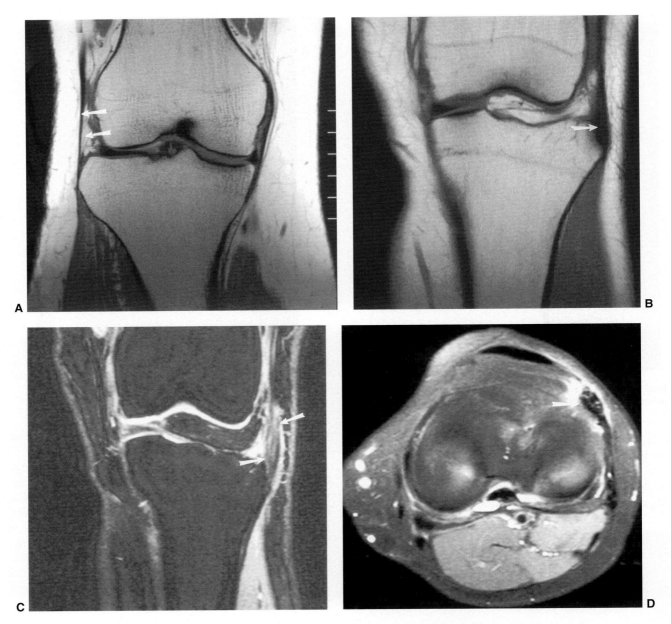

Figure 7-165   Iliotibial band syndrome. **A:** Coronal T1-weighted image demonstrating the normal iliotibial band (*arrows*). Coronal T1-weighted **(B)**, DESS **(C)**, and axial fat-suppressed proton density-weighted **(D)** images show thickening and abnormal signal intensity in the iliotibial band.

clinically less significant than a gastrocnemius tear (146). A fluid collection in the upper calf between the gastrocnemius and soleus is the most common finding in our experience (see Fig. 7-167).

Popliteal muscle tears were once considered uncommon. However, in recent years, the injury is more commonly detected. Most injuries involve the body of the muscle. However, both the muscle and tendon may be involved (360). Injuries are commonly associated with more significant structural damage that may explain why popliteal tears are less commonly reported. Bone bruises may be present in 33% of patients with popliteal muscle

tears. Tears of the ACL and PCL may be noted in 17% and 29% of patients, respectively (360).

Axial and sagittal image planes are most useful for detection of plantaris, gastrocnemius, or popliteal muscle injuries. T2-weighted or STIR sequences provide optimal contrast between normal muscle and the fluid and hemorrhage in the region of the tear (see Figs. 7-168 and 7-169).

Popliteal Artery Disorders

The popliteal artery is relatively short and affected by a unique set of pathologic conditions. Popliteal artery disease is most commonly due to atherosclerosis, but other causes

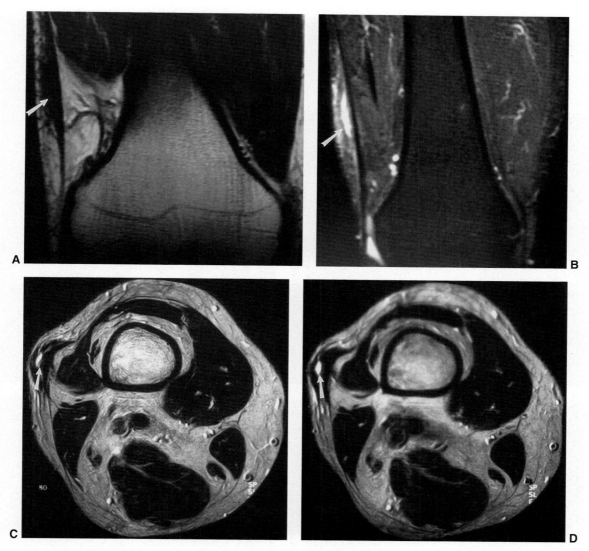

Figure 7-166   Iliotibial band syndrome. Coronal T1-weighted **(A)**, fat-suppressed, T2-weighted **(B)**, and axial proton density **(C)** and T2-weighted **(D)** images demonstrate an irregular fluid collection (*arrow*) along the iliotibial tract. The superficial location is atypical.

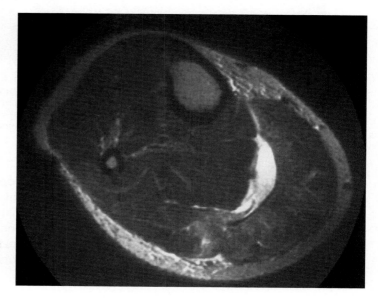

Figure 7-167   Axial T2-weighted image of the upper calf demonstrating fluid collection between the gastrocnemius and soleus due to a plantaris muscle tear.

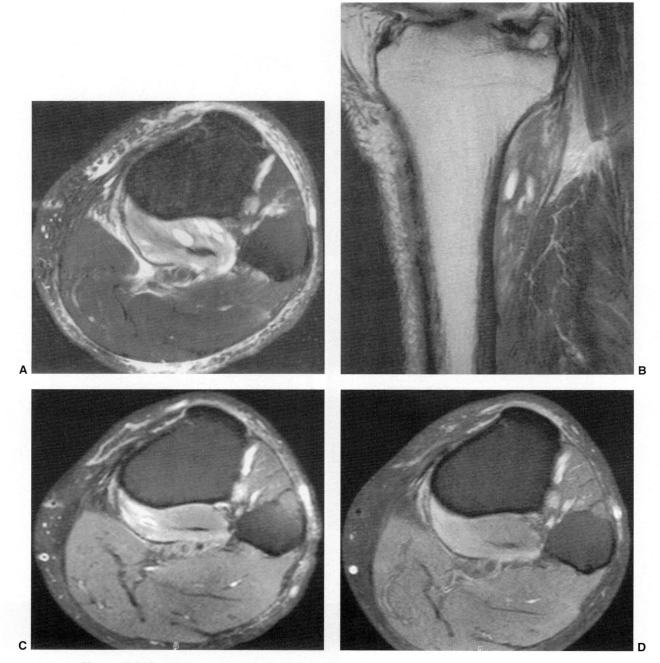

Figure 7-168 Popliteus muscle tear evolving from acute presentation **(A,B)** and at 3 months **(C)** and 6 months **(D).** Axial fast spin-echo T2-weighted sequence with fat suppression in **A** and sagittal T2-weighted **B** images demonstrate tearing and hemorrhage in the muscle belly. Axial fat-suppressed, fast spin-echo T2-weighted image at 3 months shows improvement with signal intensity returning to normal. Axial image **D** with the same sequence at 6 months shows nearly complete resolution.

including embolism, external compression from a Baker cyst, and, in young patients, there are two entities termed popliteal artery entrapment and cystic adventitial disease (361). Popliteal artery entrapment and cystic adventitial disease are of extreme clinical importance as they may produce popliteal artery occlusion and/or thrombosis (361,362).

Popliteal Artery Entrapment

This is an uncommon syndrome affecting young athletic males. Patients present with symptoms of calf claudication (362). This condition is caused by an anomalous anatomic relationship of the muscle and artery in the popliteal fossa resulting in artery compression (361). The

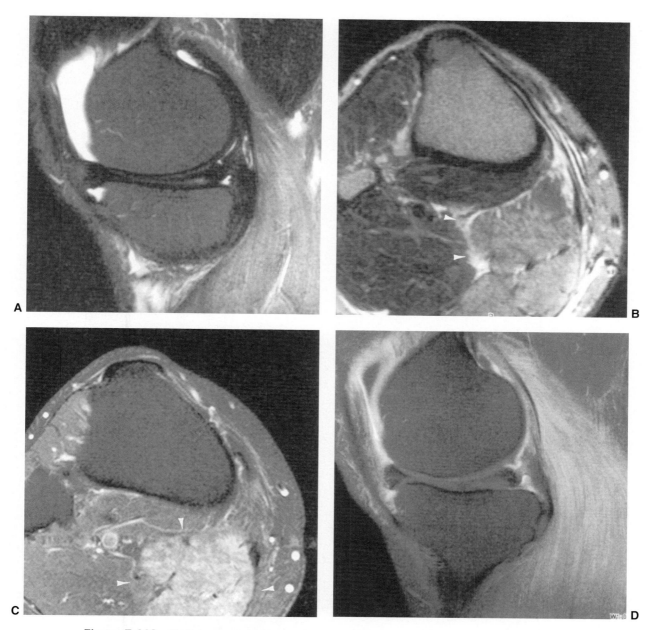

Figure 7-169 Medial gastrocnemius muscle strain demonstrated on sagittal STIR **(A)**, axial T2-weighted **(B)** (*arrowheads*), and postcontrast sagittal **(C)** (*arrowheads*) and axial **(D)** images.

condition is bilateral in 33% of cases, so both extremities should be evaluated if the condition is suspected clinically. There are five different types of popliteal artery entrapment (see Fig. 7-170) (361).

MR imaging and MR angiography now enable evaluation of popliteal fossa anatomy. MR images demonstrate the aberrant course of the popliteal artery and vein. Axial images are also quite useful for demonstrating the aberrant course of the vessels. MR angiograms demonstrate medial deviation of the popliteal arteries as well as focal stenosis or occlusion (see Fig. 7-171) (361–363).

Cystic Adventitial Disease

Cystic adventitial disease (CAD) occurs when mucin-containing cystic structures form in the popliteal artery, causing claudication (363). This disease is rare, accounting for only 0.1% of vascular occlusive disease. The entity typically affects males near the age of 40 without risk factors for atherosclerosis (103,363).

Angiograms typically demonstrate a smoothly tapered eccentric or concentric narrowing of the midpopliteal artery in an otherwise normal vascular tree. CT usually demonstrates compression of the artery by a non-enhancing soft

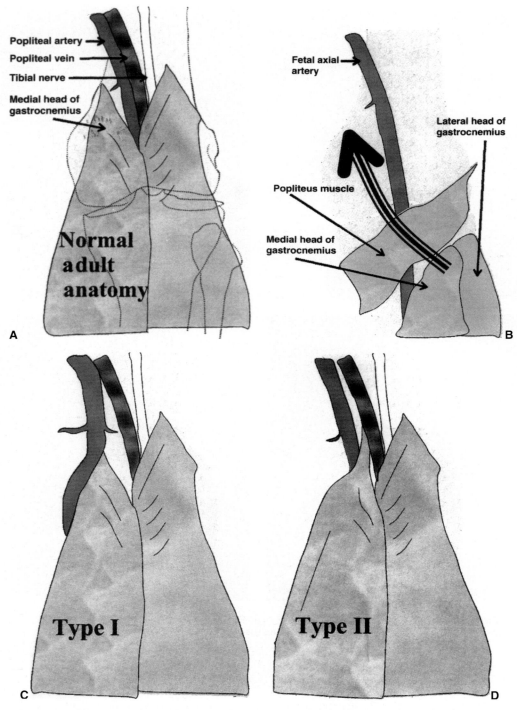

Figure 7-170 Classification of popliteal artery entrapment. **A:** Normal adult popliteal fossa anatomy. The popliteal artery, vein, and tibial nerve lie lateral to the medial gastrocnemius muscle. **B:** Embryonic development. In fetal life, medial head of the gastrocnemius initially originates from the posterior fibula and lateral tibia. However, during limb rotation and extension, its origin migrates superomedially (*large arrow*) to reach the adult attachment above the medial femoral condyle. Fetal precursor of the popliteal artery arises from the fetal axial artery and runs deep to the popliteus muscle. During development, this portion of the vessel obliterates and reforms superficial to the muscle to produce the adult form of the popliteal artery. **C:** Type I anomaly. Popliteal artery takes an aberrant course medially around the medial gastrocnemius that originates at its normal site above the medial femoral condyle. This anomaly occurs when muscle migration is delayed and therefore follows popliteal artery development. The vessel is then swept medially by muscle as the latter migrates. **D:** Type II anomaly. Medial head of the gastrocnemius has aberrant origin arising from the intercondylar notch rather than the medial femoral condyle. Popliteal artery shows little deviation from its course but is compressed by the aberrant muscle origin. This anomaly occurs when embryonic gastrocnemius migration is arrested.

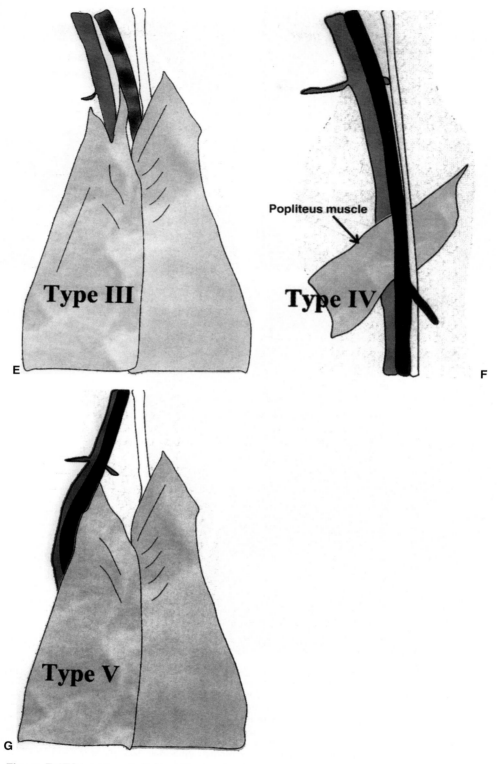

Figure 7-170 (*continued*) **E:** Type III anomaly. Accessory slip of medial gastrocnemius muscle takes origin from the intercondylar notch and forms a sling around the lateral side of the artery. This anomaly occurs when normal embryonic gastrocnemius migration is partially arrested. **F:** Type IV anomaly. Popliteal artery is entrapped as it takes an abnormal course deep to the popliteus muscle or beneath fibrous bands in the popliteal fossa. This anomaly occurs when the fetal precursor of the popliteal artery **(B)** fails to obliterate, with resulting mature popliteal artery running deep to the popliteus muscle. **G:** Type V anomaly, which is any type of entrapment that also includes the popliteal vein. (From Elias DA, White LM, Rubenstein JD, et al. Evaluation and MR imaging features of popliteal artery entrapment and cystic adventitial disease. *AJR Am J Roentgenol* 2003;180:627–632.)

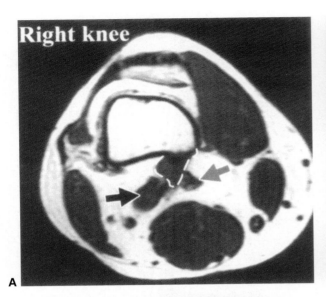

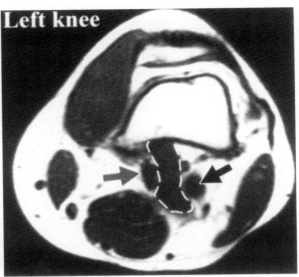

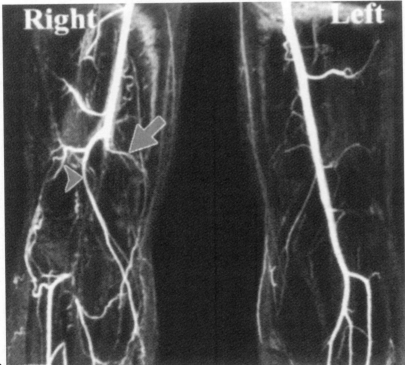

Figure 7-171 Bilateral popliteal artery entrapment in a 42-year-old who presented with calf claudication on the right for 3 months after thrombolysis for acute right foot ischemia. There were no symptoms on the left. **A:** Axial T1-weighted image of the right knee shows the popliteal artery (*right arrow*) with aberrant course that is medial to the head of the gastrocnemius (*broken lines*). Muscle origin is normally sited above the medial femoral condyle (*broken lines*) (type I anomaly). The popliteal vein (*left arrow*) is normally sited lateral to the medial head of the gastrocnemius. **B:** Axial T1-weighted image of the left knee shows the popliteal artery (*left arrow*) medial to the medial head of the gastrocnemius (*broken lines*). The muscle originates abnormally laterally at the superior intercondylar notch, consistent with a type II anomaly. The popliteal vein (*right arrow*) runs a normal course. **C:** Gadolinium enhanced MR angiogram shows the right popliteal artery occluded for 11 cm. Note reconstitution of three normal calf vessels and two collaterals, the medial superior geniculate artery (*arrow*) and sural artery (*arrowhead*). The left popliteal artery is normal caliber and has no deviation consistent with a type II anomaly. (From Elias DA, White LM, Rubenstein JD, et al. Evaluation and MR imaging features of popliteal artery entrapment and cystic adventitial disease. *AJR Am J Roentgenol* 2003;180:627–632.)

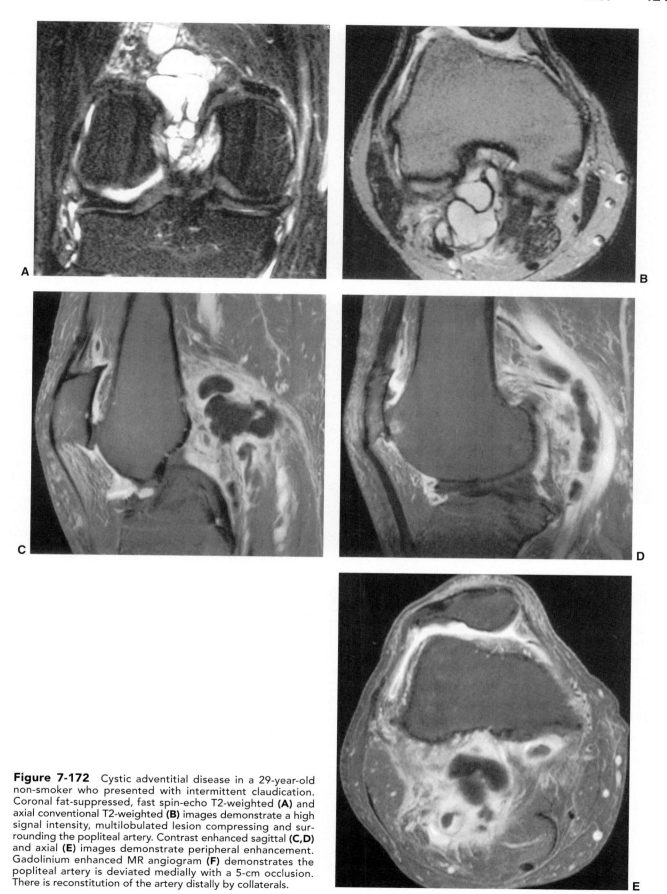

Figure 7-172 Cystic adventitial disease in a 29-year-old non-smoker who presented with intermittent claudication. Coronal fat-suppressed, fast spin-echo T2-weighted **(A)** and axial conventional T2-weighted **(B)** images demonstrate a high signal intensity, multilobulated lesion compressing and surrounding the popliteal artery. Contrast enhanced sagittal **(C,D)** and axial **(E)** images demonstrate peripheral enhancement. Gadolinium enhanced MR angiogram **(F)** demonstrates the popliteal artery is deviated medially with a 5-cm occlusion. There is reconstitution of the artery distally by collaterals.

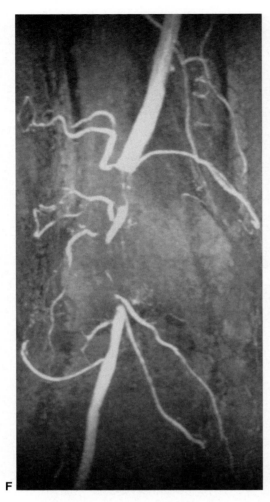

Figure 7-172 (continued)

tissue structure in close proximity to the popliteal artery wall (363). Lesions are usually high signal intensity on both T1- and T2-weighted sequences due to the mucoid protein content (see Fig. 7-172) (361,363).

Treatment consists of cyst decompression that can be performed surgically or with CT guidance. Spontaneous resolution has been reported (363).

REFERENCES

1. Berquist TH. *Imaging of sports injuries.* Garthersburg, MD: Aspen Publishing, 1992.
2. Berquist TH. Magnetic resonance imaging of musculoskeletal neoplasms. *Clin Orthop* 1989;244:101–118.
3. Berquist TH. *MRI of the musculoskeletal system,* 4th ed. Philadelphia, PA: Lippincott Williams & Wilkins, 2001.
4. Crues JV III, Ryu R. MRI of the knee: part I. *Appl Radiol* 1989;18:18–23.
5. Crues JV III, Ryu R. MRI of the knee: part II. *Appl Radiol* 1989;18:12–18.
6. Crues JV III. Magnetic resonance imaging of knee menisci. Presented at the Society of Magnetic Resonance in Medicine, Amsterdam, 1989.
7. Crues JV III. Meniscal tears: MR imaging and postoperative follow-up In: Weissman BN. *Advanced imaging of joints: theory and practice.* RSNA Categorical Course, Chicago, 1993:167–172.
8. Bergin D, Morrison WB, Carrino JA, et al. Anterior cruciate ligament ganglia and mucoid degeneration: coexistence and clinical correlation. *AJR Am J Roentgenol* 2004;182:1283–1287.
9. Bredella MA, Tirman PFJ, Peterfy CG, et al. Accuracy of T2-weighted fast spin-echo MR imaging with fat saturation in detecting cartilage defects in the knee: comparison with arthroscopy in 130 patients. *AJR Am J Roentgenol* 1999;172:1073–1080.
10. Goodwin DW, Wadghiri YZ, Zhu H, et al. Macroscopic structure of articular cartilage of the tibial plateau: influence of a characteristic matrix architecture on MRI appearance. *AJR Am J Roentgenol* 2004;182:311–318.
11. Kneeland B. Magnetic resonance imaging of articular cartilage. *Semin Roentgenol* 2000;35:249–255.
12. Laurin CA. Patellar position, patellar osteotomy, their relationship to chondromalacia—x-ray diagnosis of chondromalacia. In: Pickett JC, Radin EL, eds. *Chondromalacia patella.* Baltimore, MD: Williams & Wilkins, 1983:11–23.
13. McCarthy CL, McNally EG. The MRI appearance of cystic lesions around the knee. *Skeletal Radiol* 2004;33:187–209.
14. Munshi M, Davidson M, MacDonald PB, et al. The efficacy of magnetic resonance imaging in acute knee injuries. *Clin J Sport Med* 2000;10:34–39.
15. Recht MP, Piraino DW, Paletta GA, et al. Accuracy of fat-suppressed three-dimensional spoiled gradient-echo Flash MR imaging in detection of patellofemoral articular cartilage abnormalities. *Radiology* 1996;198:209–212.
16. Sonin AH, Fitzgerald SW, Friedman H, et al. Posterior cruciate ligament injury: MR imaging diagnosis and patterns of injury. *Radiology* 1994;190:455–458.
17. Sonin AH, Pensy RA, Mulligan ME, et al. Grading articular cartilage of the knee using fast spin-echo proton density—weighted MR imaging without fat suppression. *AJR Am J Roentgenol* 2002;179:1159–1166.
18. Magee TH, Hinson GW. MRI of meniscal bucket-handle tears. *Skeletal Radiol* 1998;27:495–499.
19. Magee T, Shapiro M, Williams D. Prevalence of meniscal radial tears of the knee revealed by MRI after surgery. *AJR Am J Roentgenol* 2004;182:931–936.
20. Muhle C, Ahn JM, Yeh LR. Iliotibial band friction syndrome: MR imaging findings in 16 patients and MR arthrographic study of six cadaver knees. *Radiology* 1999;212:103–110.
21. Munk PL, Helms CA, Genant HK, et al. Magnetic resonance imaging of the knee: current status, new directions. *Skeletal Radiol* 1989;18:569–577.
22. Uppal A, Disler DG, Short WB, et al. Internal derangements of the knee: rates of occurrence at MR imaging in patients referred by orthopedic surgeons compared with rates in patients referred by physicians who are not orthopedic surgeons. *Radiology* 1998;207:633–636.
23. Ruwe PA, McCarthy S. Cost-effectiveness of magnetic resonance imaging. In: Munk JH, Reicker MA, Crues JV III et al., eds. *MR imaging of the knee,* 2nd ed. New York: Raven Press, 1993:463–466.
24. Ruwe PA, Wright J, Randall RL, et al. Can MR imaging effectively replace diagnostic arthroscopy? *Radiology* 1992;183:335–339.
25. Maurer EJ, Kaplan PA, Dussault RG, et al. Acutely injured knee: effect of MR imaging on diagnostic and therapeutic decisions. *Radiology* 1997;204:799–805.
26. Bui-Mansfield LT, Youngberg RA, Warine W, et al. Potential cost savings of MR imaging obtained before arthroscopy of the knee: evaluation of 50 consecutive patients. *AJR Am J Roentgenol* 1997;168:913–918.
27. Vincken PWJ, Terbraak BPM, Van Erkell AR, et al. Effectiveness of MR imaging in selection of patients for arthroscopy of the knee. *Radiology* 2002;223:739–746.
28. Alioto RJ, Browne JE, Barnthouse CD, et al. The influence of MRI on treatment decisions regarding knee injuries. *Am J Knee Surg* 1999;12:91–97.
29. Munk PL, Vellet AD. Lesions of cartilage and bone around the knee. *Top Magn Reson Imaging* 1993;5:249–262.
30. Prickett WD, Ward SI, Matava MJ. Magnetic resonance imaging of the knee. *Sports Med* 2003;31:997–1019.

31. Hayes CW, Conway WF. Normal anatomy and magnetic resonance appearance of the knee. *Top Magn Reson Imaging* 1993;5(4): 207–227.

32. Antonio GE, Griffith JF, Yeung DKW. Small-field-of-view MRI of the knee and ankle. *AJR Am J Roentgenol* 2004;183:24–28.

33. Ahn JM, Kwak SM, Kang HS, et al. Evaluation of patellar cartilage in cadavers with low-field strength extremity-only magnet: comparison of MR imaging sequences with macroscopic findings as a standard. *Radiology* 1998;208:57–62.

34. Arndt WFIII, Truax AL, Barnett FM, et al. MR diagnosis of bone contusions of the knee: Comparison of coronal T2-weighted fast spin-echo with fat saturation and fast spin-echo STIR images with conventional STIR images. *AJR Am J Roentgenol* 1996;166:119–124.

35. DeSmet AA, Monu JUV, Fisher DR, et al. Signs of patellar chondromalacia on sagittal T2-weighted magnetic resonance imaging. 1992;21:103–105.

36. Disler DG, Kattapuram SV, Chew FS, et al. Meniscal tears of the knee: Preliminary three-dimensional MR reconstruction with two-dimensional MR imaging and arthroscopy. *AJR Am J Roentgenol* 1993;160:343–345.

37. Disler DG, McCauley TR, Kelman CG, et al. Fat-suppressed three-dimensional spoiled gradient-echo MR imaging of hyaline cartilage defects in the knee: comparison with standard MR imaging and arthroscopy. *AJR Am J Roentgenol* 1996;167:127–132.

38. Disler DG, McCauley TR, Wirth CR, et al. Detection of knee hyaline cartilage defects using fat-suppressed three-dimensional spoiled gradient-echo MR imaging: comparison with standard MR imaging and correlation with arthroscopy. *AJR Am J Roentgenol* 1995;165:377–382.

39. Disler DG, Peters TL, Muscoreil SJ, et al. Fat-suppressed spoiled GRASS imaging of knee hyaline cartilage: technique optimization and comparison with conventional MR imaging. *AJR Am J Roentgenol* 1994;163:887–892.

40. Disler DG. Fat-suppressed three-dimensional spoiled gradient-echo recalled imaging: assessment of articular and physeal hyaline cartilage. *AJR Am J Roentgenol* 1997;169:1117–1123.

41. Heron CW, Calvert PT. Three-dimensional gradient-echo MR imaging of the knee: comparison with arthroscopy in 100 patients. *Radiology* 1992;183:839–844.

42. Obletter N, Held P, Kett H, et al. Evaluation of 3D MR data sets in orthopedic cases. Presented at the Society of Magnetic Resonance in Medicine, Amsterdam, 1989.

43. Peterfy CG, Majundar S, Lang P, et al. MR imaging of the arthritic knee: improved discrimination of cartilage, synovium, and effusion with pulsed saturation transfer and fat-suppressed T1-weighted sequences. *Radiology* 1994;191:413–419.

44. Recht MP, White LM, Winalski CS, et al. MR imaging of cartilage repair procedures. 2003;32:185–200.

45. Rubin DA, Kneeland JB, Listerud J, et al. MR diagnosis of meniscal tears of the knee: value of fast spin-echo vs. conventional spin-echo pulse sequences. *AJR Am J Roentgenol* 1994;162: 1131–1135.

46. Smith DK, May DA, Phillips P. MR imaging of the anterior cruciate ligament: frequency of discordant findings on sagittal-oblique images and correlation with arthroscopic findings. *AJR Am J Roentgenol* 1996;166:411–413.

47. Totterman S, Simon J, Szumowski J, et al. PEACH in the detection of musculoskeletal lesions. Presented at the Society of Magnetic Resonance in Medicine, Amsterdam, 1989.

48. Totterman S, Weiss SL, Szumowski J, et al. MR fat suppression technique in the evaluation of normal structures of the knee. *J Comput Assist Tomogr* 1989;13:473–479.

49. Vandeberg BC, Lecouvet FE, Poilvache P, et al. Assessment of knee cartilage in cadavers with dual-detector spiral CT arthrography and MR imaging. *Radiology* 2002;222:430–436.

50. White LM, Schweitzer ME, Weishaupt D, et al. Diagnosis of recurrent meniscal tears: prospective evaluation of conventional MR imaging, indirect MR arthrography, and the direct MR arthrography. *Radiology* 2002;222:421–429.

51. Applegate GR, Lannigan BD, Tolin BS, et al. MR diagnosis of recurrent tears in the knee: value of intra-articular contrast material. *AJR Am J Roentgenol* 1993;161:821–825.

52. Escobedo EM, Hunter JC, Zink-Brody GC, et al. Usefulness of turbo spin-echo MR imaging in the evaluation of meniscal tears: comparison with a conventional spin-echo sequence. *AJR Am J Roentgenol* 1996;167:1223–1227.

53. Brossmann J, Preidler K-W, Daener B, et al. Imaging of osseous and cartilaginous intra-articular bodies in the knee: comparison of MR imaging and MR arthrography with CT and CT arthrography in cadavers. *Radiology* 1996;200:509–517.

54. Kaplan PA, Dussault RG. Magnetic resonance imaging of the knee: menisci, ligaments, tendons. *Top Magn Reson Imaging* 1993; 5(4):228–248.

55. Hayes CW, Conway WF. Evaluation of articular cartilage: radiographic and cross-sectional imaging techniques. *RadioGraphics* 1992;12:409–428.

56. Murphy BJ. Evaluation of grades 3 and 4 chondromalacia of the knee using T2-weighted 3D gradient echo articular cartilage imaging. 2001;30:305–311.

57. Reiser MF, Bongartz G, Erlemann R, et al. Magnetic resonance in cartilaginous lesions of the knee joint with three-dimensional gradient-echo imaging. 1988;17:465–471.

58. Smith DK, Berquist TH, An KN, et al. Validation of three-dimensional reconstructions of knee anatomy: CT vs. MR imaging. *J Comput Assist Tomogr* 1989;13:294–301.

59. McCauley TR, Disler DG. MR imaging of articular cartilage. *Radiology* 1998;209:629–640.

60. Harms SE, Flamig DP, Fisher CF, et al. 3D faster MR imaging of the knee. Presented at the Society of Magnetic Resonance in Medicine, Amsterdam, 1989.

61. Shahabpour M, Van Cauteren M, Handelberg F, et al. MRI of chondral lesions of the knee: a comparative study of 2D spin-echo and 3D gradient echo imaging. Presented at the Society of Magnetic Resonance in Medicine, Amsterdam, 1989.

62. Berquist TH. Magnetic resonance techniques in musculoskeletal diseases. *Rheum Clin North Am* 1991;17:599–615.

63. Ha TPT, Li KCP, Bergman G, et al. Anterior cruciate ligament injury: fast spin-echo MR imaging with arthroscopic correlation in 212 examinations. *AJR Am J Roentgenol* 1998;170:1215–1219.

64. Hajek PC, Sartoris DJ, Neumann CH, et al. Potential contrast agents for MR arthrography: in vitro evaluation and practical observations. *AJR Am J Roentgenol* 1987;149:97–104.

65. Hodler J, Resnick D. Current status of imaging of articular cartilage. 1996;25:703–709.

66. McCauley TR, Elfer A, Moore A, et al. MR arthrography of anterior cruciate ligament reconstruction grafts. *AJR Am J Roentgenol* 2003;181:1217–1223.

67. Wright DH, Desmet AA, Norres M. Bucket handle tears of the medial and lateral menisci of the knee: value of MR imaging in detecting displaced fragments. *AJR Am J Roentgenol* 1995;165: 621–625.

68. Drape J, Thelen P, Gay-Depassier P, et al. Intra-articular diffusion of GD-DOTA after intravenous injection in the knee: MR imaging evaluation. *Radiology* 1993;188:227–234.

69. Winalski CS, Aliabadi P, Wright RJ, et al. Enhancement of joint fluid with intravenously administered gadopenetate dimeglumine: technique, rationale and indications. *Radiology* 1993;187:179–185.

70. Winalski CS, Weissman BN, Aliabadi P, et al. Intravenous Gd-DTPA enhancement of joint fluid: a less invasive alternative for MR arthrography. *Radiology* 1991;181:304.

71. Kang HS, Resnick D. *MRI of the extremities: an anatomic atlas.* Philadelphia, PA: WB Saunders, 1991.

72. Middleton WD, Lawson TL. *Anatomy and MRI of the joints. A multiplanar atlas.* New York: Raven Press, 1989.

73. Mesgarzadeh M, Moyer R, Leder DS, et al. MR imaging of the knee: expanded classification and pitfalls to interpretation of meniscal tears. *RadioGraphics* 1993;13:489–500.

74. Mesgarzadeh M, Schneck CD, Bonakdarpour A. Magnetic resonance imaging of the knee and correlation with normal anatomy. *RadioGraphics* 1988;8:707–733.

75. Rubin DA, Kettering JM, Towers JD, et al. MR imaging of knees having isolated and combined ligament injuries. *AJR Am J Roentgenol* 1998;170:1207–1213.

76. Sick H, Burguet J. In: J Bergmann, ed. *Imaging anatomy of the knee region.* München: Verlag, 1988.

77. Rand JA, Berquist TH. The knee. In: Berquist TH, ed. *Imaging of orthopedic trauma*, 2nd ed. New York: Raven Press, 1992:333–432.

78. Rosse C, Rosse PG. *Hollinshead's textbook of anatomy*. Philadelphia, PA: Lippincott–Raven, 1997.

79. Frank LR, Wong EC, Luh W-M, et al. Articular cartilage of the knee: mapping of the physiologic parameters at MR imaging with a local gradient coil-preliminary results. *Radiology* 1999;210: 241–246.

80. Agur AMR, Lee MJ. *Grant's atlas of anatomy*, 9th ed. Baltimore, MD: Williams & Wilkins, 1991.

81. Hodler J, Haghighi P, Pathria MN, et al. Meniscal changes in the elderly: correlation with MR imaging and histologic findings. *Radiology* 1992;184:221–225.

82. Bates DG, Hresko MT, Jaramillo D. Patellar sleeve fracture: demonstration with MR imaging. *Radiology* 1994;193:825–827.

83. Hodler J, Resnick D. Chondromalacia patellae. *AJR Am J Roentgenol* 1992;158:106–107.

84. Wiberg G. Roentgenographic and anatomic studies of the femoropatellar joint with special reference to chondromalacia patella. *Acta Orthop Scand* 1941;121:319–340.

85. Lee K, Siegel MJ, Lau DM, et al. Anterior cruciate ligament tears: MR imaging-based diagnosis in a pediatric population. *Radiology* 1999;213:697–704.

86. Nemeth WC, Sanders BL. The lateral synovial recess of the knee: anatomy and role in chronic iliotibial band friction syndrome. *Arthroscopy* 1995;12:574–580.

87. Delgado-Martins H. A study of position of the patella using computerized tomography. *J Bone Joint Surg Br* 1979;61B:443–444.

88. DeMaeseneer M, Shahabpour M, Van Roy F, et al. MR imaging of the medial collateral ligament bursa: findings in patients and anatomic data derived from cadavers. *AJR Am J Roentgenol* 2001;177:911–917.

89. Rothstein CP, Laorr A, Helms CA, et al. Seimembranosus-tibial collateral ligament bursitis: MR image findings. *AJR Am J Roentgenol* 1995;155:875–877.

90. Loredo R, Hodler J, Pedowitz R, et al. Posteromedial corner of the knee: MR imaging with gross anatomic correlation. 1999;28:305–311.

91. Miller TT, Gladden P, Staron RB, et al. Posterolateral stabilizers of the knee: anatomy and injuries assessed with MR imaging. *AJR Am J Roentgenol* 1997;169:1641–1647.

92. Negendank WG, Fernandez-Madrid FR, Heilbrun LK, et al. MRI of meniscal degeneration of asymptomatic knees: evidence of a relation to clinical tears. Presented at the Society of Magnetic Resonance in Medicine, Amsterdam, 1989.

93. Sonin AH, Fitzgerald SW, Bresler ME, et al. MR imaging appearance of the extensor mechanism of the knee; functional anatomy and injury patterns. *RadioGraphics* 1995;15:367–382.

94. Stoller DW, Martin C, Crues JV, et al. Meniscal tears: pathologic correlation with MR imaging. *Radiology* 1987;163:731–735.

95. Zeiss J, Coombs RJ, Booth RL, et al. Chronic bursitis presenting as a mass in the pes anserine bursa: MR diagnosis. *J Comput Assist Tomogr* 1993;17:137–140.

96. Spritzer CE, Courneya DL, Burk LD, et al. Medial retinacular complex injury in acute patellar dislocation. MR findings and surgical implications. *AJR Am J Roentgenol* 1997;168:117–122.

97. Haims AH, Medvecky MJ, Pavlovich R, et al. MR imaging of the anatomy and injuries to the lateral and posterolateral aspects of the knee. *AJR Am J Roentgenol* 2003;180:647–653.

98. Tria AJ, Johnson CD, Zawadsky JP. The popliteus tendon. *J Bone Joint Surg Am* 1989;71:714–716.

99. Beltran J, Matityahu A, Hwang K, et al. The distal semimembranosus complex: normal MR anatomy, variants, biomechanics and pathology. 2003;32:435–445.

100. Sanders TG, Linares RC, Lawhorn KW, et al. Oblique meniscomeniscal ligament. Another potential pitfall for a meniscal tear-anatomic description and appearance at MR imaging in three cases. *Radiology* 1999;213:213–216.

101. Cho JM, Suh J-S, Na J-B, et al. Variations in meniscofemoral ligaments at anatomic study and MR imaging. *Skeletal Radiol* 1999;28:189–195.

102. De Maeseneer M, Lenchik L, Starok M, et al. Normal and abnormal medial meniscocapsular structures: MR imaging and sonography in cadavers. *AJR Am J Roentgenol* 1998;171:969–976.

103. Duc SR, Wentz KU, Kach KP, et al. First report of an accessory popliteal muscle: detection with MRI. *Skeletal Radiol* 2004;33: 429–431.

104. Watanabe AT, Carter BC, Teitelbaum GP, et al. Common pitfalls in magnetic resonance imaging of the knee. *J Bone Joint Surg Am* 1989;71A:857–862.

105. Weiss CB, Lundberg M, Hamberg P, et al. Non-operative treatment of meniscal tears. *J Bone Joint Surg Am* 1989;71A:811–822.

106. Cotton A, Flipo R-M, Herbaux B, et al. Synovial hemangioma of the knee: a frequently misdiagnosed lesion. *Skeletal Radiol* 1995;24:251–261.

107. Shellock FG, Morris E, Deutsch AL, et al. Hematopoietic bone marrow hyperplasia: high prevalence on MR images in asymptomatic marathon runners. *AJR Am J Roentgenol* 1992;158:335–338.

108. Havránek P, Lizler J. Magnetic resonance imaging in the evaluation of partial growth arrest after physeal injuries in children. *J Bone Joint Surg Am* 1991;73A:1234–1240.

109. Shankman S, Beltran J, Melamed E, et al. Anterior horn of the lateral meniscus. Another potential pitfall in MR imaging of the knee. *Radiology* 1997;204:181–184.

110. Watanabe AT, Carter BC, Teitelbaum GP, et al. Normal variations in MR imaging of the knee: appearance and frequency. *AJR Am J Roentgenol* 1989;153:341–344.

111. Noyes FR, Barter-Westin SD, Roberts CS. Use of allografts after failed treatment of rupture of the anterior cruciate ligaments. *J Bone Joint Surg Am* 1994;76A:1019–1031.

112. Herman LJ, Beltran J. Pitfalls in MR imaging of the knee. *Radiology* 1988;167:775–781.

113. Recht MP, Applegate G, Kaplan P, et al. The MR appearance of cruciate ganglion cysts: a report of 16 cases. *Skeletal Radiol* 1994;23:597–600.

114. Campos JC, Chung CB, Lektrakul N, et al. Pathogenesis of the Segond fracture: anatomic and MR imaging evidence of an iliotibial tractor anterior oblique band avulsion. *Radiology* 2001;219: 381–386.

115. Holt MD, Williams LA, Dent CM. MRI in management of tibial plateau fractures. *Injury* 1995;26:595–599.

116. Horas U, Pelinkovic D, Herr G, et al. Autologous chondrocyte implantation and osteochondral cylinder transplantation in cartilage repair of the knee joint. *J Bone Joint Surg Am* 2003;85:185–193.

117. Reicher MA, Hartzman S, Bassett LW, et al. MR imaging of the knee. Part I. Traumatic disorders. *Radiology* 1987;162:547–551.

118. Roth C, Jacobson J, Jamadar D, et al. Quadriceps fat pad signal intensity and enlargement on MRI: prevalence and associated findings. *AJR Am J Roentgenol* 2004;182:1383–1387.

119. Manaster BJ. Imaging of knee ligament reconstructions. In: Weissman GN, ed. *RSNA categorical course in musculoskeletal radiology*. Chicago, Ill: Radiology Society of North America, 1993: 211–218.

120. Tarhan NC, Chung CB, Mohana-Borges AV, et al. Meniscal tears: role of axial MRI alone and in combination with other imaging planes. *AJR Am J Roentgenol* 2004;183:9–15.

121. Tomzak RT, Hehl G, Mergo PJ, et al. Tunnel placement in anterior cruciate ligament reconstruction: MRI analysis as an important factor in the radiological report. *Skeletal Radiol* 1997;26:409–413.

122. Neuschwander DC, Drez D, Finney TP. Lateral meniscal variant with absence of the posterior coronary ligament. *J Bone Joint Surg Am* 1992;74A:1186–1190.

123. Silverman JM, Mink JH, Deutsch AL. Discoid menisci of the knee: MR imaging appearance. *Radiology* 1989;173:351–354.

124. Peterfy CG, Janzen DL, Tirman PFJ, et al. "Magic angle" phenomenon: a cause of increased signal in the normal lateral meniscus on short-TE MR images of the knee. *AJR Am J Roentgenol* 1994;163:149–154.

125. Shogry MEC, Pope TL. Vacuum phenomenon simulating meniscal or cartilaginous injury of the knee at MR imaging. *Radiology* 1991;180:513–515.

126. Turner DA, Rapoport MI, Erwin WD, et al. Truncation artifact: a potential pitfall in MR imaging of the knee. *Radiology* 1991;179: 629–633.

127. Chan WP, Peterfly C, Fritz RC, et al. MR diagnosis of complete tears of the anterior cruciate ligament of the knee: importance of anterior subluxation of the tibia. *AJR Am J Roentgenol* 1994;162:355–360.

128. Cheung Y, Magee TH, Rosenberg ZS, et al. MRI of anterior cruciate ligament reconstruction. *J Comput Assist Tomogr* 1992;16:134–137.

129. Cobby MJ, Schweitzer ME, Resnick D. The deep lateral femoral notch: an indirect sign of a torn anterior cruciate ligament. *Radiology* 1992;184:855–858.

130. Suh J-S, Jeong E-K, Shin K-H, et al. Minimizing artifacts caused by metallic implants at MR imaging: experimental and chemical studies. *AJR Am J Roentgenol* 1998;171:1207–1213.

131. Escobedo EM, Mills WJ, Hunter JC. The "Reverse Segond" fracture: association with a tear of the posterior cruciate ligament and medial meniscus. *AJR Am J Roentgenol* 2002;178:979–983.

132. Goitz HT, Rijke AM, McCue FC III. Magnetic resonance imaging of stressed anterior cruciate ligaments. Presented at the Society of Magnetic Resonance in Medicine, Amsterdam, 1989.

133. Lee J, Papakonstantinov O, Brookenthal KR, et al. Arcuate sign of posterolateral knee injuries: anatomic radiographic, and MR imaging data related to patterns of injury. *Skeletal Radiol* 2003;32:619–627.

134. McNally E. Imaging assessment of anterior knee pain and patellar mistracking. *Skeletal Radiol* 2001;30:484–495.

135. McNally EG, Nasser KN, Dawson S, et al. Role of magnetic resonance imaging in the clinical management of the acutely locked knee. *Skeletal Radiol* 2002;31:570–573.

136. Roemer FW, Bohndorf K. Long-term osseous sequelae after acute trauma of the knee joint evaluated by MRI. *Skeletal Radiol* 2002;31:615–623.

137. Hall FJ. Arthrography of the discoid lateral meniscus. *AJR Am J Roentgenol* 1977;128:993–1002.

138. Dehaven KE, Arnoczky SP. Meniscal repair: part I. Basic science, indications for repair and open repair. *J Bone Joint Surg* 1994;76A:140–152.

139. Dorsay TA, Helms CA. Bucket-handle meniscal tears of the knee: sensitivity and specificity of MRI signs. *Skeletal Radiol* 2003;32:266–272.

140. Bhattacharyya T, Gale D, Dewire P, et al. The clinical importance of meniscal tears demonstrated by magnetic resonance imaging in osteoarthritis of the knee. *J Bone Joint Surg Am* 2003;85:4–7.

141. DeSmet AA, Norris MA, Yondow DR, et al. MR diagnosis of meniscal tears of the knee: importance of high signal in the meniscus that extends to the surface. *AJR Am J Roentgenol* 1993;161:101–107.

142. DeSmet AA, Tuite MJ, Norris MA, et al. MR diagnosis of meniscal tears: analysis of causes of errors. *AJR Am J Roentgenol* 1994;163:1419–1423.

143. Huch K, Kuettner KE, Dieppe P. Osteoarthritis in ankle and knee joints. *Semin Arthritis Rheum* 1997;26:667–674.

144. Silva I, Silver DM. Tears of the meniscus as revealed by magnetic resonance imaging. *J Bone Joint Surg Am* 1988;70:199–202.

145. Van Heuzen EP, Golding RP, Van Zanten TEG, et al. Magnetic resonance imaging of meniscal lesions of the knee. *Clin Radiol* 1988;39:658–660.

146. Helms CA, Fritz RC, Garvin GJ. Plantaris muscle injury: evaluation with MR imaging. *Radiology* 1995;195:201–203.

147. Kornick J, Trefelner E, McCarthy S, et al. Meniscal abnormalities in the asymptomatic population at MR imaging. *Radiology* 1990;177:463–465.

148. Peh WCG, Chan JHM, Skek TWH, et al. The effect of using shorter echo times in MR imaging of knee menisci: a study using a porcine model. *AJR Am J Roentgenol* 1999;172:485–488.

149. Deutsch AL, Mink JH. Articular disorders of the knee. *Top Magn Reson Imaging* 1989;1:43–56.

150. Johnson RL, DeSmet AA. MR visualization of the popliteomeniscal fascicles. *Skeletal Radiol* 1999;28:561–566.

151. Reinig JW, McDevitt ER, Ove PN. Progression of meniscal degenerative changes in college football players: evaluation with MR imaging. *Radiology* 1991;181:255–257.

152. Hartzman S, Reicher MA, Bassett LW, et al. MR imaging of the knee. Part II. Chronic disorders. *Radiology* 1987;162:553–557.

153. Quinn SF, Brown TR, Szumowski J. Menisci of the knee: radial MR imaging correlated with arthroscopy in 259 patients. *Radiology* 1992;183:577–580.

154. Apple JS, Martinez S, Hardaker WT, et al. Synovial plicae of the knee. *Skeletal Radiol* 1982;7:251–254.

155. Brunner MC, Flower SP, Evancho AM, et al. MRI of the athletic knee. Findings in asymptomatic professional basketball and collegiate football players. *Invest Radiol* 1989;24:72–75.

156. Buckwalter KA, Braunstein EM, Janizek DB, et al. MR imaging of meniscal tears: narrow versus conventional window width photography. *Radiology* 1993;187:827–830.

157. Reeder JD, Matz SO, Becker L, et al. MR imaging of the knee in the sagittal projection: comparison of three-dimensional gradient-echo and spin-echo sequences. *AJR Am J Roentgenol* 1989;153:537–540.

158. Lee JHE, Singh TT, Bolton G. Axial fat-saturated FSE imaging of the knee: appearance of meniscal tears. *Skeletal Radiol* 2002;31:384–395.

159. Justice WW, Quinn SF. Error patterns in the MR imaging evaluation of menisci of the knee. *Radiology* 1995;196:617–621.

160. Yao L, Stanczak J, Boutin RD. Presumptive subarticular stress reactions of the knee: MRI detection and association with meniscal tear patterns. *Skeletal Radiol* 2004;33:260–264.

161. McCauley TR, Jee WH, Galloway MT, et al. Grade 2C signal in the meniscus on MR imaging of the knee. *AJR Am J Roentgenol* 2003;179:645–648.

162. Dillon EH, Pope CF, Jokl P, et al. Follow-up of grade 2 meniscal abnormalities in the stable knee. *Radiology* 1991;181:849–852.

163. Costa CR, Morrison WB, Carrino JA. Medial meniscus extrusion on knee MRI: is extent associated with severity of degenerative or type of tear? *AJR Am J Roentgenol* 2004;183:17–23.

164. Tuckman GA, Miller WJ, Remo JW, et al. Radial tears of the menisci: MR findings. *AJR Am J Roentgenol* 1994;163:395–400.

165. Anderson AF. Transepiphyseal replacement of the anterior cruciate ligament in skeletally immature patients. *J Bone Joint Surg Am* 2003;7:1255–1263.

166. Lacour-Petit MC, Lozeron P, Ducreux D. MRI of peripheral nerve lesions of the lower limbs. *Neuroradiology* 2003;45:166–170.

167. Cannon WD, Morgan CG. Meniscal repair: part II arthroscopic repair. *J Bone Joint Surg* 1994;76A:294–311.

168. Kaushik S, Erickson JK, Palmer WE, et al. Effect of chondrocalcinosis on the MR imaging of knee menisci. *AJR Am J Roentgenol* 2001;177:905–909.

169. Haramiti N, Staron RB, Rubin S, et al. The flipped meniscus sign. *Skeletal Radiol* 1993;22:273–277.

170. Blankenbaker DG, DeSmet AA, Smith JD. Usefulness of two indirect MR imaging signs to diagnose lateral meniscal tears. *AJR Am J Roentgenol* 2002;178:579–582.

171. Magee T, Shapiro M, Williams D. MR accuracy and arthroscopic incidence of meniscal radial tears. *Skeletal Radiol* 2002;31:686–689.

172. Soudry M, Lanir A, Angel D, et al. Anatomy of the normal knee as seen by magnetic resonance imaging. *J Bone Joint Surg Br* 1986;68A:117–120.

173. Glashow JL, Katz R, Schneider M, et al. Double-blind assessment of the value of magnetic resonance imaging in the diagnosis of anterior cruciate and meniscal lesions. *J Bone Joint Surg Am* 1989;71:113–119.

174. Newman AP, Daniels AU, Burks RT. Principles and decision making in meniscal surgery. *Arthroscopy* 1993;9:33–51.

175. Potter HG, Rodeo SA, Wickiewicz TL, et al. MR imaging of meniscal allografts: correlation with clinical and arthroscopic outcomes. *Radiology* 1996;198:509–514.

176. Recht MR, Kramer J. MR imaging of the postoperative knee: a pictorial essay. *RadioGraphics* 2002;22:765–774.

177. Lim PS, Schweitzer ME, Bhatia M, et al. Repeat tear of postoperative meniscus: potential MR imaging signs. *Radiology* 1999;210:183–188.

178. Sciulli RL, Bouten RD, Brown RR, et al. Evaluation of the postoperative meniscus of the knee: a study comparing conventional arthrography, conventional MR imaging, MR arthrography with iodinated contrast material and MR arthrography with gadolinium-based contrast material. *Skeletal Radiol* 1999;28:508–514.

179. Magee TH, Shapiro M, Rodriguez J, et al. MR Arthrography of postoperative knee: for which patients is it useful? *Radiology* 2003;229:159–163.

180. Farley TE, Howell SM, Love LF, et al. Meniscal tears: MR and orthographic findings after arthroscopic repair. *Radiology* 1991;180:517–522.

181. Burk DL Jr, Dalinka MK, Kanal E, et al. Meniscal and ganglion cysts of the knee: MR evaluation. *AJR Am J Roentgenol* 1988;150:331–336.

182. Campbell SE, Sanders TG, Morrison WB. MR imaging of meniscal cysts: incidence, location, and clinical significance. *AJR Am J Roentgenol* 2001;177:409–413.

183. Coral A, van Holsbeeck M, Adler RS. Imaging of meniscal cyst of the knee in three cases. *Skeletal Radiol* 1989;18:451–455.

184. Tyson LL, Daughters TC, Ryu RKH, et al. MRI appearance of meniscal cysts. *Skeletal Radiol* 1995;24:421:424.

185. Jansen DL, Peterfy CG, Forbes JR, et al. Cystic lesions around the knee joint: MR image findings. *AJR Am J Roentgenol* 1994;163:155–161.

186. Malghem J, Vandeberg BC, Lebon C, et al. Ganglion cysts of the knee. Articular communication revealed by delayed radiography and CT after arthrography. *AJR Am J Roentgenol* 1998;170:1579–1583.

187. Lektrakul N, Skaf A, Yeh LR, et al. Pericruciate meniscal cysts arising from tears of the posterior horn of the medial meniscus: MR imaging features that simulate posterior cruciate ganglion cysts. *AJR Am J Roentgenol* 1999;172:1575–1579.

188. Connolly B, Babyn PS, Wright JG, et al. Discoid meniscus in children: magnetic resonance imaging characteristics. *Can Assoc Radiol J* 1996;47:347–354.

189. Ryu KN, Kim IS, Kun EJ, et al. MR imaging of tears of discoid lateral menisci. *AJR Am J Roentgenol* 1998;171:963–967.

190. Dickhaut SC, DeLee JC. The discoid lateral meniscus syndrome. *J Bone Joint Surg Am* 1982;64A:1068–1073.

191. Rohren EM, Kosarek FJ, Helms CA. Discoid lateral meniscus and the frequency of meniscal tears. *Skeletal Radiol* 2001;30:316–320.

192. Ogden JA, Ganey TM, Arrington JA, et al. Meniscal ossification. *Skeletal Radiol* 1994;23:167–172.

193. Rose PM, Demlow TA, Szumowski J, et al. Chondromalacia patellae: fat-suppressed MR imaging. *Radiology* 1994;193:437–440.

194. Yu JS, Resnick D. Meniscal ossicle: MR imaging appearance in three patients. *Skeletal Radiol* 1994;23:637–639.

195. Schnarkowski P, Tirman PFJ, Tuchigami KD, et al. Meniscal ossicle: radiographic and MR imaging findings. *Radiology* 1995;196:47–50.

196. Kaye JJ. Ligament and tendon tears. secondary signs. *Radiology* 1993;188:616–617.

197. Romanini L, Calvisi V, Pappalardo S, et al. Prosthetic reconstruction of the anterior cruciate ligament of the knee: the roles of CT scan and MR. *Ital J Orthop Traumatol* 1988;14:301–310.

198. Vellet AD, Marks P, Fowler PJ, et al. Occult post-traumatic osteochondral lesions of the knee: prevalence, classification and short term sequelae evaluated on MR imaging. *Radiology* 1991;170:271–276.

199. Vellet D, Marks P, Munro T, et al. Comparative evaluation of orthogonal and non-orthogonal MRI in the evaluation of acute disruption of the anterior cruciate ligament. Presented at the Society of Magnetic Resonance in Medicine, Amsterdam, 1989.

200. Fu FH, Harner CD, Johnson DC, et al. Biomechanics of knee ligaments. *J Bone Joint Surg* 1993;75A:1716–1726.

201. Ekman EF, Pope T, Martin DF, et al. Magnetic resonance imaging of iliotibial band syndrome. *Am J Sports Med* 1994;22:851–854.

202. Pettersson H, Gillespy T, Kitchens C, et al. Magnetic resonance imaging in hemophilic arthropathy of the knee. *Acta Radiol* 1987;28:621–625.

203. Remer EM, Fitzgerald SW, Freidman H, et al. Anterior cruciate ligament injury: MR diagnosis and patterns of injury. *RadioGraphics* 1992;12:901–915.

204. Umans H, Wimpfheimer O, Haramati N, et al. Diagnosis of partial tears of the anterior cruciate ligaments of the knee: value of MR imaging. *AJR Am J Roentgenol* 1995;165:893–897.

205. Pope TL. MR imaging of knee ligaments. In: Weissman BN, ed. *Categorical course in musculoskeletal radiology.* Oak Brook, Ill: Radiological Society of North America, 1993:197–210.

206. Barry KP, Mesgarzadeh M, Triolo J, et al. Accuracy of MRI patterns in evaluating anterior cruciate ligament tears. *Skeletal Radiol* 1996;25:365–370.

207. Farooki S, Seeger LL. Magnetic resonance imaging in the evaluation of ligament injuries. *Skeletal Radiol* 1999;28:61–74.

208. Gentili A, Seeger LL, Yao L, et al. Anterior cruciate ligament tear: indirect signs at MR imaging. *Radiology* 1994;193:835–840.

209. Robertson PL, Schweitzer ME, Bartolozzi AR, et al. Anterior cruciate ligament tears: evaluation of multiple signs with MR imaging. *Radiology* 1994;193:829–834.

210. Staron RB, Haramati N, Feldman F, et al. O'Donoghue's triad: magnetic resonance imaging evidence. *Skeletal Radiol* 1994;23:633–636.

211. Yu JS, Goodwin D, Salonen D, et al. Complete dislocation of the knee: spectrum of associated soft tissue injuries depicted by MR imaging. *AJR Am J Roentgenol* 1995;164:135–139.

212. Fitzgerald SW, Remer EM, Friedman H, et al. MR evaluation of the anterior cruciate ligament. Value of supplementing sagittal images with coronal and axial images. *AJR Am J Roentgenol* 1993;160:1233–1237.

213. Haramati N, Storon RB, Cushin S, et al. Value of the coronal plane in MRI of internal derangement of the knee. *Skeletal Radiol* 1994;23:211–215.

214. Roychoudhury S, Fitzgerald SW, Sonin AH, et al. Using MR imaging to diagnose partial tears of the anterior cruciate ligament: value of axial images. *AJR Am J Roentgenol* 1997;168:1487–1491.

215. Tung GA, Davis LM, Wiggins ME, et al. Tears of the anterior cruciate ligament: primary and secondary signs at MR imaging. *Radiology* 1993;188:661–667.

216. Brandser EA, Riley MA, Berbaum KS, et al. MR imaging of anterior cruciate ligament injury: independent value of primary and secondary signs. *AJR Am J Roentgenol* 1996;167:121–126.

217. Brossmann J, Muhle C, Büll CC, et al. Evaluation of patellar tracking in patients with suspected patellar malalignment: cine MR imaging vs arthroscopy. *AJR Am J Roentgenol* 1994;162:361–367.

218. Gambari PI, Giuliani G, Poppi M, et al. Ganglion cysts of the peroneal nerve at the knee: CT and surgical correlation. *J Comput Assist Tomogr* 1990;14:801–803.

219. Murphy BJ, Hichtman KS, Uribe JW, et al. Iliotibial band friction syndrome: MR image findings. *Radiology* 1992;185:569–571.

220. Snearly WN, Kaplan PA, Dussalt RG. Lateral-compartment bone contusions in adolescents with intact anterior cruciate ligaments. *Radiology* 1996;198:205–208.

221. Yao L, Gentili A, Petrus L, et al. Partial ACL rupture: an MR diagnosis? *Skeletal Radiol* 1995;24:247–251.

222. Lee SH, Petersilge CA, Trudell DJ, et al. Extrasynovial spaces of the cruciate ligaments: anatomy, MR imaging and diagnostic implications. *AJR Am J Roentgenol* 1996;166:1433–1437.

223. Kaplan PA, Walker CW, Kilcoyne RF, et al. Occult fracture patterns of the knee associated with anterior cruciate ligament tears. Assessment with MR imaging. *Radiology* 1992;183:835–838.

224. Vahey TN, Broome DR, Kayes KJ, et al. Acute and chronic tears of the anterior cruciate ligament. Differential features of MR imaging. *Radiology* 1991;181:251–253.

225. Vahey TN, Hunt JE, Shelbourne KD. Anterior translocation of the tibia at MR imaging: a secondary sign of anterior cruciate ligament tear. *Radiology* 1993;187:817–819.

226. McCauley TR, Moses M, Kier R, et al. MR diagnosis of tears of anterior cruciate ligament of the knee: importance of ancillary findings. *AJR Am J Roentgenol* 1994;162:115–119.

227. Stallenberg B, Gevenois PA, Surtzaff SA, et al. Fractures of the posterior aspect of the lateral tibial plateau: radiographic sign of anterior cruciate ligament tear. *Radiology* 1993;187:821–825.

228. Berger PE, Ofstein RA, Jackson DW, et al. MRI demonstration of radiographically occult fractures: what have we been missing? *RadioGraphics* 1989;9:407–436.

229. Yu JS, Salonen DC, Hodler J, et al. Posterolateral aspect of the knee: improved MR imaging with a coronal oblique technique. *Radiology* 1996;198:199–204.

230. Yao L, Dungan D, Seeger LL. MR imaging of tibial collateral ligament injury: comparison with clinical examination. *Skeletal Radiol* 1994;23:521–524.

231. Schweitzer ME, Tran D, Deely DM, et al. Medial collateral ligament injuries: evaluation of multiple signs, prevalence and location of associated bone bruises and assessment with MR imaging. *Radiology* 1995;194:825–829.

232. Beltran J, Caudill JL, Herman LA, et al. Rheumatoid arthritis: MR imaging manifestations. *Radiology* 1987;165:153–157.

233. Kannus PA. Long patellar tendon: radiographic sign of patellofemoral pain syndrome—a prospective study. *Radiology* 1992;185:859–863.

234. Schweitzer ME, Mitchell DG, Ehrlch SM. The patellar tendon: thickening, internal signal buckling and other MR variants. *Skeletal Radiol* 1993;22:411–416.

235. Starok M, Lenschik L, Trudell D, et al. Normal patellar retinaculum: MR and sonographic imaging with cadaveric correlation. *AJR Am J Roentgenol* 1997;168:1493–1499.

236. Yu JS, Petersilge C, Sartoris DJ, et al. MR imaging of injuries of the extensor mechanism. *RadioGraphics* 1994;14:541–551.

237. Staeubli H-U, Bollmann C, Kreutz R, et al. Quantification of intact quadriceps tendon, quadriceps tendon insertion and

suprapatellar fat pad: MR arthrography, anatomy and cryosections in the sagittal plane. *AJR Am J Roentgenol* 1999;173: 691–698.

238. Yu JS, Popp JE, Kalding CC, et al. Correlation of MR imaging and pathologic findings in athletes undergoing surgery for chronic patellar tendinitis. *AJR Am J Roentgenol* 1995;165:115–118.

239. Deutsch AL, Shellock FG. The ext. Neck and PF joint. In: Mink JH, Reicher MA, Crues JV III et al., eds. *MRI of the knee*, 2nd ed. New York: Raven Press, 1993:189–236.

240. Scranton PE, Farrar EL. Mucoid degeneration of the patellar ligament in athletes. *J Bone Joint Surg Am* 1992;74A:435–439.

241. Kannus P, Józsa L. Histopathologic changes preceding spontaneous rupture of a tendon. *J Bone Joint Surg Am* 1991;73A:1507–1525.

242. Zeiss J, Saddemi SR, Ebraheim NA. MR imaging of the quadriceps tendon: normal layered configuration and its importance in cases of tendon rupture. *AJR Am J Roentgenol* 1992;159:1031–1034.

243. Allen GM, Tauro PG, Ostlere SJ. Proximal patellar tendinosis and abnormalities of patellar tracking. *Skeletal Radiol* 1999;28:220–223.

244. Bodne D, Quinn SF, Murray WT, et al. Magnetic resonance images of chronic patellar tendinitis. *Skeletal Radiol* 1988;17:24–28.

245. Chung CB, Skaf A, Roger B, et al. Patellar tendon-lateral femoral condyle friction syndrome: MR imaging in 42 patients. *Skeletal Radiol* 2001;30:694–697.

246. Donnelly LF, Bisset GS, Helms CA, et al. Chronic avulsive injuries of childhood. *Skeletal Radiol* 1999;28:138–144.

247. McLoughlin RF, Raber EL, Vellet AD, et al. Patellar tendinitis: MR imaging features with suggested pathogenesis and proposed classification. *Radiology* 1995;197:843–848.

248. Khan KM, Bonar F, Desmond PM, et al. Patellar tendinosis (Jumper's Knee): findings at histopathologic examination, US and MR imaging. *Radiology* 1996;200:821–827.

249. Kirsch MD, Fitzgerald SW, Friedman H, et al. Transient lateral patellar dislocation: diagnosis with MR imaging. *AJR Am J Roentgenol* 1993;161:109–113.

250. Daffner RH, Riemer BL, Lupetin AR, et al. Magnetic resonance imaging in acute tendon ruptures. *Skeletal Radiol* 1986;15:619–621.

251. Gould ES, Taylor S, Naidich JB, et al. MR appearance of bilateral, spontaneous patellar tendon rupture in systemic lupus erythematosus. *J Comput Assist Tomogr* 1987;11:1096–1097.

252. Frank CB, Jackson DW. The science of reconstruction of the anterior cruciate ligament. *J Bone Joint Surg Am* 1997;79A:1556–1576.

253. Jansson KA, Karjalainen PT, Harilainen A, et al. MRI of anterior cruciate ligament repair with patellar and hamstring tendon autografts. *Skeletal Radiol* 2001;30:8–14.

254. May DA, Snearly WN, Bents R, et al. MR imaging findings in anterior cruciate ligament reconstruction: evaluation of notchplasty. *AJR Am J Roentgenol* 1997;169:217–222.

255. Rak KM, Gillogly SD, Schaefer RA, et al. Anterior cruciate reconstruction: evaluation with MR imaging. *Radiology* 1991;178: 553–556.

256. Recht MP, Piraino DW, Applegate G, et al. Complications after anterior cruciate ligament reconstruction: radiographic and MR findings. *AJR Am J Roentgenol* 1996;167:705–710.

257. Schatz JA, Potter HG, Rodes, et al. MR imaging of anterior cruciate ligament reconstruction. *AJR Am J Roentgenol* 1997;169: 223–228.

258. Orchard JW, Fricher PA, Abud AT, et al. Biomechanics of iliotibial band friction syndrome in runners. *Am J Sports Med* 1996;24: 375–379.

259. Howell SM, Berns GS, Farley TE. Unimpinged and impinged anterior cruciate ligament grafts: MR signal intensity measurements. *Radiology* 1991;197:639–643.

260. Howell SM, Taylor MA. Failure of reconstruction of the anterior cruciate ligament due to impingement by the intercondylar roof. *J Bone Joint Surg Am* 1993;75A:1044–1055.

261. Edwards PH, Grana WA. Anterior cruciate ligament reconstruction in the immature athlete: long-term results of intra-articular reconstruction. *Am J Knee Surg* 2001;14:232–237.

262. Fayad LM, Parellada JA, Parker L, et al. MR Imaging of anterior curiciate ligament tears: is there a gender gap? *Skeletal Radiol* 2003;32:639–646.

263. Papakonstantinov O, Chung CB, Chanchairujira K, et al. Complications of anterior curiciate ligament reconstruction: MR Imaging. *Eur Radiol* 2003;13:1106–1117.

264. Huang GS, Lee CH, Chan WP, et al. Acute anterior cruciate ligament stump entrapment in anterior cruciate ligament tears: MR imaging appearance. *Radiology* 2002;225:537–540.

265. Garcia-Valtuillo R, Abascal F, Cerezal L, et al. Anatomy and MR imaging appearances of synovial plicae of the knee. *Radio Graphics* 2002;22:775–784.

266. Johnson DP, Eastwood DM, Witherow PJ. Symptomatic synovial plicae of the knee. *J Bone Joint Surg Am* 1993;75A:1485–1495.

267. Hardaker WT, Whipple TL, Bassett FH III. Diagnosis and treatment of plicae syndrome of the knee. *J Bone Joint Surg Am* 1980; 62A:221–225.

268. Patel D. Arthroscopy of the plicae—synovial folds and their significance. *Am J Sports Med* 1978;6:217–225.

269. Korasek FJ, Helms CA. The MR appearance of the infrapatellar plica. *AJR Am J Roentgenol* 1999;172:481–484.

270. Fielding JR, Franklin PD, Kustan J. Popliteal cysts: a reassessment using magnetic resonance imaging. *Skeletal Radiol* 1991;20: 433–435.

271. Brossman J, Muhle C, Schröder C, et al. Patellar tracking patterns during active and passive knee extension: evaluation with motion-triggered MR imaging. *Radiology* 1993;187:205–212.

272. Brown TR, Quinn SF. Evaluation of chondromalacia of the patellofemoral compartment with axial magnetic resonance imaging. *Skeletal Radiol* 1993;22:325–328.

273. Koskinen SK, Taimela S, Nilimarkka O, et al. Magnetic resonance imaging of patellofemoral relationships. *Skeletal Radiol* 1993;22: 403–410.

274. Virolainen H, Visuri T, Kunsela T. Acute dislocation of the patella: MR findings. *Radiology* 1993;189:243–246.

275. Lugo-Olivieri CH, Scott WW, Zerkouni EA. Fluid-fluid levels in injured knees: do they always represent lipohemarthrosis. *Radiology* 1996;198:499–502.

276. Van Leersum MD, Schweitzer ME, Gannon F, et al. Thickness of patellofemoral articular cartilage as measured on MR imaging: sequence comparison of accuracy, reproducibility, and interobserver variation. *Skeletal Radiol* 1995;24:431–435.

277. Ficat RP, Hungerford DS. *Disorders of the patellofemoral joint.* Baltimore, MD: Williams & Wilkins, 1977.

278. Miller TT, Staron RB, Feldman F. Patellar height on sagittal MR imaging of the knee. *AJR Am J Roentgenol* 1996;167:339–341.

279. Milter PR, Klein RM, Teitge RA. Medial dislocation of the patella. *Skeletal Radiol* 1991;20:429–431.

280. McCauley TR, Kier R, Lynch KJ, et al. Chondromalacia patellae: diagnosis with MR imaging. *AJR Am J Roentgenol* 1992;158:101–105.

281. Rubinstein JD, Kim JK, Heukelman RM. Effects of compression and recovery of bovine articular cartilage: appearance on MR images. *Radiology* 1996;201:843–850.

282. Outerbridge RE. The etiology of chondromalacia patellae. *J Bone Joint Surg Br* 1961;43B:752–757.

283. Kujala UM, Osterman K, Kormano M, et al. Patellar motion analyzed by magnetic resonance imaging. *Acta Orthop Scand* 1989; 60:13–16.

284. Van Leersum MD, Schweitzer ME, Gannon F, et al. Chondromalacia patellae: an invitro study. Comparison of MR criteria with histologic and macroscopic findings. *Skeletal Radiol* 1996;25:727–732.

285. Kangarloo H, Dietrich RB, Taira RT, et al. MR imaging of bone marrow in children. *J Comput Assist Tomogr* 1986;10:205–209.

286. Rao VM, Mitchell DG, Rifkin MD, et al. Marrow infarction in sickle cell anemia: correlation with marrow type and distribution by MRI. *Magn Reson Imaging* 1989;7:39–44.

287. Gagliardi JA, Chung EM, Chandnani VP, et al. Detection and staging of chondromalacia patellae: relative efficacies of conventional MR imaging, MR arthrography and CT arthrography. *AJR Am J Roentgenol* 1994;163:629–636.

288. Recht MP, Kramer J, Marcelis S, et al. Abnormalities of articular cartilage of the knee: analysis of available MR techniques. *Radiology* 1993;187:473–478.

289. Shellock FG, Deutsch AL, Mink JH, et al. Do asymptomatic marathon runners have an increased prevalence of meniscal abnormality? MR study of the knee in 23 volunteers. *AJR Am J Roentgenol* 1991;157:1239–1241.

290. Shellock FG, Foo TKF, Deutsch AL, et al. Patellofemoral joint: evaluation during active flexion with ultra-fast spoiled GRASS MR imaging. *Radiology* 1991;180:581–585.

291. Shellock FG, Mink HJ, Deutsch AL, et al. Patellar tracking abnormalities: clinical experience with kinematic MR imaging in 130 patients. *Radiology* 1989;172:799–804.

292. Shellock FG, Mink JH, Deutsch AL, et al. Patellofemoral joint: identification of abnormalities with active-movement, "unloaded" versus "loaded" kinematic MR imaging techniques. *Radiology* 1993;188:575–578.

293. Shaliriare H. Chondromalacia. *Contemp Orthop* 1985;11:27–39.

294. Hughston JC. Subluxation of the patella. *J Bone Joint Surg Am* 1968;50A:1003–1026.

295. Elias DA, White LM, Eithian DC. Acute lateral patellar dislocation at MR imaging: injury patterns of medial patellar soft-tissue restraints and osteochondral injuries of the inferomedial patella. *Radiology* 2002;225:736–743.

296. Lance E, Deutsch AL, Mink JH. Prior lateral patellar dislocation: MR image findings. *Radiology* 1993;189:905–907.

297. DeSmet AA, Ilahi O, Graf BK. Reassessment of the MR criteria for stability of osteochondritis dissecans in the knee and ankle. *Skeletal Radiol* 1996;25:159–163.

298. Delzell PB, Schils JP, Recht MP. Subtle fractures about the knee: innocuous appearing yet indicative of internal derangement. *AJR Am J Roentgenol* 1996;167:699–703.

299. Bohndorf K. Imaging of acute injuries of the articular surfaces (chondral, osteochondral and subchondral fractures). *Skeletal Radiol* 1999;28:545–560.

300. White PG, Mah JY, Friedman L. Magnetic resonance imaging of acute physeal injuries. *Skeletal Radiol* 1994;23:627–631.

301. Handelberg F, Shahabpour M, Casteleyn PP. Chondral lesions of the patella evaluated by CT, MR and arthroscopy. *J Arthrosc* 1990;6:24–29.

302. Kapelov SR, Teresi LM, Bradley WG, et al. Bone contusions of the knee: increased lesion detection with fat saturation. *Radiology* 1993;189:901–904.

303. Lee JK, Yao L. Stress fractures: MR imaging. *Radiology* 1988;169:217–220.

304. Murphy BJ, Smith RL, Uribe JW, et al. Bone signal abnormalities in the posterolateral tibia and lateral femoral condyle in complete tears of the anterior cruciate ligament: a specific sign? *Radiology* 1992;182:221–224.

305. Newberg AH. Bone bruises of the knee: MR imaging patterns and clinical importance. In: Weissman BN, ed. *Categorical course in musculoskeletal imaging*. Chicago, Ill: Radiological Society of North America, 1993;219–224.

306. Seeger LL. MR imaging of the knee: Acute ligamentous and osseous injury: chronic trauma. Presented at the Society of Magnetic Resonance in Medicine, Amsterdam, 1989.

307. Yao L, Lee JK. Avulsion of the posteromedial tibial plateau by the semimembranosus tendon: diagnosis with MR imaging. *Radiology* 1989;172:513–514.

308. Yao L, Lee JK. Occult intraosseous fractures: detection with MR imaging. *Radiology* 1988;167:749–751.

309. Stafford SA, Rosenthal DI, Gebhardt MC, et al. MRI in stress fractures. *AJR Am J Roentgenol* 1986;147:553–556.

310. Yao L, Johnson C, Gentili A, et al. Stress injuries of bone. *Acad Radiol* 1998;5:34–40.

311. Reinus WR, Fischer KC, Ritter JH. Painful transient tibial edema. *Radiology* 1994;192:195–199.

312. Weber WN, Neumann CH, Barakos JA, et al. Lateral tibial rim (Segond) fractures: MR imaging characteristics. *Radiology* 1991;180:731–734.

313. Kode L, Lieberman JM, Motto AO, et al. Evaluation of tibial plateau fractures: efficacy of MR imaging compared with CT. *AJR Am J Roentgenol* 1994;163:141–147.

314. Barrow BA, Fagman WA, Parker LM, et al. Tibial plateau fractures: evaluation of MR imaging. *RadioGraphics* 1994;14:553–559.

315. Palmer WE, Levine SM, Dupuy DE. Knee and shoulder fractures: association of fracture detection and marrow edema on MR images with mechanism of injury. *Radiology* 1997;204:395–401.

316. Nelson DW, Pipaola J, Colville M, et al. Osteochondritis dissecans of the talus and knee: prospective comparison of MR and arthroscopic classifications. *J Comput Assist Tomogr* 1990;14:804–808.

317. Seiler JG, Christie MJ, Homra L. Correlation of the findings of magnetic resonance imaging with those of bone biopsy in patients who have stage I or II ischemic necrosis of the femoral head. *J Bone Joint Surg Am* 1989;71A:28–32.

318. Lotke PA, Ecker ML. Current concepts review. Osteonecrosis of the knee. *J Bone Joint Surg Am* 1988;70:470–473.

319. Vogler JB, Murphy WA. Bone marrow imaging. *Radiology* 1988;168:679–693.

320. Craig JC, Van Holsbeeck M, Zaltz I. The utility of MR in assessing Blount disease. *Skeletal Radiol* 2003;31:208–213.

321. Resnick D, Niwayama G. *Diagnosis of bone and joint disorders*, Vol. 5. Philadelphia, PA: WB Saunders, 1988:3289–3334.

322. Rosenberg ZS, Kavelblum M, Cheung YY, et al. Osgood-Schlatter lesion: fracture or tendinitis? Scintigraphic, CT and MR imaging features. *Radiology* 1992;185:853–858.

323. Unni KK. *Dahlin's bone tumors. General aspects and data on 11,087 cases*, 5th ed. Philadelphia, PA: Lippincott–Raven, 1996.

324. Dahlin DC, Unni KK. *Bone tumors: general aspects and data on 8,542 cases*, 4th ed. Springfield, IL: Charles C. Thomas Publisher, 1986.

325. Kransdorf MJ, Moser RP, Vinh TN, et al. Primary tumors of the patella. *Skeletal Radiol* 1989;18:365–371.

326. Weiss SW, Goldblum JR. *Enzinger and weiss soft tissue tumors*, 4th ed. St. Louis, MO: Mosby, 2001.

327. Butler MG, Fuchigami KD, Chako A. MRI of posterior knee masses. *Skeletal Radiol* 1996;25:309–317.

328. Miller TT, Staron RB, Koenigsberg T, et al. MR imaging of Baker's cysts: association with internal derangement, effusion, and degenerative arthropathy. *Radiology* 1996;201:247–250.

329. Ryu KN, Jaovisidha S, Schweitzer M, et al. MR imaging of lipoma arborescenes of the knee joint. *AJR Am J Roentgenol* 1996;167:1229–1232.

330. Vilanova JC, Barcelo J, Villalon M, et al. MR imaging of lipoma aborescens and the associated lesions. *Skeletal Radiol* 2003;32:504–509.

331. Bui-Mansfield LT, Youngberg RA. Intra-articular ganglia of the knee: prevalence, presentation, etiology and management. *AJR Am J Roentgenol* 1997;168:123–127.

332. Anouchi YS, Parker RD, Seitz WH Jr. Posterior compartment syndrome of the calf resulting from misdiagnosis of a rupture of the medial head of the gastrocnemius. *J Trauma* 1987;27:678–680.

333. Ilahi OA, Younas SA, Labbe MR, et al. Prevalence of ganglion cysts originating from the proximal tibiofibular joint: a magnetic resonance imaging study. *Arthroscopy* 2003;19:150–153.

334. McIntyre J, Moelleken S, Tirman P. Mucoid degeneration of the anterior cruciate ligament mistaken for ligamentous tears. *Skeletal Radiol* 2001;30:312–315.

335. Bianchi S, Abelwahal IF, Kenan S, et al. Intramuscular ganglia arising from the superior tibiofibular joint: CT and MR evaluation. *Skeletal Radiol* 1995;24:253–256.

336. Bianchi S, Zwass A, Abdelwakah IF, et al. Diagnosis of tears of the quadriceps tendon of the knee. Value of sonography. *AJR Am J Roentgenol* 1994;162:1137–1140.

337. Sutro CT. Intraneural ganglion of the common peroneal nerve. *Bull Hosp Joint Dis* 1960;21:330–331.

338. Milgrom C, Sigal R, Robin GC, et al. MRI and CT scan compared with microscopic histopathology in osteogenic sarcoma of the proximal tibia. *Orthop Rev* 1986;15:165–169.

339. Nagamine R, Miura H, Inoue Y, et al. Malposition of the tibial tubercle during flexion in knees with patellofemoral arthritis. *Skeletal Radiol* 1997;26:597–601.

340. Nolte-Ernsting CCA, Adam G, Buhne M, et al. MRI of degenerative bone marrow lesions in experimental osteoarthritis of canine knee joints. *Skeletal Radiol* 1996;25:413–420.

341. Yamato M, Tamai K, Yamaguchi T, et al. MRI of the knee in rheumatoid arthritis: Gd-DTPA perfusion dynamics. *J Comput Assist Tomogr* 1993;17:781–785.

342. Dunn TC, Lu Y, Jin H, et al. T2 relaxation time of cartilage at MR imaging: comparison with severity of knee osteoarthritis. *Radiology* 2004;232:592–598.

343. Idy-Peretti I, Yvart J, LeBalch T. MRI of the knee: assessment and follow-up of hemophilic arthropathy. Presented at the Society of Magnetic Resonance in Medicine, Amsterdam, 1989.

344. Jacobson JA, Lenchik L, Ruboy MK, et al. MR imaging of the infrapatellar fat pad of Hoffa. *RadioGraphics* 1997;17:675–691.

345. Johnson K, Wittkop B, Haigh F, et al. The early magnetic resonance imaging features of the knee in juvenile idiopathic arthritis. *Clin Radiol* 2002;57:466–471.

346. Kulkarni MV, Droolshagen LF, Kaye JJ, et al. MR imaging of hemophiliac arthropathy. *J Comput Assist Tomogr* 1988;10:445–449.

347. Yulish BS, Lieberman JM, Newman AJ, et al. Juvenile rheumatoid arthritis: assessment of MR imaging. *Radiology* 1987;165:149–152.

348. Schweitzer ME, Falk A, Pathria M, et al. MR imaging of the knee: can changes in the intracapsular fat pads be used as a sign of synovial proliferation in the presence of an effusion? *AJR Am J Roentgenol* 1993;160:823–826.

349. Singson RD, Zalduondo FM. Value of unenhanced spin-echo MR imaging in distinguishing between synovitis and effusion of the knee. *AJR Am J Roentgenol* 1992;159:569–571.

350. Anderson SE, Bosshard C, Steinbach LS, et al. MR imaging of calcification of the lateral collateral ligament of the knee: a rare abnormality and a cause of lateral knee pain. *AJR Am J Roentgenol* 2003;181:199–202.

351. Abreu M, Johnson K, Chung CB, et al. Calcification in calcium pyrophosphate dihydrate (CPPD) crystalline deposits in the knee: Anatomic, radiographic, MR imaging and histologic study in cadavers. *Skeletal Radiol* 2004;33:392–398.

352. Huang GS, Lee CH, Chan WP, et al. Localized nodular synovitis of the knee: MR imaging appearance and clinical correlation in 21 patients. *AJR Am J Roentgenol* 2003;181:539–543.

353. Jelinek JS, Kransdorf MJ, Utz JA, et al. Imaging of pigmented villonodular synovitis with emphasis on MR imaging. *AJR Am J Roentgenol* 1989;152:337–342.

354. Spritzer CE, Dalinka MK, Kressel HY. Magnetic resonance imaging of pigmented villonodular synovitis: a report of two cases. *Skeletal Radiol* 1987;16:316–319.

355. Williamson MP, Humm G, Crisp AJ. [1]H nuclear magnetic resonance investigation of synovial fluid components in osteoarthritis, rheumatoid arthritis and traumatic effusions. *Br J Rheumatol* 1989;28:23–27.

356. Hennigan SP, Schneck CD, Mesgarzadeh M, et al. The semimembranosus-tibial collateral ligament bursa. *J Bone Joint Surg Am* 1994;76A:1322–1327.

357. Forbes JR, Helms CA, Janzen DL. Acute pes anserine bursitis: MR imaging. *Radiology* 1995;194:525–527.

358. Nishimura G, Yamamoto M, Tamai K, et al. MR findings of iliotibial band syndrome. *Skeletal Radiol* 1997;26:533–537.

359. Puig S, Dupuy DE, Sarmiento A, et al. Articular muscle of the knee: a muscle seldom recognized on MR imaging. *AJR Am J Roentgenol* 1996;166:1057–1060.

360. Brown TR, Quinn SF, Wensel JP, et al. Diagnosis of popliteus injuries with MR imaging. *Skeletal Radiol* 1995;24:511–514.

361. Elias DA, White LM, Rubenstein JD, et al. Clinical evaluation and MR imaging features of popliteal artery entrapment and cystic adventitial disease. *AJR Am J Roentgenol* 2003;180:627–632.

362. Macedo TA, Johnson M, Hallett JW, et al. Popliteal artery entrapment syndrome: role of imaging in the diagnosis. *AJR Am J Roentgenol* 2003;181:1259–1265.

363. Wright LB, Matchett WJ, Cruz CP, et al. Popliteal artery disease: diagnosis and treatment. *RadioGraphics* 2004;24:467–479.

Foot, Ankle, and Calf

8

Thomas H. Berquist

Proper application of imaging procedures is essential to obtain needed information for diagnosis and therapy on patients with suspected calf, foot, and ankle pathology (1–10). Standard radiographic views that include anteroposterior and lateral standing and oblique views are essential and provide adequate screening for most skeletal abnormalities. Special views, such as fluoroscopically positioned spot films, are also useful because of the complex osseous anatomy of the foot and ankle. Radionuclide studies are valuable for detecting subtle skeletal lesions (11–14). Computed tomography (CT) has provided valuable information regarding both osseous and soft tissue pathology in the calf, foot, and ankle. Ultrasound can be utilized to differentiate superficial soft tissue lesions and study abnormalities in certain tendons, especially the Achilles tendon (5,15,16). More invasive procedures such as arthrography, tenography, and angiography may also be required to evaluate the ligaments, tendons, and vascular structures (4,5).

Applications for magnetic resonance imaging (MRI) of the foot and ankle disorders have expanded dramatically in the last decade (17). MRI is particularly suited to evaluation of the complex bone and soft tissue anatomy of the foot, ankle, and calf because of its superior soft tissue contrast and the ability to image in multiple planes. In addition, new fast scan techniques provide improved efficiency and allow motion studies to be performed. Magnetic resonance (MR) arthrography and angiographic techniques have improved significantly in recent years, resulting in more routine use of these techniques (18,19).

TECHNIQUES

Bone and soft tissue anatomy is complex in the foot and ankle. Axial, coronal, or sagittal images adequately demonstrate the anatomy in most clinical settings. However, positioning of the foot must be carefully accomplished so the anatomy is not distorted. In some situations, off-axis oblique images may be required to optimally demonstrate anatomy (5,20–24).

Patient Positioning and Coil Selection

The patient should be studied with a closely coupled coil to achieve optimal signal-to-noise ratios and spatial resolution.(2,4,5,17,25–29) Conventional surface coils take several configurations—flat, partial volume, or circumferential (see Fig. 8-1). Different coils are suited to certain types of examinations. Generally, flat or circumferential volume coils are used for examination of the foot and ankle. In certain cases, if comparison is needed, either dual coupled coils or the head coil can be used to reduce examination time (5,26,30). The extremity coil can be used to evaluate the calf.

Patients can be examined in the supine or prone position, depending on which anatomic region is being studied (5,30,31). The prone position is useful for examination of the mid- and forefoot and assists in reducing inadvertent motion (5,30). Forefoot pathology, such as Morton neuroma, is more clearly displayed in this position (32). The prone position is also optimal for evaluating the posterior soft tissues of the calf. This avoids soft tissue compression that can distort the anatomy. However, the hindfoot soft tissues can be distorted when the patient is prone due to excessive plantar flexion of the foot (see Fig. 8-2). For example, we prefer the supine position for patients with suspected Achilles tendon pathology. In this setting, it is best to have the patient supine with the foot in neutral position so that the tendons are not collapsed or buckled, which occurs when the patient is prone or the foot is in the plantar-flexed position (Fig. 8-2B). In some cases, dorsiflexion or plantar flexion may be required to evaluate fully the origin and/or insertion of the Achilles and other tendons about the ankle (5,30). Image quality may be improved by using more numerous (smaller degrees of plantar and dorsiflexion) positions. Farooki et al. (33) used a positioning device to evaluate optimal positions for imaging the ankle tendons and ligaments. The peroneal tendons, extensor digitorum longus, and extensor hallucis longus were optimally imaged with the foot in 20° of plantar flexion and 20° of inversion. The calcaneofibular and anterior talofibular ligaments were optimally imaged with the foot in 20° of plantar flexion.

The foot and ankle should be supported with foam sponges and straps to prevent motion artifact when motion studies are not being performed. Motion studies are usually performed using flat or coupled coils (5,30).

Image Planes

Coronal, axial, and sagittal image planes are commonly used for foot and ankle examination. In the foot, coronal images are perpendicular to the metatarsals and axial images in the plane of the metatarsals (5,17,30,31). To achieve patient comfort and to optimize image planes, oblique planes are frequently used in the foot and ankle (5,17,34,35). We generally use a minimum of two image planes at 90° angles to evaluate foot and ankle disorders. Figure 8-3

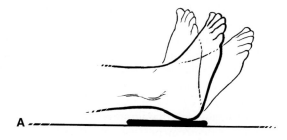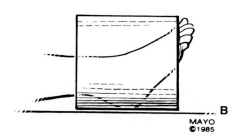

Figure 8-1 Patient positioned for examination of the foot and ankle using flat (**A**) and circumferential (**B**) coils. The former allows more flexibility with positioning and motion studies. The circumferential coil provides more uniform signal intensity but reduces positioning options.

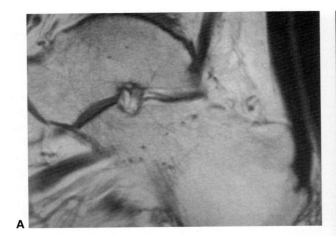

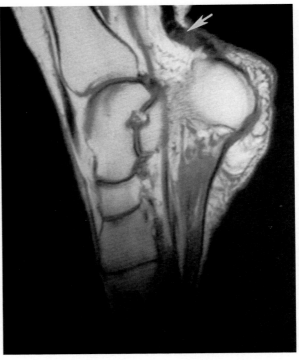

Figure 8-2 Sagittal T1-weighted MR images of the ankle with the foot in neutral **(A)** and plantar flexed (prone) **(B)** positions. Note the buckling, partial volume effects of the Achilles tendon (*arrow*), and rotation of the calcaneus in **B**.

gives examples of commonly used image planes and patient positions (5,33,35).

Pulse Sequences and Imaging Parameters

Spin-echo sequences (see Fig. 8-4) using short echo time (TE), repetition time (TR) (T1-weighted), and long TE and TR (T2-weighted) provide the necessary information for diagnosis and evaluation of most calf, foot, and ankle disorders (Table 8-1) (2,5,27,30,36). Today, proton density and T2-weighted fast spin-echo (FSE) sequences with or without fat suppression have replaced conventional spin-echo sequences in most situations. We generally perform at least two pulse sequences in at least two image planes (see Figs. 8-4 to 8-10). For example, when evaluating the ankle, T2-weighted axial images along with T1- and T2 -weighted sagittal images are usually adequate to identify and characterize pathology. Short TI inversion recovery (STIR) or T2* gradient-echo (GRE) sequences can be used in place of FSE T2-weighted images. We also add coronal dual echo steady state (DESS) images to evaluate the articular cartilage (Table 8-1). Similarly, in the foot two image planes are useful for detection and demonstrating the extent of pathology. In certain cases, special oblique images are necessary to evaluate the tendons, ligaments, and small osseous structures of the foot and ankle (5,17,30,33,35).

Additional parameters include a small field of view (FOV) (8 to 16 cm), 256 × 256 or 256 × 192 matrix, one

acquisition, and 2- to 4-mm slice thickness with 0.2- to 0.5-mm interslice gaps appear to be most useful for defining complex foot and ankle anatomy when surface coils are used. Thicker sections may be used for screening the soft tissues in the leg (Table 8-1). We initially obtain a scout view in the plane best suited to select our initial examining sequences. The sagittal or axial plane is most often used for the scout view for the foot and ankle. A coronal scout is most often used for establishing sequences for the calf. The matrix can be reduced to 256 × 128, which allows the scout image to be obtained in approximately 26 seconds using short TE/TR sequences (see Chapter 3 and Table 8-1). Most examinations of the calf or foot and ankle can be performed with imaging times of less than 30 minutes (5,17,37,38).

Three-dimensional GRE sequences are useful for reformatting in different image planes and for evaluation of bony trabeculae (5,25). Intravenous gadolinium is frequently added to the examination, especially in patients with suspected infection, inflammatory arthropathies, or neoplasm. Intravenous gadolinium does provide an arthrographic effect by 15 to 30 minutes after injection (Fig. 8-5) (39). We do not commonly perform MR arthrography, tenography, or bursography in the foot and ankle (40).

MR angiography has improved using new techniques with contrast enhancement. Distal digital arteries can be identified using contrast-enhanced three-dimensional angiography (19). Therefore, this approach is of value in patients with diabetes mellitus or peripheral vascular disease (18,19).

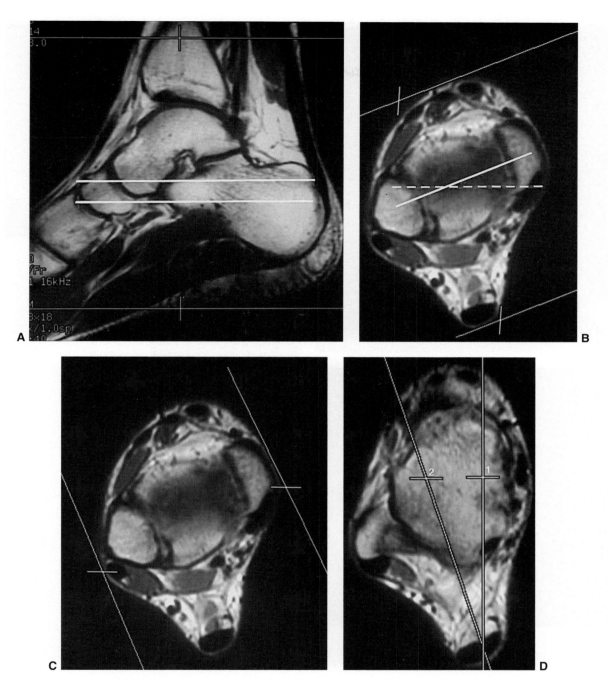

Figure 8-3 Image planes for foot and ankle MRI. **A:** Foot positioned for axial images of the ankles; *upper* and *lower lines* mark the area of coverage. Note the Achilles tendon and neutral position of the foot. With axial images, the tarsal bones (*white lines*) are sectioned out of anatomic alignment. **B:** Image planes obliqued to obtain true coronal images through the ankle mortise. The *white line* indicates planes of sections through the mortise. A conventional coronal plane (*dotted line*) would cut obliquely through the joint and anatomy. **C:** Oblique sagittal image planes to improve anatomic display of the osseous structures in the ankle. **D:** Conventional sagittal image plane (*1*) and obliqued sagittal plane (*2*) to improve evaluation of the Achilles tendon. **E:** Obliqued axial image planes to improve evaluation of the peroneal tendon. **F:** Scout sagittal image of the mid and forefoot, with the area scanned for images in the planes of the distal tarsal bones and metatarsals (*white line* indicates the image plane). **G:** Scout sagittal image for imaging perpendicular to the distal tarsal row and metatarsals (*white lines* indicate image sections). **H:** Axial forefoot scout demonstrating oblique planes (*lines*) for sagittal images of the first and second metatarsals.

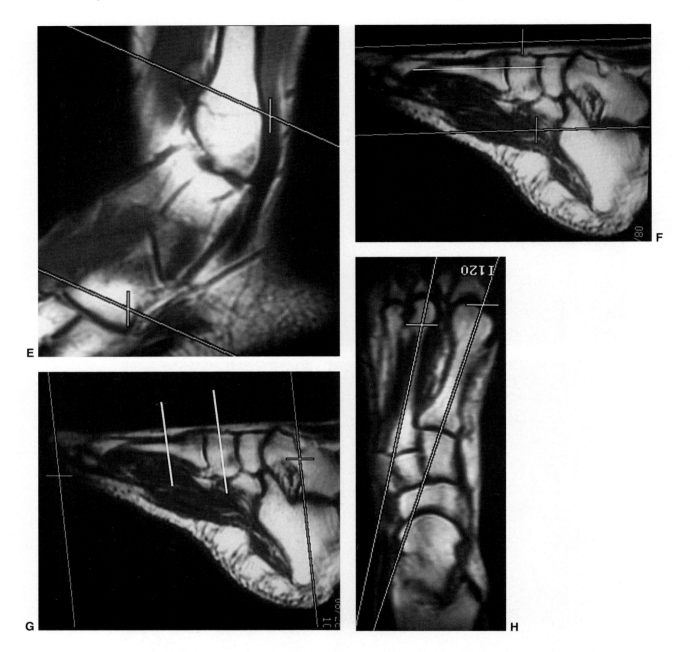

Figure 8-3 (continued)

The above general approaches can be applied to adults and children. Children younger than 5 years of age may require sedation. For this purpose, chloral hydrate is most often employed (5,9,41,42) (see Chapter 3).

Selected techniques and pulse sequences will be defined more completely later as they apply to specific clinical indications.

ANATOMY

MRI provides more diagnostic information than conventional techniques owing to improved tissue contrast and the ability to obtain multiple image planes. Therefore, a thorough knowledge of skeletal and soft tissue anatomy is even more essential than with other imaging techniques. Mastering the anatomy and biomechanics of the calf, foot, and ankle is important for evaluating MR images (Figs. 8-6 to 8-10).

Skeletal and Articular Anatomy

The ankle is composed of three osseous structures: the tibia, fibula, and talus (see Fig. 8-11) (43–46). The triangular diaphysis of the tibia, with its three surfaces (anterior, medial, and posterior), expands at the metaphysis forming the medial malleolus and the articular surface for the talus (Fig. 8-7). The articular surfaces are covered by

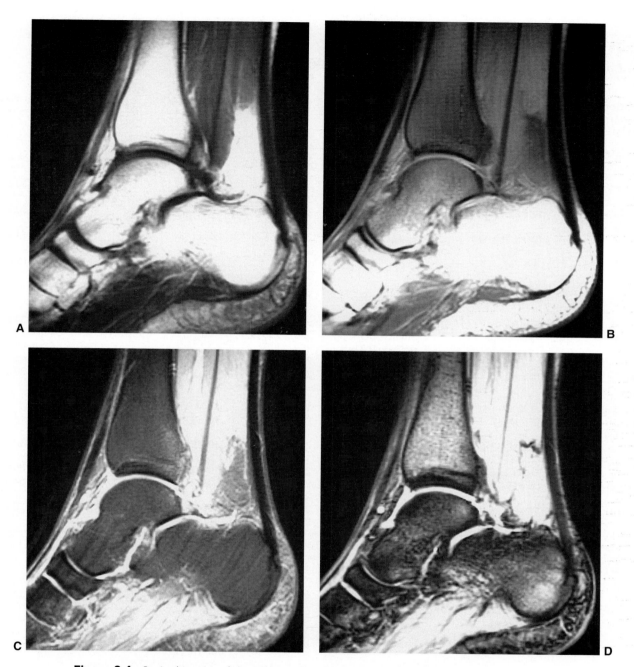

Figure 8-4 Sagittal images of the ankle and hindfoot. **A:** T1-weighted image demonstrating the high signal intensity of bone marrow and fat. Muscle is intermediate intensity and the Achilles tendon low intensity (*black*). **B:** T2-weighted fast spin-echo image with fat suppression. Note the uneven suppression with high intensity remaining in the calcaneus, certain tarsal bones, and the subcutaneous fat of the heel. Non-uniform fat suppression is not unusual in daily clinical practice. **C:** STIR sequence with low intensity in marrow and fat. Muscle signal intensity is higher than fat. The tendons remain dark. **D:** Gradient-echo sequence (700/31, flip angle 25°) shows muscle and joint fluid are higher intensity and muscle less easily separated from fat. Tendons and cortical bone remain dark or low in signal intensity.

hyaline cartilage except in the most posterior aspect of the tibia. The anterior tibia is typically smooth except for a rough anterior margin for the attachment of the anterior capsule. Posteriorly the tibia contains grooves for the flexor hallucis longus, flexor digitorum longus, and tibialis posterior tendons (Fig. 8-6) (22,44,47). Posterolaterally the

tibia articulates with the fibula and is supported by the interosseous membrane and anterior and posterior distal tibiofibular ligaments (Fig. 8-5) (5,44–49).

Supporting structures of the ankle are sometimes difficult to demonstrate with MRI, even when using off-axis oblique planes (Figs. 8-6 to 8-10) (5,35,50). These supporting

TABLE 8-1

MR EXAMINATIONS OF THE CALF, FOOT, AND ANKLE

Location	Pulse Sequence	Slice Thickness	Matrix	Field of View (FOV)	Acquisitions (NEX)	Image Time
Calf[a]						
Scout coronal	SE 200/11–20	Three 1-cm-thick	128 × 256	24–32 cm	1	26 s
Axial	SE 450/17	5 mm/skip 0.5 mm	256 × 256 or 256 × 192	24–32 cm	1	3 min 54 s
Axial	FS FSE T2 4,000/93	5 mm/skip 0.5 mm	256 × 256 or 256 × 192	24–32 cm	2	5 min 30 s
Coronal or sagittal	FS FSE T2 4,000/93	5 mm/skip 0.5 mm	256 × 256 or 256 × 192	24–32 cm	2	5 min 30 s
Or STIR	5,680/109/165	5 mm/skip 0.5 mm	256 × 256 or 256 × 192	24–32 cm	2	4 min 34 s
					Total =	19 min 14 s
Ankle						
Scout axial or sagittal	SE 200/11-20	Three 1-cm-thick	128 × 256	16–20 cm	1	26 s
Sagittal	SE 450/17	3.5 mm/skip 0.5 mm	512 × 512	12 cm	1	3 min 54 s
Sagittal	FSE PD 2,500/15	3.5 mm/skip 0.5 mm	256 × 256	12 cm	1	4 min 22 s
Coronal	DESS 23.35/7.7	1 mm/skip 0.2 mm	256 × 256	12 cm	1	6 min 00 s
Axial	FSE PD 3,170/19	3.5 mm/skip 0.5 mm	256 × 256	10 cm	2	4 min 44 s
Axial	FSE T2 4,000/93	3.5 mm/skip 0.5 mm	256 × 256	10 cm	2	5 min 30 s
Foot						
Scout sagittal	SE 200/11-20	Three 1-cm-thick	128 × 256	8–16 cm	1	26 s
Oblique axial[b] coronal	SE 450/17	3 mm/skip 0.5 mm	256 × 256 or 192 × 256	10–12 cm	1	3 min 54 s
Oblique axial[b] coronal	FS FSE T2 4,000/93	3 mm/skip 0.5 mm	256 × 256 or 192 × 256	10–12 cm	2	5 min 30 s
Oblique coronal	DESS 23.5/7.7	1 mm/skip 0.2 mm	256 × 256	10–12 cm	1	6 min 00 s
Sagittal	SE 450/17	3 mm/skip 0.5 mm	256 × 256 or 256 × 192	10–12 cm	1	3 min 54 s
Sagittal	FS FSE T2 4,000/93	3 mm/skip 0.5 mm	256 × 256 or 256 × 192	10–12 cm	2	5 min 30 s

FS, fat suppression; FSE, fast spin-echo; PD, proton density; STIR, short TI inversion recovery; DESS, dual echo steady state
[a] The body, extremity, or head coil can be used depending on the area to be studied.
[b] Image plane perpendicular to the sagittal to obtain true cross-sections of the forefoot.

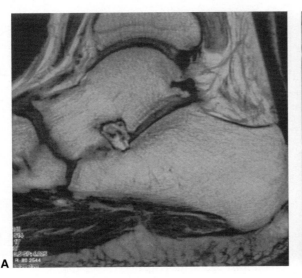
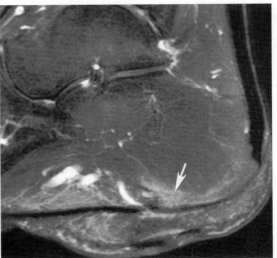

Figure 8-5   Pre- and postadministration of gadolinium intravenously. T1-weighted pre- **(A)** and post-gadolinium fat-suppressed T1-weighted image **(B)** demonstrating calcaneal enhancement due to osteomyelitis (*arrow*).

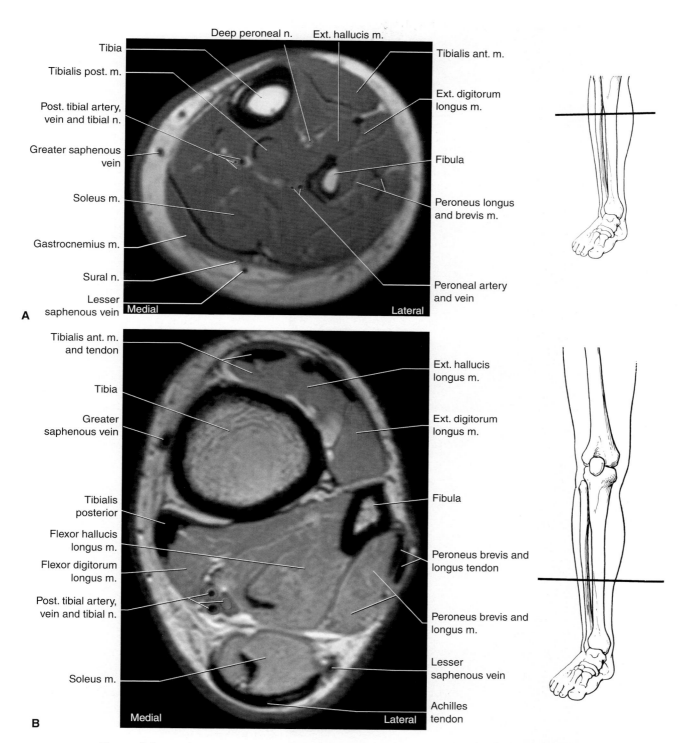

Figure 8-6   Axial T1-weighted images of the calf and ankle with level of section demonstrated. **A:** Axial image through the upper calf. **B:** Axial image through the lower calf. **C:** Axial image through the upper ankle. **D:** Axial image through the upper syndesmosis. **E:** Axial image through the lower syndesmosis. **F:** Axial image through the malleoli and talus. **G:** Axial image through the tarsal canal. **H:** Axial image through the calcaneocuboid articulation. **I:** Axial image through the plantar aspect of the foot.

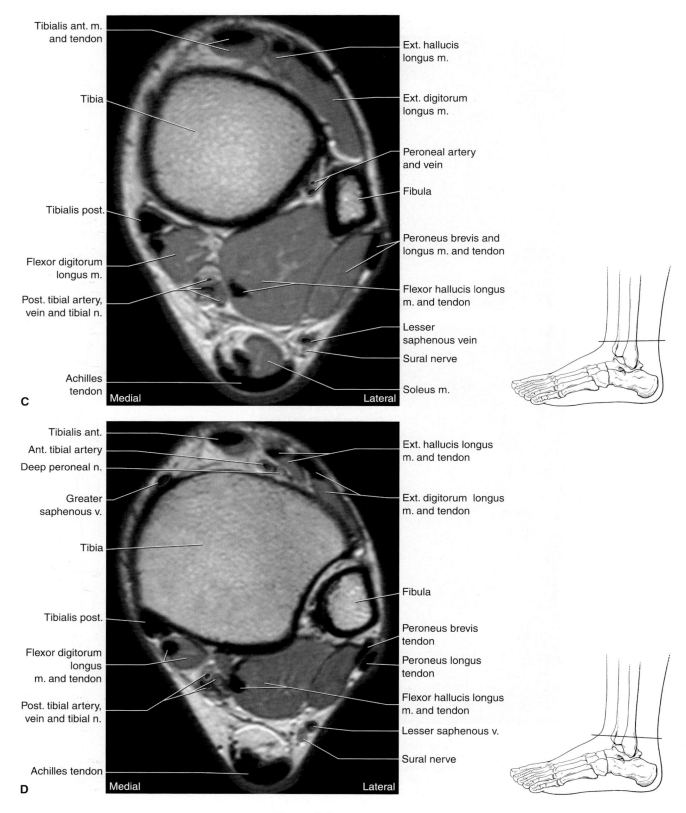

Tibialis ant. m. and tendon

Tibia

Tibialis post.

Flexor digitorum longus m.

Post. tibial artery, vein and tibial n.

Achilles tendon

Ext. hallucis longus m.

Ext. digitorum longus m.

Peroneal artery and vein

Fibula

Peroneus brevis and longus m. and tendon

Flexor hallucis longus m. and tendon

Lesser saphenous vein

Sural nerve

Soleus m.

Medial

Lateral

C

Tibialis ant.

Ant. tibial artery

Deep peroneal n.

Greater saphenous v.

Tibia

Tibialis post.

Flexor digitorum longus m. and tendon

Post. tibial artery, vein and tibial n.

Achilles tendon

Ext. hallucis longus m. and tendon

Ext. digitorum longus m. and tendon

Fibula

Peroneus brevis tendon

Peroneus longus tendon

Flexor hallucis longus m. and tendon

Lesser saphenous v.

Sural nerve

Medial

Lateral

D

Figure 8-6 *(continued)*

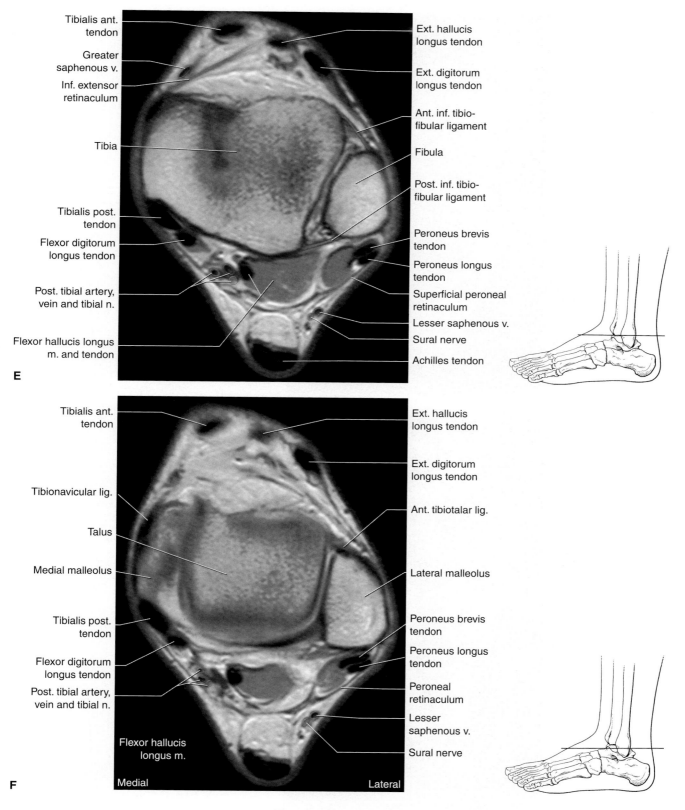

E

Tibialis ant. tendon
Greater saphenous v.
Inf. extensor retinaculum
Tibia
Tibialis post. tendon
Flexor digitorum longus tendon
Post. tibial artery, vein and tibial n.
Flexor hallucis longus m. and tendon

Ext. hallucis longus tendon
Ext. digitorum longus tendon
Ant. inf. tibio-fibular ligament
Fibula
Post. inf. tibio-fibular ligament
Peroneus brevis tendon
Peroneus longus tendon
Superficial peroneal retinaculum
Lesser saphenous v.
Sural nerve
Achilles tendon

F

Tibialis ant. tendon
Tibionavicular lig.
Talus
Medial malleolus
Tibialis post. tendon
Flexor digitorum longus tendon
Post. tibial artery, vein and tibial n.
Flexor hallucis longus m.
Medial

Ext. hallucis longus tendon
Ext. digitorum longus tendon
Ant. tibiotalar lig.
Lateral malleolus
Peroneus brevis tendon
Peroneus longus tendon
Peroneal retinaculum
Lesser saphenous v.
Sural nerve
Lateral

Figure 8-6 (*continued*)

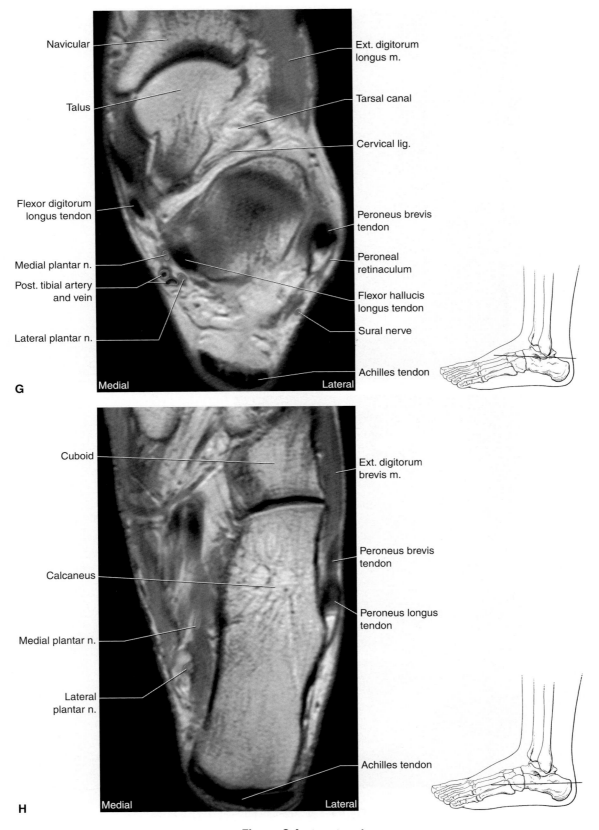

Navicular

Talus

Flexor digitorum
longus tendon

Medial plantar n.

Post. tibial artery
and vein

Lateral plantar n.

G   Medial   Lateral

Ext. digitorum
longus m.

Tarsal canal

Cervical lig.

Peroneus brevis
tendon

Peroneal
retinaculum

Flexor hallucis
longus tendon

Sural nerve

Achilles tendon

Cuboid

Calcaneus

Medial plantar n.

Lateral
plantar n.

H   Medial   Lateral

Ext. digitorum
brevis m.

Peroneus brevis
tendon

Peroneus longus
tendon

Achilles tendon

Figure 8-6   (*continued*)

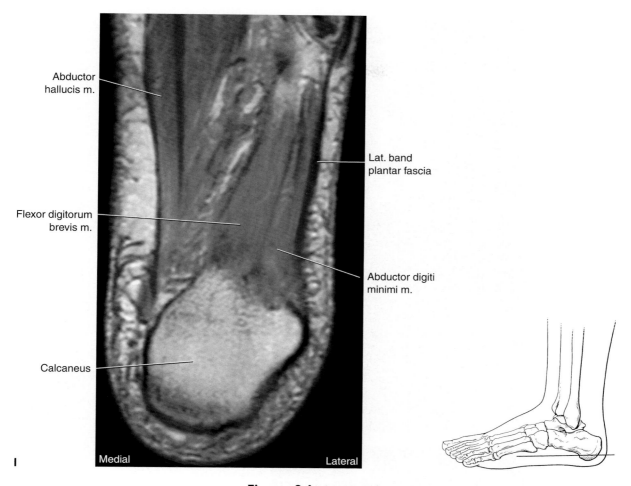

Abductor
hallucis m.

Lat. band
plantar fascia

Flexor digitorum
brevis m.

Abductor digiti
minimi m.

Calcaneus

Medial   Lateral

Figure 8-6 *(continued)*

structures include the joint capsule, medial and lateral liga-ments, and interosseous ligament (see Fig. 8-12). In addi-tion, 13 tendons cross the ankle, and there are four retinacula about the ankle (Fig. 8-6; see also Figs. 8-23 and 8-25). The interosseous ligament or membrane has obliquely oriented fibers and joins the tibia and fibula to its distal extent, which is just above the ankle joint. Projecting up between the distal tibia and fibula and below the interosseous ligaments, the syndesmotic recess is seen as an area of high signal intensity extending from the joint proper on MR images (Figs. 8-6 and 8-7). Just above the tibiotalar joint, the distal anterior and distal posterior tibiofibular ligaments provide addi-tional support as they attach to the tibia and fibula anteri-orly and posteriorly (Fig. 8-12). Just anterior to the posterior tibiofibular ligament is the transverse ligament, which makes up the fourth ligament of this syndesmotic group. This ligament lies anterior to the posterior tibiofibular liga-ment and extends from the lateral malleolus to the posterior articular margin of the tibia just lateral to the medial malle-olus (see Fig. 8-13) (5,22,27,44,46,47,51).

Medially, the deltoid ligament is a strong triangular group of fibrous tissue with its apex at the medial malleolus. As it passes caudally, the ligament fans out in a triangular

fashion and divides into superficial and deep fibers. Distal insertion of this ligament is the navicular tuberosity anteri-orly. The remaining fibers insert in the sustentaculum tali and talus (Fig. 8-12) (36,47). The spring ligament (plantar calcaneonavicular ligament) (Fig. 8-12C) is important for stabilizing the longitudinal arch. This complex structure is difficult to evaluate on MR images due to its complex multi-directional fibers. The spring ligament is important to evalu-ate in patients with posterior tibial dysfunction and will be discussed more completely later (27,44,46,47).

There are three ligaments in the lateral complex (Fig. 8-12, A and B) (47,52,53). The anterior talofibular ligament is the weakest and most frequently injured. It passes anteriorly from the fibula to insert on the anterior to the lateral talar articular facet. The posterior ligament is much stronger than the anterior and has a nearly transverse or horizontal course from the posterior aspect of the lateral malleolus to the pos-terior talar tubercle. The longest of the three ligaments is the calcaneofibular ligament, which takes a nearly vertical course from the lateral malleolus to the lateral surface of the calca-neus. The peroneal tendons lie just superficial to the calcane-ofibular ligament. Demonstration of all three of these ligaments is difficult on typical orthogonal MR images due to

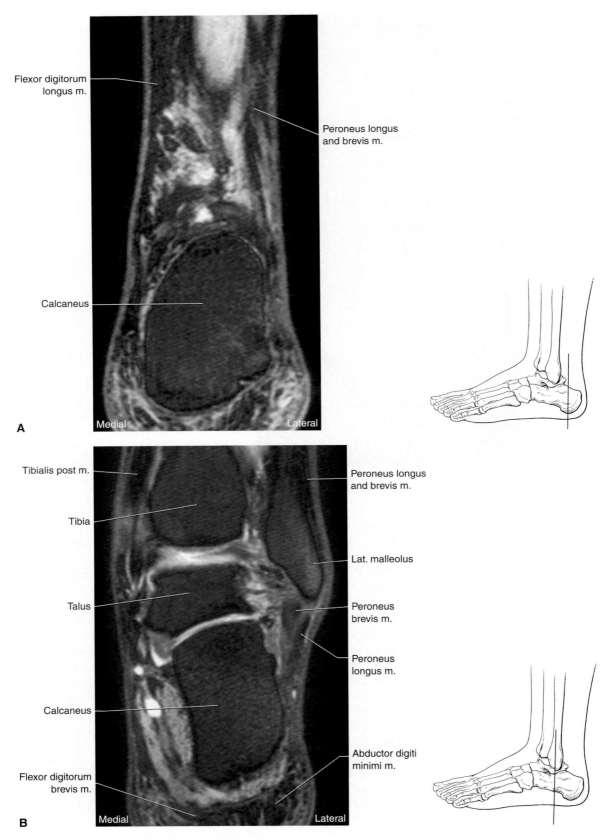

Figure 8-7 Coronal DESS images of the ankle and hindfoot from posterior to anterior with level of section demonstrated. **A:** Coronal image through the calcaneus. **B:** Coronal image through the lateral malleolus. **C:** Coronal image through the ankle mortise and sustentaculum. **D:** Coronal image through the tarsal sinus.

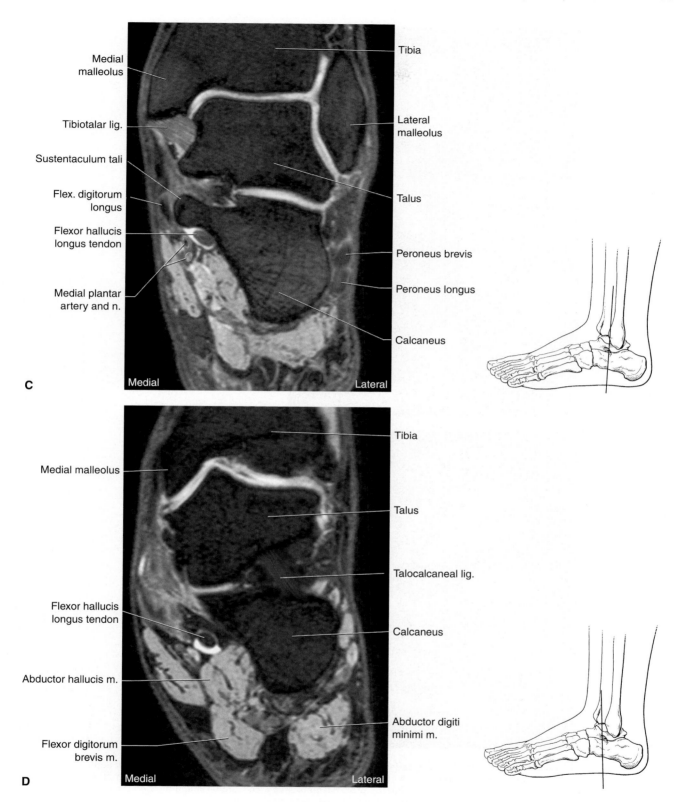

Figure 8-7 *(continued)*

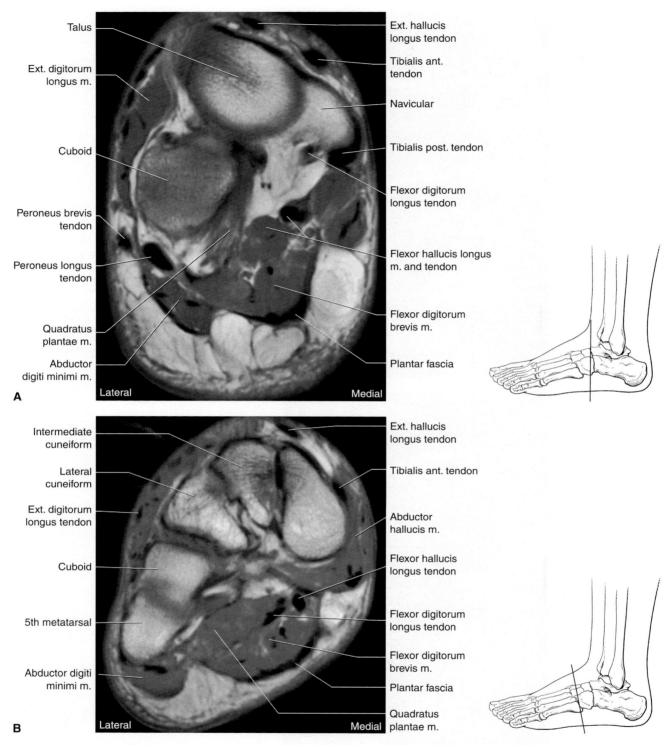

Talus

Ext. digitorum
longus m.

Cuboid

Peroneus brevis
tendon

Peroneus longus
tendon

Quadratus
plantae m.

Abductor
digiti minimi m.

A   Lateral   Medial

Ext. hallucis
longus tendon

Tibialis ant.
tendon

Navicular

Tibialis post. tendon

Flexor digitorum
longus tendon

Flexor hallucis longus
m. and tendon

Flexor digitorum
brevis m.

Plantar fascia

Intermediate
cuneiform

Lateral
cuneiform

Ext. digitorum
longus tendon

Cuboid

5th metatarsal

Abductor digiti
minimi m.

B   Lateral   Medial

Ext. hallucis
longus tendon

Tibialis ant. tendon

Abductor
hallucis m.

Flexor hallucis
longus tendon

Flexor digitorum
longus tendon

Flexor digitorum
brevis m.

Plantar fascia

Quadratus
plantae m.

Figure 8-8 Coronal T1-weighted images through the mid and forefoot with level of section demonstrated. **A:** Coronal image through the tarsal bones. **B:** Coronal image through the cuneiforms. **C:** Coronal image through the proximal metatarsals. **D:** Coronal image through the mid metatarsal region. **E:** Coronal image through the first metatarsal sesamoids.

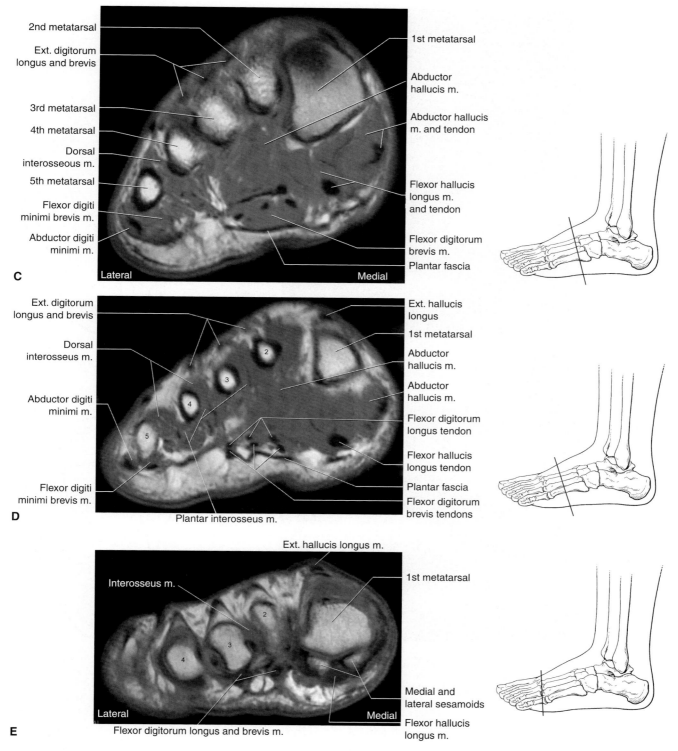

2nd metatarsal

Ext. digitorum longus and brevis

3rd metatarsal

4th metatarsal

Dorsal interosseous m.

5th metatarsal

Flexor digiti minimi brevis m.

Abductor digiti minimi m.

C   Lateral   Medial

1st metatarsal

Abductor hallucis m.

Abductor hallucis m. and tendon

Flexor hallucis longus m. and tendon

Flexor digitorum brevis m.

Plantar fascia

Ext. digitorum longus and brevis

Dorsal interosseus m.

Abductor digiti minimi m.

Flexor digiti minimi brevis m.

D   Plantar interosseus m.

Ext. hallucis longus

1st metatarsal

Abductor hallucis m.

Abductor hallucis m.

Flexor digitorum longus tendon

Flexor hallucis longus tendon

Plantar fascia

Flexor digitorum brevis tendons

Ext. hallucis longus m.

Interosseus m.

1st metatarsal

E   Lateral   Medial

Flexor digitorum longus and brevis m.

Medial and lateral sesamoids

Flexor hallucis longus m.

Figure 8-8   (*continued*)

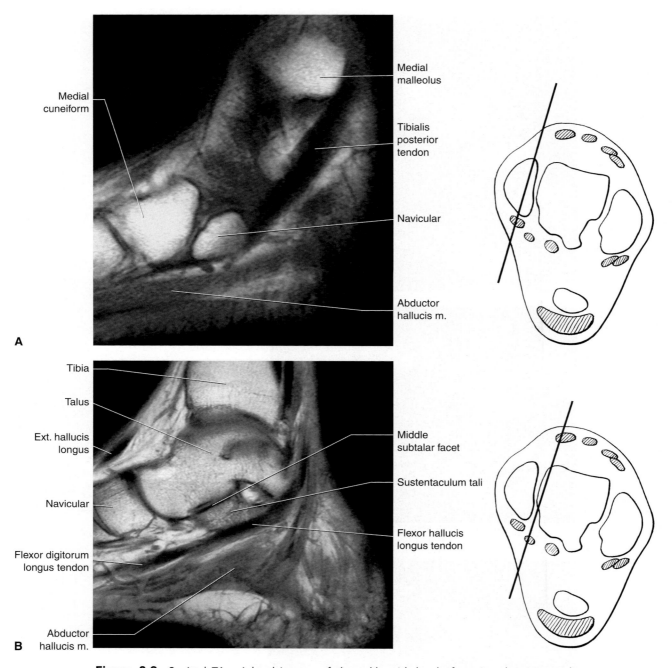

Figure 8-9 Sagittal T1-weighted images of the ankle with level of section demonstrated.
A: Sagittal image through the tibialis posterior. **B:** Sagittal image through the sustentacular level.
C: Sagittal image through the talus. **D:** Sagittal image through the peroneal tendons.

partial volume effects and the variations in the obliquity of these ligaments (Figs. 8-6 through 8-9, and 8-12) (27,44, 46,47,52). Oblique image planes, reformatted thin-section three-dimensional images, or MR arthrography are most useful for evaluating these structures.

Muhle et al. (27) found an inhomogeneous appearance of the medial collateral and the posterior talofibular ligaments on T1-weighted images that correlated with areas of fatty tissue located between ligamentous fibers.

The foot is often divided into three segments: the hindfoot, comprised of the talus and calcaneus; the midfoot, the remaining five tarsal bones; and the forefoot, comprised of the metatarsals and phalanges (44,47). The talus is the second largest of the tarsal bones and articulates with the tibia superiorly, medial and lateral malleolus and calcaneus inferiorly. The head of the talus articulates with the navicular (Figs. 8-6 through 8-9). There are three subtalar articular facets. The anterior and posterior facets articulate

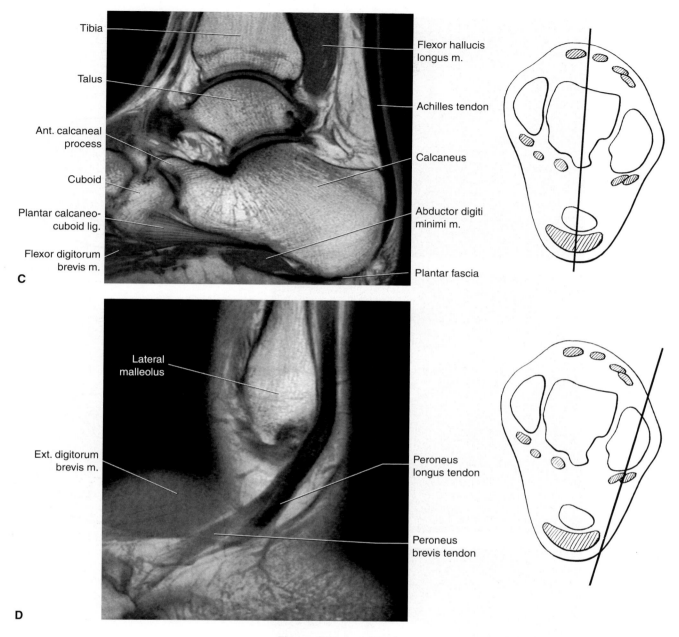

Figure 8-9 (continued)

with similarly named calcaneal facets. The middle facet is just posterior to the anterior calcaneal articular facet and articulates with the sustentaculum tali (Figs. 8-6 and 8-9) (46,47,51,54). The tarsal canal or sinus lies between the middle and anterior facets. The interosseous talocalcaneal ligament lies within this canal and is usually easily seen on sagittal MR images (Fig. 8-9). The tarsal canal has an oblique course between the talus and calcaneus measuring 10 to 15 mm in height and 5 mm in width with a length of 15 to 20 mm. This appearance on sagittal MR images can be confusing and gives the impression of synovitis with erosive changes in the talus (Fig. 8-9) (20,44,46,54,55). In addition to the three superior facets, the calcaneus articulates

anteriorly with the cuboid. There are two main ligaments that directly support the talocalcaneal joint. These are the interosseous talocalcaneal ligament, located in the tarsal canal or sinus tarsi, and the smaller lateral talocalcaneal ligaments. Ligaments of the ankle and adjacent tendons provide additional stabilization (22,44,46,47,54,55).

The remaining tarsal bones (cuboid, navicular, and three cuneiforms) make up the midfoot (46,47,51). The cuboid articulates with the calcaneus proximally and distally with the fourth and fifth metatarsals (Figs. 8-8 and 8-9). The lateral aspect of the cuboid contains a groove for the peroneus longus tendon (Fig. 8-6). The medial surface of the cuboid has an articular facet for the lateral cuneiform. Medially, the

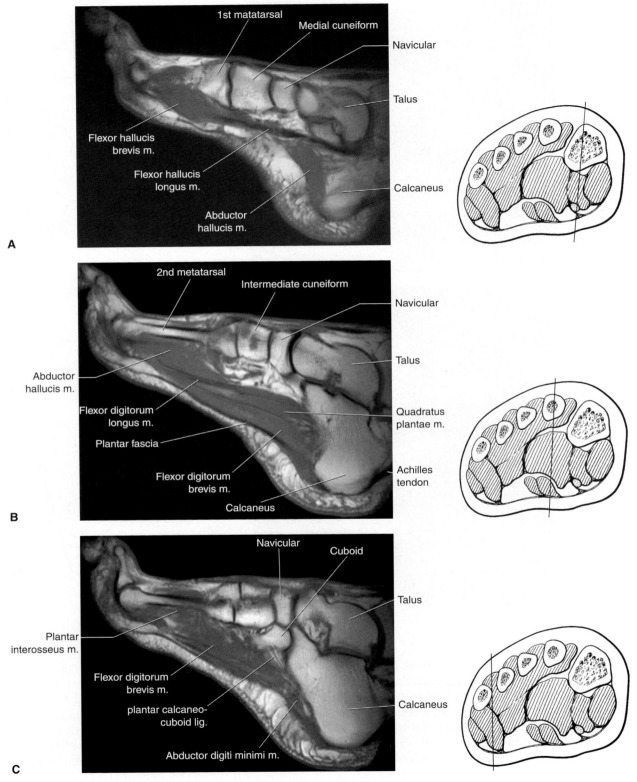

Figure 8-10 Sagittal images of the foot with level of section demonstrated. **A:** Sagittal image through the medial cuneiform and first metatarsal. **B:** Sagittal image through the second metatarsal. **C:** Sagittal image through the calcaneocuboid articulation. **D:** Sagittal image through the fifth metatarsal base.

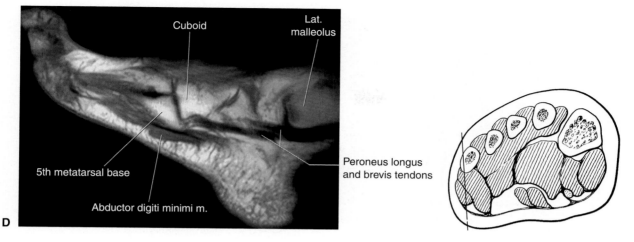

Figure 8-10 (*continued*)

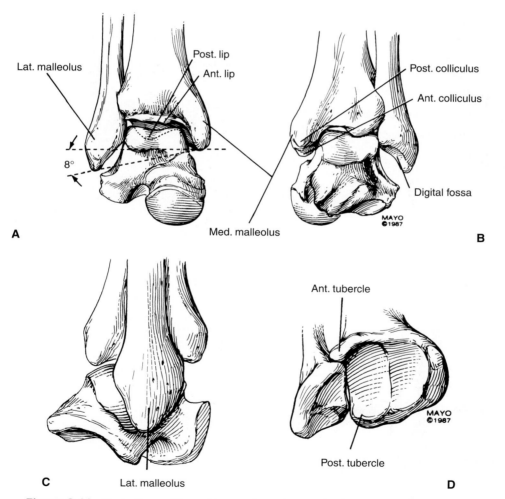

Figure 8-11 Illustrations of the ankle seen from the anterior **(A)**, posterior **(B)**, lateral **(C)**, and infratibial **(D)** surfaces. (From Berquist TH. *Radiology of the foot and ankle*, 2nd ed. Philadelphia, PA: Lippincott Williams & Wilkins, 2000.)

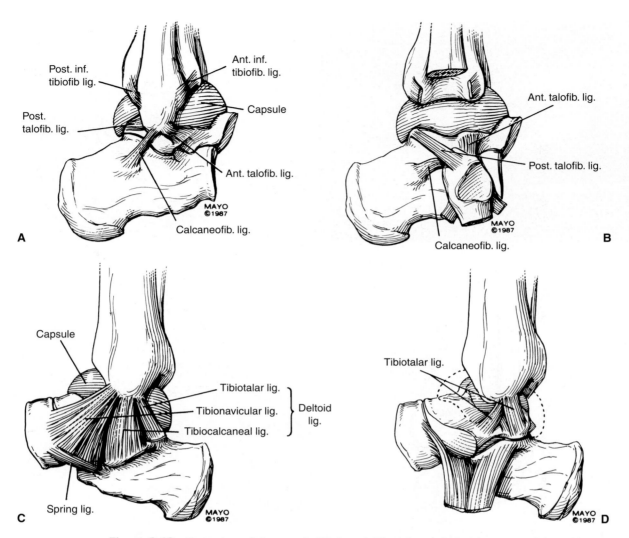

Figure 8-12 Illustrations of the capsule **(A)**, lateral **(B)**, and medial **(C,D)** ligaments of the ankle. (From Berquist TH. *Radiology of the foot and ankle*, 2nd ed. Philadelphia, PA: Lippincott Williams & Wilkins, 2000.)

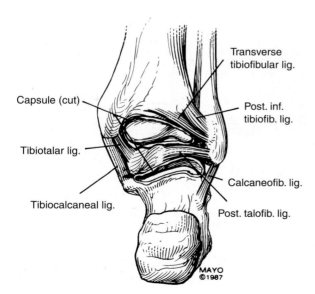

Figure 8-13 Illustrations of ligaments of the ankle seen posteriorly. (From Berquist TH. *Radiology of the foot and ankle*, 2nd ed. Philadelphia, PA: Lippincott, Williams & Wilkins, 2000.)

navicular articulates with talus proximally and anteriorly with the cuneiforms and occasionally the lateral aspect of the cuboid. An additional ligamentous structure, the spring ligament, extends from the calcaneus to the navicular tuberosity (Figs. 8-9 and 8-12). There are other interosseous ligaments both on the dorsal and plantar surfaces of the tarsal bones (44,46,47).

There are three cuneiforms located distal to the navicular and medial to the cuboid. The medial cuneiform is the largest and articulates with the navicular proximally and the intermediate cuneiform laterally. Distally, it articulates with the first and second metatarsals. Lying between medial and lateral cuneiform is the intermediate cuneiform that is the smallest of the three tarsal bones. It articulates with the latter and the navicular proximally and second metatarsal distally. The lateral cuneiform lies between the intermediate cuneiform and the cuboid. It articulates with both of these osseous structures plus the navicular proximally and the second through fourth metatarsals (46,47).

There are five metatarsals that articulate with the tarsal bones. Each has three phalanges with the exception of the great toe, which typically has two. The dorsal, plantar, and interosseous ligaments support the tarsometatarsal joints and bases of the metatarsals. Distally, the transverse metatarsal ligament connects the heads of all five metatarsals. The metatarsophalangeal joints are supported by collateral ligaments and plantar ligaments. Dorsally, the extensor tendons replace the usual dorsal ligaments seen in the midfoot (Figs. 8-6 and 8-8) (22,46,47,51,56,57).

Marrow patterns vary with age on MR images. Pal et al. (58) found that 63% of symptomatic and 57% of asymptomatic children had marrow patterns in the feet that varied from multiple distinct foci to confluent areas of low T1-weighted signal and high signal intensity on T2-weighted and STIR images. Heterogeneous bone marrow in the feet in the immature skeleton can be a normal finding (58).

Soft Tissue Anatomy

The lower extremity musculature develops from mesodermal tissues of the lower limb bud (44,46,47,51). Functional muscle groups are organized in fascial compartments. To simplify the muscular anatomy of the foot and ankle, we will discuss compartments or functional groups of muscles, including their origins, insertions, and actions. Normal variants will also be discussed.

The muscles of the leg can be divided into anterior, posterior, and lateral compartments. One of these muscles crosses only the knee, and two cross the knee and ankle. The majority arise in the leg and act on both the foot and ankle (see Fig. 8-14) (5,17,44,46,47,51,59,60).

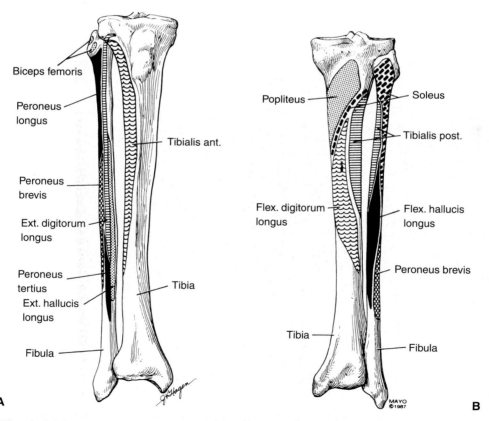

Figure 8-14 Anterior **(A)** and posterior **(B)** illustrations of the tibia and fibula demonstrating origins of muscles that insert on or affect the foot and ankle. (From Berquist TH. *Radiology of the foot and ankle*, 2nd ed. Philadelphia, PA: Lippincott Williams & Wilkins, 2000.)

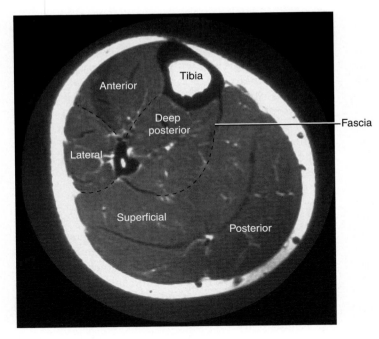

Figure 8-15 Axial MRI of the calf demonstrating the compartments with crural fascia separating the deep and superficial posterior muscle groups.

Posterior Musculature

The superficial and deep muscles of the calf are divided into compartments by the crural fascia (see Fig. 8-15) (44,47). The superficial muscle group includes the gastrocnemius, soleus, and plantaris (see Fig. 8-16). The gastrocnemius has two heads arising from the medial and lateral femoral condyles (see Fig. 8-17). The two heads unite to form the bulk of the muscle in the upper calf (Fig. 8-6A). At about the midpoint of the calf, the muscle ends in a wide, flat tendon. The soleus inserts into the anterior aspect of the gastrocnemius tendon. Below this level, the tendon narrows in

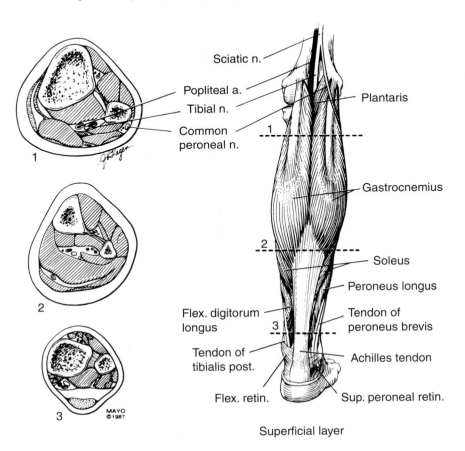

Figure 8-16 Illustrations of superficial muscles of the calf with axial correlation at three levels. (From Berquist TH. *Radiology of the foot and ankle*, 2nd ed. Philadelphia, PA: Lippincott Williams & Wilkins, 2000.)

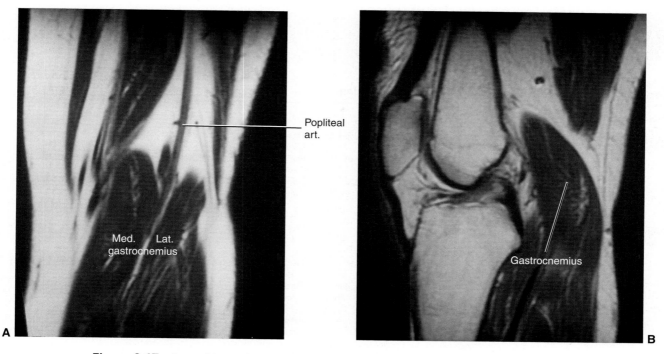

Figure 8-17 Coronal **(A)** and sagittal **(B)** T1-weighted images of the knee, demonstrating the origins of the gastrocnemius muscles.

transverse diameter and thickens forming the Achilles tendon (tendo calcaneus), which inserts on the posterior calcaneus (Figs. 8-6, 8-9 and 8-16). The gastrocnemius plantar flexes the foot and also assists in knee flexion during non-weight bearing. Innervation is by the tibial nerve and the vascular supply primarily derived from the posterior tibial artery (Table 8-2) (44,46,47).

The soleus muscle lies deep to the gastrocnemius (see Figs. 8-6 and 8-18) and also has two heads, one arising from the posterior superior fibula and the second from the popliteal line and posteromedial surface of the proximal tibia (Fig. 8-14). The popliteal vessels and tibial nerve pass deep to the body of the soleus. The soleus inserts in the anterior aspect of the gastrocnemius tendon, forming the thicker Achilles tendon (5,44,47).

The soleus muscle (Fig. 8-18) has no effect on the knee, but serves as a plantar flexor of the foot. Innervation is via the tibial nerve, with vascular supply from the posterior tibial artery (Table 8-2).

The plantaris is the third muscle included in the superficial compartment (Fig. 8-18). This small muscle takes its origin from the lateral epicondyle of the femur and the oblique popliteal ligament. The belly of the muscle is only several inches long and passes between the gastrocnemius and soleus in an oblique direction (Fig. 8-18). The long, thin tendon passes distally along the medial margin of the Achilles to insert in the calcaneus, Achilles, or flexor retinaculum. Occasionally the muscle is double and may be totally absent (46). The plantaris functions as a minor flexor of the knee and plantar flexor of the foot. Innervation and blood

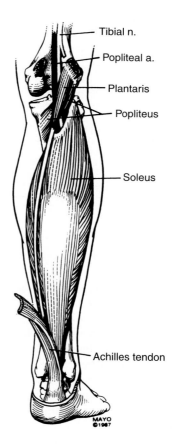

Figure 8-18 Illustration of second layer of muscles in the calf. (From Berquist TH. *Radiology of the foot and ankle*, 2nd ed. Philadelphia, PA: Lippincott Williams & Wilkins, 2000.)

TABLE 8-2
MUSCLES OF THE LEG, FOOT, AND ANKLE

Location	Muscle	Origin	Insertion	Action	Innervation (Segment)	Blood Supply
Calf						
Superficial Compartment	Gastrocnemius	Femoral condyles	Posterior calcaneus	Flexor of foot and knee	Tibial nerve (S1,S2)	Posterior tibial artery
	Soleus	Upper tibia and fibula	Gastrocnemius tendon	Plantar flexor of foot	Tibial nerve (S1,S2)	Posterior tibial artery
	Plantaris	Lateral femoral condyle and oblique popliteal ligament	Posteromedial calcaneus	Plantar flexes foot, flexes leg	Tibial nerve (L4-S1)	Posterior tibial artery
Deep compartment	Popliteus	Lateral femur and capsule of knee		Flexion and medial rotation of leg	Tibial nerve (L5,S1)	Posterior tibial artery
	Flexor hallucis longus	Posterior mid fibula	Distal phalanx great toe	Flexor great toe and ankle	Tibial nerve (L5-S2)	Posterior tibial artery
	Flexor digitorum longus	Posterior tibia	Distal phalanges second to fifth toes	Flexes toes and foot and supinates ankle	Tibial nerve (L5,S1)	Posterior tibial artery
	Tibialis posterior	Posterior tibia, fibula and interosseous membrane	Navicular, cuneiform, calcaneus, second to fourth metatarsals	Adduction of forefoot, hindfoot, inversion, plantar flexion	Tibial nerve (L5,S1)	Posterior tibial artery
Lateral compartment	Peroneus longus	Lateral fibula	First metatarsal and medial cuneiform	Evertor and weak plantar flexors	Superficial and deep peroneal nerve (L4-S1)	Peroneal artery
	Peroneus brevis	Lateral fibula	Base fifth metatarsal		Superficial peroneal nerve (L4-S1)	Peroneal artery
Anterior compartment	Extensor digitorum longus	Upper tibia, fibula, and interosseous membrane	Lateral four toes	Dorsiflexes toes, everts foot	Deep peroneal nerve (L4-S1)	Anterior tibial artery
	Peroneus tertius	Distal fibula and interosseous membrane	Base fifth metatarsal	Dorsiflexes and everts foot	Deep peroneal nerve (L4-S1)	Anterior tibial artery
	Extensor hallucis longus	Distal fibula and interosseous membrane	Distal phalanx great toe	Extends great toe, weak invertor and dorsiflexion of foot	Deep peroneal nerve (L4-S1)	Anterior tibial artery
	Tibialis anterior	Lateral tibia and interosseous membrane	Medial cuneiform and first metatarsal	Strong dorsiflexion and invertor of foot	Deep peroneal nerve (L4-S1)	Anterior tibial artery

From references 5, 22, 44, 46, and 47.

supply are from the tibial nerve and posterior tibial artery (Table 8-2) (44,46).

The deep compartment of the calf contains the popliteus, tibialis posterior, flexor hallucis longus, and flexor digitorum longus muscles (see Figs. 8-6 to 8-10, and 8-19) (44,46,47).

The popliteus is a small triangular muscle forming a portion of the floor of the popliteal fossa (see Fig. 8-19). Its origin is from the lateral femoral condyle, the arcuate popliteal ligament, and capsule of the knee. The insertion is the posterior surface of the upper tibia above the origin of the soleus (Fig. 8-19). The popliteus acts on the knee and leg as a flexor and medial rotator. Neurovascular supply is by the tibial nerve and posterior tibial artery (Table 8-2) (44,46,47,59).

The flexor hallucis longus is the most lateral of the three remaining deep muscles of the leg (flexor hallucis longus,

flexor digitorum longus, and tibialis posterior) (Figs. 8-6 and 8-19). It arises from the lateral aspect of the middle half of the posterior fibula (Fig. 8-14) (46,47,59). Its tendon begins above the malleoli of the ankle and courses medially behind the ankle deep to the flexor retinaculum (Fig. 8-19). The tendon is posterior to the tendons of the tibialis posterior and flexor digitorum longus behind the medial malleolus (Fig. 8-6 and 8-19). The posterior aspect of the talus contains an oblique groove (see Fig. 8-20) for the flexor hallucis longus tendon (22,44). The tendon passes along the plantar aspect of the foot to insert in the distal phalanx of the great toe (Figs. 8-6 and 8-29). The flexor hallucis longus is a flexor of the great toe and assists in ankle flexion. The muscle is innervated by the tibial nerve and receives its blood supply from the posterior tibial artery (Table 8-2) (44,46,59).

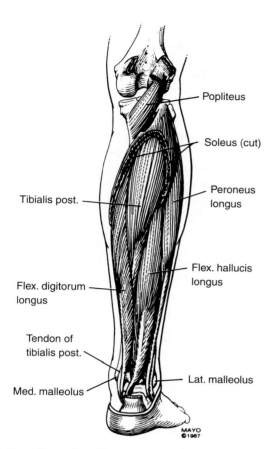

Figure 8-19 Illustration of the deep muscles of the calf. (From Berquist TH. *Radiology of the foot and ankle*, 2nd ed. Philadelphia, PA: Lippincott Williams & Wilkins, 2000.)

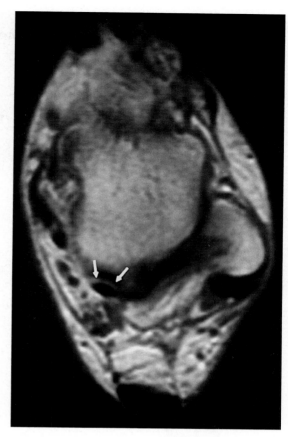

Figure 8-20 Axial MRI demonstrating the talar groove for the flexor hallucis longus tendon (*arrows*).

The flexor digitorum longus lies medially in the deep compartment of the calf (Fig. 8-6). It arises from the upper half of the posteromedial aspect of the tibia (Fig. 8-14). Along its caudad course it passes posterior to the tibialis posterior so that at the ankle it lies between the flexor hallucis longus and tibialis posterior (Fig. 8-6). The tendon passes through the flexor retinaculum, posterior to the medial malleolus, and then divides into four slips that insert in the distal phalanges of the lateral four digits (see Figs. 8-19 and 8-29). On the plantar aspect of the foot, these four tendon slips are associated with the lumbrical muscles and pass through the divided slips of the flexor digitorum brevis prior to inserting on the distal phalanges (5,46,59).

The flexor digitorum longus flexes the lateral four toes and also plantar flexes the foot and supinates the ankle. The muscle is innervated by branches of the tibial nerve and receives its vascular supply from posterior tibial artery branch (Table 8-2) (22,44).

The tibialis posterior is the deepest and most centrally located muscle in the deep posterior compartment (Figs. 8-6 and 8-19). It arises from the upper posterior aspects of the tibia and fibula and the interosseous membrane (Fig. 8-14). Thus, it is positioned between the flexor hallucis longus and flexor digitorum longus. Therefore, it is the most anterior of the three tendons as it passes behind the medial malleolus (Fig. 8-6). The tendon flares to insert in the navicular, tarsal bones, and bases of the two to three metatarsals (see Figs. 8-6, 8-21, and 8-31) (46,47,59).

The tibialis posterior aids in adduction, inversion, and plantar flexion of the foot. The muscle is innervated by branches of the tibial nerve and receives its blood supply from the posterior tibial artery (Table 8-2) (44). Table 8-2 summarizes the muscles of the calf and their functions.

Neurovascular Anatomy of the Calf

The tibial nerve is a continuation of the sciatic nerve at the level of the popliteal fossa. As the nerve passes inferiorly it enters the calf between the heads of the gastrocnemius muscle, passing deep to the soleus to lie between the soleus and tibialis posterior in the deep compartment (see Figs. 8-6 and 8-22) (44,46). The tibial nerve sends branches to all of the superficial and deep muscles of the calf (Table 8-2). At the ankle level, the nerve generally lies between the flexor hallucis longus and flexor digitorum longus tendons (Fig. 8-4). Distal to the flexor retinaculum it divides, forming the medial and lateral plantar nerves (46,47).

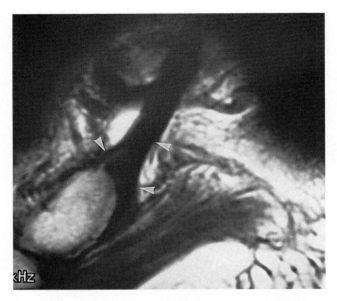

Figure 8-21 Sagittal MRI demonstrating the normal flare or widening (*arrowheads*) of the tibialis posterior tendon as it inserts onto the navicular.

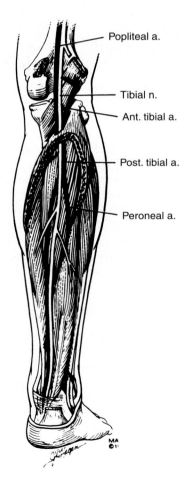

Figure 8-22 Illustration of the major neurovascular structures in the calf. (From Berquist TH. *Radiology of the foot and ankle*, 2nd ed. Philadelphia, PA: Lippincott Williams & Wilkins, 2000.)

The popliteal artery is a direct continuation of the superficial femoral artery as it passes through the adductor canal (Fig. 8-22). It divides into anterior and posterior tibial branches at the level of the popliteus muscle. The anterior tibial artery enters the anterolateral leg above the upper margin of the interosseous membrane while the posterior tibial artery joins the tibial nerve in the deep compartment of the calf (see Figs. 8-22 and 8-26). In the leg it provides muscular branches to all of the calf muscles and a nutrient artery to the tibia. Its largest branch, the peroneal artery arises high in the leg and passes deep to the flexor hallucis longus near the interosseous membrane and fibula (Figs. 8-6 and 8-22). At the ankle level it forms anastomotic branches with the posterior tibial artery and perforates the interosseous membrane to supply the dorsal aspect of the foot. Generally, paired veins accompany the arteries. These veins are more variable and enter the popliteal vein superiorly (46,47).

Anterolateral Musculature

The peroneus longus and brevis are the two muscles of the lateral compartment. Both arise from the superior lateral surface of the fibula. The origin of the peroneus longus is more superior, with the muscle passing superficial to the peroneus brevis (Fig. 8-14). The muscles progress caudad in the lateral compartment, with their tendons entering a common tendon sheath above the ankle (see Figs. 8-6, 8-9, and 8-23). The tendons pass posterior to the lateral malleolus and deep to the superior and inferior peroneal retinacula. The tendons diverge on the lateral surface of the foot (see Fig. 8-24) with the peroneus brevis inserting on the base of the fifth metatarsal. The peroneus longus takes an inferior course passing under the lateral aspect of the foot where it inserts on the base of the 1st metatarsal and medial cuneiform (Fig. 8-31) (22,44,46).

These muscles serve as evertors of the foot and assist in plantar flexion. Innervation is from the superficial peroneal nerve, with branches of the common or deep peroneal nerve supplying a portion of the peroneus longus. Vascular supply is via the peroneal artery (Table 8-2) (61).

Anterior Compartment Musculature

There are four muscles in the anterior compartment. These include the extensor digitorum longus, peroneus tertius, extensor hallucis longus, and tibialis anterior (see Figs 8-6 and 8-25) (Table 8-2).

The extensor digitorum longus is the most lateral muscle in the anterior compartment (Figs. 8-6 and 8-25). It arises from the lateral tibial condyle, anterior fibula, and interosseous membrane (Fig. 8-14). The tendon passes deep to the superior and inferior extensor retinaculae prior to dividing into four slips that insert and the dorsal aspects of the four lateral toes (Fig. 8-25). The insertions are divided such that portions insert in the middle and distal phalanges (53,62,63). The extensor digitorum longus dorsiflexes the

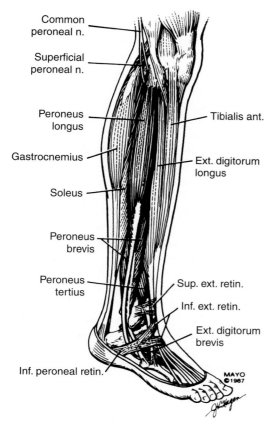

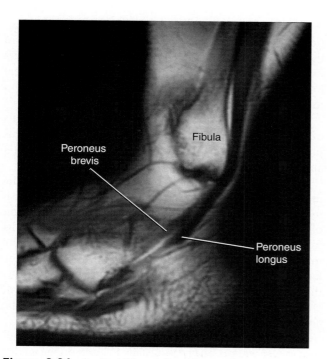

toes and also assists in eversion of the foot. It is innervated by the deep peroneal nerve and receives its vascular supply from the anterior tibial artery (Table 8-2). Variations in its origin and distal insertions are not uncommon, but these rarely cause confusion on MR images (44,46).

The peroneus tertius is closely associated with the extensor digitorum longus, and may be considered a portion of the latter (44). It arises from the distal anterior fibula, interosseous membrane, and membrane of the peroneus brevis (Fig. 8-14). Its tendon passes deep to the extensor retinaculae to insert on the dorsal aspect of the base of the fifth metatarsal (Fig. 8-25). Neurovascular supply to the peroneus tertius is via the deep peroneal nerve and anterior tibial artery. This muscle varies in size and may be absent (Table 8-2) (22,44,47).

The tibialis anterior muscle arises from the lateral tibia surface, deep fascia, and interosseous membrane (Fig. 8-14). It passes inferiorly, becoming tendonous in the lower leg; it is the most medial tendon as it passes deep to the extensor retinaculae (Fig. 8-6). It passes along the medial foot to insert in the medial cuneiform and plantar portion of the first metatarsal (Fig. 8-25) (46,47). This muscle is a strong dorsiflexor and inverter of the foot. Neurovascular supply is via the deep peroneal nerve and anterior tibial artery (Table 8-2) (44).

Figure 8-23 Illustration of the lateral muscle group of the leg. (From Berquist TH. *Radiology of the foot and ankle*, 2nd ed. Philadelphia, PA: Lippincott, Williams & Wilkins 2000.)

Figure 8-24 Sagittal T1-weighted image demonstrating the peroneus brevis and longus as they separate after passing inferior to the lateral malleolus.

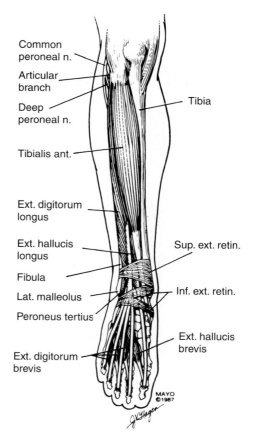

Figure 8-25 Illustration of the anterior compartment muscles. (From Berquist TH. *Radiology of the foot and ankle*, 2nd ed. Philadelphia, PA: Lippincott Williams & Wilkins, 2000.)

Neurovascular Anatomy of the Anterolateral Muscles

The common peroneal nerve is a branch of the sciatic nerve and courses laterally in the popliteal fossa. It is subcutaneous and relatively unprotected just below the fibular head (see Fig. 8-26). Therefore, it is susceptible to direct trauma in this area (5,46). As it descends between the fibula and peroneus longus it divides into two or three branches. These are the superficial, deep, and articular branches of the peroneal nerve. The superficial peroneal nerve lies between the peroneus longus and brevis and supplies these muscles and the subcutaneous tissues. The deep peroneal nerve courses anteriorly, deep to the peroneus longus, to supply the anterior muscles of the leg (Table 8-2). It joins the anterior tibial artery on the anterior aspect of the interosseous membrane (44,46).

The anterior tibial artery passes superior to the interosseous membrane in the upper leg and then lies with the deep peroneal nerve along the anterior aspect of the interosseous membrane (Fig. 8-26). It supplies the anterior muscles and continues as the dorsalis pedis artery on the dorsum of the foot (see Fig. 8-33) (44,46). Table 8-2 summarizes the muscles of the leg, their functions, and neurovascular supply.

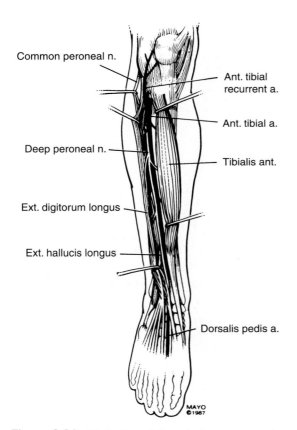

Common peroneal n.

Ant. tibial recurrent a.

Ant. tibial a.

Deep peroneal n.

Tibialis ant.

Ext. digitorum longus

Ext. hallucis longus

Dorsalis pedis a.

MAYO ©1987

Figure 8-26 Illustration of the anterior neurovascular anatomy. (From Berquist TH. *Radiology of the foot and ankle*, 2nd ed. Philadelphia, PA: Lippincott Williams & Wilkins, 2000.)

Foot Musculature

The muscles of the foot are considered in layers instead of compartments (see Fig. 8-27) (44,46,47,64).

The superficial layer of plantar muscles includes the abductor hallucis, flexor digitorum brevis, and abductor digiti minimi. The abductor hallucis arises from the medial process of tubercle of the calcaneus, the flexor retinaculum, and plantar aponeurosis. Its insertion is the medial side of the flexor surface of the proximal phalanx of the great toe (see Figs. 8-6, 8-8, and 8-28) (44,46). The medial and lateral plantar vessels and nerves (Fig. 8-6) pass deep to the proximal position of the muscle as they enter the foot. The muscles are supplied by branches of the medial plantar nerve and artery. The abductor hallucis functions weakly as an abductor of the metatarsophalangeal joint of the great toe (Table 8-3) (44,46).

The flexor digitorum brevis is the most central of the superficial plantar muscles (Figs. 8-6, 8-7, and 8-28). It arises from the medial tubercular process of the calcaneus and plantar fascia. Four tendons pass distally and divide into two slips at the level of the proximal phalanx. The tendons of the flexor digitorum longus pass through the divided brevis tendons. The divided tendon slips insert on the middle phalanx (44). The muscle flexes the lateral four toes. The flexor digitorum brevis receives its neurovascular supply from the medial plantar nerve and artery. The lateral plantar nerve and artery pass deep to this muscle. It is not uncommon for the tendon to the fifth toe to be absent (38%) (Table 8-3) (44).

The abductor digiti minimi is the most lateral muscle in the superficial layer (Figs. 8-6 and 8-28). It arises from the lateral process of the calcaneal tubercle and the distal portion of the medial process. It inserts in the lateral aspect of the base of the proximal phalanx of the fifth toe and serves to flex and abduct the toe at the metatarsal phalangeal joint. This muscle receives its neurovascular supply from the lateral plantar nerve and artery (Table 8-3) (63).

The second layer of the foot is composed of the tendons of the flexor hallucis longus and flexor digitorum longus plus the quadratus plantae and lumbrical muscles (Figs. 8-8 and 8-29) (44,46,47).

The quadratus plantae has two heads that arise from the medial and lateral plantar aspects of the calcaneal tuberosity. The muscle inserts in the lateral and posterior margin of the flexor digitorum longus just before it divides into its four tendon slips (Figs. 8-7, 8-8, and 8-29) (5,44). The muscle assists the flexor digitorum longus in flexing the lateral four toes. The neurovascular supply is provided by the lateral plantar nerve and artery. Occasionally, the lateral head or, in certain cases, the entire muscle may be absent (Table 8-3) (44,46).

The four lumbrical muscles arise from the flexor digitorum longus tendon. They pass distally to insert on the medial side of metatarsophalangeal joints of the four lateral toes (Fig. 8-29). They act as flexors of the metatarsophalangeal

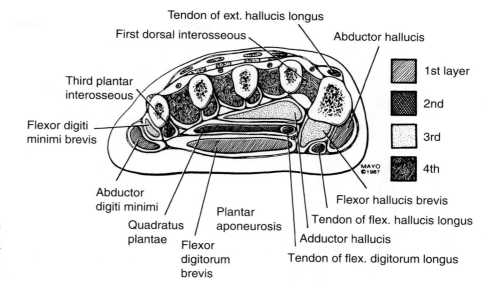

First dorsal interosseous
Tendon of ext. hallucis longus
Abductor hallucis
Third plantar interosseous
Flexor digiti minimi brevis
1st layer
2nd
3rd
4th
MAYO ©1987
Abductor digiti minimi
Quadratus plantae
Plantar aponeurosis
Flexor digitorum brevis
Flexor hallucis brevis
Tendon of flex. hallucis longus
Adductor hallucis
Tendon of flex. digitorum longus

Figure 8-27 Illustration of the muscle layers in the foot. (From Berquist TH. *Radiology of the foot and ankle*, 2nd ed. Philadelphia, PA: Lippincott Williams & Wilkins, 2000.)

TABLE 8-3
MUSCLES OF THE FOOT

Location	Muscle	Origin	Insertion	Action	Innervation (Segment)	Blood Supply
Plantar						
Superficial first layer	Abductor hallucis	Medial calcaneus, plantar aponeurosis, and flexor retinaculum	Proximal phalanx great toe	Flexor and abductor MTP joint great toe	Medial plantar nerve (L5,S1)	Medial plantar artery
	Flexor digitorum brevis	Medial calcaneus plantar fascia	Middle phalanges second to fifth toes	Flexor of toes	Medial plantar nerve (L5,S1)	Medial plantar artery
	Abductor digiti minimi	Lateral process calcaneal tubercle	Lateral base proximal phalanx small toe	Abductor and flexor small toe	Lateral plantar nerve (S1,S2)	Lateral plantar artery
Second layer	Quadratus plantae	Medial and lateral calcaneal tuberosity	Flexor digitorum longus tendon	Flexes terminal phalanges two to five	Lateral plantar nerve (S1,S2)	Lateral plantar artery
	Lumbricals	Flexor digitorum longus tendon	MTP joints two to five	Flexes MTP joints	Medial and lateral plantar nerve (S1,S2)	Medial and lateral plantar arteries
Third layer	Flexor hallucis brevis	Cuboid, cuneiform	Great toe	Flexor great toe	Medial plantar nerve (L5,S1)	Medial and lateral artery
	Adductor hallucis	Second to fourth metatarsal bases and third to fifth capsules transverse leg	Great toe	Adductor great toe, maintains transverse arch	Lateral plantar nerve (L5,S1)	Lateral plantar artery
	Flexor digiti minimi brevis	Cuboid and fifth metatarsal base	Proximal phalanx fifth toe	Flexes fifth toe	Lateral plantar nerve (S1,S2)	Lateral plantar artery
Fourth layer	Interossei dorsal	Metatarsal bases	Bases of second to fourth proximal phalanges	Abduct toes	Lateral plantar nerve (S1,S2)	Lateral plantar artery
	Plantar	Metatarsal bases	Bases of third to fifth proximal phalanges	Abduct toes	Lateral plantar nerve (S1,S2)	Lateral plantar artery
Dorsal	Extensor digitorum brevis	Superior calcaneus, lateral talocalcaneal ligament, extensor retinaculum	Lateral first to fourth toes	Extends toes one to four	Deep peroneal nerve (L5,S1)	Dorsalis pedis artery

From references 5, 44, 46, and 47.

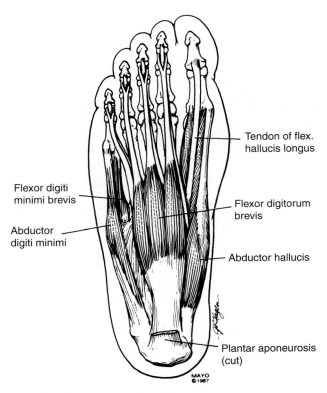

Figure 8-28 Illustration of the superficial muscle layers of the foot. (From Berquist TH. *Radiology of the foot and ankle*, 2nd ed. Philadelphia, PA: Lippincott Williams & Wilkins, 2000.)

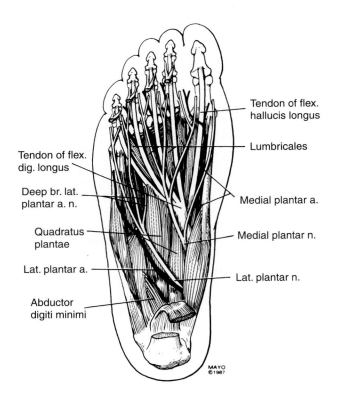

Figure 8-29 Illustration of the second muscle layer of the foot with neurovascular structures. (From Berquist TH. *Radiology of the foot and ankle*, 2nd ed. Philadelphia, PA: Lippincott Williams & Wilkins, 2000.)

joints. The most medial muscle is innervated by the medial plantar nerve, while the lateral plantar nerve supplies the lateral three muscles. Blood supply is via the medial and lateral plantar arteries. Absence of one or more of the lumbricals has been reported. Occasionally, two muscles insert on the fourth and fifth toes (Table 8-3) (44).

The third layer of plantar muscles includes the flexor hallucis brevis, adductor hallucis, and flexor digiti minimi brevis (see Figs. 8-6 and 8-30). The flexor hallucis brevis has two bellies arising from the plantar aspect of the cuboid and adjacent cuneiform (Fig. 8-30). The tendons insert at the sides of the base of the great toe and the sesamoids. The muscle serves as a flexor of the great toe and is supplied by the medial plantar nerve and artery (5,46,47).

The adductor hallucis muscle has oblique and transverse heads (Fig. 8-30). The oblique head arises from the long plantar ligament, and the second through fourth metatarsal bases (59,63). The smaller transverse head arises from the capsules of the third through fifth metatarsophalangeal joints and the deep transverse ligaments. The two heads join lateral to the great toe to insert with the lateral head of the flexor hallucis brevis. The adductor hallucis adducts and flexes the great toe. In addition, it assists in flexion of the proximal phalanx and maintaining the transverse arch. It is supplied by the lateral plantar arteries and nerves (Table 8-3) (44).

The flexor digiti minimi brevis arises from the cuboid and base of the fifth metatarsal and inserts in the lateral base of the proximal phalanx of the fifth toe (Fig. 8-30). The muscle serves as a flexor of the small toe and is supplied by branches of the lateral plantar nerve and artery (44,46).

The fourth and deepest layer of plantar muscles consists of seven interosseous muscles—three plantar and four dorsal (Figs. 8-8 and 8-31). The four dorsal interossei muscles arise with two heads from the adjacent aspects of the metatarsal bases (Figs. 8-8 and 8-31). The tendons insert into the bases of the proximal phalanges with the two medial bellies inserting on the medial and lateral side of the second and the third and fourth inserting on the lateral sides of the third and fourth proximal phalanges. The three plantar interosseous muscles arise from the bases of the third through fifth metatarsals and insert on the medial sides of the proximal phalanges of the third, fourth, and fifth toes. Thus, the dorsal interossei are abductors and the plantar interossei adductors. All interossei muscles are supplied by branches of the lateral plantar artery and nerve (Table 8-3) (44,47).

The extensor digitorum brevis (Figs. 8-8 and 8-25) is the dorsal muscle of the foot. This broad, thin muscle arises from the superior calcaneus, lateral talocalcaneal ligament, and extensor retinaculum. It takes a medial oblique course ending in four tendons that insert in the lateral aspect of the proximal phalanx of the great toe and the lateral aspect of the extensor digitorum longus tendons of the second to fourth toes. The muscle extends the great toe and second through fourth toes. Neurovascular supply is provided by the deep peroneal nerve and dorsalis pedis artery (5,44,46). The muscles of the foot are summarized in Table 8-3.

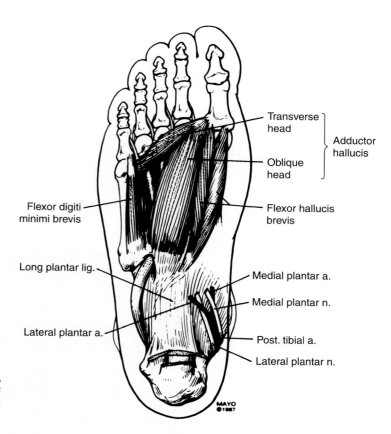

Figure 8-30 Illustration of the third *muscle layer of the foot with plantar nerves. (From Berquist TH. Radiology of the foot and ankle,* 2nd ed. Philadelphia, PA: Lippincott Williams & Wilkins, 2000.)

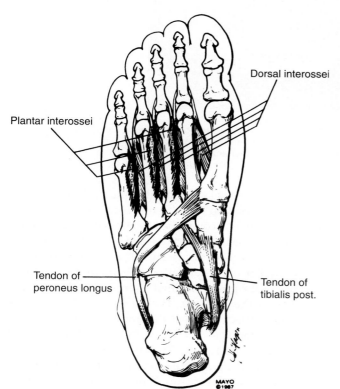

Figure 8-31 Illustration of the deepest (fourth) layer of muscles in the foot, with peroneus longus and posterior tibial tendon insertions. (From Berquist TH. *Radiology of the foot and ankle,* 2nd ed. Philadelphia, PA: Lippincott Williams & Wilkins, 2000.)

Soft tissue contrast provided by MRI and, to a lesser degree, CT has popularized the compartment concept for evaluating soft tissue infection and neoplasms in the foot (65–70). Although this concept is controversial, most clinicians consider that the plantar compartments of the foot are divided by intermuscular septa that extend dorsally from the plantar aponeurosis (see Fig. 8-32) (44,66, 68–70). The medial septum (Fig. 8-32) courses dorsally from the aponeurosis to attach to the navicular, the medial cuneiform, and the lateral planter aspect of the first metatarsal. The lateral septum (Fig. 8-32) extends from the aponeurosis to the medial aspect of the fifth metatarsal. Thus, the lateral, central or intermediate, and medial compartments are created (Fig. 8-32) (46,66,68). The medial compartment contains the abductor hallucis and flexor hallucis and flexor hallucis brevis muscles and the flexor hallucis longus tendon. The lateral compartment contains the flexor digiti minimi brevis and abductor digiti minimi. The central compartment contains three layers described earlier, including the flexor digitorum brevis, the flexor digitorum longus tendon, the quadratus plantae, the lumbrical muscles, and the adductor hallucis (44,66). Spread of infection tends to follow these compartments.

Neurovascular Supply of the Foot

The anterior tibial artery continues over the midanterior aspect of the tibia passing deep to the extensor tendons

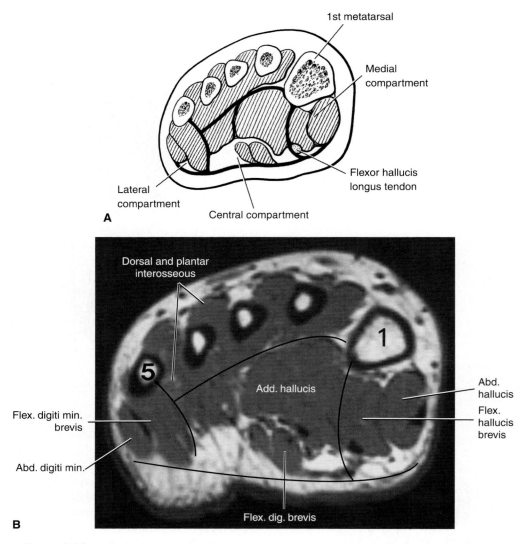

Figure 8-32 **A:** Axial illustration through the proximal metatarsals demonstrating the lateral, central, and medial compartments. The medial compartment contains the flexor hallucis longus tendon. **B:** Axial MRI demonstrating the compartments of the foot with muscular anatomy.

and retinaculae of the ankle (Fig. 8-33). At the ankle, the anterior tibial artery anastomosis with the perforating branch of the peroneal artery both supply the periarticular structures of the ankle. As the anterior tibial artery emerges from the extensor retinaculum it becomes the more superficial dorsalis pedis artery. After giving off the deep plantar artery, it becomes the first dorsal metatarsal artery. This vessel courses distally, ending in digital branches of the first and second toes. Dorsal branches of the foot include medial and lateral tarsal arteries and the arcuate artery with its dorsal metatarsal branches (Fig. 8-33) (44,46).

The deep peroneal nerve accompanies the anterior tibial, dorsalis pedis, and first dorsal metatarsal arteries. It supplies the anterior muscles of the foot and leg. The superficial peroneal nerve runs over the anterior aspect of the fibula supplying the peroneal muscles and the lateral aspect of the foot (Fig. 8-32) (18,46,47).

The posterior tibial artery divides into medial and lateral plantar branches deep to the flexor retinaculum. The posterior tibial artery is accompanied by similarly named nerves and veins. The neural branches (medial and lateral plantar nerves) are branches of the tibia nerve (see Fig. 8-34) (44,46).

The medial plantar artery is the smaller of the two branches of the posterior tibial artery and ends in digital branches to the first toe. The lateral plantar artery is larger and forms an arch at the midfoot level that gives off four metatarsal arteries with their distal digital branches (Fig. 8-34) (63). The lateral plantar artery also gives off perforating muscular branches that form anastomoses with the dorsal arteries. Numerous minor variations in the digital arteries have been described (18,44,46).

The peroneal artery passes inferior to the lateral malleolus and ends on the calcaneal surface in the lateral calcaneal artery (44,46).

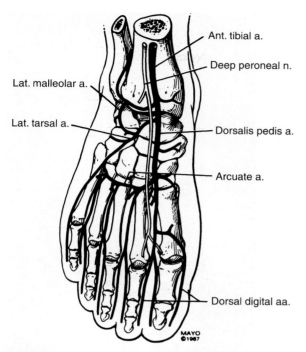

Figure 8-33 Illustration of the dorsal neurovascular anatomy of the foot. (From Berquist TH. *Radiology of the foot and ankle*, 2nd ed. Philadelphia, PA: Lippincott Williams & Wilkins, 2000.)

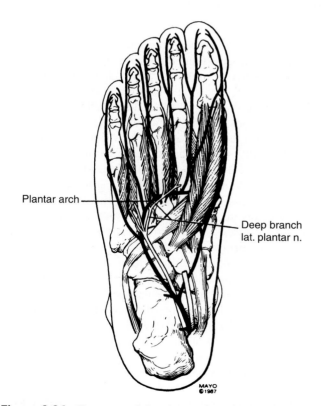

Figure 8-34 Illustration of the plantar neurovascular anatomy of the foot. (From Berquist TH. *Radiology of the foot and ankle*, 2nd ed. Philadelphia, PA: Lippincott Williams & Wilkins, 2000.)

Table 8-3 summarizes the neurovascular supply to the muscles of the foot.

PITFALLS AND NORMAL VARIANTS

Misinterpretation of MR images can be related to partial volume effects, flow and other artifacts, failure to review associated radiographs, and normal anatomic variants. Recognition of these nonpathologic conditions is important to prevent misinterpretation of images and unnecessary treatment (5,38,63,71–74).

There are numerous soft tissue variants in the calf, foot, and ankle (38,71,74–76). Muscle variations can cause particular confusion when accessing subtle changes on MR images. For example, the gastrocnemius may have only one head, typically the medial head (44,46). The popliteus may originate from the inner aspect of the fibular head and insert above the oblique tibial line in 14% of cases. The normal origin and insertion are demonstrated in Fig. 8-17. A fairly common accessory flexor muscle, the accessorius longus digitorum, arises from the lower tibia and fibula and interosseous membrane and passes anterior to the flexor retinaculum to insert with the flexor digitorum longus and quadratus plantae tendons (44). Cheung et al. (77) found a 6% prevalence of the flexor digitorum accessorius longus in a group of 100 asymptomatic volunteers. Eberle et al. (72) reported this accessory muscle in 8% of the population. Flexor hallucis syndrome can occur when this accessory muscle is present.

Several variations may cause confusion on MR or CT images. The muscles may fuse to form one unit, and occasionally the peroneus longus insertion expands to include the bases of the three to five metatarsals. An accessory peroneal muscle may arise from the fibula between the peroneus longus and brevis. Its tendon generally inserts in the peroneus longus tendon on the plantar aspect of the foot (5,44,46).

The peroneus quadratus is present in about 10% to 13% of patients (38,71,78). This anomalous muscle is three times as common in males compared with females. This arises from the posterior fibula between the longus and brevis. Three variations of the peroneus quadratus have been described based on their insertions. One of this subgroup inserts on the calcaneus (perocalcaneus externum), one on the cuboid (peroneocuboideus), and the third variation inserts on the peroneal tendon (long peroneal) (44). The peroneus quadratus has been associated with clinical symptoms (pain and instability), and it is associated with peroneal tendon subluxation. On MRI (see Fig. 8-35), the peroneus quadratus tendon is posterior to the brevis and longus tendons (44,78).

The peroneus digiti minimi is rare. It arises from the lower fibula and inserts on the extensor surface of the fifth toe (5,44).

An important variant is the accessory soleus muscle. This muscle bundle extends into the pre-Achilles fat

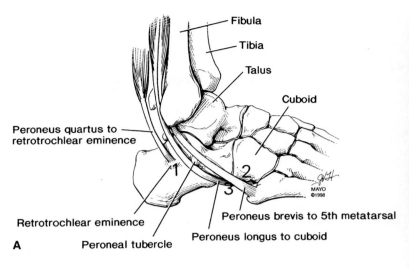

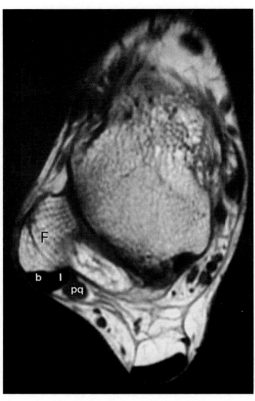

Figure 8-35   **A:** Illustration of the peroneus quadratus, which may insert on the retrotrochlear eminence (*1*), cuboid (*2*), or peroneus longus tendon (*3*). **B:** Axial MRI demonstrating peroneus quadratus (*pq*) medial and posterior to the peroneus brevis (*b*) and longus (*l*) tendons. *F*, fibula.

(Kager's fat pad) (79–82). This muscle may be noted incidentally or cause clinical symptoms. Patients may present with pain after exercise or a soft tissue mass. MRI (see Figs. 8-36 and 8-37) can confirm the presence of this normal variant and differentiate normal muscle from a muscle tear or neoplasm (5,75).

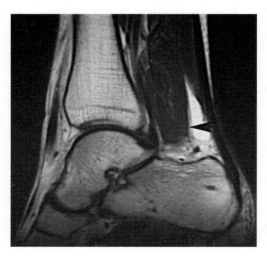

Figure 8-36   Accessory soleus muscle. Sagittal MR image of the ankle on a patient with an accessory soleus muscle (*arrowhead*). Compare to normal sagittal images in Fig. 8-9.

Another accessory muscle, the peroneocalcaneus internus, occurs in 1% of asymptomatic patients (83). In up to 75% of cases this accessory muscle is bilateral. The muscle arises from the lateral flexor hallucis longus and the posterior fibula. It lies posterolateral to the flexor hallucis longus as it courses inferiorly to the sustentaculum tali to insert on the calcaneus (44). Both tendons may be visible on sagittal and axial MR studies as they pass inferiorly to the sustentaculum tali (see Figs. 8-38 and 8-39) (84). The peroneocalcaneus internus muscle does not present as a soft tissue mass or cause neurovascular compression, which can occur with other accessory muscles (38,71,79). However, in some cases, it may displace the flexor hallucis longus muscle and may cause indirect neurovascular compression.

One must also be familiar with accessory ossicles and variations in bony anatomy (see Fig. 8-40) (47). Ossicles are easily detected and characterized on routine radiographs and CT. However, ossicles may cause confusion on MR images (see Fig. 8-41). This is one of several reasons why it is important to compare MRI with routine radiographs before interpreting MRI studies (5). Common ossicles include the accessory navicular, os peroneum, os subfibulare (Fig. 8-41), and os sustentactuli (38,71). The os sustenculi is seen in 1% of patients. The ossicle lies at the posterior margin of the sustentaculum tali. This ossicle can become symptomatic, but should not be confused with a fracture (71).

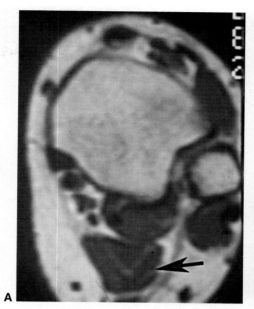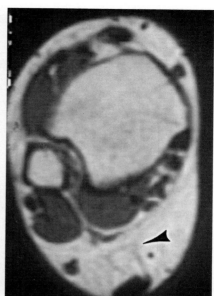

Figure 8-37 Patient with ankle pain and fullness posteriorly. Examination is performed in the head coil to allow comparison and improved detection of subtle lesions. Axial T1-weighted images of the ankles demonstrate an accessory soleus muscle on the left **(A)** (*arrow*) that may have been overlooked if the opposite ankle were not available for comparison. Note the normal pre-Achilles fat on the right **(B)** (*arrowhead*).

There are three types of accessory navicular. Type I is round to oval and imbedded in the distal posterior tibial tendon. Type II is more triangular and maintains a fibrocartilagenous attachment to the navicular (see Fig. 8-42). Overuse can lead to symptoms at the fibrocartilagenous junction. Type III is cornuate and incompletely incorporated into the navicular. Both type II and type III are frequently seen in patients with posterior tibial tendon dysfunction (5,71).

A pseudodefect in the posterior talar articular surface is a common finding on MR images (see Fig. 8-43). The defect is seen as an area of irregularity at the posterior articular margin (Fig. 8-43). Signal intensity is reduced on both T1- and T2-weighted sequences. Both tali are involved in 86% of patients. The pseudodefect should not be confused with bone erosion or an osteochondral fracture (85).

There are two areas of prominence on the lateral calcaneus. The peroneal tubercle is seen in 40% of the general population and is part of the fibro-osseous tunnel for the peroneal tendons. Posterior to the peroneal tubercle is the retrotrochlear eminence that is evident in 98% of patients. The accessory penoneus quadradus muscle may attach on this eminence (Fig. 8-35A) (38,71,82,86).

Pseudo-osteochondral defects have also been reported in the distal tibia (groove for the posterior tibiofibular ligament) and talus that should not be confused with erosions or osteochondral fractures (38,71,82,87).

Noto et al. (88) reviewed normal variants on MR images in 30 patients. Common variations included an irregularity of the posterior tibiotalar joint (27/30 cases), variations in signal intensity at points of tendon insertions (not to be confused with tendon rupture), and small amounts of fluid in the tendon sheath surrounding otherwise normal tendons. The latter may be particularly difficult to differentiate from early tenosynovitis.

There is normally a small amount of fluid in the tendon sheaths of the foot and ankle. This finding is more common in the flexors than the extensor (38,71). The presence of asymptomatic fluid is more common in active or athletic individuals. A small amount of fluid in the retrocalcaneal bursa is evident in 53% to 68% of patients. Increased fluid in the joints (18% to 34%) and peritendinous regions (22%) is also common (38,89,90).

The posterior intermalleolar ligament is a normal variant that lies between the posterior tibiofibular ligament and the posterior talofibular ligament (see Fig. 8-44). The posterior intermalleolar ligament has received some attention in the orthopedic literature because of its association with posterior impingement syndrome (60,91). Rosenberg et al. (91) studied MR features of this ligament and found that it was most easily detected on axial or coronal images (Fig. 8-44B). The ligament was identified on 19% of clinical MRI studies (91). This ligament may be more easily studied using three-dimensional GRE images.

Fiorella et al. (92) evaluated MR imaging features of the posterior intermalleolar ligament in patients with posterior impingement syndrome of the ankle. They found a prominent intermalleolar ligament as the most probable cause of posterior impingement syndrome in these patients in the absence of other structured causes. Ankle arthroscopy was performed in one of these patients in which arthroscopic resection of the intermalleolar ligament resulted in resolution of the posterior impingement syndrome in this patient (92).

Partial volume effects can also create apparent abnormalities. This is a particularly significant problem when evaluating the complex ligament anatomy and the variations in signal intensity created by the "fanned" insertions and multidirectional slips of the ligaments (5,38,88). Use

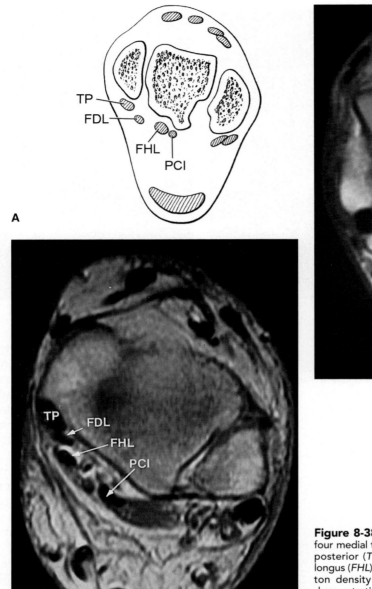

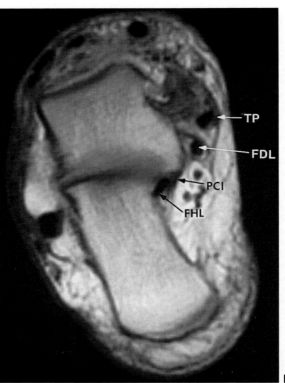

Figure 8-38 **A:** Axial illustration of the ankle demonstrating four medial tendons instead of the usual three tendons: tibialis posterior (*TP*), flexor digitorum longus (*FDL*), flexor hallucis longus (*FHL*), and peroneocalcaneus internus (*PCI*). **B:** Axial proton density image just proximal to the sustentaculum tali demonstrating two tendons in the usual location of the flexor hallicis longus. **C:** Axial image of the tibiotalar junction shows four tendons instead of three. The PCI is most lateral.

of multiple image planes can be helpful in minimizing this problem.

The "magic angle" effect can create apparent pathology when structures (tendons or ligaments) are oriented 55° to the magnetic field (B_0) (82,93,94). Signal intensity is increased maximally at 55° with intermediate signal intensity within 10° (45° to 65°) of the magic angle (94). This phenomenon is most commonly associated with short TE spin-echo or GRE sequences (see Fig. 8-45). Signal intensity aberrations can also be detected at ligament or tendon insertions where diverging fibrous structures enter the magic angle (93,94). In our experience

(Fig. 8-45), this phenomenon and partial volume effects can have a similar MR appearance.

CLINICAL APPLICATIONS

The applications for MRI of the calf, foot, and ankle have expanded dramatically in the last decade (1,25,59, 65,89,95–109). Ease of positioning, multiple image planes, and the superior contrast afforded by MR are ideal for examination of many foot and ankle disorders. In our practice, the most common applications are

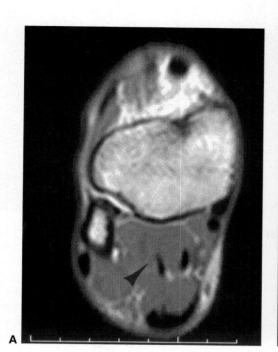
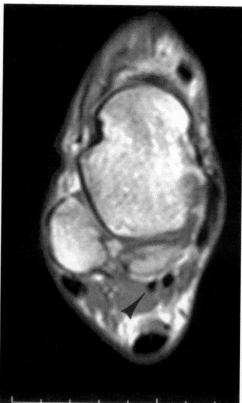

Figure 8-39 T1-weighted images **(A,B)** demonstrating the peroneocalcaneus internus (*arrowheads*) lateral to the flexor hallucis longus.

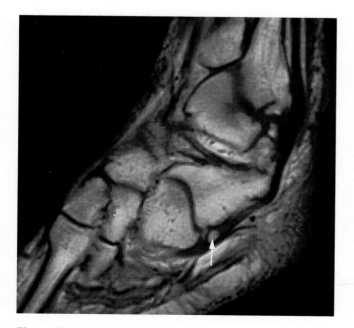

Figure 8-40 Sagittal MRI of the os peroneum (*arrow*).

trauma, specifically soft tissue trauma, neoplasms, infection, avascular necrosis (AVN), nerve compression syndromes, and diabetic foot disorders.

TRAUMA

Foot and ankle injuries account for 10% or more of emergency room visits (9,27,110). Routine radiographs and conventional techniques are still best suited for evaluation of patients with acute skeletal injuries. Chronic posttraumatic syndromes and certain soft tissue injuries may be more ideally suited to MRI evaluation (Fig. 8-42). Karasick et al. (111) demonstrated that MRI is important for evaluating painful conditions of the forefoot when conventional radiography is not diagnostic.

Fractures

Most skeletal injuries are still easily detected with routine radiographs. However, subtle fractures, bone contusions, and complete assessment of fracture patterns, physeal, and

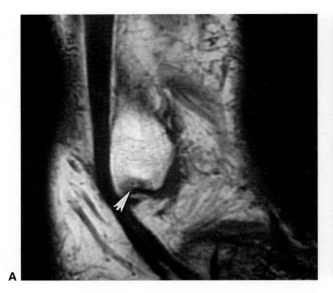
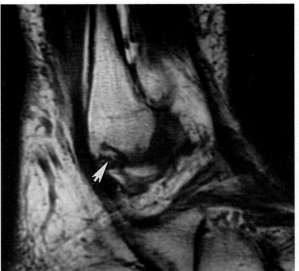

Figure 8-41 Sagittal T1-weighted images **(A,B)** demonstrating a small os subfibulare (*arrow*). Determining whether an abnormality or an ossicle is present can be difficult, depending on the size and marrow content of the ossicle.

associated soft tissue injuries is more easily accomplished with MRI (4,5,7,17,112). Subtle marrow injuries (bone bruises and marrow edema) can be detected that may go undiagnosed with conventional imaging techniques (see Figs. 8-46 and 8-47) (102,112–115).

Bone marrow edema and bone bruises may occur in multiple settings. Areas of low signal intensity on T1- and high signal intensity on T2-weighted sequences are commonly seen in the foot (115). The etiology is unclear, but may be traumatic or related to stress response (see Fig. 8-48)

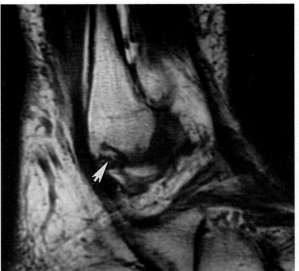

Figure 8-42 Type II accessory navicular. Sagittal T1-weighted image shows the posterior tibial tendon (*PTT*) attaching to the triangular accessory navicular with fibrous (*arrow*) attachment.

(113,115). Symptoms may be present with these findings for up to one year, but generally respond to conservative therapy (102,115). Bone bruises are typically associated with acute trauma. Seven to 25% of patients with ankle sprains have associated bone bruises (116). Axial loading injuries can result in bilateral calcaneal bone bruises (112). Bone bruises have a similar appearance to marrow edema. Signal intensity changes are likely related to microfracture and hemorrhage. If continued stress is applied to the involved area a complete fracture can result (17,102).

Stress fractures and insufficiency fractures are common in the foot and ankle. The former is related to repetitive stress to normal bone structure. Insufficiency fractures occur when normal stress is applied to abnormal bone (5,17,114). In the foot, stress fractures most commonly involve the second through fourth metatarsal shafts and necks (see Fig. 8-49). The metatarsal bases are more commonly involved in ballet dancers (117,118). The navicular and base of the fifth metatarsal may also be involved (117,118). Stress response is the first stage of stress fractures (17,113). Edema, hyperemia, and increased osteoclastic activity in the involved region show a poorly defined area of signal abnormality with low signal intensity on T1- and high signal intensity on T2-weighted or STIR sequences (17,113). Over time, a linear fracture line may be evident, especially in the navicular and calcaneus (see Fig. 8-50). Periosteal callus forms early around metatarsal stress fractures (Fig. 8-49C). This can be easily identified on axial and coronal or sagittal MR images. MRI is more sensitive and specific than radionuclide scans, particularly in the elderly or osteopenic population (17,114).

Robbins et al. (119) found that MR was valuable in detecting subtle fractures of the anterosuperior calcaneal process. If these fractures are not immobilized early, painful nonunion may result. Marrow edema confined to

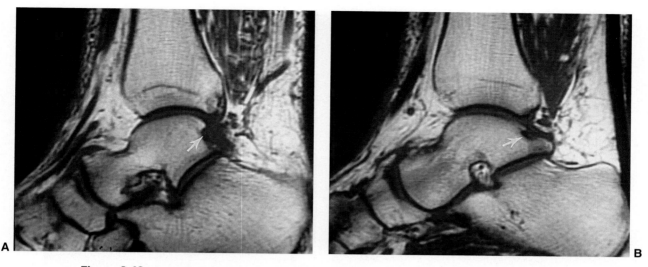

Figure 8-43 Sagittal T1-weighted images **(A,B)** demonstrating a low-signal-intensity pseudodefect near the posterior articular margin of the talus (*arrow*).

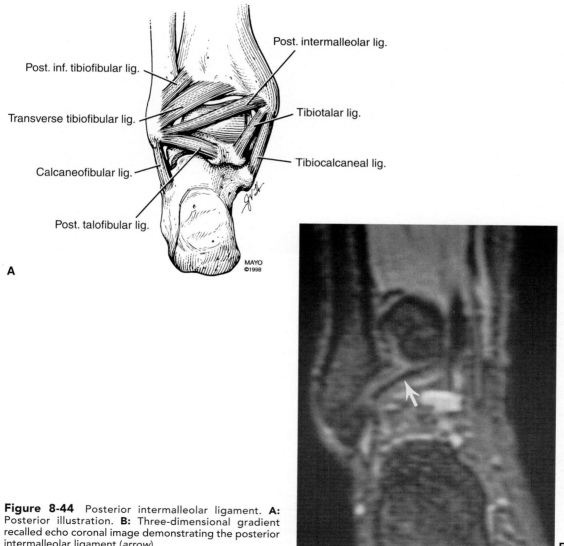

Post. inf. tibiofibular lig.

Transverse tibiofibular lig.

Calcaneofibular lig.

Post. talofibular lig.

Post. intermalleolar lig.

Tibiotalar lig.

Tibiocalcaneal lig.

MAYO
©1998

A

B

Figure 8-44 Posterior intermalleolar ligament. **A:** Posterior illustration. **B:** Three-dimensional gradient recalled echo coronal image demonstrating the posterior intermalleolar ligament (*arrow*).

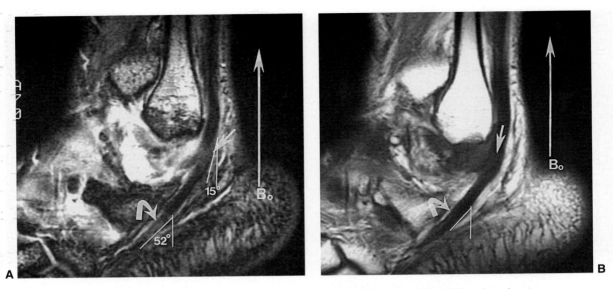

Figure 8-45 Gradient echo **(A)** and T1-weighted **(B)** sagittal images of the peroneal tendons in a patient with synovitis and areas of increased signal intensity in the tendon proximally (*straight arrow*) and inferiorly (*curved arrow*). The angle of the tendon is 52° inferiorly and increased signal is due to magic angle effect. Partial volume effects create increased signal proximally due to inflammation in the adjacent tissues.

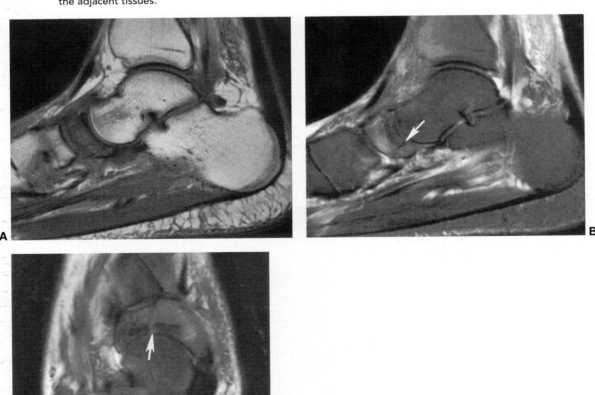

Figure 8-46 Patient with midfoot pain and normal radiographs. Sagittal T1- **(A)** and T2-weighted **(B)** and axial T2-weighted **(C)** images demonstrate marrow edema and a fracture in the navicular (*arrow*). The axial image **(C)** more clearly demonstrates the fracture.

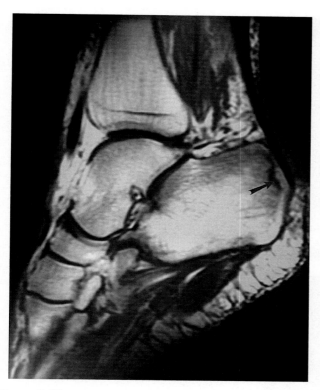

Figure 8-47 Sagittal proton density-weighted image of a subtle calcaneal fracture (*arrow*).

the anterosuperior calcaneal process is consistent with a bifurcate ligament avulsion. Marrow edema seen in both the anterosuperior calcaneal process and the cuboid is an impaction type fractures called the "nutcracker lesion," which is seen in athletes such as gymnasts (119).

Osteochondral fracture can be related to an acute injury or chronic repetitive trauma (osteochondritis dissecans)

(17,120,121). Both lesions are easily detected and classified using MRI. The talar dome (see Fig. 8-51) is most commonly involved and accounts for 4% of cases of osteochondritis dissecans (120).

Berndt and Harty (122) classified osteochondral lesions of the talar dome based upon cartilage integrity and fragment position. Stage I lesions involve subchondral bone with intact cartilage. Stage II lesions have partially detached osteochondral fragments, and stage III lesions are completely detached but undisplaced. Stage IV lesions are completely detached and displaced.

Magee et al. (10) reviewed MR images in 30 patients with persistent ankle pain 6 weeks after injury and with normal findings on conventional radiographs. They found that limited MR studies are valuable for identification of talar dome injuries (see Fig. 8-52). MR images were positive in 57% of patients with normal radiographs. Early recognition of talar dome injuries is important for early immobilization (Figs. 8-51 and 8-52) (10). MR imaging can accurately detect and stage talar dome lesions. Two image planes are essential to evaluate the size and location of the lesion. Coronal and sagittal DESS images provide excellent cartilage detail. Thin-section three-dimensional spoiled GRE and proton density or T2-weighted FSE fat-suppressed sequences may also be considered (17,120). High-signal-intensity fluid extends into stage II and surrounds stage III lesions using the above sequences. Intraarticular or intravenous gadolinium is usually not required unless one needs to differentiate granulation tissue from high-signal-intensity fluid in chronic lesions (17).

Treatment is conservative for early stages. Surgical treatment with lesion curettage and debriding is more commonly performed for stage III and IV lesions (17,120,122).

Growth plate injuries are easily detected and followed with MRI. T2- or T2*-weighted, STIR and DESS images are

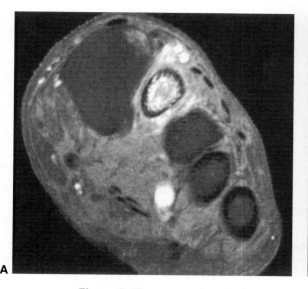

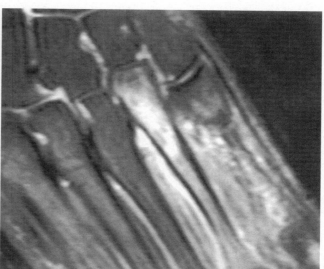

Figure 8-48 Stress response. Fat-suppressed T2-weighted fast spin-echo axial **(A)** and coronal **(B)** images demonstrate marrow edema in the proximal second metatarsal without cortical disruption.

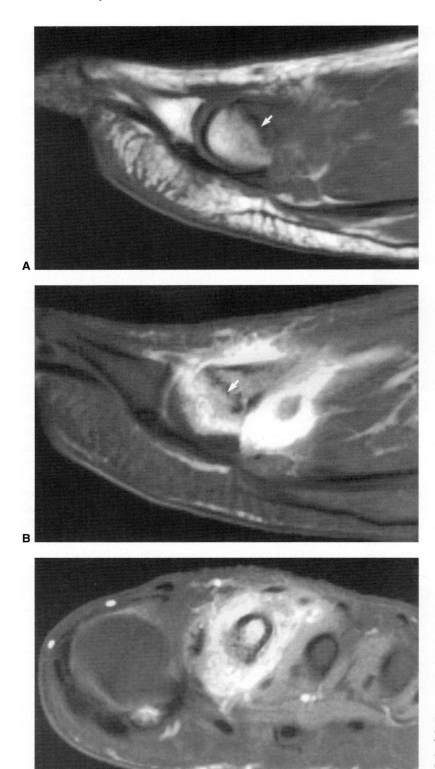

Figure 8-49 Stress fracture of the second metatarsal neck. Sagittal T1- **(A)** and fat-suppressed fast spin-echo T2-weighted **(B)** images demonstrate a fracture line (*arrow*) with marked soft-tissue edema. Axial T2-weighted fast spin-echo image **(C)** shows the extensive soft tissue reaction and early callus formation.

most useful to evaluate early closure or bone bar formation. Physeal injuries will be discussed more completely in Chapter 15. Associated soft tissue injuries, specifically involving the tendons and ligaments, can also be assessed with MRI.

Ligament Injuries

Athletic ankle injuries are common (52,53,116,123). Lateral ankle sprains are reported in 45% of basketball players. In addition, 17% to 25% of lost participation is

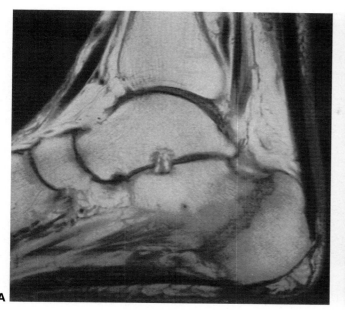 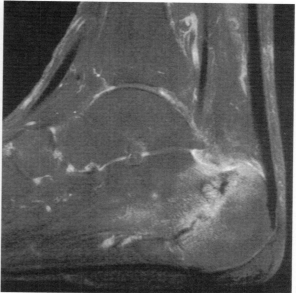

A   B

Figure 8-50 Calcaneal stress fracture. Sagittal T1- **(A)** and fast spin-echo T2-weighted **(B)** images demonstrate a fracture line with marrow edema.

related to ankle sprains. Medial ankle injuries account for 5% and syndesmotic sprains 10% of ankle sprains (114,116). Syndesmotic injury with ankle mortise asymmetry is often associated with a high fibular fracture (4). Ligament injuries are graded 1 to 3. Grade 1 injuries have minimal fiber disruption; grade 2, approximately 50% of the fibers are disrupted; and with grade 3 injuries there is a complete ligament tear (4,37,124,125).

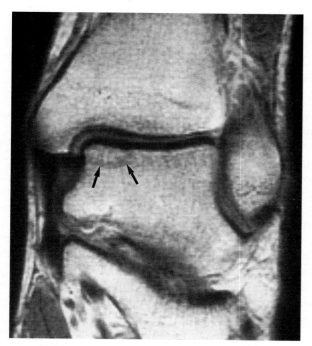

Figure 8-51 Coronal T1-weighted image of the ankle in a patient with a suspected soft tissue injury. The stage I talar dome fracture (*arrows*) is easily identified.

The ligaments, capsule, and major supporting structures of the ankle have been discussed in the anatomic section of this chapter. The anatomic position of the tendons and ligaments in the foot and ankle makes it difficult to align these structures properly in a single MR image plane. Partial volume and magic angle effects can create false positive MR examinations (33,126). Thin section (1 mm) three-dimensional imaging techniques or oblique image planes should be considered (5,33,35). However, in our practice, MRI may not be the initial study used to identify typical ligament sprains and tears about the ankle (5,127).

Before selecting the imaging technique (arthrography, tenography, MRI, or MR arthrography), we must consider the clinical features, type of injury suspected (i.e., one vs. two of lateral ligament complex), and whether operative intervention would be performed if two ligaments were injured in a given patient. Conservative management is selected in most patients even when both the anterior talofibular and calcaneofibular ligaments are injured. Therefore, MRI or invasive studies are only performed in a select group of patients, predominantly athletes (4,114,127).

Conventional MR imaging can be accomplished using coronal and axial images with T2-weighted sequences or three-dimensional, thin-section GRE images. Discontinuity of the ligament is most easily detected (grade 3) (17,128). Thickening and detachment may also be identified with ligament tears. Grade 1 injuries present with subtle thickening and slightly increased signal intensity. Grade 2 lesions are thickened with increased signal intensity involving about 50% of the ligament (5,45,129). Conventional MR imaging is 94% accurate for detection of anterior talofibular and calcaneofibular ligament tears (17). However, accuracy decreases to 59% with chronic tears. Fluid in the peroneal

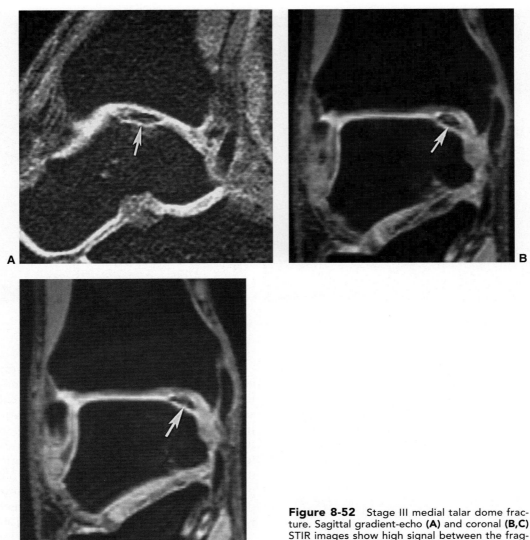

Figure 8-52 Stage III medial talar dome fracture. Sagittal gradient-echo (**A**) and coronal (**B,C**) STIR images show high signal between the fragment and the talus indicating that fluid (*arrow*) extends between the fragment and the talus.

tendon sheaths is commonly seen with lateral ligament tears and fluid in the posterior tibial tendon sheath with medial ligament disruptions (17).

Oae et al. (124) evaluated syndesmotic injury and distal tibiofibular ligament tears. Two criteria were used: ligament discontinuity, and a wavy or nonvisualized ligament. Using the first criteria alone, the sensitivity was 100%, specificity 94%, and accuracy 84% for the distal anterior tibiofibular ligament and 100%, 94%, and 95%, respectively, for the posterior distal tibiofibular ligament. When both criteria were used, the sensitivity was 100% for both the anterior and posterior ligaments. Specificity and accuracy were 100% posteriorly and 93% and 97%, respectively, for the anterior distal tibiofibular ligament (124).

Secondary findings are commonly associated with ankle sprains and chronic instability. These include osseous injuries (bone bruise, etc.), osteochondral fractures, anterolateral and anteromedial impingement, sinus tarsi syndrome, and

tendon tears (116,125,130). Osteochondral injuries most commonly involve the talar dome (Fig. 8-51) (4,116,125).

DiGiovanni et al. (37) identified 15 associated findings in patients with chronic ankle instability. Peroneal tendonitis was noted in 77%, anterolateral impingement in 67%, attenuated retinaculum in 54%, and ankle synovitis in 49%. Loose bodies were evident in 26%, peroneus brevis tears in 25%, and talar dome fractures in 23%.

The value of conventional or MR arthrography is detection and grading of ligament injuries and the frequently associated osseous and tendon injuries (37,124,125,130). Chandnani et al. (21) found MR arthrography superior to conventional MRI and stress radiography for detection of lateral ligament injuries.

Superior flexor retinaculum injuries may be acute or chronic (37). The structure forms the posterior lateral border of the peroneal tunnel and maintains the normal relationship of the peroneal tendons to the fibular groove

(Fig. 8-6) (131). Abnormalities in the retinaculum can result in tendon tears, subluxation, or dislocation.

The normal retinaculum originates from the distal fibula (see Fig. 8-53). With a type I injury, a portion of the retinaculum is stripped from the fibula. Type II injuries are avulsions of the retinaculum. Type III injury demonstrates displacement of the avulsed bone fragment, and with type IV injury there is a retinacular tear (Fig. 8-53).

Axial T2-weighted images can accurately identify the anatomy and categorize the injury (131). The retinaculum should be carefully evaluated in patients with suspected lateral ligament or peroneal tendon injuries (5).

Tendon Injuries

There are 13 tendons that cross the ankle. These include the peroneus brevis and longus laterally; the Achilles tendon posteriorly; the tibialis posterior, flexor digitorum longus, and flexor hallucis longus medially; and anteriorly the tibialis anterior, extensor hallucis longus, tendons of the extensor digitorum longus, and peroneus tertius. All of these tendons are enclosed within tendon sheaths, except the Achilles tendon. Tendon injury may occur as an isolated event, in association with a fracture, or because of previous fracture with degenerative joint disease. Tendons may also rupture on patients undergoing steroid therapy (systemic or direct injection) or with chronic inflammatory diseases. We typically evaluate suspected tendon pathology with T1-weighted spin-echo and FSE T2-weighted sequences in the sagittal and axial planes. The extremity coil is used with the foot in neutral position for evaluation of the Achilles tendon. Excessive plantar flexion buckles the tendon (Fig. 8-2), which exaggerates partial volume effects. Slight plantar flexion (20°) or oblique image planes can be used for examination of the remaining tendons (33,35). T2-weighted sequences clearly demonstrate the high signal intensity of blood or fluid in or about the normally dark tendons. Normally, minimal fluid is noted around these tendons on T2-weighted MR images. For purposes of discussion, it is best to consider each of the tendons separately.

Peroneal Tendons

Peroneal muscles assist in pronation and eversion of the foot. Peroneus brevis tendon is anterior to the peroneus longus as they pass posterior to the lateral malleolus (Figs. 8-3 and 8-23). In approximately 80% of patients, there is a notch in the fibula posteriorly that accommodates a portion of the peroneus brevis. In 20%, this notch is either shallow or absent which may lead to peroneal tendon subluxation. The two peroneal tendons are immediately adjacent to the calcaneofibular ligament between the superior and inferior retinacula, through which they also pass (Fig. 8-23)

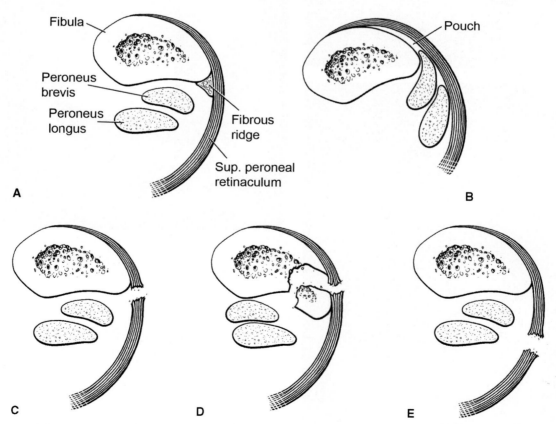

Figure 8-53 Superior peroneal retinacular injuries. **A:** Normal. **B:** Type I, retinaculum stripped from the distal fibula. **C:** Type II, retinacular tear. **D:** Type III, avulsed retinaculum with bone fragment. **E:** Type IV, tear of the posterior attachment.

(44,46,131). Both tendons have a common sheath to the inferior margin of the superior retinaculum. At this point, the sheath divides so that the peroneus longus and peroneus brevis each have their own tendon sheath (see Fig. 8-54). The peroneus brevis passes inferior to the lateral malleolus to insert on the base of the fifth metatarsal (Figs. 8-9 and 8-23). Rademaker et al. (132) reviewed the ankles of 12 adult asymptomatic volunteers in dorsiflexion and plantarflexion.

They found distal extension of the peroneus brevis muscle to or beyond the fibular groove in 11 ankles in dorsiflexion and in seven ankles in plantarflexion. It was concluded extension of the muscle belly of the peroneus brevis into and distal to the fibular groove in part of the normal motion of the muscle (see Fig. 8-55) (132). The peroneus longus progresses inferior to the peroneal tubercle of the calcaneus and passes to the plantar aspect of the foot,

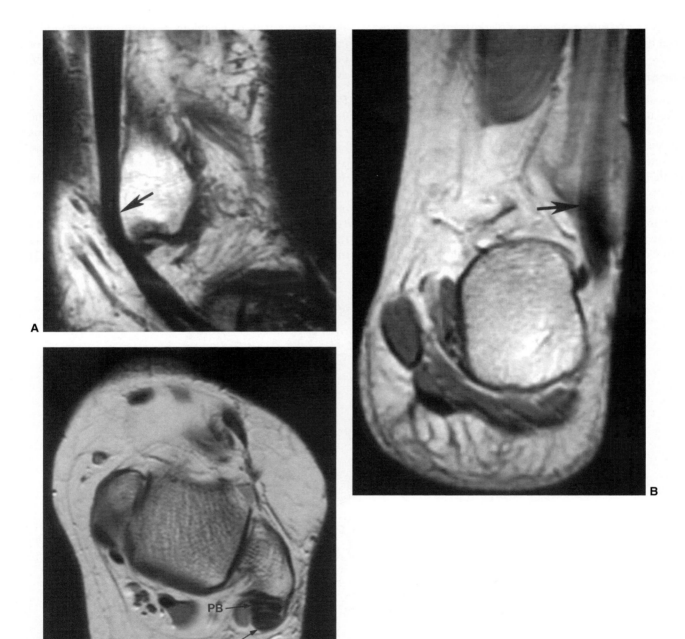

Figure 8-54 MR images of the peroneal tendons in the sagittal **(A),** coronal **(B),** and axial **(C)** planes (*arrow*). *PB*, peroneus brevis; *PL*, peroneus longus.

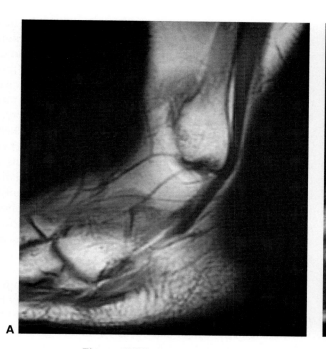
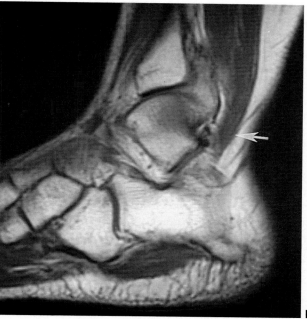

Figure 8-55 Position of the peroneus brevis muscle may vary with foot position. **A:** Normal-appearing tendons with foot slightly plantar flexed. **B:** The muscle extends distally (*arrow*) when the foot is dorsiflexed.

where it inserts in the base of the first metatarsal and medial cuneiform (Fig. 8-31) (5,22,133,134). This portion of the tendon can be difficult to evaluate on MR because of its oblique position. Both peroneal tendons proximal to the base of the fifth metatarsal are easily demonstrated on the axial and sagittal planes using MRI. Oblique planes may be required to evaluate fully the entire extent of the tendons. Diagnosis of inflammatory changes such as tendonitis and subluxation or complete or incomplete disruption can be easily accomplished (5,35,133,134).

Diagnosis of subluxation or dislocation of the peroneal tendons is difficult (see Fig. 8-56). Many patients present with "ankle sprain" or recurrent "giving way" (22,95). Dislocations usually occur with inversion dorsiflexion or abduction dorsiflexion injuries. Patients present with pain and swelling over the lateral malleolus, similar to an ankle sprain. Swelling can make tendon palpation difficult. Though small avulsion fractures of the lateral malleolus have been described, MRI, CT, or tenography are typically required to confirm the diagnosis (4,5,135). There is an increased incidence of subluxation in patients with a deficient superior retinaculum, shallow or convex fibular groove, or prior calcaneal fracture (31,114,129,131). Subluxation is more common in basketball players, skiers, skaters, and soccer players (Fig. 8-56) (17). MRI is most useful as it can also identify the multiple peroneal tendon disorders most effectively.

T2-weighted or T2* GRE sequences are most useful for detection of subtle subluxations or dislocations (4,5). Axial images with internal and external rotation of the foot

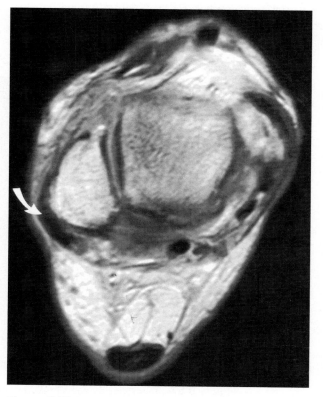

Figure 8-56 Axial proton density-weighted image of the ankle in a patient with chronic peroneal tendon subluxation (*curved arrow*). The tendons lie lateral to the malleolus.

can be accomplished quickly with GRE techniques. Cine images can be produced to simulate motion that allows detection of subtle lesions. This permits tendon pathology and position changes with regard to the fibular notch to be easily assessed. In some cases, comparison with the opposite ankle is useful (5).

Peroneal tenosynovitis is a common overuse injury in athletic individuals (see Fig. 8-57) (129). This condition, along with stenosing tenosynovitis, may also result from displaced calcaneal fractures, enlargement of the peroneal tubercle, and foot deformities (flat foot, tarsal coalition) (17,86,129). MR images demonstrate fluid in the tendon sheath with normal signal intensity in the tendons (see Figs. 8-57 and 8-58). In the case of stenosing tenosynovitis, motion studies may be required to confirm the diagnosis. Tenosynovitis may progress to tendinosis, which demonstrates subtle intermediate signal intensity in the tendon in addition to fluid in the tendon sheath (5,17,31,114).

Ruptures of the peroneal tendon are uncommon. However, this injury is easily overlooked so the true incidence is not known (5,114,131,136–138). Patients present acutely with ankle sprain symptoms or with chronic instability. The latter is more common in patients with arthropathy or patients on systemic steroids. Cavovarus foot deformities and compartment syndromes have also been reported with peroneal tendon rupture. When completely torn, patients are unable to evert the foot (95,139,140).

Peroneal tendon tears have been classified as degenerative, partial, and complete (see Fig. 8-59 and Table 8-4). Most tears are partial with a longitudinal configuration. The mechanism of injury and clinical features for the peroneus longus

and peroneus brevis may vary. Peroneus longus injury may be acute or chronic (see Figs. 8-60 to 8-62). Acute injuries are uncommon and are most often seen in patients with an os peroneum who have inversion injuries with the foot supinated (138). The tear is usually distal to the os peroneum. When the os peroneum is present, the sesamoid may be displaced or avulsed (see Fig. 8-63). In long distance runners, longitudinal tears are more common (114,129). These chronic peroneus longus injuries are usually due to degeneration, resulting in a longitudinal split that usually begins at the lateral malleolar margin and extends proximally and distally. The tear may also occur at the level of the peroneal tubercle on the calcaneus. In addition to tendon morphology and signal intensity changes, one may also see marrow edema in the lateral calcaneus (31,129). Systemic diseases such as diabetes mellitus may also lead to degeneration and peroneus longus tears (139,140).

Peroneus brevis tendon tears are usually longitudinal splits that may extend 2.5–5.0 cm. Multiple splits may be identified at surgery. Schweitzer et al. (50) reviewed MR images of surgically proven peroneal brevis split in 20 ankles. They concluded that peroneal split syndrome (see Fig. 8-64) shows with a high frequency a bisected peroneus brevis tendon, flat or convex fibular groove, and spur on the posterolateral aspect of the fibular groove. Shallow or convex fibular grooves are seen in 95% of peroneus brevis splits (31). Increased fluid in the peroneal tendon sheath was seen in only 55% of these ankles and an hypertrophied peroneus longus tendon in only 15% of these ankles (50). Khoury et al. (140) reviewed MR findings of surgically proven peroneal tendon tears. Increased internal tendon

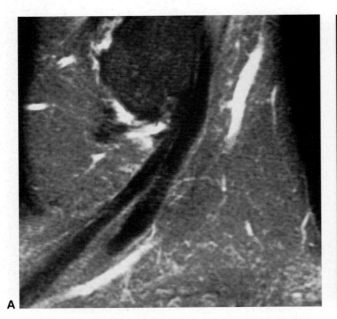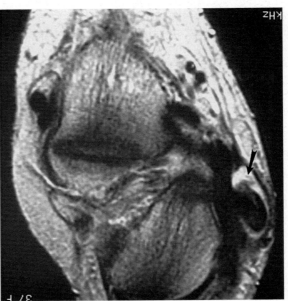

Figure 8-57 Tenosynovitis due to tendon microtrauma. Sagittal fat-suppressed fast spin-echo T2-weighted image **(A)** of the peroneal tendons with minimal fluid in the tendon sheaths. Axial T2-weighted image **(B)** shows fluid about the tendon (*arrow*) with slightly increased signal in the tendon (*arrow*).

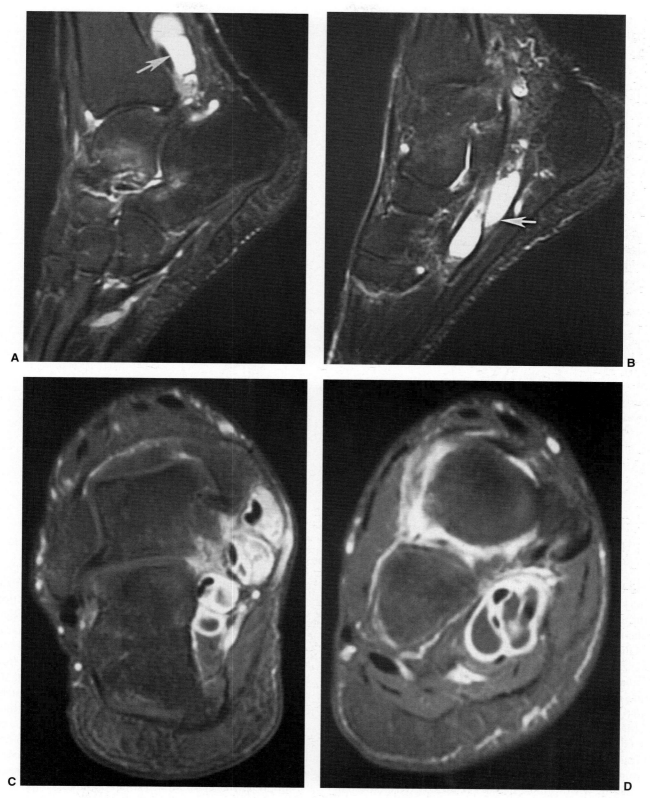

Figure 8-58 Advanced fluid distension of the tendon sheaths. **A,B**: Sagittal fat-suppressed fast spin-echo T2-weighted images demonstrate marked tendon sheath distension (*arrows*). **C**: Axial fat-suppressed fast spin-echo T2-weighted image demonstrates inhomogeneous signal intensity and distension of the tendon sheaths. **D**: Axial fat-suppressed T1-weighted image after gadolinium shows synovial enhancement with low-signal-intensity fluid.

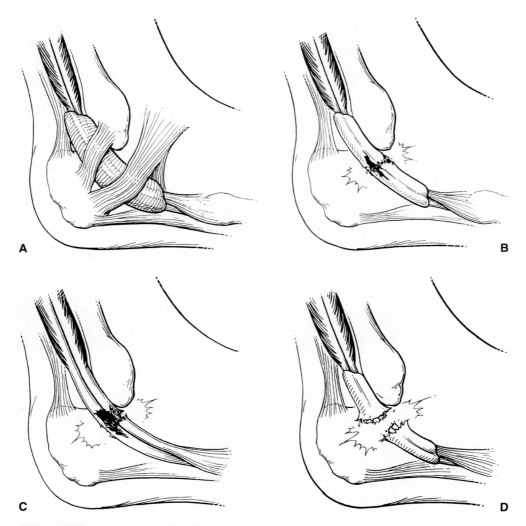

Figure 8-59   Classification of tendon tears. **A:** Tendons intact with tenosynovitis. **B:** Grade 1 tear; minimal fiber disruption. **C:** Grade 2 tear; approximately 50% of fibers are disrupted. **D:** Grade 3 tear; complete disruption of the tendon. (From Berquist TH. Radiology *of the foot and ankle*, 2nd ed. Philadelphia, PA: Lippincott Williams & Wilkins, 2000.)

signal intensity on T1- and T2-weighted images (see Fig. 8-65) was the most common finding in these peroneal tendon tears. Marrow edema in the fibula is not unusual on patients with active pain (31).

Ultrasonography, CT, MRI, and tenography can be used to evaluate peroneal tendon disorders (5,16). For purposes of anatomic display and grading the injury, we find axial and sagittal T2-weighted sequences most useful (Figs. 8-60 and 8-64). Complete ruptures can be identified by absence of the tendon on the axial and sagittal images, with high signal intensity replacing the normally black tendon. Thickening and retraction of the separated tendon ends is commonly noted. Incomplete tears are demonstrated as thickening with variable degrees of increased signal intensity on T2-weighted sequences (Fig. 8-65).

Achilles Tendon

The Achilles tendon is the longest and strongest tendon in the foot and ankle. It originates where the gastrocnemius and soleus tendons join and inserts on the posterior calcaneus (Figs. 8-6, 8-16, and 8-18). In its axial presentation, the tendon thickens as it passes caudally, becoming elliptical with a slightly concave anterior and convex posterior surface (Fig. 8-6). Solia et al. (29) found a wavelike bulge in the anterior aspect of the Achilles tendon that shifted from lateral to medial in the craniocaudal direction in 56 of 100 clinically asymptomatic volunteers (29). The average anteroposterior thickness, measured at the level of greatest thickness, was 5.2 ± 0.73 and the average width measured at 3 cm above the calcaneal corner was 14.7 ± 2.06 (see Fig. 8-66). Two to 6 cm above the ankle, the fibers in the tendon cross. It is at the same level that there is some reduction in the vascular supply. Therefore, many tears of the Achilles tendon occur at this level (5,23,104,141).

There have been multiple approaches to classification of Achilles tendon injuries (17,31,141). Noninsertional (2 to 6 cm proximal to calcaneal insertion) injuries include diffuse acute and chronic peritendinosis, tendinosis, and

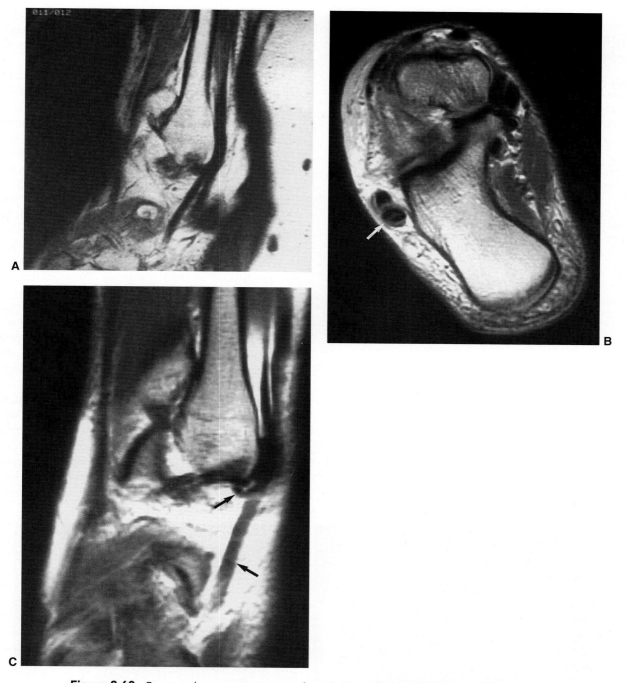

Figure 8-60 Peroneus longus rupture—complete. **A:** Normal sagittal MRI showing the peroneus brevis and longus tendons. **B:** Axial T2-weighted image demonstrates thickening of the peroneus longus (*arrow*). **C:** Sagittal T1-weighted image with complete rupture of the peroneus longus shows the normal peroneus brevis (*lower arrow*) and ruptured end of the peroneus longus (*upper arrow*).

rupture. Insertional Achilles tendinosis may be associated with Haglund deformity (see Fig. 8-67) (17,141).

The Achilles tendon has no sheath. However, there is a vascular peritenon that extends into the tendon substance. Inflammation of the peritenon results in edema in the pre-Achilles fat and linear increased signal intensity about the tendon, usually anteriorly. Inflammation may be associated with conditions such as rheumatoid arthritis. Inflammation

may also be associated with retrocalcaneal bursitis (see Fig. 8-68). These inflammatory changes are easily appreciated on axial and sagittal T2-weighted sequences (5,17,141).

Tendinosis is preferred to tendonitis due to the degenerative nature of the process. Four degenerative histologic patterns have been described (17,31,141). These include hypoxic fibromatosis, lipoid, myxoid, and calcific or ossific degeneration. The first is the most common and occurs in

TABLE 8-4
MRI FEATURES OF TENDON INJURIES

Injury Category	MR Features
Acute complete tear (grade 3)	Tendon ends separated completely with ↑ signal intensity between segments on T2-weighted sequences. Fluid in tendon sheaths.
Acute partial tear (grades 1–2)	Tendon thickening with increased signal intensity ≤50% of tendon thickness on T2-weighted sequences.
Chronic partial tear or tendinosis	Tendon thickened with intermediate signal on T1-weighted and proton density images that does not ↑ significantly on T2-weighted images.
Tenosynovitis	Tendon normal to slightly thickened. Fluid in tendon sheath with ↑ signal surrounding tendon on T2-weighted sequences.

the critical zone related to vascular ischemia (31,104,141). This results in low-signal-intensity thickening proximal (2 to 6 cm) to the calcaneal insertion (see Fig. 8-69).

Myxoid degeneration is the second most common tendinosis. Patients are frequently asymptomatic. MR images demonstrate thickening with areas of increased signal intensity on T2-weighted and STIR sequences (see Fig. 8-70) (141).

Lipoid degeneration occurs in older patients and is also frequently asymptomatic. This form of degeneration must be differentiated from xanthomas. The latter is related to metabolic disorders, such as lipoproteinemias (141).

Calcific or ossific tendinosis is only seen in about 3% of patients with tendon tears. Calcification or ossification in the tendon may be obvious radiographically (141).

The Achilles tendon, though one of the strongest, is commonly torn (4,5,23,104,141). Tears may be microscopic, interstitial, partial, or complete. Ruptures are usually the result of indirect trauma. The injury can occur during any athletic activity and at any age. Generally, ruptures occur in strenuous activities while the foot is plantar flexed or during raising up on the toes such as with pushing off or jumping with the knee extended. In nonathletes, the injury is most common in 30- to 50-year-old patients (5,31,104). Certain systemic and local conditions may also predispose to tendon rupture. These include gout, systemic lupus erythematosus, rheumatoid arthritis, hyperparathyroidism, chronic renal failure, systemic or local steroids, and diabetes mellitus (5,142–145). Patients on systemic steroids or with systemic diseases may have spontaneous rupture of both Achilles tendons. Local steroid injections may also lead to partial or complete disruption of the Achilles tendon (5,142).

Clinically, patients generally present with pain, local swelling, and inability to raise up on their toes on the affected side. If completely torn, a palpable defect may be noted on physical exam; however, clinical exam is not always accurate. Misdiagnosis of complete tears occurs in 25% of patients (17). Failure to diagnose these lesions clinically occurs because a gap in the tendon may not be

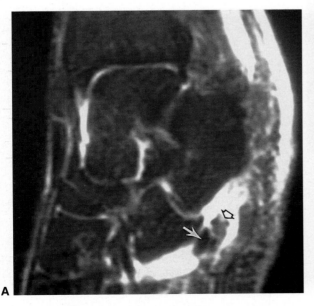
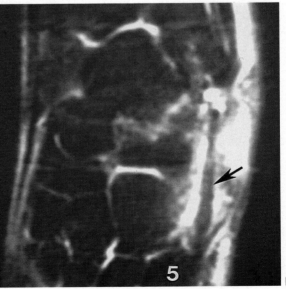

Figure 8-61 Oblique coronal STIR image **(A)** demonstrates extensive soft tissue injury with a torn peroneus longus (*open arrow*) near the os peroneum (*white arrow*). Oblique STIR image **(B)** on different plane demonstrates the intact peroneus brevis (*arrow*) inserting on the base of the fifth metatarsal (5).

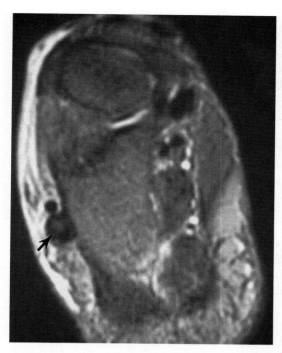

Figure 8-62 Axial T2-weighted image demonstrates thickening with increased signal intensity in the peroneus longus tendon (*arrow*).

palpable and patients may be able to plantar flex the foot with the toes. Differentiation from venous thrombosis, gastrocnemius, and plantaris tears may be difficult (5,140). Therefore, examination of the calf may be required when images of the Achilles tendon are normal.

Imaging of the Achilles tendon can be accomplished using several approaches, including soft tissue radiographic techniques, ultrasound (see Fig. 8-71), CT, and MRI (5,17, 31,142). Astrom et al. (146) compared ultrasonography, MRI, and surgical findings in 27 histologically verified cases of chronic Achilles tendinopathy. Ultrasonography was positive in 21 of 26 and MRI in 26 of 27 cases. Evaluation of the peritenon was unreliable with ultrasound and MRI in their series. Though all of these techniques can be useful in given situations, we find MRI most useful for detection of subtle lesions and also in following the healing process on patients with partial or complete tears (5).

T1- and T2-weighted (with or without fat suppression) or STIR axial and sagittal images provide excellent anatomy and good contrast (fluid, hemorrhage, high intensity against normal black appearance of tendons) with normal soft tissue structures (5,104,141). We usually begin with a sagittal scout, choose the axial levels, and then use the axial images to obtain optimal sagittal images of the tendon (5).

MRI is accurate in demonstrating partial (see Figs. 8-72 to 8-74) and complete (see Figs. 8-75 and 8-77) tears, following healing (see Figs. 8-77 to 8-79), and differentiating tendon tears from venous thrombosis (see Fig. 8-80) or gastrocnemius muscle tears. The latter should be excluded in

patients with clinically suspected Achilles tendon tear and normal MR examinations of the ankle. T1- and T2-weighted axial images of both calves in the prone position (avoids tissue compression) and contrast-enhanced images provide a complete screening examination in this clinical setting. New MR angiographic techniques are more effective for demonstrating thrombus (18,19,147).

Conservative (cast immobilization in plantar flexion) or surgical management is based upon the extent of tear and tendon retraction. Baseline MR images are important with either approach to optimize follow-up evaluations. Also, if the tendon ends are not approximated with cast immobilization, the treatment will fail (Fig. 8-79). With healing, the signal intensity returns to normal, though thickening persists (17,141).

Medial Tendons

The posterior tibial, flexor digitorum longus, and flexor hallucis longus tendons make up the medial tendon group. These tendons are located anterior to posterior in the above order (see Figs. 8-6, 8-9, and 8-81). The posterior tibial tendon (PTT), with its tendon sheath, passes just posterior to the medial malleolus, lateral to the flexor retinaculum, and broadens at its insertion in the navicular tuberosity and base of the medial cuneiform (see Figs. 8-31, 8-42, and 8-82). Keep in mind the magic angle effect can cause subtle signal intensity increase in areas where tendons expand at the insertion (126). The flexor digitorum longus takes a similar course proximally, lying between the posterior tibial tendon and posterior tibial artery (Fig. 8-81). As it turns toward the plantar aspect of the foot, it passes superficially to the flexor hallucis longus before dividing into tendon slips that insert in the bases of the second through fifth distal phalanges (Figs. 8-6, 8-9, and 8-29). The flexor hallucis longus tendon is located more posteriorly and laterally (Fig. 8-81). It passes through a fibro-osseous tunnel beneath the sustentaculum tali and along the medial plantar aspect of the foot to insert in the base of the distal phalanx of the great toe (Figs. 8-6, 8-9, and 8-29) (31,44,46).

The PTT is the most commonly injured of the three medial tendons (5,55,139,148–150). Risk factors include obesity, hypertension, gout, rheumatoid arthritis, and Reiter syndrome (31). Patients with an accessory navicular are also at risk (129).

PTT dysfunction is a continuum of processes that include tenosynovitis, tendinosis, and partial and complete tears (31,55,151). Tenosynovitis is the initial phase due to chronic overuse. Fluid of 2 mm or more surrounding the tendon sheath is identified on MR images with normal signal intensity in the tendon (see Fig. 8-83). With continued overuse, tendinosis occurs, resulting in subtle increased signal intensity in the PTT at the level of the medial malleolus on T1- and proton density images (see Fig. 8-84). Signal intensity does not increase or may be less evident on T2-weighted images. With progression, partial or complete tears may develop (5,31,129,151).

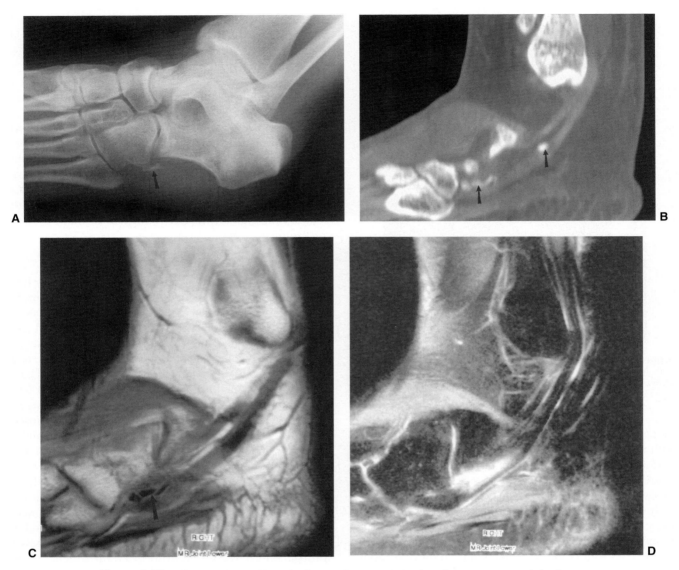

Figure 8-63   Oblique radiograph **(A)** and sagittal CT image **(B)** show fragmentation and displacement of the os peroneum (*arrows*). Sagittal T1- **(C)** and T2-weighted **(D)** MR images demonstrate abnormal signal intensity in the peroneus longus with low intensity (*arrow*) fragments due to a peroneus longus tear.

Patients generally present with pain, local tenderness, and swelling, and physical examination may reveal a non-palpable tendon. Rupture of the PTT can lead to progressive flatfoot deformity, inability to raise up on the toes, and weakness on inversion of the foot (5,31,140,149).

Standing lateral radiographs of the foot may demonstrate collapse of the arch on patients with medial tendon injuries (4,5). Tenography can be accomplished, though this is difficult depending upon the experience of the examiner. Evaluation of the medial tendons can be accomplished with ultrasound, CT, and MRI. As with the other tendons, in our experience MRI has been most useful in assessing the nature and degree of tendon pathology (4,5,22).

PTT tears (see Fig. 8-85) have been classified by Rosenberg et al. (152) using MRI and CT findings. Type 1

tears are incomplete with tendon thickening and vertical slits in the tendon. The tendon appears thickened with scattered areas of high signal intensity on T2-weighted images (Fig. 8-85). Type 2 injuries are partial tears with areas of attenuation in the tendon. This has the appearance of a thinned area on axial and sagittal images. When the tendon is completely torn (type 3) (see Fig. 8-86), there is a gap in the tendon that will be seen clearly on axial and sagittal images. The tendon will be absent on axial images (see Fig. 8-87). Older tears may have reduced signal intensity, for granulation tissue begins to form about 2 weeks after injury (153). This has more intermediate signal intensity on T2-weighted sequences. Axial and sagittal images (see Fig. 8-88) can be obtained on both feet and ankles using the head coil. Comparison (Fig. 8-88) is useful for

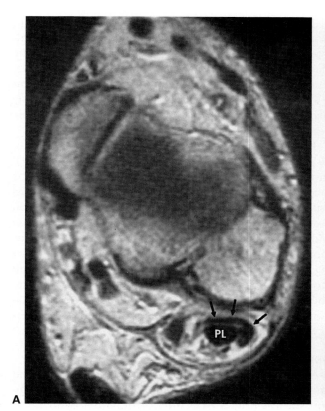

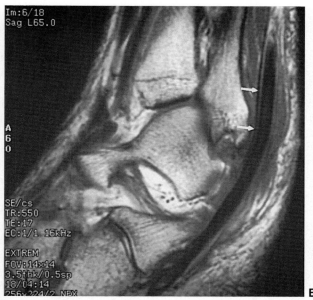

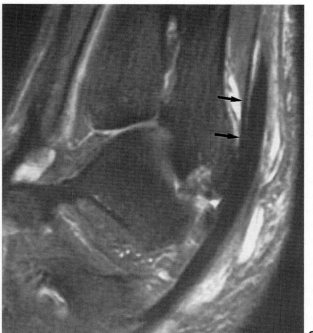

Figure 8-64 **(A)** Axial proton density-weighted image demonstrates a peroneus brevis split with flattening (*arrows*) anterior to the peroneus longus (*PL*). Sagittal T1-weighted **(B)** and fat-suppressed T2-weighted **(C)** images show the thin peroneus brevis (*arrows*) and soft tissue inflammation.

subtle injuries and to evaluate bilateral involvement that is not uncommon (5,16,152).

Bencardino et al. (154) looked at the MR imaging appearance of seven cases of PTT dislocation and subluxation. The tendon was dislocated medial to the medial malleolus in five of the seven patients. The flexor retinaculum was torn from its medial malleolar insertion in five patients and torn in two patients. A shallow retromalleolar groove can be a cause for PTT dislocation.

The spring ligament (plantar calcaneonavicular ligament) is not routinely identified on axial and sagittal MR images. However, this ligament is important to assess when

evaluating patients with PTT dysfunction, as it provides additional stability for the longitudinal arch (see Fig. 8-89) (5,44,55). Therefore, the status of the spring ligament is important for surgical planning (4,5,55).

Yao et al. (155) evaluated MR images of 13 cases of surgically proven spring ligament insufficiency and in 18 control volunteers. They found increased heterogeneous signal on short TE spin-echo images and increase in thickness of the medial portion of the spring ligament in spring ligament insufficiency. The sensitivity and specificity of MRI for the diagnosis of spring ligament insufficiency was 54% to 77% and 100%, respectively.

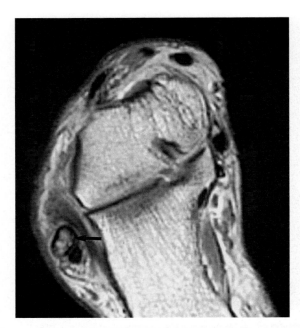

Figure 8-65 Incomplete tear of the peroneus brevis tendon. Axial proton density-weighted image shows local thickening with increased signal intensity (*arrow*) in the tendon.

Secondary signs of posterior tibial tendon dysfunction have also been described. A talonavicular fault results in excessive plantar flexion of the navicular that can be identified on lateral radiographs or sagittal MR images (31,156). Heel valgus may also be evident on coronal MR images (see Fig. 8-90). Tibial–calcaneal alignment is normally 0° to 6° valgus. Focal tibial osteophytes and an unopposed peroneus brevis leading to lateral shift of the midfoot may also be evident (156). The presence of an accessory navicular also predisposes patients to posterior tibial tendon dysfunction (129). Patients may also have associated sinus tarsi syndrome. Patients with advanced posterior tibial tendon dysfunction also have spring ligament abnormalities (97%), sinus tarsi syndrome (77%) and plantar fasciitis (37%). Two or more of these features were evident in 80% of patients (55).

Flexor Digitorum Longus and Flexor Hallucis Longus Tendons

Injuries to the flexor hallucis longus and flexor digitorum longus occur less frequently compared to the PTT (31,114). Flexor hallucis tenosynovitis occurs in the talar tunnel as the tendon passes between the medial and lateral talar tubercles. Tenosynovitis occurs most commonly after repetitive full plantar flexion. This activity is common in ballet dancers and soccer players (17,129). Left untreated, stenosing tenosynovitis and fibrosis may develop. Inflammatory changes may also occur as the tendon passes between the sesamoids at the level of the first metatarsal head (17,114).

T2-weighted images demonstrate significant fluid around the tendon. The medial tendon sheaths communicate with the ankle joint in 20% of patients. Therefore, the diagnosis should be made with caution unless there is distention of the tendon sheath or no ankle effusion (17,129). Tenosynovitis of the flexor hallucis longus may also be associated with os trigonum syndrome and the flexor digitorum longus accessory muscle (17).

Ruptures of the flexor digitorum longus and flexor hallucis longus tendons (see Fig. 8-91) are uncommon (157). However, Garth did report rupture of the flexor hallucis longus in ballet dancers and soccer players (157). Patients usually present with swelling, tenderness, and crepitation near the sustentaculum tali. Symptoms generally increase with flexion and extension of the great toe. Tenography, though possible for the posterior tibial tendon and flexor digitorum longus, is much more difficult for the deep and more posteriorly located flexor hallucis longus tendon. Therefore, MRI (Fig. 8-91) is the ideal technique for evaluation of this structure. Image features are similar regardless of which tendon is being evaluated (5,157).

Anterior Tendons

Anteriorly, the anterior tibial, extensor hallucis longus, and extensor digitorum longus tendons are all enclosed in tendon sheaths (Fig. 8-81). Anterior tibial tenosynovitis is uncommon and ruptures are rare (158). Tenosynovitis is seen in downhill runners and hikers (129).

The anterior tibial tendon accounts for 80% of dorsiflexion of the foot. However, following disruption weakness may be difficult to detect clinically and a limp is unusual. Therefore, diagnosis is often delayed or overlooked (158,159).

Anterior tibial tendon tears are categorized as acute or chronic. Acute tears are related to laceration or tibial shaft fractures. Acute on chronic are associated with tendon degeneration due to overuse, inflammatory arthropathies, or prior steroid injections (158,159). Tears occur with forced plantar flexion in middle-age or elderly patients. The tear is typically located at the level of the inferior extensor retinactulum 0.5 to 3 cm proximal to the insertion. The proximal remnant retracts and appears thickened on MR images (5,129,158,159). Clinically patients present with pain and swelling over the anterior ankle. There may also be decreased ability to dorsiflex the foot on physical examination (5,129,158,159).

Though other radiographic techniques can be utilized to demonstrate the anterior tendons, specifically ultrasound, we prefer MRI (see Figs. 8-92 to 8-94) to determine the extent of injury and also follow patients who are treated conservatively and surgically. T2-weighted or STIR sequences in the axial and sagittal planes are preferred. The increased signal intensity of the fluid and hemorrhage seen against the black or low signal of the tendon makes identification and staging easier to accomplish (5,158,159).

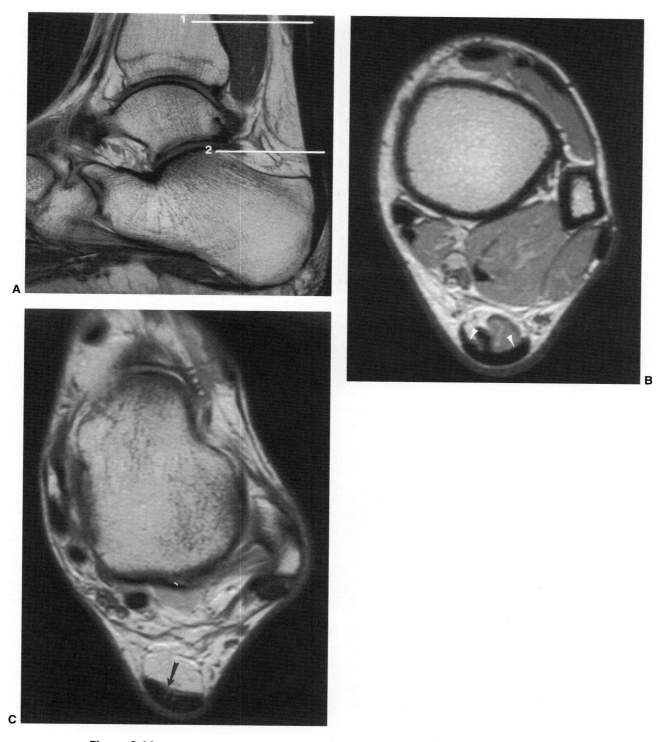

Figure 8-66   Normal MR anatomy of the Achilles tendon. Sagittal MR image **(A)** demonstrating levels for axial images of the Achilles tendon. Axial image at level 1 **(B)** shows a concave anterior border (*white arrowheads*). The soleus muscle is still evident. Axial image at level 2 **(C)** shows the tendon (*arrow*) contrasted against the high-intensity pre-Achilles fat.

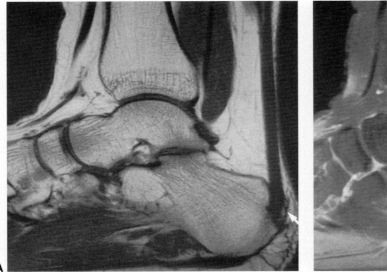

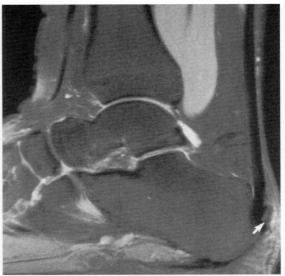

Figure 8-67 Retro-Achilles bursitis. Sagittal T1-weighted **(A)** and fat-suppressed fast spin-echo T2-weighted **(B)** images demonstrate heterotopic ossification and calcification in the retro-Achilles bursa (*arrow*) with associated soft-tissue inflammation.

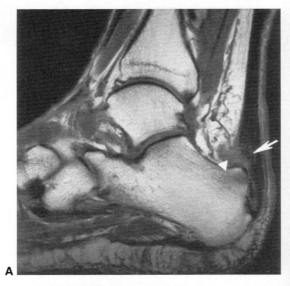

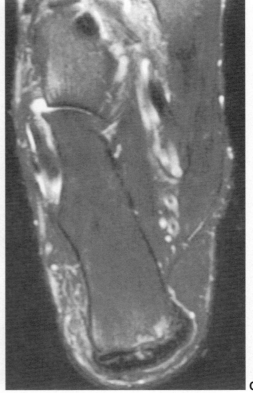

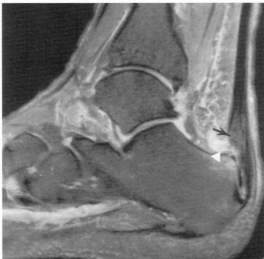

Figure 8-68 Retrocalcaneal bursitis with Achilles tendon thickening and inflammation. Sagittal T1-weighted **(A)** and sagittal **(B)** and axial **(C)** T2-weighted images demonstrate an inflamed distended bursa (*arrowhead*) and thickening and increased signal intensity in the adjacent Achilles tendon (*arrow*).

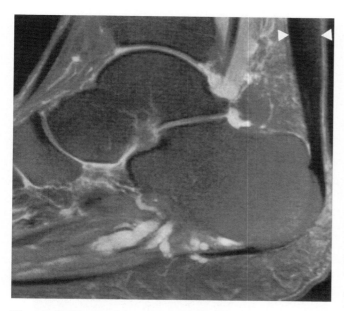

Figure 8-69 Tendinosis (hypoxic fibromatosis). Sagittal fat-suppressed fast spin-echo T2-weighted image shows low-signal-intensity thickening (*arrowheads*) proximal to the insertion.

Surgical repair is optimal for treatment of anterior tibial tendon ruptures. Left untreated, 25.5% of patients have long-term adverse results. Sequelae include neuromas and extensor substitution with claw and hammer toe deformities (158).

MISCELLANEOUS DISORDERS AND OVERUSE SYNDROMES

There are numerous syndromes and traumatic conditions that involve the ankle, hindfoot, midfoot, and forefoot. Disorders will be reviewed by location, since symptoms related to anatomic regions may be caused by multiple conditions that can be confused clinically (5,139,160–162).

Heel Pain

There are numerous causes of heel pain (160). Etiologies include trauma, neoplasms, inflammatory disorders, and systemic diseases (Table 8-5) (4,5,106).

Bursitis

There are two bursae (see Fig. 8-95) near the Achilles insertion (5,46,47,106). The retrocalcaneal bursa lies between the Achilles and posterior calcaneal angle. The retro-Achilles or subcutaneous bursa is subcutaneous just posterior to the Achilles tendon (44,46,106). Calcaneal bursae inflammation is not uncommon (Fig. 8-95) (5,163). MRI is very useful for detection of these inflammatory changes. As noted previously, T2-weighted axial and sagittal images need to be obtained with the foot in neutral and plantar flexed positions. Normally, the pre-Achilles fat fills in the space between the tendon and calcaneus during plantar flexion (see Fig. 8-96). When the anterior bursa is inflamed, this does not occur (Fig. 8-68). Also, a well-defined area of high signal intensity may be seen due to a fluid-filled distended bursa (163). Bursal calcification or ossification is seen as a defined focus of "no signal intensity" (5). MRI is preferred to evaluate the bursae, Achilles tendon, and adjacent bony changes. Early changes with only small amounts of fluid in the bursa are most easily detected with the foot slightly plantar flexed (see Fig. 8-97). Sagittal and axial T2-weighted images are optimal for evaluating the bursa, Achilles tendon, and associated osseous changes (see Figs. 8-98 to 8-99) (5,106,163).

Plantar Fasciitis

The plantar aponeurosis is composed of medial, lateral and central components (5,44,47,66,164). The plantar fascia (aponeurosis) extends distally from its origin on the posteromedial calcaneal tuberosity (see Fig. 8-100). The central component is the thickest (2 to 4 mm) and strongest. The central portion divides into five bands at the mid-metatarsal level. Proximal to the metatarsal heads, these bands divide into superficial and deep tracts. Distally, the tracts attach to the flexor tendons. The medial component extends to form the fascia of the abductor hallucis. The lateral band consists of four distinct bands. The peroneal component extends toward the cuboid where it divides into medial and lateral components. The lateral component is stronger and inserts on the base of the fifth metatarsal. The medial band extends distally to insert on the plantar plate of the third or fourth metatarsophalangeal joint. The lateral band may also be incomplete or absent (44,46,165).

Prolonged pronation stresses and repetitive microtrauma during heel strike lead to degeneration and inflammation of the central component (164,165). Plantar fasciitis is a chronic, potentially disabling condition that must be differentiated from other causes of posterior heel pain. It is the most common cause of plantar heel pain (5,164–167). Calcaneal stress fractures, tarsal tunnel syndrome, or medial calcaneal neuritis and seronegative arthropathies must be considered in the differential diagnosis (5,166).

Plantar fasciitis is a common overuse injury in running and jumping athletes. The condition accounts for 7% to 9% of all running injuries (129). Repetitive microtrauma leads to microtears near the calcaneal attachment, resulting in an inflammatory response with angiofibroblastic hyperplasia and eventually calcification in the affected fascia (129,165,167). Predisposing factors include pes planus, pes cavus, a tight Achilles tendon, and suboptimal foot wear (129,166). Systemic diseases including rheumatoid arthritis, gout, and spondyloarthropathies also cause inflammation of the plantar fascia (166).

Radiographs may demonstrate plantar enthesophytes, distortion of tissue planes, and fascial calcification (see Fig. 8-101) (5,17,114). Enthesophytes are common (25% to 37%) in patients with fasciitis, but many asymptomatic

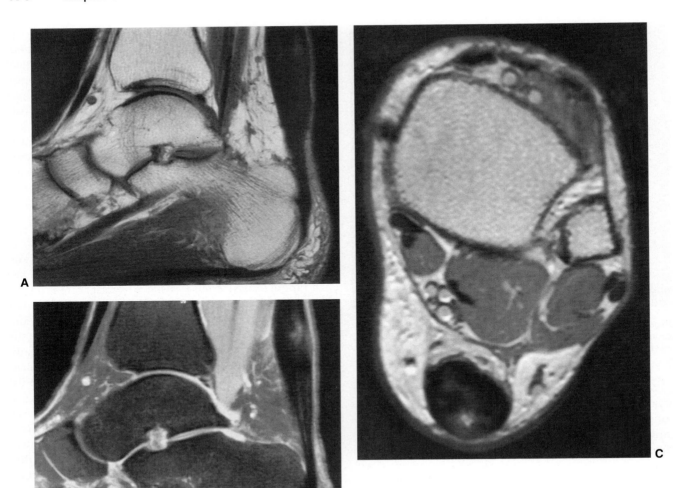

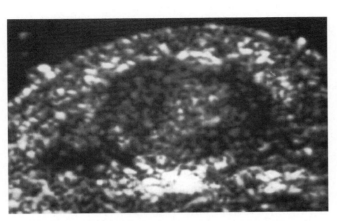

Figure 8-70 Myxoid tendinosis. Sagittal T1- **(A)** and T2-weighted **(B)** and axial proton density-weighted **(C)** images demonstrate thickening 6 cm proximal to the insertion with central increased signal intensity.

Figure 8-71 Transverse sonogram of an acute Achilles tendon tear with hemorrhage.

patients also demonstrate this finding (see Fig. 8-102) (17,114). Though radionuclide bone scans may demonstrate increased tracer, MRI is superior for diagnosis (see Figs. 8-103 and 8-104) of plantar fasciitis and to exclude other conditions that may mimic plantar fasciitis (5,114,166). The foot should be in neutral position for the examination (5,164). Coronal and sagittal images using T2-weighted or STIR sequences are most useful (see Figs. 8-100 and 8-105) (5,164,166). Plantar fasciitis is demonstrated by the infiltrative high signal intensity in the plantar fascia (Figs. 8-103 through 8-105). There is also increased signal intensity in the tissues superior and inferior to the fascia (5,17).

Grasel et al. (164) reviewed the MR imaging findings of plantar fasciitis in 25 patients with clinical diagnosis, MR examinations, and clinical follow-up. They found the most

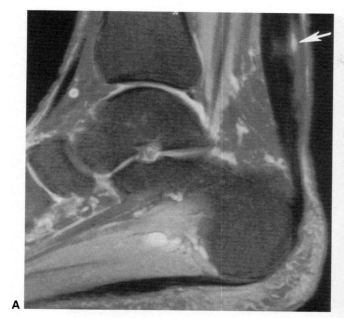

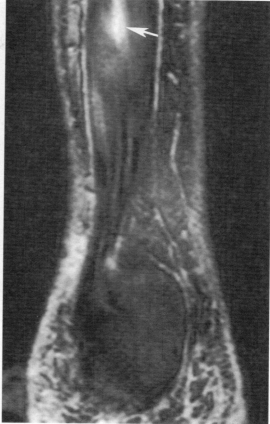

B

Figure 8-72 Sagittal fast spin-echo T2-weighted **(A)** and coronal DESS **(B)** images demonstrate thickening of the Achilles tendon with focal increased signal intensity (*arrow*) due to a low grade tear.

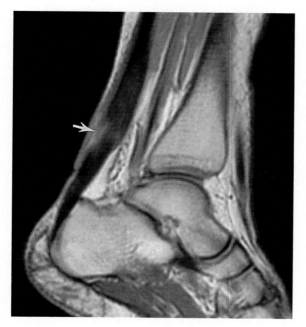

Figure 8-73 Sagittal proton density-weighted image demonstrating thickening of the Achilles tendon with a grade 1 (few fibers torn) tear (*arrow*) in the Achilles tendon.

common MR finding of plantar fasciitis was perifascial edema, superficial and deep to the plantar fascia (Figs. 8-104 and 8-105). The second most common finding was abnormal marrow edema in the calcaneus at the plantar insertion site. The third most common finding was increased signal intensity within the plantar fascia on STIR images. The least common finding in their series was plantar fascia thickening (>5mm) (see Fig. 8-106).

Partial or complete rupture of the plantar fascia is easily appreciated on T2-weighted or STIR images (see Fig. 8-107). Contrast enhancement is usually of little value (5,165).

Treatment of fasciitis is usually conservative. Surgical repair is reserved for patients that fail conservative approaches and athletes. Surgical success is reported at 90% to 95% (129,167–169).

Yu et al. (167,169) studied the MR appearance of subjects with previous fasciotomies for treatment of chronic plantar fasciitis. They found the mean thickness of the plantar fascia at the site of surgery in these asymptomatic subjects after surgery was two to three times that of normal. However, the changes in signal intensity were most prominent at the enthesis. There was absence of edema in the fascia and perifascial soft tissues in the asymptomatic volunteers (169). Up to 25% demonstrate a persistent gap after fasciotomy. Patients with recurrent symptoms

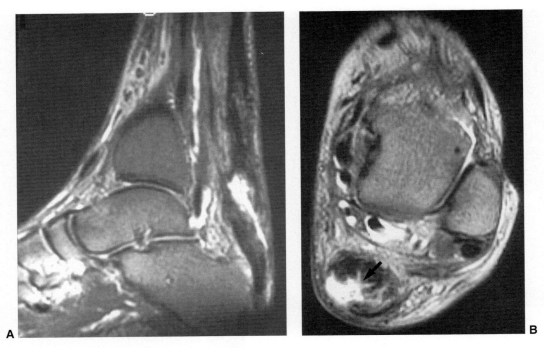

Figure 8-74 Sagittal **(A)** and axial **(B)** T2-weighted images demonstrating a high grade tear of the Achilles tendon (*arrow*).

demonstrate MR features similar to pre-operative fasciotomy findings (167).

Tarsal Tunnel Syndrome

Tarsal tunnel syndrome is a compression neuropathy of the posterior tibial nerve as it passes through the tarsal tunnel.

The tarsal tunnel (see Fig. 8-108) is bordered medially by the flexor retinaculum and laterally by the calcaneus and talus. The tunnel extends from above the medial malleolus to the abductor hallucis muscle inferiorly (103,106,170).

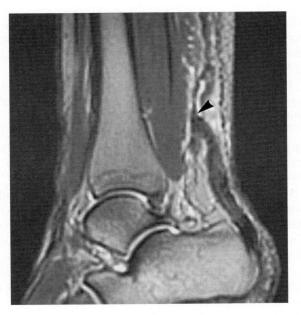

Figure 8-75 Sagittal T2-weighted image shows a "wavy," lax Achilles tendon (*arrowhead*) due to a complete tear.

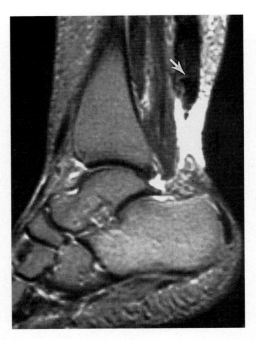

Figure 8-76 Complete Achilles tendon tear. Sagittal T2-weighted image of the ankle demonstrates high signal intensity with thickening and retraction of the proximal fragment (*arrow*) commonly seen with complete tears.

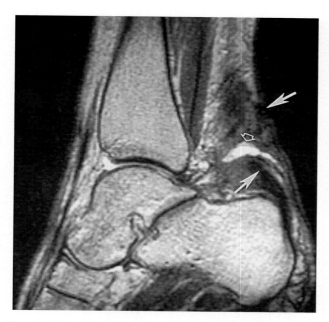

Figure 8-77 Old complete tear of the Achilles tendon. Note the distal end (*lower arrow*), proximal end (*upper arrow*) with inflammatory changes in the fat, and active hemorrhage or edema (*open arrow*) in the tendon gap.

The posterior tibial nerve can be compressed by varicosities, ganglion cysts, edema, synovial hypertrophy, tarsal coalition, muscle anomalies, or acquired (including trauma) bone and soft tissue abnormalities (119,171–173). There are several septi within the tarsal tunnel that reduce the volume of the compartments so that smaller lesions can also compress the nerve (103).

The diagnosis of tarsal tunnel syndrome is usually made on the basis of history and physical examination. Pain, paresthesias, and motor function reduction in muscles supplied by the posterior tibial nerve are usually present. Unlike carpal tunnel syndrome, the condition is most often unilateral. Pressure on the nerve, percussion of the nerve, or sustained inversion and eversion of the foot may reproduce the symptoms (17,103,106). Electromyographic techniques and MRI are useful confirmatory studies. Axial T1-weighted MR images (see Fig. 8-109) provide excellent anatomic detail. The axial plane with supplementary sagittal and/or coronal images may provide additional information. T2-weighted or STIR images are required to identify and characterize the pathology (see Figs. 8-110 and 8-111) (53,86). Gadolinium can be used to differentiate solid from cystic lesions and better define varicosities (Fig. 8-111).

Pfeiffer and Cracchiolo (173) found dilated veins (Fig. 8-110) to be the most frequent operative explanation for nerve compression. Identification of a definite space-occupying lesion is the best indication for operative intervention (106). In 50% of cases, no cause can be identified.

Sinus Tarsi Syndrome

The tarsal canal and sinus extend in a posteromedial to anterolateral course at an angle of approximately 45 degrees to the calcaneal axis (see Fig. 8-112) (20,128). The tarsal canal and sinus is a cone-shaped structure, larger laterally, that lies between the posterior subtalar joint and the talocalcaneonavicular joint anteriorly (Fig. 8-112) (24, 162,174). The contents of the canal include fat, neurovascular structures, and five ligaments that support talocalcaneal alignment and restrict inversion (174). The ligaments include the medial, intermediate, and the cervical ligament and the ligament of the tarsal canal (Fig. 8-113) (162,174). Sinus tarsi syndrome is usually due to inversion injuries (70%), and 79% have associated lateral ligament tears (162,174,175). Also, 10% of patients with lateral ankle instability have subtalar instability (116,123).

Seventy percent of patients with sinus tarsi syndrome have a history of trauma. The remaining 30% develop the syndrome secondary to inflammatory arthropathies, gout, ganglion cysts, and foot deformities (129). There are also commonly associated injuries. Tears in the anterior talofibular ligament are seen in 43% and posterior tibial tendon tears in 47% of patients with sinus tarsi syndrome (148). Patients with advanced posterior tibial tendon dysfunction have associated spring ligament tears (95%) and sinus tarsi syndrome (72%) (55).

Patients with sinus tarsi syndrome usually present with a history of inversion injury, lateral foot pain, and tenderness to palpation over the tarsal canal. Identification of ligament injury in the tarsal canal and sinus is especially important if surgical repair of the lateral ankle ligaments is planned (162,174,176). Other conditions such as arthropathy, subtalar capsular hypertrophy, and space-occupying lesions must be excluded.

Imaging of the tarsal canal and sinus can be accomplished with routine radiographs, subtalar arthrography, CT, and MRI (4,5). Subtalar arthrography and diagnostic injections are useful to localize the symptoms to the tarsal canal (5). In our practice, we prefer MRI, which can be accomplished using T1- and T2-weighted sequences.

Klein and Spreitzer (174) described the normal and abnormal MR features of this condition (see Fig. 8-113). Images in all three planes (axial, coronal, and sagittal) may be required to define the anatomy (see Fig. 8-114). Both T1- and T2-weighted sequences should be obtained. Infiltrative changes in the tarsal canal and sinus were evident using these sequences (see Figs. 8-115 through 8-117). A calcaneofibular ligament tear was evident in 80% and fluid collections in the tarsal sinus in 15% of patients (174).

Breitenseher et al. (36) compared MRI and stress radiography to evaluate the extent of recent lateral ankle inversion injuries in 60 athletic patients. Surgery demonstrated MR to have 74% sensitivity and 100% specificity for the detection of complete lateral ankle ligament tears. Their study revealed

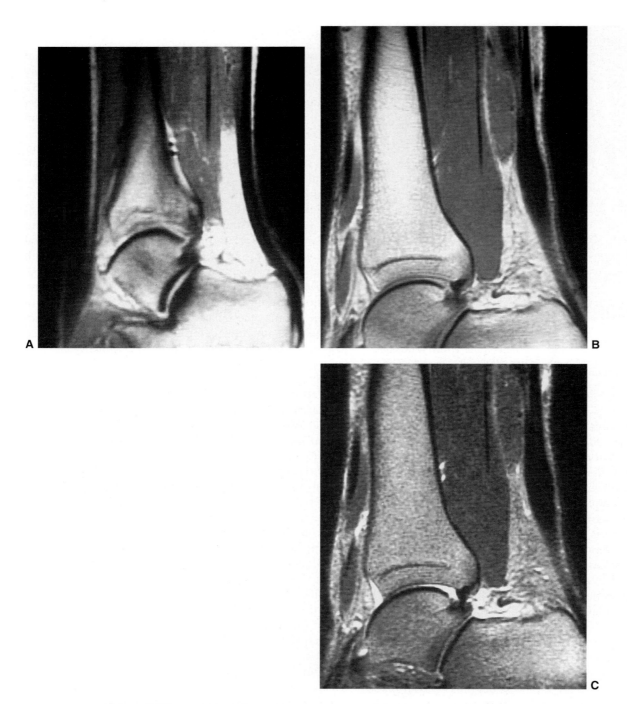

Figure 8-78   Healed Achilles tendon tear. **A:** Normal Achilles tendon. T1- (**B**) and T2-weighted (**C**) images show thickening (*arrow*) but no increased signal intensity in the healed Achilles tendon.

there is bad correlation of the talar tilt angle on stress radiography and the severity of ligament injury on MRI. They concluded that MRI should be utilized in young patients if surgery is debated, especially in patients with a 6° to 14° talar tilt on stress radiography, since stress radiography can under- or overestimate lateral ligament injury.

More recently, Lekrakul et al. (176) stressed the importance of MR arthrography with reformatting to define ligament tears in the tarsal canal and sinus. Accurate knowledge of the status of these ligaments is critical for surgical planning.

Os Trigonum Syndrome

The os trigonum is analogous to a secondary ossification center. It is formed in a cartilaginous posterior extension of

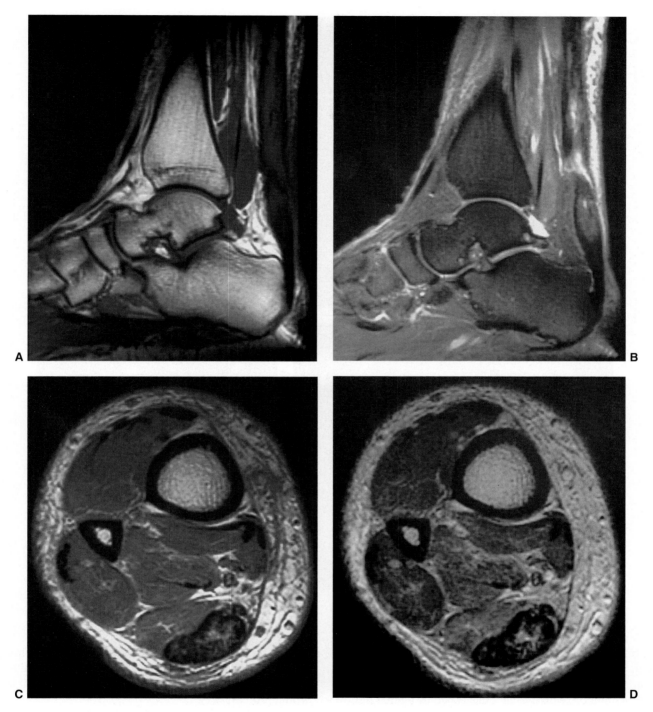

Figure 8-79 Sagittal T1- **(A)**, sagittal T2-weighted **(B)**, axial proton density-weighted **(C,D)** images demonstrate diffusely abnormal signal and thickening of the Achilles tendon consistent with a healing complete tear of the midtendon and a diffuse partial tear. The tendon is satisfactorily aligned without a gap.

the talus (see Fig. 8-118) (5,47,139,161). The os trigonum is connected to the talus by a cartilaginous synchondrosis. Ossification of this process occurs between the ages of 7 and 13 years. Fusion usually occurs within a year of ossification, forming Stieda's process (Fig. 8-118B). A separate ossicle remains in 7% to 14% of patients. The presence on

an os trigonum is frequently bilateral. In the adult, the ununited ossification center may be difficult to differentiate from an old fracture (161).

Os trigonum syndrome may be due to acute trauma or overuse (repetitive microtrauma). The syndrome includes process fracture, flexor hallucis longus tendinitis, and

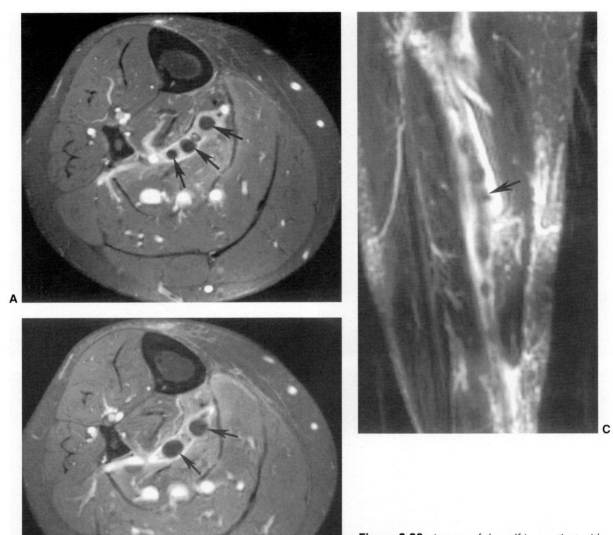

Figure 8-80 Images of the calf in a patient with a suspected Achilles tendon injury. The Achilles tendon was normal. Contrast-enhanced fat-suppressed T1-weighted **(A,B)** and coronal **(C)** images demonstrate no contrast in the veins (*arrows*) with thrombosis.

posterior tibiotalar impingement (177). Patients present with posterior ankle pain and swelling. Physical examination reveals posterior ankle tenderness anterior to the Achilles tendon. Pain is often exaggerated by plantar flexion of the foot (161,177).

Os trigonum syndrome is difficult to diagnose clinically. Therefore, the role of imaging to suggest or confirm the diagnosis is important (161,177). The identification of an os trigonum radiographically is not sufficient to make the diagnosis. However, irregularity at the margins or associated distortion of the pre-Achilles fat may suggest acute fracture or inflammation (see Fig. 8-119) (177). Stress views or plantar flexion studies may demonstrate posterior impingement and recreate the patient's symptoms. Bone

scanning may be useful as increased tracer in the region of the os trigonum should at least indicate further study. A normal bone scan excludes the diagnosis trigonum syndrome (20,161,177).

CT may be useful for detection of acute fractures or fragmentation of the lateral talar tuberosity or os trigonum (Fig. 8-118) (178). However, MRI is most useful to detect soft tissue changes (edema, flexor hallucis longus tenosynovitis) and subtle osseous changes due to impingement (5, 161,177). MR imaging should be performed using a small (10 to 14 cm) FOV. Both T1- and T2-weighted sequences are used (see Fig. 8-120). We use axial and sagittal image planes (Fig. 8-120). However, specifically for os trigonum syndrome, images with the foot plantar flexed or

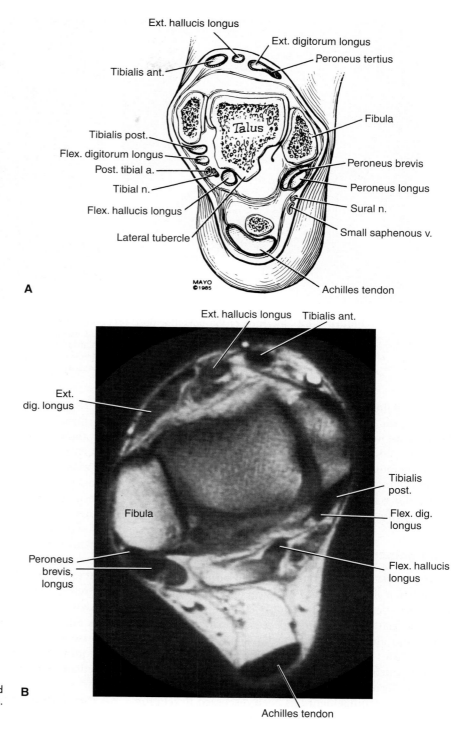

Figure 8-81 **A:** Illustration of tendon and neurovascular relationships about the ankle. **B:** Axial MRI with anatomy labeled.

sagittal GRE motion studies are useful. Impingement and motion of the os trigonum are more clearly demonstrated using the latter approach (5,177).

Bureau et al. (178) reviewed MR features in seven patients with posterior impingement. All patients demonstrated marrow contusions in the os trigonum or lateral talar tubercle. Fragmentation of these structures also occurred. The latter

may be more easily appreciated on CT examinations. Soft tissue features included distention of the posterior subtalar and tibiotalar recesses and fluid in the flexor hallucis longus tendon sheath (Fig. 8-120) (178).

Treatment of os trigonum syndrome is conservative in most cases. Direct injection of the synchondrosis or space between the talus and os trigonum is useful to confirm the

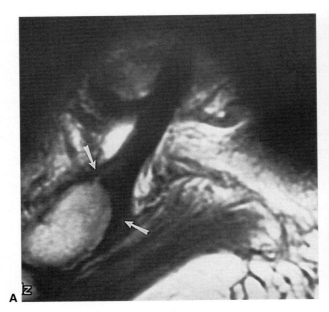
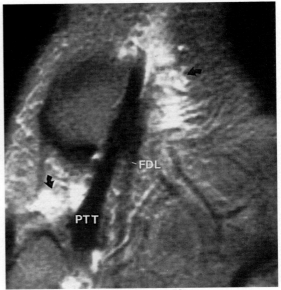

Figure 8-82   Insertion of the posterior tibial tendon on the navicular. **A:** Sagittal T1-weighted image demonstrates the normal fanning of the tendon at its insertion (*arrows*). The foot is slightly plantar flexed. **B:** Sagittal T2-weighted image with foot plantar flexed shows the posterior tibial tendon (*PTT*) and flexor digitorum longus tendon (*FDL*). *Arrows* indicate edema. (See also Fig. 8-42, where the posterior tibial tendon inserts on a type II accessory navicular.)

source of pain and provide therapy. We use a mixture of Marcaine and celestone (5,161). Immobilization with a short leg cast for 4 to 6 weeks may also be selected for initial treatment. When conservative measures fail, resection of the os trigonum is indicated. Results of resection are excellent in the majority of patients. When there is associated flexor hallucis longus tendinitis (Fig. 8-120), some surgeons will also perform a tendon release (161).

Impingement Syndromes

Impingement syndromes in the ankle may be related to bone or soft tissue abnormalities. Five categories of impingement have been described based upon clinical findings and anatomic features. Symptoms are caused by friction of joint tissues and altered biomechanics related to prior injury (98,129,156,179–181). Impingement syndromes include anterior, anterolateral, anteromedial, posteromedial, and posterior (98,181).

Posterior impingement has been discussed in relation to os trigonum syndrome (Fig. 8-120). Additional causes of posterior impingement syndrome include an elongated lateral talar tubercle (Stieda's process), downward sloping posterior tibial margin and loose bodies (98).

Anterior Impingement Syndrome

Anterior impingement syndrome is common. The syndrome is frequently seen in athletes required to perform repetitive dorsiflexion. Osseous beaklike changes in the anterior tibia with secondary deformity of the talar neck may be obvious on lateral radiographs or CT (see Fig. 8-121)

(98,181). Osteophytes form at the site of capsular attachment. There is usually associated synovial hypertrophy and scarring. Osteophytes alone may be asymptomatic in 45% to 59% of athletes (181).

Patients present with anterior ankle pain, swelling, and "blocking" on dorsiflexion. Osseous changes may be best identified with radiographs or CT (Fig. 8-121). Soft tissue changes are optimally demonstrated on T2-weighted axial and sagittal MR images. Synovial hypertrophy may be more obvious with intravenous or intraarticular contrast studies. These approaches are especially useful in the absence of a joint effusion (5,179).

Treatment of anterior impingement syndrome is initially conservative. Surgical treatment is reserved for nonresponders. Surgical success is related to the degree of degenerative disease in the remainder of the ankle. Patients with a normal joint space and minimal degeneration generally have excellent results (181).

Anterolateral Impingement Syndrome

The anterolateral recess is bordered by the tibia and fibula. Anterolaterally, the recess is limited by the joint capsule, anterior talofibular ligament, calcaneofibular ligament, and the anterior tibiofibular ligament (179,181, 182). The condition is believed to be related to previous inversion plantar flexion injuries. Tears in the capsule and ligaments without significant mechanical instability result in chronic anterolateral ankle pain (98,181–183). Repetitive minor trauma may also lead to thickening of the anterior tibiofibular ligament and osteophyte formation (see Fig. 8-122) (181).

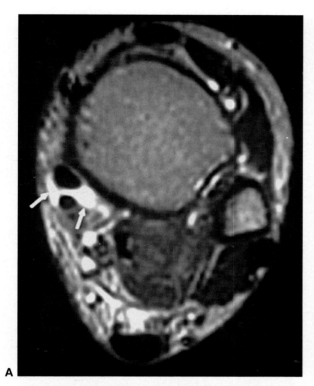

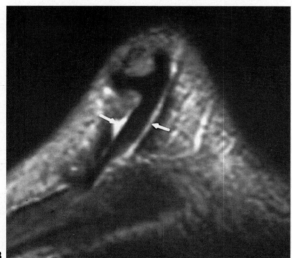

Figure 8-83 A middle-aged woman with medial ankle pain. Axial **(A)** and sagittal **(B)** T2-weighted images demonstrate fluid in the tendon sheaths (*arrows*) of the posterior tibial and flexor digitorum longus tendons resulting from tenosynovitis. The tendon size and signal intensity are normal.

Patients present with anterolateral ankle pain and swelling that is aggravated by pronation and supination of the foot. There is absence of instability on examination (98,182). Axial and sagittal T2-weighted MR images demonstrate soft tissue abnormalities in the anterolateral gutter (see Fig. 8-123). Conventional MR images have produced inconsistent results (sensitivity 39% to 100% and specificity of 50% to 100%). MR arthrography may be more specific (98,179).

Anteromedial Impingement Syndrome

The etiology of anteromedial impingement is felt to be related to eversion injuries with partial tearing of the deltoid (tibiotalar) ligament (98,181,184). However, the exact mechanism is not completely clear (181).

Patients typically demonstrate capsular thickening, thickening of the anterior deltoid ligament, and osteophytes. Associated lateral ligament injuries are not uncommon (98). Medial talar dome defects may be present in 55% of cases (181).

Patients present with chronic anteromedial ankle pain aggravated by dorsiflexion. There is local tenderness and limited dorsiflexion and inversion on physical examination (181).

MR imaging features have not been clearly defined. However, soft tissue thickening, osteophytes, and osteochondral lesions anteromedially have been described. MR arthrography is more accurate than conventional MRI (98,179,181).

Posteromedial Impingement Syndrome

The posterior and anterior tibiotalar ligaments form the deep portion of the deltoid ligament. The superficial complex is composed of the tibiocalcaneal, tibiospring, spring, and tibionavicular ligaments (156).

Posteromedial impingement is uncommon but has been described following severe ankle injuries with crushing of the deep fibers of the deltoid ligament. This may lead to chronic inflammation and hypertrophy of the ligament (98). Koulouris et al. (156) reviewed 25 patients with posteromedial impingement and all had prior posterior inferior tibiofibular ligament injuries. There was also associated tendon encasement in 12 of 25 cases, and bony avulsion in five of 25 cases.

Diagnosis is difficult clinically and arthroscopically. Early diagnosis is essential, as surgical repair provides excellent results (156). Conventional MR using T2-weighted sequences demonstrates capsular and ligament thickening in the posteromedial gutter along with tenosynovitis and marrow edema (98,156).

Midfoot and Forefoot Syndromes

Osseous and soft tissue overuse syndromes in the midfoot and forefoot are not uncommon (Table 8-6). Stress fractures in the tarsal and metatarsal regions are common (5,12, 185–187). Two conditions have been described—stress response and actual stress fractures. These conditions were discussed in the fracture section of this chapter. Therefore, we will not expand upon stress fractures in this section.

Midfoot injuries may be due to ligament injury or in association with fractures, especially Lisfranc injuries. The oblique Lisfranc ligament is the major supporting structure preventing lateral subluxation of the metatarsals. The second metatarsal joint is susceptible due to lack of a ligamentous attachment to the first metatarsal (44,118).

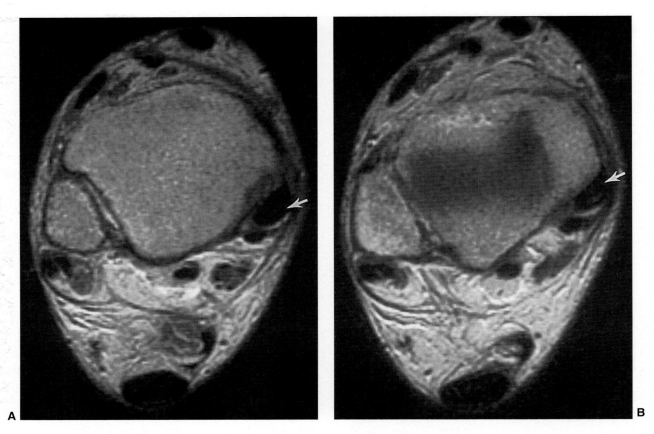

Figure 8-84 Axial proton density-weighted images **(A,B)** demonstrate thickening (*arrow*), with slight increased signal intensity in the posterior tibial tendon at the level of the medial malleolus.

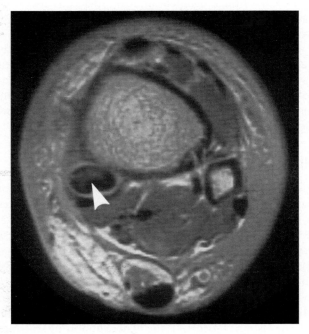

Figure 8-85 Axial T2-weighted image demonstrating an incomplete tear of the posterior tibial tendon. Note the high signal intensity in the substance of the thickened tendon (*arrowhead*) and the fluid in the tendon sheath.

Lisfranc injuries are usually related to significant trauma with obvious fracture/dislocation. Subtle injuries also occur after trauma or in diabetics with neurotrophic arthropathy. In these situations, early diagnosis is important to prevent rapid onset degenerative arthritis (5,118).

MR imaging is reserved for situations where symptoms are present and radiographs and CT are inconclusive. Oblique coronal and axial T2-weighted or STIR images demonstrate discontinuity of the ligament fibers and slight subluxation of the second metatarsal (118).

Tenosynovitis is common in the midfoot. The posterior tibial and peroneal tendons are most commonly symptomatic. Fluid surrounding the tendons is obvious on axial and sagittal T2-weighted images (5,118).

Many forefoot syndromes are diagnosed clinically and do not require imaging when they respond to conservative therapy. Imaging plays a more significant role when conservative measures fail. In this setting, properly selected imaging techniques are necessary to better define the nature of the disorders (5,17,114,118). Table 8-6 summarizes common forefoot syndromes (5,12,185).

Forefoot pain is a common problem in athletes and patients with occupational activity that involves weight bearing for long periods of time. Metatarsalgia may be related to

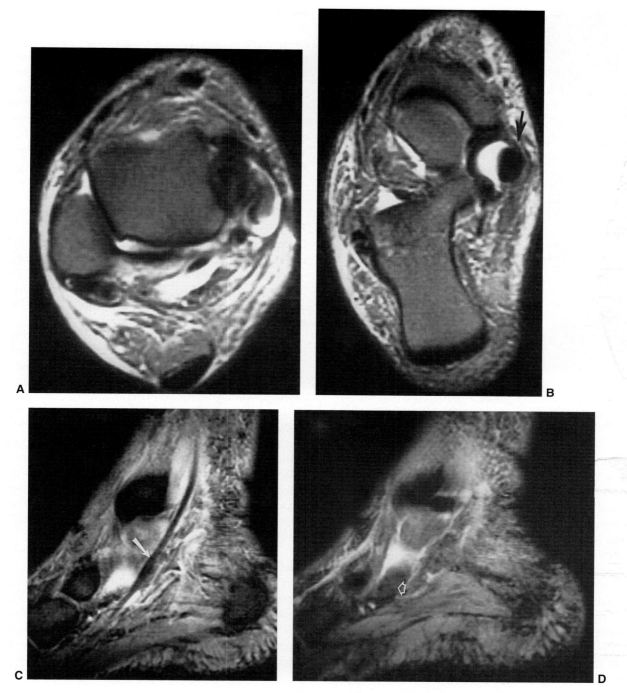

Figure 8-86 Posterior tibial tendon tear (type 3). Axial T2-weighted images at the level of the talus **(A)** and distally near the navicular **(B)** show fluid around the tendon or tendon bed with no definite tendon proximally in **A** and thickening in **B** distally *(arrow)*. Sagittal gradient-echo images **(C,D)** show the isolated flexor digitorum longus *(arrow)* with high signal intensity in the region of the posterior tibial tendon. The distal tendon remnant is visible on image **D** *(open arrow)*.

a long second metatarsal or hypermobile first metatarsal. More generalized metatarsal pain may be evident in athletes with a tight Achilles tendon or anterior ankle impingement (160). Routine radiographs are usually adequate for identifying metatarsal length.

Sesamoiditis

Sesamoid pain syndromes are common in runners (5,113,188). The medial and lateral sesamoids lie in the medial and lateral slips of the flexor hallucis brevis. The sesamoids function to elevate the first metatarsal head,

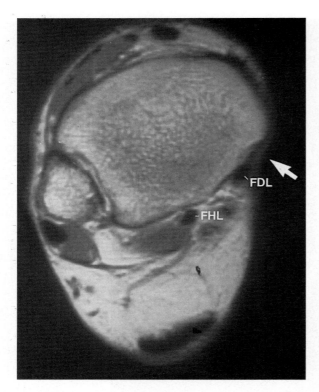

Figure 8-87 Axial T1-weighted image of the ankle in a patient with a complete tear of the posterior tibial tendon. Note the complete absence (*arrow*) of the posterior tibial tendon. *FDL,* flexor digitorum longus; *FHL,* flexor hallucis longus.

disperse impact forces, to protect the flexor hallucis tendon, and to increase the mechanical advantage of the flexor hallucis brevis (44,46,188). Sesamoids may become inflamed, fracture, or undergo osteonecrosis. In addition to pain, physical examination may cause discomfort with dorsiflexion of the great toe (113,118,188).

Routine radiographs including anteroposterior, oblique, lateral, and sesamoid views may be diagnostic (4). The sesamoids may be fragmented, sclerotic, or fractured (see Fig. 8-124). Soft tissue swelling over the involved sesamoid is usually present, as well. In subtle cases, radionuclide bone scans are useful. Increased tracer occurs in the presence of sesamoid pathology. A normal scan excludes the diagnosis. In some cases, MRI is required for evaluating unresponsive sesamoid pain (118,188). MR images may demonstrate marrow edema (↓ signal intensity on T1- and ↑ signal intensity on T2-weighted images); fracture; or, in the case of fragmentation and necrosis, low signal intensity on both T1- and T2-weighted sequences. Sesamoiditis is frequently associated with tenosynovitis and bursitis (113).

Treatment of sesamoid disorders is usually conservative initially. Footwear changes, a sesamoid pad, and antiinflammatory medications may be sufficient. When conservative measures fail, surgical resection is recommended (5,160).

Freiberg Infraction

Osteochondritis may also lead to forefoot pain. Osteonecrosis of the second metatarsal head occurs most frequently. However, the third to fifth metatarsals may also be involved (5). Women are affected more often than men (113). Routine radiographs are usually diagnostic. However, when indicated, MRI is useful to confirm the diagnosis and exclude other conditions such as synovitis. In the latter, intravenous gadolinium may be useful to detect early synovial changes. Synovitis, like osteonecrosis, also more commonly involves the second metatarsophalangeal joint (5,160). MR features of osteonecrosis of the metatarsal heads are similar to changes described in the hip (Chapter 6).

Plantar Plate

Disruption of the plantar plates of the second through fifth metatarsophalangeal joints occurs most commonly in women. Hyperextension forces and increased weight bearing from footwear (high heels and pointed toes) are predisposing factors. The second metatarsophalangeal joint is most often involved (113).

MR imaging in the axial and sagittal planes using T2-weighted sequences will demonstrate increased signal intensity in the plantar aspect of the joint or actual disruption of the plantar plate. Associated hyperextension and tenosynovitis are common (113).

Hallux Rigidus

Hallux rigidus usually occurs due to chronic trauma. Athletes involved in track and football are commonly affected (5). Joint space narrowing without hallux valgus deformity may be the only radiographic finding initially. If left untreated, marked narrowing and prominent osteophytes may develop. Surgical resection may be indicated in advanced cases. MR imaging is rarely indicated.

Turf Toe

Turf toe is a hyperextension injury of the first metatarsophalangeal joint with plantar ligament sprain. This is a clinical diagnosis in most cases (114). MR images in the axial and sagittal planes demonstrate increased signal intensity in the plantar capsule and, occasionally, bone bruises on T2-weighted sequences (5,114).

Bursitis

The intermetatarsal bursa lies between the metatarsal heads deep to the transverse metatarsal ligament (44,46). When inflamed, the bursa can distend and can compress the interdigital nerve if distention exceeds 3 mm. This causes severe local pain (118). The submetatarsal bursa directly below the metatarsal head may also be involved. Axial T2-weighted or STIR images demonstrate a well-defined high-signal-intensity structure regardless of which bursa is involved. Peripheral enhancement occurs with intravenous gadolinium (5,113,118).

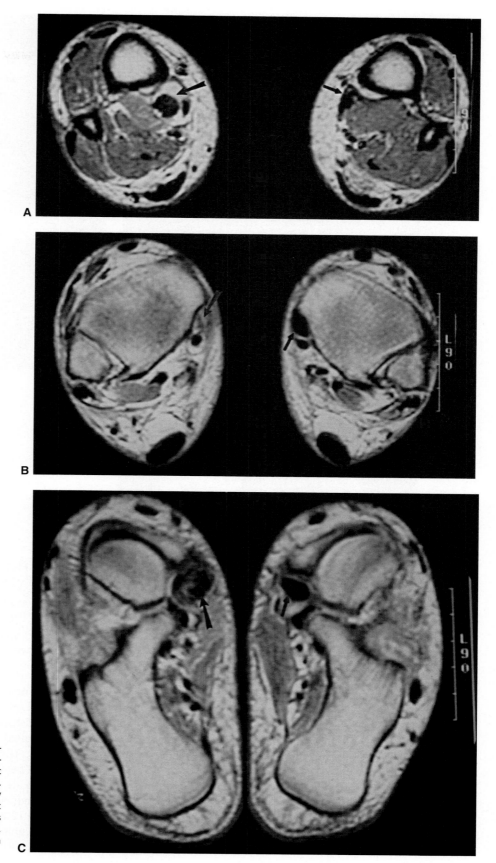

Figure 8-88 Axial proton density-weighted images comparing the normal left (*smaller arrows*) and torn right posterior tibial tendon (*large arrows*). The tendon is thickened proximally with fluid in the tendon sheath **(A)**. At the level of the tear **(B)**, the tendon is absent. Distally near the insertion **(C)**, the distal remnant is thickened with increased signal intensity.

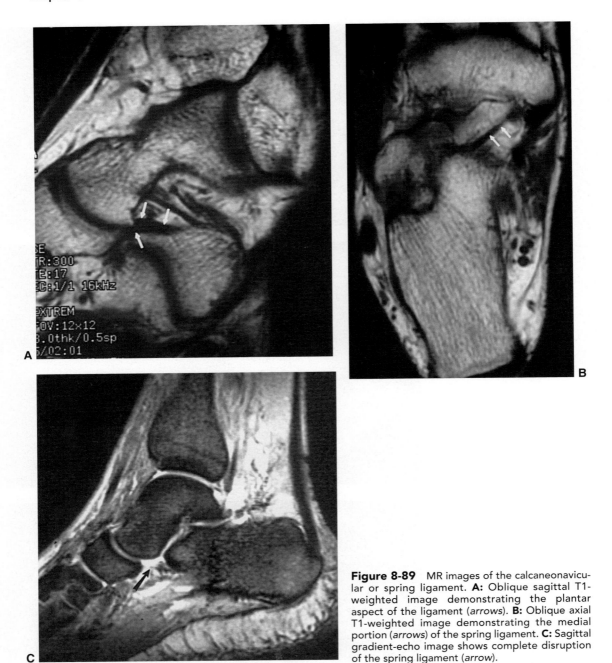

Figure 8-89 MR images of the calcaneonavicular or spring ligament. **A:** Oblique sagittal T1-weighted image demonstrating the plantar aspect of the ligament (*arrows*). **B:** Oblique axial T1-weighted image demonstrating the medial portion (*arrows*) of the spring ligament. **C:** Sagittal gradient-echo image shows complete disruption of the spring ligament (*arrow*).

Morton's Neuroma

Morton's neuromas occur due to fibrous degeneration following chronic trauma to the plantar interdigital nerve (17,113,118). Symptoms are classically described between the third and fourth metatarsal heads (see Fig. 8-125), though any of the intermetatarsal spaces can be involved. Paresthesia and numbness of the sensory distribution of the nerve are common. Clinical history and physical examination are usually diagnostic. MRI or ultrasound (see Figs. 8-126 and 8-127) are useful in selected cases (5,189). Confidence in diagnosis is increased significantly and treatment plans may be modified in 57% of patients with

suspected Morton's neuroma after MR studies have been performed (190). Axial MR images (Figs. 8-125 through 8-127) are most useful. Weishaupt et al. (32) demonstrated that the prone position resulted in the lesion appearing larger and more conspicuous. The neuroma is typically dumbbell-shaped and located between the metatarsal heads (17,191). Morton's neuromas are usually small, interdigital, and low intensity on T1-weighted images. Signal intensity may also be low or mixed on T2-weighted images (Fig. 8-127) (5,113, 118,191). Contrast enhancement is variable (Fig. 8-125), but may be intense (17,118). Size is important, as neuromas less than 5 mm are felt to be insignificant (118,192).

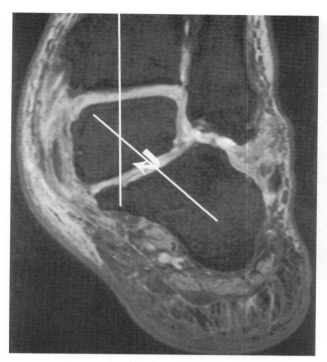

Figure 8-90 Posterior tibial tendon dysfunction. Coronal DESS image shows marked swelling medially with the edema. The tibiocalcaneal angle (normal 0° to 6°) measures 40° (*curved arrow*).

Differentiation from bursitis can be accomplished by demonstrating peripheral enhancement of an inflamed bursa on fat-suppressed postgadolinium T1-weighted images. Keep in mind that associated bursitis is not uncommon (17).

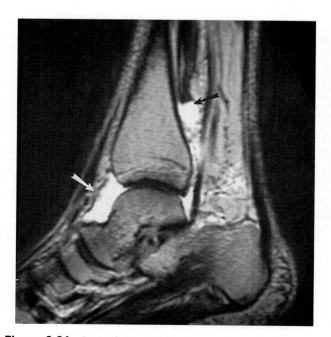

Figure 8-91 Sagittal T2-weighted image demonstrating a tear and retraction of the flexor hallucis longus (*arrow*). There is a large effusion (*white arrow*).

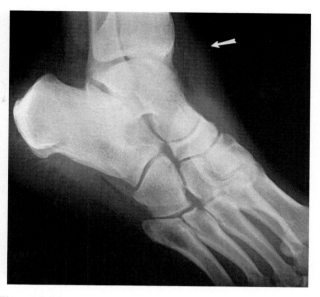

Figure 8-92 Oblique radiograph in a patient with anterior tibial tendon rupture. There is focal anterior soft tissue swelling (*arrow*).

Calf Trauma

Trauma to the calf may lead to contusion, intramuscular hemorrhage or hematoma formation, compartment syndrome, muscle herniation or, when chronic, overuse syndromes (5,114,193–195). Neurovascular injury and compartment syndrome may also result from direct trauma or secondary to undiagnosed muscle tears (5,195). Muscle tears, particularly in the gastrocnemius and plantaris muscles, are not uncommon. Muscle tears occur in 10% to 11% of runners. Medial gastrocnemius tears are commonly seen in tennis players (5,193,196).

Physical examination and history are important in defining the region and severity of injury. Until recently, imaging studies were usually not obtained except when venous thrombosis was suspected. It may be difficult to differentiate deep venous thrombosis from dissecting popliteal cysts, muscle tears, and Achilles tendon injuries clinically (5,126,193,194,197). Staging of muscle injuries (strains) is graded based on the extent of injury and function.

First-degree strains have minor muscle fiber injury with no loss of strength. Second-degree strains are partial tears with some degree of strength reduction. Third-degree strains are complete tears with functional loss, and there are typically fluid collections between the torn muscle segments (5,193,194,198).

A first-degree strain (stretch injury) has high-signal-intensity edema and hemorrhage surrounding the myotendinal junction that spreads into the adjacent muscle on T2-weighted and STIR images. In a second-degree strain (partial tear), the myotendinous junction is partially torn and MR shows irregular thinning of the tendon fibers with

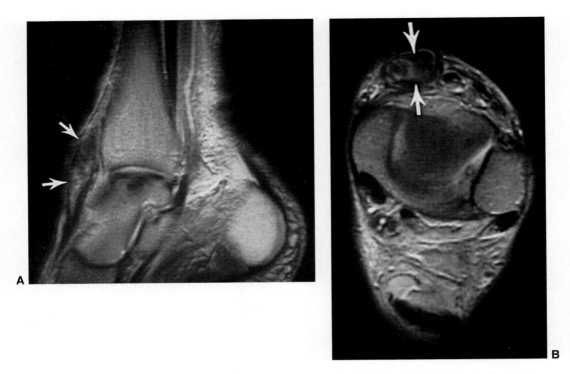

Figure 8-93 Sagittal **(A)** and axial **(B)** T2-weighted images demonstrate focal thickening (*arrows*) between the retinacula with increased signal intensity resulting from a partial tear in the anterior tibial tendon.

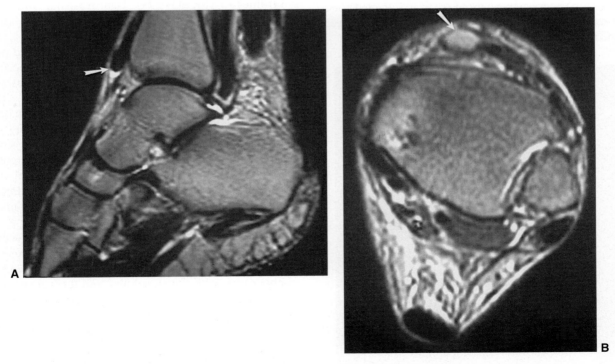

Figure 8-94 Sagittal **(A)** and axial **(B)** T2-weighted images demonstrate a complete tear in the anterior tibial tendon (*arrow*).

TABLE 8-5
HEEL PAIN

Differential Diagnoses

Local osseous etiologies

    Calcaneal stress fracture
    Calcaneal periostitis
    Calcaneal spurs
    Sever disease
    Arthropathies
    Os trigonum syndrome
    Tarsal coalition
    Haglund deformity

Local soft tissue etiologies

    Subcalcaneal pain syndrome
    Painful heel pad
    Nerve entrapment
    Plantar fasciitis
    Retrocalcaneal bursitis
    Retro-Achilles bursitis
    Tarsal tunnel syndrome
    Achilles tendon syndrome
    Flexor hallucis longus tendon injury
    Peroneal tendon injury

Systemic causes[a]

    Ankylosing spondylitis
    Reiter syndrome
    Psoriatic arthritis
    Rheumatoid arthritis
    Gout

[a]16% of patients with heel pain.
From Berquist TH. *Radiology of the foot and ankle*, 2nd ed. Philadelphia, PA: Lippincott Williams & Wilkins, 2000 and Narvaez JA, Narvaez J, Ortega R, et al. Painful heel: MR image findings. *Radiographics* 2000;20:333–352.

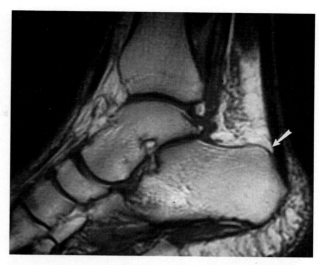

Figure 8-96 Sagittal T1-weighted image of the ankle demonstrating extension of the fat (*arrow*) between the calcaneus and Achilles tendon during plantar flexion.

more prominent muscle edema and hemorrhage than first-degree strains. Third-degree strain is a complete myotendinous rupture with MR evidence of muscle and tendon retraction, and later, muscle fatty infiltration and atrophy.

MR examinations are generally performed with the patient prone to prevent compression of the soft tissues in the posterior compartments. The patient can be supine for lateral or anterior compartment injuries. An extremity coil or,

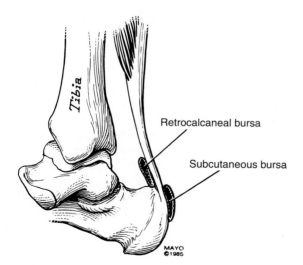

Figure 8-95 Sagittal illustration of the calcaneal bursae. (From Berquist TH. *Radiology of the foot and ankle*. New York: Raven Press, 1989.)

Retrocalcaneal bursa

Subcutaneous bursa

Tibia

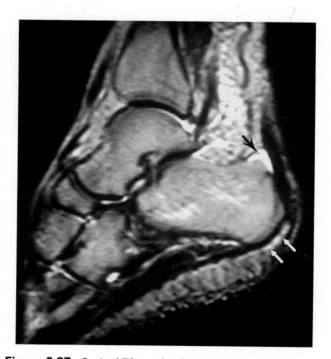

Figure 8-97 Sagittal T2-weighted image with the foot slightly plantar flexed. The retro calcaneal bursa contains fluid (*arrow*). There is also slight inflammation in the deep heel pad (*small arrows*).

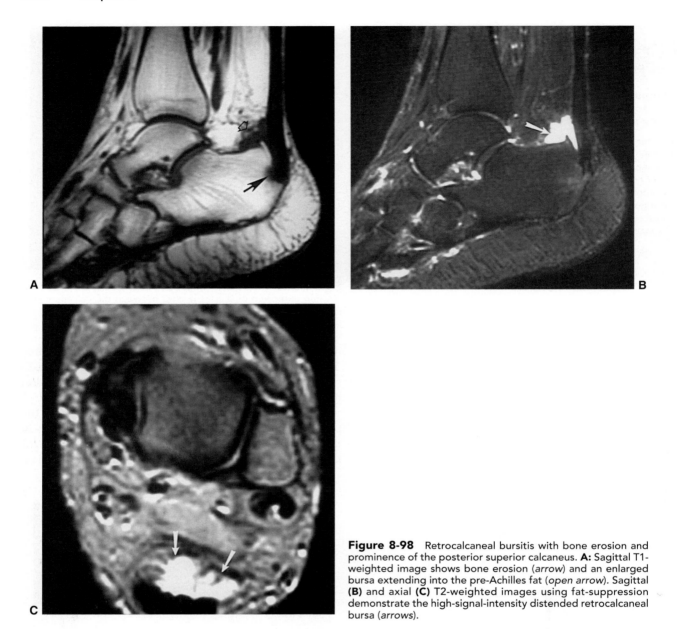

Figure 8-98 Retrocalcaneal bursitis with bone erosion and prominence of the posterior superior calcaneus. **A:** Sagittal T1-weighted image shows bone erosion (*arrow*) and an enlarged bursa extending into the pre-Achilles fat (*open arrow*). Sagittal **(B)** and axial **(C)** T2-weighted images using fat-suppression demonstrate the high-signal-intensity distended retrocalcaneal bursa (*arrows*).

when comparison is needed, the torso coil are most often used (5). Section thickness is varied depending on the anatomic area that needs to be imaged. Axial images with 0.5- to 1-cm-thick slices using T1- and STIR or fat-suppressed FSE T2-weighted images in two image planes (axial and coronal or sagittal) are usually adequate to identify and grade the injury. T2-weighted or STIR sequences are most useful, as acute hemorrhage or hematoma can be isointense with muscle on T1-weighted sequences (see Fig. 8-128) (5,114,198).

Certain vascular abnormalities can be detected with conventional sequences (Fig. 8-80) (199). However, flow phenomenon may cause intraluminal signal, leading to false diagnosis of thromboses (5). Contrast-enhanced images or

new angiographic techniques are most useful to exclude associated vascular injuries or thrombosis (18).

We have noted different responses to therapy and prolonged recovery on patients with hematomas. Hematomas may develop between muscle bundles or in third-degree strains. Patients with intramuscular hemorrhage (see Figs. 8-129 and 8-130) tend to recover weeks to months earlier than patients with hematomas (see Figs. 8-130 and 8-131). In addition, chronic changes (see Fig. 8-132) with persistent fluid collections and/or scar formation (see Fig. 8-133) appear to occur more frequently in patients with well-defined hematomas (5,200). This would suggest a more aggressive approach, such as evacuation, should be

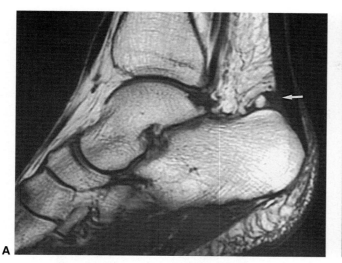
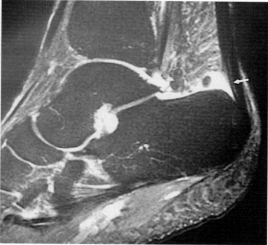

Figure 8-99 Sagittal SE 500/11 (**A**) and fat-suppressed FSE (**B**) images demonstrate bursitis and inflammation in the adjacent Achilles tendon (*arrows*).

considered when hematomas are identified with MRI. (See Chapter 2 for discussion of image features of blood.) (5,201)

Complications of muscle tears include acute and chronic compartment syndrome, neurovascular injury, fatty replacement, fibrosis (Fig. 8-133), and myositis ossificans (5,193). MRI is well suited for imaging all with the exception of myositis ossificans where CT features may be more easily interpreted.

Compartment syndrome results from muscle enlargement, hemorrhage, hematoma, or inflammation leading to increased intracompartmental pressure (59,195,202,203).

Elevated pressure can lead to neurovascular compromise and ischemia if left untreated (59,193,202,203).

The leg is typically divided into four compartments (see Fig. 8-134). The anterior compartment contains the tibialis anterior, extensor hallucis longus, and extensor digitorum longus muscles. The peroneus longus and brevis are in the lateral compartment. There are two posterior compartments, superficial and deep. The soleus and gastrocnemius are in the superficial and the tibialis posterior, flexor hallucis longus, and flexor digitorum longus make up the deep compartment (44,46,195).

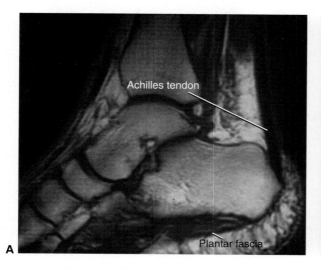
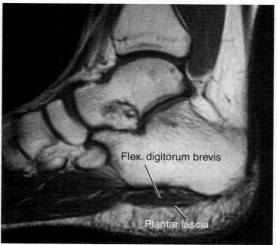

Figure 8-100 Normal MR images of the heel. **A,B:** Sagittal MRIs demonstrating the heel, plantar fascia, and Achilles tendon insertion. **C:** Coronal illustration localizing coronal images. **D:** Coronal image at the Achilles insertion. **E:** Coronal images just anterior to the Achilles tendon. **F:** Coronal image through the calcaneus.

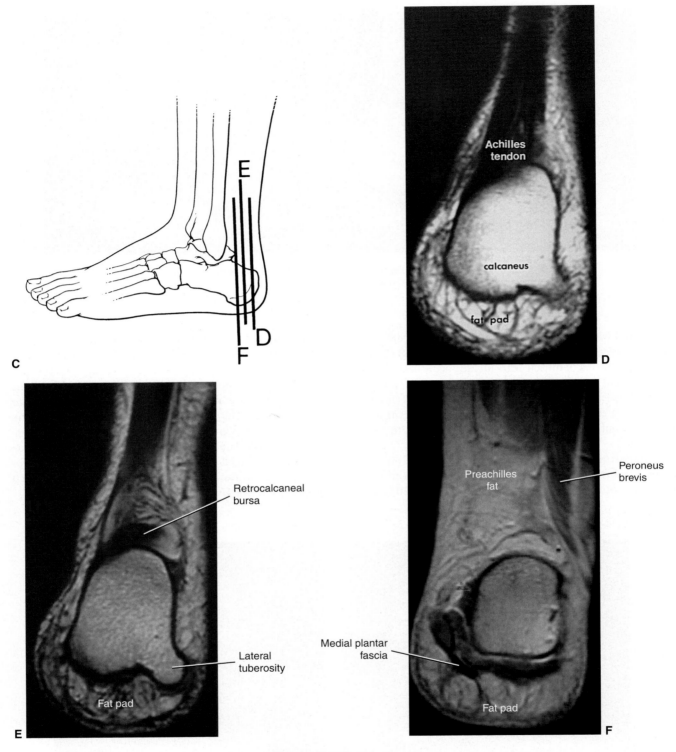

C

D

E

F

Achilles tendon

calcaneus

fat pad

Retrocalcaneal bursa

Lateral tuberosity

Fat pad

Preachilles fat

Peroneus brevis

Medial plantar fascia

Fat pad

Figure 8-100 (*continued*)

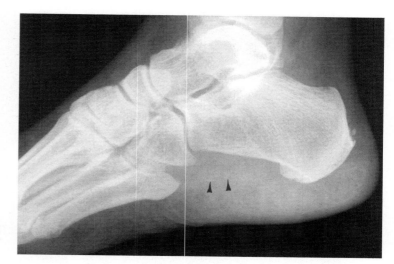

Figure 8-101 Plantar fasciitis. Lateral radiograph demonstrates plantar soft tissue edema with faint calcification (*arrowheads*) in the plantar fascia.

Acute compartment syndrome is usually due to fracture or blunt trauma. There is severe pain, neurovascular symptoms, and ischemia that can lead to necrosis if not treated with fasciotomy (203,204).

Chronic compartment syndrome (see Fig. 8-135) is most commonly seen in the anterior and lateral compartments in military recruits and runners (195,203,205). Muscle volume increases and pressure rises up to 20% after exercise (206). Normal resting compartment pressure is 5 mm Hg. After exercise, pressures increase dramatically but usually return to normal quickly. Pressures of 40 to 45 mm

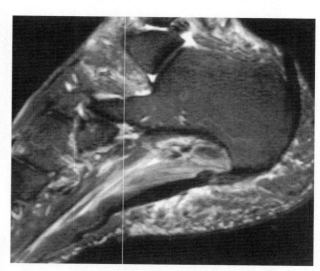

Figure 8-103 Sagittal T2-weighted image demonstrates thickened fascia with proximal thickening, inflammation, and edema along the plantar aspect of the fascia.

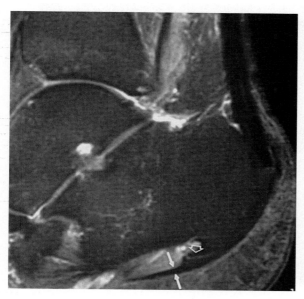

Figure 8-102 Chronic fascial changes. Fat-suppressed T2-weighted fast spin-echo sequence demonstrates an osteophyte (*open arrow*) and fascial thickening (*small arrows*). There is no increased signal intensity to suggest active inflammation.

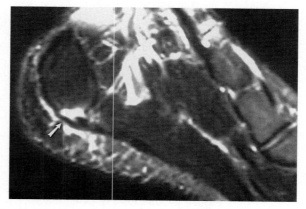

Figure 8-104 Sagittal fat-suppressed T2-weighted image demonstrates fasciitis with fascial irregularity and edema superior and inferior to the fascia (*arrow*).

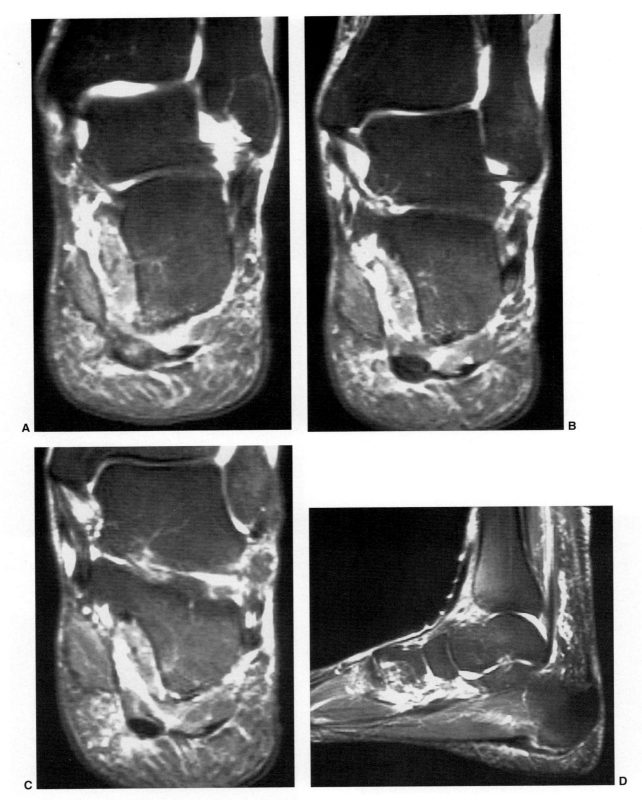

Figure 8-105 Coronal **(A–C)** and sagittal **(D)** fast spin-echo T2-weighted images demonstrate mild thickening and increased T2-weighted signal of the proximal plantar fascia near its origin, consistent with plantar fasciitis.

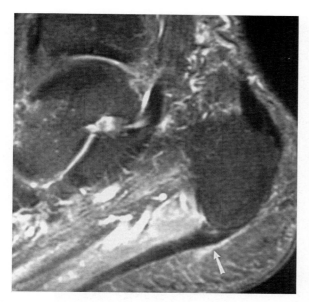

Figure 8-106 Chronic fasciitis. Sagittal fat-suppressed T2-weighted image demonstrates marked thickening with proximal inflammation (*arrow*).

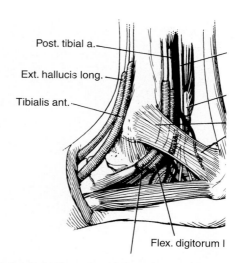

Figure 8-108 Illustration of the medial ankle and hindfoot demonstrating the course of the neurovascular structures through the tarsal tunnel.

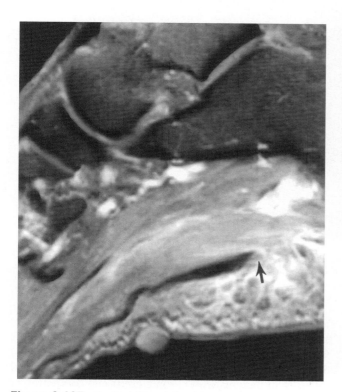

Figure 8-107 Sagittal T2-weighted image demonstrates complete disruption of the plantar fascia (*arrow*) with distal retraction.

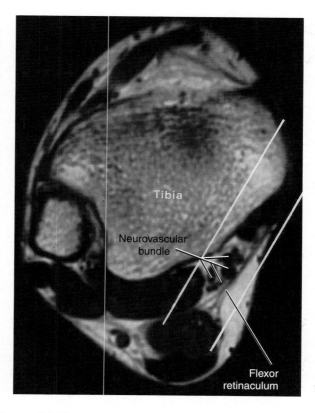

Figure 8-109 Axial T1-weighted image demonstrating structures in the tarsal tunnel. In addition to axial images, oblique sagittal images (*white lines*) can be obtained.

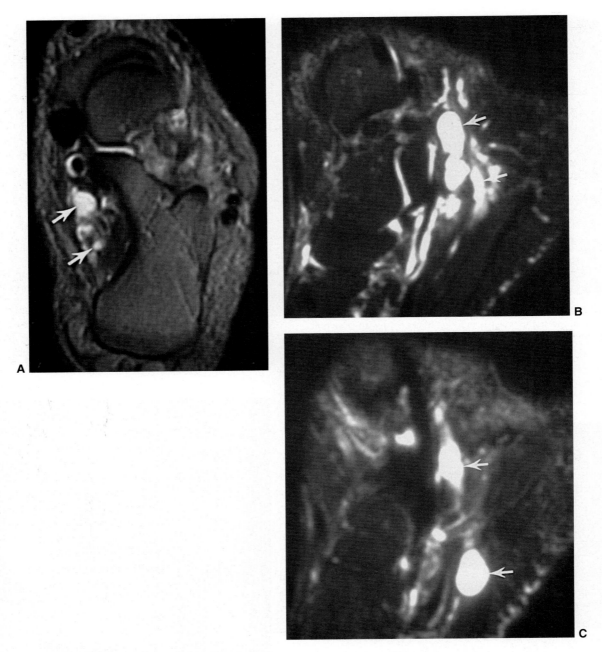

Figure 8-110 Axial **(A)** and sagittal **(B,C)** T2-weighted images with fat suppression demonstrate multiple high-signal-intensity varicose veins (*arrows*) causing tarsal tunnel syndrome.

Hg or within 30 mm Hg of diastolic blood pressure are diagnostic of compartment syndrome. Chronic compartment syndromes are almost always bilateral (203,206).

Symptomatic variations occur in compartment syndrome. Some patients present with pain only at rest, while others present with pain during exercise that is relieved by rest. Therefore, pre- and post-exercise axial images may be required to evaluate these patients fully (193,205). Axial T2-weighted (with or without fat suppression) or STIR images demonstrate infiltrative high signal intensity in the muscle with bulging of the fascia on patients with compartment syndrome. Verleisdonk et al. (195) demonstrated significant increase in T2-weighted signal intensity in patients with chronic exertional compartment syndrome. This finding was significantly more useful in the anterior compartment than the posterior or lateral compartments. Signal intensity returned to normal after fasciotomy.

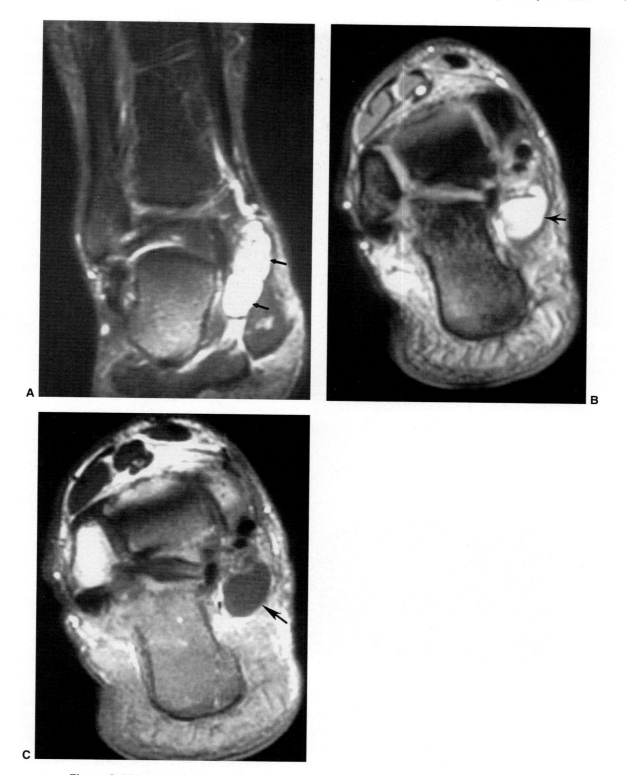

Figure 8-111   Multilobulated ganglion cyst. Coronal **(A)** and axial **(B)** T2-weighted images demonstrate a high intensity well-defined mass (*arrows*). T1-weighted fat-suppressed postcontrast image **(C)** shows no enhancement (*arrow*), a finding indicating a cyst.

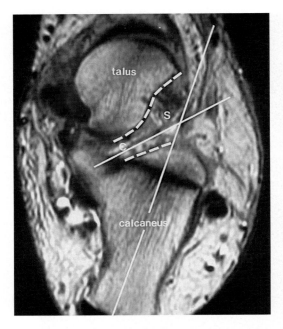

Figure 8-112 Axial T1-weighted image demonstrating the configuration (*broken lines*) of the tarsal canal and sinus. The relationship to the calcaneal axis (*white lines*) is about 45°. *C*, canal; *S*, sinus.

Spectroscopy (P-31) may be useful in evaluating muscle ischemia and metabolism. However, to date this has not been used frequently in the clinical setting (207–209).

Axial images are usually best when evaluating neurovascular injury. The course of the vessels and nerves varies so that contiguous slices can be followed to determine if hematomas or other posttraumatic changes effect the neurovascular structures. Chronic injuries can result in formation of neurofibromas (5).

NEOPLASMS

Soft tissue neoplasms in the calf are not uncommon (see Chapter 12) (99,210–215). Bone and soft tissue neoplasms of the foot and ankle do not occur commonly. Osseous neoplasms involving the foot and ankle (Table 8-7) account for only about 3% of all primary skeletal tumors (67,216–220). In a series of 255 cases from the Armed Forces Institute of Pathology, 83.5% were benign. The metatarsals were most commonly involved, followed by the calcaneus (221). Skeletal metastasis and multiple

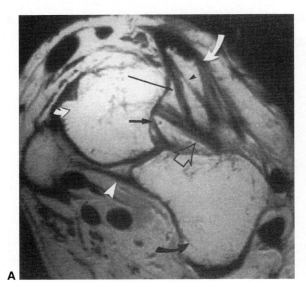

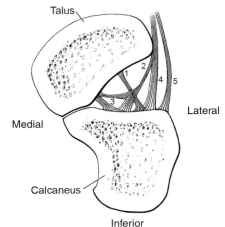

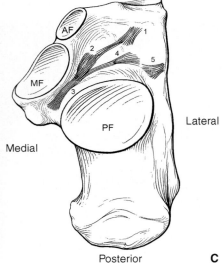

Figure 8-113 **A:** Coronal SE 600/15 image of the tarsal sinus and canal. Ligament of the tarsal canal (*short black arrow*), intermediate (*small black arrowhead*) and lateral (*curved white arrow*) bands of the inferior extensor retinaculum. Talus (*short curved white arrow*) and calcaneus (*curved black arrow*) are demonstrated along with the plantar calcaneonavicular ligament (*white arrowhead*). Coronal **(B)** and axial **(C)** illustrations demonstrating attachment sites for the cervical ligament (*1*); ligament of the tarsal canal (*3*); and the medial (*2*), intermediate (*4*), and lateral (*5*) segments of the inferior extensor retinaculum. *AF*, anterior facet; *MF*, middle facet; *PF*, posterior facet. (**A** is from Klein MA, Spreitzer AM. MR imaging of the tarsal sinus and canal: Normal anatomy, pathologic findings, and features of sinus tarsi syndrome. *Radiology* 1993;186:223–240.)

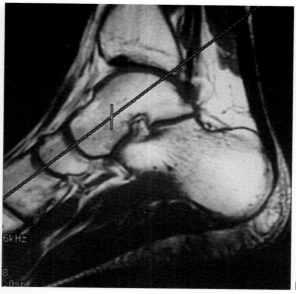

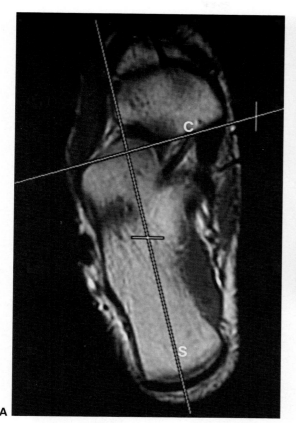

Figure 8-114 MR imaging approaches to the tarsal canal and sinus. **A:** Axial image demonstrating oblique sagittal *(S)* and oblique coronal *(C)* image planes selected. **B:** Sagittal scout demonstrating the plane for oblique axial images.

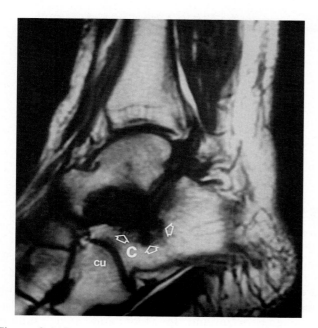

Figure 8-115 Sagittal T1-weighted image at the lateral margin of the tarsal sinus near the calcaneocuboid articulation. *C,* calcaneus; *cu,* cuboid. The normal high-intensity fat is replaced by low-signal-intensity inflammatory tissue and there are erosions *(open arrows)* in the calcaneus.

myeloma (0.2%) occur even less frequently than primary bone neoplasms. Benign lesions are slightly more common than malignant (Table 8-7) (219,222,223). All lesions summarized in Table 8-7 are more common in the ankle (tibia and fibula) than the foot (67,153,219, 222,224). Of benign lesions throughout the entire skeleton, nonossifying fibromas, chondromyxoid fibromas, and interosseous lipomas most commonly involve the foot and ankle (67,222,223). Interosseous lipoma deserves mention here. This lesion is composed of mature fat cells with fibrovascular components. Over time, involution with infarction, cyst formation, and dystrophic calcification occurs (see Fig. 8-136). Thirty-two percent of interosseous lipomas involve the calcaneus (Fig. 8-136) (222). Radiographically, the lesion may resemble a nonossifying fibroma, aneurysmal bone cyst, infarct, or chondroid lesion (153,222,224).

Seventy percent of patients present with pain. This may be due to microfracture. MR images demonstrate the lesion to be completely or partially fatty with signal intensity similar to subcutaneous fat on all pulse sequences. Marginal low signal intensity with central low intensity foci (calcifications) is common. Malignant degeneration is rare. Therefore, surgery is reserved for patients that are at

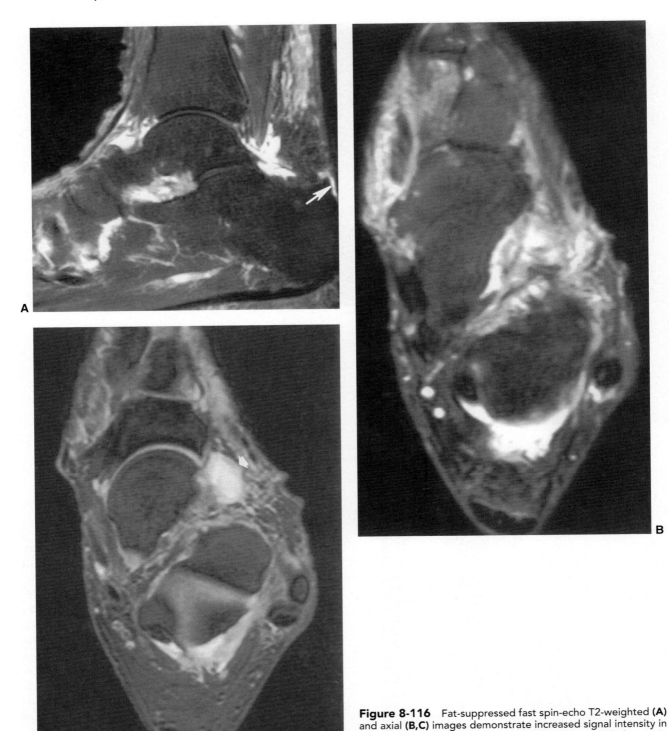

Figure 8-116 Fat-suppressed fast spin-echo T2-weighted **(A)** and axial **(B,C)** images demonstrate increased signal intensity in the tarsal canal with a localized fluid collection (*thick arrow*). Note the retrocalcaneal bursitis (*arrow*).

risk for pathologic fracture (222,224). Routine radiographs are still the most useful screening technique on patients with suspected skeletal neoplasms. The features of many lesions can be characterized accurately using routine radiographic techniques (see Figs. 8-137 to 8-140). Therefore, MRI is reserved mainly for those patients whose tumors are equivocal or as a staging technique for patients with suspected malignancy. MRI has essentially replaced CT as a staging technique for foot and ankle tumors (5,67,99,213,225,226). We use T1- and T2-weighted and postcontrast fat-suppressed T1-weighted imaging routinely when evaluation skeletal neoplasms.

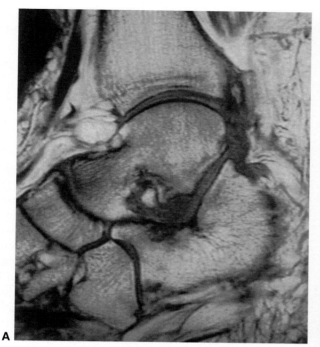

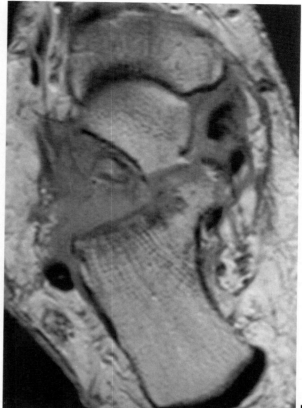

Figure 8-117 Sagittal **(A)** and axial **(B)** T1-weighted images show osseous fragments and decreased signal intensity in the tarsal canal and sinus.

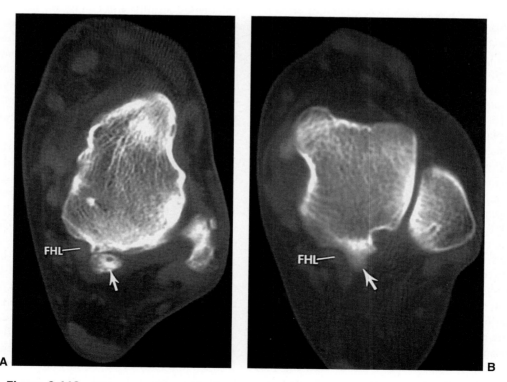

Figure 8-118 CT images of the ankle demonstrating the os trigonum (*arrow*) **(A)** and a fused Stieda process (*arrow*) **(B).** Note the relationship of the flexor hallucis longus tendon (*FHL*). There are degenerative changes along the synchondrosis of the os trigonum in **A.**

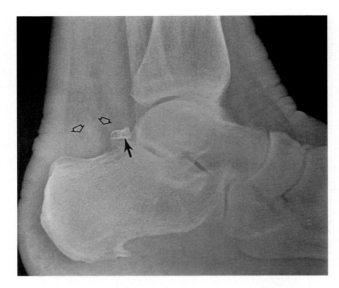

Figure 8-119 Lateral computed radiographic image *(CR)* of the calcaneus shows an ostrigonum *(black arrow)* and edema *(open arrows)* in the pre-Achilles fat due to os trigonum syndrome.

Soft tissue masses in the foot and ankle are also uncommon (67,211,225–228). In fact, most soft tissue masses are non-neoplastic, such as ganglion cysts and Morton neuromas (221). Table 8-8 lists the soft tissue tumors of the foot and ankle in a series of 736 tumors (228). Kirby et al. (213) reviewed 83 soft tissue masses in the foot and ankle. Eighty-seven percent were benign and 13% were malignant. The majority of masses were related to inflammation. Therefore, it is not surprising that most benign lesions were ganglion cysts (see Fig. 8-141) or fibromatosis (see Fig. 8-142) (212,229). Fibromatosis relates to various proliferating fibrous tissue lesions that include benign fibromatosis, nodular fasciitis, aggressive fibromatosis (desmoid tumors) (see Figs. 8-142 through 8-144), and fibrosarcoma (5,212,230). Fibromatoses occur most frequently in the plantar region of the midfoot (213,226,230). Plantar fibromatosis is a benign lesion involving the superficial medial plantar fascia (113). MR images demonstrate thickening and irregularity of the fascia. T1-weighted images show the lesion to be isointense to slightly higher signal intensity compared to muscle. Signal intensity on T2-weighted or STIR sequences varies from low to intermediate or, in some cases, high signal intensity (Fig. 8-142). Contrast enhancement is typically nonuniform (113,118).

The majority of malignant lesions in the series reported by Kirby were synovial sarcomas (see Fig. 8-145) (213). Most malignant lesions were located in the heel region. Other large series also report synovial sarcoma as most common followed by clear cell sarcoma, epitheliod sarcoma and liposarcoma (Table 8-8) (228).

We generally perform both T1- and T2-weighted sequences in two image planes to optimally characterize and stage (extent) lesions. Gadolinium may be useful to characterize certain lesions (5,216). A more complete discussion of musculoskeletal neoplasms can be found in Chapter 12.

ARTHRITIS/INFECTION

Imaging of inflammatory conditions in the calf, foot, and ankle has traditionally been accomplished using routine radiography (see Fig. 8-146), CT, and radionuclide studies. Over the years, the role of MRI for evaluating arthropathies has become more established. MR imaging is useful for early detection of synovial changes (active vs. inactive pannus) as well as osseous and articular changes in the small bones of the foot and ankle (58,143,144, 231–233). Early synovial changes and effusions are easily demonstrated, even in small joints of the foot that may be difficult to evaluate clinically (25,143,234–236). Joint effusions are easily detected on T2-weighted sequences. However, the signal intensity of joint fluid is not useful in differentiating effusion from infection (see Fig. 8-147) (5,30,231,237).

The role of MRI in non-infectious arthropathies has become more clearly defined. This is particularly true for detection, staging, and monitoring treatment response in patients with rheumatoid arthritis (30,143,238). T1- and T2-weighted sequences are still useful. However, intravenous gadolinium (conventional or dynamic bolus injections) permits more effective evaluation of active synovial inflammation and subtle cartilage abnormalities. Patients with rheumatoid arthritis also commonly have Achilles and PTT involvement. In fact, PTT tears occur most commonly on patients with rheumatoid arthritis. The bursae about the Achilles tendon are also commonly involved (143,238).

Karasick et al. (239) found that the fibular notch is a frequent finding in rheumatoid arthritis. This scalloped fibular defect probably results from chronic erosion from adjacent synovial proliferation and pannus in a "bare area" of the fibula without articular cartilage.

On patients with Reiter syndrome tenosynovitis involving the PTT, flexor digitorum longus and flexor hallucis longus is characteristic. Retrocalcaneal bursitis and plantar calcaneal erosions are also common. Both psoariatic arthritis and Reiter's typically involve the distal phalangeal joints. Uniform swelling of the digit (sausage digit) may also be evident on MR images (143).

Gout is the most common arthropathy in males over 30 years of age (143). Yu et al. (144) reviewed 13 MR examinations on nine patients with gouty arthritis. They concluded the MR appearance of tophi was constant on T1- but variable on T2-weighted images (see Figs. 8-148 and 8-149). Almost all the tophi had intermediate T1-weighted signal intensity. T2-weighted images demonstrated a homogeneous increase in signal intensity of the tophi in three sites and heterogeneous decrease in signal intensity in the tophi of ten sites. The variability of signal intensity on T2-weighted images

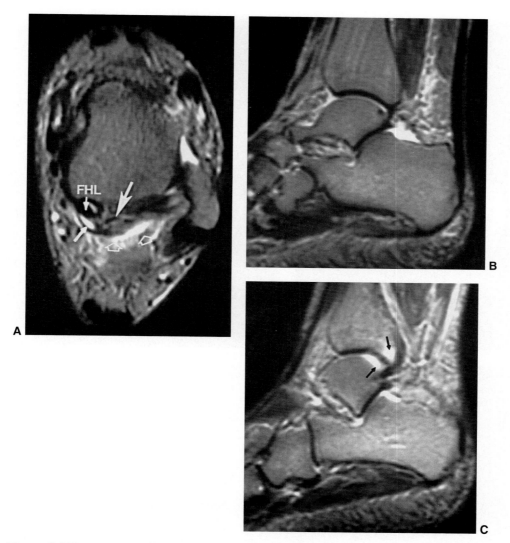

Figure 8-120 Os trigonum syndrome. **A:** Axial fat-suppressed T2-weighted image demonstrates edema (*open arrows*) and fluid (*small white arrow*) around the flexor hallucis longus tendon (*FHL*). The irregular-appearing ostrigonum (*large white arrow*) is not clearly demonstrated on this section. Sagittal T2- (**B**) and proton density-weighted (**C**) images demonstrate fluid posteriorly and marginal tibiotalar edema (*arrows*) due to associated impingement.

could be secondary to calcium in a tophus. Homogeneous enhancement was seen in all of the tophi except for one.

Pigmented villonodular synovitis (PVNS) is characterized by synovial proliferation with hemosiderin deposition (17,240). Changes may be intraarticular or involve bursae and tendon sheaths. When the tendon sheath is affected, the condition is termed giant cell tumor of the tendon sheath (5,17,241).

Patients are typically 20 to 50 years of age. The hip, knee, ankle, and elbow are most commonly involved (17). Large bone erosions may be evident radiographically (see Fig. 8-150). MR features are characteristic with decreased signal intensity on T1- and T2-weighted sequences due to hemosiderin deposition (see Fig. 8-151). Following resection, recurrence approaches 50%. Therefore, baseline postoperative

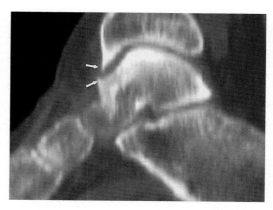

Figure 8-121 Sagittally reformatted CT image demonstrates an anterior tibial osteophyte with secondary deformity of the talus (*arrows*).

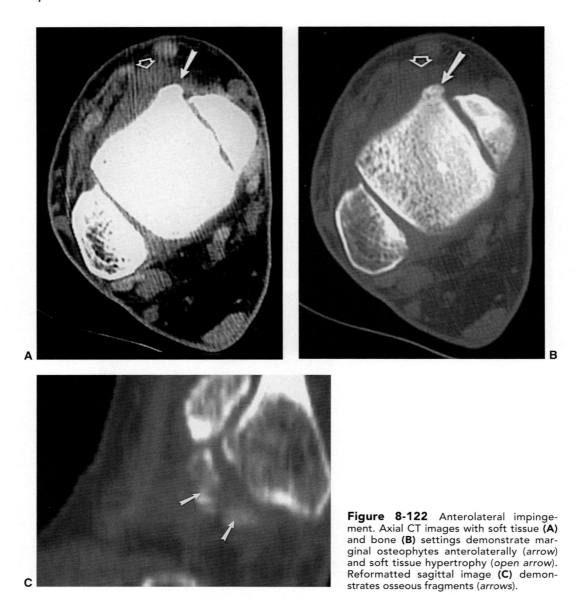

Figure 8-122 Anterolateral impingement. Axial CT images with soft tissue **(A)** and bone **(B)** settings demonstrate marginal osteophytes anterolaterally (*arrow*) and soft tissue hypertrophy (*open arrow*). Reformatted sagittal image **(C)** demonstrates osseous fragments (*arrows*).

TABLE 8-6

FOREFOOT PAIN SYNDROMES

Stress fractures
Lisfranc injuries
Metatarsalgia
Sesamoiditis
Osteochondritis
Metatarsophalangeal subluxation/synovitis
Hallux rigidus
Neuromas
Turf toe
Plantar plate injuries
Freiberg infraction
Bursitis

From references 5, 17, 114, and 118.

studies should be obtained to optimize detection of residual or recurrent lesions (17,143,240).

Infections in the foot and ankle may result from direct implantation (puncture wound or surgery), spread from a contiguous source (i.e., soft tissue to bone or joint) or via the hematogenous route (5,13,68,101,234,242). In the hindfoot, infections tend to remain localized. However, in the midfoot and forefoot, infection can spread along tendon sheaths and different compartments despite fascial separation (69,70). The majority of infections are bacterial. However, tuberculosis, atypical mycobacterial, and fungal infections are becoming more common, especially in immunocompromised patients (5,23,243). Only 10% of skeletal tuberculosis involves the foot. Therefore, diagnosis is often delayed because of insidious onset and lack of physician awareness (23).

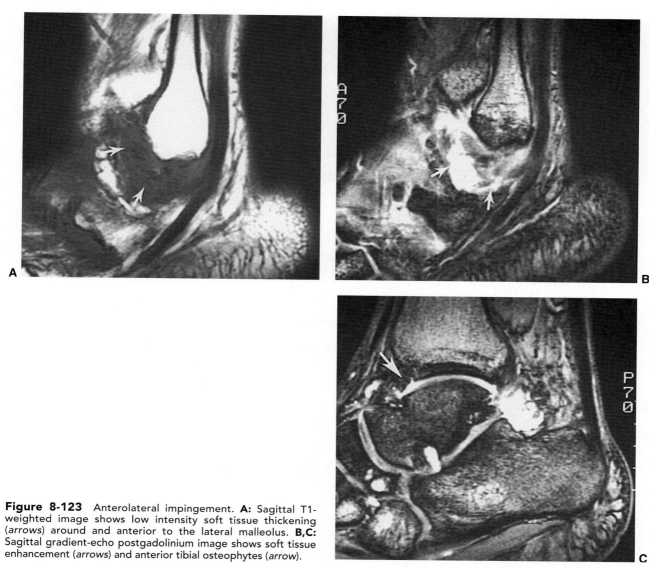

Figure 8-123 Anterolateral impingement. **A:** Sagittal T1-weighted image shows low intensity soft tissue thickening (*arrows*) around and anterior to the lateral malleolus. **B,C:** Sagittal gradient-echo postgadolinium image shows soft tissue enhancement (*arrows*) and anterior tibial osteophytes (*arrow*).

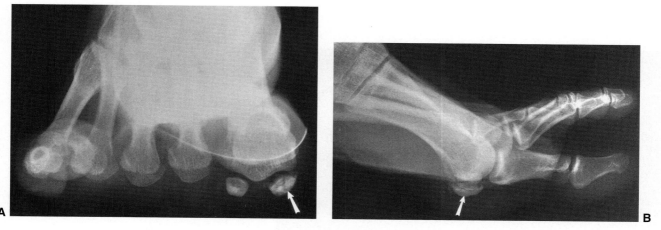

Figure 8-124 Sesamoid view **(A)** and lateral **(B)** radiographs demonstrate sclerosis and fragmentation of the medial sesamoid (*arrow*).

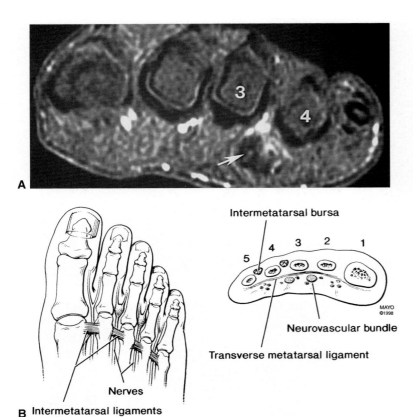

Intermetatarsal bursa

Neurovascular bundle

Transverse metatarsal ligament

Nerves

B Intermetatarsal ligaments

Figure 8-125 **A:** Axial fat-suppressed postgadolinium image demonstrates a large Morton neuroma (*arrow*) between the third (*3*) and fourth (*4*) metatarsal heads. **B:** Illustration of the location of Morton neuroma and bursae with relation to the transverse metatarsal ligament.

T1- and T2-weighted or STIR sequences along with contrast-enhanced fat-suppressed T1-weighted images are important to detect and stage infections (5,143).

A more thorough discussion of infection can be found in Chapter 13. However, because of complex problems, including infection in the diabetic foot, a more thorough discussion of diabetic foot disorders is warranted.

DIABETIC FOOT

There are 15 million diabetic patients in the United States. Problems involving the feet occur in 10% of diabetics and 15% to 20% will be hospitalized at some point for foot and ankle complications (105,172, 232,244). There are 50,000 lower extremity amputations

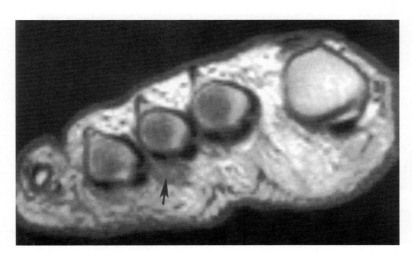

Figure 8-126 Morton neuroma. Axial T1-weighted image shows an intermediate-signal-intensity neuroma (*arrow*) between the third and fourth metatarsal heads.

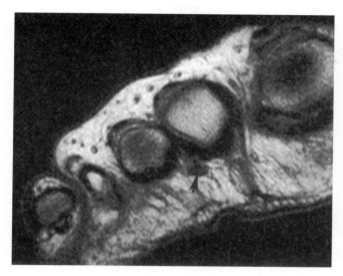

Figure 8-127 Morton's neuroma. Axial T1-weighted image demonstrates a low-signal-intensity neuroma (*arrow*) between the second and third metatarsal heads.

in diabetic patients each year, resulting in costs that exceed $1 billion (172).

Diabetic patients have numerous problems that make detection and characterization complex on imaging studies (1,5,14,232,245–247). Cellulitis, neurotrophic and ischemic ulceration, vascular insufficiency, bone infarction, infection, and neurotrophic arthropathy may all be present to varying degrees (1,5,172).

Both large- and small-vessel disease lead to ischemic changes with poor wound healing and ulceration (172,246,

247). Neuropathy may affect the motor nerves, resulting in muscle atrophy and altered biomechanics that then cause foot calluses and ulceration. Sensory neuropathy leads to decreased perception resulting in soft tissue injury and neurotrophic arthropathy (105,172,232,246,247).

Neurotrophic arthropathy is most often seen in diabetics during the fifth through seventh decades (1,232,247). Radiographically, the earliest changes include soft tissue swelling, juxta-articular osteopenia due to hyperemia, and joint effusions. Later, changes progress to include joint subluxation and osteoarticular destructive changes (Fig. 8-152). Tarsometatarsal involvement is often severe, leading to metatarsal displacement resembling a Lisfranc injury (1,5,232).

Infection can be difficult to differentiate from neurotrophic changes. Both conditions can cause cartilage destruction, bone resorption, bone proliferation, and subluxation (see Figs. 8-152 and 8-153). The presence of sequestra and periosteal reaction are more suggestive of infection (232,247).

Numerous imaging techniques have been employed to solve these difficult foot problems in diabetic patients. Three-phase bone scans are sensitive and useful for patients with suspected infection (14,245). Seldin et al. (245) described focal hyperemic changes on early (vascular and blood pool) ^{99m}Tc-methylene diphosphonate (MDP) bone scans with associated focal increased tracer on delayed images were 94% sensitive and 79% specific for osteomyelitis. Combined studies using ^{99m}Tc-MDP with ^{67}Ga-citrate or ^{111}In-labeled white blood cells may be more specific (11). Though reports vary to some degree, Merkel et al. (13) reported a sensitivity of 48%, specificity of 86%,

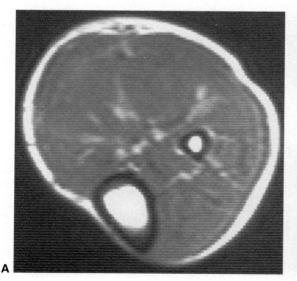

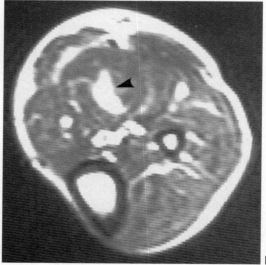

A   B

Figure 8-128 Prone axial images of the calf in a patient with a tear in the medial head of the gastrocnemius. Axial T1-weighted image **(A)** does not demonstrate the lesion, as the hemorrhage is isointense with muscle. The tear is only evident on the T2-weighted image **(B)** (*arrowhead*).

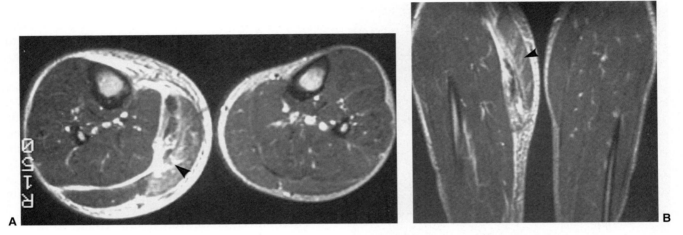

Figure 8-129 Athlete with acute calf pain. Axial **(A)** and coronal **(B)** T2-weighted images show infiltrative high signal intensity (*arrowheads*) due to hemorrhage into the medial gastrocnemius.

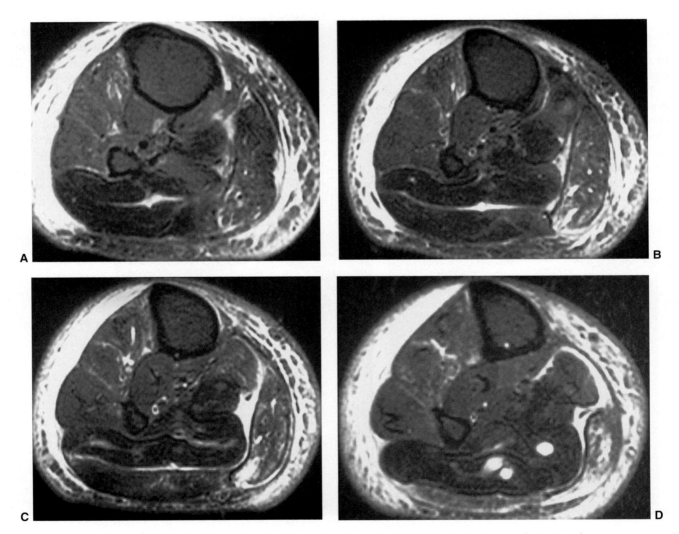

Figure 8-130 Axial fast spin-echo T2-weighted images **(A–D)** demonstrate abnormally increased T2-weighted signal within and surrounding the proximal and midportions of the medial head of gastrocnemius muscle, consistent with partial tear and hematoma.

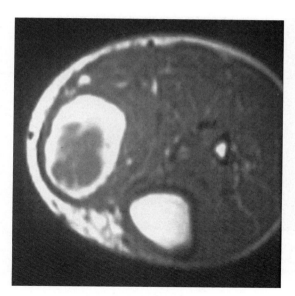

Figure 8-131 Axial T2-weighted image of the calf in a patient with a large gastrocnemius hematoma.

and accuracy of 57% for combined ^{99m}Tc-MDP and ^{67}Ga-citrate and sensitivity of 86%, specificity of 83%, and accuracy of 83% for combined ^{99m}Tc-MDP and [111]-labeled white blood cell studies in patients with low-grade infection. Multiple series compared three-phase bone scans combined with ^{111}In-labeled white blood cells from 1986 through 1993. Sensitivities varied from 73% to 90% and specificities from 55% to 91% in diabetic patients (105). CT can also be useful, especially for evaluation of bone loss and sequestra formation (11,232).

MRI offers significant advantages over other techniques for evaluating bone, soft tissue, and vascular disease (1,5,105,246–249). Early marrow abnormalities are easily detected due to low signal intensity on T1-weighted images and high signal intensity on T2-weighted and STIR sequences (see Figs. 8-153 to 8-154) (5,172). Signal intensity changes in marrow were 98% sensitive and 75% specific for infection in a series reported by Erdman et al. (101) Contrast-enhanced fat-suppressed T1-weighted images are used routinely and improve accuracy for detection and

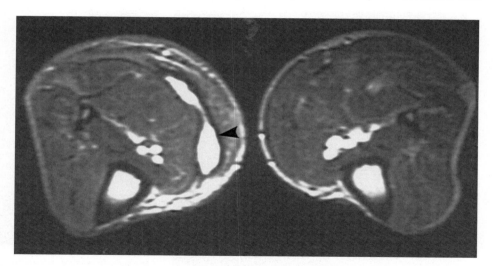

Figure 8-132 Prone axial T2-weighted image in a patient with a muscle tear 2 years ago. Note the fluid collection (*arrowhead*) with surrounding fibrous capsule.

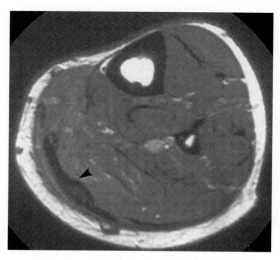

Figure 8-133 Old gastrocnemius tear with scar tissue (*arrowhead*) replacing the muscle in the region of injury.

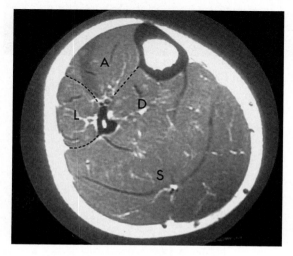

Figure 8-134 Axial T1-weighted image of the calf demonstrating the four compartments of the leg. *A*, anterior; *L*, lateral; *D*, deep posterior; *S*, superficial posterior.

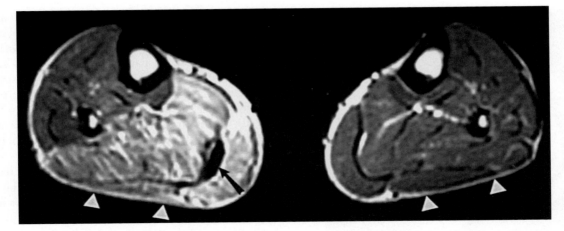

Figure 8-135 Axial T2-weighted images of the calves in a patient with chronic compartment syndrome. There is fibrosis (*arrow*) due to an old tear and increased signal intensity posteriorly due to chronic edema. Note the compression of soft tissue (*arrowheads*) due to failure to use prone instead of supine positioning.

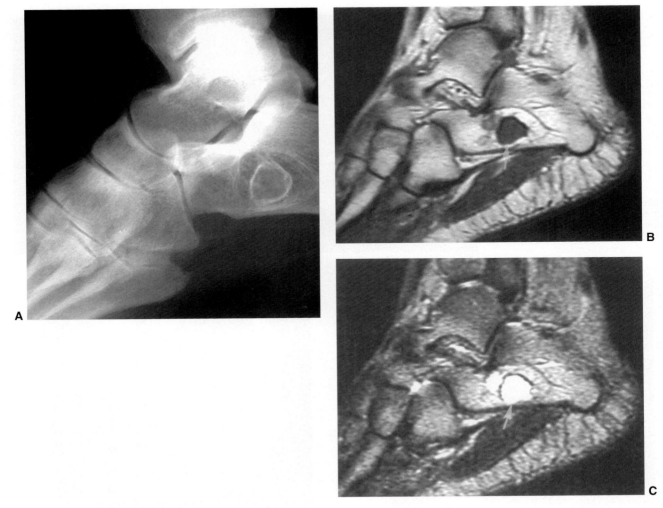

Figure 8-136 Interosseous lipoma. **A:** Radiograph demonstrates a lucent area in the calcaneus with calcification. Sagittal T1- **(B)** and T2-weighted **(C)** images demonstrate cystic involution (*arrow*).

TABLE 8-7

BONE TUMORS OF THE FOOT AND ANKLE (11,087 PRIMARY BONE TUMORS)

Lesions	#/% Foot and ankle
Benign (299)	
Interosseous lipoma	66/32%
Osteochondroma	45/5%
Nonossifying fibroma	38/30%
Osteoid osteoma	33/10%
Giant cell tumor	35/6%
Aneurysmal bone cyst	25/9%
Enchondroma	25/9%
Chondromyxoid fibroma	11/24%
Chondroblastoma	11/9%
Osteoblastoma	7/8%
Malignant (176)	
Osteogenic sarcoma	62/4%
Ewing sarcoma	43/8%
Chondrosarcoma	32/4%
Hemangioendothelial sarcoma	13/16%
Fibrosarcoma	11/4%
Lymphoma	12/2%
Adamantinoma	6/18%
Multiple myeloma	2/0.2%

From Campbell RSD, Grainger AJ, Beggs I, et al. Intraosseous lipoma: report of 35 new cases and a review of the literature. *Skeletal Radiol* 2003;32:209–222; Kiegley BA, Haggar AM, Gaba A, et al. Primary tumors of the foot: MR imaging. *Radiology* 1989;171:755–759; and Unni KK. *Dahlin's bone tumors: general aspects and data on 11,087 cases,* 5th ed. Philadelphia, PA: Lippincott–Raven, 1996.

staging of infections (105,250). As noted above, joint fluid or soft tissue ulceration over an osseous structure (see Figs. 8-155 through 8-157) without marrow signal abnormality usually do not indicate osseous infection.

MRI is also more useful than isotope studies in demonstrating the extent of soft tissue inflammation and abscess involvement of specific compartments in the foot (see Figs. 8-157 to 8-159). Soft tissue contrast provided by MRI is superior to CT in this regard. Delineation of the extent and compartments (Fig. 8-158) involved with infection is especially important if operative debridement is to be accomplished successfully.

Ledermann et al. (69,70,250,251) evaluated several aspects of infection including bone, joint, tendon involvement, and dissemination of infection. Tendon involvement occurs in 50% of foot infections, with evidence of dissemination along the tendon sheath in 20% of cases (69). Spread through fascial compartments also occurred, indicating compartments do not serve as a barrier to dissemination of infections. Ninety-seven percent of abscesses occurred adjacent to skin ulcerations (250).

Morrison et al. (105) compared the cost effectiveness of MRI with other imaging modalities for diagnosis of osteomyelitis in 27 diabetic and 35 nondiabetic patients. The cost of MRI was felt to be competitive related to changes in and effectiveness of treatment plans. MRI showed a sensitivity of 82% and specificity of 80% in diabetics and 89% and 94%, respectively, in nondiabetic patients (see Figs. 8-160 and 8-161) (105).

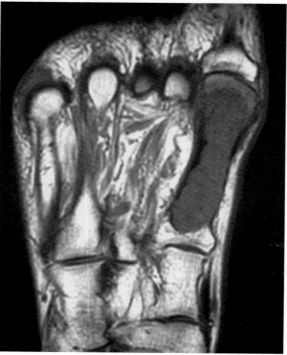

Figure 8-137 Enchondroma. Axial T2-weighted image **(A)** shows a high intensity lesion in the first metatarsal with no soft tissue extension. Coronal proton density-weighted image **(B)** shows a low intensity lesion involving the majority of the first metatarsal. Radiographically an enchondroma was the more obvious diagnosis.

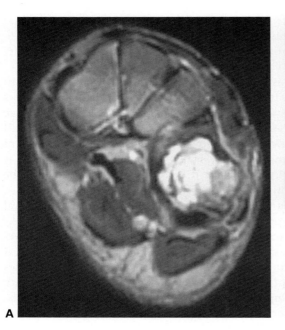

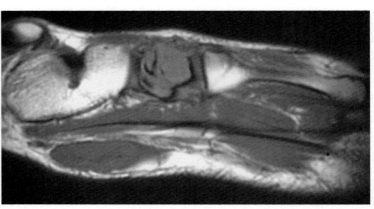

Figure 8-138 Giant cell tumor of the cuboid. Axial T2- **(A)** and sagittal T1-weighted **(B)** images show an expanding inhomogeneous lesion that could be difficult to differentiate from malignancy based on MR features. However, the soft tissues are clearly spared.

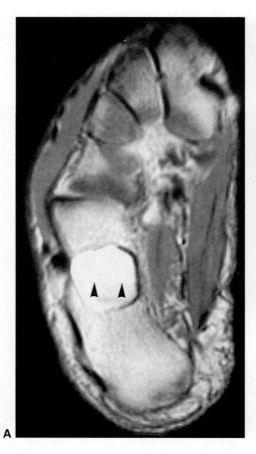

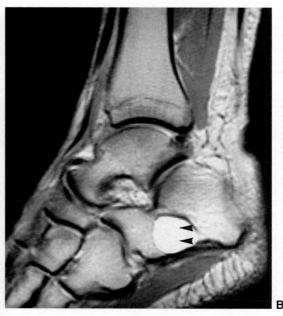

Figure 8-139 Simple cyst. Axial **(A)** and sagittal **(B)** proton density-weighted images demonstrate a cystic lesion in the calcaneus with a fluid–fluid level (*arrowheads*). This is nonspecific and can be noted in giant cell tumors, aneurysmal bone cysts, simple cysts, chondroblastomas, and telangiectatic osteosarcomas.

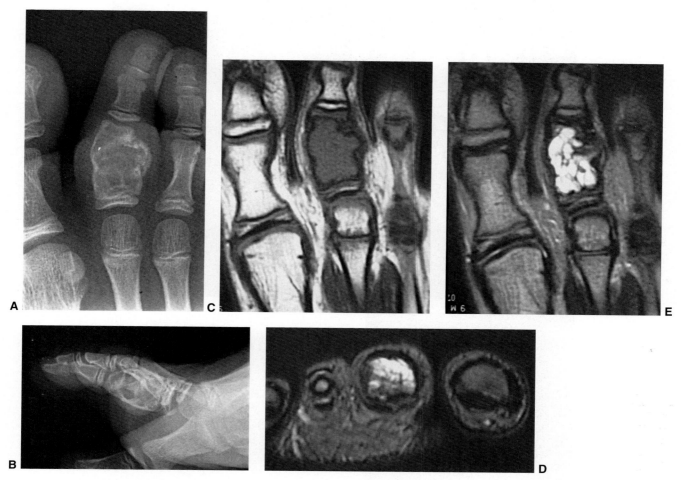

Figure 8-140 Aneurysmal bone cyst of the second proximal phalanx. The growth plates are still open, effectively excluding giant cell tumor from the differential diagnosis. Anteroposterior **(A)** and lateral **(B)** radiographs show the expanded septated appearance. Coronal T1-weighted image **(C)** demonstrates a lesion with signal intensity slightly higher than muscle. Axial **(D)** and coronal **(E)** T2-weighted images show high signal intensity with septation and small fluid-fluid levels. (From Berquist TH. *Radiology of the foot and ankle*, 2nd ed. Philadelphia, PA: Lippincott, Williams & Wilkins, 2000.)

TABLE 8-8

SOFT TISSUE TUMORS OF THE FOOT AND ANKLE (736 CASES)

Fibrohistiocytic tumors (inter. malign.)	170
Glomus tumor	98
Synovial sarcoma	78
Clear cell sarcoma	54
Epithelioid sarcoma	50
Liposarcoma	49
Angiosarcoma with and without lymphedema	47
Rhabdomyosarcoma	40
Hemangiopericytoma	37
Glomangioma	29
Alveolar sarcoma (soft part)	21
Fibromatoses	18
Extraskeletal Ewing sarcoma	18
Glomangiomyoma	14
Giant cell tumor (tendon sheath)	13

From Weiss SW, Goldblum JR. *Enzinger and Weiss's soft tissue tumors*, 4th ed. St. Louis, MO: Mosby, 2001.

Both conventional and MR angiography can be used to evaluate vascular disease in diabetic patients (5,18,19,172). Both are effective for large vessel disease to evaluate potential bypass procedures. Dynamic bolus gadolinium techniques can be used to improve demonstration of small vessel disease. Vascular changes and reduction in soft tissue enhancement indicate lack of tissue perfusion (18,19).

Chomel et al. (18) used three-dimensional contrast-enhanced MR angiography to evaluate diabetic vascular disease. Both feet were evaluated using a phased array head coil. Images were acquired in the oblique coronal plane using FLASH (4.6/1.8, a 420 rectangular field of view, 310 × 512 matrix, slice-thickness of 92 mm divided into 46 parts. and an acquisition time of 52 s). Three-dimensional mask images were obtained prior to injection. A double dose (0.2 mmol/kg) of gadolinium was administered at 1 mm/sec. Macro- and microvascular changes were clearly demonstrated using this technique.

MRI is also capable of demonstrating soft tissue ulceration (Figs. 8-155 and 8-160) and callus formation.

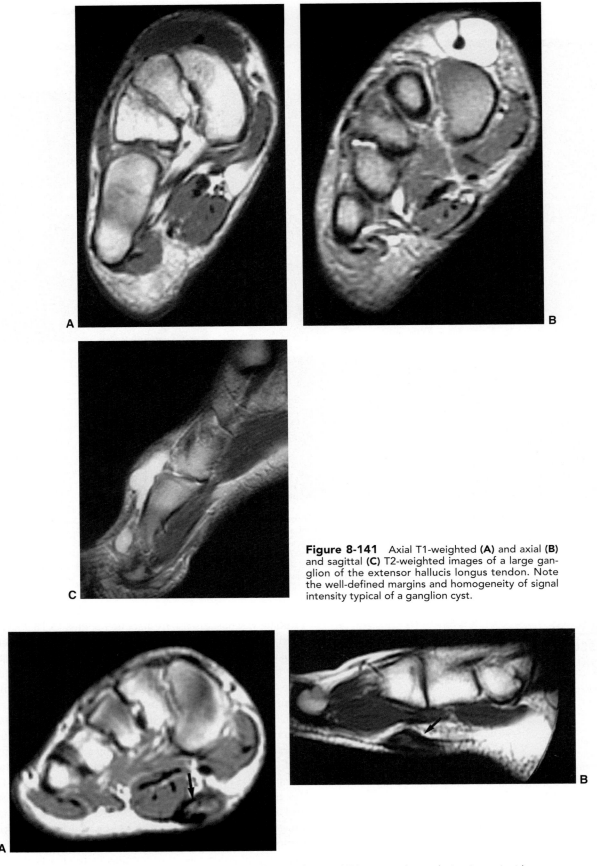

Figure 8-141 Axial T1-weighted **(A)** and axial **(B)** and sagittal **(C)** T2-weighted images of a large ganglion of the extensor hallucis longus tendon. Note the well-defined margins and homogeneity of signal intensity typical of a ganglion cyst.

Figure 8-142 Plantar fibromatosis. Axial **(A)** and sagittal **(B)** images show a lesion (*arrow*) with a large amount of scar or collagen (*black*) and central increased signal intensity. Findings are typical of fibromatosis or desmoid tumor.

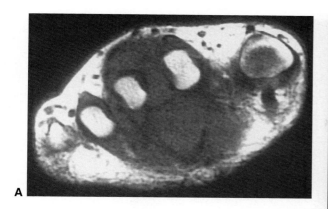

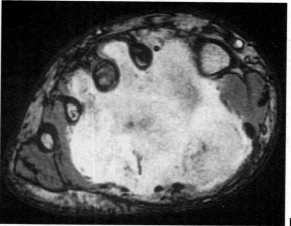

Figure 8-143 Desmoid tumor. Axial T1- **(A)** and T2-weighted **(B)** images demonstrate a large lesion involving multiple plantar and dorsal compartments. There are areas of low intensity on the T2-weighted sequence in **B**.

Calluses are common beneath the metatarsal heads. There is skin thickening with low signal intensity in the subcutaneous fat on both T1- and T2-weighted sequences (see Fig. 8-162). Enhancement can occur on postcontrast images (172).

MARROW EDEMA AND OSTEONECROSIS

Not unlike the hip, marrow edema and osteonecrosis in the foot and ankle have similar presentations. Edema may involve single or multiple osseous structures (252). Fernandez-Canton et al. (102) reported edema in an average of four osseous structures. All patients had associated soft tissue edema and one third had joint effusions. In 72% of cases, the pain and edema improved. There was partial improvement in 20%, no improvement in 8%, and the edema developed in the contralateral foot in 24%.

Zanetti et al. (115) described three marrow edema patterns. Type one was a simple edema pattern; type 2, edema plus necrotic zones; and type 3, edema with linear fracture-like zones. Symptoms were slow to resolve with edema only (type 1).

Specific areas of interest in the foot and ankle include posttraumatic AVN of the talus, which is a significant problem following fractures of this structure (5,253). Additional areas where AVN occur include the metatarsal heads (Freiberg infraction) and the navicular (Köhler disease) (see Fig. 8-163) (41,180). The MR patterns of AVN or osteonecrosis of bone in the foot and ankle are similar to those described elsewhere (see Chapter 6).

AVN in the tarsal bones, particularly the talus, is more common and generally follows significant trauma (5,253). Necrosis occurs because of the tenuous vascular supply of the talus, which has extensive articular surface area and few entrance sites for blood supply. AVN following talar neck injury is most common after complex fracture dislocations (Hawkins type III and IV) (253). The body of the talus is more prone to osteonecrosis than the head or neck. The earliest radiographic signs do not occur for 6 to 8 weeks. In the presence of a fracture, radionuclide studies may not be as useful because of the increased uptake due to normal fracture healing.

MRI is a sensitive technique for early detection of AVN. Both T1- and T2-weighted sequences should be performed to assist in differentiating areas of hyperemia or revascularization (high signal intensity on T1-weighted sequences) from new bone or sclerotic areas (low signal intensity on both T1- and T2-weighted sequences) (see Figs. 8-163 and 8-164) (5,102,115). Contrast enhancement is useful to evaluate perfusion. Comparison with routine radiographs is very useful, especially when areas of bone sclerosis are present. Comparison affords more accurate interpretation of MR images (Fig. 8-163).

The morphologic features vary slightly depending on the osseous structure (tarsals vs. metatarsals) involved. Patterns of osteonecrosis in the talus are geographic (Fig. 8-164) similar to those described in the femoral head (Chapter 6). Involvement of the smaller tarsal bones tends to be more diffuse. Uniform loss of signal intensity on T1-weighted sequences is common in Köhler disease and spontaneous osteonecrosis of the navicular (5,61).

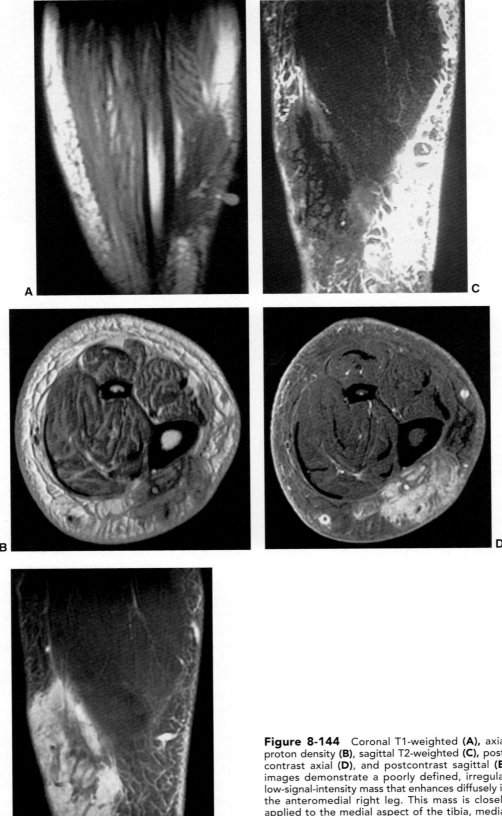

Figure 8-144 Coronal T1-weighted **(A)**, axial proton density **(B)**, sagittal T2-weighted **(C)**, post-contrast axial **(D)**, and postcontrast sagittal **(E)** images demonstrate a poorly defined, irregular low-signal-intensity mass that enhances diffusely in the anteromedial right leg. This mass is closely applied to the medial aspect of the tibia, medial gastrocnemius muscle, and shows extension to the superficial dermis. Mild subcutaneous edema is seen throughout the leg. Findings are consistent with desmoid tumor.

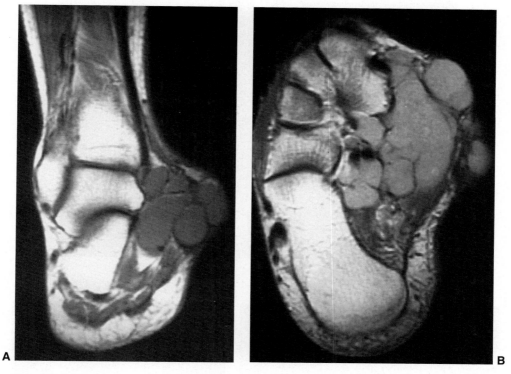

Figure 8-145 Synovial sarcoma. Coronal T1- **(A)** and axial proton density-weighted **(B)** images demonstrate a large multicystic or septated lesion. Cystic appearance is common with synovial sarcomas and could lead one to think this was a benign lesion.

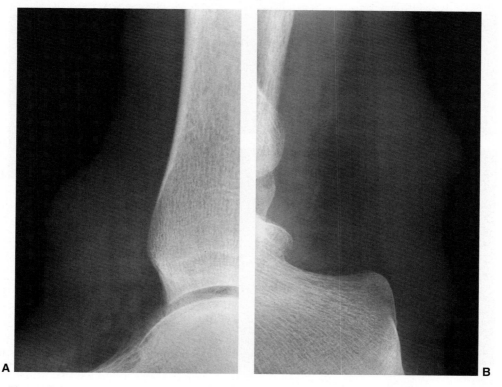

Figure 8-146 Rheumatoid nodules. **A,B:** Lateral images of the ankle demonstrate soft tissue nodules both anteriorly and in the region of the Achilles tendon. Coronal T1-weighted **(C)** and T1-weighted fat-suppressed image with gadolinium enhancement **(D)** in a different patient display a biopsy-proven rheumatoid nodule. The low signal intensity on T1-weighted imaging and intense heterogeneous enhancement has been reported in rheumatoid nodules, but these findings are nonspecific and must be correlated with the clinical history.

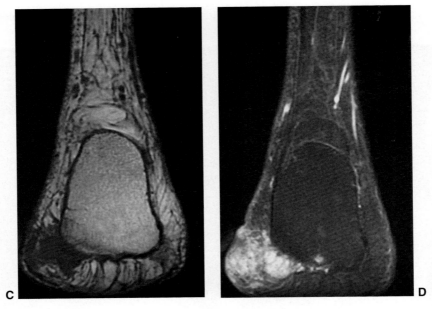

C

D

Figure 8-146 *(continued)*

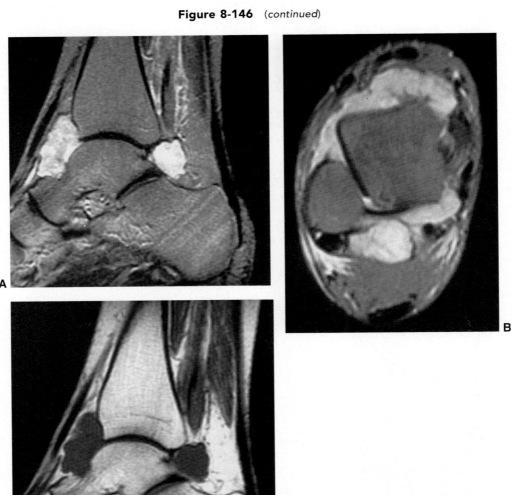

A

B

C

Figure 8-147 T2-weighted sagittal **(A)** and axial **(B)** images of the ankle demonstrate a large high-signal-intensity effusion in the ankle. The T1-weighted sagittal image **(C)** shows the fluid as homogeneous low signal intensity. There are no erosions. The appearance of this fluid is nonspecific. Diagnosis: posttraumatic.

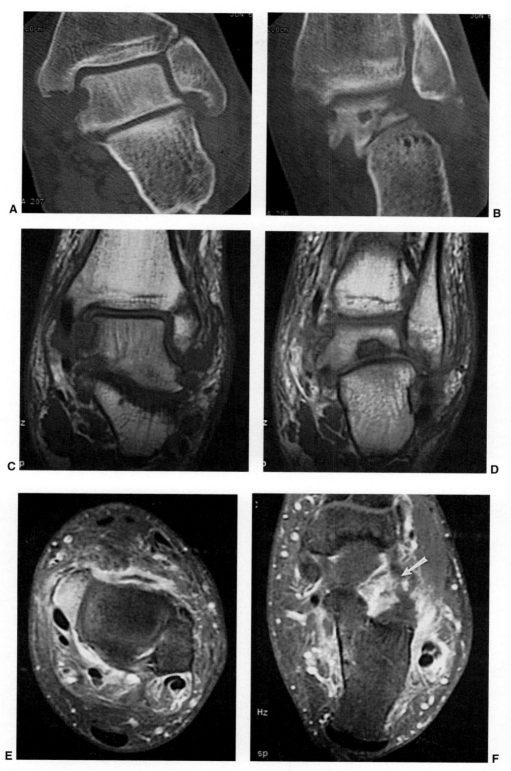

Figure 8-148 Gouty arthritis of the ankle. Coronal CT images displayed in bone windows through the **(A)** medial and **(B)** posterior ankle joint display the extensive erosions involving the medial and lateral malleoli and the medial and posterior talus. **C,D:** Coronal T1-weighted images through the corresponding regions demonstrate low-signal-intensity soft tissue foci associated with the erosive changes. These abnormalities proved to be gouty tophi at arthroscopy. Axial T1-weighted, fat-suppressed, gadolinium-enhanced images of the levels of the ankle joint **(E)** and sinus tarsi **(F)** demonstrate marked enhancement of the tophi throughout the ankle, with associated synovial enhancement of the extensor and peroneal tendon sheaths. Also notice the marked enhancement within the sinus tarsi (*arrow*).

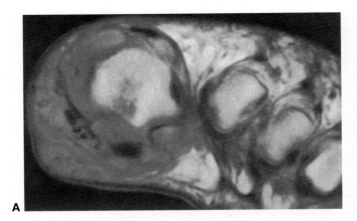

A

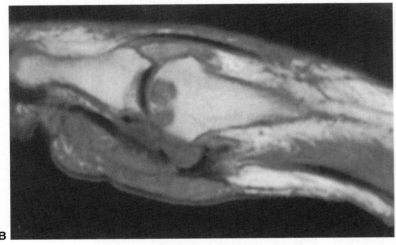

B

Figure 8-149 Gout. Axial **(A)** and sagittal **(B)** T1-weighted images of the great toe demonstrate erosions with intermediate-signal-intensity tophi about the joint.

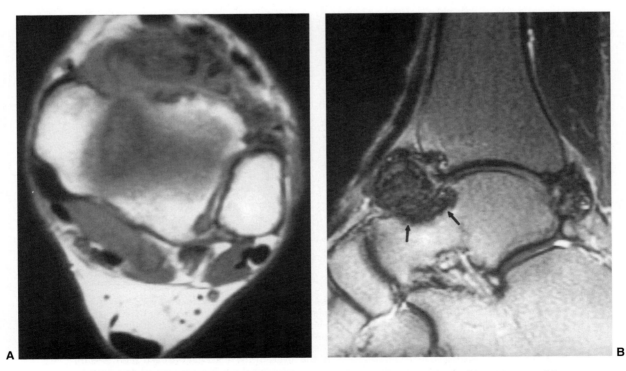

A

B

Figure 8-150 Axial T1- **(A)** and sagittal T2-weighted **(B)** images show low-signal-intensity synovial proliferation with talar erosion (*arrows*) due to pigmented villonodular synovitis.

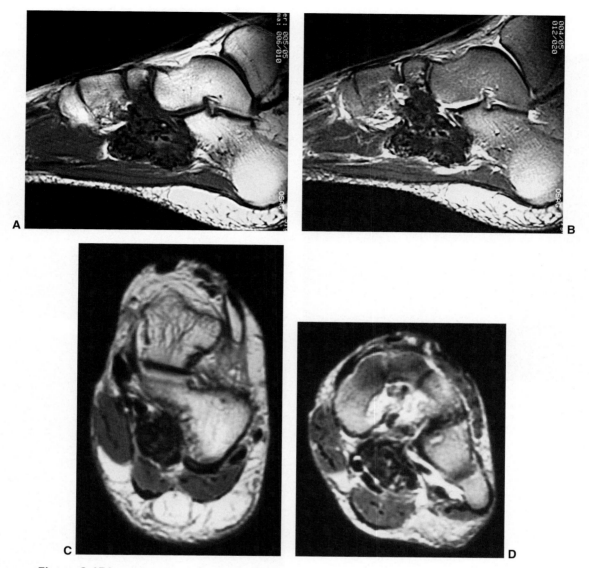

Figure 8-151 Sagittal T1- **(A)** and T2-weighted **(B)** and coronal T1- **(C)** and T2-weighted **(D)** images demonstrate a large low-signal-intensity lesion due to pigmented villonodular synovitis.

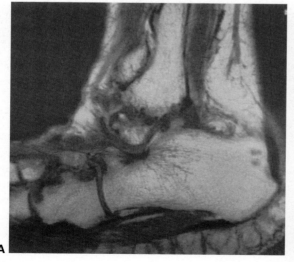

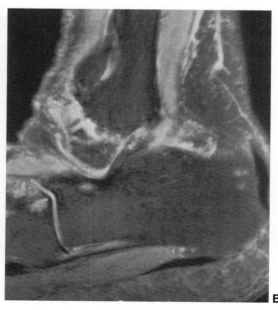

Figure 8-152 Sagittal T1- **(A)** and fast spin-echo T2-weighted **(B)** images demonstrate neurotrophic arthropathy involving the ankle with arch collapse.

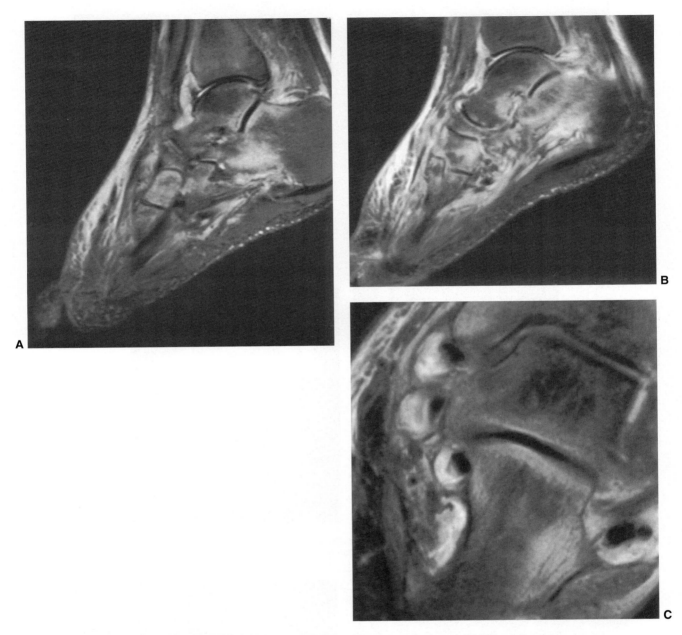

Figure 8-153 Neurotrophic arthropathy. Sagittal **(A,B)** and coronal **(C)** T2-weighted images demonstrate soft tissue and marrow edema with tenosynovitis in **C.** Diabetic foot infections are usually focal compared to the diffuse marrow changes seen in this case.

The latter is a condition that occurs primarily in older women. Patients may have debilitating pain. Bilateral navicular involvement is common. Haller (61) reported uniform low signal intensity on T1-weighted MR images with more subtle changes on T2 weighted sequences. MR features are not specific, and differentiation from trauma and other inflammatory diseases may be difficult (61).

Osteonecrosis of the metatarsal heads (Freiberg infraction) most commonly involves the second metatarsal, but the third metatarsal and, less frequently, the fourth and fifth may also be involved. Females outnumber males 4:1 (5). MR images reveal changes similar to those described in the femoral head (Chapter 6), with a wedge-shaped area of low signal intensity on T1-weighted images. Progression

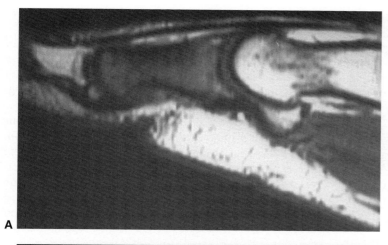

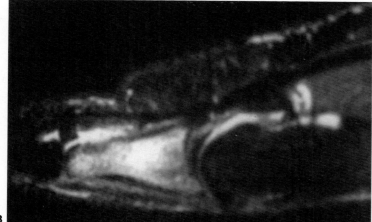

Figure 8-154 Diabetic patient with osteomyelitis of the great toe. Sagittal T1- **(A)** and T2-weighted **(B)** images demonstrate abnormal signal intensity in the first proximal phalanx due to osteomyelitis.

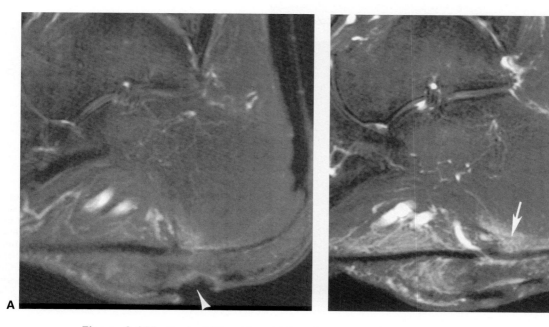

Figure 8-155 Sagittal T2-weighted **(A)** and contrast-enhanced fat-suppressed T1-weighted **(B)** images demonstrate a large ulcer (*arrowhead*) and calcaneal enhancement (*arrow*) due to osteomyelitis.

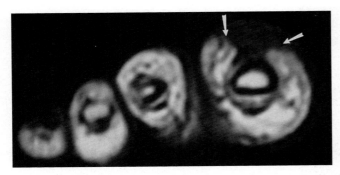

Figure 8-156 Soft tissue ulceration over the great toe. Axial T1-weighted image shows an area of low signal intensity in the soft tissues (*arrows*) but no bone involvement.

to subchondral collapse and degenerative arthritis also occurs (5,17).

Bone infarction has a similar appearance to other areas of the skeleton (Fig. 8-164). Typically, there are well-marginated areas of low to normal signal intensity on T1-weighted sequences and areas of well-defined high signal intensity on T2-weighted sequences (5,61).

Abrahim-Zadeh et al. (96) reviewed six calcanei (in four patients) that contained areas of calcaneal bone infarction. In five of the six calcanei, the foci of bone infarction were entirely or predominantly in the posterior half of the calcaneus (Fig. 8-164). They proposed two theories for bone infarction predominantly seen in the posterior calcaneus: Convergence of the recurrent intraosseous calcaneal artery

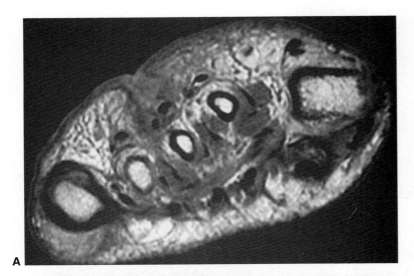

A

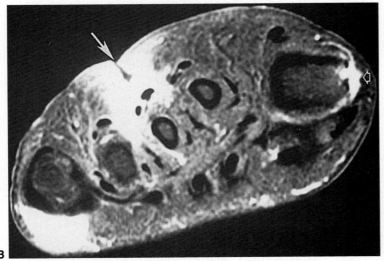

B

Figure 8-157 Proton density **(A)** and fat-suppressed T2-weighted **(B)** images of the foot demonstrate a dorsal sinus tract with soft tissue inflammation best seen on the T2-weighted image in **B** (*arrow*). There is an enlarged plantar bursa beneath the fifth metatarsal and fluid with degenerative erosion (*open arrow*) in the first metatarsal. There is cortical thickening in the fifth metatarsal but no increased signal to suggest infection.

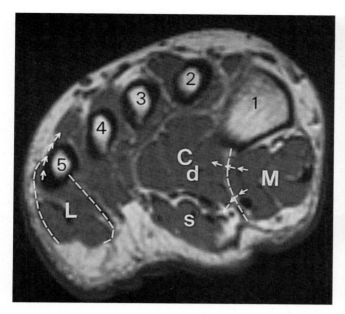

Figure 8-158 Axial T1-weighted image of the foot demonstrating the compartments and direction infections spread (*arrows*). *1–5*, metatarsals; *M*, medial compartment; *C*, central (intermediate) compartment with deep (*d*) and superficial (*s*) sections; *L*, lateral compartment.

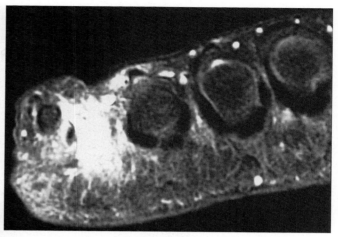

Figure 8-159 Axial postgadolinium fat-suppressed images demonstrate a large area of soft tissue enhancement between the metatarsals resulting from infection. No abscess is present.

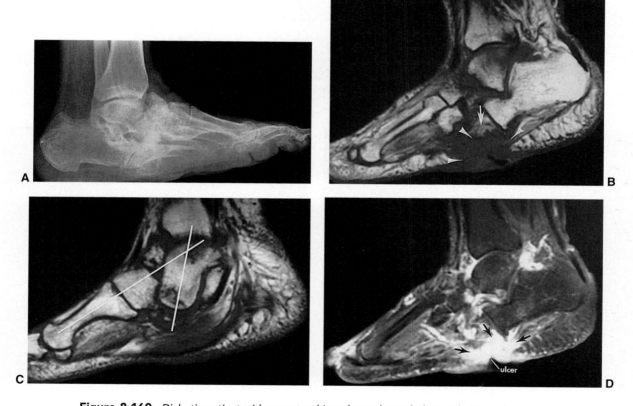

Figure 8-160 Diabetic patient with neurotrophic arthropathy and plantar draining ulcer. Lateral **(A)** radiograph demonstrates midfoot fragmentation with increased bone density and rocker bottom deformity. No destructive lesions or erosions are present. T1-weighted images **(B,C)** demonstrate normal marrow, except for areas of avascular necrosis in the talus and abnormal cuboid (*arrow*). The soft tissue inflammation with the ulceration is of low intensity (*arrowheads*). The talus is vertically oriented (*white lines*). Sagittal fat-suppressed T2-weighted fast spin-echo image **(D)** demonstrates high-signal-intensity soft tissue near the ulcer (*arrows*) with an absent cuboid. The signal intensity in the other visualized osseous structures is normal.

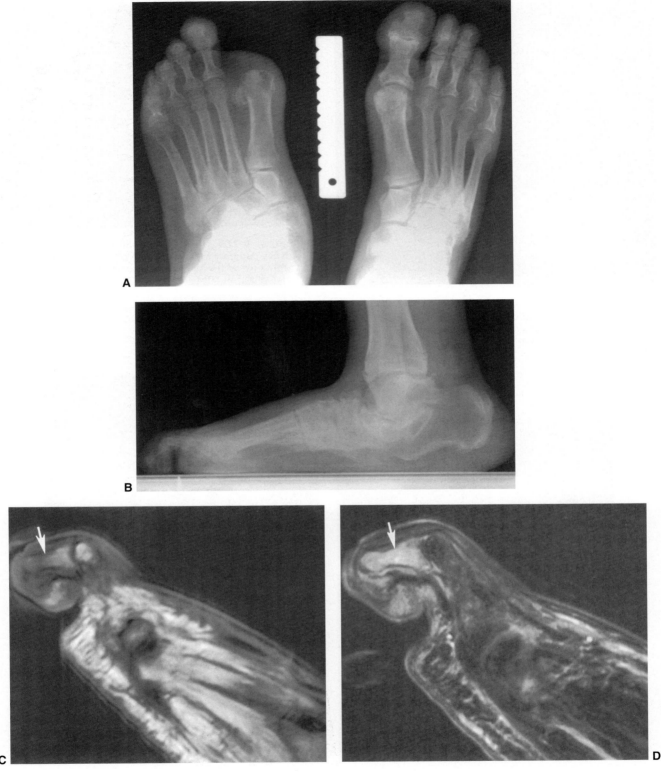

Figure 8-161 Anteroposterior (**A**) and lateral (**B**) radiographs demonstrate neurotrophic changes, amputation of the left great toe, and hammertoe deformities. Sagittal T1- (**C**) and T2-weighted (**D**) images show signal intensity abnormality in the second digit (*arrow*) due to osteomyelitis.

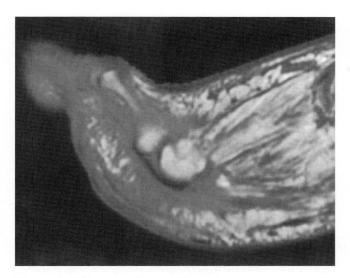

Figure 8-162 Callus. Sagittal T1-weighted images shows skin thickening and low signal intensity in the subcutaneous fat due to a large callus under the metatarsal head.

may act as single dominant artery that is more susceptible to vascular injury; and a watershed zone may be found between the recurrent and the epiphyseal arteries.

Complications of AVN in the foot and ankle do occur. The most common problem is degenerative arthritis resulting in anatomic deformity of the articular surface. Ligament degeneration is a rare complication, but has been described in bone infarcts in the distal tibia. Fibrosarcoma, osteosarcoma, and malignant fibrous histiocytoma have been reported in association with bone infarcts in the ankle (214).

Ischemic changes in the soft tissues are primarily related to vascular diseases and diabetes mellitus. The utility of MRI in determining the extent of ischemic change and the viability of the soft tissues has improved significantly with new MR angiographic techniques (18,19). Spectroscopy may play a role in the future in determining the extent of viable tissue in the leg and foot and following both surgical and medical therapy of soft tissue ischemic disorders (53).

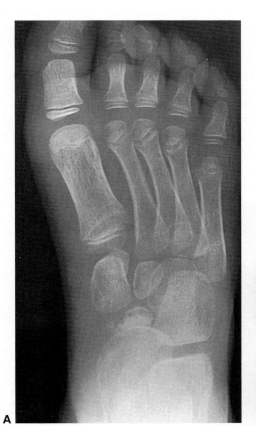

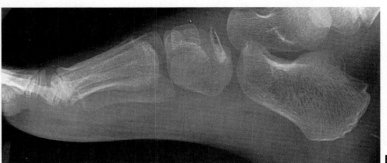

A

B

Figure 8-163 Köhler disease. **A:** Anteroposterior radiograph of the foot demonstrates an irregular sclerotic navicular in a patient with focal pain. **B:** Lateral radiograph taken 4 days later demonstrates progressive collapse of the navicular. **C:** T1-weighted sagittal image demonstrates complete loss of signal of the navicular, consistent with known collapse. **D:** Fast spin-echo T2-weighted fat-suppressed sagittal image shows a hypointense navicular with some focal areas of increased signal (*arrows*).

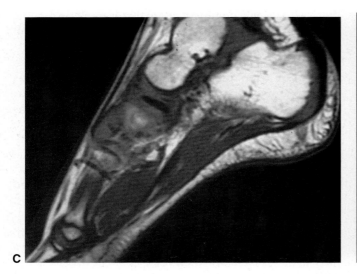

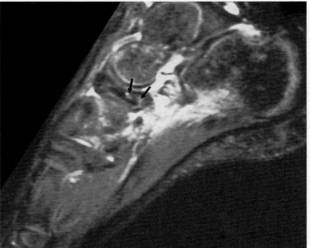

C   D

Figure 8-163 *(continued)*

MEDIAL TIBIAL STRESS SYNDROME

Medial tibial stress syndrome (MTSS) is an exercise-induced syndrome presenting with pain along the tibia. The pain typically occurs during running and is relieved by rest (193,207,254,255). MTSS accounts for 13% of injuries in runners and 22% of injuries in aerobic dancers (255). The syndrome may be due to osseous, periosteal, or deep muscle inflammation (256). Detmer (256) classified this syndrome into three categories. Type I is primarily an

osseous problem. Type II syndromes involve the periosteum or periosteal-fascial junction, and type III injuries are similar to deep chronic compartment syndrome primarily due to muscle inflammation (see Fig. 8-165).

Patients present with pain in the mid- to distal tibia along the posteromedial border. Pain typically persists for hours after the activity is discontinued (255,256). Axial and coronal or sagittal T2-weighted or STIR images are best suited to identify the subtle tibial, periosteal, or soft tissue changes (see Fig. 8-166).

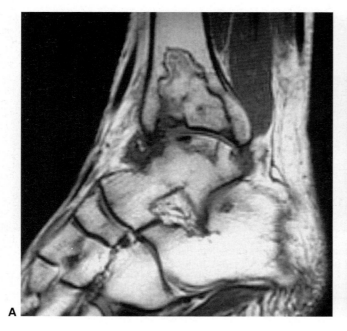

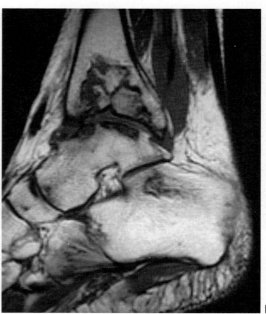

A   B

Figure 8-164 Sagittal images of the ankle in a patient with infarcts in the tibia and calcaneus and avascular necrosis of the talus. T1- **(A,B)** and T2-weighted **(C,D)** images demonstrate the classic well-marginated changes of infarction.

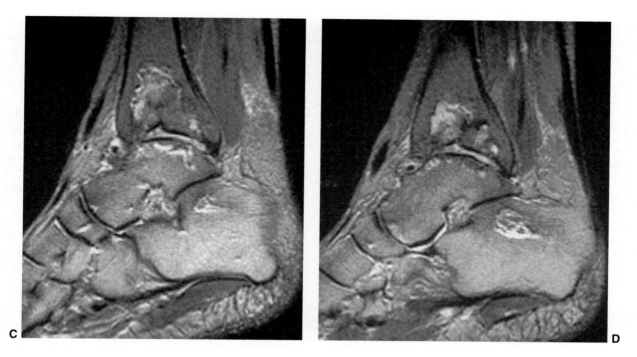

Figure 8-164   (continued)

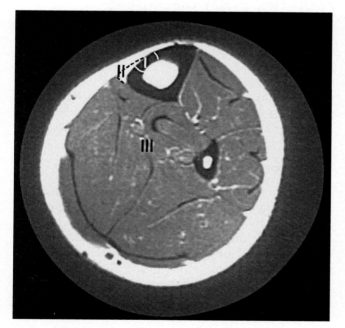

Figure 8-165   Axial T1-weighted image demonstrating the sites of involvement of medial tibial stress syndrome (53). Type I, stress or microfracture of the medial tibia; type II, periosteal-fascial inflammation (dotted lines); type III, inflammation of deep muscles of the posterior tibia.

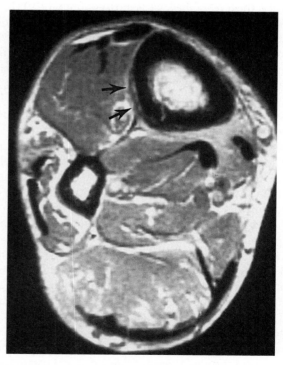

Figure 8-166   Axial T2-weighted image of the leg demonstrating periosteal inflammation along the tibia (arrows).

Treatment is conservative in most cases. However, surgical decompression can provide excellent results in patients who do not respond to rest, steroid injection, antiinflammatory medications, or changes in footwear (255).

More recently, Reinius et al. (84) described a painful tibial condition described as transient tibial edema. MR features and clinical features differ significantly from MTSS (84,256). The four patients described with transient tibial edema were middle-aged or older white females with no history of exercise-induced symptoms or trauma. MR images show diffuse marrow edema (low signal intensity on T1-weighted and increased marrow signal on T2-weighted or STIR sequences) in the tibia. Marrow signal abnormality can be impressive with stress fractures, as well. However, with tibial edema, nearly the entire shaft is involved. Patients with transient tibial edema typically improve spontaneously over 2 to 13 months (84).

NERVE COMPRESSION SYNDROMES

Nerve compression syndromes can occur in the calf, foot, and ankle. Tarsal tunnel syndrome was discussed earlier and will not be repeated in this section. In the calf, nerve injuries or compression may be related to muscle herniation, ganglion cysts, hematomas, and other soft tissue masses. Impingement of the common, deep, or superficial peroneal nerves at the level of the knee is most common (4,193).

Nerve entrapment in the foot and ankle is commonly related to acute or chronic trauma, but space-occupying lesions may also be involved (17,103,106,257). Clinical and electromyographic diagnosis are not always reliable. Therefore, there is a role for high resolution MR imaging and ultrasound in these patients (257). The posterior tibial nerve and branches are often affected in the tarsal tunnel. However, we will focus on other nerve entrapment syndromes.

The medial calcaneal nerve arises from the lateral plantar of posterior tibial nerve (see Fig. 8-167). It passes through the flexor retinaculum to supply the cutaneous region medial to the Achilles tendon and the posteromedial heel (44,46,257). Chronic heel trauma in runners or fat pad atrophy in diabetic patients can result in medial calcaneal nerve injury (257).

The inferior calcaneal nerve branches from the lateral plantar nerve at the level of the medial malleolus (Fig. 8-167). The nerve then passes between the abductor hallucis and quadratus plantae to send motor branches to the abductor digiti quinti and a sensory branch to the anterior calcaneal tubercle (44,46). Heel pain mimics plantar fasciitis. Nerve injury may result from calcaneal osteophytes, foot deformities, or plantar fasciitis. Atrophy of the abductor digiti quinti muscle may occur over time (257).

The sural nerve (Figs. 8-6 and 8-167) follows the lateral margin of the Achilles tendon and continues distally inferior to the peroneal tendon sheath. The nerve divides into medial and lateral branches at the level of the fifth metatarsal base. The sural nerve provides sensory fibers to the lateral heel, foot, and ankle (44,46). Injury may result from fractures of the base of the fifth metatarsal; calcaneus, cuboid, peroneal tendon disorders; or in patients with chronic lateral ankle instability (62,257).

The deep peroneal nerve passes under the extensor retinaculum between extensor digitorum longus and extensor hallucis longus (Fig. 8-167). Distally, there is a medial sensory and lateral motor branch. Compression can occur in the tarsal tunnel or over the dorsum of the foot (257). Tight footwear, foot deformity, or dorsal soft tissue trauma are responsible for the latter (257).

The superficial peroneal nerve passes through the deep fascia of the leg well above the lateral malleolus (Fig. 8-167). The nerve supplies motor branches to the peroneal muscles and sensory branches to the dorsal lateral ankle and foot (Fig. 8-167) (44,46,257). Nerve injury may occur with inversion or plantar flexion injuries (257).

MR imaging with axial or oblique axial planes is optimal for following the course of neural structures. Both T1- and T2-weighted images should be obtained. Contrast-enhanced images are useful for evaluating perfusion and nerve inflammation. Contrast enhancement is especially useful in the absence of obvious pathology in the region of the nerve (5).

PEDIATRIC FOOT DISORDERS

MR imaging provides valuable information regarding evolving osseous and cartilaginous structures in infants and children (8,41,258–260). Trauma, osteochondritis dissecans, neoplasms, and Köhler disease (Fig. 8-63) were discussed in earlier sections of this chapter. Therefore, we will focus on the utility of MRI for evaluation of tarsal coalition and congenital foot deformities.

Tarsal Coalition

Tarsal coalition occurs in 2% of the general population. It is a common cause of hindfoot pain in adolescents. The condition is bilateral in 50% of patients. Tarsal coalitions involve two or more tarsal bones with fibrous, cartilaginous, or osseous fusion. The condition may be posttraumatic, but most believe this is a congenital condition inherited as an autosomal dominant trait with variable penetration (41,261). Calcaneonavicular or talocalcaneal coalitions account for 90% of cases. Fusion of the other tarsal bones occur less frequently (see Figs. 8-169 and 8-170) (41).

Radiographs may demonstrate characteristic features such as the talar beak and "C" sign. The latter is seen as a C-shaped bony density projecting over the midcalcaneus (see Fig. 8-168A) (261). Differentiation of the type of coalition and talar anatomy is better accomplished with CT or MRI (262). T1- and T2-weighted MR images in the sagittal,

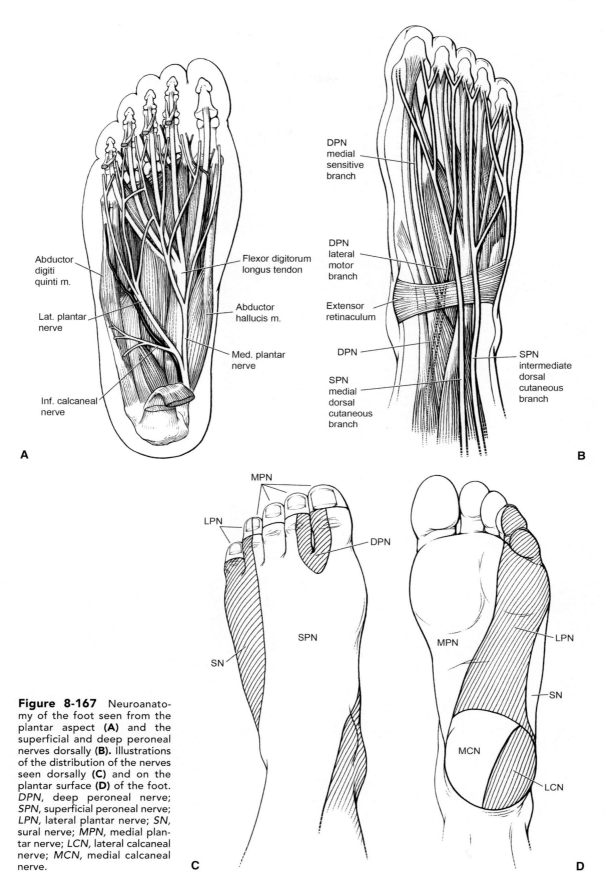

Figure 8-167 Neuroanatomy of the foot seen from the plantar aspect (**A**) and the superficial and deep peroneal nerves dorsally (**B**). Illustrations of the distribution of the nerves seen dorsally (**C**) and on the plantar surface (**D**) of the foot. *DPN*, deep peroneal nerve; *SPN*, superficial peroneal nerve; *LPN*, lateral plantar nerve; *SN*, sural nerve; *MPN*, medial plantar nerve; *LCN*, lateral calcaneal nerve; *MCN*, medial calcaneal nerve.

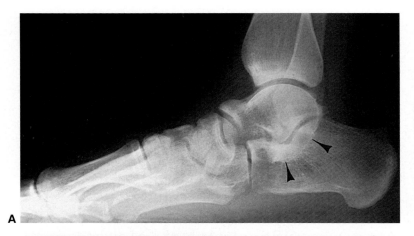

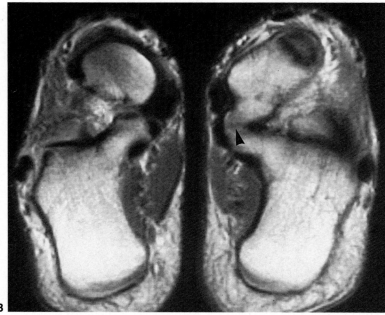

Figure 8-168 Patient with foot pain and suspected tarsal coalition. **A:** Weight-bearing lateral radiograph of the foot demonstrates a talar beak and C-shaped overlap (*arrowheads*) indicating tarsal coalition. **B:** Bony coalition demonstrated on T1-weighted image (*arrowhead*).

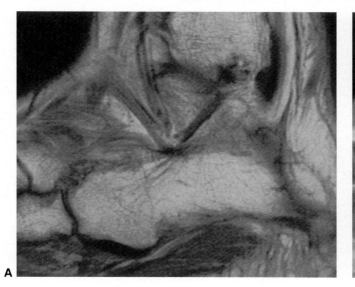

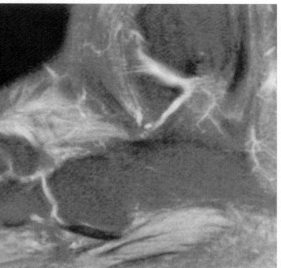

Figure 8-169 Sagittal T1- **(A)** and T2-weighted **(B)** images demonstrate osseous calcaneocuboid coalition.

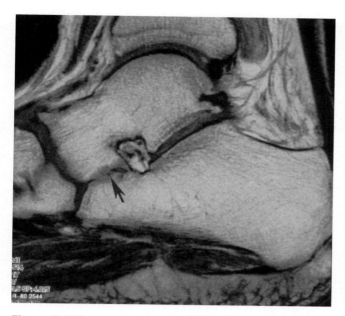

Figure 8-170 Sagittal T1-weighted image shows talocalcaneal coalition anteriorly (*arrow*) that is partially osseous and partially fibrocartilagenous.

coronal, and axial plane or thin-section three-dimensional three- images provide anatomic data and also can differentiate the type of fusion based upon the signal intensity of the coalition. Osseous coalitions have marrow signal intensity (see Fig. 8-169), fibrous low signal intensity on both T1- and T2-weighted sequences, and cartilaginous coalitions have intermediate signal intensity (see Fig. 8-170). The presence of high-signal-intensity fluid between the osseous structures excludes the diagnosis.

Treatment is conservative unless pain is nonresponsive to therapy or range of motion is significantly restricted (41,261).

Congenital Foot Deformities

The use of MRI for congenital foot deformities has been limited due to cost, patient cooperation, and use of radiographs to detect and follow treatment response. In recent years, more attention has been given to MRI due to the multiplanar or three-dimensional capabilities and the ability to evaluate unossified structures effectively. Clubfoot, metatarsus adductus, skewfoot, flatfoot, and congenital vertical talus have been evaluated using MRI (8,42,193).

Clubfoot (talipes equinovarus) disorders have been divided into multiple categories. Congenital clubfoot is the most common, occurring in 1 per 1,000 births. It occurs most commonly in males and is bilateral in 50% of cases (41). Clubfeet can also be related to *in utero* fetal position, associated with other congenital disorders, arthrogryposis, or myelodysplasia (8,41).

Traditionally, measurements and osseous relationships have been obtained using radiographs (5). However, recently

MRI has been used to evaluate hindfoot relationships before and after surgical correction. MRI using conventional coronal, sagittal, and axial images or three-dimensional techniques is useful to measure rotation and subluxation of the tarsal bones as well as postoperative complications (8,42).

The role of MRI in metatarsus adductus, skewfoot, and congenital vertical talus should be similar. However, to date, the MR literature in these areas is not extensive (41).

MISCELLANEOUS CONDITIONS

There are still numerous conditions in which the role of MRI remains unclear. For example, there has been little utility for MRI in evaluation of many metabolic disorders (5,25,263). Recently, studies have been performed to evaluate the role of MR imaging on patients with osteoporosis (25). However, it is unlikely that MR imaging will replace current bone mineral density techniques due to cost and availability.

Hemoglobinopathies and anemias can be detected due to the changes created in the signal intensity of bone marrow on MRI (5,264). However, these changes are not specific and do not allow clear definition of the type of infiltrative process. An exception might be sickle cell anemia, where MRI can detect early changes in the marrow such as infarction (264).

REFERENCES

1. Beltran J, Campanini DS, Knight C, et al. The diabetic foot: magnetic resonance imaging evaluation. *Skeletal Radiol* 1990;19: 37–41.
2. Beltran J, Noto AM, Mosure JC, et al. Ankle: surface coil MR imaging at 1.5 T. *Radiology* 1986;161:203–210.
3. Berger PE, Oftein RA, Jackson DW, et al. MRI demonstration of radiographically occult fractures: what have we been missing? *Radiographics* 1989;9(3):407–436.
4. Berquist TH. *Imaging of orthopedic trauma*, 2nd ed. New York: Raven Press, 1992:453–557.
5. Berquist TH. *Radiology of the foot and ankle*, 2nd ed. Philadelphia: Lippincott Williams & Wilkins, 2000.
6. Erickson SJ, Rosengarten JL. MR imaging of the forefoot: normal anatomic findings. *AJR Am J Roentgenol* 1993;160:565–571.
7. Futami T, Foster BK, Morris LL. Magnetic resonance imaging of growth plate injuries: the efficacy and indications for surgical procedures. *Arch Orthop Trauma Surg* 2000;120:390–396.
8. Kamegaya M, Shinohara Y, Kokuji Y, et al. Evaluation of pathologic abnormalities of clubfoot by magnetic resonance imaging. *Clin Orthop* 2000;379:218–223.
9. Lohman M, Kivisaari A, Kallio P, et al. Acute pediatric ankle trauma: MRI versus plain radiography. *Skeletal Radiol* 2001;30: 504–511.
10. Magee TH, Hinson GW. Usefulness of MR imaging in the detection of talar dome injuries. *AJR Am J Roentgenol* 1998;170: 1227–1230.
11. Gold RH, Hawkins RA, Kats RD, et al. Bacterial osteomyelitis: findings on plain radiography, and scintigraphy. *AJR Am J Roentgenol* 1991;157:365–370.
12. Lee JK, Yao L. Stress fracture: MR imaging. *Radiology* 1988;169: 217–220.
13. Merkel KD, Brown MD, Dewanjee MK, et al. Comparison of indium-labeled leukocyte imaging with sequential technetium-gallium scanning in diagnosis of low grade musculoskeletal sepsis. *J Bone Joint Surg Am* 1985;67A:465–476.

14. Segall GM, Nino-Murcia M, Jacobs T, et al. The role of bone scan and radiography in the diagnostic evaluation of suspected pedal osteomyelitis. *Clin Nucl Med* 1989;14:255–260.

15. Myerson MS, McGarvey W. Disorders of the insertion of the Achilles tendon and Achilles tendinitis. *J Bone Joint Surg* 1999;80A:1814–1824.

16. Premkumar A, Perry MB, Dwyer AJ, et al. Sonography and MR imaging of posterior tibial tendinopathy. *AJR Am J Roentgenol* 2002;178:223–232.

17. Rosenberg ZS, Beltran J, Bencardino JT. MR imaging of the foot and ankle. *Radiographics* 2000;20:S153–S179.

18. Chomel S, Douek P, Moulin P, et al. Contrast enhanced MR angiography of the foot: anatomy and clinical application in patients with diabetes. *AJR Am J Roentgenol* 2004;182:1435–1442.

19. Sharafuddin MJ, Stolpen AH, Sun S, et al. High-resolution multiphase contrast-enhanced three-dimensional MR angiography compared to two-dimensional time-of-flight MR angiography for identification of pedal vessels. *J Vasc Interv Radiol* 2002;13:695–702.

20. Cahill DR. Anatomy and function of the contents of the human tarsal sinus and canal. *Anat Rec* 1965;153:1–18.

21. Chandnani VP, Harper MT, Ficke JR, et al. Chronic ankle instability: evolution with MR arthrography, MR imaging and stress radiography. *Radiology* 1994;192:189–194.

22. Cheung Y, Rosenberg ZS, McGee T, et al. Normal anatomy and pathologic conditions of ankle tendons: current imaging techniques. *Radiographics* 1992;12:429–444.

23. Deutsch AL, Mink JH, Kear R. *MRI of the foot and ankle.* New York: Raven Press, 1992.

24. Klein MA. Reformatted three-dimensional fourier transform gradient-recalled echo MR imaging of the ankle: spectrum of normal and abnormal findings. *AJR Am J Roentgenol* 1993;161:831–836.

25. Boutry N, Cortet B, Dubois P, et al. Trabecular bone structure of the calcaneus: preliminary in vivo MR imaging assessment of men with osteoporosis. *Radiology* 2003;227:708–717.

26. Hardy CJ, Katzberg RW, Frey RL, et al. Switched surface coil system for bilateral MR imaging. *Radiology* 1988;167:835–838.

27. Muhle C, Frank LR, Rand T, et al. Collateral ligaments of the ankle: high-resolution MR imaging with a local gradient coil and anatomic correlation in cadavers. *Radiographics* 1999;19:673–683.

28. Sierra A, Potchen EJ, Moore J, et al. High field magnetic resonance imaging of aseptic necrosis of the talus. *J Bone Joint Surg Am* 1986;68A:927–928.

29. Soila K, Karjalainen PT, Aronen NJ, et al. High-resolution MR imaging of the asymptomatic Achilles tendon: new observations. *AJR Am J Roentgenol* 1999;173:323–328.

30. Berquist TH. Magnetic resonance techniques in musculoskeletal diseases. *Rheum Dis Clin North Am* 1991;17:599–615.

31. Tuite MJ. MR imaging of the tendons of the foot and ankle. *Semin Musculoskelet Radiol* 2002;6:119–131.

32. Weishaupt D, Treiber K, Kundert H-P, et al. Morton neuroma: MR imaging in prone, supine and upright weight-bearing positions. *Radiology* 2003;226:849–856.

33. Farooki A, Sokoloff RM, Theodorou DJ, et al. Visualization of ankle tendons and ligaments with MR imaging: influence of passive positioning. *Foot Ankle Int* 2002;23:554–559.

34. Rosenberg ZS, Chueng Y, Jahss MH. Computed tomography scan and magnetic resonance imaging of the ankle tendons. An overview. *Foot Ankle Int* 1988;8:297–307.

35. Rubin DA, Towers JB, Britton CA. MR imaging of the foot. Utility of complex oblique imaging planes. *AJR Am J Roentgenol* 1996;166:1079–1084.

36. Breitenseher MJ, Trattnig S, Kukla C, et al. MRI versus lateral stress radiography in acute lateral ankle ligament injuries. *J Comput Assist Tomogr* 1997;21(2):280–285.

37. DiGiovanni BF, Fraga CJ, Cohen BE, et al. Associated injuries found in chronic lateral ankle instability. *Foot Ankle Int* 2000;21:809–815.

38. Pfirrmann CWA, Zanetti M, Hodler J. Joint magnetic resonance imaging. Normal variants and pitfalls related to sports injury. *Radiol Clin North Am* 2002;40:167–180.

39. Winalski CS, Aliabadi P, Wright RJ, et al. Enhancement of joint fluid with intravenously administered gadopenetate and meglumine: techniques, rationale and implication. *Radiology* 1993;187: 179–185.

40. Mohana-Borges AVR, Theumann NH, Pfirrmann CWA, et al. Lesser metatarsophalangeal joints: standard MR imaging, MR arthrography, bursography-initial results in 48 cadaver joints. *Radiology* 2003;227:175–182.

41. Harty MP, Hubbard AM. MR imaging of pediatric abnormalities in the ankle and foot. *Magn Reson Imaging Clin N Am* 2001;9:579–601.

42. Pekindil G, Aktas S, Saridogan K, et al. Magnetic resonance imaging in follow-up of treated clubfoot during childhood. *Eur J Radiol* 2001;37:123–129.

43. Goergen TG, Danzig LA, Resnick D, et al. Roentgen evaluation of the tibiotalar joint. *J Bone Joint Surg Am* 1977;59A:874–877.

44. Gray H, Williams PL. *Anatomy of the human body,* 38th ed. New York: Churchill-Livingstone, 1995.

45. Morrey BF, Cass JR, Johnson KA, et al. Foot and ankle. In: Berquist TH, ed. *Imaging of orthopedic trauma and surgery,* Philadelphia, PA: WB Saunders, 1986.

46. Rosse C, Rosse PG. *Hollinshead's textbook of anatomy,* Philadelphia, PA: Lippincott–Raven Publishers, 1997.

47. Berquist TH. Anatomy, normal variants, and basic biomechanics. In: Berquist TH ed. *Radiology of the foot and ankle,* 2nd ed. Philadelphia: Lippincott Williams & Wilkins, 2000:1–40.

48. Schneck CD, Mesgarzadeh M, Bonakdorpour A, et al. MR imaging of the most commonly injured ankle ligaments. Part I: normal anatomy. *Radiology* 1992;184:499–506.

49. Schneck CD, Mesgarzadeh M, Bonakdorpour A. MR imaging of the most commonly injured ankle ligaments. Part II: ligament injuries. *Radiology* 1992;184:507–512.

50. Schweitzer ME, Ed ME, Deely D, et al. Using MR imaging to differentiate peroneal splits from other peroneal disorders. *AJR Am J Roentgenol* 1997;168:129–133.

51. Vallejo JM, Jaramillo D. Normal imaging anatomy of the ankle and foot in the pediatric population. *Magn Reson Imaging Clin N Am* 2001;9:435–657.

52. Blanchard KS, Finlay DBL, Scott DJA, et al. A radiological analysis of lateral ligament injuries of the ankle. *Clin Radiol* 1986;37:247–251.

53. Bleichrodt RP, Kingma LM, Binnendijk B, et al. Injuries of the lateral ankle ligaments: classification with tenography and arthrography. *Radiology* 1989;173:347–349.

54. Resnick D. Radiology of the talocalcaneal articulations. *Radiology* 1974;111:581–586.

55. Balen PF, Helms CA. Association of posterior tibial tendon injury with spring ligament injury, sinus tarsi abnormality and plantar fasciitis on MR imaging. *AJR Am J Roentgenol* 2001;176:1137–1143.

56. Ferkel RD, Scranton PE. Arthroscopy of the foot and ankle. *J Bone Joint Surg Am* 1993;75A:1233–1242.

57. Fetto JF. Anatomy and physical examination of the foot and ankle. In: Nicholas JA, Hershman EB, eds. *The lower extremity and spine in sports medicine,* Vol. I. St. Louis, MO: C.V. Mosby, 1986:371–395.

58. Pal CP, Tasker AD, Osttere SJ, et al. Heterogeneous signal in bone marrow on MRI of children's feet: a normal finding? *Skeletal Radiol* 1999;28:274–278.

59. Anouchi YS, Parker RD, Seitz WH. Posterior compartment syndrome of the calf resulting from misdiagnosis of a rupture of the medial head of the gastrocnemius. *J Trauma* 1987;27:678–680.

60. Khoury NJ, El-Khoury GY, Saltzman CL, et al. MR imaging of posterior tibial tendon dysfunction. *AJR Am J Roentgenol* 1996;167:675–682.

61. Haller J, Sartoris DJ, Resnick D, et al. Spontaneous osteonecrosis of the tarsal navicular in adults: imaging findings. *AJR Am J Roentgenol* 1988;151:355–358.

62. Chien AJ, Jacobson JA, Famadar DA, et al. Imaging appearances of lateral ankle ligament reconstruction. *Radiographics* 2004;24:999–1008.

63. Hecker P. Study on the peroneus of the tarsus. *Anat Rec* 1923;26:79–82.

64. Wood Jones F. *Structure and function as seen in the foot.* Baltimore, MD: Williams & Wilkins, 1944.

65. Berkowitz JF, Kier R, Rudicel S. Plantar fasciitis: MR imaging. *Radiology* 1991;179:665–667.

66. Goodwin DW, Salonen DC, Yu SS, et al. Planter components of the foot. MR appearance in cadavers and diabetic patients. *Radiology* 1995;196:623–630.
67. Kiegley BA, Haggar AM, Gaba A, et al. Primary tumors of the foot: MR imaging. *Radiology* 1989;171:755–759.
68. Ledermann HP, Morrison WB, Schweitzer ME. MR image analysis of pedal osteomyelitis: distribution, patterns of spread, and frequency of associated ulceration and septic arthritis. *Radiology* 2002;223:747–755.
69. Ledermann HP, Morrison WB, Schweitzer ME, et al. Tendon involvement in pedal infection: MR analysis of frequency, distribution and spread of infection. AJR *Am J Roentgenol* 2002;179:939.
70. Ledermann HP, Morrison WB, Schweitzer ME. Is soft-tissue inflammation in pedal infection contained by fascial planes? MR analysis of compartmental involvment in 115 feet. *AJR Am J Roentgenol* 2002;178:605–612.
71. Bencardino JT, Rosenberg ZS. Normal variants and pitfalls in MR imaging of the ankle and foot. *Magn Reson Imaging Clin N Am* 2001;9:447–463.
72. Eberle CF, Moran B, Gleason T. The accessory flexor digitorum longus as a cause of flexor hallicus syndrome. *Foot Ankle Int* 2002;23:51–55.
73. Yu JS, Resnick D. MR imaging of the accessory soleus muscle appearance in six patients and review of the literature. *Skeletal Radiol* 1994;23:525–528.
74. Zammit J, Sigh D. The peroneus quadratus muscle. Anatomy and clinical relevance. *J Bone Joint Surg* 2003;85B:1134–1137.
75. Mellado JM, Rosenberg ZS, Beltran J. Low incorporation of soleus tendon. A potential diagnostic pitfall on MR imaging. *Skeletal Radiology* 1998;27:222–224.
76. Moorman CT III, Monto RR, Bassett FH III. So-called trigger ankle due to an aberrant flexor hallicus longus muscle in a tennis player. *J Bone Joint Surg* 1992; 74A:294–296.
77. Cheung YY, Rosenerg ZS, Colon E, et al. MRI imaging of flexor digitorum accessory longus. *Skeletal Radiology* 1999;28:130–137.
78. Cheung YY, Rosenberg ZS, Raamsinghavi R, et al. Peroneus quadratus muscle. MR imaging features. *Radiology* 1997;202:745–750.
79. Dunn AW. Anomalous muscle simulating soft tissue tumors in the lower extremities. *J Bone Joint Surg Am* 1965;47A:1397–1400.
80. Kokter G, Linclau LA. The accessory soleus muscle: symptomatic soft tissue tumor or accidental finding. *Neth J Surg* 1981;33(3):146–149.
81. Romanus B, Lindahl S, Stener B. Accessory soleus muscle: a clinical and radiographic presentation of 11 cases. *J Bone Joint Surg Am* 1986;68A:731–734.
82. Vogler JB, Helmes CA, Callan PW. Normal Variants and Pitfalls in Imaging, Philadelphia: W.B. Saunders, 1986.
83. Mellado JM, Rosenberg ZS, Beltran J, et al. The peroneocalcaneus internus muscle. MR imaging features. *AJR Am J Roentgenol* 1997;169:585–588.
84. Reinus WR, Fischer KC, Ritter JH. Painful transient tibial edema. *Radiology* 1994;192:195–199.
85. Miller TT, Bucchieri JS, Joshi A, et al. Pseudodefect of the talar dome. Anatomic pitfall of ankle MR imaging. *Radiology* 1997;203:857–858.
86. Boles MA, Lomasney LM, Denos TC, et al. Enlarged peroneal process with peroneus longus tendon entrapment. *Skeletal Radiol* 1997;26:313–315.
87. Mintz DN, Tashjian S, Connell DA, et al. Osteochondral lesions of the talus: a new magnetic resonance grading system with arthroscopic correlation. *Arthroscopy* 2003;19:353–359.
88. Noto AM, Cheung Y, Rosenberg ZS, et al. MR imaging of the ankle: normal variants. *Radiology* 1989;170:121–124.
89. Friedman MJ. Injuries of the leg in athletes. In: Nichols JA, Hershman EB, eds. *The lower extremity and spine in sports medicine.* St. Louis, MO: CV Mosby, 1986:601–655.
90. Cohen JM, Weinreb JC, Maravilla KR. Fluid collections in the intraperitoneal and extraperitoneal spaces: comparison of MR and CT. *Radiology* 1985;155:705–708.
91. Rosenberg ZS, Cheung YY, Beltran J, et al. Posterior intermalleolar ligament of the ankle. Normal anatomy and MR imaging features. *AJR Am J Roentgenol* 1995;165:387–390.
92. Fiorella D, Helms CA, Nunley JA II. The MR imaging features of the posterior intermalleolar ligament in patients with posterior

93. impingement syndrome of the ankle. *Skeletal Radiology* 1999;28:573–576.
93. Erickson SJ, Prost RW, Timins ME. The "magic angle" effect: background physics and clinical relevance. *Radiology* 1993;188:22–25.
94. Link SC, Erickson SJ, Timins ME. MR imaging of the ankle and foot: normal structures and anatomic variants that may simulate disease. *AJR Am J Roentgenol* 1993;161:607–612.
95. Abraham E, Stirnaman JE. Neglected rupture of the peroneal tendons causing recurrent sprains of the ankle. *J Bone Joint Surg Am* 1979;61A:1247–1248.
96. Abrahim-zadeh R, Klein RM, Leslie D, et al. Characteristics of calcaneal bone infarction: an MR imaging investigation. *Skeletal Radiol* 1998;27:321–324.
97. Alexander IJ, Johnson KA, Berquist TH. Magnetic resonance imaging in diagnosis of disruption of the posterior tibial tendon. *Foot Ankle Int* 1987;8:144–147.
98. Cerezal L, Abascal F, Canga A, et al. MR imaging of ankle impingement syndromes. *AJR Am J Roentgenol* 2003;181:551–559.
99. Cohen JM, Weinreb JC, Redman HC. Arteriovenous malformations of the extremities: MR imaging. *Radiology* 1986;158:475–479.
100. Daffner RH, Reimer BL, Lupetin ARE, et al. Magnetic resonance imaging in acute tendon ruptures. *Skeletal Radiol* 1986;15:619–621.
101. Erdman LOA, Tomburro F, Jayson HT, et al. Osteomyelitis: characteristics and pitfalls of diagnosis with MR imaging. *Radiology* 1991;180:533–539.
102. Fernandez-Canton G, Casado O, Capelastegui A, et al. Bone marrow edema syndrome of the foot: one-year follow-up with MR imaging. *Skeletal Radiol* 2003;32:273–278.
103. Ho VW, Peterfly C, Helms CA. Tarsal tunnel syndrome caused by strain of an anomalous muscle: an MRI-specific diagnosis. *J Comput Assist Tomogr* 1993;17:822–823.
104. Karjalainen P, Soila K, Aronen HJ, et al. MR imaging of overuse injuries of the Achilles tendon. *AJR Am J Roentgenol* 2000;175:251–260.
105. Morrison WB, Schweitzer ME, Wapner KL, et al. Osteomyelitis in feet of diabetics: clinical accuracy, surgical utility and cost-effectiveness of MR imaging. *Radiology* 1995;196:557–564.
106. Narvaez JA, Narvaez J, Ortega R, et al. Painful heel: MR image findings. *Radiographics* 2000;20:333–352.
107. Stafford SA, Rosenthal DI, Gebhardt MC, et al. Case report—MRI in stress fracture. *AJR Am J Roentgenol* 1986;147:553–556.
108. Schmid MR, Pfirrmann CWA, Hodler J, et al. Cartilage lesions in the ankle joint: comparison of MR arthrography and CT arthrography. *Skeletal Radiol* 2003;32:259–265.
109. Hubbard AM, Meyer JS, Davidson RS, et al. Relationship between the ossification center and cartilaginous cartilage in the normal hindfoot in children: study with MR imaging. *AJR Am J Roentgenol* 1993;161:849–853.
110. Cass JR, Morrey BF. Ankle instability: current concepts, diagnosis and treatment. *Mayo Clin Proc* 1984;59:165–170.
111. Karasick D, Schweitzer ME. Disorders of the hallux sesamoid complex: MR features. *Skeletal Radiology* 1998;27:411–418.
112. Dienst M, Blauth M. Bone bruise of the calcaneus. *Clin Orthop* 2000;378:202–205.
113. Ashman CJ, Klecker RJ, Yu JS. Forefoot pain involving the metatarsal region: differential diagnosis with MR imaging. *Radiographics* 2001;21:1425–1440.
114. Dunfee WR, Dalinka MK, Kneeland JB. Imaging of athletic injuries to the foot and ankle. *Radiol Clin North Am* 2002;40:289–312.
115. Zanetti M, Steiner SCL, Seifert B, et al. Clinical outcomes of edema-like bone marrow abnormalities of the foot. *Radiology* 2002;222:184–188.
116. Narvaez JA, Cerezal L, Narvaez J. MRI of sports-related injuries of the foot and ankle: Part I. *Curr Probl Diagn Radiol* 2003;32:139–155.
117. Theodorou DJ, Theodorou SJ, Kakitsubata Y, et al. Fractures of the proximal portion of the fifth metatarsal bone: anatomic and imaging evidence of a pathogenesis of avulsion of the plantar aponeurosis and the short peroneal muscle tendon. *Radiology* 2003;226:857–865.
118. Yu JS, Tanner JR. Considerations in metatarsalgia and midfoot pain: an MR imaging perspective. *Semin Musculoskelet Radiol* 2002;6:91–104.

119. Robbins MI, Wilson MG, Sella EJ. MR imaging of anterosuperior calcaneal process fractures. *AJR Am J Roentgenol* 1999;172: 475–479.

120. Bui-Mansfield LT, Kline M, Chew FS, et al. Osteochondritis dissecans of the tibial plafond: imaging characteristics and a review of the literature. *AJR Am J Roentgenol* 2000;175:1305–1308.

121. Yulish BS, Mulopulos GP, Goodfellow DB, et al. MR imaging of osteochondral lesions of the talus. *J Comput Assist Tomogr* 1987;11:296–301.

122. Berndt AL, Harty M. Transchondral fractures (osteochondritis dissecans) of the talus. *J Bone Joint Surg Am* 1959;41A:988–1020.

123. Myer JM, Garcia J, Hoffmeier P, et al. The subtalar sprain: a roentgenographic study. *Clin Orthop* 1988;266:169–173.

124. Oae K, Takao M, Naito K, et al. Injury of the tibiofibular syndesmosis: value of MR imaging for diagnosis. *Radiology* 2003; 227:155–161.

125. Uys HD, Rijke AM. Clinical association of acute lateral ankle sprain with syndesmotic involvement. A stress radiography and magnetic resonance imaging study. *Am J Sports Med* 2002;30: 816–822.

126. Ehman RL, Berquist TH. Magnetic resonance imaging of trauma. *Radiol Clin North Am* 1986;24:291–319.

127. Zanetti M, DeSimoni C, Wetz HH, et al. Magnetic resonance imaging of injuries to the ankle joint: can it predict clinical outcomes? *Skeletal Radiol* 1997;26:82–88.

128. Cardone BW, Erickson SJ, Den Hartog BD, et al. MRI of injury of the lateral collateral ligamentous complex of the ankle. *J Comput Assist Tomogr* 1993;17:102–107.

129. Narvaez JA, Cerezal L, Narvaez J. MRI of sports-related injuries of the foot and ankle: Part II. *Curr Probl Diagn Radiol* 2003; 32: 177–193.

130. Brown KW, Morrison WB, Schweitzer ME, et al. MRI findings associated with distal tibiofibular syndesmosis injury. *AJR Am J Roentgenol* 2004;182:131–136.

131. Rosenberg ZS, Bencardino J, Astion D, et al. MRI features of chronic injuries of the superior peroneal retinaculum. *AJR Am J Roentgenol* 2003;181:1551–1557.

132. Rademaker J, Rosenberg ZS, Beltran J, et al. Alterations in the distal extension of the musculous peroneus brevis with foot movement. *AJR Am J Roentgenol* 1997;168:787–789.

133. Basset FH, Speer KP. Longitudinal rupture of the peroneal tendons. *Am J Sports Med* 1993;21:354–357.

134. Zeiss J, Saddemi SR, Ebraheim NA. MR imaging of the peroneal tunnel. *J Comput Assist Tomogr* 1989;13(5):840–844.

135. Church CC. Radiographic diagnosis of acute peroneal tendon dislocation. *AJR Am J Roentgenol* 1977;129:1065–1068.

136. Kier R, McCarthy S, Dietz MJ, et al. MR appearance of painful conditions of the ankle. *Radiographics* 1991;11:401–414.

137. Kingston S. Magnetic resonance imaging of the ankle and foot. *Clin Sports Med* 1988;7:15–28.

138. Rademaker J, Rosenberg ZS, Delfaut EM, et al. Tear of the peroneus longus tendon: MR image features in nine patients. *Radiology* 2000;214:700–704.

139. Kelikian H, Kelikian AS. *Disorders of the ankle.* Philadelphia, PA: WB Saunders, 1985.

140. Khoury NJ, El-Khoury GY, Saltzman CL, et al. Peroneus longus and brevis tendon tears: MR imaging evaluation. *Radiology* 1996;200:833–841.

141. Schweitzer ME, Karasick D. MR imaging of disorders of the Achilles tendon. *AJR Am J Roentgenol* 2000;175:613–625.

142. Kleinman M, Grass AE. Achilles tendon rupture following steroid injection. *J Bone Joint Surg Am* 1983;65A:1345–1347.

143. Weishaupt D, Schweitzer ME, Alam F, et al. MR imaging of inflammatory joint diseases of the foot and ankle. *Skeletal Radiol* 1999;28:663–669.

144. Yu JS, Chung C, Recht M, et al. MR imaging of tophaceous gout. *AJR Am J Roentgenol* 1997;168:523–527.

145. Yu JS, Witte D, Resnick D, et al. Ossification of the Achilles tendon: imaging abnormalities in 12 patients. *Skeletal Radiol* 1994;23:127–131.

146. Astrom M, Gentz C, Nilsson P, et al. Imaging in chronic Achilles tendinopathy: a comparison of ultrasonography, magnetic resonance imaging and surgical findings in 27 histologically verified cases. *Skeletal Radiol* 1996;25:615–620.

147. Moody AR, Pollock JG, O'Connor AR, et al. Lower-limb deep venous thrombosis: direct MR imaging of thrombus. *Radiology* 1998;209:349–355.

148. Anderson MW, Kaplan PA, Dussault RG, et al. Association of posterior tibial tendon abnormalities with abnormal signal intensity in the sinus tarsi on MR imaging. *Skeletal Radiol* 2000;29:514–519.

149. Rule J, Yao L, Seeger LL. Spring ligament of the ankle: normal MR anatomy. *AJR Am J Roentgenol* 1993;161:1241–1244.

150. Schweitzer ME, Karasick D. MR imaging of disorders of the posterior tibialis tendon. *AJR Am J Roentgenol* 2000;175: 627–635.

151. Tjin A, Ton ER, Schweitzer ME, et al. MR imaging of peroneal tendon disorders. *AJR Am J Roentgenol* 1997;168:135–140.

152. Rosenberg ZS, Cheung Y, Jahss MH, et al. Rupture of posterior tibial tendon: CT and MR imaging with surgical correlation. *Radiology* 1988;169:229–235.

153. Hatori M, Hosaka M, Ehara S. Imaging features of intraosseous lipomas of the calcaneus. *Arch Orthop Trauma Surg* 2001;121: 429–432.

154. Bencardino J, Rosenberg ZS, Betltran J, et al. MR imaging of dislocation of the posterior tibial tendon. *AJR Am J Roentgenol* 1997;169:1109–1112.

155. Yao L, Gentili A, Cracchiolo A. MR imaging findings in spring ligament insufficiency. *Skeletal Radiology* 1999;28:245–250.

156. Koulouris G, Connell D, Schneider T, et al. Posterior tibiotalar ligament injury resulting in posteromedial impingement. *Foot Ankle Int* 2003;24:575–583.

157. Garth WP. Flexor hallucis tendonitis in a ballet dancer. *J Bone Joint Surg Am* 1981;63A:1489.

158. Gallo RA, Kolman BH, Daffner RH, et al. MRI of tibialis anterior tendon rupture. *Skeletal Radiol* 2004;33:102–106.

159. Khoury NJ, El-Khoury GY, Saltzman CL, et al. Rupture of the anterior tibial tendon: diagnosis by MR imaging. *AJR Am J Roentgenol* 1996;167:351–354.

160. Jahss MH. *Disorders of the foot*, 2nd ed. Philadelphia, PA: WB Saunders, 1991.

161. Karasick D, Schweitzer ME. The os trigonum syndrome: imaging features. *AJR Am J Roentgenol* 1996;166:125–129.

162. Kjaersgaard-Anderson P, Anderson K, Soballe K, et al. Sinus tarsi syndrome: presentation of seven cases and review of the literature. *J Foot Surg* 1989;28:3–6.

163. Carroso JJ, Liu N, Traill MR, et al. Physiology of the retrocalcaneal bursa. *Ann Rheum Dis* 1988;47:910–912.

164. Grasel RP, Schweitzer ME, Kovalovich AM, et al. MR imaging of plantar fasciitis: edema, tears and occult marrow abnormalities correlated with outcome. *AJR Am J Roentgenol* 1999;173: 699–701.

165. Theodorou DJ, Theodorou SJ, Kakitsubata Y, et al. Plantar fasciitis and fascial rupture: MR image findings in 26 patients supplemented with anatomic data in cadavers. *Radiographics* 2000;20:S181–S197.

166. Theodorou DJ, Theodorou SJ, Farooki S, et al. Disorders of the plantar aponeurosis: a spectrum of MR imaging findings. *AJR Am J Roentgenol* 2001;176:97–104.

167. Yu JS. Pathologic and post-operative conditions of the plantar fascia: review of MR imaging appearances. *Skeletal Radiol* 2000; 29:491–501.

168. Jarde O, Diebold P, Havet E. Degenerative lesions of the plantar fascia: surgical treatment by fasciectomy and excision of the heel spur: a report of 38 cases. *Acta Orthop Belg* 2003;69:267–274.

169. Yu JS, Smith G, Ashman C, et al. The plantar fasciotomy: MR imaging findings in asymptomatic volunteers. *Skeletal Radiol* 1999;28:447–452.

170. Sammarco GJ, Conti SF. Tarsal tunnel syndrome caused by an anomalous muscle. *J Bone Joint Surg Am* 1994;76A:1306–1314.

171. Mirra JM, Bullough PG, Marcove RC, et al. Malignant fibrous histiocytoma and osteosarcoma in association with bone infarcts. *J Bone Joint Surg Am* 1979;56A:932–940.

172. Morrison WB, Ledermann HP, Schweitzer ME. MR imaging of the diabetic foot. *Magn Reson Imaging Clin N Am* 2001;9: 603–613.

173. Pfeiffer WH, Cracchiolo A III. Clinical results after tarsal tunnel decompression. *J Bone Joint Surg Am* 1994;76A:1222–1231.

174. Klein MA, Spreitzer AM. MR imaging of the tarsal sinus and canal: normal anatomy, pathologic findings and features of sinus tarsi syndrome. *Radiology* 1993;186:223–240.

175. Lowe A, Schilero J, Kanat IO. Sinus tarsi syndrome: a postoperative analysis. *J Foot Surg* 1985;24:108–112.

176. Lektrakul N, Chung CB, Lai Y, et al. Tarsal sinus: arthrographic, MR imaging, and pathologic findings in cadavers and retrospective study data in patients with sinus tarsi syndrome. *Radiology* 2001;219:802–810.

177. Wakely CD, Johnson CP, Watt I. The value of MR imaging in the diagnoses of os trigonum syndrome. *Skeletal Radiol* 1996;25: 133–136.

178. Bureau NJ, Cardinal E, Hobden R, et al. Posterior ankle impingement syndrome: MR imaging findings in seven patients. *Radiology* 2000;215:497–503.

179. Robinson P, White LM, Salonen DC, et al. Anterolateral ankle impingement: MR arthrographic assessment of the anterolateral recess. *Radiology* 2001;221:186–190.

180. Robinson P, White LM, Salonen DC, et al. Anteromedial impingement of the ankle: using MR arthrography to assess the anteromedial recess. *AJR Am J Roentgenol* 2002;178:601–604.

181. Robinson P, White LM. Soft-tissue and osseous impingement syndromes of the ankle: role of imaging in diagnosis and management. *Radiographics* 2002;22:1457–1471.

182. Jordan LK, Helms CA, Cooperman AE, et al. Magnetic resonance imaging findings in anterolateral impingement of the ankle. *Skeletal Radiol* 2000;29:34–39.

183. Hauger O, Moinard M, Lasalarie JC, et al. Anterolateral compartment of the ankle in the lateral impingement syndrome: appearance on CT arthrography. *AJR Am J Roentgenol* 1999;173: 685–690.

184. Klein MA. MR imaging of the ankle: normal and abnormal findings in the medial collateral ligament. *AJR Am J Roentgenol* 1994;162:337–383.

185. Marti B, Vader VP, Minder CE, et al. On the epidemiology of running injuries. *Am J Sports Med* 1988;16:285–294.

186. Preidler KW, Brossmann J, Daenen B, et al. MR Imaging of the tarsometatarsal joint: analysis of injuries in 11 patients. *AJR Am J Roentgenol* 1996;167:1217–1222.

187. Yao L, Lee JK. Occult intraosseous fracture: detection with MR imaging. *Radiology* 1988;167:749–751.

188. Taylor JAM, Sartoris DJ, Huang G, et al. Painful conditions of the first metatarsal sesamoid bones. *Radiographics* 1993;13:817–830.

189. Sharp RJ, Wade CM, Hennessy MS, et al. The role of MRI and ultrasound imaging in Morton's neuroma and the effect of size of lesions on symptoms. *J Bone Joint Surg Br* 2003;85:999–1005.

190. Zanetti M, Strehle JK, Kundert H-P, et al. Morton neuroma: effect of MR imaging on diagnostic thinking and therapeutic decisions. *Radiology* 1999;213:583–588.

191. Erickson SJ, Canale PB, Carrera GF, et al. Interdigital (Morton) neuroma: high resolution imaging with a solenoid coil. *Radiology* 1991;181:833–836.

192. Bencardino J, Rosenberg ZS, Beltran J, et al. Morton's neuroma: is it always symptomatic. *AJR Am J Roentgenol* 2000;175: 649–653.

193. Brown RR, Rosenberg ZS. MR imaging of exercise induced lower leg pain. *Magn Reson Imaging Clin N Am* 2001;9:533–551.

194. DeSmet AA. Magnetic resonance findings in skeletal muscle tears. *Skeletal Radiol* 1993;22:479–484.

195. Verleisdonk EJMM, van Gils A, van der Werken C. The diagnostic value of MRI scans for the diagnosis of chronic exertional compartment syndrome of the lower leg. *Skeletal Radiol* 2001;30: 321–325.

196. Logigan EL, Berger AR, Bhagwan TS, et al. Injury to the tibial and peroneal nerves due to hemorrhage in the popliteal fossa. *J Bone Joint Surg Am* 1989;71A:768–770.

197. Stevens MA, El-Khoury GY, Kathol MH, et al. Imaging features of avulsion injuries. *Radiographics* 1999;19:655–672.

198. Garrett WE. Muscle strain injuries: clinical and basic aspects. *Med Sci Sports Exerc* 1990;22:436–443.

199. Spritzer CE, Sussman SK, Blunder RA, et al. Deep venous thrombosis evaluation with limited flip-angle, gradient refocused MR imaging: preliminary experience. *Radiology* 1988;166:371–375.

200. Matsusue Y, Yamamuro T, Ohta H, et al. Fibrotic contracture of the gastrocnemius muscle. *J Bone Joint Surg Am* 1994;76A:739–743.

201. Pakter RL, Fishman EK, Zerhouni EA. Calf hematoma–computed tomographic and magnetic resonance findings. *Skeletal Radiol* 1987;16:393–396.

202. Fleckenstein JL, Canby RC, Parkey RW, et al. Acute effects of exercise on MR imaging of skeletal muscle in normal volunteers. *AJR Am J Roentgenol* 1988;151:231–237.

203. Halpern AA, Nagel DA. Anterior compartment pressures in patients with tibial fractures. *J Trauma* 1980;20:786–790.

204. Stack C. Superficial posterior compartment syndrome of the leg with deep venous compromise. *Clin Orthop* 1987;220:223–236.

205. Jones DC, James SL. Overuse injuries of the lower extremity: shin splints, iliotibial band friction syndrome, and exertional compartment syndrome. *Clin Sports Med* 1987;6:273–290.

206. Reneman RS. The anterior and lateral compartment syndrome of the leg due to intensive use of muscles. *Clin Orthop* 1975; 113:69–80.

207. Beck BR, Osternig LR. Medial tibial stress syndrome: the location of muscles in the leg in relation to symptoms. *J Bone Joint Surg Am* 1994;76A:1057–1061.

208. Keller U, Oberhansli R, Huber P, et al. Phosphocreatine content and intracellular pH of calf muscle measured by phosphorus NMR spectroscopy in occlusive arterial disease of the legs. *Eur J Clin Invest* 1985;15:382–388.

209. Mancini DM, Ferraro N, Tuchler M, et al. Detection of abnormal calf muscle metabolism on patients with heart failure using phosphorus-31 NMR. *Am J Card* 1988;62:1234–1240.

210. Cohen EK, Kressel HY, Perosio T, et al. MR imaging of soft-tissue hemangiomas: correlation with pathologic findings. *AJR Am J Roentgenol* 1988;150:1079–1081.

211. Dooms GC, Hricak H, Sollitto RA, et al. Lipomatous tumors and tumors with fatty component: MR imaging potential and comparison of MR and CT results. *Radiology* 1985;157:479–483.

212. Feld R, Burg DL, McCue P, et al. MRI of aggressive fibromatosis: frequent appearance of high signal intensity of T2 weighted images. *Magn Reson Imaging* 1990;8:583–588.

213. Kirby EJ, Shereff MJ, Lewis MM. Soft-tissue tumors and tumorlike lesions of the foot. An analysis of eighty-three cases. *J Bone Joint Surg Am* 1989;71:621–626.

214. Mahajan H, Kim EE, Wallace S, et al. Magnetic resonance imaging of malignant fibrous histiocytoma. *Magn Reson Imag* 1989; 7:283–288.

215. Mahajan H, Lorigan JG, Shirkhoda A. Synovial sarcoma: MR imaging. *Magn Reson Imag* 1989;7:211–216.

216. Erlemann R, Reiser MF, Peters PE, et al. Musculoskeletal neoplasms: static and dynamic Gd-DTPA-enhanced MR imaging. *Radiology* 1989; 171:767–773.

217. Hottya GA, Steinbach LS, Johnston JO, et al. Chondrosarcoma of the foot: imaging, surgical and pathological correlation of three new cases. *Skeletal Radiol* 1999;28:153–158.

218. Kaplan PA, Murphey M, Greeway G, et al. Fluid levels in giant cell tumors of bone: report of two cases. *J Comput Tomogr* 1987; 11:151–155.

219. Lee GK, Kang IW, Lee ES, et al. Osteoid osteoma of the tarsal cuboid mimicking osteomyelitis. *AJR Am J Roentgenol* 2004; 183:341–342.

220. Yeager BA, Schiebler ML, Wertheim SB, et al. Case report—MR imaging of osteoid osteoma of the talus. *J Comput Assist Tomogr* 1987;11:916–917.

221. Maldjian C, Rosenberg ZS. MR imaging features of tumors in the ankle and foot. *Magn Reson Imaging Clin N Am* 2001;9:639–657.

222. Campbell RSD, Grainger AJ, Beggs I, et al. Intraosseous lipoma: report of 35 new cases and a review of the literature. *Skeletal Radiol* 2003;32:209–222.

223. Unni KK. *Dahlin's bone tumors: general aspects and data on 11,087 cases,* 5th ed. Philadelphia, PA: Lippincott–Raven Publishers, 1996.

224. Hirata M, Kusuzaki K, Hirasawa Y. Eleven cases of intraosseous lipoma of the calcaneus. *Anticancer Res* 2001;21:4099–4104.

225. Tachibana R, Hatori M, Hosaka M, et al. Glomus tumors with cystic changes around the ankle. *Arch Orthop Trauma Surg* 2001;121: 540–543.

226. Waldt S, Rechl H, Rummeny EJ, et al. Imaging of benign and malignant soft tissue masses of the foot. *Eur Radiol* 2003;13:1125–1136.

227. Russel WO, Cohen J, Enzinger F, et al. A clinical and pathologic staging system for soft tissue sarcomas. *Cancer* 40:1562–1570.

228. Weiss SW, Goldblum JR. *Enzinger and Weiss's soft tissue tumors*, 4th ed. St Louis, MO: Mosby, 2001.

229. Morrison WB, Schweitzer ME, Wapner KL, et al. Plantar fibromatosis: a benign aggressive neoplasm with characteristic appearance on MR images. *Radiology* 1994;193:841–845.

230. Leung LYJ, Shu SJ, Chan ACL, et al. Nodular fasciitis: MRI appearance and literature review. *Skeletal Radiol* 2002;31:9–13.

231. Schweitzer ME, van Leersum M, Erlich SS, et al. Fluid in normal and abnormal ankle joints: amount and distribution as seen on MR images. *AJR Am J Roentgenol* 1994;162:111–114.

232. Unger E, Moldofsky P, Gatenby R, et al. Diagnosis of osteomyelitis by MR imaging. *AJR Am J Roentgenol* 1988;1509:605–610.

233. Yuh W, Corson J, Baraniewski HM, et al. Osteomyelitis of the foot in diabetic patients: evaluation with plain film 99mTc MDP bone scintigraphy and MR imaging. *AJR Am J Roentgenol* 1989;152:795–800.

234. Dhillon MS, Singh P, Sharma R, et al. Tuberculous osteomyelitis of the cuboid: a report of four cases. *Foot Ankle Int* 2000;39:329–335.

235. Sugimoto K, Iwai M, Kawate K, et al. Tenosynovial osteochondromatosis of the tarsal tunnel. *Skeletal Radiol* 2003;32: 99–102.

236. Yulish BS, Lieberman JM, Newman AJ, et al. Juvenile rheumatoid arthritis: assessment with MR imaging. *Radiology* 1987;165: 149–152.

237. Yulish BS, Lieberman JM, Strandjord SE, et al. Hemophilic arthropathy: assessment with MR imaging. *Radiology* 1987;164: 759–762.

238. Bouysset M, Tebib J, Tavernier T, et al. Posterior tibial tendon and subtalar joint complex in rheumatoid arthritis: magnetic resonance imaging study. *J Rheumatol* 2003;30:1951–1954.

239. Karasick D, Schweitzer ME, O'hara BJ. Distal fibular notch: a frequent manifestation of the rheumatoid ankle. *Skeletal Radiology* 1997;26:529–532.

240. Spritzer CE, Dalinka MK, Kressel HY. Magnetic resonance imaging of pigmented villonodular synovitis. *Skeletal Radiol* 1987; 16:316–319.

241. Sherry CS, Harms SE. MR evaluation of giant cell tumors of the tendon sheath. *Magn Reson Imaging* 1989;7:195–201.

242. Chaudhuri R, McKeown B, Harrington D, et al. Micromycosis osteomyelitis causing avascular necrosis of the cuboid bone: MR image finding. *AJR Am J Roentgenol* 1992;159:1035–1037.

243. Zacharia TT, Shah JR, Patkar JR, et al. MRI in ankle tuberculosis: review of 14 cases. *Australas Radiol* 2003;47:11–16.

244. Tang JSH, Gold RH, Bassett LW, et al. Musculoskeletal infection of the extremities: evaluation with MR imaging. *Radiology* 1988;166:205–209.

245. Seldin DW, Heiken J, Feldman F, et al. Effect of soft-tissue pathology on detection of pedal osteomyelitis in diabetics. *J Nucl Med* 1985;26:988–993.

246. Yuh WTC, Corson JD, Baraniewski HM, et al. Osteomyelitis of the foot in diabetic patients: evaluation with plain film, 99m Tc-MDP bone scintigraphy, and MR imaging. *AJR Am J Roentgenol* 1989;152:795–800.

247. Zlatkin MB, Pathria M, Sartoris DJ, et al. The diabetic foot. *Radiol Clin North Am* 1987;25:1095–1105.

248. Moore TE, Yuh WTC, Kathol MH, et al. Abnormalities of the foot in patients with diabetes mellitus: findings on MR imaging. *AJR Am J Roentgenol* 1991;157:813–816.

249. Quinn SF, Murray W, Clark RA, et al. MR imaging of chronic osteomyelitis. *J Comput Assist Tomogr* 1988;12:113–117.

250. Ledermann HP, Morrison WB, Schweitzer ME. Pedal abscesses in patients suspected of having pedal osteomyelitis: analysis with MR imaging. *Radiology* 2002;224:649–655.

251. Ledermann HP, Schweitzer ME, Morrison WB. Non-enhancing tissue on MR imaging of pedal infection: characterization of necrotic tissue and associated limitations for diagnosis of osteomyelitis and abscess. *AJR Am J Roentgenol* 2002;178:215–222.

252. Judd DB, Kim DH, Hrutkay JM. Transient osteoporosis of the talus. *Foot Ankle Int* 2000;21:134–137.

253. Hawkins LG. Fractures of the neck of the talus. *J Bone Joint Surg* 1970;52A:991–1002.

254. Mubarak SJ, Gould RN, Lee FF, et al. The medial tibial stress syndrome. *Am J Sports Med* 1982;10:201–205.

255. Yates B, Allen MJ, Barnes MR. Outcome of surgical treatment of medial tibial stress syndrome. *J Bone Joint Surg Am* 2003;85A: 1974–1980.

256. Detmer DE. Chronic shin splints: classification and management of medial tibial stress syndrome. *Sports Med* 1986;3: 436–446.

257. Delfaut EM, Demondion X, Bieganski A, et al. Imaging of foot and ankle nerve entrapment syndromes: from well-demonstrated to unfamiliar sites. *Radiographics* 2003;23:613–662.

258. Lewis OJ. The joints of the evolving foot. I. The ankle joint. *J Anat* 1980;13:527–543.

259. Vanhoenacker F, Bernaerts A, Gielen J, et al. Trauma of the pediatric foot and ankle. *JBR-BTR* 2002;85:212–218.

260. Lee MS, Harcke HT, Kumer SJ, et al. Subtalar joint coalition in children: new observations. *Radiology* 1989;172:635–639.

261. Newman JS, Newberg A. Congenital tarsal coalition: Multimodality evaluation with emphasis on CT and MR imaging. *Radiographics* 2000;20:321–332.

262. Wechsler RJ, Schweitzer ME, Deely DM, et al. Tarsal coalition: depiction and characterization with CT or MR images. *Radiology* 1994;193:447–452.

263. Holder LE, Cole LA, Myerson MS. Reflex sympathetic dystrophy of the foot. Clinical and scintigraphic criteria. *Radiology* 1992;184:531–535.

264. Rao VM, Fishman M, Mitchell DG, et al. Painful sickle cell crisis: bone marrow patterns observed with MR imaging. *Radiology* 1986;161:211–215.

Shoulder and Arm

Thomas H. Berquist   Jeffrey James Peterson

There are numerous clinical problems relating to the shoulder, arm, and brachial plexus. The last has been partially discussed in Chapter 5; however, a more detailed discussion of brachial plexus lesions will be covered in this chapter. There is some overlap in clinical syndromes relating to the shoulder, upper extremity, and brachial plexus, but for purposes of discussion, each area will be considered separately.

Most patients with shoulder pathology present with pain and/or pain with reduced range of motion. For many years, shoulder evaluation has been based on clinical data as well as findings from routine radiographs (1–7). Routine radiographs are still an important part of the workup of patients with shoulder pain, as subtle changes in both the bone and soft tissues can lead to appropriate selection of additional imaging techniques (8). This may include ultrasound, computed tomography (CT), or magnetic resonance imaging (MRI) (8–13). In recent years, MRI or MR arthrography have frequently replaced other techniques for evaluating shoulder disorders. Similarly, soft tissue problems involving the upper arm are easily assessed with MRI. An additional benefit of MRI is the ability to image the shoulder and arm in any orthogonal or off-axis oblique plane (14–21).

The brachial plexus can be evaluated with myelography and CT. However, the complex anatomy, along with inability to clearly demonstrate all neurovascular structures, has reduced the effectiveness of these techniques to some degree (22–25). Myelography only demonstrates the spinal canal and nerve root sheaths. Though it demonstrates soft tissue pathology to some degree, CT myelography has difficulty in clearly differentiating all neurovascular structures. In addition, there may be artifact in the shoulder region on many CT scanners, which makes examination of this area suboptimal. Examination of the brachial plexus using MRI can be accomplished in the axial, sagittal, and coronal planes, which allows more complete evaluation of neurovascular structures as they exit the paraspinal tissues and extend into the axillary and shoulder region (10,23,26).

This chapter will discuss techniques, anatomy, and applications for evaluation of the shoulder, brachial plexus, and upper arm. Techniques vary depending upon the clinical setting. Anatomy in sagittal, coronal, and axial planes, especially with regard to the course of the neural structures, will be stressed.

TABLE 9-1
MR EXAMINATIONS OF THE SHOULDER, ARM, AND BRACHIAL PLEXUS

	Pulse Sequence	Slice Thickness/gap	Field of View (cm)	Matrix	Excitations (NEX)	Image Time
Shoulder						
Three-plane scout	Fl 15/5	3 1 cm/no skip	24	256 × 192	1	16 s
Axial	SE 634/16	4 mm/skip 0.5 mm	14 (12–16)	256 × 256	1	3 min 39 s
Axial	GRE 613/19, FA 20°	4 mm/0 skip	14 (12–16)	256 × 256	1	2 min 43 s
Oblique coronal	TSE PD 2,000/19	4 mm/skip 0.5 mm	14 (12–16)	256 × 256	1	3 min
Oblique coronal	TSE 3,500/91 2F5	4 mm/skip 0.5 mm	14 (12–16)	256 × 256	1	4 min 22 s
Oblique sagittal	TSE PD with FS 3,050/26	4 mm/skip 0.5 mm	14 (12–16)	256 × 256	2	3 min
Arthrography						
Three-plane scout	Fl 15/5	3 1 cm	24	256 × 192	1	16 s
Axial	SE 500/12 with FS	4 mm/skip 0.5 mm	14	256 × 256	1	3 min 16 s
Sagittal	SE 544/12 with FS	4 mm/skip 0.5 mm	14	256 × 256	1	3 min 33 s
Coronal oblique	SE 525/12 with FS	4 mm/skip 0.5 mm	14	256 × 256	1	3 min 25 s
Coronal oblique	TSE PD 2,000/19	4 mm/skip 0.5 mm	14	256 × 256	1	3 min 30 s
Coronal oblique	TSE T2 4,140/19 with FS	4 mm/skip 0.5 mm	14	256 × 256	1	3 min 20 s
ABER	SE 500/12 with FS	4 mm/skip 0.5 mm	14	256 × 256	1	3 min 16 s
Arm						
Three-plane scout	Fl 15/5	3 1 cm/no skip	30–48	256 × 192	1	16 s
Axial	TSE PD 3,050/26	0.5–1 cm/0.5–1.0 mm skip	~24	156 × 256	1	3 min
Axial	TSE T2 3,500/91	0.5–1 cm/0.5–1.0 mm skip	~24	256 × 256	1	4 min 22 s
Axial, coronal or sagittal	SE 634/23	0.5–1 cm/0.5–1.0 mm skip for axial; 3–5 mm /0 skip for coronal or sagittal of humerus	~24	256 × 256	1	3 min 39 s
Brachial Plexus						
Three-plane scout	Fl 15/5	3 1 cm/0 skip	30–48	256 × 256	1	16 s
Coronal	TSE 400/17	1.5 mm/0 skip	36	256 × 256	1	5 min 16 s
Axial (right and left)	SE 419/17	5 mm/1.5 mm skip	18	256 × 256	2	4 min 47 s × 2 if bilateral
Sagittal (right and left)	SE 500/13	5 mm/1.5 mm skip	22	256 × 256	1	3 min 40 s × 2 if bilateral
Axial bilateral	TIR 5950/99/TI160	5 mm/1.5 mm skip	36	256 × 256	1	4 min 5 s
Coronal bilateral	TIR 5950/99/TI160	5 mm/1.5 mm skip	36	256 × 256	1	4 min 5 s

SE, spin echo; TSE, turbo spin-echo; Fl, flash; FS, fat suppression; PD, proton density; T2, T2-weighted; ABER, abduction–external rotation; TIR, turbo inversion recovery

TECHNIQUES

Techniques for MR examination of the shoulder, brachial plexus region, and arm vary depending upon the clinical symptoms. For purposes of discussion, it is best to consider the shoulder, arm, and the brachial plexus regions separately, as there are significant differences in the methods for MR examination (Table 9-1).

Glenohumeral and Acromioclavicular Joints

Obtaining quality MR images of the upper extremity can be more challenging than evaluation of the lower extremity. High-field imaging gantries limit positioning to a certain extent. This varies with patient size. Larger patients may have to be rotated slightly (see Fig. 9-1). Positioning for shoulder imaging should assure patient comfort and avoid motion artifact (1,8,27,28). Low-field open gantries are less confining and provide more flexibility for patient positioning.

The arm is at the side in most cases, and a neutral to slightly external rotated position is preferred (see Fig. 9-2) (28–30). Towels or bolsters can be used to improve comfort and reduce motion. Full external rotation makes soft tissue structures, specifically the labrum, easier to evaluate, but this position may be uncomfortable or difficult to maintain, resulting in motion artifact (27,31,32). We prefer to tailor our examination to the comfort of the patient but avoid internal rotation whenever possible (28). Internal rotation causes overlap of the supraspinatus and infraspinatus, which may mimic a lesion (29,33). Tirman et al. (34) advocated abduction and external rotation (arm above the head) to more easily evaluate partial tears. This position may also improve detection of labral pathology (35,36). This technique is not often used in our practice except for MR

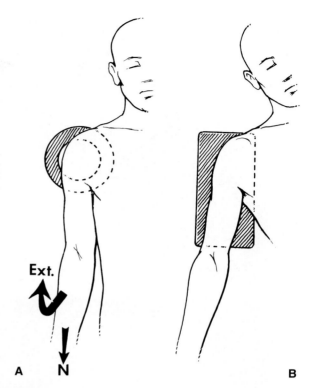

Figure 9-2 Illustration of patient positioned for examination of the shoulder **(A)** and arm **(B)**. The arm is neutral to externally rotated (*arrows*) in **A**. A larger phased-array coil or a wraparound coil is used for the arm **B**. *N*, neutral; *Ext*, external rotation.

arthrography. Patients frequently complain of shoulder pain, and problems with motion artifact occur with greater frequency than when the arm is at the side (28,37). Up to one fourth of patients are unable to tolerate this position (28,35,38).

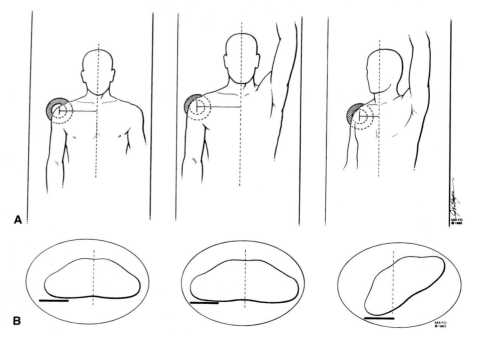

Figure 9-1 Illustration of patient positioned for shoulder examination using a circular coil. Changes in patient position are demonstrated in the frontal **(A)** and axial **(B)** planes to indicate the relationship of the shoulder to the gantry center. The position on the left in **A** is most comfortable. However, larger patients may have to be rotated or have one arm elevated to allow optimal positioning.

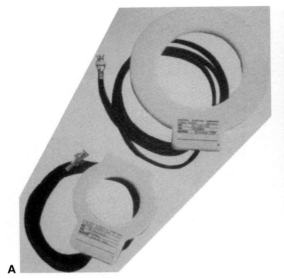

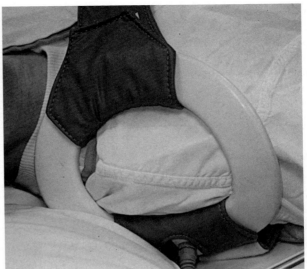

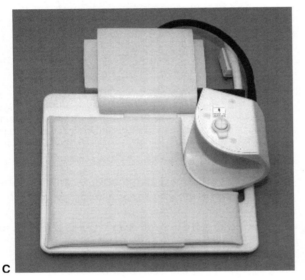

Figure 9-3 Photographs of coils used for the shoulder. **A:** General purpose flat circular coils. **B:** Shoulder coil with chest strap demonstrated on a patient. **C:** Phased array shoulder coil.

New software and coil (see Fig. 9-3) techniques have greatly enhanced the ability of MRI examinations to more optimally evaluate patients with shoulder symptoms. A dedicated phased-array shoulder coil (Fig. 9-3C) is placed over the shoulder to be examined (27,28). New coil technology continues to evolve (27,29).

Our routine shoulder examination begins with a three-plane scout image [15/5, 24 cm field of view (FOV), 256 × 192 matrix, and one acquisition] that can be obtained in 16 seconds (Table 9-1).

Axial images should include from above the acromioclavicular joint through the axillary region (see Fig. 9-4). Two sequences are obtained using 4-mm-thick sections, 256 × 256 or 256 × 192 matrix, a 14-cm FOV, and one acquisition. The first sequence is T1-weighted spin-echo (634/16) and the second a gradient-echo (GRE) [613/19/flip angle (FA) 20°] sequence. The latter is useful

for labral evaluation and the reduced image time can also decrease motion artifact (8,28,29).

Axial images or scout images are used to select the oblique coronal plane along the scapula or supraspinatus and perpendicular to the glenohumeral articulation (see Fig. 9-5) (39). Using the same general parameters, we obtain fast spin-echo (FSE) proton density [2,000/19, echo time (ET) 5] and T2-weighted (3,500/90, ET 7) images. Fat suppression is used with the T2-weighted FSE series. Use of both proton density and T2-weighted images provides excellent anatomic detail and allows joint fluid (high signal intensity on T2-weighted images) abnormalities in the glenoid labrum and rotator cuff to be more easily appreciated and classified. Signal intensity in the rotator cuff increases from proton density to T2-weighted images when partial or complete cuff tears are present. Signal intensity does not increase significantly in areas of tendinosis on T2-weighted sequences (28,40–42).

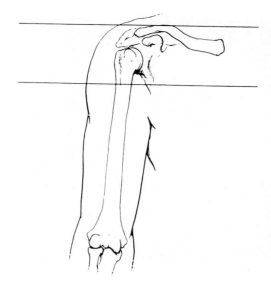

A

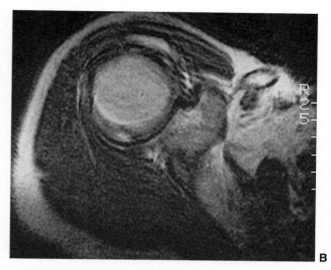

B

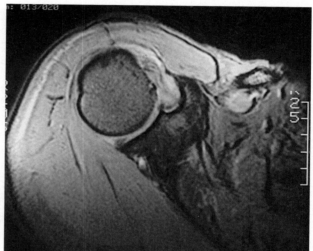

C

Figure 9-4   A: Coronal illustration demonstrating the region studied (*between lines*) with axial images. The area from above the acromioclavicular joint to below the axillary recess should be included. **B:** Axial SE 2,000/80 image degraded by motion artifact. **C:** Multiplanar gradient-echo (700/31, flip angle 25°) image in the same patient. There is no motion artifact.

Sagittal images are obtained using axial scout images to select sections perpendicular to the coronal plane and aligned with the glenohumeral articulation (8,43). We obtain 4-mm thick sections from proximal to the spinoglenoid notch to beyond the lateral margin of the humeral head (see Fig. 9-6). Using a 14-cm FOV, 256 × 256 or 256 × 192 matrix, and one acquisition, we obtain a FSE proton density (3,050/26, ET 7) sequence (28,44). Sagittal images are useful for evaluation of the acromioclavicular joint, acromial configuration, and quantifying the size and location of rotator cuff tears (17,27,28,45).

In some situations, additional sequences or image planes may be indicated, but the above technique is generally appropriate for most shoulder or glenohumeral joint pathology (1,27,46,47). In certain cases, subtle marrow abnormalities may be more easily detected using short TI inversion recovery sequences (STIR) or when the glenoid labrum is not optimally noted with the routine examination, radial GRASS interleaved (GRIL) images may be used to further define this anatomy (28,48–51).

MR Arthrography

MR arthrography is commonly performed today to evaluate articular cartilage, the biceps-labral complex, and capsular ligamentous complex (46,52–58). Both direct (intraarticular) and indirect (intravenous) approaches have been used (59–63). We prefer the direct approach except for evaluation of synovial enhancement. Direct arthrography results in more homogenous signal intensity throughout the joint fluid and provides capsular distention that aids delineation of the labroligamentous structures.

Optimally, patients should be selected for MR arthrography before they present to the MR suite to assure accurate scheduling. In some cases, conventional MR images are obtained initially. If patients are referred for specific

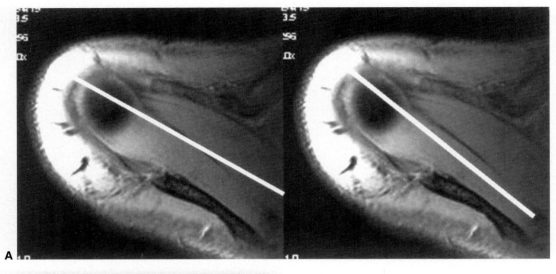

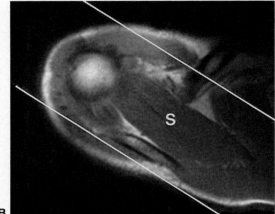

Figure 9-5   A: Image planes selected for coronal images along the axis of the supraspinatus muscle (*left*) or central supraspinatus tendon (*right*). **B:** Axial MR image demonstrating the area covered along the axis of the supraspinatus (*S*).

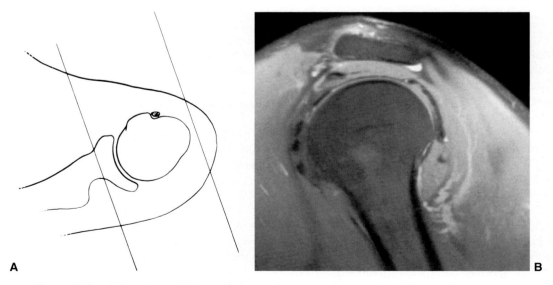

Figure 9-6   A: Illustration of the image plane and area covered with sagittal images. **B:** Sagittal SE 450/16 image demonstrating a normal supraspinatus muscle. The acromion is straight.

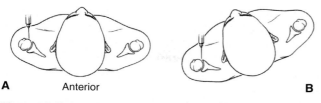

Figure 9-7 Illustrations of anterior injection sites with the patient supine **(A)** and slightly rotated **(B)**.

indications or when conventional images have been previously obtained, an MR arthrogram may be performed as the only procedure. Injections may be performed using fluoroscopic, ultrasound, open MR monitoring, or palpation of the glenohumeral joint with the arm abducted 45° (64–66). We prefer fluoroscopic guidance to assure proper needle position and to monitor the contrast injection.

There are several anterior injection approaches (see Fig. 9-7). Selection of injection approach may vary due to the patient's anatomy or location of suspected pathology (67). For the conventional injection, the patient is supine on the fluoroscopic table with the arm externally rotated (Fig. 9-7A). The patient may be rotated with the involved side down to open the joint (Fig. 9-7B). The shoulder is prepared using sterile technique. The injection site is localized directly over the medial margin of the humeral head, at the junction of the middle and lower third of the glenoid (see Fig. 9-8). Local anesthetic is injected into the superficial tissues over the site selected for joint entry. Needle placement is confirmed with a small amount of iodinated contrast medium. Using the conventional anterior approach, it is not unusual to cause extravasation in the soft tissues anteriorly (see Fig. 9-9).

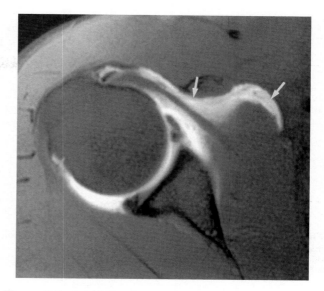

Figure 9-9 Axial MR arthrogram image demonstrating anterior contrast extravasation (*arrows*).

Dépelteau et al. (68) have suggested an alternative anterior approach to avoid contrast extravasation in the anterior supporting structures of the shoulder. This is accomplished by injecting higher on the humeral head (see Fig. 9-10). Again, the patient is supine with the arm externally rotated to avoid the long head of the biceps tendon. Anesthetic is injected over the upper medial humeral head close to the articular margin. A direct vertical or slightly medially angulated approach is used. When the needle contacts the humeral head, the intraarticular location is confirmed with iodinated contrast (68).

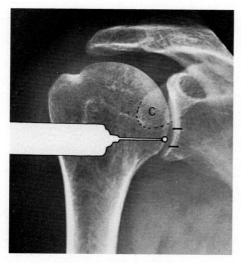

Figure 9-8 Illustration of injection site for MR arthrography. (From Berquist TH. *Imaging of orthopedic trauma*, 2nd ed. New York: Raven Press, 1992.)

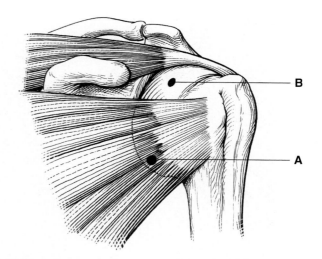

Figure 9-10 Illustration of the typical anterior injection site **(A)** through the subscapularis and higher **(B)** in the rotator cuff interval between the subscapularis and supraspinatus.

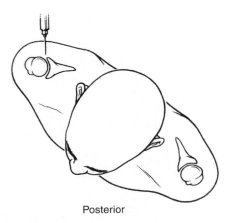

Posterior

Figure 9-11 Illustration of patient positioned for posterior injection.

Anatomically, the needle enters between the supraspinatus and subscapularis and may traverse the coracohumeral ligament and potentially the superior glenohumeral ligament (67,68). The injection site avoids the subscapularis, inferior glenohumeral ligament, and anterior inferior labrum (Fig. 9-10) (68).

The posterior approach is advocated in certain situations and avoids distortion of anterior supporting structures (see Fig. 9-11). Many radiologists are less familiar with this technique. However, it can be quite useful in certain instances. The patient is prone, with the involved shoulder rotated superiorly to align the glenohumeral articular surface. Patient position is supported by bolsters. After sterile preparation, the skin is marked over the lower medial humeral head. Following anesthetic injection, a spinal needle is advanced vertically until it contacts the humeral

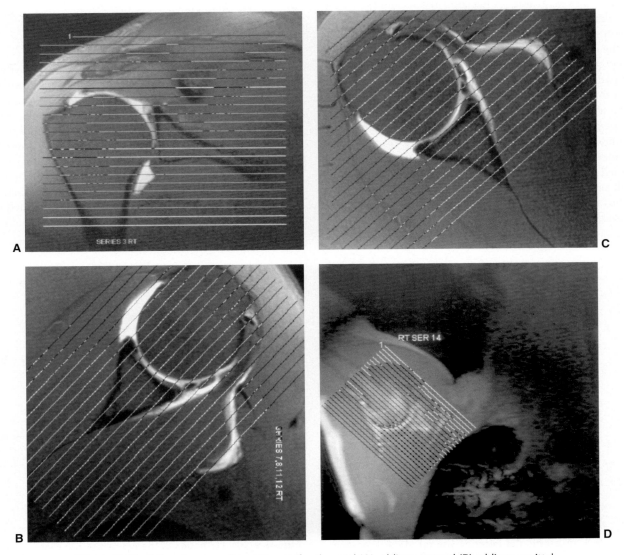

Figure 9-12 MR arthrogram. Scout images for the axial **(A)**, oblique coronal **(B)**, oblique sagittal **(C)**, and abduction–external rotation (ABER) view **(D)**. Normal axial **(E–G)**, coronal **(H,I)**, sagittal **(J–L)**, and ABER **(M)** images.

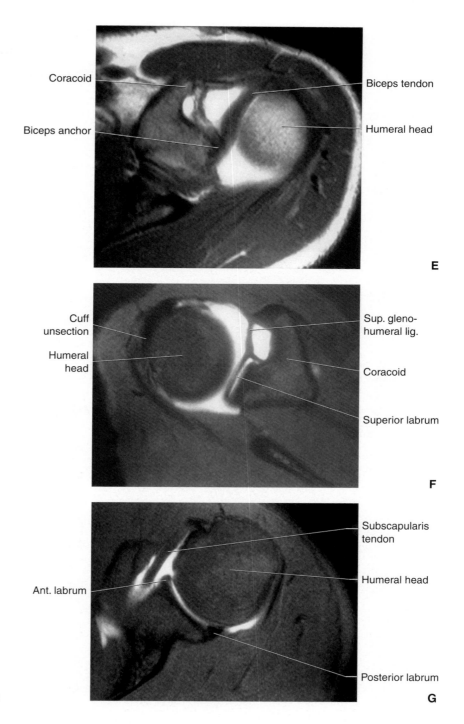

Figure 9-12 *(continued)*

head. Intraarticular position is confirmed with iodinated contrast (67,69).

At our institution, we most commonly use the conventional anterior approach. Regardless of the entry site we confirm needle position and inject 10 to 15 mL of gadolini um diluted in a mixture of 50% iodinated contrast, and Marcaine is injected (0.1 mL of gadopentetate dimeglumine in 20 mL solution).

Other alternative combinations of injection solutions may be utilized (52,54,56,62,70). It has been demonstrated

that mixing iodinated contrast with gadolinium is safe (71). The syringe and tubing must be checked for air. If air is introduced into the joint, it may mimic a loose body (54). Using fluoroscopic guidance, the shoulder is exercised to distribute the contrast medium. Radiographic image can be obtained prior to moving the patient to the MR suite. Lee et al. (72) have recommended the Grashey view (oblique with beam tangential to the glenohumeral articular) for evaluation of the superior labrum. This may increase the level of confidence when evaluating coronal

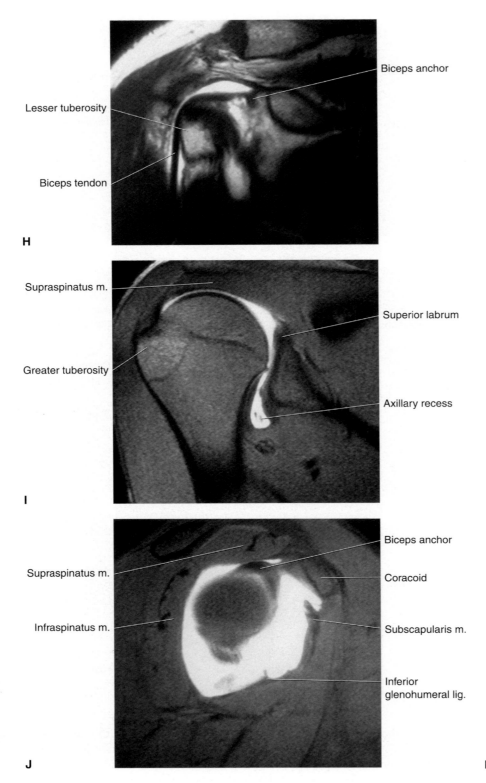

Lesser tuberosity

Biceps tendon

Biceps anchor

H

Supraspinatus m.

Greater tuberosity

Superior labrum

Axillary recess

I

Supraspinatus m.

Infraspinatus m.

Biceps anchor

Coracoid

Subscapularis m.

Inferior
glenohumeral lig.

J

Figure 9-12 *(continued)*

oblique images. MR images are obtained 30 to 45 minutes following the injection.

Table 9-1 summarizes pulse sequences and image planes used for MR arthrography. We routinely obtain fat-suppressed T1-weighted axial, sagittal, and coronal oblique images. Oblique coronal images are also obtained using turbo (fast) spin-echo (TSE) proton density and T2-weighted images. In many cases, we also perform the abduction–external rotation view (ABER, elbow flexed with hand behind the head of involved shoulder) (see Fig. 9-12). This

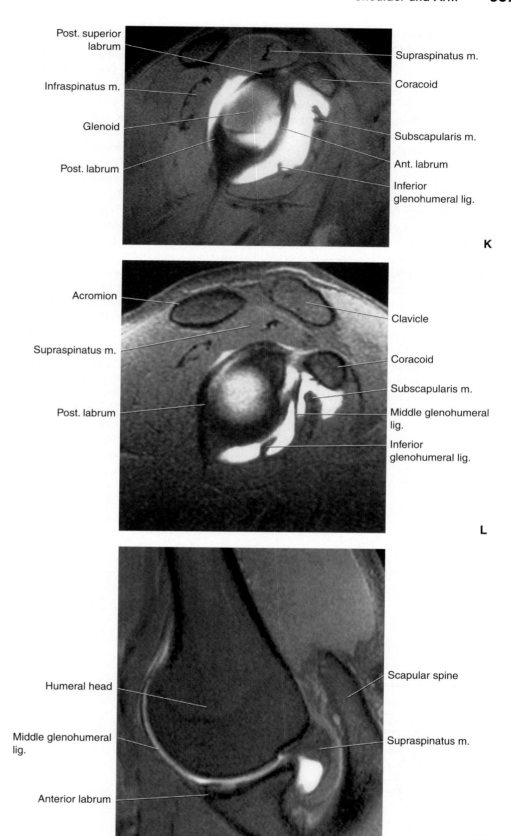

Post. superior labrum
Infraspinatus m.
Glenoid
Post. labrum
Supraspinatus m.
Coracoid
Subscapularis m.
Ant. labrum
Inferior glenohumeral lig.

K

Acromion
Supraspinatus m.
Post. labrum
Clavicle
Coracoid
Subscapularis m.
Middle glenohumeral lig.
Inferior glenohumeral lig.

L

Humeral head
Middle glenohumeral lig.
Anterior labrum
Scapular spine
Supraspinatus m.

M

Figure 9-12 (*continued*)

image series is useful for evaluating the anterior labrum and the extent of partial tears of the rotator cuff (36,48,73,74).

Arm

MR evaluation of the arm may be included as a portion of the shoulder examination or performed separately. The patient should be supine (Fig. 9-2B). Patients with suspected bone or soft tissue pathology in the arm are usually examined with axial T2-weighted images with either 1-cm or 5-mm slice thicknesses depending upon the area of interest (Table 9-1). Fat suppression techniques are useful for subtle pathology. Axial TSE proton density and TSE T2-weighted sequences provide an excellent screening examination. This sequence can be followed by T1-weighted axial images if soft tissue pathology is suspected. Comparing similar sections on both T1- and T2-weighted sequences is useful for more accurate lesion characterization. A second T1-or T2-weighted sequence is performed in the coronal or sagittal plane depending upon the suspect pathology and extent of the lesion. When marrow pathology is suspected, sagittal or coronal images should be selected along the plane of the humerus using either T1-weighted spin-echo sequences and STIR or fat-suppressed TSE T2-weighted images to evaluate subtle changes in the marrow. Contrast-enhanced fat-suppressed T1 or TSE T2-weighted sequences in similar planes are commonly added to our examination. Table 9-1 lists the different examinations for the shoulder and arm as well as the parameters and examination times.

Brachial Plexus

Examination of the brachial plexus requires a different approach (Table 9-1). The cervical spine is examined as part of the study (see Chapter 5). Routine cervical spine examination may be done first to exclude any spinal canal or proximal nerve root abnormalities. These techniques are fully discussed in Chapter 5. Evaluation of the brachial plexus requires images from the midcervical spine to the humerus, so a large FOV is necessary (see Fig. 9-13). A torso coil is commonly employed. If symptoms are unilateral a smaller off-center FOV can be used. Comparison is helpful, so we often examine both brachial plexus regions simultaneously. The axial images (right, left, or bilateral) are obtained using cardiac and respiratory gating to minimize the artifact from respiratory and cardiac motion. Slice thickness of 5 mm with 1.5-mm skip and an 18- (unilateral) or 36±- (bilateral) cm FOV with 256 × 256 matrix and 1 to 2 acquisitions are commonly used. Axial images are usually obtained from the midcervical level (C3–C4) to the midhumerus, which allows the lower neck, shoulder, and upper arm to be completely included in the FOV (see Fig. 9-14).

There is considerable fat along the course of the neurovascular bundle of the brachial plexus. Therefore, sagittal T1-weighted images (see Fig. 9-15) provide optimal evaluation of the nerve roots as they exit the spinal foramina and extend into the soft tissues of the neck and arm (23,26). The nerve roots appear as small, low-signal-intensity structures with this sequence and are accompanied by the larger arteries and veins as they extend peripherally.

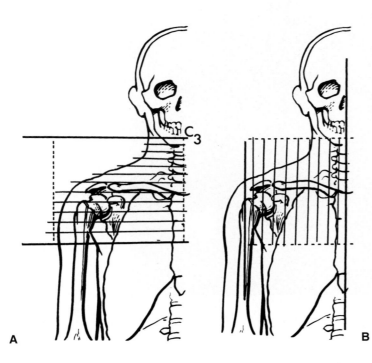

Figure 9-13 Illustration of area studied with axial **(A)** and sagittal **(B)** imaging of the brachial plexus.

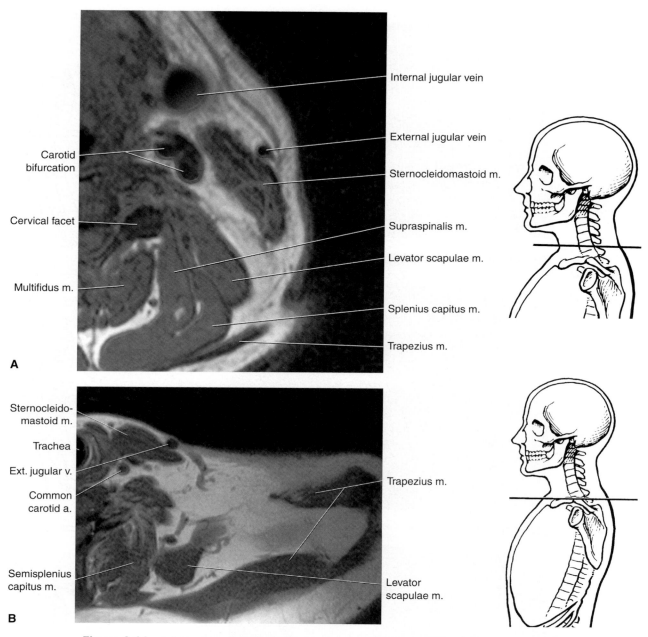

Figure 9-14 Axial images of the brachial plexus region with anatomic levels indicated. **A:** Axial image through the lower cervical region. **B:** Axial image at the base of the neck. **C:** Axial image through the upper humeral head. **D:** Axial image through the glenohumeral level. **E:** Axial image through the upper arm and axilla.

Soft tissue masses in the brachial plexus region are seen as low intensity areas and are clearly separated from the fat around the neurovascular bundle. In most situations, the axial and sagittal images provide an adequate screening examination for brachial plexus pathology. We typically add coronal and axial STIR images (see Fig. 9-16). Postcontrast fat-suppressed T1-weighted images are useful for evaluation of neural inflammation and characterizing adjacent masses or soft tissue abnormalities. Technical details will be discussed more completely in the clinical applications section of this chapter.

ANATOMY

It is important to have a thorough knowledge of anatomy in the commonly used conventional (see Figs. 9-17 to 9-19) MR image planes and those used for MR arthrography (Fig. 9-12).

Osseous Anatomy

The shoulder is comprised of three bony structures—the clavicle, scapula, and humerus (75,76). The glenohumeral

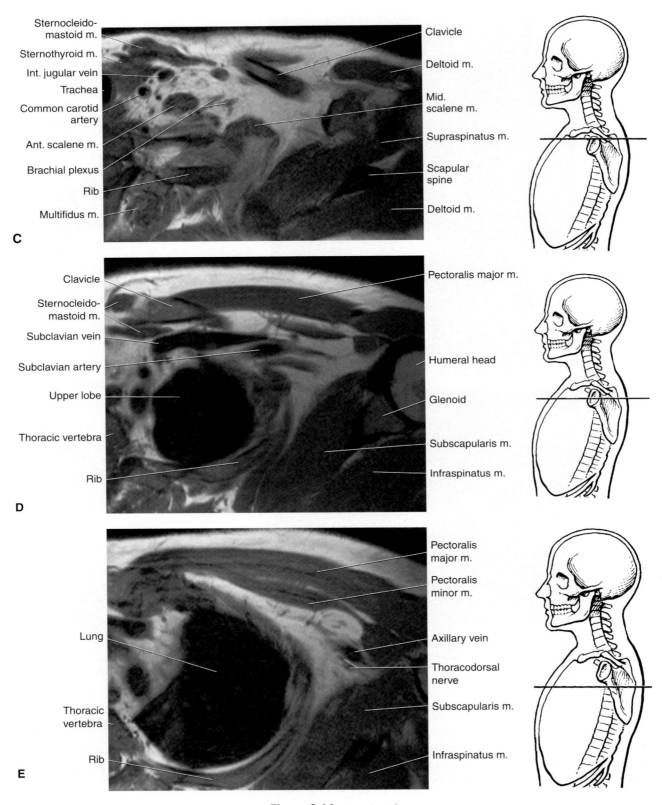

Sternocleido-
mastoid m.

Sternothyroid m.

Int. jugular vein

Trachea

Common carotid
artery

Ant. scalene m.

Brachial plexus

Rib

Multifidus m.

C

Clavicle

Deltoid m.

Mid.
scalene m.

Supraspinatus m.

Scapular
spine

Deltoid m.

Clavicle

Sternocleido-
mastoid m.

Subclavian vein

Subclavian artery

Upper lobe

Thoracic vertebra

Rib

D

Pectoralis major m.

Humeral head

Glenoid

Subscapularis m.

Infraspinatus m.

Lung

Thoracic
vertebra

Rib

E

Pectoralis
major m.

Pectoralis
minor m.

Axillary vein

Thoracodorsal
nerve

Subscapularis m.

Infraspinatus m.

Figure 9-14 (continued)

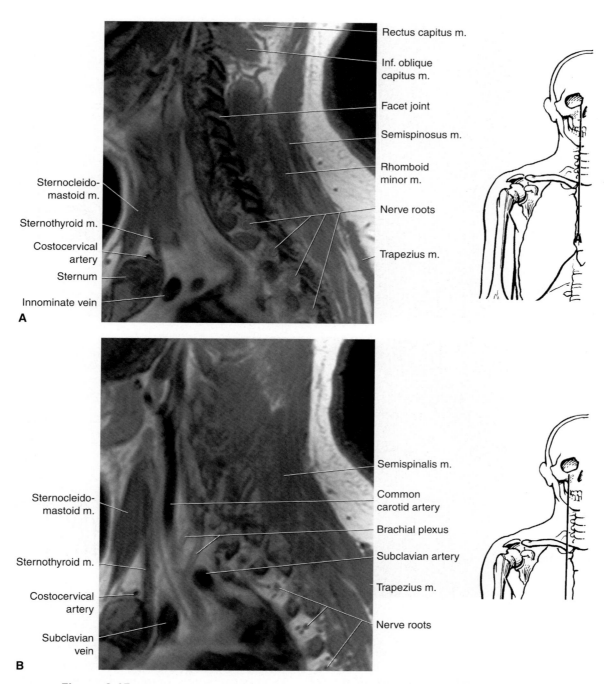

Figure 9-15 Sagittal images of the brachial plexus region with anatomic levels indicated. **A:** Sagittal image through the facets and intervertebral foramina. **B:** Sagittal image through the carotid artery. **C:** Sagittal image through the lateral neck. **D:** Sagittal image through the lateral chest.

joint is a ball and socket joint. The humeral head is four times larger than the glenoid fossa of the scapula. This permits significant range of motion but also results in an increased susceptibility to instability. The majority of the muscles acting on the humerus are for adduction. Therefore, the clavicle and the sternoclavicular articulation provide important support in maintaining the muscular efficiency of the shoulder (4,8,76).

There are two main articulations in the shoulder region, the acromioclavicular joint and the glenohumeral joint (see Figs. 9-18 and 9-20). The acromioclavicular articulation is a synovial joint formed by the capsule about the clavicle and acromion. In some cases, the joint is divided by a small articular disk. Motion at this articulation is limited to slight gliding movements between the scapula and clavicle. Supporting structures of the acromion of the

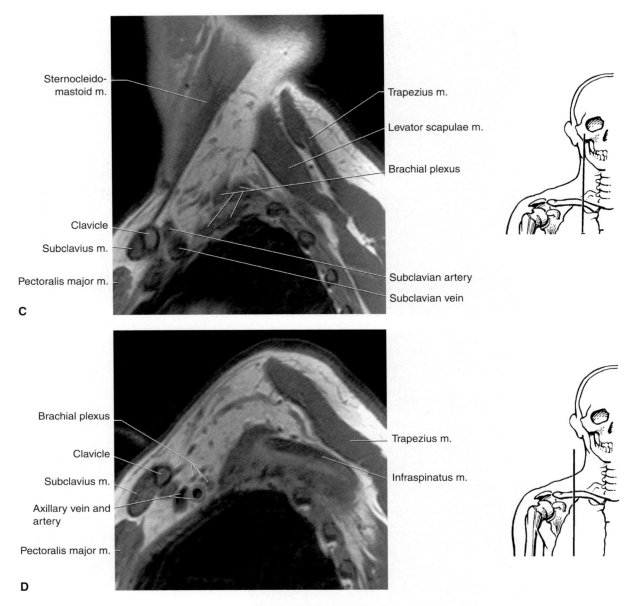

Figure 9-15   (continued)

scapula, the distal clavicle, and coracoid include the acromioclavicular ligament and the coracoacromial ligament, which extends from the coracoid process to the undersurface of the acromion just distal to the acromioclavicular joint. The coracoclavicular ligament is divided into the coronoid and trapezoid bands (see Fig. 9-21). These ligaments prevent upward displacement of the clavicle by the muscle forces of the trapezius and sternocleidomastoid muscles (4,76).

The glenohumeral articulation is formed by the shallow glenoid cavity, which is surrounded by a cartilaginous labrum (see Figs. 9-12 and 9-22) (4,50). The labrum is composed of fibrocartilage similar to the meniscus in the knee and is, therefore, seen as a triangular dark or low-intensity structure on MR images (Figs. 9-12 and 9-17). The labrum is somewhat blunted or rounded posteriorly and generally more triangular and sharper-appearing anteriorly (77–79). The capsule of the shoulder is lined with synovial membrane that arises from the margin of the glenoid labrum and extends around the head of the humerus anteriorly and posteriorly, where it attaches at about the level of the physeal line or anatomic neck (76,80). The capsule, therefore, usually closely approximates the margins of the articular cartilage of the humeral head (see Fig. 9-23). There are variations in the anterior capsular attachment that may play a role in recurrent dislocations. Type I attaches in or near the labrum (Fig. 9-23). Types II and III attach to the scapula more proximally. Capsules that attach more

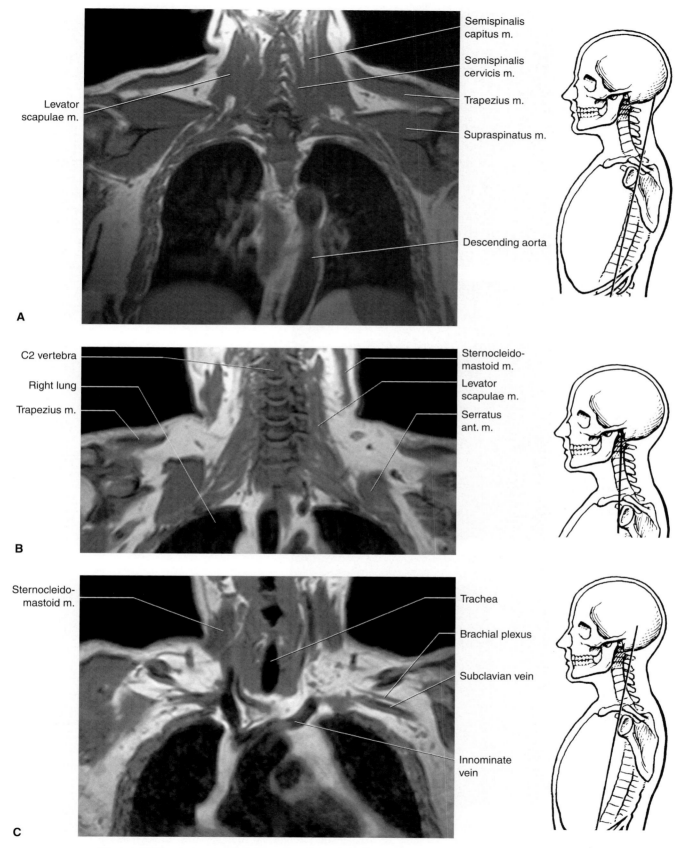

Figure 9-16 Coronal images of neck and shoulders with anatomic levels indicated. **A:** Coronal image through the descending aorta. **B:** Coronal image through the cervical spine. **C:** Coronal image through the neurovascular region.

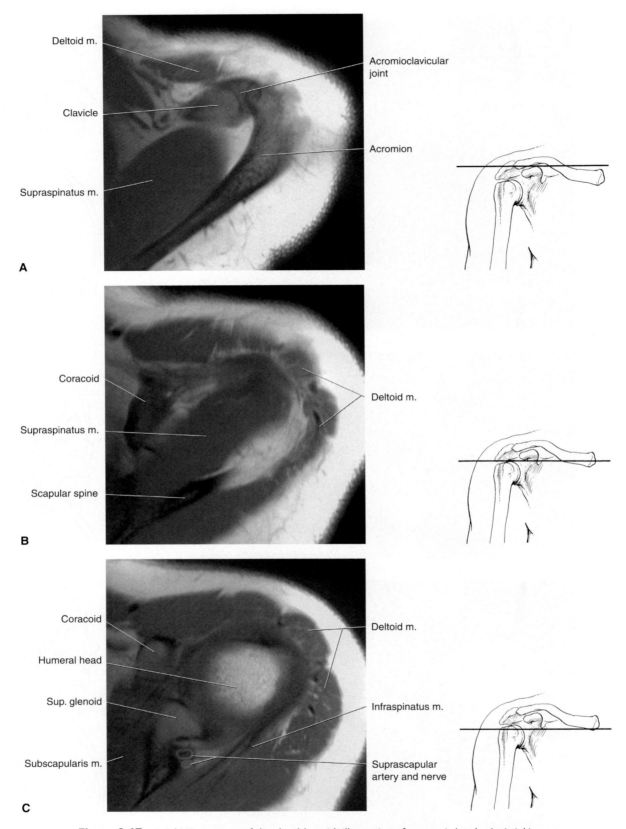

Figure 9-17   Axial MR anatomy of the shoulder with illustration of anatomic levels. **A:** Axial image through the acromioclavicular joint. **B:** Axial image through the supraspinatus. **C:** Axial image through the upper glenoid and coracoid. **D:** Axial image through the humeral head and glenoid demonstrating the normal labrum. **E:** Axial image through the lower glenoid.

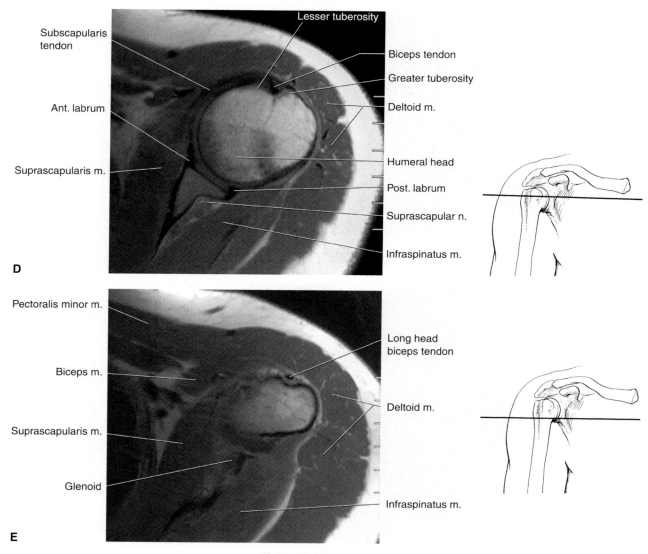

D

Subscapularis tendon
Ant. labrum
Suprascapularis m.

Lesser tuberosity
Biceps tendon
Greater tuberosity
Deltoid m.
Humeral head
Post. labrum
Suprascapular n.
Infraspinatus m.

E

Pectoralis minor m.
Biceps m.
Suprascapularis m.
Glenoid

Long head biceps tendon
Deltoid m.
Infraspinatus m.

Figure 9-17 (*continued*)

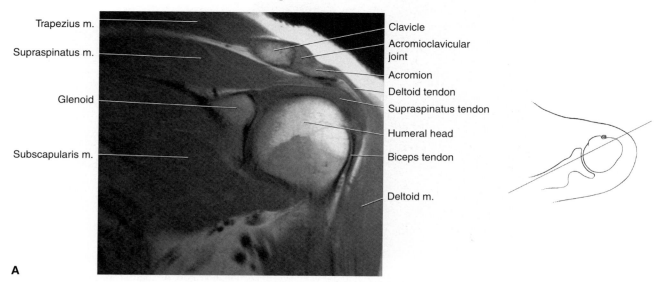

A

Trapezius m.
Supraspinatus m.
Glenoid
Subscapularis m.

Clavicle
Acromioclavicular joint
Acromion
Deltoid tendon
Supraspinatus tendon
Humeral head
Biceps tendon
Deltoid m.

Figure 9-18 Coronal MR images of the shoulder with illustration of the section levels. **A:** Coronal image through the humeral head and acromioclavicular joint. **B:** Coronal image through the gleno-humeral joint.

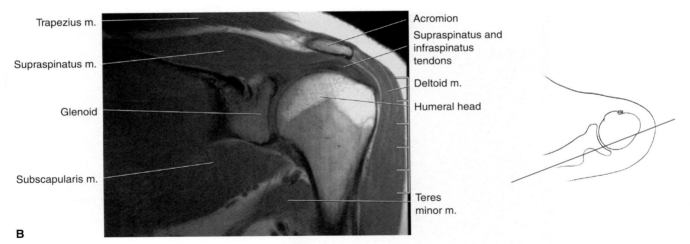

B

Figure 9-18 (*continued*)

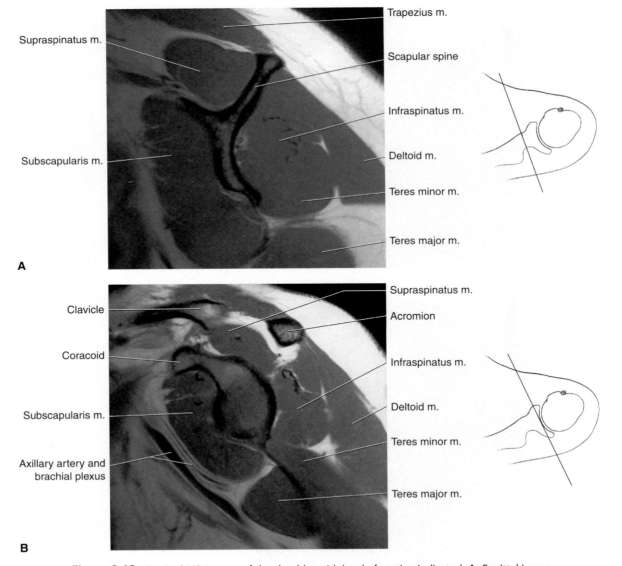

A

B

Figure 9-19 Sagittal MR images of the shoulder with level of section indicated. **A:** Sagittal image through the scapular spine. **B:** Sagittal image through the coracoid. **C:** Sagittal image through the glenoid articular surface. **D:** Sagittal image through the humeral head and acromioclavicular joint. **E:** Sagittal image through the lateral humeral head.

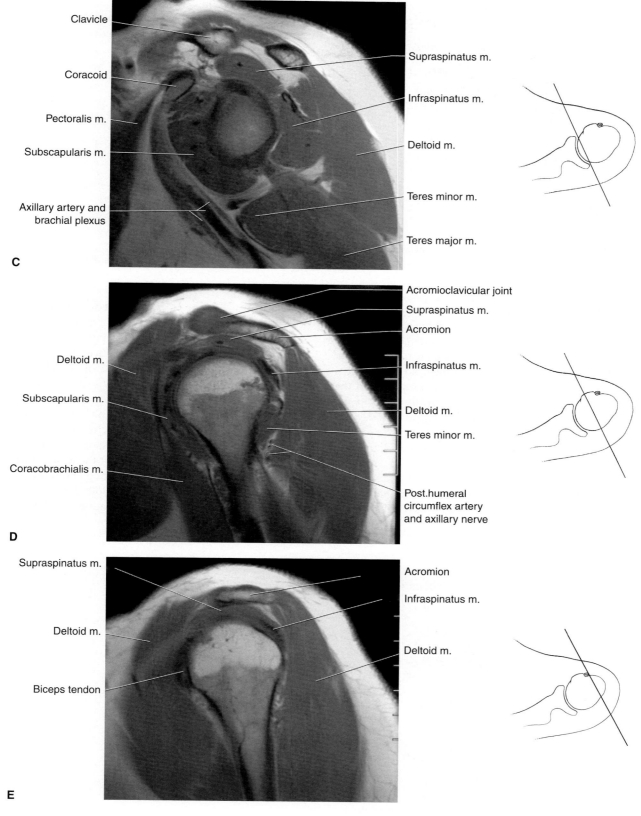

Clavicle

Coracoid

Pectoralis m.

Subscapularis m.

Axillary artery and
brachial plexus

C

Supraspinatus m.

Infraspinatus m.

Deltoid m.

Teres minor m.

Teres major m.

Deltoid m.

Subscapularis m.

Coracobrachialis m.

D

Acromioclavicular joint

Supraspinatus m.

Acromion

Infraspinatus m.

Deltoid m.

Teres minor m.

Post. humeral
circumflex artery
and axillary nerve

Supraspinatus m.

Deltoid m.

Biceps tendon

E

Acromion

Infraspinatus m.

Deltoid m.

Figure 9-19   (*continued*)

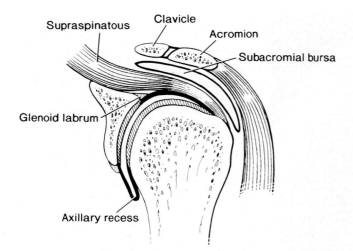

Figure 9-20 Illustration of the shoulder, demonstrating the glenohumeral and acromioclavicular joints and surrounding structures.

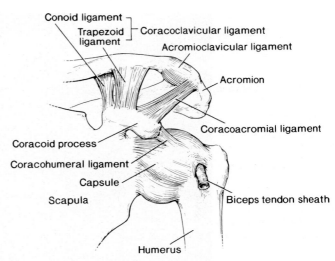

Figure 9-21 Illustration of the ligaments of the shoulder.

medially (type III) either predispose to, or are the result of, recurrent dislocations (17,18). Similar changes may be seen posteriorly when there is posterior instability (28). The synovial membrane continues between the greater and lesser tuberosities, forming a sheath for the long head of the biceps tendon. This sheath extends for variable lengths into the upper arm. Extension of the tendon sheath distal to the groove should not be confused with disruption (52). The synovium also extends through a small defect in the capsule anteriorly to form the subscapular or subcoracoid bursa (see Fig. 9-24) (8,17,18,81,82).

The capsule of the shoulder is supported by several fibrocapsular ligaments. The most consistent of these ligaments is the coracohumeral ligament (Fig. 9-21), which is a strong band arising from the most lateral edge of the coracoid process and extending over the superior aspect of the shoulder to attach to the greater tuberosity. The glenohumeral ligaments vary in thickness and may be difficult to appreciate on conventional MR images (see Fig. 9-25)(58). The inferior glenohumeral ligament is usually the most obvious; it extends from the middle anterior margin of the glenoid labrum to the lower medial aspect of the humeral neck. The middle glenohumeral ligament is attached somewhat superior to this, extending from both the labrum and the coracoid attaching to the anterior aspect of the lesser tuberosity (Fig. 9-25) (76,80,82,83). The superior glenohumeral ligament arises at the same level as the middle glenohumeral ligament and extends in a parallel manner to the middle

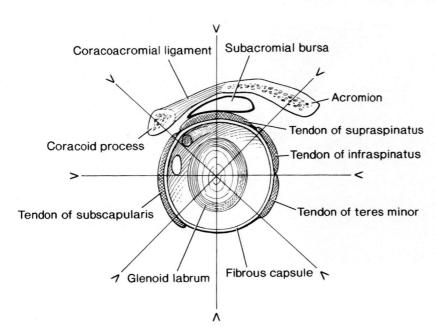

Figure 9-22 Illustration of the shoulder, demonstrating the glenoid articular surface, labrum, and supporting structures. Radial image planes and labral configuration are demonstrated.

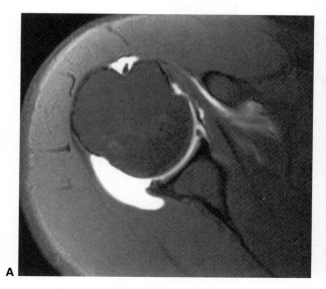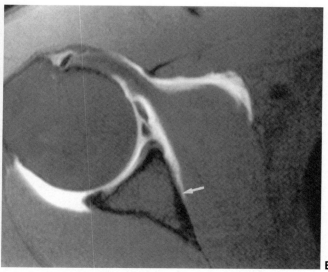

Figure 9-23 Capsular attachments. **A:** Axial MR arthrogram image of the shoulder demonstrating the capsular attachments. There is a type I attachment anteriorly and more medial type II attachment posteriorly with capsular distention. **B:** Axial MR arthrogram image demonstrating a type I posterior attachment and type III anterior attachment (*arrow*).

glenohumeral ligament. The transverse ligament extends across the greater and lesser tuberosities, enclosing the synovial sheath and long head of the biceps tendon (82–84).

Muscular Anatomy

There are numerous muscles that act upon the scapula, shoulder, and glenohumeral articulation. The most important of these, from a clinical standpoint, are the intrinsic muscles of the shoulder comprises the deltoid and rotator cuff group. The deltoid is a large muscle covering the shoulder superficially that arises from the lateral third of the clavicle, the acromion, and the spine of the scapula

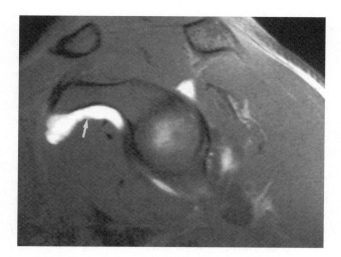

Figure 9-24 Sagittal MR arthrogram shows the subcoracoid bursa (*arrow*).

(see Figs. 9-17 to 9-19, and 9-26). The fibers of the deltoid all converge distally and laterally to insert on the deltoid tuberosity on the lateral aspect of the upper humerus (Fig. 9-26). The deltoid serves as a powerful abductor of the humerus (Table 9-2) (76,82).

The supraspinatus muscle (Figs. 9-17 to 9-19, and 9-26) is a critical muscle and tendon unit in evaluating patients with rotator cuff tears (8,21,79,85). The supraspinatus muscle arises from the supraspinous fossa of the scapula and is covered by the trapezius in its proximal portion. As the muscle extends peripherally, it passes under the acromion, coracoclavicular ligament, and acromioclavicular (AC) joint (Fig. 9-26) to insert on the most superior of the three facets of the greater tuberosity. Tendon of the supraspinatus is broad, covering the top of the shoulder and blending with the capsule superiorly. The primary function of the supraspinatus is to assist the deltoid in abduction of the humerus (Table 9-2) (76,82, 86,87).

The infraspinatus arises from the infraspinous fossa of the scapula (Fig. 9-26B). As it passes laterally, it is often separated from the scapula by a bursa that sometimes communicates with the shoulder joint (Table 9-3). The infraspinatus is separated from the supraspinatus by the scapular spine (Figs. 9-17 to 9-19). Its tendon forms the upper posterior portion of the rotator cuff and inserts in the greater tuberosity posterior and inferior to the supraspinatus tendon (82,85,88–91).

The teres minor arises from the middle half of the lateral scapular border, extends in an oblique upward direction to insert as a large flat tendon on the most posterior and inferior of the three facets of the greater tuberosity

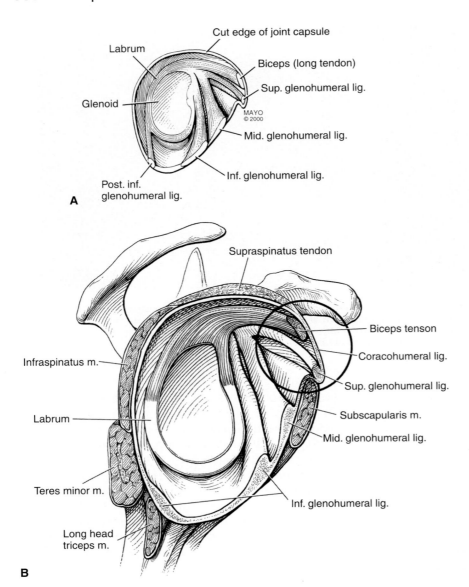

A

Cut edge of joint capsule
Labrum
Biceps (long tendon)
Sup. glenohumeral lig.
Glenoid
MAYO © 2000
Mid. glenohumeral lig.
Inf. glenohumeral lig.
Post. inf. glenohumeral lig.

B

Supraspinatus tendon
Biceps tenson
Coracohumeral lig.
Infraspinatus m.
Sup. glenohumeral lig.
Subscapularis m.
Labrum
Mid. glenohumeral lig.
Teres minor m.
Inf. glenohumeral lig.
Long head triceps m.

Figure 9-25 Illustration of the gleno-humeral ligaments **(A)** and their relationship to the coracohumeral ligament **(B)**.

(Figs. 9-19 and 9-26B). Like the infraspinatus, the teres minor is primarily an external rotator of the humerus (82).

Along with the supraspinatus, infraspinatus, and teres minor, the subscapularis makes up the fourth of the rotator cuff muscles (8,82,85). The subscapularis arises from the anterior subscapular surface of the scapula with its fibers converging and extending laterally to insert in a broad tendon or band along with the capsule on the lesser tuberosity of the humerus and the crest below this tuberosity (Figs. 9-17 to 9-19). This large, triangle-shaped muscle forms the posterior wall of the axilla with the axillary vessels and brachial plexus passing across and anterior to the muscle (see Fig. 9-27). The subscapularis bursa or recess lies between the muscle and the neck of the scapula and can communicate with the shoulder joint (Table 9-3). The primary function of the subscapularis is internal rotation of the humerus (Table 9-2) (76,82).

The teres major (Fig. 9-26B) arises on the dorsal aspect of the scapula from its lower lateral border and extends anteriorly to insert below the subscapularis on the medial aspect of the intertubercular groove. The teres major is an additional internal rotator of the humerus and when acting with the latissimus dorsi also serves as an extensor and adductor of the humerus. The muscle is innervated by the subscapular nerve, which receives its branches from the C5–C6 levels (82,85).

The extrinsic muscles of the shoulder arise from the vertebral column or thoracic cage and attach to the scapula or humerus (Fig. 9-26B). Two of these muscles, the trapezius and latissimus dorsi, completely cover the deep musculature of the back as they course to insert in the shoulder region (Fig. 9-26B). The trapezius has a long, broad origin from the upper superior nuchal line of the occipital bone, ligamentum nuchae, and upper thoracic spinous processes

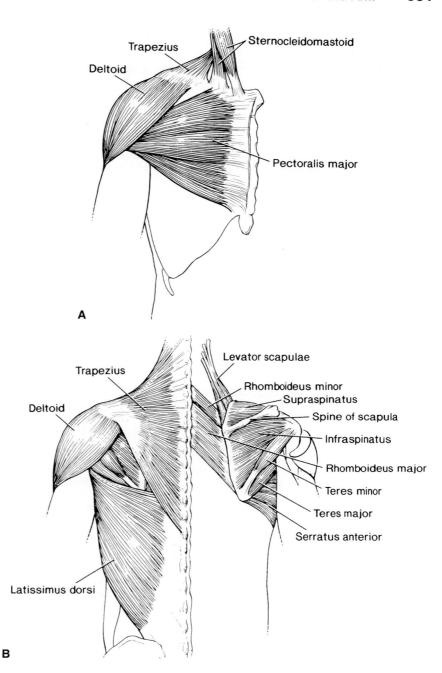

Figure 9-26 Illustrations of the extrinsic shoulder muscles from anterior **(A)** and posterior **(B)**.

(Figs. 9-18 and 9-26B). The upper fibers insert on the posterior superior aspect of the distal clavicle while the middle fibers insert more inferiorly on the border of the acromion and spine of the scapula. The lower fibers insert on a more clearly defined tendon at the base of the scapular spine. There is commonly a small bursa between the tendon of the lower fibers and the spine of the scapula. The trapezius serves as a retractor of the scapula and an elevator of the scapula. It is innervated by the accessory spinal nerve and roots from C3 and C4 (76,82).

The latissimus dorsi is a second very broad-based muscle taking its origin from the lower six thoracic spinous

processes and the spinous processes of the lumbar and upper sacral vertebrae (Fig. 9-26B). Superiorly, the muscle origin is covered by the lower fibers of the trapezius. This broad, triangular muscle extends superiorly to its insertion along the medial wall of the intertubercular or bicipital groove. There is a bursa between the tendons of latissimus dorsi and the teres major that, when inflamed, can be seen as an area of well-defined high intensity on MR images. The chief actions of the latissimus dorsi are adduction, internal rotation, and extension of the humerus. The muscle is supplied by the thoracodorsal nerve with roots from C6 through C8 (Table 9-2) (76,82).

TABLE 9-2
MUSCLES OF THE SHOULDER AND UPPER ARM

Muscles	Origin	Insertion	Action	Innervation
Intrinsic				
Deltoid	Lateral clavicle, acromion, scapular spine	Deltoid tuberosity humerus	Abductor of humerus	Axillary nerve (C5, C6)
Supraspinatus	Supraspinous fossa of scapula	Greater tuberosity superiorly	Abductor of humerus	Suprascapular nerve (C5, C6)
Infraspinatus	Infraspinous fossa of scapula	Posterior inferior greater tuberosity	Lateral rotation humerus	Suprascapular nerve (C5, C6)
Teres minor	Lateral midscapular border	Lateral inferior facet, greater tuberosity	External rotator of humerus	Axillary nerve (C5, C6)
Subscapularis	Suprascapular fossa	Lesser tuberosity	Internal rotator of humerus	Subscapular nerves (C5–C7)
Teres major	Inferior lateral scapula	Medial intertubercular groove	Internal rotation, adduction, extensor of humerus	Subscapular nerve (C5–C6)
Extrinsic				
Trapezius	Ligamentum nuchae, thoracic spinous processes	Distal clavicle, acromion, scapular spine	Retractor and elevator of scapula	Spinal accessory and C2, C3
Latissimus dorsi	Spinous processes T6–T12, lumbar, upper sacrum	Medial intertubercular groove	Adductor, internal rotator, and extensor of humerus	Thoracodorsal nerve (C6–C8)
Levator scapulae	Posterior tubercles, C1–C4 transverse processes	Upper medial scapul	Elevates medial scapula	Cervical plexus (C3–C4)
Rhomboidei				
Major	C2–T5 spinous processes	Posterior medial scapula	Retractor of scapula	Dorsal scapular nerve (C5)
Minor	Ligamentum nuchae C7 and T1 spinous processes	Posterior medial scapula at base of scapular spine		
Serratus anterior	Anterior ribs 1–9	Anterior medial scapula	Protractor, anterior drawing of scapula	Long thoracic nerve (C5–C7)
Pectoral Region				
Pectoralis major	Inferomedial clavicle, sternum, and costochondral junctions	Lateral intertubercular groove	Adductor of humerus	Medial and lateral anterior thoracic nerves (C5–T1)
Pectoralis minor	Anterior ribs 2–5	Coracoid of scapula	Depress angle of scapula	Medial pectoral nerve (C8–T1)
Subclavius	Anteromedial rib 1	Midinferior clavicle	Stabilize sternoclavicular joint	Subclavian nerve

From Carter BL, Morehead J, Walpert JM, et al. *Cross-sectional anatomy: computed tomography and ultrasound correlation.* New York: Appleton-Century Crofts, 1977; Iannotti JP, Gabriel JP, Schneck SL, et al. The normal glenohumeral relationship. *J Bone Joint Surg* 1992;74A:491–500; and Rosse C, Rosse PG. *Hollinsheads textbook of anatomy.* Philadelphia, PA: Lippincott-Raven, 1997.

The levator scapulae (Fig. 9-26B) originates from the posterior tubercles of the upper first through fourth transverse processes of the cervical spine. The muscle then passes in an oblique posteroinferior direction to insert on the superior angle of the medial scapular border. It is deep to the sternocleidomastoid superiorly and trapezius inferiorly. The main function of this muscle is to elevate the scapular border. The muscle is innervated by the deep cervical plexus from the third and fourth roots (Table 9-2) (76,82).

The rhomboid muscles (Fig. 9-26) are often divided into minor and major groups; however, in reality, especially on MR images, the muscle is difficult to separate into two groups. The muscles take a broad origin from the ligamentum nuchae and spinous processes of C2 through T5 to pass laterally and insert on the posterior medial aspect of the scapula near the base of the scapular spine. The chief functions of these muscles are to retract the scapula and they are innervated by the dorsoscapular nerve, which is primarily derived from the C5 root (Table 9-2) (76).

TABLE 9-3
SHOULDER BURSAE

Bursa	Location	Normal Joint Communication
Subscapular	Between subscapulosus tendon and capsule	Yes
Infraspinatus	Between capsule and infraspinatus tendon	Inconsistent
Subdeltoid	Between deltoid and rotator cuff	No
Subacromial	Between acromion and rotator cuff (usually contiguous with subdeltoid)	No
Supraacromial	Superior to acromion	No
Subcoracoid	Between coracoid and subscapularis (may be contiguous with subacromial)	~20% of cases
Coracoclavicular	Between the coronoid and trapezius fascicles of the coracoclavicular ligament	No
Coracobrachialis	Between coracobrachialis and subscapularis	No
Latissimus dorsi	Between latissimus and teres major	No
Teres major	Between teres and humeral insertion	No
Pectoralis major	Between pectoralis and humeral insertion	No

From references 8, 81, 82, and 92.

The serratus anterior (Figs. 9-26B) is a large, flat muscle that covers the thoracic cage laterally and acts primarily on the scapula. It arises from the outer surfaces of the proximal eight or nine ribs and extends around the lateral aspect of the thoracic cage to insert on the anterior medial aspect of the scapula. The chief function of this muscle is to protract or draw the scapula anteriorly. The muscle is supplied by the long thoracic nerve that typically arises from cervical nerves (Table 9-2) (76).

Three muscles constitute the musculature of the pectoral region. These include the pectoralis major, pectoralis minor, and subclavius muscles (Figs. 9-17 and 9-26A). The pectoralis major is a large, triangular, flat muscle covering much of the upper thorax. The pectoralis major has an extensive origin from the medial inferior aspect of the clavicle, the lateral margin of the sternum, and the chondral junctions of the upper ribs. The fibers of this muscle converge to form a broad tendon that passes just anterior to coracobrachialis and biceps brachii. The muscle then passes deep to the anterior margin of the deltoid to insert on the crest of the greater tubercle or lateral aspect of the intertubercular groove. The pectoralis major is a strong adductor of the humerus and is innervated by two nerves, the lateral and medial (anterior thoracic) nerves (Table 9-2) (76,82).

The pectoralis minor is deep to the pectoralis major and arises from the anterior aspects of the second through fifth ribs. The muscle passes in a superior and oblique direction to insert on the coracoid process of the scapula. Its chief action is to depress the angle of the scapula. Nerve supply is via the medial pectoral nerve (C8–T1) (Table 9-2) (76).

The subclavius is a small muscle that takes its origin from the junction of the first rib and its articular cartilage and passes upward and laterally to insert on the inferior aspect of the midclavicle. This muscle is covered by the pectoralis major and is innervated by a small branch of the subclavian nerve. It is often seen as a small, intermediate-density structure beneath the clavicle on the sagittal images (Fig. 9-19) and should not be confused with a soft tissue mass (Table 9-2) (76,82).

Bursae

There are numerous bursae about the shoulder that are of importance in identification and excluding significant pathology (81). Table 9-3 summarizes these bursae and their locations. It is important to note that the subscapular bursa normally communicates with the shoulder joint. The infraspinatus bursa inconsistently communicates with the shoulder joint, and the remaining bursae should not, in normal patients, communicate with the glenohumeral joint (52,76,81,82). Most important of these bursae are the subdeltoid and subacromial bursae (Fig. 9-20), which are normally contiguous, do not communicate with the shoulder joint, but can be inflamed. Inflammation does not generally occur in the absence of impingement and rotator cuff tear (52,82).

Neurovascular Anatomy

Because of its complexity and significant clinical implications, the brachial plexus will be discussed separately from the arterial and venous anatomy of the shoulder and upper arm. The brachial plexus (see Fig. 9-28) arises from the anterior rami of the fifth, sixth, seventh, and eighth cervical and first thoracic nerves. In some situations, C4 also forms a portion of the brachial plexus. In most situations, the C5 and C6 roots form the upper, C7 the middle, and C8 and T1 the lower trunks of the brachial plexus. Each trunk then divides to form anterior and posterior divisions. The anterior divisions of the upper and middle trunks form the lateral cord (Fig. 9-28). The anterior division of the lower trunk continues as the medial cord. The posterior divisions of the upper, middle, and lower trunks unite to form the posterior cord (Fig. 9-28). The branches arising from these

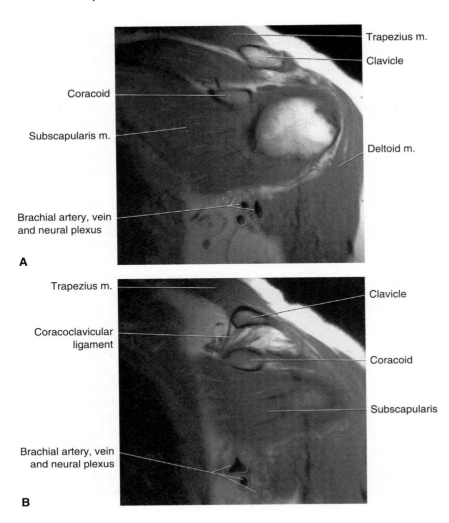

A

B

Figure 9-27 **A,B:** Coronal T1-weighted images through the anterior shoulder, demonstrating the subscapularis and adjacent neurovascular structures.

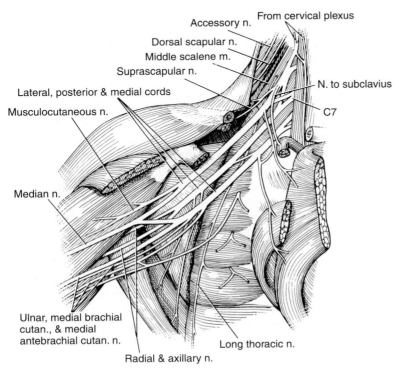

Figure 9-28 Illustration of the brachial plexus and branches.

cords are demonstrated in Figure 9-28. Sagittal MR images usually clearly define the nerve roots as they exit the intervertebral foramen (Fig. 9-15). As one passes peripherally, it is more difficult to identify the individual cords and branches of the brachial plexus. However, there are certain relationships that can be easily identified and followed on MR images (23,26,82).

In the lower neck, the brachial plexus lies above the subclavian artery, except for the lower trunk, which lies posterior to this vessel. This relationship is maintained as the brachial plexus crosses the first rib and enters the axilla. Upon entering the axillary region, the brachial plexus is more closely grouped to the axillary artery and vein (Figs. 9-15 and 9-16). At this level, the lateral cord and a major portion of the posterior cord lie lateral and superior to the axillary artery. The lower trunk of the medial cord is posterior to the artery, with the major continuation of the other groups closely approximately to the vessel (Figs. 9-16 and 9-28). On sagittal images, this forms a closely approximated group of low-intensity structures (Fig. 9-15) (23,26,76,82).

Figure 9-29 demonstrates the major vascular supply of the shoulder. The subclavian artery, along with the transverse cervical and subscapular arteries, is generally clearly demonstrated on MR images. These are most easily demonstrated in the coronal plane (Fig. 9-16). The smaller branch vessels are more difficult to identify on

conventional spin-echo sequences (93). However, new angiographic techniques clearly define the major branch vessels, including the circumflex vessels, thoracodorsal artery, and other branch vessels around the glenohumeral articulation (see Fig. 9-30). The nerve branches of the brachial plexus generally closely follow the courses of the subclavian and axillary artery branches (Fig. 9-15) (26,76,82).

PITFALLS

Pitfalls in MR imaging and MR arthrography may be related to hardware or software artifacts, motion and/or flow artifacts, and normal anatomic variants (1,28,94,95). Additional problems occur with partial volume effects and improper positioning (8,28,33,50,51,96,97).

Technique

Technical factors may include choice of imaging parameters, injection technique and approaches in MR arthrography, and patient positioning (28,67,94,98). Motion and flow artifacts occur less frequently in the shoulder compared to the elbow and wrist. Motion artifacts may be related to pain, tremor, respiratory motion, or forced external or abduction–external rotation, which may be difficult

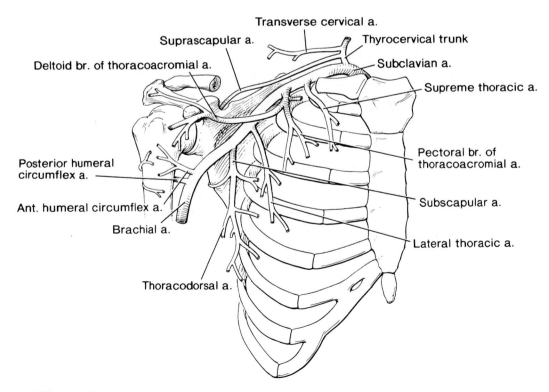

Figure 9-29 Illustration of the vascular anatomy in the axillary region.

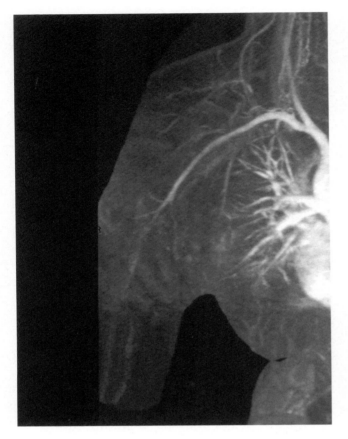

Figure 9-30 Coronal MR angiogram of the neck and shoulder.

and may cause increased signal in the supraspinatus in the region of the critical zone (28,97,100). This is not a problem with T2-weighted (long TE) sequences. Therefore, if one compares short and long TE images, the signal intensity will return to normal. Also, changing the position of the arm alters the location of the signal intensity changes confirming that it is magic angle phenomenon (97).

Errors in arthrographic techniques can also create pitfalls. Improper injection of contrast can result in extravasation, which can be confused with pathology (67,94). Inadvertent injection of air bubbles may cause areas of low signal intensity on MR arthrograms that mimic loose bodies. "Blooming" may cause the air bubble to appear larger due to magnetic susceptibility artifact. This phenomenon is more common on GRE images (94).

Improper positioning may result in apparent signal intensity abnormality in the rotator cuff or capsule. Davis et al. (102) demonstrated abnormal signal intensity in the rotator cuff when the arm is internally rotated. This apparent abnormal signal intensity is due to overlap or narrowing of the supraspinatus and infraspinatus. Internal rotation may also cause overlap of anterior capsule and soft tissue structures, which can result in perceived labral or capsular abnormalities. The degree of internal or external rotation can be determined by the position of the biceptal groove on axial images (see Fig. 9-34) (94).

Anatomic

Anatomic pitfalls and variants have been described by several authors and contribute significantly to difficulties in interpreting MR images of the shoulder (10,21,33, 50,96,103,104). The most frequently encountered pitfalls involve variations in or adjacent to the rotator cuff, labral configuration, marrow patterns, and fluid collections (33,96,104,105).

Rotator Cuff

Normal tendons have uniformly low signal intensity (17–21,28,79,94). Unfortunately, in many adults there is an area of increased signal intensity (intermediate intensity compared to low signal intensity) in the supraspinatus tendon about 1 cm proximal to its insertion. This area of increased signal intensity corresponds to the critical zone (hypovascular area in the cuff). The signal intensity increase is usually 5 to 10 mm and round or oval in appearance (21). Several theories have been proposed for this signal intensity change. Abnormal signal may represent tendon degeneration (106–108). In cadaver studies, Kjellen et al. (109) found that similar abnormal signal intensity represented mucoid degeneration. Though signal intensity was increased on proton density images, it did not increase further on the second echo or a T2-weighted spin-echo sequence, as do rotator cuff tears (see Fig. 9-35) (109).

positions to maintain (see Fig. 9-31) (28,33). Motion artifacts can be reduced by increasing patient comfort, positioning, and using faster sequences to reduce imaging time (21,28). Flow artifacts are a less significant problem. Artifact occurs in the phase encoding direction. Therefore, phase encoding directions should be selected based upon the suspected pathology. A transverse phase encoding should be selected for rotator cuff disease (see Fig. 9-32) to reduce confusion that may occur when flow artifact is in the superior–inferior direction that would pass through the rotator cuff (28,99).

Nonuniform signal intensity or fat suppression also can cause confusion when interpreting MR images. The former is not common today with new shoulder phased-array coils compared to circular or flat coils used previously (Fig. 9-3). Nonuniform fat suppression can result in spurious high signal intensity due to marrow or subcutaneous fat. This is a particular problem with FSE T2-weighted sequences. Metal may also cause nonuniform fat suppression (28,94). Carroll and Helms (94) have recommended the use of inversion recovery sequences in these situations.

Erickson et al. described the magic angle phenomenon (see Fig. 9-33) that can be seen with tendons oriented approximately 55° to the magnetic field (B_o) (97,100,101). This phenomenon occurs with short TE pulse sequences

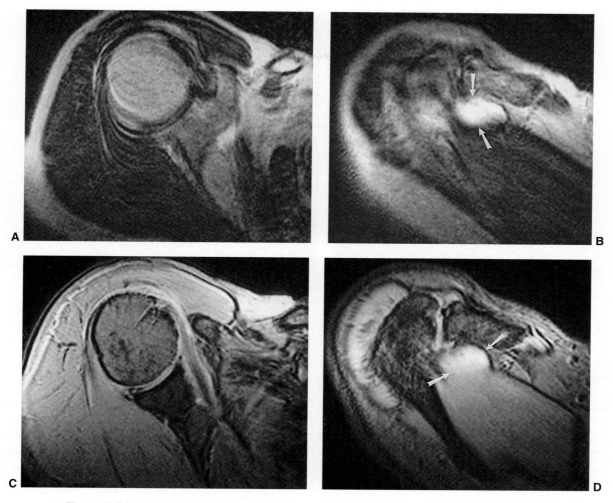

Figure 9-31   Axial T2-weighted **(A,B)** and gradient-echo **(C,D)** images in a patient with a rotator cuff tear (*arrows*). There is motion artifact that degrades image quality on conventional spin-echo sequences **A,B**. No significant artifact is evident on the gradient-echo sequences **C,D**.

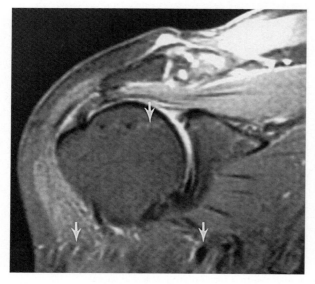

Figure 9-32   Coronal T2-weighted fast spin-echo image with fat suppression. The flow artifact (*arrows*) runs transversely.

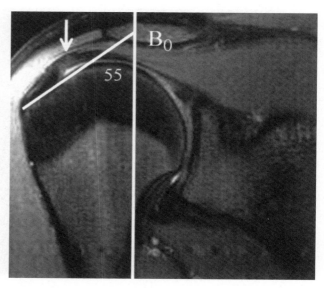

Figure 9-33   Coronal SE 500/11 sequence demonstrating increased signal (*white arrow*) in the supraspinatus that is angled at 55° to the magnet bore (*white line*).

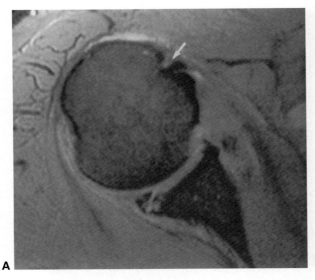
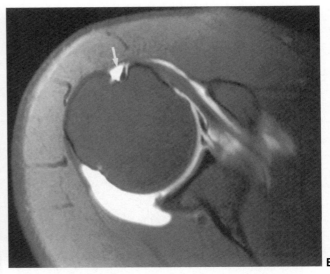

Figure 9-34 Axial gradient-echo image **(A)** with the bicipital groove (*arrow*) position indicating slight internal rotation. Axial MR arthrogram **(B)** shows more external rotation with the groove (*arrow*) more lateral and a stretched subscapularis.

Vahlensieck et al. (110) noted similar increased signal intensity in 85% of normal patients. Explanations for these signal intensity changes included mucoid degeneration, positioning artifacts and partial volume effects, and magic angle effect (35,111). Liou et al. (112) noted intermediate signal intensity in most shoulders, abnormal features in the subdeltoid fat in 95%, and degenerative changes in the AC joint in 48% of asymptomatic patients.

Secondary signs of rotator cuff tear including an abnormal subdeltoid–subacromial fat plane and fluid in the bursa (see Fig. 9-36) can also create pitfalls (39). Specifically,

abnormalities (thinning, irregularity, partial obliteration) in the fat plane are the rule rather than the exception in patients with normal rotator cuffs. Abnormal fat planes are noted in up to 95% of normal patients (112). Fluid in the subacromial or subdeltoid bursa can also be detected in patients without an associated rotator cuff tear (86,113). However, other conditions such as impingement, bursitis, and tendinitis may be associated with fluid in the bursa (65). Fat-suppression techniques may be useful to reduce problems caused by chemical shift artifacts that occur at fat–water interfaces (86,113).

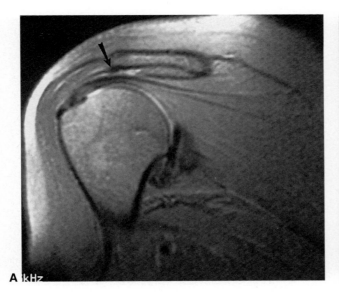
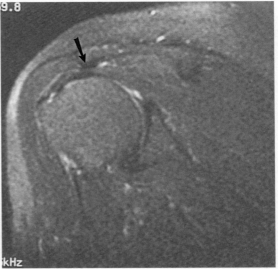

Figure 9-35 Fat-suppressed coronal spin-echo sequences with intermediate increased signal intensity that does not increase between the first **(A)** and second **(B)** echoes. Note the dark deltoid tendon slip (*arrow*) that can be mistaken for an osteophyte.

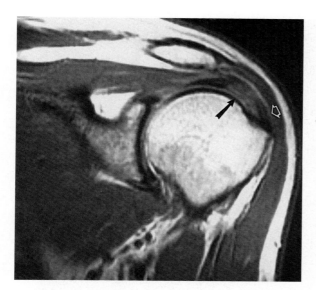

Figure 9-36 Coronal proton density image with increased signal in the supraspinatus (*arrow*) and loss of the fat plane (*open arrow*). No rotator cuff tear.

Labral–Capsular Complex

The glenoid labrum is a fibrous extension of the glenoid rim that has an MR appearance similar to the acetabular labrum or knee meniscus in that it is low signal intensity and typically triangular in shape. This structure is important for maintaining glenohumeral stability (114–116).

Anatomic variations in the labrum, labral–biceps complex, and adjacent capsule can create confusion and simulate a labral tear (21,50,54,94,116–120). Neumann et al. (118) described multiple labral configurations in asymptomatic shoulders. The most frequent configuration is a triangular anterior (45%) and posterior (73%) labrum. However, in our experience the posterior labrum is frequently more rounded (see Fig. 9-37) than the sharper anterior labrum. A rounded appearance (19% anteriorly, 12% posteriorly) (Fig. 9-37) was the second most common appearance reported by Neumann et al. (118) Cleaved (frayed appearance) and notched labra were reported in 15% and 8% of cases, respectively. Flat labra were noted in 6% to 7%, and absence of the labrum was seen anteriorly in 6% and posteriorly in 8% (121). In our experience, we have not seen an absent labrum in the normal shoulder.

A normal cleft is usually seen between the articular cartilage and labrum (Fig. 9-37B). This does not transverse the entire length of the labrum and should not be mistaken for a tear (96,112). The proximity of the middle glenohumeral ligament to the anterior labrum (Fig. 9-37C) can also be confusion with a tear (54,96,112).

There are other clinically significant variations in the ligaments, capsule, and labrum that deserve mention in

Figure 9-37 Normal variations in the glenoid labrum. **A:** Illustrations of variations in the anterior labrum at the midglenoid level. *a,* triangular; *b,* small but triangular; *c,* rounded; *d,* crescentic; *e,* recess between the labrum and cartilage; *f,* middle glenohumeral ligament proximal to the labrum; *g,* small anterior labrum with adjacent thick middle glenohumeral ligament. **B:** MR arthrogram demonstrating triangular (*arrows*) anterior and posterior labra. The posterior capsule is distended with a type II or III attachment (*open arrow*). **C:** MR arthrogram demonstrating near-complete absence of the anterior labrum (*arrow*) and a rounded posterior labrum (*bracket*). **D:** MR arthrogram depicting rounded anterior and posterior labra. **E:** MR arthrogram demonstrating a rounded posterior labrum and intermediate signal intensity and deformity of the anterior labrum (*arrow*) due to a prior Bankart repair.

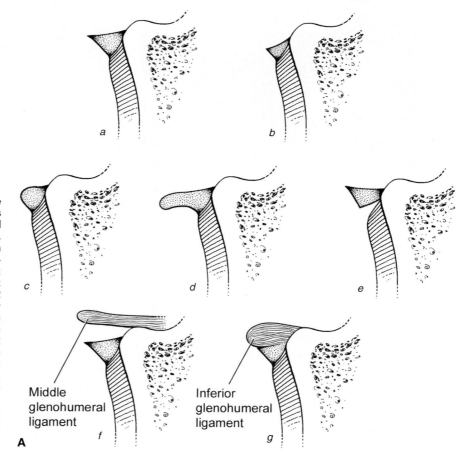

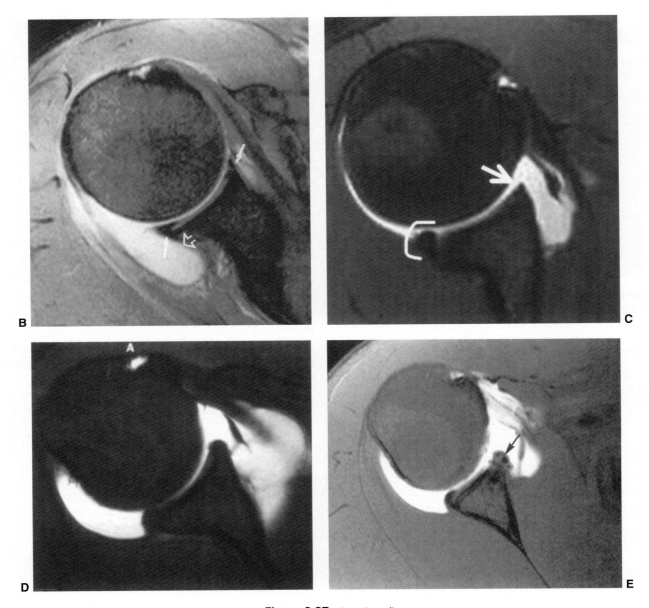

Figure 9-37   (continued)

this section. Most common variations occur in the ligaments and capsular attachment (21,54,116).

The superior glenohumeral ligament originates at the superior glenoid margin anterior to the long head of the biceps tendon. This ligament may originate separately or with the biceps tendon or middle glenohumeral ligament (see Fig. 9-38) (54,76). The superior glenohumeral ligament can be identified in 98% of patients on MR arthrograms (54). Variations in thickness of the superior and middle glenohumeral ligaments is common. The superior glenohumeral ligament is usually thinner than the middle glenohumeral ligament. When the superior ligament is thicker, the middle glenohumeral ligament may be absent or thinner (21,54,116). The superior glenohumeral ligament may be absent in up to 10% of patients (54).

The middle glenohumeral ligament is the most variable. It may be thick or thin and is absent in up to 30% of specimens (54). The middle glenohumeral ligament originates at the anterosuperior labrum (Fig. 9-38), where it may blend with the superior and/or inferior glenohumeral ligament. The ligament blends with the capsule and inserts on the humerus at the base of the greater tuberosity (21,54,76). The middle glenohumeral ligament may be thick and associated with absence of the anterior superior labrum (see Fig. 9-39). This anatomic configuration is called the Buford complex (21,54,94,116,122). This anatomic variation is seen in about 1.5% of the general population (94) This differs from the sublabral foramen, which consists of a normal anterosuperior labral detachment (see Fig. 9-40). The sublabral foramen is present in 8% to 12% of individuals (21,94,122). The middle

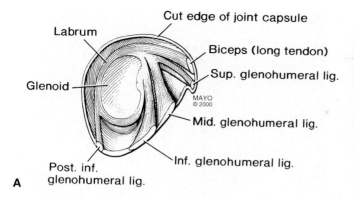

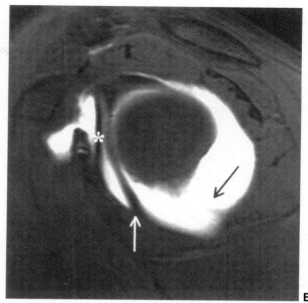

Figure 9-38 **A:** Illustration of glenohumeral ligaments, labrum, and capsule seen in the sagittal plane. **B:** Sagittal MR arthrogram demonstrating the middle glenohumeral ligament (*), the anterior band of the inferior glenohumeral ligament (*white arrow*) and the posterior band of the inferior glenohumeral ligament (*black arrow*).

glenohumeral ligament is not thickened and isolated labral tears in this region are rare (54).

The inferior glenohumeral ligament has anterior and posterior bands with an interposed axillary recess. The anterior and posterior bands arise from the inferior labrum anteriorly and posteriorly and extend to the respective regions on the surgical neck of the humerus (21,76) The anterior band is typically thicker than the posterior bands (Fig. 9-38A) (54).

Duplication of the long head of the biceps tendon may be seen in up to 10% of individuals. This results from a third or fourth head of the biceps brachii muscle (76,94). This creates the appearance of a longitudinal tendon split (94).

Fluid Collections

There is usually a small amount of fluid in the glenohumeral joint in normal subjects. Recht et al. (105) reported only

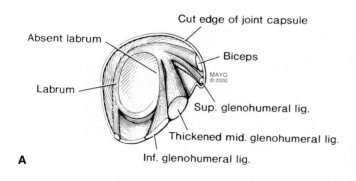

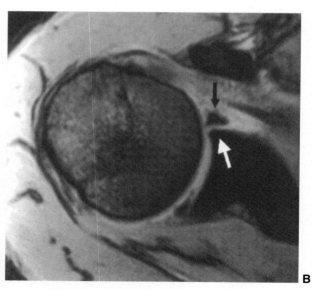

Figure 9-39 **A:** Illustration of the Buford complex with absent anterior superior labrum and thickening of the middle glenohumeral ligament. **B:** Axial MR image demonstrating an absent anterior labrum (*white arrow*) and thickening of the middle glenohumeral ligament (*black arrow*).

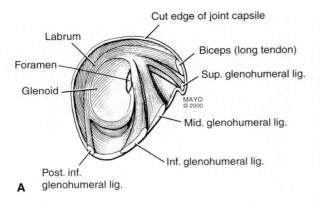

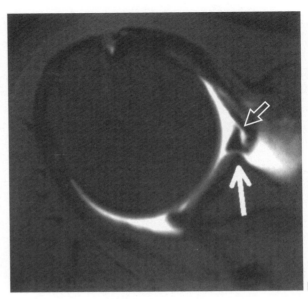

Figure 9-40 **A:** Illustration of the anterior labral foramen. **B:** MR arthrogram demonstrating a sublabral foramen with a small focal area of the anterior labrum (*open arrow*) that is not adherent to the underlying anterior superior glenoid (*white arrow*).

about 2 mL of fluid in normal shoulders. Schweitzer et al. (123) reported that sufficient fluid to be identified as more than a fine line in the joint or bursa should be considered an effusion and is usually associated with degenerative disease or rotator cuff tears.

There are numerous bursae about the shoulder (Table 9-3). Most do not communicate with the joint. Therefore, fluid in these bursae is usually abnormal and indicates inflammation or communication with the joint via a rotator cuff tear or capsular defect (Fig. 9-20) (21,52,76).

Fluid may also be demonstrated in the biceps tendon sheath. Kaplan et al. (96) reported a small amount of fluid in the tendon sheath in 14 of 15 normal subjects. In addition, a rounded fluid density was noted in 19 of 30 cases. This proved to be the anterolateral branch of the anterior circumflex artery and not fluid.

Fluid in the biceps tendon sheath should not be considered abnormal unless the tendon is completely surrounded by fluid (see Fig. 9-41) (96).

Fluid in the subcoracoid bursa is commonly seen, as this bursa communicates with the joint in 20% of cases (21,76,94). The subscapularis bursa is seen in 90% of cases (Table 9-3) (21). Fluid may be evident in the subacromial subdeltoid bursae if inflammation is present or following

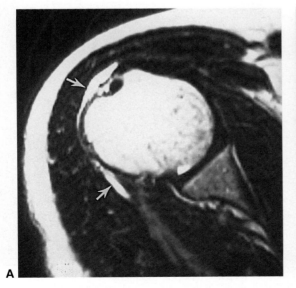

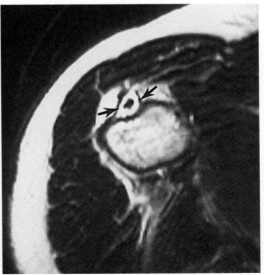

Figure 9-41 Axial SE 2,000/80 images of the shoulder in a patient with fluid in the subdeltoid bursa **(A)** (*arrows*) and completely surrounding and distending the biceps tendon sheath **(B)** (*arrows*). Features are due to bursitis and tendinitis.

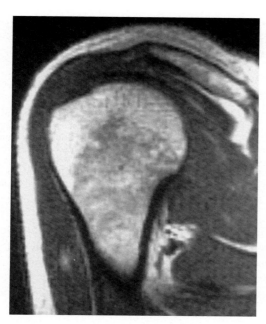

Figure 9-42 Coronal proton density image demonstrating yellow marrow in the epiphysis with mixed red and yellow marrow (predominantly red) in the metaphysis in a 19-year-old male. The marrow pattern in the clavicle is also mixed.

therapeutic injections. Fluid typically remains up to 48 hours after an injection (94,124).

Marrow/Osseous Variants

Variations in red and yellow marrow and other anatomic osseous variants may also create confusion on MR images. There is considerable variation in the amount of red and yellow marrow in the metaphysis (see Fig. 9-42). With age, there is generally conversion of red to yellow marrow. Richardson and Patten (125) evaluated marrow patterns on patients 15 to 69 years of age. Each of five regions (glenoid, acromion, epiphysis, metaphysis, and diaphysis) was graded (see Fig. 9-43) from 1 to 7, with 1 representing 100% red marrow, 2 to 6 indicating reducing percentages of red marrow, and 7 representing 0% red marrow (all yellow marrow). Marrow was graded as homogeneous (red), geographic, mottled, or all yellow (see Fig. 9-44) (125). Marrow patterns changed with age in all five regions in a fairly predictable fashion. However, red marrow can persist beyond the previously reported 15-year age range. For example, subchondral red marrow can be seen in 88% of patients in their 20s and up to 23% of patients in the seventh decade of life. Therefore, signal inhomogeneity in the shoulder may be due to red–yellow marrow variations. Normal marrow patterns can mimic marrow abnormalities. However, errors can be avoided by comparison with the contralateral shoulder (marrow patterns are usually symmetrical). Also, marrow variations are not associated with cortical bone destruction or soft tissue changes (104,125–127).

There is a groove in the posterior lateral humeral head which can be confused with a Hill-Sachs lesion. This normal finding is usually located more distally than a Hill-Sachs lesion (see Fig. 9-45) (104,127). In our experience, most Hill-Sachs lesions are much larger (Figs. 9-45B).

Another osseous variant that may be related to clinical symptoms is the os acromiale. This is due to a developmental abnormality of ossification involving the anterior acromion (94,128–130). This is usually evident on all MR image planes but is typically most obvious on axial images (see Fig. 9-46). The deltoid may displace the os acromiale resulting in impingement (21,94,131).

Recently, Morgan et al. (95) described pseudotumor deltoideus, an anatomic variant at the deltoid insertion on the humerus. This variant is a spectrum of changes at the deltoid insertion that may present as a lucent area or with prominence or irregularity in the corticoperiosteal region on radiographs. Bone scans may demonstrate a focal area of increased tracer. There is mixed increased and decreased signal intensity on MR images (see Fig. 9-47) (95).

Miscellaneous Variants

Interpreters of MR images must also become familiar with other artifacts or variants created by technique, positioning, anatomy, and equipment problems. In the shoulder, the rotator cuff, labrum, fluid changes, and marrow

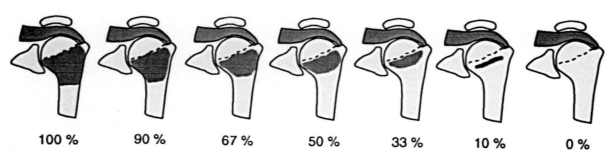

100 %   90 %   67 %   50 %   33 %   10 %   0 %

Figure 9-43 Grading system for conversion from red (100% *left*) to yellow marrow with no residual red marrow in grade 7. (From Richardson ML, Patten RM. Age-related changes in marrow distribution in the shoulder: MR image findings. *Radiology* 1994;192:209–215.)

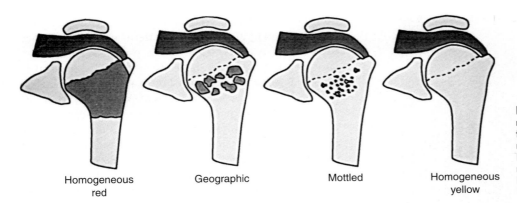

Homogeneous red   Geographic   Mottled   Homogeneous yellow

Figure 9-44 Illustration of marrow pattern categories progressing from homogeneous red to homogeneous yellow. (From Richardson ML, Patten RM. Age-related changes in marrow distribution in the shoulder: MR image findings. *Radiology* 1994;192:209–215.)

changes are most frequently discussed in the literature as noted above. Other variants, such as tendon attachments (Fig. 9-36A), can be confused with osteophytes (96). Confusion can be avoided by comparing MR findings with radiographic features. Other findings such as soft tissue

calcifications (see Fig. 9-48) provide additional value for radiographic comparison when interpreting MR images.

Vacuum phenomenon can be noted in the shoulder as well as the knee and other joints. In the shoulder, this finding is particularly common when the arm is positioned in

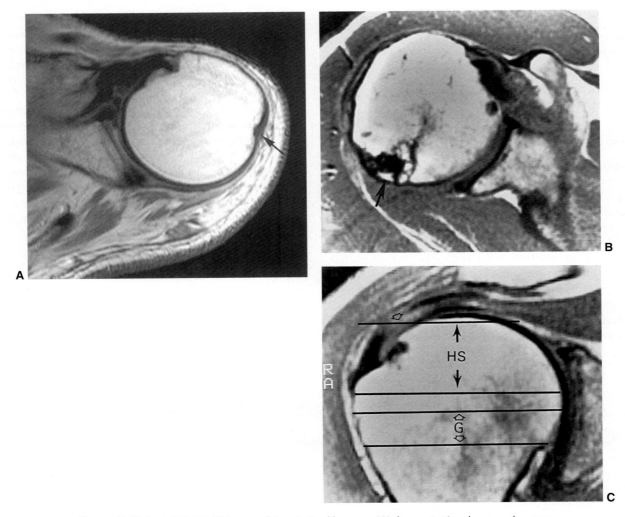

Figure 9-45 Axial SE 450/15 image of the proximal humerus **(A)** demonstrating the normal posterolateral groove (*arrow*). Axial **(B)** and coronal **(C)** proton density images demonstrating a Hill-Sachs lesion (*arrow*) and a rotator cuff tear (*open arrow*). The levels of the usual Hill-Sachs (*HS*) lesion and normal groove (*G*) are indicated with transverse lines to show where they would be seen on axial images.

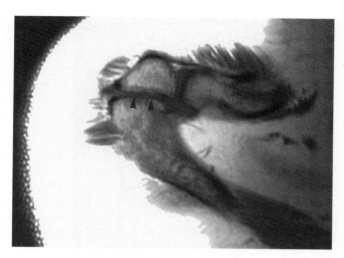

Figure 9-46 Axial proton density image shows an os acromiale (*arrowheads*).

external rotation (10). The MR finding appears to occur most frequently on gradient echo sequences (see Fig. 9-49). Patten (10) reported the vacuum phenomenon in up to 20% of cases. Awareness of this artifact is important to avoid misinterpretation of intraarticular air as loose bodies or chondrocalcinosis (10).

APPLICATIONS

Routine radiography is an important initial examination for screening patients with shoulder, arm, and suspected brachial plexus lesions (8,53,132–134). Other techniques, including radionuclide studies, CT, and arthrography, also have an important role in evaluating these patients (8,37,135–138). In recent years, ultrasound has become a useful tool in some institutions for screening patients with suspected rotator cuff tears and other abnormalities in the shoulder region (139–144). Because of the clinical presentations and anatomic and examination differences, we will discuss the shoulder and arm separate from brachial plexus examinations.

SHOULDER AND ARM

The majority of patients who are referred for MRI of the shoulder or arm present with pain or restricted range of motion in the shoulder. Most commonly, patients are referred for MRI because of suspected rotator cuff tears or impingement, defects in the glenoid–labrum, or instability, osteonecrosis, biceps tendon abnormalities, suspected soft tissue or bony neoplasms, and infectious or inflammatory disorders (21,79,145).

Osseous Trauma

Routine radiography and radionuclide studies are usually sufficient for identifying subtle and/or complete fractures and other osseous injuries in the shoulder and humerus. Occasionally, CT is needed to clearly identify the position of the fracture fragments (8,52). MRI also plays a significant role in evaluating isolated osseous trauma. Subtle fractures can be easily identified with MRI. Also, any associated soft tissue injuries are easily detected (see Fig. 9-50) (99, 146–149). Osseous injuries are frequently associated with soft tissue injury and/or instability. Hill-Sachs lesions (see Fig. 9-51) and other fractures or osteochondral injuries may also provide valuable clues to additional soft tissue pathology and shoulder instability (see Fig. 9-52) (27,99,147,148,150). Both Hill-Sachs and Bankart lesions are commonly associated with anterior dislocations. However, tuberosity fractures may also be evident in 15% of patients with anterior dislocations (Fig. 9-50). Fractures of the greater tuberosity may also follow forced abduction or direct trauma. Symptoms may mimic a rotator cuff tear (151). This injury is often subtle. However, when displaced, greater tuberosity fractures may result in biceps tendon entrapment (8,152). Avulsion of the lesser tuberosity along with the capsule (see Fig. 9-53) or subscapularis tears are also noted with anterior dislocations (16).

Injuries to the distal clavicle and AC joint are common (129,153–158). Acromioclavicular dislocations account for 10% of shoulder injuries (153). Routine radiographs or stress views are usually adequate for diagnosis and classification (107,159).

The classification system for AC joint injuries was developed by Buckholtz and Hickman (160). This classification is based upon mechanism of injury and extent of ligament and osseous injury. MR features may provide additional information regarding both soft tissue and osseous injuries (153). However, patient age is important, as articular and soft tissue degenerative changes are common in older adults and may not be related to clinical symptoms (131,153). Table 9-4 summarizes AC joint injuries and MR features. Keep in mind MR features are most useful in children and young adults that have not yet developed degenerative changes.

Type I injury is a sprain of the AC ligaments (160,161). Radiographs are normal. MR images using T2-weighted or STIR sequences may demonstrate increased signal intensity in the periarticular tissues and early marrow edema (27). Type II injuries result in disruption of the AC ligaments and coracoclavicular sprain. Stress radiographs demonstrate subluxation of the joint. MR images demonstrate increased signal in the AC ligaments and marrow edema in the acromion and clavicale. There may also be increased signal intensity I the coracoclavicular ligament (153). Axial and sagittal image planes are most useful. Type III injuries result in disruption of the AC and coracoclavicular ligaments. The joint dislocates radiographically. MR images demonstrate increased signal intensity in both ligament complexes (Table 9-4) and

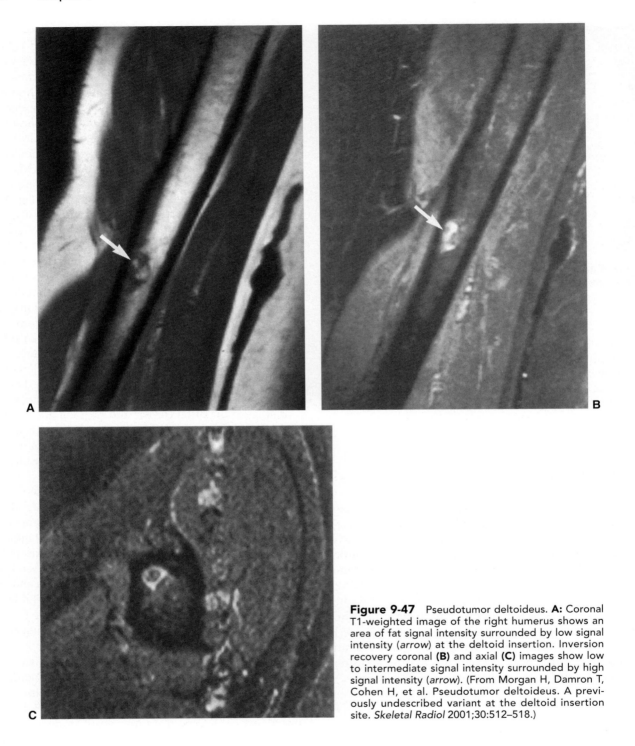

Figure 9-47 Pseudotumor deltoideus. **A:** Coronal T1-weighted image of the right humerus shows an area of fat signal intensity surrounded by low signal intensity (*arrow*) at the deltoid insertion. Inversion recovery coronal (**B**) and axial (**C**) images show low to intermediate signal intensity surrounded by high signal intensity (*arrow*). (From Morgan H, Damron T, Cohen H, et al. Pseudotumor deltoideus. A previously undescribed variant at the deltoid insertion site. *Skeletal Radiol* 2001;30:512–518.)

widening with varying degrees of joint subluxation or dislocation (153,160). The deltoid and trapezius muscles may be detached from the distal clavicle (153). All three image planes may be required to assess the soft tissue and articular changes completely. A fracture at the base of coracoid has also been reported instead of coracoclavicular ligament disruption (160). Fractures of the coracoid base are most obvious on sagittal images. Type IV dislocations result in posterior displacement of the clavicle which is most easily appreciated on axial images (153). Sternoclavicular dislocations may also occur with this injury. Therefore, both medial and lateral ends of the clavicle should be imaged (153,160). Type IV dislocations are similar to type III except the trapezius and deltoid muscles are stripped from the ends of the clavicle and acromion. The clavicle is significantly elevated by cephalad traction of the sternocleidonastoid muscle. This feature is best appreciated on coronal images. Type

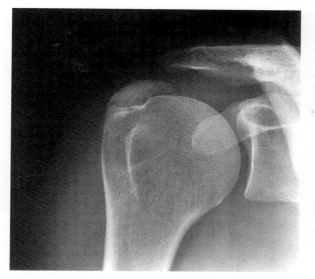

Figure 9-48 Anteroposterior radiograph demonstrates dense calcification in the supraspinatus tendon.

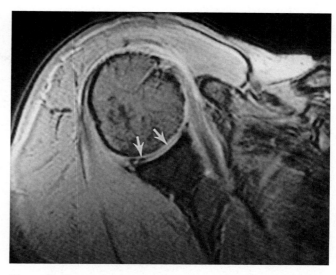

Figure 9-49 Axial gradient-echo image of the shoulder with linear and globular areas of intraarticular decreased signal intensity (*arrows*) due to vacuum phenomenon. Joint fluid would be high signal intensity. Loose bodies tend to be located in recesses or areas of articular abnormality.

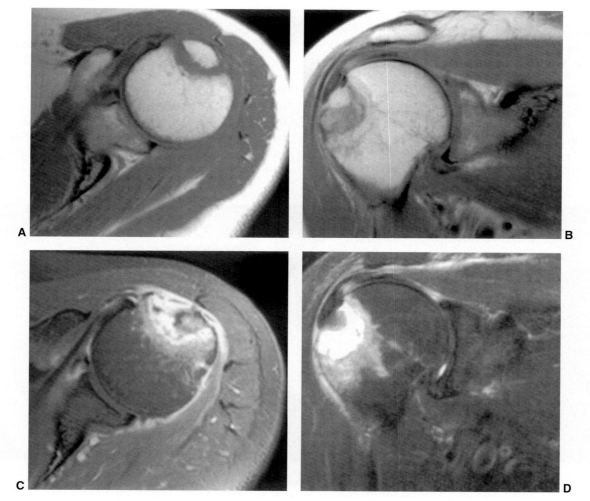

Figure 9-50 Patient with posttraumatic shoulder pain. Routine radiographs were normal. Axial (**A**) and coronal (**B**) T1-weighted and axial (**C**) and coronal (**D**) T2-weighted images demonstrate a fracture of the greater tuberosity with fluid between the fragments on the T2-weighted images **C,D**.

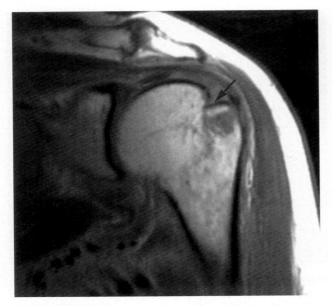

Figure 9-51 Coronal proton density-weighted image demonstrating a Hill-Sachs lesion (*arrow*) not evident on routine radiographs.

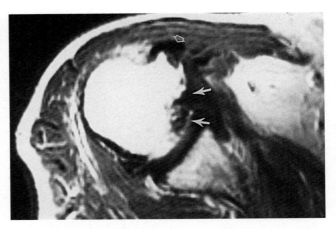

Figure 9-52 Axial T1-weighted image in a patient with chronic pain and reduced motion in the shoulder. There is an anteromedial osteochondral fracture (*arrows*) due to a previous posterior dislocation. The biceps tendon (*open arrow*) is subluxed medially.

VI dislocations result from severe force from superior to the clavicle with the humerus abducted (160). Type IV injuries may be most easily identified on coronal or sagittal images.

Posttraumatic osteolysis is another condition that may mimic fracture or rotator cuff tear clinically (8,162). This condition typically follows acute trauma to the AC joint usually due to falling on the point of the shoulder. Osteolysis may also follow repeated microtrauma in laborers, throwing athletes and individuals involved in weight training (27,155,163,164). Patients present with pain and tenderness over the AC joint and weakness on arm abduction (8,163). Radiographs demonstrate subtle resorption of the distal clavicle.

MR images in the coronal, sagittal and axial planes will demonstrate irregularity of the clavicle with increased signal intensity on T2- and decreased signal on T1-weighted images. The acromion is relatively spared. There may be fluid in the joint and increased signal intensity in the surrounding soft tissues (see Fig. 9-54) (163). Conservative therapy may result in complete recovery with image features returning to normal. Residual chronic changes may remain (see Fig. 9-55). If left untreated, extensive joint hypertrophy and instability of the joint may develop (see Fig. 9-56).

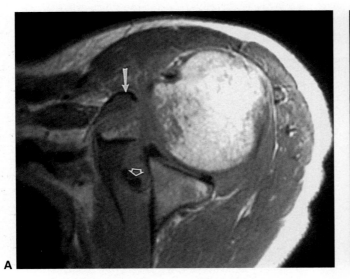
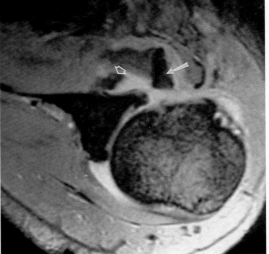

Figure 9-53 Lesser tuberosity avulsion and tears in the capsule and middle glenohumeral ligament. Axial proton density (**A**) and gradient-echo (**B**) images show the displaced lesser tuberosity (*arrow*) and ligament tear (*open arrow*).

TABLE 9-4

ACROMIOCLAVICULAR JOINT INJURIES

Classification	Description	MR Features (T2 or STIR)
Type I	Acromioclavicular ligament sprain	↑ Signal intensity in periarticular soft tissues
Type II	Acromioclavicular ligament tear with coracoclavicular sprain	Marrow edema, ↑ signal intensity in AC ligaments. Type I coracoclavicular
Type III	Acromioclavicular dislocation, disruption coracoclavicular ligament	↑ Signal intensity both ligaments, joint widening and/or displacement
Type IV	Same as type III, but posterior clavicular dislocation	Same as type III plus posterior clavicle position
Type V	Same as type III, with deltoid and trapezius muscles stripped from the acromion and clavicle	Same as type III with soft tissue changes
Type VI	Inferior clavicle dislocation	Same as type III with clavicle inferior to acromion or coracoid

From references 8, 129, 154, and 161.

Patients that do not respond to conservative therapy may be treated by resection of the distal clavicle.

Interpretation of AC abnormalities is more complex in older adults. The presence of osteophytes, capsular hypertrophy, and joint space changes, including effusion, may not correlate with clinical symptoms. Jordan et al. (131) found some correlation with high signal intensity in the distal clavicle and a trend toward the presence of an effusion and a positive clinical examination. Other changes did not correlate with clinical findings (131). Schweitzer et al. (165) reported joint effusions in 66% of patients with grade 2 or 3 impingement compared to 12% in normal volunteers.

Rotator Cuff Tears

The primary application of MRI for shoulder and upper arm trauma is evaluation of soft tissue injuries. Most of these injuries are chronic in nature.

There are numerous causes of shoulder pain. Most are related to rotator cuff pathology or instability; however, other lesions may also be evaluated with MRI (163,166–168).

The most common indication for MRI is evaluation of patients with suspected rotator cuff tear or impingement syndrome (8,19,21,169–171).

The rotator cuff is comprised of the supraspinatus, infraspinatus, teres minor, and suprascapularis tendons. The supraspinatus, infraspinatus, and teres minor insert on the superior, middle, and inferior facets of the greater tuberosity. The subscapularis inserts on the lesser tuberosity, with fibers extending over the bicipital groove to the greater tuberosity. This forms the transverse ligament (21,76,172). The space between the supraspinatus and subscapularis is the rotator cuff interval. The coracoid projects into this space medially. Within this space are the medial and lateral bundles of the coracohumeral ligament. Deep to the ligament, the interval contains the superior glenohumeral ligament (21,71).

The rotator cuff provides 33% to 50% of the muscle effort required for abduction, and 80% to 90% for external rotation (173,174). Multiple etiologies have been implicated in development of rotator cuff tears (Table 9-5). Zlatkin (21) categorized etiologies of rotator cuff tears as extrinsic (impingement, impingement with instability, subcoracoid, etc.) and primary cuff degeneration, which may be ischemic.

Primary extrinsic impingement occurs when the rotator cuff is entrapped beneath the subacromial arch. The arch is composed of the clavicle, anterior acromion, AC arch, anterior or distal coracoid, and the coracoacromial ligament (see Fig. 9-57) (175–182). This includes acromial abnormalities, AC joint osteophytes, and thickening of the coracoacromial ligament. This mechanism for pathophysiology of rotator cuff tears has been most popular over the years.

Neer proposed that the majority (95%) of rotator cuff tears were the result of chronic impingement of the supraspinatus tendon against the acromial arch (2,21,175,183). Impingement can occur due to abnormalities or variants in the coracoacromial arch. Abnormalities in the osseous, ligamentous, or soft tissues within the arch may cause impingement. The os acromiale is due to failure to fuse of one of three acromial ossification centers (184–186). The os acromiale may be one or more infused segments. The incidence has been reported to be 1% to 15% of the general population. Sammarco (186) evaluated 2,367 cadaver specimens and reported the incidence of os acromiale to be 0.8%. The variant was bilateral in 33%. Others have reported bilateral involvement in up to 60 % (185). Os acromiale are more common in males than females and in African-Americans than whites (186). This variant, along with abnormalities in the osseous and soft tissue structures of the arch, can result in impingement of the rotator cuff (see Fig. 9-58) (21,27,130,180,187,188). Acromial configuration has also been implicated in impingement (see Fig. 9-59) and rotator cuff tears (9,130,179,189). A type 1 acromial configuration is straight; type 2, curved; type 3, hooked; and type 4 has a convex inferior surface (Fig. 9-59) (21,31). Anterior or lateral angulation of the acromion may also cause impingement (see Fig. 9-60) (179,189). Type 1 acromions occur in 18% to 23%; type 2, in 42% to 68%; and type 3, 10% to 39% of patients. Type 4 acromia

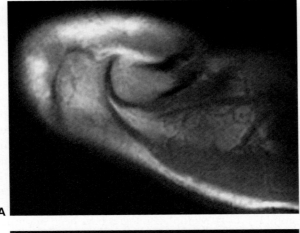

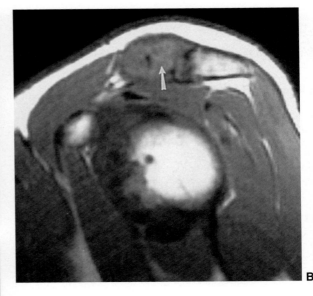

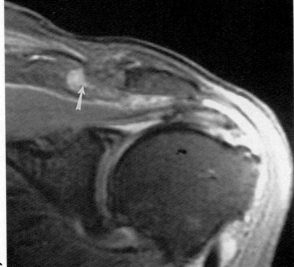

Figure 9-54 Posttraumatic osteolysis. **A:** Axial SE 500/10 image of the normal acromioclavicular joint. The bone margins are sharp and there is no joint effusion or soft tissue edema. Proton density sagittal (**B**) and coronal (**C**) images demonstrate irregularity and abnormal signal in the distal clavicle (*arrow*) with sparing of the acromion.

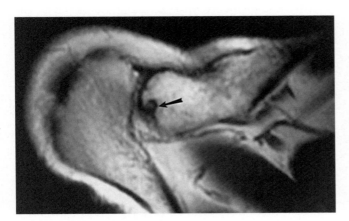

Figure 9-55 Axial T1-weighted image shows residual erosive changes (*arrow*) in the distal clavicle after traumatic osteolysis.

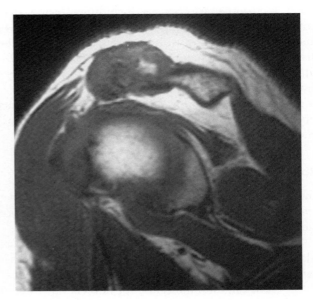

Figure 9-56 Chronic untreated traumatic osteolysis with marked joint hypertrophy on this sagittal T1-weighted image.

TABLE 9-5

ETIOLOGIES OF ROTATOR CUFF TEARS

Primary extrinsic impingement
Acromial configuration
Lateral/downsloping acromion
Acromioclavicular joint osteophytes or hypertrophy
Acromial osteophytes
Low-lying acromion
Os acromiale
Thickened coracoclavicular ligament
Secondary extrinsic impingement
Instability in throwing athletes
Posterosubglenoid impingement
Throwing athletes
Subcoracoid impingement
Primary cuff degeneration
Ischemia
Trauma

From references 21, 27, 175, and 176.

occur in 7% of the general population (21,31,189). Type 3 or hooked acromia are more common in males (190). Zlatkin and Falchook (18) reported rotator cuff tears in 51% of patients with type 3 acromia, os acromiale, or anterior inferior acromial bone spurs (see Fig. 9-61). More recent studies noted type 3 acromia in 70% to 80% of rotator cuff tears. Only 3% of patients with rotator cuff tears had type 1 acromia (191).

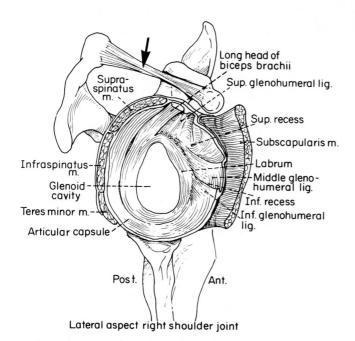

Figure 9-57 Illustration demonstrating the coracoacromial arch and supporting structures of the shoulder. Note the coracoacromial ligament (*arrow*).

Consistent categorization of the acromial shape (Figs. 9-59 to 9-61) is not always possible on MR images (192). In fact, Haygood et al. (192) indicated that routine radiography may be more accurate (6,133,134,180,193,194). The important feature is not so much the shape but the impact of the underlying tissues and humeroacromial distance (see Fig. 9-62). Additional causes of primary extrinsic impingement alone or in combination include anterior acromial osteophytes, AC osteophytes and joint hypertrophy, low lying acromia and thickening of the coracoacromial ligament (9,18,21,191).

Neer (175) divided rotator cuff disease into three stages (see Fig. 9-63). The initial stage (Stage I) consists of edema or hemorrhage in the rotator cuff, specifically the supraspinatus tendon. During stage II there is progression of the inflammatory stage to a more fibrotic process. The final stage, stage III, results in a tear of the rotator cuff. The most susceptible area in the cuff is approximately 1 cm from the insertion of the supraspinatus tendon into the greater tuberosity. This "critical zone" is where the majority of tendon ruptures occur. Chronic impingement of this avascular area leads to tendinitis or inflammation during the first stage of the degeneration period (180,195,196). This most commonly stage occurs in younger patients (<25 years) (19). This abnormality is identifiable on MR images, which is important since inflammatory changes may be reversible. As the degenerative process continues to stage II (25-45 years of age) and stage III (>45 years of age), progressive change in the supraspinatus tendon and AC joint region occur (18,21,166,175,176,180). Therefore, when evaluating MR images of the shoulder it is important to compare them with routine radiographs to detect secondary osseous changes, especially around the AC joint, as well as the position of the humeral head in relation to the AC joint and the acromial shape (see Fig. 9-64) (1,52,53,193). On the normal AP radiograph in external rotation the distance between the under surface of the acromion and humeral head should measure 7 mm or more. When this space is reduced to less than 7 mm, a rotator cuff tear (Fig. 9-62 and 9-64)) is almost certainly present. The angled AP view and supraspinatus outlet views are also useful for evaluating secondary osseous changes (91,197). Recently, Stallenberg et al. (193) evaluated the soft tissue contour, muscle density and heterogeneity of the supraspinatus on the scapular Y view. Atrophy, fatty infiltration and morphologic changes predicted a full thickness tear in 80% to 85% of patients.

Secondary extrinsic impingement (Table 9-5) occurs with glenohumeral or scapulothoracic instability (21,27). This form of impingement occurs in young athletes who perform repetitive overheard or throwing movements. The result is labral and anterior ligament laxity leading to increased work load and wear in the rotator cuff muscles. Over time, this results in anterior superior migration of the humeral head and rotator cuff tears (27,198).

Impingement of the rotator cuff on the posterior superior glenoid (internal impingement) has also been recognized in

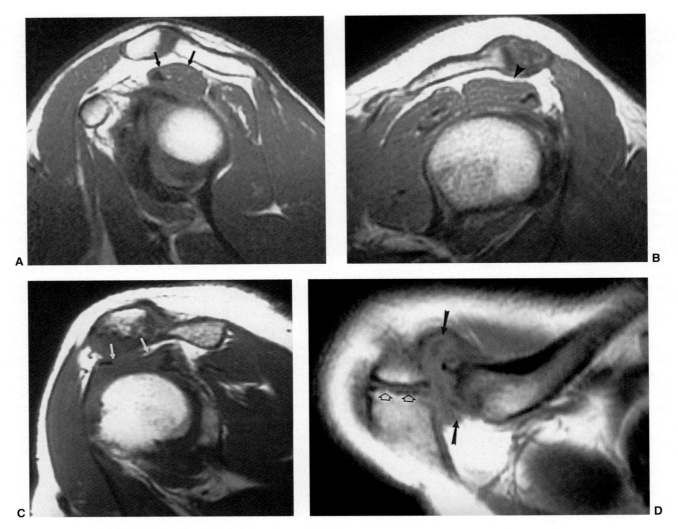

Figure 9-58 Impingement of the rotator cuff. **A:** Sagittal T1-weighted image of a normal acromio-clavicular joint region. There is fat between the bone and the upper surface (*arrows*) of the supraspinatus is convex. **B:** Sagittal T1-weighted image demonstrating degenerative change in the acromioclavicular joint causing mild impingement with a concave upper surface (*arrowhead*) on the supraspinatus muscle. There is still fat between the muscle and joint. **C:** Sagittal T1-weighted image demonstrating moderate to marked impingement due to AC joint hypertrophy (*arrows*). **D:** Axial proton density-weighted image demonstrating acromioclavicular joint degeneration (*arrows*) and an os acromiale (*open arrows*).

throwing athletes. This occurs during the cocking phase of the throwing motion (21,199).

Subcoracoid impingement results from encroachment of the subscapularis tendon on the lesser tuberosity (21,200). This occurs with narrowing of the space between the coracoid and humeral head. Narrowing of this space may be due to developmental elongation of the coracoid, previous fracture of the coracoid or lesser tuberosity or coracoid osteotomy (21,201). The distance between the coracoid and lesser tuberosity with the arm in internal rotation should be ≥11mm (202). Changes are most easily appreciated on axial images. Remember, on most MR examinations, the area is neutral to externally rotated. Therefore, this condition must be considered prior to performing the MR examination.

Other causes of impingement include fracture callus adjacent to the tuberosities and supraspinatus hypertrophy (21).

Primary rotator cuff degeneration is another consideration (Table 9-5) for the pathogenesis of rotator cuff tear (21,27,203). Ischemia in the critical zone about 1 cm from the supraspinatus insertion leads to degeneration and rotator cuff tears. Cadaver studies have documented cuff tears in this location without associated features of impingement described above (203).

Trauma may be associated with rotator cuff tears. This may be chronic microtrauma or acute injury such as anterior dislocation. The incidence is still higher in older patients who may already have rotator cuff pathology (21,175).

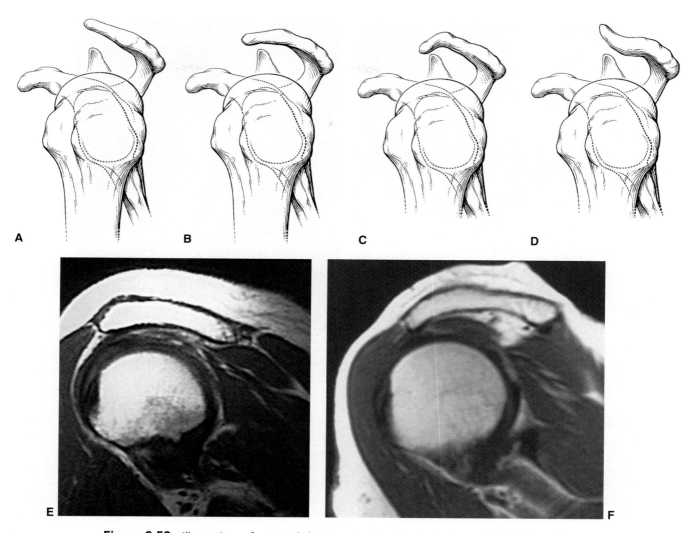

A   B   C   D

E   F

Figure 9-59   Illustrations of acromial shapes and orientations as seen on oblique sagittal MR images. **A:** Flat. **B:** Curved. **C:** Hooked. **D:** Convex inferior surface. **E:** Sagittal SE 500/20 image of a curved (type 2) acromion. **F:** Sagittal SE 500/20 image of a curved, anteriorly angled acromion compressing the supraspinatus.

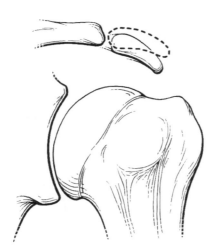

Figure 9-60   Illustration of an inferiorly angulated, downsloping acromion (*dotted line, normal*).

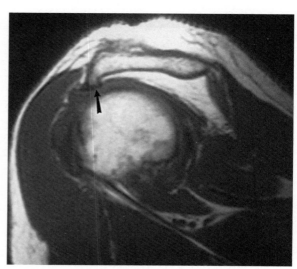

Figure 9-61   Sagittal SE 500/11 image demonstrating a type 3 hooked acromion (*arrow*) with impingement.

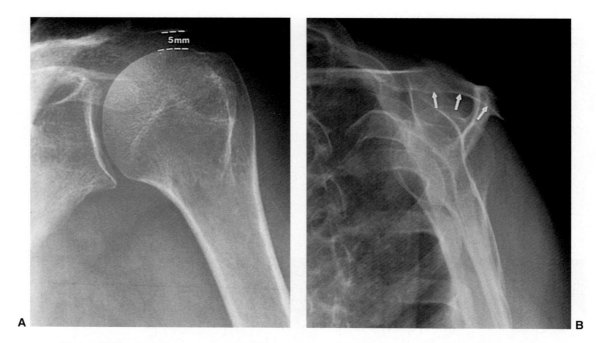

Figure 9-62 True anteroposterior **(A)** and scapular Y views **(B)** demonstrate a curved acromion (*arrows* in **B**) and reduced humeroacromial distance (*dashed lines* in **A**). Normal humeroacromial distance is >7 mm.

Most rotator cuff tears begin in the anterior supraspinatus near the greater tuberosity insertion and biceps tendon (204). This may explain the frequent association of biceps tendon tears and rotator cuff tears (205). As the tears enlarge other portions of the cuff, they may also become involved.

The incidence of rotator cuff tears increases with age. Most studies have been based upon cadaver data (203). Sher, et al, (142) studied 100 asymptomatic volunteers and found partial tears in 22% and complete tears in 14%. Partial tears were uncommon (4%) in individuals less

than 40 years of age. Complete tears were noted in patients 60 years of age or older. In asymptomatic volunteers over 60 years of age, 54% had a rotator cuff tear (142).

Most tears are chronic (92%) but 8% of tears may occur with acute injuries (19,167,206). Patients with rotator cuff tears generally present with chronic pain. On examination the pain increases with 70° to120° of abduction and external rotation if impingement is the etiology (175,176,207). Pain is typically located over the anterolateral aspect of the shoulder and increases with forward flexion or abduction of

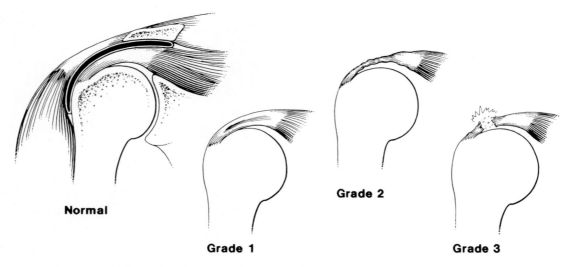

Figure 9-63 Illustration of the Neer classification for rotator cuff tears. Grade 1, edema and hemorrhage in the cuff; grade 2, thinning and fibrosis; grade 3, complete tear.

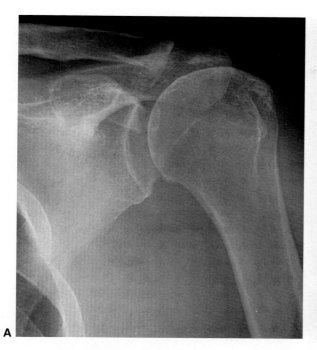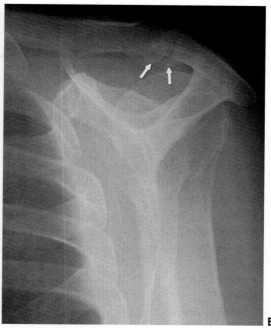

Figure 9-64 Chronic rotator cuff tear with cuff arthropathy. **A:** Anteroposterior radiograph demonstrates superior humeral migration with marked reduction in the humeroacromial space and widening of the glenohumeral joint suggesting multidirectional instability. **B:** Scapular Y view shows narrowing of the humeroacromial space with osteophytes projecting inferiorly from the AC joint (*arrows*).

the arm. Night pain that prevents sleep is a common problem. Strength reduction and crepitus are also commonly noted during physical examination (167).

When imaging patients with suspected rotator cuff tear it is important to evaluate the cuff and surrounding structures. The size of the tear, extent of tendon involvement, tendon margins, muscle atrophy and osseous changes should all be noted (Table 9-6) (21,208).

TABLE 9-6

MRI CLASSIFICATION FOR ROTATOR CUFF TEARS

Grade	MR Features
0	Normal—uniform low signal intensity
1	Diffuse or linear increased signal intensity on T1WI and PDWI. Normal morphology. No signal intensity ↑ on T2WI
2	Increased signal intensity on T1WI or PDWI with thinning or irregularity
3	Intermediate signal intensity on PDWI that increases on T2WI involving full tendon thickness

T1WI, T1-weighted image; PDWI, proton density image; T2WI, T2-weighted image.
From references 53, 110, 204, 209, and 210.

Partial Tears

Partial cuff tears are classified by depth or vertical tendon thickness effected. Grade 1 partial tears are <3 mm in depth, Grade 2 3-6 mm (see Fig. 9-65) and Grade 3 partial tears are >6 mm (177). Partial tears may involve the articular surface (33%), bursal surface (28%) or both aspects of the rotator cuff (39%) (203).

Horizontal intrasubstance tears have also been classified (36). Intrasubstance tears have treatment implications based upon the type of tear. Type A tears (17%) are horizontal intrasubstance tears with no surface involvement. Type B tears (21%) are horizontal with irregularity at the articular surface. Type C tears (62%) have a flap lesion on the articular surface (see Fig. 9-66) (36).

Conventional MR imaging (Fig. 9-65A) is less sensitive and less accurate for evaluation of partial tears (45,108, 111,211–213) (Table 9-7). In fact, ultrasound and conventional MRI are relatively the same in their utility for detecting partial tears (144,214). Partial tears tend to occur in the critical zone. Articular surface tears are seen as focal areas of intermediate signal on proton density sequences that increased in signal intensity on T2-weighted sequences. Fat suppressed FSE T2 sequences or STIR sequences make the lesion more conspicuous (21). This assumes joint fluid is present (see Fig. 9-67). Diagnosis is even more difficult if there is little joint fluid or the tear has filled in with granulation tissue or scar (27,191).

MR arthrography is the technique of choice for diagnosis of partial articular surface tears (36,211,219–223). The

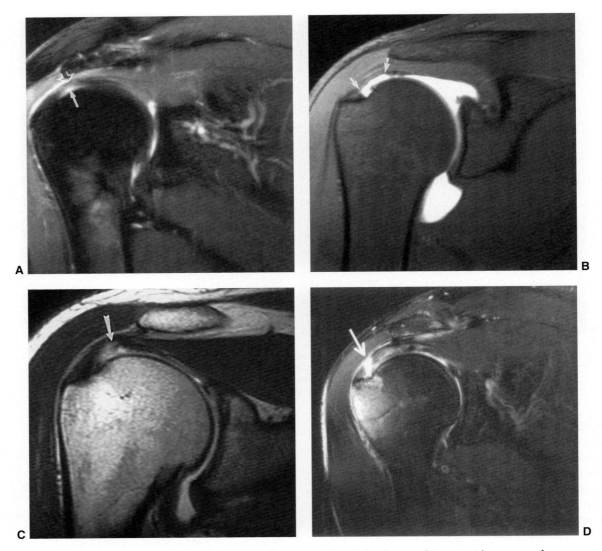

Figure 9-65 MR images of rotator cuff tears. **A:** T2-weighted coronal image with an area of tendinopathy (*open arrow*) and a grade 1 partial articular surface tear (*arrow*). **B:** Coronal MR arthrogram with a grade 1 partial tear (*arrows*). **C:** MR arthrogram with a small partial tear (*arrow*) involving 3 to 6 mm of cuff thickness, grade 2. **D:** Coronal T2-weighted image with fat suppression revealing a full-thickness tear of the distal supraspinatus (*arrow*).

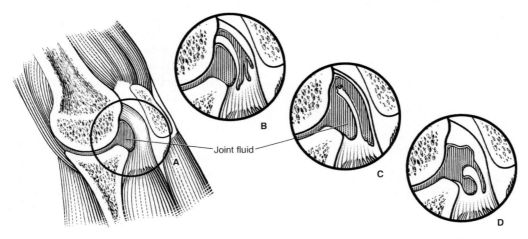

Figure 9-66 Horizontal intrasubstance tears on the abduction–external rotation view. **(A)** normal; **(B)** type A, horizontal with no surface involvement; **(C)** type B, horizontal with surface irregularity; and **(D)** type C, horizontal with articular flap lesion.

TABLE 9-7

SIGNAL INTENSITY OF NORMAL AND ABNORMAL ROTATOR CUFF TENDONS AND ADJACENT SOFT TISSUE STRUCTURES

Categories	T1WI Spin-echo	PDWI SE or FSE	T2 (SE or FSE) or T2*WI	Subdeltoid Fat Plane	Joint Fluid	Bursal Fluid	Tendon/muscle Retraction
Normal	Low	Low	Low	Normal	Minimal	±	None
Tendon degeneration	Intermediate 1 cm from insertion	Intermediate 1 cm from insertion	No ↑ signal intensity compared to T1WI or PDWI	Usually normal	Minimal	±	None
Tendinitis	Intermediate	Intermediate	Slight, usually linear increased intensity	May be abnormal	Small	±	None
Partial tear	Intermediate	Intermediate	↑ signal involving inferior superior surface or both	Abnormal	Small-moderate	±	None
Complete tears–small to moderate	Intermediate	Intermediate	↑ signal in full thickness of tendon; may fill in with scar or granulation	Abnormal	Moderate	+	Slight or none
Complete tears–large to massive	Intermediate	Intermediate	↑ signal with large gap of >4 cm, tendon retraction	Abnormal	Moderate to large	+	Yes

T1WI, T1-weighted image; SE, spin echo; PDWI, proton density-weighted image; FSE, fast spin-echo; T2 or T2*WI, T2- or T2*-weighted image. From references 40, 123, 179, 181, 182, 191, and 215–218.

ABER view displaces the undersurface of the cuff from the humeral head, which allows the tear and horizontal extension into the cuff to be more clearly classified (see Fig. 9-66 and 9-68) (36).

Bursal surface tears may be difficult to diagnose if there is no fluid in the subacromial bursa. MR arthrography is not helpful in this setting. Bursography is not commonly performed to confirm these tears (21,27). On fat-suppressed

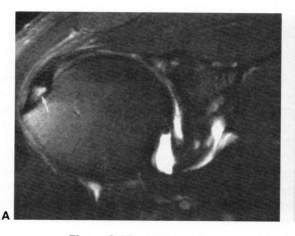
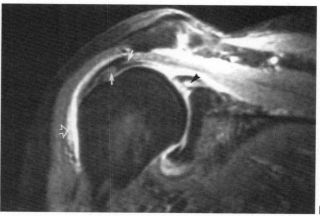

Figure 9-67   A: Coronal fat-suppressed fast spin-echo T2-weighted image demonstrates a peripheral intrasubstance tear with high-signal intensity (*arrow*). **B:** T2-weighted coronal image shows high-signal intensity fluid in the superior labrum anterior posterior (SLAP) lesion (*arrowhead*). There are areas of intermediate signal intensity in the supraspinatus (*arrows*) due to degeneration and granulation tissue. There is also fluid in the subdeltoid bursa (*open arrow*).

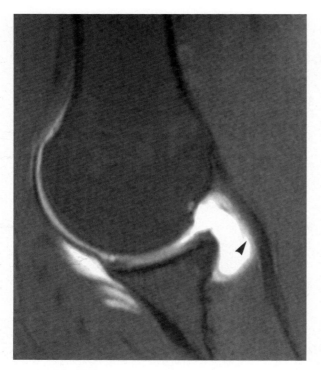

Figure 9-68 Abduction–external rotation view from an MR arthrogram shows a low-grade partial tear (*arrowhead*).

T2-weighted images, these tears have the same appearance as articular surface tears (27,191).

Intersubstance tears that do not communicate with the tendon surface are seen as linear areas of increased signal intensity that increase in intensity from proton density to the T2-weighted image. MR arthrography is not useful unless there is a small defect in the articular surface. These lesions are difficult to confirm even arthroscopically unless the tendon is incised (19).

Arthroscopic classification of partial tears is grade 1 if <25% of the tendon fibers are involved, grade 2 if <50% (Fig. 9-65, A and B), and grade 3 if >50% (Fig. 9-65C) of fibers are involved. These categories are similar to the MR classification scheme. Indications for surgery for impingement or partial cuff tears depend upon the patient's age, activity, expectations, and compliance (31,36,167,211,224). vary Philosophy and aggressiveness with different orthopedic surgeons. Therefore, it is critical that we understand the approach used by the surgeons we work with to optimize our technique, interpretations, and patient care (164,175, 176,225,226). Repair is typically reserved for younger or active patients. Multiple approaches alone or in combination may be used. These include arthroscopic or open subacromial decompression, cuff debridement, open division of the coracoacromial ligament, and open excision and repair of the defect (21,36).

Meister et al. (211) demonstrated a sensitivity of 84%, specificity of 96%, and accuracy of 91% for partial articular surface tears using T1-weighted fat-suppressed oblique coronal MR arthrogram images. T2-weighted sequences did not improve the data. Most were arthroscopic grade 2 (<50%) lesions. Arthroscopic debridement improved symptoms and returned athletes to their sport in the majority of patients (211).

Complete (Full-Thickness) Tears

Conventional MR imaging is capable of diagnosing most full-thickness tears of the rotator cuff (21,191). Axial (GRE and T1-weighted), oblique coronal (fat-suppressed FSE proton density and T2-weighted) images (Table 9-1) allow detection and grading of rotator cuff tears. The ABER view is usually not necessary for medium to large full-thickness tears (191). Full-thickness tears are considered small if they are <1 cm, moderate (medium) if 1 to 3 cm, large if 3 to 5 cm, and massive if >5 cm (27,191). MR arthrography is useful for demonstrating small full-thickness tears.

Fluid signal intensity extending through the tendon is the most useful feature on conventional MR images (see Figs. 9-69 and 9-70) (21,27,191). Tendon retraction is also a useful feature and common with larger tears (see Fig. 9-71). Farley et al. (179) demonstrated that the normal myotendinous junction should be no farther than 15° from a line through the 12 o'clock position in the humeral head. Keep in mind there can be anatomic variation and arm position may also change the location of the myotendinous junction (17–21,79). In chronic tears, the defect may scar, resulting in thinning but low signal intensity on T2-weighted sequences. This can occur in up to 10% of chronic tears (12). In this setting, retraction of the myotendinous junction is a very useful MR feature (179).

Secondary signs of rotator cuff tear have been described for conventional MR imaging (Table 9-8). As mentioned earlier, reduction of humeroacromial space to ≤7 mm on the anteroposterior radiograph with the humerus in external rotation indicates a rotator cuff tear (Fig. 9-71) (1,191). Loss of the bursal fat plane was a useful sign in early MR experience. This was usually related to inflammation, granulation tissue, or fluid in the subacromial subdeltoid bursae (21). This finding, along with fluid in the bursa, is evident in 92% to 94% of patients with complete tears of the rotator cuff (17–21). Though fluid in the bursa is sensitive (93%), tendon discontinuity remains the most specific (96%) MR feature of complete rotator cuff tear (179,181). Patients with symptomatic shoulder may have fluid in the bursa due to impingement (43%), labral abnormalities or instability (29%), bursitis (19%), or tendonitis (14%) (218).

Muscle atrophy is common with complete rotator cuff tears (see Fig. 9-72) (179). Atrophy may involve multiple muscles in addition to the supraspinatus. Tears larger then 2.5 cm in anteroposterior dimension typically extend into the infraspinatous and subscapularis (27,228). Muscle atrophy is typically seen with large chronic tears. This, along with tendon retraction, is of primary importance to the orthopedic surgeon. Open versus

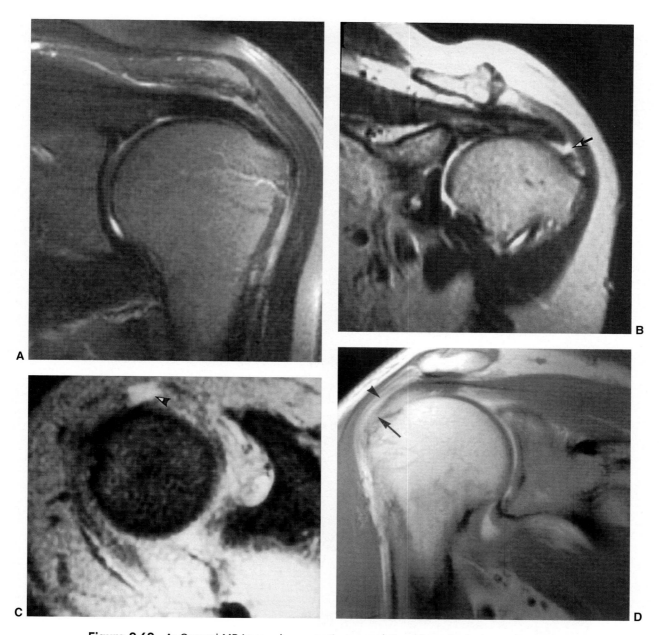

Figure 9-69 **A:** Coronal MR image demonstrating normal signal intensity in the supraspinatus. Coronal **(B)** and axial **(C)** T2-weighted images of a small rotator cuff tear (*arrowhead*) without tendon retraction. **D:** Coronal T1-weighted arthrogram shows a large partial tear with a small peripheral complete tear (*arrow*) and fluid in the bursa (*arrowhead*).

arthroscopic repair and the likelihood of a good result are impacted by the presence of these MR features. Muscle atrophy can also be seen with adhesive capsulitis and nerve compression syndromes (24,32,229,230).

Acromiclavicular joint communication and cystic changes in the muscle are also described with full-thickness rotator cuff tears (see Fig. 9-73). Communication of the glenohumeral and AC joint typically occur with impingement and joint degeneration. Fluid is seen contiguous with the glenohumeral joint, bursa, and AC joint (165). However, MR arthrography is most accurate for demonstrating this finding (15,191).

Over the years, there have been numerous studies evaluating the accuracy of conventional MRI for rotator cuff tears. Studies compared pulse sequences, surgical and arthroscopic findings, and conventional MR with arthrograms (14,17,41,171,231).

Kneeland et al. (232) reviewed 25 patients with suspect rotator cuff tear. MRI detected 20 of 22 tears demonstrated by arthrography or surgery. Evanco et al. (171) confirmed the difficulty with detecting partial tears compared to complete cuff tears. MRI demonstrated a sensitivity of 80%, specificity of 94%, and accuracy of 89% for complete rotator cuff tears. If one included both partial

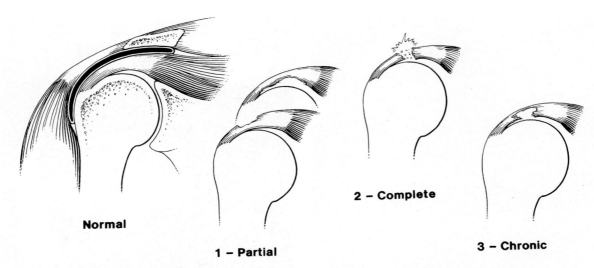

Figure 9-70 Illustration of rotator cuff tears. Partial tears may involve the superior or inferior tendon surface. Complete tears result in separation of the tendon ends. Chronic tears may be partially filled in with fibrous or granulation tissue.

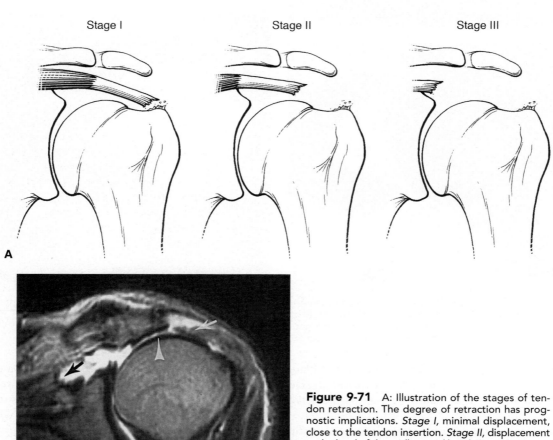

Figure 9-71 A: Illustration of the stages of tendon retraction. The degree of retraction has prognostic implications. *Stage I*, minimal displacement, close to the tendon insertion. *Stage II*, displacement at the level of the midhumeral head. *Stage III*, retraction to the glenoid margin. **B:** Coronal T2-weighted image of a chronic large complete rotator cuff tear in the left shoulder. The humeroacromial space (*arrowhead*) is nearly obliterated due to the cuff tear and superior humeral migration. This feature could be seen on routine radiographs. There is marked supraspinatus retraction (*black arrow*) (stage III) and a long, irregular distal remnant (*white arrow*) with granulation tissue and thickening distally.

TABLE 9-8

CONVENTIONAL MR IMAGING SECONDARY SIGNS OF ROTATOR CUFF TEAR

Tendon retraction
Loss of bursal fat plane
Fluid in subacromial bursa
Fluid in AC joint and subacromial bursa
Muscle atrophy
Cysts in muscle or AC joint
Superior humeral migration

AC, acromioclavicular.
From references 19, 20, 79, 179, 187, and 227.

and complete tears, the sensitivity decreased to 69%, specificity remained at 94%, but accuracy decreased to 84% (171).

Rafii et al. (233) reported sensitivity of 97%, specificity of 94%, and accuracy of 95% for complete tears. Sensitivity was 89%, specificity 84%, and accuracy 85% for partial thickness tears.

Multiple pulse sequence approaches were also evaluated (40,194,234). Tuite et al. (204) evaluated T2-weighted spin-echo and T2* GRE sequences. The sensitivity was 91% and specificity 95% compared with 75% and 87% for partial tears. Fat-suppression technique with T2-weighted sequences improved the accuracy for detection of both complete and partial tears (235). Somewhat later, Sonin et al. (42) demonstrated conventional spin-echo and FSE techniques provided similar results (sensitivity 89%, specificity 94%, accuracy 92%) for full-thickness cuff tears. FSE sequences reduced examination time and increased spatial resolution.

Increased experience and increased utilization of MR arthrography have improved diagnostic accuracy for rotator cuff tears (8,21,34,211,219,236). MR arthrography is particularly useful for small full-thickness tears, partial tears of the articular surface of the cuff, and evaluating intrasubstance extension (41,237). The sensitivity and specificity for MR arthrography is nearly 100% for full-thickness tears (see Fig. 9-74) (34). Fat-suppression techniques (Table 9-1) improve accuracy and assist in differentiating contrast from the peribursal fat (211,236).

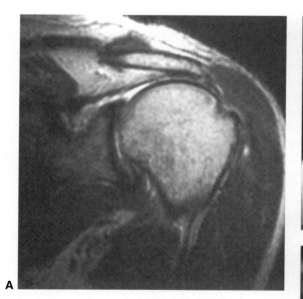

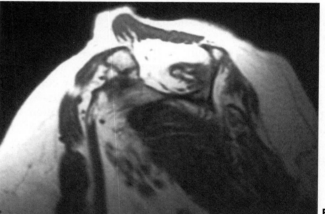

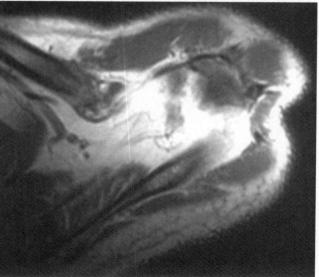

Figure 9-72 Massive rotator cuff tear with supraspinatus atrophy. Coronal T1-weighted image **(A)** shows the tear with loss of humeroacromial space. Sagittal **(B)** and axial **(C)** T1-weighted images demonstrate marked atrophy with fatty replacement.

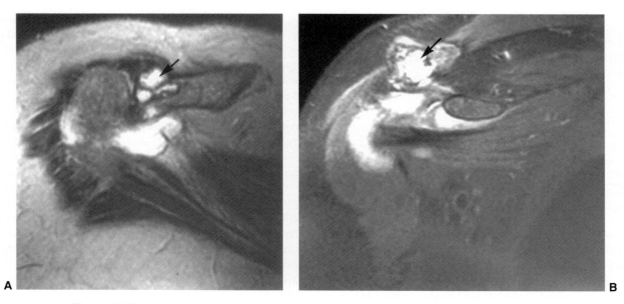

Figure 9-73 Axial **(A)** and coronal **(B)** T2-weighted images in a patient with a large rotator cuff tear demonstrate fluid and cystic change in the acromioclavicular joint (*arrows*).

Zanetti et al. (223) demonstrated that MR arthrography has a significant impact on clinical decisions. Clinical diagnosis was changed in 34% and totally new diagnoses made in 13% after MR arthrography. Treatment approaches were modified in 49% after MR arthrography.

Low field (<0.5 T) and open-bore magnets are commonly used in imaging centers and orthopedic practices. Imaging time is longer and motion artifact more often occurs. However, MR arthrography performed is low and high field (≥1.5 T) units are fairly comparable for full-thickness cuff tears (218,238).

Indirect (intravenous) MR arthrography may also be selected as an approach for evaluating the rotator cuff. Patient scheduling and the less invasive approach may be advantageous. However, joint fluid volumes, lack of joint distention, and vessel specification are potential disadvantages. Partial tears are also more difficult to separate from tendon degeneration (218).

Treatment of rotator cuff tears varies with surgical philosophy, patient age, activity level, expectations, and the size of the tear along with muscle atrophy and AC joint changes. Repairing tendon defects by suturing adjacent

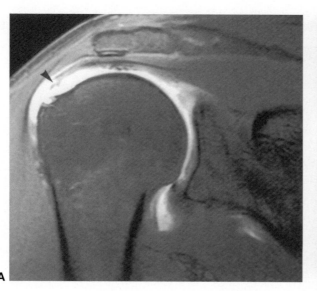
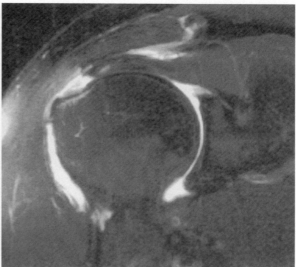

Figure 9-74 Complete rotator cuff tears. MR arthrogram images in different patients demonstrate a small peripheral tear (*arrowhead*) without retraction **(A)** and a larger tear with slight retraction **(B)**.

tendinous tissue or into bone are common. Larger tears may require subscapularis, biceps, or other tendon allografts (197,239–241).

Tendinosis/Tendinopathy

Tendon abnormalities without surface involvement were once considered tendinitis (21). Most now prefer the term tendinosis or tendinopathy (12,27,109,242). Etiology may include degeneration, overuse, trauma, or underlying systemic disorders that weaken the tendon (27). MR signal intensity changes without surface involvement are characteristic (12,21,40). Tendons are often thickened with increased signal intensity on T1- and proton density sequences with no or little signal intensity increase on T2-weighted sequences (see Fig. 9-75) (27,109). Some reports indicate that any signal intensity increase on T2-weighted

sequences indicates more severe tendon breakdown (242). Fluid in the subacromial–subdeltoid bursa and fat plane distortion may also indicate more advanced disease, with conservative therapy less likely to result in improvement (12).

Signal intensity abnormalities in patients with tendinosis frequently involve the critical zone, which is about 1 cm proximal to the supraspinatus insertion (Fig. 9-75) (18–21,112,175,243). Differential diagnosis includes magic angle and partial volume effects (12,27). When fluid is present in the subacromial subdeltoid bursa, one must also consider bursitis or recent therapeutic injection. MR imaging should not be performed until at least 3 days after shoulder injection (21,124,244).

Calcific tendinitis or peritendinitis also deserves mention. Both tendinosis and calcific tendinitis may lead to rotator cuff tear (245,246). Calcific tendinitis or peritendinitis is most common in the fourth through sixth

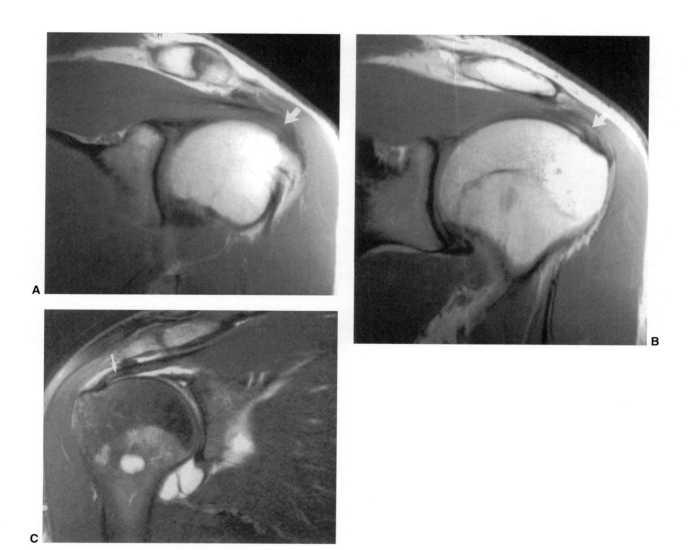

Figure 9-75 Tendinosis. Coronal T1-weighted images **(A,B)** demonstrate increased signal intensity peripherally (*arrow*). Note the normal musculature. T2-weighted arthrogram image **(C)** in a different patient shows intermediate signal intensity in the supraspinatus (*arrow*) without a tear.

decades. Females and manual laborers are most often affected. Calcification is often obvious on radiographs or CT (Fig. 9-48) (246). MR images may demonstrate a focal area of low signal intensity on both T1- and T2-weighted sequences (28). There may be associated marrow and soft tissue edema that can be confused with infection or neoplasm if radiographs are not available for comparison (28,246). Aspiration or resection of the calcified region may be needed in patients with symptoms not responding to conservative therapy (28,246,247).

Postoperative Changes

Surgical procedures to correct or repair rotator cuff tears and impingement may include direct repair of the rotator cuff defect and/or decompression of the acromial arch (139,166,180,224,248–251). Cofield reported pain relief in 87% of patients after cuff repair (139). Though results are usually satisfactory, up to 26% of patients may have recurrent symptoms (Table 9-9) (196,252). Inadequate acromial resection, hardware failure, adhesive capsulitis, and recurrent cuff tear should be considered in patients with recurrent symptoms.

Postoperatively, normal osseous and soft tissue anatomy is distorted. To interpret postoperative imaging studies properly, it is critical that we understand the common arthroscopic or open procedures used for treatment of impingement and/or rotator cuff tears (70,177,256,257).

Procedures consist of decompression of the acromial arch or a combination of decompression and cuff repair (see Figs. 9-76 and 9-77). Patients with impingement may be approached with open, mini-open, or arthroscopic procedures (21,31,139). The anterior acromion is resected (Fig. 9-76). The subacromial–subdeltoid bursa is also removed in most cases, as it is typically chronically inflamed. A portion of the coracoacromial ligament may also be resected. In patients with AC joint hypertrophy and osteophytes, the distal 2.5 cm of the clavicle is removed. Any areas of fraying in partial cuff tears are debrided and/or repaired (139,166,176).

TABLE 9-9
COMPLICATIONS AFTER ROTATOR CUFF REPAIR

Intraoperative

Acromial fracture
Arthroscopy portal-induced cuff tear
Axillary nerve injury

Short term

Infection
Hematoma
Physical therapy-induced capsular tendon avulsion

Long term

Recurrent rotator cuff tears
Impingement
Bursitis
Tendinitis
Synovitis
Suprascapular nerve palsy
Adhesive capsulitis
Deltoid dehiscence
Scarring
Biceps tendon subluxation
Hardware failure
Heterotropic ossification

From references 21, 31, 196, 241, 250, and 252–255.

Cuff repair may be performed for partial or complete tears of the rotator cuff. Again, open, mini-open (anterior superior deltoid incision), or arthroscopic approaches may be used. Arthroscopic approaches are anterior, lateral, and posterior bursal portals (139,197,258). Partial tears are repaired if they involve ≤50% of the tendon thickness. Tendon to tendon or tendon to bone sutures are used for full-thickness tears, depending upon the size of the tear. For the latter, a trough is created in the bone and the cuff is sutured to bone (21,177,257). Large or massive tears require open repair. The long head of the biceps tendon, subscapularis, or allograft may be incorporated to close the

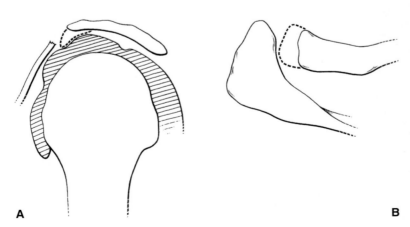

A   **B**

Figure 9-76 Sagittal **(A)** and axial **(B)** illustrations of resection of the distal clavicle and anterior acromion (*broken lines*) for impingement.

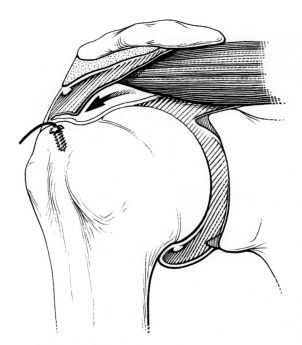

Figure 9-77 Coronal illustration of reattachment of the supraspinatus using a soft tissue anchor. A portion of the acromion (*speckled region*) has been resected.

defect (139,197). Soft tissue anchors are often used, especially with arthroscopic procedures. Anchors may contain fibromagnetic material, titanium, plastic, or absorbable polymers (177,254,256,257). Up to 87% of patients have pain relief after rotator cuff repair (139). Rehabilitation for patients with large or massive tears may require up to 1 year (224). Recurrent symptoms following cuff repair may be due to inadequate decompression, repair failure, poor tendon quality leading to a new cuff tear, or partial placement in arthroscopic repairs (139,177,255,257).

Imaging of patients postoperatively can be difficult. Radiographs can be used to assess changes in the osseous structures and for evaluating soft tissue anchor failure (see Fig. 9-78) (254,259). Ultrasound is useful for evaluating recurrent tears (31,195). CT or CT arthrography may also play a role. However, MRI, or more often MR arthrography, is most useful. Postoperative features can be confusing and may not cause symptoms. Baseline radiographs and MR studies are important to make evaluation of later complications less difficult (21,28).

Postoperative changes involve osseous and soft tissue (granulation, inflammation, fluid in the bursal region) structures (21,31,260,261). There is flattening of the undersurface of the acromion with resection of the anterior acromion (Fig. 9-76). There may also be absence of the distal clavicle when a Mumford procedure has been performed. Marrow signal intensity in the operative site may be low on both T1- and T2-weighted sequences due to fibrosis (21,31). Granulation tissue around suture material in the cuff or bone trough may cause intermediate to high signal intensity that can be confused with recurrent cuff tear. Also, it is not unusual to identify slight superior humeral migration. This might be most easily followed on anteroposterior external rotation radiographs of the shoulder (8,28). Mild bone marrow edema may be evident for up to 5 years (21,262,263).

The region of the subacromial subdeltoid bursa is often distorted in postoperative patients. The fat plane is lost and there may be scarring, granulation tissue, or fluid in this region. Evaluation of the tendons is particularly difficult due to scarring, granulation tissue, and fluid. Identification of partial or full thickness tears is more difficult, especially with conventional MR techniques. Small full-thickness defects may be asymptomatic if repairs are not watertight. Therefore, even using MR arthrography, fluid may extend superior to the tendons into the bursal space (Fig. 9-78) (21,260,261,263,264).

Metal artifact from soft tissue anchors or microscopic metal fragments from drilling add additional problems (Fig. 9-78) (8,28,254). Local image distortion may be related to misregistration that affects spatial geometry. This artifact is most evident on spur-echo (long TE) and GRE sequences. There may also be signal loss (T2* effect) due to the absence of the 180° refocusing pulse on GRE sequences (103). Blooming artifact may also be seen on GRE images resulting in size exaggeration of osseous structures and reduction in soft tissues (181). Field inhomogeneity also reduces the effectiveness of fat saturation techniques (31,103). Image artifact can be reduced by using FSE and inversion recovery sequences instead of spin-echo or GRE sequences (21,31,103,258).

If conventional MR imaging is used one should perform FSE proton density and T2-weighted images in the axial, oblique, coronal, and oblique sagittal planes after surgery to obtain a baseline. Inversion recovery sequences may be useful in the presence of metal artifact (21,31). Sagittal images are most useful to evaluate the acromial changes and coracoacromial ligament (21,31,252,260). Evaluation of recurrent rotator cuff tears is particularly difficult due to scarring and granulation tissue (252,260,263). Fluid signal intensity involving the entire thickness of the cuff or absence of tendon may be the only accurate features for recurrent cuff tear on conventional MR images (see Fig. 9-79). Partial tears are even more difficult to diagnose unless MR arthrography is used for the baseline study and in follow-up (21).

Multiple studies have evaluated postoperative MR findings in asymptomatic and symptomatic patients. Spielman et al. (260) studied asymptomatic patients and found only 10% had normal low-signal intensity tendons. Fifty-three percent had mildly increased signal intensity, and greater than 33% demonstrated features similar to partial or complete rotator cuff tears.

Zanetti et al. (261,263) evaluated asymptomatic and symptomatic patients after rotator cuff repair. Follow-up was 27 to 53 months after surgery. Bursal abnormalities

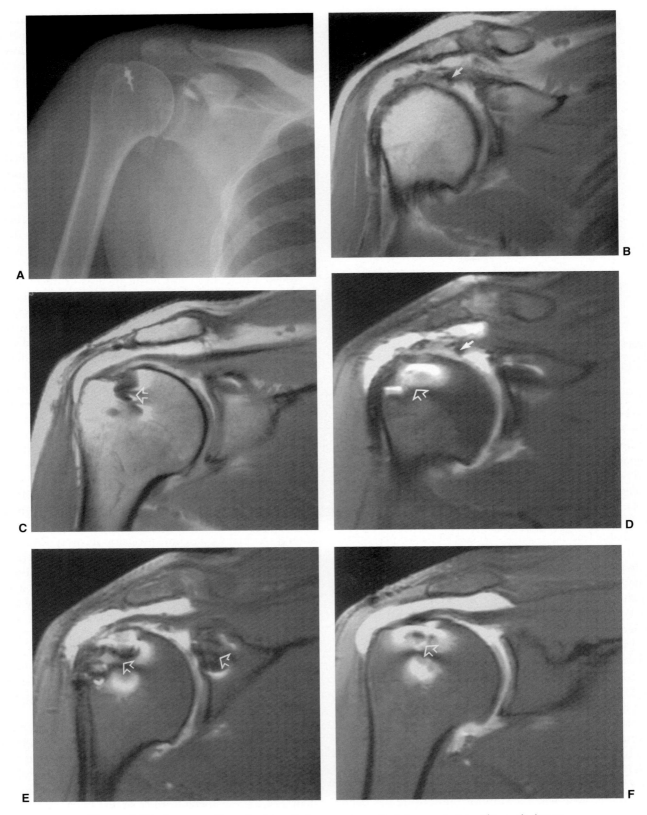

Figure 9-78 Rotator cuff repair with soft tissue anchors. **A:** Anteroposterior radiograph demonstrates the soft tissue anchors. MR arthrogram with coronal T1- **(B,C)** and fat-suppressed T1-weighted **(D–I)** and sagittal **(J,K)** demonstrate metal artifact (*open arrows*) and an intact rotator cuff despite fluid in the subdeltoid bursa.

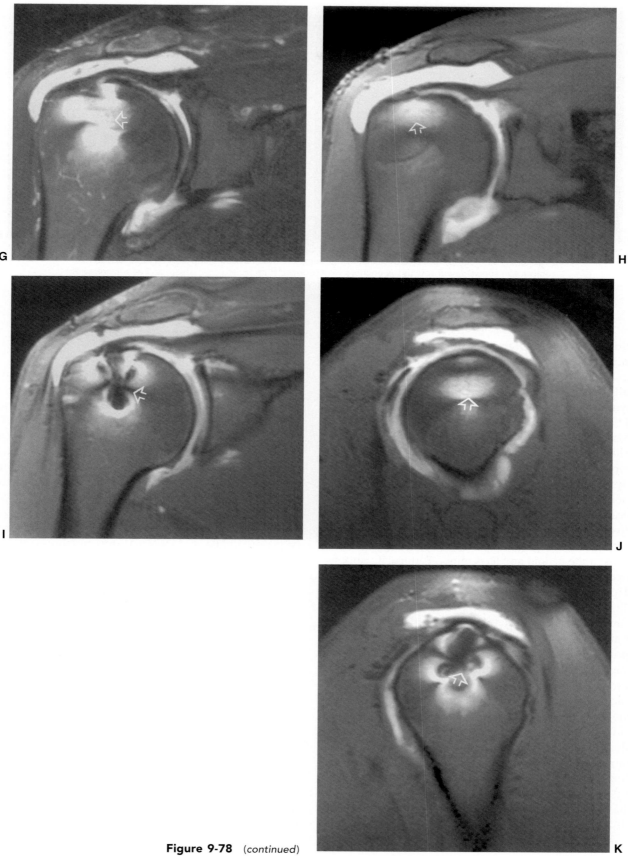

Figure 9-78 *(continued)*

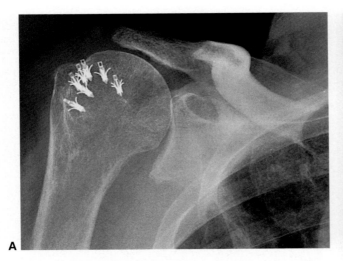
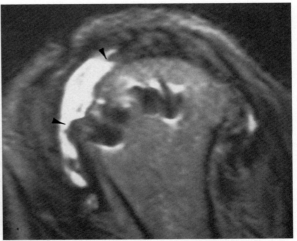

A B

Figure 9-79 Postoperative rotator cuff repair with soft tissue anchors in place. **A:** Anteroposterior radiograph shows seven soft tissue anchors with reduced humeroacromial distance. Fat-suppressed T2-weighted sagittal image **(B)** shows artifact from the soft tissue anchors with increased signal intensity (*arrowheads*) due to a large recurrent tear.

(fluid, scarring, granulation tissue) were evident in all asymptomatic patients. Residual tendon defects or tears were evident in 21% to 33% of symptomatic patients. Small cuff defects (<1cm) were not always symptomatic. In symptomatic patients, cuff defects were evident in 47% and bursal abnormalities in 97% (261).

Magee et al. (252) showed conventional MRI had an 83% sensitivity and 83% specificity for partial tears and 86% sensitivity and 92% specificity for complete tears postoperatively. Tendon retraction and muscle atrophy are useful secondary signs (21). However, even these findings may be difficult to interpret unless preoperative or baseline postoperative studies are available for comparison. For example, intraoperative auxiliary nerve injury (Table 9-9) may cause atrophy of the deltoid and teres minor. Fortunately, atrophy related to rotator cuff tear usually involves the supraspinatus and infraspinatus (21,31).

Table 9-9 summarizes complications associated with acromial decompression and rotator cuff tears. Baseline MR arthrograms and follow-up studies are increasingly important to evaluate the rotator cuff more effectively. Remember, rotator cuff repairs may not be watertight, so arthrographic contrast can extend into the subacromial–subdeltoid region. Also, small defects may not be symptomatic (261,263).

Adhesive capsulitis requires intraarticular contrast to evaluate capsular volume. Therefore, conventional or MR arthrography is essential to exclude this diagnosis. There are no new specific features described using MR arthrography (230).

Baseline and follow-up radiographs are also useful to evaluate hardware failure, heterotopic ossification, and progressive reduction in humeroacromial distance (8,28).

INSTABILITY

As noted in the anatomy section, the capsular structures of the shoulder consist of the synovial membrane, the capsule, the associated glenohumeral ligaments, glenoid labrum, and associated bursa and recesses (31,76,188, 265–270). The subscapularis muscle and tendon are also closely applied to the anterior capsule (52,76,252,271). Shoulder stability is dependent upon the capsule, labrum, pericapsular soft tissues, and glenohumeral osseous structures (78,81,265,272,273). Instability can be anterior (95%), posterior (~ 3%), or multidirectional (2%) (239,274–281). Anteriorly, the capsule and three glenohumeral ligaments (superior, middle, and inferior), anterior labrum, and subscapularis muscle and tendon maintain stability. Posteriorly, support is maintained by the capsule, posterior labrum, and muscles of the rotator cuff (Figs. 9-21 and 9-22) (239,275, 276,278,280,281).

Iannotti (82) described four types of glenohumeral instability. Type I is involuntary unidirectional (usually anterior) instability due to trauma. Associated injuries include labral, capsular, or rotator cuff tears and Bankart and Hill-Sachs lesions (see Fig. 9-80). Recurrent dislocation or subluxation is reported in 50% to 90% of patients (145,282,283). Type II instability is due to overuse or repetitive trauma such as seen with swimmers or throwing athletes (82,271,275,280). Capsular laxity and subtle glenoid labral tears may be evident (82). Type III instability is multidirectional (see Fig. 9-81) and due to generalized ligament laxity. This type of instability is more often bilateral and invariably has an inferior component. Type IV instability is voluntary. Patients generally have intermittent symptoms that include pain or a sensation of abnormal joint motion (82,251).

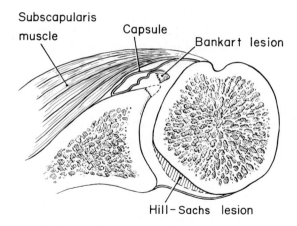

Figure 9-80 Axial illustration of Bankart and Hill-Sachs lesions.

Matsen et al. (284) proposed a useful classification based upon etiology and treatment. One category is traumatic and the second atraumatic. The acronym for the traumatic form of instability is TUBS, where T is for trauma, U for unidirectional, B for associated Bankart lesion, and S because surgery is usually required for successful treatment (21,284). In the second category, A is for atraumatic, M for multidirectional, B for bilateral, R for rehabilitation as conservative therapy, and I for inferior capsular shift if surgical therapy is required. Therefore, the acronym is AMBRI (279,284).

Anterior Instability

Anterior dislocations account for 50% of all joint dislocations (8,31,279). Dislocation occurs when the extended arm is abducted and externally rotated, forcing the humeral head against the anterior capsule and supporting structures of the shoulder. Less severe translation of the humeral head may result in subluxation (8,257). Anterior dislocation is frequently followed by recurrent subluxations or dislocations. In younger patients (<40 years of age), recurrence approaches 90% (8,257). In patients older than 40 years of age at the time of initial dislocation, the incidence of recurrent dislocation is only about 15%. The incidence may be higher in very active older patients (21,257,279).

Anterior instability is associated with osseous and soft tissue supporting structure injuries. The most common osseous injuries are the Hill-Sachs and Bankart lesions (Fig. 9-80), though tuberosity fractures occur in up to 15% of patients with anterior dislocations (8,17,79,257,285).

Hill-Sachs lesions are reported in 74% of patients with recurrent anterior dislocations (8,79,257). Radiographically, a line of condensation is seen extending inferiorly on the anteroposterior view. A notch defect may be seen on axillary or Stryker-Wotch views. The latter is most accurate, detecting over 90% of Hill-Sachs lesions (8). Hill-Sachs lesions are obvious on axial CT and MR images and located in the posterolateral aspect of the humeral head. Workman et al. (148) reported sensitivity of 97%, specificity of 91%, and accuracy of 94% for Hill-Sachs lesion detection using MRI.

Osseous Bankart lesions involve the anterior inferior glenoid margin (8,279). The injury may be seen on anteroposterior radiographs. However, the West Point view (prone axillary with tube angles 15° to 20°) is more optimal for lesion detection (8). The lesion is also well-demonstrated

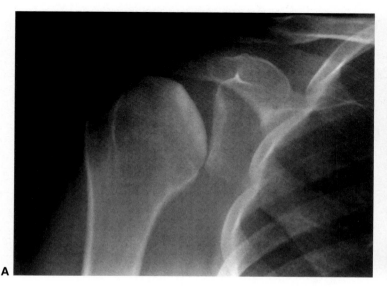

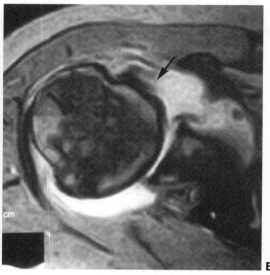

Figure 9-81 **A:** Anteroposterior radiograph demonstrates inferior subluxation with sclerosis and deformity of the humeral head. **B:** Axial arthrogram image shows a large capsule anteriorly and posteriorly with posterior subluxation and a subscapularis tear (*arrow*).

on CT and MRI (27,108,158). Bankart lesions are noted in 50% of patients with anterior dislocations (8).

Soft Tissue Injuries

Anterior instability is associated with injury or avulsion of the anterior inferior labroligamentous complex. Injury may involve the glenoid attachment (70% to 75%), ligament capsular substance (15% to 20%), or humeral attachment (5% to 10%) (21,50).

When evaluating the labrocapsular complex, the labrum is usually discussed based upon localization by the face of a clock. Twelve o'clock is superior, 6 o'clock inferior, 3 o'clock anterior, and 9 o'clock posterior (see Fig. 9-82) (265). The labrum may also be divided in six segments (Fig. 9-82B). The Bankart lesion involves the labroligamentous complex from 3 to 6 o'clock or anterior inferior segment. The normal anterior labrum is triangular, measuring 4 mm at the glenoid attachment and extending 3 mm to the triangular apex (28,265). Intermediate signal intensity between the articular cartilage of the glenoid and labrum (transitional zone) should not be confused with a labral tear (49). Variations in labral configuration were discussed in the Pitfalls section and will not be reviewed.

Labral tears may present with altered configuration (deformed, truncated, or absent) and/or abnormal signal intensity or both (17–21,28,79,94). Labral appearance can be classified similar to the meniscus of the knee. Low signal intensity is normal. Increased signal intensity not communicating with the articular surface represents degeneration. Abnormal signal intensity extending to the articular surface indicates a tear. This finding along with subtle surface changes (i.e., fraying) is most easily appreciated using MR arthrography (see Fig. 9-83) (173,222). However, conventional MR images using fat-suppressed proton density and T2-weighted FSE sequences may also demonstrate labral tears (Fig. 9-83A) (279,286,287). Chandnami et al. (288) reported detection of labral tears using conventional MRI in 93%, and 96% with MR arthrography. Labral detachment was detected on MR images in 46% and on MR arthrograms in 96%. Others have reported similar findings with sensitivities of 89% to 91% and specificities of 93% to 98% for detection of labral tears with MR arthrography (21,289).

Labral tears are commonly accompanied by capsular–ligament injuries (see Fig. 9-84) (28,285,289). The anterior capsule may have three types of attachment. A type I capsule inserts at the labrum, type II just medial (≤1cm) to the labrum, and type III >1 cm from the labral margin (46). A type III capsule may predispose to subluxation or it may be related to prior dislocation and capsular strapping (46). More recent studies question the usefulness of type III capsules for evaluating instability (16,194,273). Unless there is a significant joint effusion, MR arthrography may be necessary to more completely evaluate the anterior inferior capsule and associated inferior glenohumeral ligament (273,289). Contrast will demonstrate a labral tear or detachment with associated capsular or periosteal stripping (279,286,287).

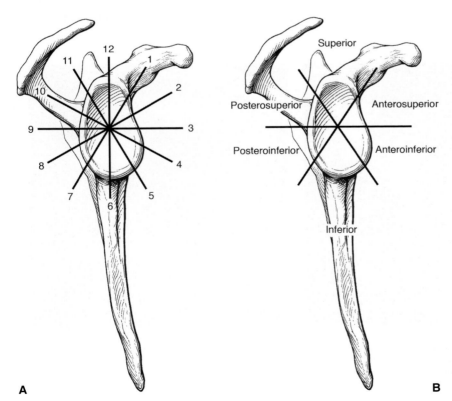

A

B **Figure 9-82** Illustration of the labral segments based upon the face of a clock **(A)** and the six-segment approach **(B)**.

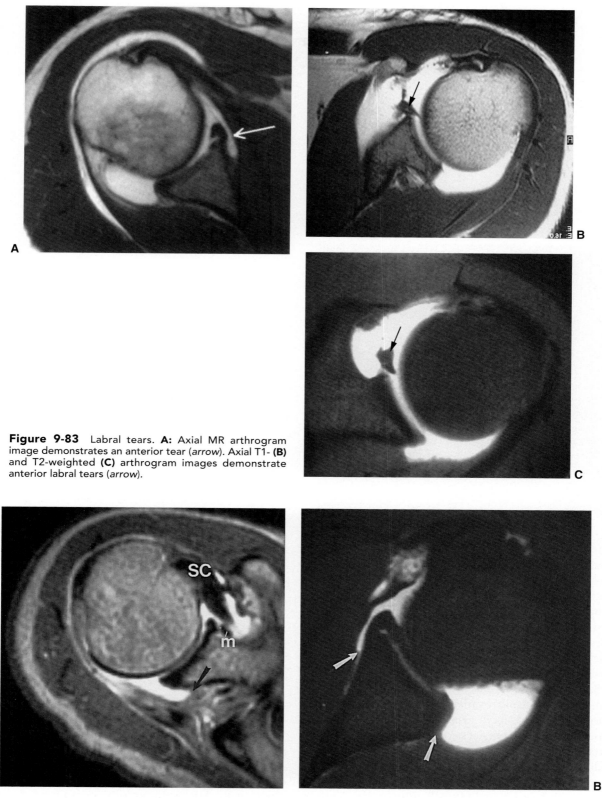

Figure 9-83 Labral tears. **A:** Axial MR arthrogram image demonstrates an anterior tear (*arrow*). Axial T1- **(B)** and T2-weighted **(C)** arthrogram images demonstrate anterior labral tears (*arrow*).

Figure 9-84 **A:** Axial T2-weighted image demonstrates attachment of the posterior capsule medial to the labral margin (*arrow*). The anterior capsule is type II. Note the subscapularis tendon (*SC*) and middle glenohumeral ligament (*m*). **B:** Axial MR arthrogram demonstrates capsular attachments more clearly (*arrows*).

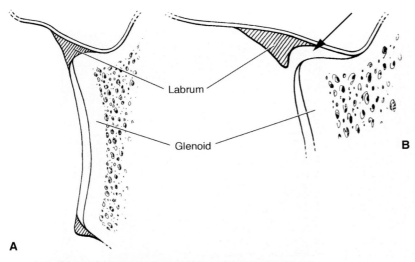

A

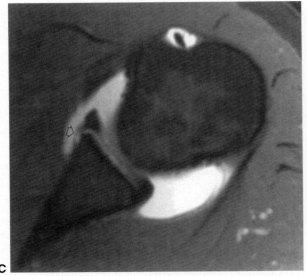

C

Figure 9-85 Illustration of the normal labrum and its bony insertion **(A)** and the Perthes lesion (*arrow* in **B**). Axial MR arthrogram **(C)** shows stripped periosteum (*open arrow*) with contrast extending under the labrum.

The Perthes lesion (see Fig. 9-85) is a variant of the Bankart lesion. The periosteum of the scapular is stripped medially, but remains intact. The labrum may be detached or in normal anatomic position (Fig.9-85). Therefore, diagnosis may be difficult to establish even arthroscopically if not suspected in advance (287). Wischer et al. (287) demonstrated this lesion is most easily appreciated with a fluid-filled capsule or MR arthrography using the ABER position. The lesion may also be seen on axial images. However, this was true in only 50% of patients.

An additional Bankart variant is the anterior labroligamentous periosteal sleeve avulsion (ALPSA) (290). The periosteum is stripped but does not rupture, resulting in inferior rotation of the labroligamentous structures. If undiagnosed, it may heal in this position, resulting in a redundant labrum and chronic instability. This lesion is also difficult to diagnose with conventional MR. MR arthrography demonstrates this lesion more effectively. This lesion, also termed the medial Bankart lesion, requires a different repair compared to a conventional Bankart lesion (290).

Humeral osteochondral or ligament avulsions occur less frequently but must be considered in the spectrum of anterior instability (16,21,285). Avulsion of the glenohumeral ligament (HAGL) may be purely soft tissue or involve bony avulsion (BHAGL). The latter is rare. This lesion is seen on 7.5% to 9.4% of patients with anterior instability. The HAGL lesion typically occurs in patients over 30 years of age. Up to 68% of patients have associated injuries. Rotator cuff tears and greater tuberosity fractures may be associated (16,21,285). Other associated injuries include Bankart, Hill-Sachs, distal clavicle fractures, and partial tears of the long head of the biceps tendon (285). Prior anterior dislocation is reported in 67% (285). On conventional MR images, the glenohumeral ligament may appear thickened, wavy, or irregular, with increased signal intensity on T2-weighted sequences in the ligament gap. MR arthrography demonstrates contrast extravasation at the humeral attachment and capsular stripping (see Fig. 9-86). Though rare, osseous avulsion may be difficult to detect if the osseous fragment is small

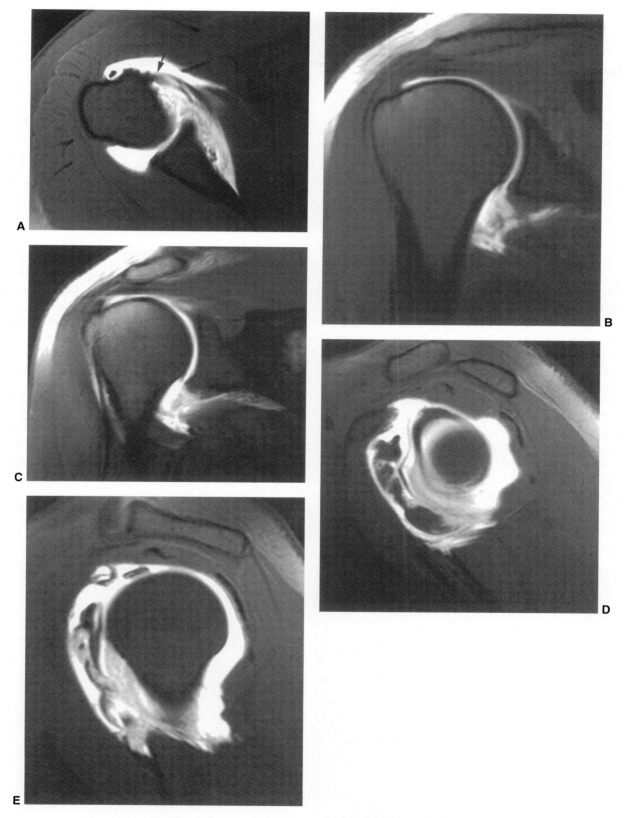

Figure 9-86   Humeral avulsion of the glenohumeral ligament (HAGL). Axial **(A)**, coronal **(B,C)** and sagittal **(D,E)** arthrogram images demonstrate anterior inferior capsular ligament avulsion with a subscapularis tear (*arrow*).

(21,285). Uncommonly, the glenohumeral ligament complex may avulse from the glenoid and humerus (21).

Posterior Instability

Posterior instability is much less common than anterior instability. Posterior shoulder dislocations account for 2% to 4% of shoulder dislocations (see Fig. 9-87) (8). Bilateral posterior dislocations are associated with electroconvulsive therapy. Recurrent dislocations occur following atraumatic and traumatic dislocations with reverse Hill-Sachs bony lesions and posterior glenoid defects. Lesions in the humeral head involve the anteromedial aspect. Lesser tuberosity fractures may also occur with posterior dislocations (8). Dysplastic changes in the posterior glenoid may also contribute to recurrent subluxation or dislocation (21). Osseous lesions may be evident on radiographs. However, CT or MRI are more definitive (8,21,291,292).

Posterior subluxation is much more common than posterior dislocation (Fig. 9-81B). This is a particular problem in athletes involved in swimming and throwing sports. Recurrent subluxation is due to repetitive microtrauma (267,292). Instability occurs with injury to the posterior capsule and labroligamentous complex (279,292). Posterior labrocapsular periosteal sleeve avulsion (POLPSA) has also been described as a cause of posterior instability (see Fig. 9-88) (292). Yu et al. (292) noted this injury in six athletes. There were four football players, one wrestler, and a weight lifter. The condition was bilateral in the weight lifter. Patients presented with pain and joint effusion. The labrum is detached but remains with the capsule and stripped periosteum (similar to the Perthes lesion).

This creates a redundant recess that communicates with the joint. This defect may fill in with fibrous tissue over time. The POLPSA lesion can be identified on axial MR images in the presence of a joint effusion. However, MR arthrography is the preferred technique (292).

Patients may have associated posterior rotator cuff tears involving the infraspinatous and teres minor. This is not unexpected, as the POLPSA lesion is related to the Bennett lesion (292).

The Bennett lesion is a posterior labral injury commonly seen in overhead-throwing athletes. Patients have injury to the posterior rotator cuff and ossification of the posterior inferior soft tissues at the glenoid margins (293). Radiographs or CT may demonstrate the soft tissue calcification or ossification. MR arthrography is most useful to define all aspects of this lesion (see Fig. 9-89).

Multidirectional Instability

Multidirectional instability is typically atraumatic and accounts for 2% of cases of shoulder instability (239,274–278,280,281,294). The labrum is approached like the face of the clock. It is also divided into six quadrants (Fig. 9-82). Multidetectional instability occurs with a labrocapsular injury to segments 3 and 4 or 3 and 5 (274,295) Instability may be anterior and posterior or include inferior and superior components (Fig. 9-81).

Patients develop multidirectional instability due to reported microtrauma or episodes of more significant trauma (21). The capsule is typically enlarged, with labral injuries in multiple quadrants (274). Other than capsular distention, the labral injuries may be minor or degenerative superior labrum anterior posterior (SLAP) lesions (296–298).

SLAP was introduced by Snyder as a term defining injuries to the labral–biceps complex (299). The biceps–labral

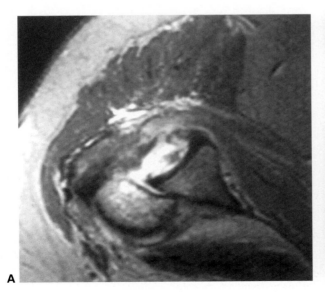
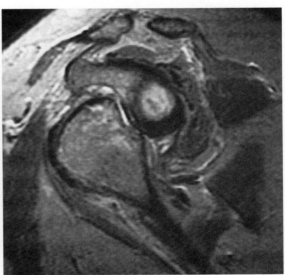

Figure 9-87 Axial **(A)** and sagittal **(B)** T2-weighted images in a patient with fixed posterior dislocation and an anteromedial humeral defect.

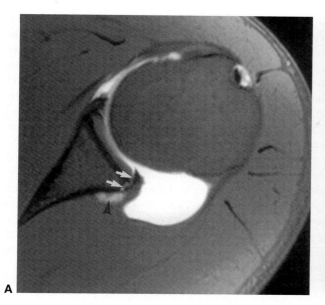 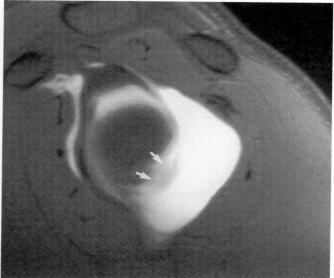

Figure 9-88   Axial **(A)** and sagittal **(B)** arthrogram images demonstrate a large posterior capsule and avulsed labrum (*arrows*) with a paralabral cyst (*arrowhead*).

complex forms the superior portion of the labrum. Three types of complexes have been described. A type 1 complex is firmly attached to the glenoid rim. A type 2 complex attaches several millimeters medial to the glenoid rim. A type 3 complex has a meniscus-shaped labrum with a large sublabral recess that extends under the labrum (see Fig. 9-90). Sublabral recesses are common, occurring in 73% of patients (see Fig. 9-91) (299). Recesses have been graded according to size and depth.

SLAP lesions may be related to acute or chronic trauma. Falls on the outstretched arm with abduction and forward

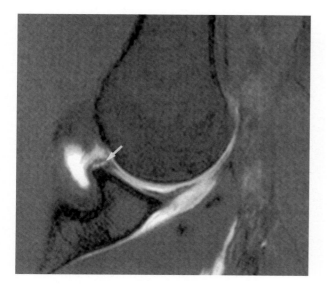

Figure 9-89   Abduction–external rotation arthrogram image demonstrating a posterior labral tear (*arrow*).

flexion of the arm may cause acute injury. Repetitive overuse such as baseball, tennis, swimming, or volleyball may result in SLAP lesions. Patients present with pain, increased with overhead motion and snapping or catching (299,300). These lesions are detected in 3.9% to 6% of all patients undergoing arthroscopy (265).

Snyder et al. (299) originally described four types of injury (see Fig. 9-92-1). A Type I injury results in superior labral fraying or degeneration. The labrum remains attached to the glenoid. Type I lesions account for 10% to 21% of SLAP lesions and are usually not clinically relevant unless they occur in young overhead-throwing athletes (73,265,299). Type II lesions (Fig. 9-92-2) have fraying of the labrum with stripping of the labrum and biceps tendon from the glenoid cartilage (265,299,300). The superior labrum is more loosely attached which may make diagnosis of the Type II SLAP lesions more difficult (265). Type II lesions account for 41% to 55% of SLAP lesions (265,299,300). Type III lesions comprise 6% to 33% of SLAP injuries. Type IV lesions are bucket-handle tears with a split tear of the biceps tendon. Type IV lesions account for 3% to 15% of SLAP lesions (265,299,300).

Several revisions or modifications have occurred since Snyder's original classification of SLAP lesions. In 1995, Maffet et al. (301) added three more categories of injury. Type V is a Bankart lesion (Fig. 9-92-5) that extends superiorly to involve the biceps tendon and superior labrum, thus involving the first through fourth quadrants of the labrum (Fig. 9-82). Type VI lesions (Fig. 9-92-6) consist of an anterior or posterior flap tear with separation of the biceps tendon superiorly. Type VII lesions (Fig. 9-92-7) consist of separation of the biceps tendon and labrum with anterior extension to include the middle glenohumeral ligament (301).

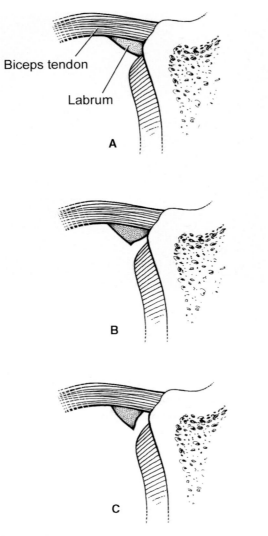

Biceps tendon

Labrum

A

B

C

Figure 9-90 Illustration of a tightly attached type 1 recess **(A)**, small type 2 recess **(B)**, and large type 3 **(C)** labral recess.

Morgan et al. (302) and Burkhart et al. (154) subdivided type II lesions into 2A, anterior superior; 2B, posterior superior; and 2C, both anterior and posterior extension. Posterior (2B) and combined (2C) lesions result in increased disability for overhead-throwing athletes due to posterior superior instability and anterior inferior pseudolaxity (21,154) Posterior (2B) and combined (2C) lesions are also commonly associated with rotator cuff tears (154).

Though somewhat controversial, three more SLAP lesions have been added in recent years. A Type VIII lesion (Fig. 9-92-8) is similar to a Type 2B, but there is greater posterior extension. A Type IX lesion (Fig. 9-92-9) has severe anterior and posterior extension resulting in near to complete detachment of the glenoid labrum. Type X lesions (Fig. 9-92-10) involve the anterior superior labrum with extension into the rotator cuff interval (265).

Etiology of SLAP lesions varies to some extent with the classification. Types I and II lesions (2A–C) occur in overhead-throwing athletes and with atraumatic instability. Falls on the outstretched hand may result in types III–V. Type V and VII lesions occur in patients with instability after acute trauma (21,154,301,302). In a series of 544 patients, Kun et al. (232) noted SLAP lesions in 26%. Using the Snyder classification, 74% were type I, 21% type II, 0.7% type III, and 4% type IV. Type II lesions in patients younger than 40 years of age had associated Bankart lesions. Type II lesions in patients over 40 years of age had rotator cuff tears.

Treatment also varies with the type of lesion, requiring accurate preoperative classification. Type I lesions are not always clinically significant and can be treated conservatively with arthroscopic debridement (Fig. 9-92-1) (73). Type II lesions are treated with biceps anchor repair. Types III and IV (Figs. 9-92, 3 and 4) are usually treated with resection of the bucket handle fragment and biceps tenodesis with labral

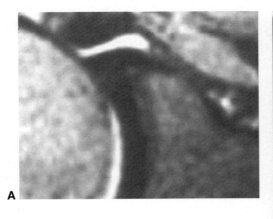

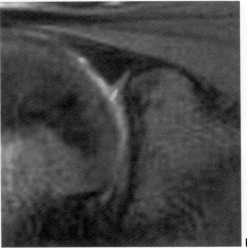

Figure 9-91 Coronal T1- **(A)** and T2-weighted **(B)** images demonstrating a firmly attached labrum **(A)** and type 3 complex with a grade III recess (*arrow*) in **B**.

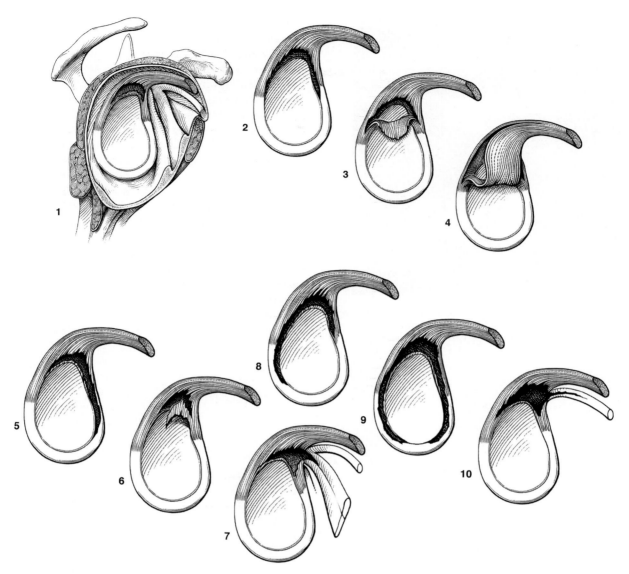

Figure 9-92 Illustration of the categories of SLAP lesions. *1*, fraying of the superior labrum; *2*, stripping of superior labrum and biceps tendon from the glenoid; *3*, bucket-handle tear of the labrum with intact biceps; *4*, bucket-handle tear extending into the biceps; *5*, Bankart with superior extension to include the superior labrum and biceps; *6*, anterior and posterior flap tear with superior biceps involvement; *7*, biceps labral complex tear extending into the middle glenohumeral ligament; *8*, superior labral tear with posterior extension; *9*, nearly complete labral detachment; *10*, SLAP lesion with extension of tear to rotator interval and involved structures.

repair. Types V and VI are treated with labral and biceps anchor repair. Type VII lesions (Fig. 9-92-7) are treated with biceps anchor repair and repair of the middle glenohumeral ligament (265,303).

SLAP lesions can be difficult to evaluate on conventional MR images. The superior labrum is not well seen on the axial plane, but is better visualized on oblique coronal and sagittal images (see Fig. 9-93) (304). Normal variants described early can cause confusion, specifically the superior recesses (Figs. 9-90 and 9-91) (265,305). Tuite et al. (305) reviewed three signs for effectiveness on diagnosing SLAP lesions with T2-weighted images. These signs included: (i) a high-signal intensity linear defect extending to the articular surface posterior to the biceps anchor; (ii) an irregular or laterally curve area of high signal intensity; and (iii) two linear areas of high signal intensity (double "Oreo cookie" sign) (see Fig. 9-94) (52,305,306). Signs (i) and (ii) were most useful. Multiple observers noted linear increased signal extending to the articular surface posterior to the anchor with sensitivities of 48% to 61%, specificities of 81% to 94%, and accuracies of 72% to 74%. Laterally curved increased signal intensity demonstrated sensitivities of 56% to 65%, a specificity of 84%, and accuracy of 72% to 76% (305).

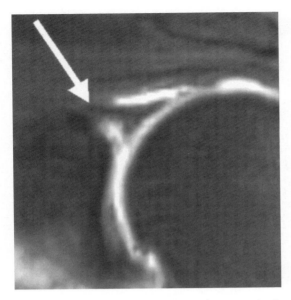

Figure 9-93 Coronal MR arthrogram image demonstrating irregular globular extension of contrast into the substance of the superior labrum (*arrow*) compatible with a tear. Compare to Fig. 9-91.

MR arthrography provides improved visualization of intraarticular structures, including SLAP lesions of all types (21,73,265,292,307). Contrast enters the labrum, allowing detection and classification to be more accurate. Demonstrating intralabral contrast may be facilitated by using arm traction during the MR examination (308). However, motion artifact may be a problem with this technique. On coronal images, tears extend laterally; this may alleviate confusion with the sublabral recess, which is oriented medially (see Fig. 9-95) (52,305). Most use the Snyder (type I–IV) classification for image interpretation. The labrum should be described as intact, detached, a tear without displacement, or with displacement if there is a flap or bucket-handle component (see Fig. 9-96) (52,73,265,309). The extent of tear and associated abnormalities to the rotator cuff, capsule, and ligaments should also be described.

Recently another potential cause of multidirectional instability was reported. Chung et al. (291) described MR arthrographic features of 17 patients with humeral avulsion of the posterior band of the inferior glenohumeral ligament. This lesion may occur as an isolated injury or in

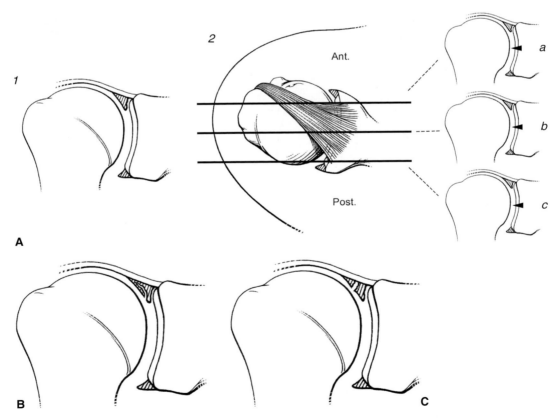

Figure 9-94 **A:** Illustration of the normal recess (*1*) and biceps anchor with increased signal in the labrum anterior and posterior (*a–c*) to the anchor (*arrowheads*). **B:** Illustration of a laterally directed area of increased signal intensity that is easily differentiated from a recess. **C:** Illustration of two linear areas of increased signal intensity (double "Oreo cookie" sign) in the superior labrum.

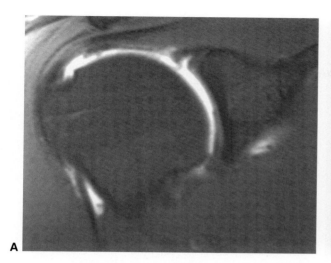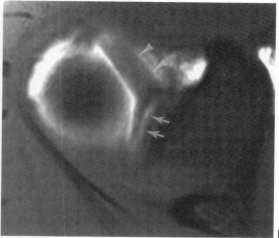

A B

Figure 9-95 Coronal **(A)** and axial **(B)** MR arthrogram images demonstrate a superior labral tear. Contrast is seen extending into the substance of the superior labrum in **A** compatible with a tear. Incidental note is made of an articular surface tear in the distal supraspinatus. Axial image in **B** demonstrates the extent of the tear (*arrows*) that extends posterior to the attachment of the long head of the biceps tendon (*arrowheads*). Compare to Figs. 9-91 and 9-92.

association with other posterior capsular injuries. This injury is less common than the anterior inferior lesion.

Patients present with a history of trauma, prior posterior dislocation, or chronic repetitive microtrauma. Multidirectional instability is evident on physical examination (291). The injury may involve the glenoid or humeral insertion or the midsubstance of the ligament (293). In this series, all 17 patients demonstrated avulsion of the posterior band of the inferior glenohumeral ligament from the humeral attachment. MR arthrograms demonstrated contrast extending along the humeral shaft and discontinuity of ligament fibers (see Fig. 9-97) (291).

Postoperative Evaluation of Instability Repair

Repairs for instability may be anatomic (do not alter anatomy) or nonanatomic. Most common procedures are designed for anterior instability, as they account for 95% of cases of instability (27,279,287,310). Direct repair of the labrum and capsular structures is most often performed. The Bankart repair (see Fig. 9-98) is designed to repair the anterior inferior labral ligament complex. This requires suturing the tissues back to the glenoid margin. Soft tissue anchors are commonly used. This procedure is anatomic but may reduce external rotation (20,31,311) Other procedures are nonanatomic and rely upon capsular tightening. These procedures [Putti-Platt (see Fig. 9-99) and Magnuson-Stack] usually focus on subscapularis tightening. The result is significant reduction in external rotation (20,21,31). Other procedures involve bone blocks. The Bristow-Helfet procedure (see Fig. 9-100) involves resecting

the coracoid with attached tendons to the scapular neck. Bone block osteomy accomplishes a similar goal. Both prevent anterior displacement of the humeral head. Again, motion, specifically external rotation, is reduced (11,20). The Neer capsular shift procedure (see Fig. 9-101) is used for multidirectional instability. This procedure is intended to tighten the capsule by placing the inferior capsule more superiorly and overlapping it by placing the superior capsule antero inferiorly. The overlapping portions of the capsule are also sutured together. This procedure tightens and thickens the capsule (19,21,31).

Posterior instability and SLAP lesions are also treated with debridement and reattaching the labraligamentous structures or biceps anchor in SLAP lesions (see Fig. 9-102) (73,257,303).

MR imaging experience after instability repair has lagged behind rotator cuff repair. Success rates for repair of anterior instability are excellent with open procedures. Recurrence rates are only 1% to 10% (21,257). Arthroscopic procedures have a higher recurrence rate (15% to 20%) (20,21,31).

Interpretation of MR images may be difficult due to anchor artifacts, scarring, capsular thickening, and unrepaired labral defects that may be interpreted as new injuries (see Fig. 9-103) (20,286). Baseline postoperative images are useful to evaluate later complications (Table 9-10). MR arthrography is the preferred technique. Osseous, cartilaginous, and soft tissue structures are more easily evaluated (286,310). Also, capsular volume can be accurately measured and new capsular changes detected. For example, overcorrection for anterior instability can result

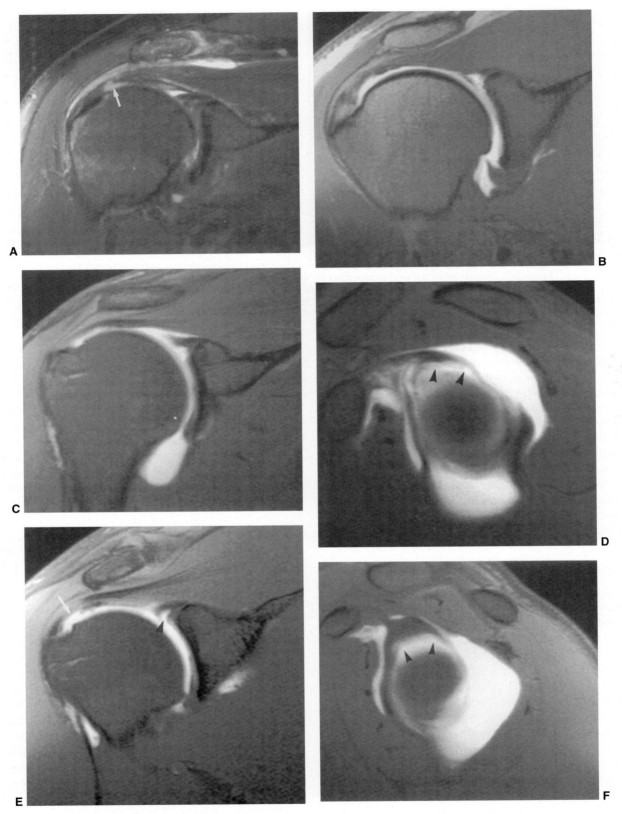

Figure 9-96 SLAP lesions. **A:** Coronal fat-suppressed T2-weighted image with diffuse intermediate signal intensity in the labrum due to degeneration. There is also a partial rotator cuff tear (*arrow*). **B:** Coronal arthrogram image of a type III tear (see Fig. 9-92-3). **C,D:** Coronal in **C** and sagittal in **D** images of a tear extending into the biceps and posteriorly (*arrowheads*). **E,F:** Coronal in **E** and sagittal in **F** arthrogram images demonstrate a labral tear (*arrowheads*) and partial tear in the supraspinatus (*arrow*).

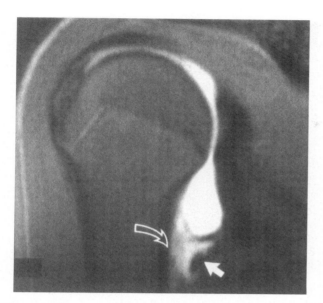

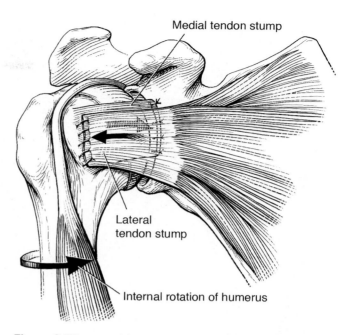

Figure 9-97 Humeral avulsion of the posterior band of the inferior glenohumeral ligament. Teenage athlete with multidirectional instability on physical examination. Coronal fat-suppressed T1-weighted arthrogram image shows discontinuous retracted fibers (*straight arrow*) of the posterior band of the inferior glenohumeral ligament and abnormal contrast distribution (*curved arrow*) that extends distally along the shaft. (From Chung CB, Sorenson S, Dwek JR, et al. Humeral avulsion of the posterior band of the inferior glenohumeral ligament: MR arthrography and clinical correlation in 17 patients. *AJR* 2004;183:355–359.)

Figure 9-99 Putti-Platt repair. The anterior capsule and tendons are shortened. The lateral tendon remnant is attached to the glenoid (*medial arrow*) and the subscapularis (*lateral arrow*) is attached to the lesser tuberosity with the humerus in internal rotation.

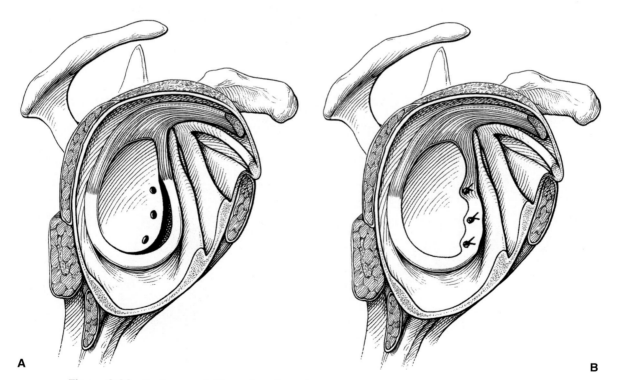

Figure 9-98 Bankart repair. Illustration of anterior repair with drill holes at 3, 4, and 5 o'clock positions **(A)** and suture anchors inserted **(B)** for labral reattachment.

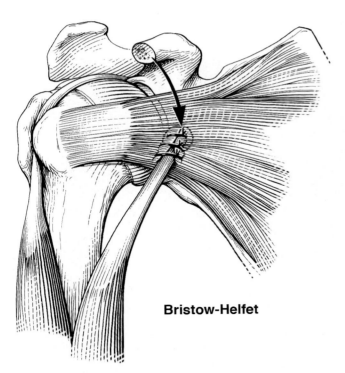

Bristow-Helfet

Figure 9-100 Bristow-Helfet repair. The coracoid and short head of the biceps are transferred to the anterior inferior glenoid rim through a subscapularis split.

in posterior capsular changes. Wagner et al. (310) reported overall accuracy of 79% for recurrent labral tears and 88% for recurrent cuff tears when evaluating MRI, indirect MR arthrography, and MR arthrography.

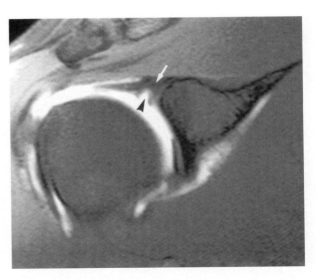

Figure 9-102 SLAP repair with suture anchors. Coronal arthrogram image shows thickening in the region of the repair (*arrow*) and a persistent labral defect (*arrowhead*).

BICEPS TENDON

MRI is an excellent technique for evaluating the normal osseous groove, biceps tendon anatomy, and pathology (see Fig. 9-104). The biceps muscle has two bellies. The tendon of the short head of the biceps attaches to the coracoid. The tendon of the long head of the biceps passes through the bicipital groove in the upper humerus, where it is hooded by the transverse humeral ligament. Superior to the bicipital groove within the rotator interval, the tendon is stabilized by the coracohumeral and

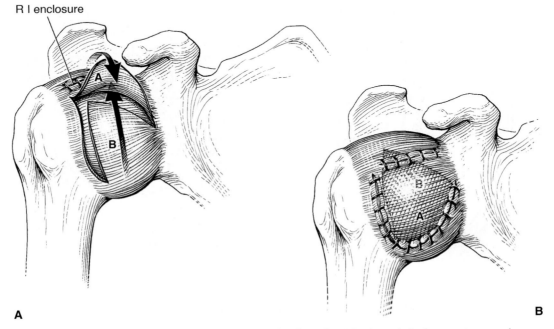

A

B

Figure 9-101 Capsular shift repair. A horizontal L-shaped incision is made in the anterior capsule **(A).** The inferior capsule is shifted superiorly and the superior portion inferiorly. The overlapping capsule is sutured at the margins **(B).**

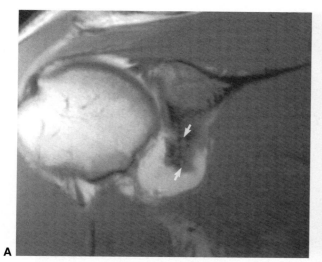

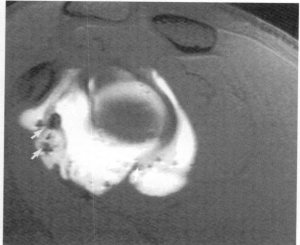

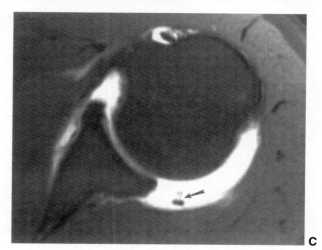

Figure 9-103 Bankart repair. Coronal **(A)** and sagittal **(B)** arthrogram images demonstrate anchor artifacts (*arrows*) and a prominent axillary recess **A.** There is apparent separation of the anterior labrum **B.** Axial MR **(C)** arthrogram image in a patient with prior repair and a loose soft tissue anchor (*arrow*) floating freely in the joint space.

TABLE 9-10

COMPLICATIONS OF INSTABILITY REPAIR

Short Term

Infection
Hematoma
Nerve injury

Long Term

Recurrence
Overtightening
Degenerative arthritis
Adhesive capsulitis
Nonunion (Bristow-Helfet, bone lock–osteotomy)
Anchor pullout
Paralabral cysts

From references 20, 21, 31, 52, 257, 286, 292, 307, and 311.

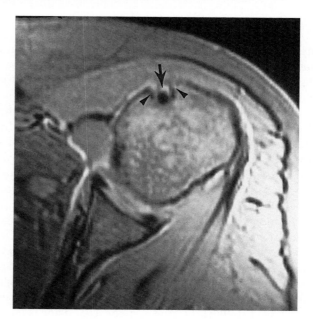

Figure 9-104 Axial gradient-echo image of the shoulder demonstrating the biceps groove (*arrowheads*) and the normal low-signal-intensity tendon (*arrow*). Note there is no fluid around the tendon.

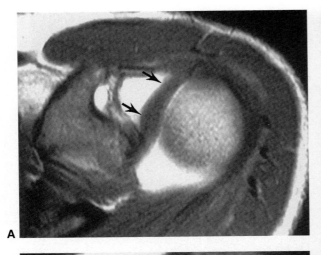

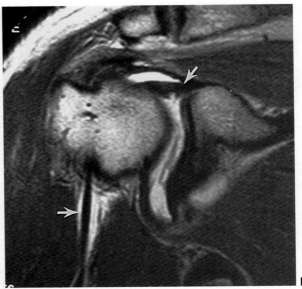

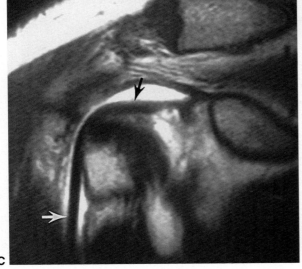

Figure 9-105 MR arthrogram with axial **(A)** and coronal **(B,C)** images demonstrating the course of the biceps tendon (*arrows*).

superior glenohumeral ligaments (312). The tendon arches over the humeral head, taking an intraarticular course (see Fig. 9-105) before attaching to the glenoid tubercle and/or labrum superiorly (96,101,313).

Conventional or CT arthrography can be used to study the biceps tendon. However, it is not unusual to fail to fill the tendon sheath with contrast resulting in suboptimal evaluation. MRI can be used to evaluate the substance of the tendon, osseous pathology, inflammatory changes, and associated injuries such as rotator cuff tears can be evaluated as well (8,101,262,312).

The biceps tendon can be identified on multiple image planes (axial, oblique coronal, oblique sagittal). On oblique coronal images, the tendon is oriented approximately 55° to the magnetic field as it passes over the lateral aspect of the humeral head. Therefore, magic angle effect may be noted on short TE (≤ 20 ms) sequences (Fig. 9-33) (21,100,101). However, the axial plane is most useful (see Figs. 9-104 through 9-106) (1,8,28).

The biceps tendon is normally a smooth round or slightly elliptical low intensity structure that nearly completely fills the biceps groove on axial MR images (Fig. 9-104). The width and depth of the groove and length of the tendon sheath vary, which must be kept in mind when evaluating anatomy and suspected tendon or osseous abnormality. All contiguous images (Fig. 9-106) should be evaluated with this in mind. Cone et al. (314) evaluated the bicipital groove on radiographs. They reported an average medial wall angle (Fig. 9-106) of 48° with average width of 11 mm and depth of 4.6 mm. Medial wall angles of 90° or greater were associated with stenosis and angles 30° or less were reported with subluxation (see Fig. 9-107). Bone spurs, especially along the medial wall, were reported in 33% of cases. These features should be kept in mind when evaluating MR images.

Tendinopathy/Tears

Tendinopathy may be due to impingement, subluxation, or attrition. The latter is due to inflammation in the groove leading to stenosis, osteophyte formation, or thinning of the tendon (262). Tendinosis or tenosynovitis is classified as impingement or attrition. The first is associated with

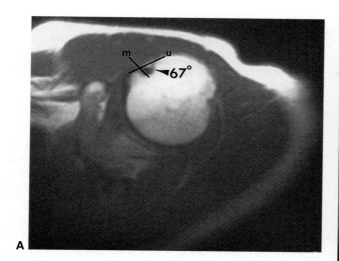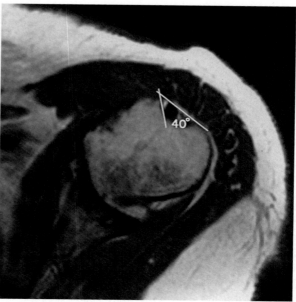

Figure 9-106 Axial images of the bicipital groove and tendon of the long head of the biceps. **A:** T1-weighted image demonstrates the normal tendon that nearly completely fills the groove at its narrower upper extent. There is normally a small amount of fat, vascular structures, and perhaps a small amount of fluid. The medial wall angle [lines along upper margin (*u*) and medial wall (*m*) form the angle] measures 67° at this level of the groove. **B:** Axial image through a lower level of the bicipital groove. The groove is shallower with an angle of 40°. The tendon is normal in size and signal intensity.

impingement and rotator cuff tears. Attritional lesions occur in the bicipital groove (21,101,313).

Tenosynovitis is the most frequent abnormality noted in our practice (Table 9-11). A fluid-filled tendon sheath (see Fig. 9-108) with normal-appearing substance and signal intensity of the tendon is most often noted. We do not make this diagnosis unless fluid completely surrounds the tendon

(96). It is difficult to be certain if fluid entered the tendon sheath from the joint in some cases (313). Tenosynovitis is commonly seen in patients with rotator cuff tears (101). Tendinitis frequently accompanies fluid or synovitis in the tendon sheath. Increased signal intensity and thickening may be noted on T1- and T2-weighted sequences. This finding is most easily detected on oblique sagittal images (313).

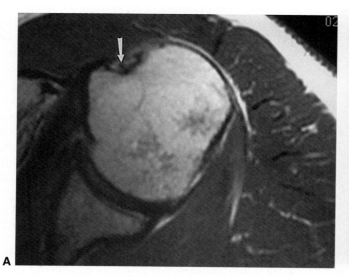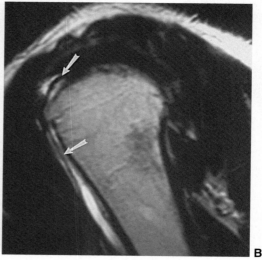

Figure 9-107 Axial T1- **(A)** and sagittal T2-weighted **(B)** images show an atrophic thinned biceps tendon (*arrows*). Note the shallow groove with low intensity margins (bone sclerosis) suggesting recurrent subluxation as the etiology.

TABLE 9-11

BICEPS TENDON ABNORMALITIES

Tendinitis
Tendinosis
Rupture
Subluxation/dislocation
Osseous groove (too shallow, constricted)
Bicipital osteophytes

From references 1, 96, 101, 205, 262, 312, 313, and 315.

Ruptures of the biceps tendon account for only 3% of all tendon ruptures (315). Ninety-six percent of ruptures occur in the proximal tendon. Several types of tears have been described. Longitudinal splits in the tendon can occur in the bicipital groove. The tendon may appear double with high signal intensity between the fragments and fluid in the tendon sheath or thickened with increased signal intensity in the tendon on T2-weighted sequences. A bifid long head of the biceps is a normal variant and can be confused with a longitudinal split (94).

Complete rupture may be associated with tendon retraction. Patients typically describe a loud pop. The displaced biceps muscle is palpable on physical examination (21,313). Tendon rupture without retraction may also occur. Most ruptures are intraarticular and associated with rotator cuff tears. Beall et al. (205) reported associated tears in the supraspinatus in 96.2% of biceps tears. Tears of the infraspinatus were evident in 34.6% and subscapularis tears in 47.1% of cases. Axial and sagittal T2-

or T2*-weighted images will show an absent tendon (empty bicipital groove) with retraction of the muscle distally. The tendon is thickened with areas of increased signal intensity on T2-weighted images when a partial tear is present (96,101,262,313).

Subluxation/Dislocations

The long head of the biceps tendon is stabilized by the coracohumeral ligament, subscapularis tendon, and transverse ligament, which covers the bicipital groove (205,312,316). An abnormally shallow bicipital groove predisposes to subluxation or dislocation (8,314).

Diagnosis is difficult clinically, as symptoms are overshadowed by rotator cuff tears. It is important to establish the diagnosis preoperatively in patients undergoing rotator cuff repair. Full range of motion may not be recovered if biceps tenodesis is not performed with the rotator cuff repair (21,312,314).

Biceps dislocations (see Figs. 9-109 and 9-110) are characterized as anterior to the subscapularis (subscapularis tendon intact) or posterior to the subscapularis, in which case the tendon displaces medially to an intraarticular location (21,147,312).

Biceps tendon dislocation may be appreciated on conventional MR images. MR arthrography is not usually required. However, in cases of subluxation, axial images in multiple degrees of internal and external rotation using FSE or GRE T2 and T2*-weighted sequences may be required to establish the diagnosis (Fig. 9-109) (8,80,314).

Spritzer et al. (312) evaluated biceps instability on oblique coronal, oblique sagittal, and axial images. Specific features that may be related to instability were reviewed by three musculoskeletal radiologists. Features included: tendon shape; tendon perching on the lesser tuberosity; abrupt change in angulation; tendinosis or tear; fluid in the joint and tendon sheath; subscapularis integrity; and acute (<90°) or obtuse (<90°) angles of the bicipital groove. They concluded that the presence of a flat tendon perched on the lesser tuberosity and an obtuse bicipital groove angle are most useful for predicting instability. Perching of the tendon on the lesser tuberosity resulted in a sensitivity of 89%, specificity of 90%, positive predictive value of 89%, and negative predictive value of 90%. A flat (normal round or elliptical) tendon resulted in a sensitivity of 89%, specificity of 60%, positive predictive value of 67%, and negative predictive value of 86%. An obtuse bicipital groove resulted in 89% sensitivity, 70% specificity, 73% positive predictive value, and 88% negative predictive value. The other features were not useful for suggesting instability (312).

Surgical repair of the biceps tendon includes debridement, repair of partial and complete tears, tenodesis in the bicipital groove, and inspection of the rotator cuff interval to avoid misdiagnosis of medial displacement (201).

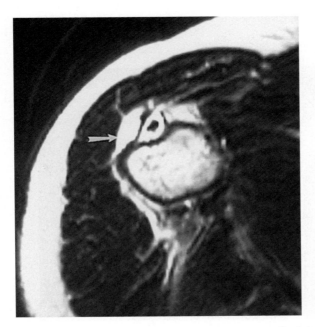

Figure 9-108   Axial T2-weighted image demonstrating fluid distending the tendon sheath. There is also fluid in the subdeltoid bursa (*arrow*).

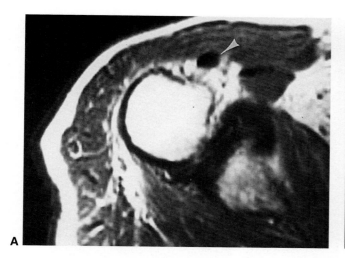
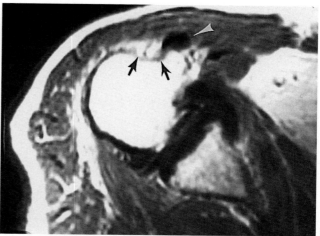

Figure 9-109 Axial proton density images **(A,B)** demonstrating dislocation of the biceps tendon. The tendon is thickened due to recurrent dislocation and healed inflammation with scarring. The biceps groove (*arrows*) is shallow but the medial wall angle is normal.

Miscellaneous Disorders

Subscapularis

Subscapularis tendon tears are difficult to diagnose clinically and can be overlooked with arthroscopy or open procedures if the tendon is not specifically inspected (27,317).

Three patterns of subscapularis tears have been described. Tears may be isolated to the subscapularis, associated with large rotator cuff tears, or associated with anterior superior rotator cuff lesions (317). Isolated subscapularis tears are rare. They may result from forced abduction and external rotation anterior dislocations, or from anterior instability (21,27).

Subscapularis tears are most often seen in association with rotator cuff tears (317,318). The incidence of subscapularis involvement with rotator cuff tears is 2% to 8%

(201,319). Li et al. (319) found subscapularis involvement in 2% of rotator cuff tears. Rotator cuff tears were complete in 73% and partial in 27%. Almost all extended from the supraspinatus (79%). Tears extended into the infraspinatus in 56%, teres minor in 49%, and complete biceps tears were seen in 7% (319).

Subscapularis tears may also be associated with anterior superior lesions that involve the glenohumeral and superior glenohumeral ligaments (27,317). Degenerative tears may be noted in patients with anterior superior impingement (69).

MR imaging of the subscapularis is optimized using fat-suppressed T2-weighted FSE sequences in the oblique sagittal and axial planes (see Fig. 9-111) (317,319). MR arthrography is useful for partial tears and to demonstrate contrast extravasation on to the lesser tuberosity. However,

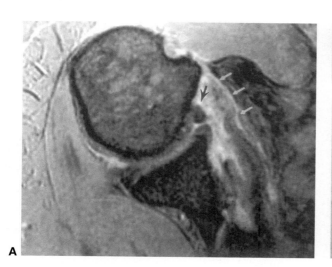
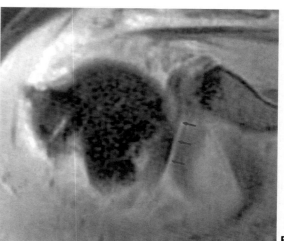

Figure 9-110 **A:** Axial image demonstrates a subscapularis tear (*white arrows*) with associated intraarticular dislocation of the long head of the biceps tendon (*black arrow*). Coronal image **(B)** shows the medially dislocated tendon (*black arrows*).

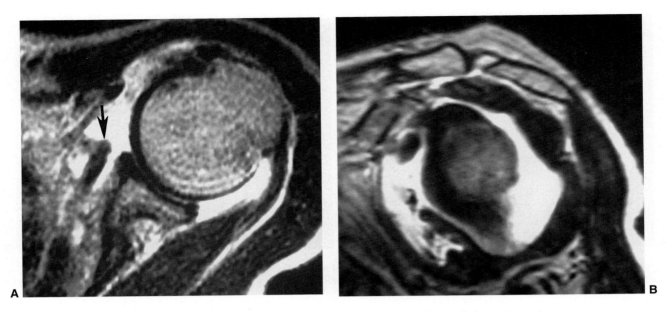

Figure 9-111 Axial **(A)** and sagittal **(B)** T2-weighted images of a subscapularis tear (*arrow*).

a posterior injection site is suggested for cases of suspected subscapularis tears. Pfirrmann et al. (317) demonstrated sensitivity of 91% and specificity of 86% using combined axial and sagittal image planes.

Treatment of subscapularis tears is conservative for patients with low functional demand. This may include antiinflammatory agents or steroid injections and arthroscopic debridement. Open repair with pectoralis transfer is reserved for patients with high functional demand (21,317).

Adhesive Capsulitis

Adhesive capsulitis or frozen shoulder may develop after trauma or surgery, or may present as an idiopathic condition with spontaneous onset (8,178,282). In the latter setting, the condition is most frequent in women in their 60s and most often involves the nondominant shoulder. The condition is bilateral in 34% of patients. There are associated medical problems in 13% (diabetes mellitus, hyperthyroid) and cervical spine symptoms in 11% (282). Though much of the literature indicates that idiopathic frozen shoulder is self-limited, Shaffer et al. (282) noted persistent restricted motion and symptoms in 45% of 62 patients on long-term follow-up.

Radiographs are most often normal. However, in our experience, 20% of patients have osteopenia and other chronic nonspecific radiographic findings (8). Arthrograms (conventional or MR arthrography) are most useful for measuring capsular volume (<10 mL can be injected) and evaluating the other features (small axillary recess and subscapularis bursa, synovitis, lymphatic filling, irregular capsular margins) of adhesive capsulitis (8). Distention

arthrography can be performed following the diagnostic portion of the examination (see Fig. 9-112) to treat selected cases.

MRI is not as effective for diagnosing this condition unless contrast is injected and the amount of fluid measured. Some features, such as limited fluid in the glenohumeral joint, thickened axillary recess, and lack of fluid in the biceps tendon sheath may be suggestive of adhesive capsulitis (see Fig. 9-113). Emig et al. (178) found the thickness of the capsule and synovium in the axillary recess measured 3.5 to 7.4 mm (mean 5.2 mm) in patients with capsulitis, compared to 2.0 to 3.8 mm (mean 2.9 mm) in normal patients. However, in our practice, if there are no features to explain shoulder symptoms with conventional MR imaging, we consider the possibility of frozen shoulder and suggest arthrography with distention technique (Fig. 9-112) if the diagnosis is confirmed. In a clinical setting of previous trauma or clinically suspected frozen shoulder (female 60 years, restricted motion, etc.), we may use conventional arthrography as the initial technique (8).

Pectoralis Muscle Tears

Pectoralis muscle tears are uncommon and difficult to diagnose. Most injuries occur during weight lifting, specifically the bench press maneuver (320). Patients are usually athletic males 20 to 40 years of age. Patients typically describe hearing a pop with burning pain in the shoulder region. There may be swelling and ecchymoses in the chest. When tears are complete, the retracted muscle may be visible and palpable (320,321).

Anatomically, the pectoralis is a thick triangular muscle with progressive increase in fiber length from cephalad to caudad (Fig. 9-26A) (76). The muscle takes its origin from

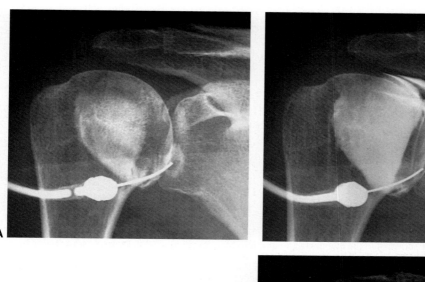

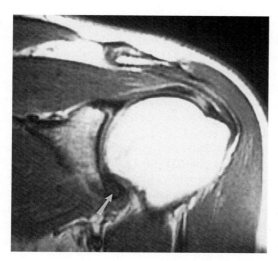

Figure 9-112 Adhesive capsulitis. **A:** There is marked reduction in capsular volume with no filling of recesses. The joint is distended with contrast and anesthetic **(B)** until rupture of the capsule occurs **(C).**

Figure 9-113 Coronal proton density image with increased signal in the supraspinatus tendon but no full-thickness cuff tear. There is no fluid in the glenohumeral joint and the axillary recess (*arrow*) is thickened.

the clavicle, sternum, and upper six coastal cartilages. There are two heads, clavicular and sternal. Muscle fibers converge to insert on the lateral margin of the bicipital groove along the upper humeral diaphysis (Fig. 9-17 and 9-26A). The pectoralis muscle adducts the arm and also serves as a medial rotator. The clavicular head assists with flexion of the humerus. The pectoralis is supplied by the medial and lateral pectoral nerves that arise from the medial and lateral cords of the brachial plexus (76,320).

Classification of pectoral muscle tears includes the extent of disruption (partial or complete) and location of the tear (tendon attachment, myotendinous junction, or muscle belly). MRI can provide valuable pretreatment information regarding the presence and extent of muscle or tendon injury (see Fig. 9-114). Axial fat-suppressed FSE T2-weighted or STIR sequences make edema and hemorrhage more conspicuous. Comparison of both pectoral muscles is useful for more subtle or partial lesions.

The ABER view may be useful for stretching the muscle fibers to make a tear more conspicuous. This also allows

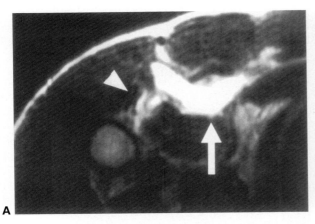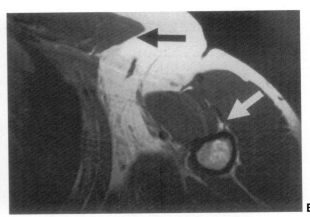

Figure 9-114 Pectoralis muscle tears. **A:** Complete tear at the myotendinous junction. Axial T2-weighted image shows fluid (*arrow*) due to a complete tear. Residual tendon (*arrowhead*) adheres to the anterior musculature. **B:** Chronic tear. Axial T1-weighted image shows the detached pectoralis tendon (*white arrow*) and atrophy (*black arrow*) of the pectoralis major. Fat fills the area of muscle atrophy. (From Carrino JA, Chandnanni VP, Mitchell DB, et al. Pectoralis major muscle tears: diagnosis and grading using magnetic resonance imaging. *Skeletal Radiol* 2000;29:305–313.)

better visualization of the tendon insertion on the humerus (320). In a series of 10 patients reported by Carrino et al. (320), the majority of tears involved the tendinous insertion.

The same criteria applied to tears of other myotendinous units can be applied to pectoralis tears. A complete tear involves the entire thickness with increased signal intensity extending through the structure on T2-weighted images. Muscle retraction may be present. Partial tears involve only a portion of the myotendinous unit (28,80,320).

Nerve Entrapment Syndromes

Neurovascular injury is a well-known potential complication of fractures and dislocations of the shoulder (8,83,269). However, until recently, imaging of other nerve compression syndromes as a cause of shoulder pain received little attention. With the increased utilization of MRI for shoulder imaging, two nerve compression syndromes have been given more attention in the radiology literature. These two syndromes are the quadrilateral space compression syndrome and suprascapular nerve entrapment (32,322–325).

The axillary nerve and posterior humeral circumflex artery and vein pass between the teres minor and teres major (Figs. 9-28 and 9-29 and Table 9-2) in the quadrilateral space (76,323). Nerve compression can occur in this region resulting in pain, paresthesias in the axillary nerve distribution, and muscle atrophy of the teres minor and major muscles. Pain is frequently exacerbated by abduction and external rotation of the arm (32,323). This syndrome (quadrilateral space compression syndrome) should be kept in mind when evaluating MR images on patients with shoulder pain. All too frequently, our attention is focused on rotator cuff pathology. When atrophy of the teres muscles with normal deltoid muscles is detected on MR images, this syndrome should be considered (323).

The suprascapular nerve contains motor and sensory fibers. This branch is derived from the fourth through sixth cervical roots of the brachial plexus (Table 9-2). The nerve enters the supraspinatus fossa via the suprascapular notch and passes beneath the superior transverse scapular ligament (see Fig. 9-115) (76,228,229,322). The suprascapular nerve courses posteriorly beneath the supraspinatus muscle entering the infraspinatus fossa and passing anterior to the inferior transverse scapular ligament (Fig. 9-115) (322). The nerve supplies both the supraspinatus and infraspinatus muscles (Table 9-2) (76). Compression of the nerve anteriorly will result in atrophy of both muscles, while posterior compression results in infraspinatus atrophy (see Fig. 9-116) (228,322).

Patients with suprascapular nerve entrapment present with pain and muscle atrophy. Compression may result from trauma, thickening of the scapular ligaments, or soft tissue masses (Fig. 9-116) (322). The abnormalities described are easily appreciated on conventional MR images even when screening examinations for rotator cuff tears or more common pathology are performed. Abnormalities (Fig. 9-116A), as expected, are most easily demonstrated using T2-weighted sequences.

Nerve compression may be due to soft tissue masses, paralabral cysts, or dilated veins (32,228,229,326,327). Paralabral cysts may be synovial, ganglion cysts, or pseudocysts. Synovial cysts result from evagination of the joint capsule or bursae. These cysts are lined by synovial cells. Ganglion cysts may arise from the joint capsule, bursae, ligaments, or tendons. A pseudocyst forms when fluid extravasates into the periarticular or soft tissues through a capsular or ligament tears. The walled-off fluid forms a pseudocyst (327). Tung et al. (327) reviewed 2,211 MR studies and found paralabral cysts in 2.3%. Fifty-seven percent of cysts were adjacent to the

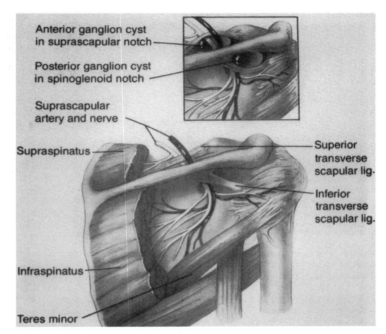

Figure 9-115 The anatomy of the suprascapular nerve with insert demonstrating anterior (proximal) and posterior compression by ganglia. (From Fritz RC, Helms CA, Steinbach LS, Genant HK. Suprascapular nerve entrapment: evaluation with MR imaging. *Radiology* 1992;182:437–444.)

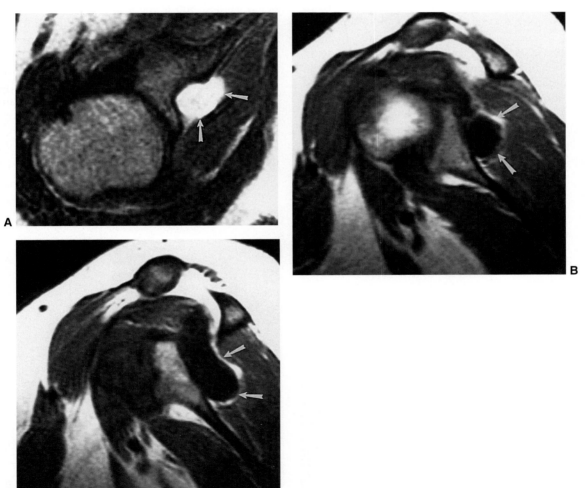

Figure 9-116 Patient with severe chronic shoulder pain thought to be due to rotator cuff pathology. Axial T2-weighted **(A)** and sagittal T1-weighted **(B,C)** images demonstrate a well-defined ganglion (*arrows*) compressing the suprascapular nerve posteriorly.

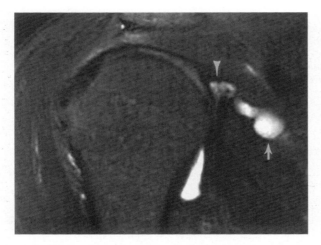

Figure 9-117 Coronal T2-weighted image demonstrating a superior labral tear (*arrowhead*) with associated paralabral cyst in the suprascapular notch (*arrow*).

posterior labrum (see Fig. 9-117), 21% the anterior labrum, 14% superior labrum, and 8% were adjacent to the inferior labrum. There were associated labral tears in 88% of cases. Cysts were simple in 41% and multiloculated in 59%. Multiloculated cysts were larger. Cysts can be clearly identified on T2-weighted sequences. Paralabral cysts typically do not communicate with the joint. Therefore, T2-weighted sequences should also be obtained with MR arthrograms (see Fig. 9-118) (327).

Carroll et al. (229) described nerve compression secondary to dilated veins in the spinoglenoid notch resulting in suprascapular nerve compression (see Fig. 9-119). The veins

were 6 to 10 mm (avg. 8.4 mm) compared to 1 to 4 mm (avg. 2.2 mm) in normal patients. All cases demonstrated infraspinatous atrophy.

In some cases, no soft tissue or osseous abnormality is evident. Trauma, stretching, or contusion may also cause neuropathy. MRI may demonstrate inflammatory or fatty change in the involved muscle (see Fig. 9-120) (228). When a specific abnormality (i.e., mass) cannot be defined, conservative therapy may be preferred over surgical exploration and decompression (328). Cyst aspiration provides temporary relief of symptoms (327).

Infection and Inflammatory Diseases

The shoulder, specifically the glenohumeral joint, is frequently involved in osteoarthritis and other types of inflammatory arthropathies (8,21,123,329–331). Soft tissue changes as well as early changes in the articular and osseous structures of the shoulder are more easily defined using MRI than conventional radiography. Chronic synovial changes such as proliferative synovitis can also be demonstrated. Subtle changes in the synovium or articular cartilage are more easily demonstrated with intraarticular or intravenous gadolinium studies (331).

Arthropathies involving the shoulder may be bilateral and symmetrical (rheumatoid arthritis), bilateral but asymmetrical (osteoarthritis), or involve only the shoulder (infection, pigmented villonodular synovitis) (28). Inflammatory arthropathies are discussed in Chapter 15. However, certain common shoulder arthropathies deserve mention.

Crystal deposition diseases commonly involve the shoulder. The shoulder is the most common site for calcium

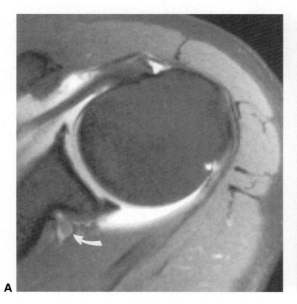

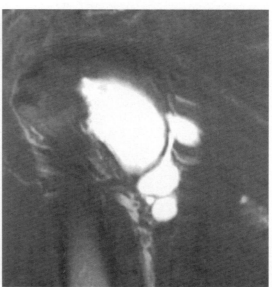

Figure 9-118 **A:** Axial MR arthrogram with a nonfilling multiloculated cyst (*curved arrow*) near the suprascapular nerve. **B:** Coronal T2-weighted arthrogram image demonstrates the high-signal intensity loculated cyst.

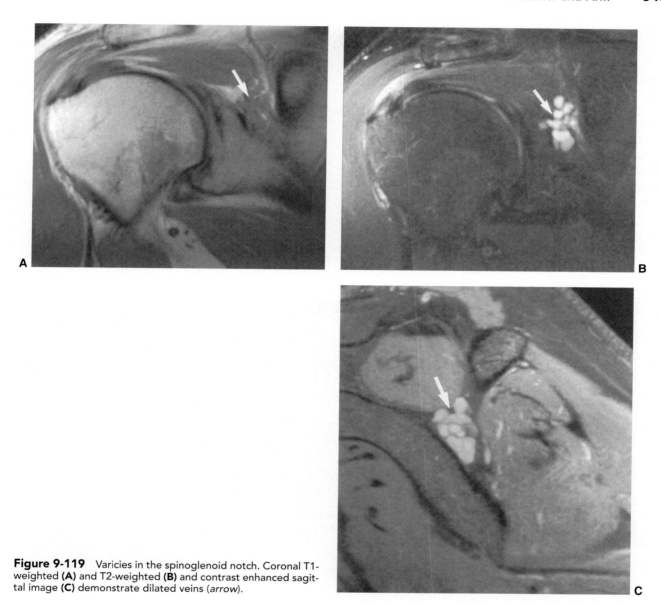

Figure 9-119 Varicies in the spinoglenoid notch. Coronal T1-weighted **(A)** and T2-weighted **(B)** and contrast enhanced sagittal image **(C)** demonstrate dilated veins (*arrow*).

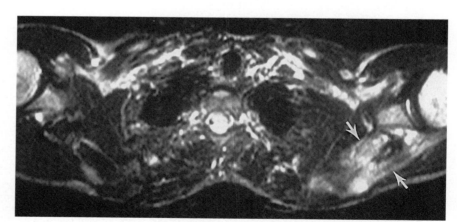

Figure 9-120 Axial MR image demonstrating signal abnormality (*arrows*) but no mass or etiology for nerve compression.

hydroxyapatite deposition disease (HADD) (332). Patients may be asymptomatic even though calcific deposits are evident on radiographs or CT images. Up to 45% of patients have associated pain. This condition is most often seen after 40 years of age. Both shoulders may be affected in up to 50% of patients (21,332). The bursae and tendons are most often involved. The supraspinatus tendon is affected in 52% of cases (332,333).

Radiographs demonstrate amorphous or dense, well-defined calcifications in the region of the supraspinatus and subacromial subdeltoid bursa. This feature, coupled with clinical symptoms, is usually diagnostic (79,247,332,333).

MR imaging is not necessary for diagnosis. However, it is not uncommon to image patients for other shoulder problems such as rotator cuff tear or instability. MR features can

be confusing if radiographs are not available for comparison (28,333). Calcium deposits may be difficult to identify if small. Larger calcifications are low signal intensity on all sequences (see Fig. 9-121) and may cause the supraspinatus to appear thickened near its attachment. Hydroxyapatite crystals cause inflammation in the bursa and soft tissues resulting in fluid-filled bursae and soft tissue inflammation. These changes are easily appreciated on T2-weighted images (21,28,332–334).

Hydroxyapatite deposition disease may occur with calcium pyrophosphate deposition disease. Also, McCarty et al, (335) describe the "Milwaukee shoulder," which is a more destructive arthropathy with hydroxyapatite deposition, rotator cuff tear, and high collagenase levels in synovial fluid. Differential diagnosis for aggressive shoulder arthropathies

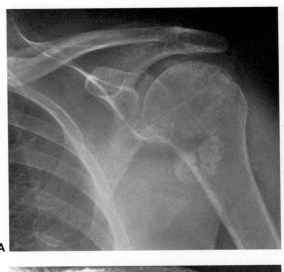

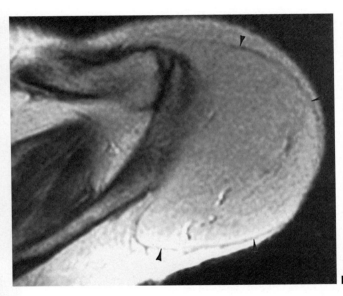

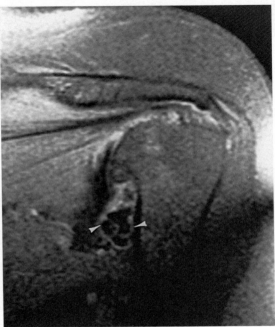

Figure 9-121   Patient with a superficial soft tissue mass and shoulder pain. **A:** Routine anteroposterior radiograph demonstrates degenerative changes with large osteocartilaginous loose bodies in the inferior joint space. Axial **(B)** and coronal **(C)** T2-weighted images show a large lipoma (*black arrowheads*) and low-signal intensity loose bodies (*white arrowheads*) in the axillary recess.

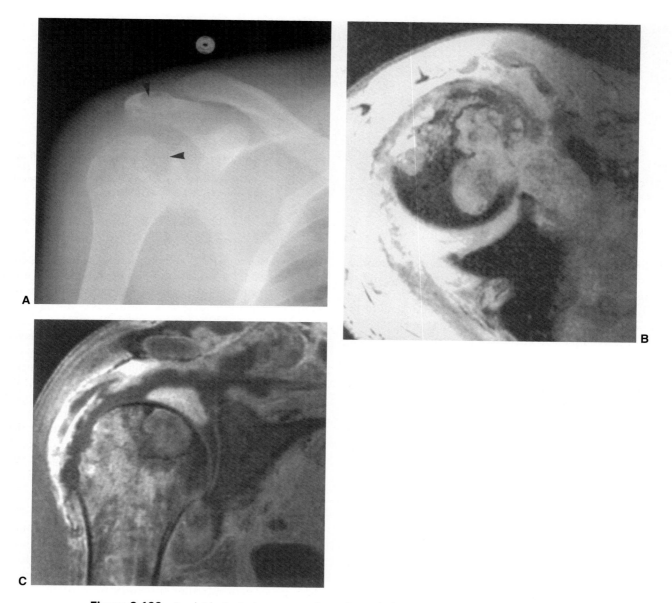

Figure 9-122 Amyloidosis. **A:** Anteroposterior radiograph demonstrates obvious erosions in the humeral head and acromion (*arrowheads*) and soft tissue swelling. Axial gradient-echo **(B)** and coronal postgadolinium T1-weighted image **(C)** demonstrate large erosions with extensive synovitis.

also includes neurotrophic arthropathy idiopathic chondrolysis, amyloidosis (see Fig. 9-122), rheumatoid arthritis, pyogenic arthritis, and osteonecrosis.

Rheumatoid arthritis commonly involves the shoulder. Resorption of the distal clavicle glenohumeral erosions and synovial proliferation are easily detected with MR images. Postintravenous studies are optimal for evaluating early synovial inflammation and proliferation. Fluid in the bursa and associated rotator cuff tears are also common (28).

Osteoarthritis in the shoulder is typically related to prior trauma or underlying conditions such as crystal deposition disease.

Pyogenic arthritis in the shoulder is most common in infants and the elderly. Osteomyelitis and infectious arthritis involving the shoulder can be detected early with MRI (28). Tuberculosis or atypical mycobacterial infections are uncommon in the shoulder. The extent of bone and soft tissue involvement can be more clearly defined using MRI than conventional radiographs or radionuclide scans (1,336). Contrast-enhanced images are generally added to the conventional shoulder series (Table 9-1). Infections are discussed more completely in Chapter 13.

Osteonecrosis

Detection of early AVN or osteonecrosis of the humeral head can be difficult with routine radiographs and radionuclide

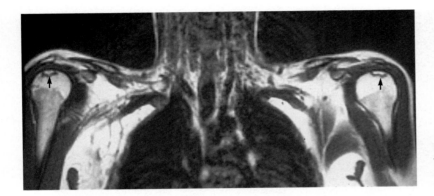

Figure 9-123 Renal transplant patient on systemic steroid therapy. Screening T1-weighted coronal images of the shoulders show classic MR features of avascular necrosis (*arrows*).

studies (8,28). Later, once these changes have become obvious, the radiographic appearance is typical and MRI is not usually indicated.

The appearance of osteonecrosis in the humeral head does not differ significantly from the hip (see Fig. 9-123) (28,337). A complete discussion of the etiology and pathophysiology of osteonecrosis is included in Chapter 6 and will not be repeated here.

Screening for AVN in the shoulder can be accomplished with coronal T1-weighted images. Early or subtle changes may require surface coils to delineate more clearly the changes in one or both shoulders. In this setting, coronal and sagittal images are useful to evaluate the articular cartilage and the area of involvement. T2-weighted or STIR images are added in more difficult cases. Gadolinium is useful for evaluating the revascularization of involved bone.

Neoplasms

MRI has become the technique of choice for staging of musculoskeletal neoplasms, whether they are primary or metastatic (28,102,114,127,336,338). Soft tissue and bony lesions in the shoulder are no exception.

Characterization of bony lesions is still most easily accomplished using routine radiographs (see Fig. 9-124) (1,339). Scapular lesions are divided into S1 (wing) and S2 (glenoid–acromial complex). Benign lesions more commonly involve S2 and malignant S1 segment of the scapula (338). However, T1-weighted sequences or, in certain situations STIR sequences, provide valuable information regarding the extent of bony involvement in primary, metastatic, and infiltrative lesions such as lymphoma or leukemia (102,127,339). We routinely use T1-, T2-weighted, or STIR and contrast-enhanced fat-suppressed T1-weighted images for staging skeletal neoplasm (28). Table 9-12 lists the incidence of common benign and malignant osseous lesions in the shoulder and upper humerus (340).

Data on soft tissue tumors in the shoulder region are also important to note here (Table 9-13) (114,341–343). There are not many soft tissue lesions that more commonly occur in the shoulder region except subcutaneous or superficial lipomas (Fig. 9-121) and extraabdominal desmoid tumors. Subcutaneous lipomas are most common in the shoulder, upper arm, and back. Desmoids occur most frequently in the shoulder (20% to 22%) (28,343). Malignant lesions that commonly involve the shoulder are summarized in Table 9-13.

Soft tissue tumors can be identified and classified using T1- and T2-weighted or STIR sequences (28,114,336). We also obtain contrast-enhanced fat-suppressed T1-weighted images in two image planes to further characterize soft tissue lesions. Specific soft tissue lesions, especially those that are benign, are more often histologically predictable on MRI than malignant lesions. Image characteristics of specific lesions are discussed more fully in Chapter 12.

Brachial Plexus Lesions

The brachial plexus is a difficult area to image with most radiographic techniques. CT has significant limitations, including restriction of imaging planes and artifacts from the shoulder (23,344). In addition, it is more difficult to distinguish neurovascular structures from nodes in the brachial plexus region using conventional CT techniques. The superior soft tissue contrast and multiple image planes available with MRI provide significant advantages in this regard (22–24,26). Subtle cases may require gadolinium studies (dynamic or static fat-suppressed T1-weighted images) for more optimal evaluation.

Wiltenberg and Adkins reported that radiation, primary and metastatic lung cancer (see Fig. 9-125), and breast metastasis account for 75% of cases of brachial plexopathy (25). Numerous other metastatic tumors may also involve the brachial plexus (24). Trauma and other inflammatory disorders may also result in brachial plexopathy.

Radiation fibrosis is the most common cause of brachial plexopathy (31%). Radiation is most often related to treatment of breast cancer patients (see Fig. 9-126). Patients present with shoulder weakness, parasthesias, and pain. Radiation doses resulting in plexopathy are typically 60 Gy or greater. Symptoms can occur months to years after therapy (25).

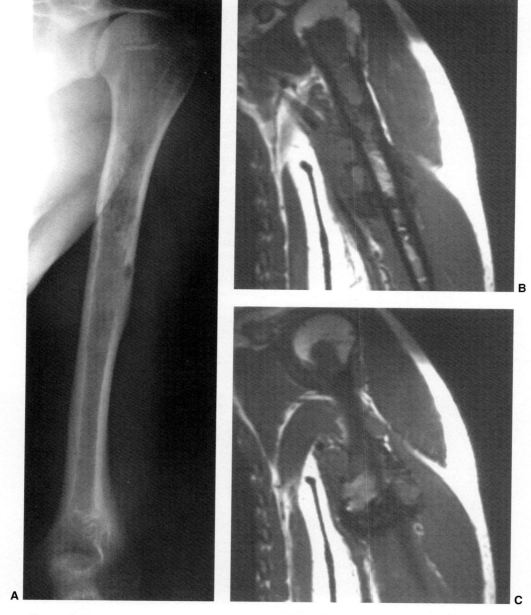

Figure 9-124 Osseous malignant fibrous histiocytoma. **A:** Radiograph demonstrates a permeative lesion in the midhumerus. T1-weighted coronal images **(B,C)** demonstrate the extent of marrow involvement and a large soft tissue mass. The extent of the mass would be demonstrated more effectively on T2-weighted or contrast-enhanced images.

MR features are useful for differentiating radiation change from tumor infiltration. T1-, T2- and contrast-enhanced fat-suppressed images are utilized. At least two image planes, axial and sagittal or coronal should be performed. Comparison with the uninvolved plexus is also useful (Table 9-1) (28). Metastatic lesions are demonstrated as soft tissue masses adjacent to the plexus in most cases, but can infiltrate the plexus (Fig. 9-125), as well. Tumors or infiltration are high signal intensity on T2-weighted and contrast-enhanced images. Radiation

fibrosis will result in thickening of the cords and roots with low signal intensity on T1- and T2-weighted sequences. There is diffuse contrast enhancement without focal mass lesions (24,25,345).

Both benign (BPNST) and malignant (MPNST) peripheral nerve sheath tumors may involve the brachial plexus (343). Roughly 20% of nerve sheath tumors (Table 9-13) involve the brachial plexus. Patients present with symptoms similar to those described above. Pain at rest is suggestive of MPNST (24). About one third of patients with

TABLE 9-12
SKELETAL NEOPLASMS OF THE SHOULDER

Lesion	# Shoulder/ total Lesions	% of Total
Benign		
Chondroblastoma	25/119	21
Osteochondroma	159/872	18
Chondroma	43/290	15
Giant cell tumor	22/568	4
Osteoid osteoma	13/331	4
Hemangioma	4/108	4
Osteoblastoma	1/83	1.2
Malignant		
Chondrosarcoma	144/895	16
Ewings sarcoma	57/512	11
Osteosarcoma	159/1649	10
Lymphoma	70/694	10
Fibrosarcoma	21/255	8
Myeloma	57/814	7

From Chan TW, Dalinka MK, Kneeland BJ, et al. Biceps tendon dislocation: evaluation with MR imaging. *Radiology* 1991;179:649–652; and Unni KK. Dahlin's bone tumors. *General aspects and data on 11,087 cases*, 5th ed. Philadelphia, PA: Lippincott-Raven, 1996.

TABLE 9-13
SOFT TISSUE TUMORS OF THE SHOULDER

Tumor	% in Shoulder
Benign	
Lipoma	28–50
Desmoids	20–22
Myxoma	4–5
Fibromatosis	4–8
Hemangioma	3–4
Benign nerve sheath tumors	3–4
Malignant	
Malignant fibrous histiocytoma	33–35
Liposarcoma	16–21
Malignant nerve sheath tumors	9–12
Fibrosarcoma	2–4
Leiomyosarcoma	2–7
Synovial sarcoma	2–4

From Berquist TH. *MRI of the musculoskeletal system*, 4th ed. Philadelphia, PA: Lippincott Williams & Wilkins, 2001; and Weiss SW, Goldblum JP. *Enzinger and Weiss's soft tissue tumors*, 4th ed. St. Louis: Mosby, 2001.

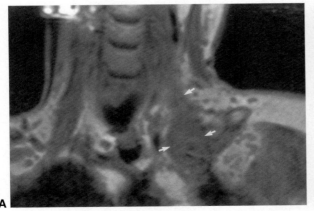

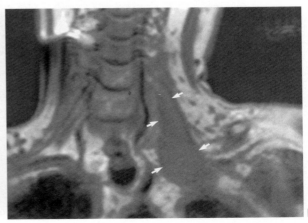

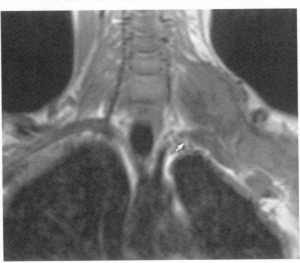

Figure 9-125 Metastasis involving the brachial plexus. Coronal T1-weighted images **(A,B)** show lung metastasis (*arrows*) infiltrating the brachial plexus. Coronal T1-weighted images in a different patient **(C)** show encasement of the nerve roots by lung metastasis (*arrow*).

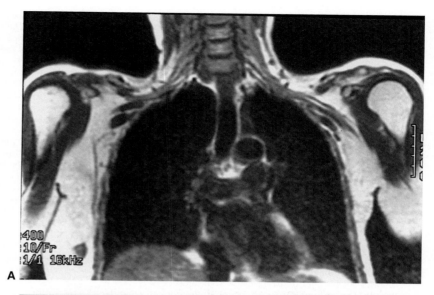

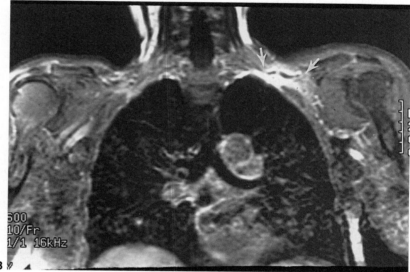

Figure 9-126 Left brachial plexus lesion suspected after mastectomy and radiation therapy. **A:** Coronal T1-weighted image shows postoperative changes in the *left* chest wall (reduced fat and muscle compared to the *right*). **B:** T1-weighted fat-suppressed image with gadolinium shows enhancement along the left brachial plexus (*arrows*) due to radiation.

BPNST have neurofibromatosis type I. Neurofibromatosis type I is diagnosed with two or more of the following features: (i) six or more café'-au-lait skin lesions; (ii) two or more neurofibromas or one plexiform neurofibroma; (iii) inguinal or axillary freckling; (iv) optic glioma; (v) two or more iris hematomas; (vi) osseous lesions; and (vii) parent, sibling, or child with type I. Neurofibromas account for 75% of lesions in patients with neurofibromatoses type I. If this condition is not present, 50% of lesions are schwannomas (24). Schwannoma is a well-encapsulated lesion that displaces but does not infiltrate nerve fascicles. Plexiform neurofibromas infiltrate the fascicles and, therefore, it is difficult to avoid nerve injury during surgery (24,25).

Solitary neurofibromas (nonplexiform) and schwannomas typically are well-defined, oval with the line of the nerve, with high signal intensity on T2- and intermediate signal intensity on T1-weighted sequences. A low-signal intensity center (target sign) may be evident on T2-weighted sequences. There is traumatic enhancement on postcontrast images. In some cases, signal intensity and enhancement are inhomogeneous. When necrosis occurs in schwannomas, they may be difficult to differentiate from MPNST (24,346).

MPNSTs have no specific characteristics and cannot be differentiated from sarcomas. Margins are irregular, signal intensity is inhomogeneous, and enhancement is not uniform. The target sign will not be seen in MPNSTs (345,346). Neurofibromatosis type I is associated in 3% to 13% (25).

Other primary benign and malignant tumors may also involve the brachial plexus. Common benign lesions include desmoid tumors and lipomas (Table 9-13). Malignant lesions include fibrosarcoma, synovial sarcoma, and radiation induced sarcoma (55). The image features of these lesions are discussed in Chapter 12.

Another condition affecting the brachial plexus is Parsonage-Turner syndrome (acute brachial neuritis) (106). Patients present with sudden-onset severe shoulder pain and no history of trauma. Pain decreases over several weeks, followed by muscle weakness. The etiology is unknown, but viral or immunological causes have been postulated. The condition is bilateral in 33% of patients (347).

MR image features include diffuse high signal intensity in the involved nerves on T2-weighted sequences. The supra and infraspinatous muscles are most commonly involved (348). MR imaging is also useful to exclude other sources of shoulder pain.

REFERENCES

1. Berquist TH. Magnetic resonance techniques in musculoskeletal diseases. *Rheum Dis Clin North Am* 1991;17:599–615.
2. Brandt TD, Cardone BW, Grant TH, et al. Rotator cuff sonography: a reassessment. *Radiology* 1989;173:323–327.
3. Goldman AB, Gehlman B. The double contrast shoulder arthrogram: a review of 158 studies. *Radiology* 1978;127:655–663.
4. Huber DJ, Sauter R, Mueller E, et al. MR imaging of the normal shoulder. *Radiology* 1986;158:405–408.
5. Jones MW, Matthews JP. Rupture of pectoralis major in weightlifters: a case report and review of the literature. *Injury* 1988;19:219.
6. Kornguth PJ, Salazar AM. The apical oblique view of the shoulder: it's usefulness in acute trauma. *AJR Am J Roentgenol* 1987;149:113–116.
7. Ohoshi K, El-Khoury GY, Albright JP, et al. MRI of complete rupture of the pectorales major muscle. *Skeletal Radiol* 1996;25:625–628.
8. Berquist TH. *Imaging of orthopedic trauma*, 2nd ed. New York: Raven Press, 1992.
9. Getz JD, Recht MP, Piraino DW, et al. Acromial morphology: relation to sex, age, symmetry, and subacromial enthesophytes. *Radiology* 1996;1996:737–742.
10. Patten RM. Vacuum phenomenon: a potential pitfall in the interpretation of gradient-recalled-echo MR images of the shoulder. *AJR Am J Roentgenol* 1994;162:1383–1386.
11. Rafii M, Firooznia H, Sherman O, et al. Rotator cuff lesions: signal patterns at MR imaging. *Radiology* 1990;177:817–823.
12. Rafii M, Firooznia H, Sherman O, et al. Rotator cuff lesions: signal patterns at MR imaging. *Radiology* 1991;181:837–841.
13. Taljanovic MS, Carlson KL, Kuhn JE, et al. Sonography of the glenoid labrum: a cadaveric study with arthroscopic correlation. *AJR Am J Roentgenol* 2000;174:1717–1722.
14. Burk LD, Karasick D, Kurtz AB, et al. Rotator cuff tears: prospective comparison of MR imaging with arthrography, sonography and surgery. *AJR Am J Roentgenol* 1989;153:87–92.
15. Cvitanic O, Schimalde J, Cruse J, et al. The acromioclavicular joint cyst: glenohumeral joint communication revealed by MR arthrography. *J Comput Assist Tomogr* 1999;23:141–143.
16. Tirman PFJ, Steinbach LS, Feller JF, et al. Humeral avulsion of the anterior shoulder stabilizing structures after anterior shoulder dislocation: demonstration by MRI and MR arthrography. *Skeletal Radiol* 1996;25:743–748.
17. Zlatkin MB, Dalinka MK. The glenohumeral joint. *Top Magn Reson Imaging* 1989;1(3):1–13.
18. Zlatkin MB, Falchook FS. Magnetic resonance pathology of the rotator cuff. *Top Magn Reson Imaging* 1994;6:94–120.
19. Zlatkin MB, Iannotti JP, Roberts MC, et al. Rotator cuff disease. Diagnostic performance of MR imaging. *Radiology* 1989;172:223–229.
20. Zlatkin MB. MRI of the post-operative shoulder. *Skeletal Radiol* 2002;31:63–80.
21. Zlatkin MB. *MRI of the shoulder*. Philadelphia, PA: Lippincott Williams & Wilkins, 2003.
22. Blaire DN, Rapoport S, Sostman HD, et al. Normal brachial plexus: MR imaging. *Radiology* 1988;165:763–767.
23. Rapoport S, Blair DN, McCarthy SM, et al. Brachial plexus: correlation of MR imaging with CT and pathologic findings. *Radiology* 1988;167:161–165.
24. Saifuddin A. Imaging tumors of the brachial plexus. *Skeletal Radiol* 2003;32:375–387.
25. Wittenberg KH, Adkins MC. MR imaging of nontraumatic brachial plexopathies: frequency and spectrum of findings. *Radiographics* 2000;20:1023–1032.
26. Castagno AA, Shuman WP. MR imaging in clinically suspected brachial plexus. *AJR Am J Roentgenol* 1987;149:1219–1222.
27. Bencardino JT, Garcia AI, Palmer WE. Magnetic resonance imaging of the shoulder: rotator cuff. *Top Magn Reson Imaging* 2003;14(1):51–68.
28. Berquist TH. *MRI of the musculoskeletal system*, 4th ed. Philadelphia, PA: Lippincott Williams & Wilkins, 2001.
29. Recht MP, Resnick D. Magnetic resonance imaging studies of the shoulder. *J Bone Joint Surg Am* 1993;75A:1244–1253.
30. Tuite MJ, DeSmet AA, Norris MA, et al. MR diagnosis of labral tears of the shoulder: value of T2*-weighted gradient-recalled echo images made in external rotation. *AJR Am J Roentgenol* 1995;164:941–944.
31. Mohana-Borges AVR, Chung CB, Resnick D. MR imaging and MR arthrography of the post-operative shoulder: spectrum of normal and abnormal findings. *Radiographics* 2004;24:69–85.
32. Robinson P, White LM, Lox M, et al. Quadrilateral space syndrome caused by glenoid labral cyst. *AJR Am J Roentgenol* 2000;175:1103–1105.
33. Davis SJ, Teresi LM, Bradley WG, et al. Effect of arm rotation on MR imaging of the rotator cuff. *Radiology* 1991;181:265–268.
34. Tirman PFJ, Bost FW, Steinbach LS, et al. MR arthrographic depiction of tears of the rotator cuff: benefit of abduction and external rotation of the arm. *Radiology* 1994;192:851–856.
35. Cvitanic O, Tirman PFJ, Feller JF, et al. Using abduction and external rotation of the shoulder to increase the sensitivity of MR arthrographies revealing tears of the anterior glenoid labrum. *AJR Am J Roentgenol* 1997;169:837–844.
36. Lee SY, Lee JK. Horizontal component of partial thickness tears of the rotator cuff: imaging characteristics and comparison of the ABER view with oblique coronal view at MR arthrography. *Radiology* 2002;224:470–476.
37. Pennes DR, Jonsson K, Buckwalter K, et al. Computed arthrotomography of the shoulder: comparison of examinations made with internal and external rotation of the humerus. *AJR Am J Roentgenol* 1989;153:1017–1019.
38. McGee KP, Grimm RO, Felmlee JP, et al. The shoulder: adoptive motor correction of MR images. *Radiology* 1997;205:541–545.
39. Dibb MJ, Noble DJ, Wong LLS, et al. Comparison of supraspinatus tendon and glenohumeral joint axes in MR imaging of the shoulder. *Skeletal Radiol* 2000;29:397–401.
40. Carrino JA, McCauley TR, Katz LD, et al. Rotator cuff: evaluation with fast spin-echo versus conventional spin-echo imaging. *Radiology* 1997;202:533–539.
41. Hodler J, Kursunoglu-Brahme S, Snyder SJ, et al. Rotator cuff disease: assessment with MR arthrography versus standard imaging in 36 patients with arthroscopic confirmation. *Radiology* 1992;182:431–436.
42. Sonin AH, Peduto AJ, Fitzgerald SW, et al. MR imaging of the rotator cuff mechanism: comparison of spin-echo and turbo spin-echo sequences. *AJR Am J Roentgenol* 1996;167:333–338.
43. Huber DJ, Mueller E, Heribes A. Oblique magnetic resonance imaging of the normal shoulder. *Radiology* 1986;158:405–408.
44. Tuite MJ, Yandow DR, DeSmet AA, et al. Effect of field of view on MR diagnosis of rotator cuff tears. *Skeletal Radiol* 1995;24:495–498.
45. Hattrup S, Cofield RH, Berquist TH, et al. Shoulder arthrography for determination of size of rotator cuff tear. *J Shoulder Elbow Surg* 1992;1:98–105.
46. Moseley HG, Overgaard B. The anterior capsular mechanism in recurrent anterior dislocation of the shoulder: morphological and clinical studies with special reference to the glenoid labrum and the glenohumeral ligaments. *J Bone Joint Surg* 1962;44:913–927.

47. Munk PL, Holt RG, Helms CA, et al. Glenoid labrum: preliminary work with use of radial sequences MR imaging. *Radiology* 1989;173:751–753.

48. Beltran J, Jbara M, Miamon R. Shoulder: labrum and biceps tendon. *Top Magn Reson Imaging* 2003;14(1):35–49.

49. Loredo R, Longo C, Salonen D, et al. Glenoid labrum MR imaging with histologic correlation. *Radiology* 1995;196:33–41.

50. Marsengill AD, Seeger LL, Yao L, et al. Labrocapsular ligamentous complex of the shoulder: normal anatomy, anatomic variation and pitfalls of MR imaging and arthrography. *Radiographics* 1994;14:1211–1223.

51. McCauley TR, Pope CF, Jokl P. Normal and abnormal glenoid labrum: assessment with multiplanar gradient-echo MR imaging. *Radiology* 1992;183:35–37.

52. Beltran J, Bercardino J, Mellado J, et al. MR arthrography of the shoulder: variants and pitfalls. *Radiographics* 1997;17:1403–1412.

53. Beltran J, Gray LA, Bools JC, et al. Rotator cuff lesions of the shoulder: evaluation by direct sagittal CT arthrography. *Radiology* 1986;160:161–165.

54. Bencardino JT, Beltran J, Rosenberg ZS, et al. Superior labrum criteria—posterior lesions: diagnosis with MR arthrography of the shoulder. *Radiology* 2000;214:267–271.

55. Hall FM, Rosenthal DI, Goldberg RP, et al. Morbidity from shoulder arthrography: etiology, incidence and prevention. *AJR Am J Roentgenol* 1981;136:56–62.

56. Kottal RA, Vogler JB III, Matamoros A, et al. Pigmented villonodular synovitis: a report of MR imaging in two cases. *Radiology* 1987;163:551–553.

57. Kwak SM, Brown RR, Resnick D, et al. Anatomy, anatomic variations and pathology of the 11-to-3 o'clock position of the glenoid labrum: findings on MR arthrography and anatomic sections. *AJR Am J Roentgenol* 1998;171:235–238.

58. Chandnani VP, Gagliardi JA, Murnane TG, et al. Glenohumeral ligaments and shoulder capsular mechanism: evaluation with MR arthrography. *Radiology* 1995;196:27–32.

59. Willemsen UF, Wiedemann E, Brunner U, et al. Prospective evaluation of MR arthrography performed with high-volume intra articular saline enhancement in patients with recurrent anterior dislocations of the shoulder. *AJR Am J Roentgenol* 1998;170:79–84.

60. Winalski CS, Aliabadi P, Wright RJ, et al. Enhancement of joint fluid with intravenously administered gadopenetate dimeglumine: technique, rationale and implications. *Radiology* 1993;187:179–185.

61. Binkert CA, Zanetti M, Gerber C, et al. MR arthrography of the glenohumeral joint: two concentrations of gadoteradol versus ringers solution as intraarticular contrast material. *Radiology* 2001;220:219–224.

62. Kopka L, Funke M, Fischer A, et al. MR arthrography of the shoulder with pentetate dimeglumine: influence of concentration, iodinated contrast material and time on signal intensity. *AJR Am J Roentgenol* 1994;163:621–623.

63. Bergin D, Schweitzer ME. Indirect magnetic resonance arthrography. *Skeletal Radiol* 2003;32:551–558.

64. De Mouy EH, Menendez CV, Bodin CJ. Palpation-directed (nonfluoroscopically guided) saline-enhanced MR arthrography of the shoulder. *AJR Am J Roentgenol* 1997;169:229–231.

65. Miller TT. MR arthrography of the shoulder and hip after fluoroscopic landmarking. *Skeletal Radiol* 2000;29:81–84.

66. Valls R, Melloni P. Sonographic guidance of needle position for MR arthrography of the shoulder. *AJR Am J Roentgenol* 1997;169:845–847.

67. Chung CB, Dwek JR, Feng S, et al. MR arthrography of the glenohumeral joint: a tailored approach. *AJR Am J Roentgenol* 2001;177:217–219.

68. Dépelteau H, Bureau NJ, Cardinal E, et al. Arthrography of the shoulder: a simple fluoroscopically guided approach to target the rotator cuff interval. *AJR Am J Roentgenol* 2004;182:329–332.

69. Gerber C, Hersche O, Farron A. Isolated rupture of the subscapularis tendon. *J Bone Joint Surg Am* 1996;78A:1015–1023.

70. Birkert CA, Zanetti M, Gerber C, et al. MR arthrography of the glenohumeral joint: two concentrations of gadoteridol versus ringer solution as the intra-articular contrast material. *Radiology* 2001;220:219–224.

71. Brown RR, Clarke DW, Daffner RH. Is a mixture of gadolinium and iodinated contrast material safe during MR arthrography. *AJR Am J Roentgenol* 2000;175:1087–1090.

72. Lee JHE, van Raalte V, Malian V. Diagnosis of SLAP lesions with Grashey-view arthrography. *Skeletal Radiol* 2003;32:388–395.

73. Jee W-H, McCauley TR, Katz LD, et al. Superior labral anterior posterior (SLAP) lesions of the glenoid labrum: reliability and accuracy of MR arthrography for diagnosis. *Radiology* 2001;218:127–132.

74. Kwak SM, Brown RR, Trudell D, et al. Glenohumeral joint: comparison of shoulder positions at MR arthrography. *Radiology* 1998;208:375–380.

75. Brossmann J, Stabler A, Preidler KW, et al. Sternoclavicular joint: MR imaging—anatomic correlation. *Radiology* 1996;198:193–198.

76. Rosse C, Rosse PG. *Hollinsheads textbook of anatomy.* Philadelphia, PA: Lippincott-Raven, 1997.

77. Cooper DE, Arnoczky SP, O'Brien SJ, et al. Anatomy, histology and vascularity of the glenoid labrum. *J Bone Joint Surg Am* 1992;74A:46–52.

78. Pappas AM, Goss TP, Kleiman PK. Symptomatic shoulder instability due to lesions of the glenoid labrum. *Am J Sports Med* 1983;11:279–288.

79. Zlatkin MB, Dalinka MK, Kressel HY. Magnetic resonance imaging of the shoulder. *Magn Reson Q* 1989;5(1):3–22.

80. Beltran J, Bencardiro J, Padrou M, et al. The middle glenohumeral ligament: normal anatomy, variants and pathology. *Skeletal Radiol* 2002;31:253–262.

81. Bureau NJ, Dussault RG, Keats TE. Imaging of bursae of the shoulder joint. *Skeletal Radiol* 1996;25:513–517.

82. Iannotti JP, Gabriel JP, Schneck SL, et al. The normal glenohumeral relationship. *J Bone Joint Surg Am* 1992;74A:491–500.

83. Totterman SM, Miller RJ, Meyers SP. Basic anatomy of the shoulder by magnetic resonance imaging. *Top Magn Reson Imaging* 1994;6:86–93.

84. Carter BL, Morehead J, Walpert JM, et al. *Cross-sectional anatomy: computed tomography and ultrasound correlation.* New York: Appleton-Century Crofts, 1977.

85. Clark JM, Harryman DTII. Tendons, ligaments and capsules of the rotator cuff. *J Bone Joint Surg* 1992;74A:713–725.

86. Middleton WD, Kneel and JB, Carrera GF, et al. High-resolution MR imaging of the normal rotator cuff. *AJR Am J Roentgenol* 1987;148:559–564.

87. Seeger LL, Gold RH, Bassett LW, et al. Shoulder impingement syndrome: MR findings in 53 shoulders. *AJR Am J Roentgenol* 1988;150:343–347.

88. Kieft GH, Bloem JL, Rozing PM, et al. MR imaging of recurrent anterior dislocation of the shoulder: comparison with CT arthrography. *AJR Am J Roentgenol* 1988;150:1083–1087.

89. Kieft GJ, Bloem JH, Obermann WR, et al. Normal shoulder: MR imaging. *Radiology* 1986;159:741–745.

90. Kieft GJ, Sartoris DJ, Bloem JL, et al. Magnetic resonance imaging of glenohumeral joint disease. *Skeletal Radiol* 1987;16:285–290.

91. Kilcoyne RF, Reddy PK, Lyons F, et al. Optimal plain film imaging of the shoulder impingement syndrome. *AJR Am J Roentgenol* 1989;153:795–797.

92. Applegate GR. Three-dimensional MR arthrography of the shoulder: an intra articular perspective. *AJR Am J Roentgenol* 1998;171:239–241.

93. Andary JL, Peterson SA. The vascular anatomy of the glenohumeral capsule and ligaments: an anatomic study. *J Bone Joint Surg Am* 2002;84A:2258–2265.

94. Carroll KW, Helms CA. Magnetic resonance imaging of the shoulder: a review of potential sources of diagnostic errors. *Skeletal Radiol* 2002;31:373–383.

95. Morgan H, Damron T, Cohen H, et al. Pseudotumor deltoideus: a previously undescribed anatomic variant at the deltoid insertion. *Skeletal Radiol* 2001;30:512–518.

96. Kaplan PA, Bryans KC, Davick JP, et al. MR imaging of the normal shoulder: variants and pitfalls. *Radiology* 1992;184:519–524.

97. Timins ME, Erickson SJ, Estkowski LD, et al. Increased signal in the normal supraspinatus tendon on MR imaging: diagnostic pitfall caused by the magic-angle effect. *AJR Am J Roentgenol* 1995;164:109–114.

98. Farmer KD, Hughes PM. MR arthrography of the shoulder: fluoroscopically guided technique using a posterior approach. *AJR Am J Roentgenol* 2002;178:433–434.

99. Berger PE, Ofstein RA, Jackson DW, et al. MRI demonstration of radiographic occult fractures: what have we been missing? *Radiographics* 1989;9:407–436.

100. Erickson SJ, Cox IH, Hyde JS, et al. Effect of tendon orientation on MR imaging signal intensity: a manifestation of the "magic angle" phenomenon. *Radiology* 1991;181:389–392.

101. Erickson SJ, Fitzgerald SW, Quinn SF, et al. Long bicipital tendon of the shoulder: normal anatomy and pathologic findings on MR imaging. *AJR Am J Roentgenol* 1992;158:1091–1096.

102. Daffner RH, Lupetin AR, Dash N, et al. MRI in the detection of malignant infiltration of bone marrow. *AJR Am J Roentgenol* 1986;146:353–358.

103. Peh WCG, Chan JHM. Artifacts in musculoskeletal magnetic resonance imaging: identification and correction. *Skeletal Radiol* 2001;30:179–191.

104. Richards RD, Sartores DJ, Pathrea MN, et al. Hill-Sachs lesion and normal humeral groove: MR imaging features allowing their differentiation. *Radiology* 1994;190:665–668.

105. Recht MP, Kramer J, Petersilge CA, et al. Distribution of normal and abnormal fluid collections in the glenohumeral joint: implications for MR arthrography. *J Magn Reson Imaging* 1994;4:173–177.

106. Parsonage MJ, Turner JWA. Neurologic amyotrophy: the shoulder girdle syndrome. *Lancet* 1948;1:973–978.

107. Strobel K, Pfirrmann CWA, Zanetti M, et al. MRI features of the acromioclavicular joint that predict pain relief from intra-articular injection. *AJR Am J Roentgenol* 2003;181:755–760.

108. Surgson RD, Huang T, Dan S, et al. MR evaluation of rotator cuff pathology using T2-weighted fast spin-echo technique with and without fat suppression. *AJR Am J Roentgenol* 1996;166:1061–1065.

109. Kjellin I, Ho CP, Cervilla V, et al. Alterations in e supraspinatus tendon at MR imaging: correlation with histopathologic findings in cadavers. *Radiology* 1991;181:837–841.

110. Vahlensieck M, Pollock M, Lang P, et al. Two segments of the supraspinatus muscle: cause of high signal intensity at MR imaging. *Radiology* 1993;18b:449–454.

111. Sans N, Richardi G, Railhac J-J, et al. Kinematic MR imaging of the shoulder: normal patterns. *AJR Am J Roentgenol* 1996; 167:1517–1522.

112. Liou JTS, Wilson AJ, Totty WG, et al. The normal shoulder: common variations that simulate pathologic conditions at MR imaging. *Radiology* 1993;186:435–441.

113. Mirowitz SA. Normal rotator cuff: MR imaging with conventional and fat-suppression techniques. *Radiology* 1991;180:735–740.

114. Kallas KM, Vaughan L, Haghitbi P, et al. Hibernoma of the left axilla: a case report and review of MR imaging. *Skeletal Radiol* 2003;32:290–294.

115. Tirman PFJ, Feller JF, Janzen DL, et al. Association of glenoid labial cysts with labral tears and glenohumeral instability. Radiographic findings and clinical significance. *Radiology* 1994;190:653–658.

116. Tirman PFJ, Feller JF, Palmer WE, et al. The Buford complex—a variation of normal shoulder anatomy: MR arthrographic imaging features. *AJR Am J Roentgenol* 1996;166:869–873.

117. Krietner K-F, Botchen K, Rude J, et al. Superior labrum and labral-bicipital complex: MR imaging with pathologic-anatomic and histologic correlation. *AJR Am J Roentgenol* 1998;170:599–605.

118. Neumann CH, Petersen SA, Jahnke AH. MR imaging of the labral-capsular complex: normal variations. *AJR Am J Roentgenol* 1991;157:1015–1021.

119. Tuite MF, Orwur JF. Anterosuperior labral variants of the shoulder: appearance on gradient recalled-echo and fast spin-echo MR images. *Radiology* 1996;199:537–540.

120. Yeh LR, Kwak S, Kun Y-S, et al. Anterior labroligamentous structures of the glenohumeral joint: correlation of MR arthrography and anatomic dissection in cadavers. *AJR Am J Roentgenol* 1998;171:1229–1236.

121. Ly JQ, Beall DP, Bond DF, et al. Incidence of pathologic shoulder conditions found by magnetic resonance imaging in patients with shoulder pain. *Radiologist* 2002;9(4):191–208.

122. Tuite MJ, Blanken Vaher DG, Seifert M, et al. Sublabral foramen and buford complex; inferior extent of the unattached or absent labrum in 50 patients. *Radiology* 2002;223:137–142.

123. Schweitzer ME, Magbalon MJ, Fenlin JM, et al. Effusion criteria and clinical importance of glenohumeral joint fluid: MR imaging evaluation. *Radiology* 1995;194:821–824.

124. Major NM. MR imaging after therapeutic injection of the subacromial bursa. *Skeletal Radiol* 1999;28:268–671.

125. Richardson ML, Patten RM. Age-related changes in marrow distribution in the shoulder: MR image findings. *Radiology* 1994;192:209–215.

126. Mirowitz SA. Hemopoeitic bone marrow within the proximal humeral epiphysis in normal adults. Investigation with MR imaging. *Radiology* 1993;188:689–693.

127. McKinstry CS, Steiner RE, Young AT, et al. Bone marrow in leukemia and aplastic anemia: MR imaging before, during and after treatment. *Radiology* 1987;162:701–707.

128. Uri DS, Kneeland JB, Herzog R. Os acromiale: evaluation of markers for identification on sagittal and coronal oblique MR images. *Skeletal Radiol* 1997;26:31–34.

129. Väätainen U, Pirinen A, Mäkelä A. Radiological evaluation of the acromio clavicular joint. *Skeletal Radiol* 1991;20:115–116.

130. Morrison DS, Bigliani LU. The clinical significance of variations in acromial morphology. *Orthop Trans* 1986;11:234–240.

131. Jordan LK, Kenter K, Griffiths HL. Relationship between MRI and clinical findings in the acromioclavicular joint. *Skeletal Radiol* 2002;31:516–521.

132. Goldman AB. Calcific tendonitis of the long head of the biceps brachii distal to the glenohumeral joint: plain film radiographic findings. *AJR Am J Roentgenol* 1989;153:1011–1016.

133. Newhouse KE, El-Khoury GY, Nepola JV, et al. The shoulder impingement view: a fluoroscopic technique for the detection of subacromial spurs. *AJR Am J Roentgenol* 1988;151:539–541.

134. Newhouse KE, El-Khoury GY, Nepola JV, et al. The shoulder impingement view: a fluoroscopic technique for detection of subacromial spurs. *AJR Am J Roentgenol* 1988;155:539–541.

135. Aisen AM, Martel W, Braunstein EM, et al. MRI and CT evaluation of primary bone and soft tissue tumors. *AJR J Roentgenol* 1986;146:749–756.

136. Cahill BR. Osteolysis of the distal part of the clavicle in male athletes. *J Bone Joint Surg Am* 1982;64A:1053–1058.

137. Calvert PT, Packer NP, Stoker DJ, et al. Arthrography of the shoulder after operative repair of the torn rotator cuff. *J Bone Joint Surg Br* 1986;68:147–150.

138. McNiesh LM, Callaghan JJ. CT arthrography of the shoulder: variations of the glenoid labrum. *AJR Am J Roentgenol* 1987;149:963–966.

139. Cofield RH. Rotator cuff disease of the shoulder. *J Bone Joint Surg Am* 1985;67:974–979.

140. Hodler J, Fretz CJ, Terrier F, et al. Rotator cuff tears: correlation of sonographic and surgical findings. *Radiology* 1988;169:791–794.

141. Mack LA, Matsen FA III, Kilcoyne RF, et al. US evaluation of the rotator cuff. *Radiology* 1985;157:205–209.

142. Sher JS, Uribe JW, Murphy BJ, et al. Abnormal findings on magnetic resonance images of asymptomatic shoulder. *J Bone Joint Surg Am* 1995;77A:10–15.

143. Wohlwend JR, Van Holesbeeck M, Craig K, et al. The association between irregular greater tuberosities and rotator cuff tears: a sonographic study. *AJR Am J Roentgenol* 1998;171:229–233.

144. Miller TT, Adler RS. Sonography of tears of the distal biceps tendon. *AJR Am J Roentgenol* 2000;175:1081–1086.

145. Schweitzer ME. MR arthrography of the labral-ligamentous complex of the shoulder. *Radiology* 1994;190:641–643.

146. Yu JS, Greenway G, Resnick D. Osteochondral defect of the glenoid fossa: cross-sectional imaging features. *Radiology* 1998;206:35–40.

147. Cervilla V, Schweitzer ME, Hu C, et al. Medial dislocation of the biceps brachii tendon: appearance at MR imaging. *Radiology* 1991;180:253–256.

148. Workman TL, Burkhard TK, Resnick D, et al. Hill-Sachs lesion: comparison of detection with MR imaging, radiography and arthroscopy. *Radiology* 1992;185:847–852.

149. Donnelly LF, Helms CA, Biosett GS. III Chronic avulsive injury of the deltoid insertion in adolescents: imaging findings in three cases. *Radiology* 1999;211:233–236.

150. Rowe CR. Prognosis in dislocations of the shoulder. *J Bone Joint Surg Am* 1956;38A:957–977.

151. Reinus WR, Hatem SF. Fractures of the greater tuberosity presenting as rotator cuff abnormality. Magnetic resonance demonstration. *J Trauma* 1998;44(4):670–675.

152. Mason BJ, Kier R, Bindleglass DF. Occult fractures of the greater fiberosity of the humerus. Radiographic and MR imaging findings. *AJR Am J Roentgenol* 1999;172:469–473.

153. Antonio GE, Cho JH, Chang CB, et al. MR imaging appearance and classification of acromioclavicular joint injury. *AJR Am J Roentgenol* 2003;180:1103–1110.

154. Burkhart SS, Morgan D, Kibler WS. Shoulder injuries in over hand athletes. The "dead arm" revisited. *Clin Sports Med* 2000; 19:125–128.

155. Fiorella D, Helms CA, Speer KP. Increased T2 signal intensity in the distal clavicle: incidence and clinical implications. *Skeletal Radiol* 2000;29:697–702.

156. Kaplan PA, Resnick D. Stress-induced osteolysis of the clavicle. *Radiology* 1986;158:139–140.

157. Keats TE, Pope TL. Jr. The acromioclavicular joint: normal variation and diagnosis of dislocation. *Skeletal Radiol* 1988;17:159–162.

158. Kellman GM, Kneeland JB, Middleton WD, et al. MR imaging of the supraclavicular region: normal anatomy. *AJR Am J Roentgenol* 1987;148:77–82.

159. Strizak AM, Danzig L, Jackson DW, et al. Subacromial bursography. *J Bone Joint Surg Am* 1982;64:196–201.

160. Buckholz RW, Hickman JD. *Rockwood and Green's fractures in adults*, 5th ed. Philadelphia, PA: Lippincott Williams & Wilkins, 2001:1210–1244.

161. Tirman PFJ, Bost FW, Garvin GJ, et al. Posterosuperior glenoid impingement of the shoulder: finding at MR imaging and MR arthrography with arthroscopic correlation. *Radiology* 1994;193:431–436.

162. Levine AH, Pais MJ, Schwartz EE. Posttraumatic osteolysis of the distal clavicle with emphasis on early radiologic changes. *AJR Am J Roentgenol* 1976;126:781–784.

163. de la Puente R, Boutin RD, Theodorou DJ, et al. Post traumatic and stress induced osteolysis of the distal clavicle: MR imaging findings in 17 patients. *Skeletal Radiol* 1999;28:202–208.

164. Roach NA, Schweitzer ME. Does osteolysis of the distal clavicle occur following spinal cord injury? *Skeletal Radiol* 1997;26:16–19.

165. Schweitzer ME, Magbalon MJ, Frieman BG, et al. Acromioclavicular joint fluid: determination of clinical significance with MR imaging. *Radiology* 1994;192:205–207.

166. Depalma AF. *Surgery of the shoulder*. Philadelphia, PA: J.B. Lippincott, 1983.

167. Iannotti JP. Clinical evaluation of shoulder pain. In: Zlatkin MB, ed. *MRI of the shoulder*. New York: Raven Press, 1991:41–54.

168. Lie S, Mast WA. Subacromial bursography: techniques and clinical application. *Radiology* 1982;144:626–630.

169. Brossmann J, Preidler DW, Pedowitz RA, et al. Shoulder impingement syndrome: influence of shoulder position on rotator cuff impingement—an anatomic study. *AJR Am J Roentgenol* 1996;167:1511–1515.

170. Buirski G. Magnetic resonance imaging in acute and chronic rotator cuff tears. *Skeletal Radiol* 1990;19:109–111.

171. Evancho AM, Stiles RG, Fajman WA, et al. MR imaging diagnosis of rotator cuff tears. *AJR Am J Roentgenol* 1988;151:751–754.

172. Ko J-Y, Shih C-H, Chen W-J, et al. Coracoid impingement caused by a ganglion from the subscapularis tendon. *J Bone Joint Surg Am* 1994;76A:1709–1711.

173. Gusmer PB, Potter HG, Schatz JA, et al. Labral injuries: accuracy of detection with unenhanced MR imaging of the shoulder. *Radiology* 1996;200:519–524.

174. Wiener SN, Sietz WH. Sonography of the shoulder in patients with tears of the rotator cuff: accuracy and value in selecting surgical options. *AJR Am J Roentgenol* 1993;160:103–107.

175. Neer CE. III Impingement lesions. *Clin Orthop* 1983;173:70–77.

176. Neer CS. III Anterior acromioplasty for the chronic impingement syndrome of the shoulder: a preliminary report. *J Bone Joint Surg Am* 1972;54:41–50.

177. Ellman H, Kay SP, Wirth M. Arthroscopic treatment of full thickness rotator cuff tears: 2 to 7 year follow-up study. *Arthroscopy* 1993;9:195–200.

178. Emig EW, Schweitzer ME, Karasick D, et al. Adhesive capsulitis of the shoulder: MR diagnosis. *AJR Am J Roentgenol* 1995;164: 1457–1459.

179. Farley TE, Newman CH, Steinbach LS, et al. Full thickness tears of the rotator cuff of the shoulder: diagnosis with MR imaging. *AJR Am J Roentgenol* 1992;158:347–351.

180. Needell SD, Zlatkin MB, Sher JS, et al. MR imaging of the rotator cuff: peri tendon and bone abnormalities in an asymptomatic population. *AJR Am J Roentgenol* 1996;166:863–867.

181. Parsa M, Tuite M, Norris M, et al. MR imaging of rotator cuff tendon tears: comparison of T2*-weighted gradient-echo and conventional dual-echo sequences. *AJR Am J Roentgenol* 1997;168: 1519–1524.

182. Robertson PL, Schweitzer ME, Mitchell DG, et al. Rotator cuff disorders: interobserver and intraobserver variations in diagnosis with MR imaging. *Radiology* 1995;194:831–835.

183. Farin PU, Jaroma H. Acute traumatic tears of the rotator cuff: value of sonography. *Radiology* 1995;197:269–273.

184. Owen RS, Iannotti JP, Kneeland JB, et al. Shoulder after surgery: MR imaging with surgical validation. *Radiology* 1993;186: 443–447.

185. Park JG, Lee JK, Phelps CT. Os acromiale associated with rotator cuff impingement: MR imaging of the shoulder. *Radiology* 1994; 193:255–257.

186. Sammarco VJ. Os acromiale: frequency, anatomy and clinical implications. *J Bone Joint Surg Am* 2000;82A:394–400.

187. Gold RH, Seeger LL, Yao L. Imaging shoulder impingement. *Skeletal Radiol* 1993;22:555–561.

188. Turkel SJ, Panio MW, Marshall JL, et al. Stabilizing mechanisms prevent anterior dislocation of the glenohumeral joint. *J Bone Joint Surg Am* 1981;63:1208–1217.

189. Epstein RE, Schweitzer ME, Frieman BG, et al. Hooked acromion: prevalence on MR images of painful shoulders. *Radiology* 1993;187:479–481.

190. Edelman RR, Stark DD, Sairi S, et al. Oblique planes of selection in MR imaging. *Radiology* 1986;159:807–810.

191. Bigliani LU, Morrison DS, April EW. The morphology of the acromion and its relationship to rotator cuff tears. *Orthop Trans* 1986;10:228–234.

192. Haygood TM, Langlotz CP, Kneeland JB, et al. Categorization of acromial shape: interobserver variability with MR imaging and conventional radiology. *AJR Am J Roentgenol* 1994;162:1377–1382.

193. Stallenberg B, Rommeris J, Leground C, et al. Radiographic diagnosis of rotator cuff tear based on the supraspinatus muscle radiodensity. *Skeletal Radiol* 2001;30:31–38.

194. Tuite MJ, Toivonen DA, Orwin JF, et al. Accurial angle on radiographs of the shoulder: correlation with impingement syndrome and rotator cuff tears. *AJR Am J Roentgenol* 1995;165: 609–613.

195. Mack LA, Nyberg DA, Matsen FR III, et al. Sonography of the postoperative shoulder. *AJR Am J Roentgenol* 1988;150: 1089–1093.

196. MacNab I, Hastings D. Rotator cuff tendinitis. *Can Med Assoc J* 1968;99:91–98.

197. Neviaser TJ. Tears of the rotator cuff. *Orthop Clin North Am* 1980;11:295–303.

198. Fritz RC. Magnetic resonance imaging of sports related shoulder: impingement and rotator cuff. *Radiol Clin North Am* 2002; 40:217–234.

199. Edelson G, Teitz C. Internal impingement in the shoulder. *J Shoulder Elbow Surg* 2000;9:308–315.

200. Dines DM, Warren RE, Inglis AE, et al. The coracoid impingement syndrome. *J Bone Joint Surg* 1990;72B:314–316.

201. Deutch A, Altchek DW, Veltri DM, et al. Traumatic tears of the subscapularis tendon: clinical diagnosis, MRI findings and operative treatment. *Am J Sports Med* 1997;25:13–22.

202. Bonutti PM, Norfray JF, Friedman RJ, et al. Kinematic MRI of the shoulder. *J Comput Assist Tomogr* 1993;17:666–669.

203. Ozaki J, Fujiuroto S, Nakagawa Y, et al. Tears of the rotator cuff of the shoulder associated with pathologic changes in the acromion. *J Bone Joint Surg Am* 1988;70A:1224–1230.

204. Tuite MJ, Yandow DR, DeSmet AA, et al. Diagnosis of partial and complete rotator cuff tears using combined gradient echo and spin-echo imaging. *Skeletal Radiol* 1994;23:541–546.

205. Beall DP, Williamson EE, Ly JQ, et al. Association of biceps tendon tears with rotator cuff abnormalities: degree of correlation with tears of the anterior and superior portions of the rotator cuff. *AJR Am J Roentgenol* 2003;180:633–639.

206. Resnick DR. Shoulder arthrography. *Radiol Clin North Am* 1981;19:243–255.

207. Paavolainen P, Ahovuo J. Ultrasonography and arthrography in diagnosis of tears of the rotator cuff. *J Bone Joint Surg Am* 1994;76A: 335–340.

208. Zanetti M, Weishaespt D, Jost B, et al. MR imaging for traumatic tears of the rotator cuff: high prevalence of greater tuberosity fractures and subscapulares tendon tears. *AJR Am J Roentgenol* 1999;172:463–467.

209. Balich SM, Sheley RC, Brown TR, et al. MR imaging of the rotator cuff tendon: interobserver agreement and analysis of interpretive errors. *Radiology* 1997;204:191–194.

210. Vahlensieck M, Lang P, Sommer T, et al. Indirect MR arthrography: techniques and applications. *Semin. Ultrasound CT MR* 1997;18:302–306.

211. Meister K, Thesing J, Montgomery WJ, et al. MR arthrography of partial thickness tears of the undersurface of the rotator cuff: an arthroscopic correlation. *Skeletal Radiol* 2004;33:136–141.

212. Resendes M, Helms CA, Eddy R, et al. Double-echo MPGR imaging of the rotator cuff. *J Comput Assist Tomogr* 1991;15:1077–1079.

213. Sahin-Akyar G, Miller TT, Staron RB, et al. Gradient-echo versus fat-suppressed fast spin-echo MR imaging of rotator cuff tears. *AJR Am J Roentgenol* 1998;171:223–227.

214. Teefey SA, Rubin DA, Middleton WD, et al. Detection and quantification of rotator cuff tears. *J Bone Joint Surg Am* 2004;86A:708–716.

215. Karzel RP, Snyder SJ. Magnetic resonance arthrography of the shoulder. A new technique of shoulder imaging. *Clin Sports Med* 1993;12:123–136.

216. Kneeland JB, Middleton WD, Carrera GF, et al. MR imaging of the shoulder: diagnosis of rotator cuff tears. *AJR Am J Roentgenol* 1987;149:333–337.

217. Middleton WD. Sonographic detection and quantification of rotator cuff tears. *AJR Am J Roentgenol* 1993;160:109–110.

218. Monu JUV, Pruett S, Vanarthos WJ, et al. Isolated subacromial bursal fluid on MRI of the shoulder in symptomatic patients: correlation with arthroscopic findings. *Skeletal Radiol* 1994;23: 529–533.

219. Brenner ML, Morrison WB, Carrino JA, et al. Direct MR arthrography of the shoulder: is exercise prior to imaging beneficial or detrimental? *Radiology* 2000;215:491–496.

220. Güchel C, Nidecher A. The rope ladder: an uncommon artifact and potential pitfall in MR arthrography of the shoulder. *AJR Am J Roentgenol* 1997;168:947–950.

221. Guntern DJ, Pfirrmann CWA, Schmid MR, et al. Articular cartilage lesions of the glenohumeral joint: diagnostic effectiveness of MR arthrography and prevalence in patients with subacromial impingement syndrome. *Radiology* 2003;226:165–170.

222. Steinbach LS, Palmer WE, Schweitzer ME. MR arthrography. *Radiographics* 2002;22:1223–1246.

223. Zanetti M, Jost B, Lustenberger A, et al. Clinical impact of MR arthrography of the shoulder. *Acta Radiol* 1999;40:296–302.

224. Rokito AS, Cuomo F, Gallagher MA, et al. Long term functional outcome of repair of large and massive chronic tears of the rotator cuff. *J Bone Joint Surg* 1999;81A:991–997.

225. Bosley RC. Total acromioectomy. *J Bone Joint Surg* 1991;73A: 961–969.

226. Traughber PD, Goodwin TE. Shoulder MRI: arthroscopic correlation with emphasis on partial tears. *J Comput Assist Tomogr* 1992;16:129–133.

227. Farley TE, Neumann CH, Steinbach LS, et al. The coracoacromial arch: MR evaluation and correlation with rotator cuff pathology. *Skeletal Radiol* 1994;23:641–645.

228. Yao L, Mehta U. Infra spinatus muscle atrophy: implications. *Radiology* 2003;226:161–164.

229. Carroll KW, Helms CA, Otte MT, et al. Enlarged spine glenoid notch views causing suprascapular nerve compression. *Skeletal Radiol* 2003;32:72–77.

230. Manton GL, Schweitzer ME, Weishaupt D, et al. Utility of MR arthrography in diagnosis of adhesive capsulitis. *Skeletal Radiol* 2001;30:326–330.

231. Patten RM. Tears of the anterior portion of the rotator cuff the subscapularis tendon: MR imaging finding. *AJR Am J Roentgenol* 1994;162:351–354.

232. Kim TK, Queale WS, Cosgarea AJ, et al. Clinical feature of the different types of SLAP lesions. *J Bone Joint Surg* 2003;85A:66–71.

233. Prato N, Banderali A, Neumaier CE, et al. Calcific tendinitis of the rotator cuff as a cause of drooping shoulder. *Skeletal Radiol* 2003;32:82–85.

234. Thomas J, Colby M. Radiation-induced or metastatic brachial plexopathy. *JAMA* 1971;222:1392–1395.

235. Reinus WR, Shaky XL, Mirowitz S, et al. MR diagnosis of rotator cuff tears of the shoulder: value of using T2-weighted fat saturated images. *AJR Am J Roentgenol* 1995;164:1451–1455.

236. Palmer WE, Brown JH, Rosenthal DI. Rotator cuff evaluation with fat-suppressed MR arthrography. *Radiology* 1993;188:683–687.

237. Lazarus MD, Sidles JA, Harryman DT, et al. Effect of chondral-labral defect on glenoid concavity and glenohumeral stability. *J Bone Joint Surg Am* 1996;78A:94–102.

238. Loew R, Kreitner KF, Runkel M, et al. MR arthrography of the shoulder: comparison of low field (0.2 T) vs high field (1.5 T) imaging. *Eur Radiol* 2000;10:989–996.

239. Coumas JM, Howard BA, Guilford WB. Instability: CT and MR imaging of the shoulder. In: Weissman BN, ed. *RSNA categorical course.* Chicago, IL: RSNA, 1993:113–125.

240. Wolfgang GL. Surgical repair of tears of the rotator cuff of the shoulder. *J Bone Joint Surg Am* 1974;56A:14–26.

241. Gaenslen ES, Satterlee CG, Hinson GW. Magnetic resonance imaging for evaluation of failed repairs of the rotator cuff. *J Bone Joint Surg Am* 1996;78A:1391–1396.

242. Tyson LL, Crues JV III. Pathogenesis of rotator cuff disorders: magnetic resonance imaging characteristics. *Magn Reson Imaging Clin N Am* 1993;1:37–56.

243. Kieft GJ, Bloem JL, Rozing PM, et al. Rotator cuff impingement syndrome: MR imaging. *Radiology* 1988;166:211–214.

244. Wright RW, Fritts HM, Tierney GS, et al. MR imaging of the shoulder after an impingement test: how long to wait. *AJR Am J Roentgenol* 1998;171:769–773.

245. Gotch M, Higuchi F, Suzuki R, et al. Progression from calcifying tendinitis to rotator cuff tear. *Skeletal Radiol* 2003;32:86–89.

246. Kraemer EJ, El-Khoury GY. Atypical calcific tendinitis with cortical erosions. *Skeletal Radiol* 2000;29:690–696.

247. Aina R, Cardinal E, Bureau NJ, et al. Calcific shoulder tendinitis: treatment with modified US-guided fine-needle technique. *Radiology* 2001;221:455–461.

248. Hawkins RJ. The rotator cuff and biceps tendon. In: Evarts CM, ed. *Surgery of the musculoskeletal system.* New York: Churchill Livingstone, 1983.

249. Nixon JE, Distefano V. Ruptures of the rotator cuff. *Orthop Clin North Am* 1975;6:423–447.

250. Rand T, Trattnig S, Breitenseher M, et al. The post-operative shoulder. *Top Magn Reson Imaging* 1999;10(4):203–213.

251. Rothman RH, Marvel JP, Heppenstall RB. Anatomic considerations in the glenohumeral joint. *Orthop Clin North Am* 1975;6:341–352.

252. Magee TH, Gaenslen ES, Seitz R, et al. MR imaging of the shoulder after surgery. *AJR Am J Roentgenol* 1997;168:925–928.

253. Gusmer PB, Potter HG, Donovan WD, et al. MR imaging of the shoulder after rotator cuff repair. *AJR Am J Roentgenol* 1997;168:559–563.

254. Major NM, Banks MC. MR imaging of complications of loose surgical tacks in the shoulder. *AJR Am J Roentgenol* 2003;180:377–380.

255. Norwood L, Fowler EH. Rotator cuff tear: a shoulder arthroscopy complication. *Am J Sports Med* 1989;17:837–841.

256. Baker CL, Liu SH. Comparison of open and arthroscopically assisted rotator cuff repairs. *Am J Sports Med* 1995;23:99–104.

257. Matsen FA, Avtnz CT, Lippitt SB. Rotator cuff. In: Rockwood CE, Matson FA, eds. *The Shoulder.* Philadelphia, PA: WB Saunders, 1998:755–795.

258. Rand T, Freilinger W, Breitenseher M, et al. Magnetic resonance arthrography (MRA) in the post-operative shoulder. *Magn Reson Imaging* 1999;17:843–850.

259. Rockwood CA, Lyons FR. Shoulder impingement syndrome: diagnosis, radiographic evaluation, and treatment with modified neer acromioplasty. *J Bone Joint Surg Am* 1993;75A:409–424.

260. Speilman AL, Forster BB, Koban P, et al. Shoulder after rotator cuff repair: MR findings in asymptomatic individuals—initial experience. *Radiology* 1999;213:705–708.

261. Zanetti M, Jost B, Hodler J, et al. MR imaging after rotator cuff repair: full thickness defects and bursitis-like subacromial abnormalities in asymptomatic subjects. *Skeletal Radiol* 2000;29:314–319.

262. Zanetti M, Weishaupt D, Gerber C, et al. Tendinopathy and rupture of the tendon of the long head of the biceps brachii muscle: evaluation with MR arthrography. *AJR Am J Roentgenol* 1998;170:1557–1561.

263. Zanetti MD, Jost B, Hodler J. MR findings in asymptomatic patients after supraspinatus reconstruction. *Radiology* 1999;213(P):517.

264. De Maeseneer M, Von Roy F, Lenchick L, et al. CT and MR arthrography of normal and pathologic anterosuperior labrum and labral bicipital complex. *Radiographics* 2000;20:S67–S81.

265. Mohana-Borges AYR, Chung CB, Resnick D. Superior labral antero posterior tear: classification and diagnosis on MRI and MR arthrography. *AJR Am J Roentgenol* 2003;181:1449–1462.

266. Oveson J, Sojbjerg JO. Lesions in different types of anterior glenohumeral joint dislocations. *Arch Orthop Trauma Surg* 1986;105:216–218.

267. Shankman S, Bercardino J, Beltran J. Glenohumeral instability: evaluation using MR arthrography of the shoulder. *Skeletal Radiol* 1999;28:365–382.

268. Tockman GA, Devlin TC. Axillary nerve injury after anterior glenohumeral dislocation: MR findings in three patients. *AJR Am J Roentgenol* 1996;167:695–697.

269. Townley CO. The capsular mechanism in recurrent dislocation of the shoulder. *J Bone Joint Surg Am* 1950;32:370–380.

270. Harryman DTII, Sidles JA, Harris SL, et al. The role of the rotator interval capsule in passive motion and stability of the shoulder. *J Bone Joint Surg Am* 1992;74A:53–66.

271. Rose CO, Patel D, Southnayd WW. The Bankart procedure. *J Bone Joint Surg* 1978;60:1–16.

272. Palmer WE, Caslowitz PL, Chew FS. MR arthrography of the shoulder: normal intra-articular structures and common abnormalities. *AJR Am J Roentgenol* 1995;164:141–146.

273. Palmer WE, Caslowitz PL. Anterior shoulder instability: diagnostic criteria determined from prospective analysis of 121 MR arthrograms. *Radiology* 1995;197:819–825.

274. Coumas JM, Waite RJ, Goss TP, et al. CT and MR evaluation of the labral capsular ligamentous complex of the shoulder. *AJR Am J Roentgenol* 1992;158:591–597.

275. Fischbach TJ, Seeger LL. Magnetic resonance imaging of the glenohumeral instability. *Top Magn Reson Imaging* 1994;6:121–132.

276. Flatow EL, Warner JJP. Instability of the shoulder: complex problems and failed repairs. *J Bone Joint Surg* 1998;80A:122–140.

277. Hottya GA, Tirman PFJ, Bost FW, et al. Tear of the posterior stabilizers after posterior shoulder dislocation: MR imaging and MR arthrographic findings with arthroscopic correlation. *AJR Am J Roentgenol* 1998;178:763–768.

278. Huang LF, Rubin DA, Britton CA. Greater tuberosity changes as revealed by radiography: lack of clinical usefulness in patients with rotator cuff disease. *AJR Am J Roentgenol* 1999;172:1381–1388.

279. Ly JQ, Beall DP, Sanders TG. MR imaging of glenohumeral instability. *AJR Am J Roentgenol* 2003;181:203–213.

280. Roger B, Skaf A, Hooper AW, et al. Imaging findings in the dominant shoulder of throwing athletes: comparison of radiography, arthrography, CT arthrography, and MR arthrography with arthroscopic correlation. *AJR Am J Roentgenol* 1999;172:1371–1380.

281. Seeger LL, Gold RH, Bassett LW. Shoulder instability: evaluation with MR imaging. *Radiology* 1988;168:695–697.

282. Shaffer B, Tibone JE, Kerlan RK. Frozen shoulder. *J Bone Joint Surg Am* 1992; 74A:738–746.

283. Schraner AB, Major NM. MR imaging of the subcoracoid bursa. *AJR Am J Roentgenol* 1999;172:1567–1571.

284. Matsen FA, Harryman DT, Sidles JA. Mechanics of glenohumeral stability. *Clin Sports Med* 1991;10:783–792.

285. Bui-Mansfield LT, Taylor DC, Uhorchak JM, et al. Humeral avulsions of the glenohumeral ligament: imaging features and review of the literature. *AJR Am J Roentgenol* 2002;179:649–655.

286. Sugimoto H, Suzuki K, Mihara K, et al. MR arthrography of shoulder after suture-anchor Bankart repair. *Radiology* 2002;224:105–111.

287. Wischer TK, Bredella MA, Genant HK, et al. Perthes lesion (a variant of the Bankart lesion): MR imaging and MR arthrographic findings with surgical correlation. *AJR Am J Roentgenol* 2002;178:233–237.

288. Chandnani VP, Yeager TD, DeBerardino T, et al. Glenoid labral tears: prospective evaluation with MR imaging, MR arthrography and CT arthrography. *AJR Am J Roentgenol* 1993;161:1229–1235.

289. Palmer WE, Brown JH, Rosenthal DI. Labral-ligamentous complex of the shoulder: evaluation with MR arthrography. *Radiology* 1994;190:645–651.

290. Neviaser TJ. The anterior labroligamentous periosteal sleeve avulsion injury: a cause of anterior instability of the shoulder. *Arthroscopy* 1993;9:17–21.

291. Chung CB, Sorenson S, Dwek JR, et al. Humeral avulsion of the posterior band of the inferior glenohumeral ligament: MR arthrography and clinical correlation in 17 patients. *AJR Am J Roentgenol* 2004;183:355–359.

292. Yu JS, Ashman CJ, Jones G. The POLPSA lesion: MR imaging findings with arthroscopic correlation in patients with posterior instability. *Skeletal Radiol* 2002;31:396–399.

293. Ferrari DJ, Ferrari DA, Coumas J, et al. Posterior ossification of the shoulder: the Bennett lesion. Etiology, diagnosis and treatment. *Am J Sports Med* 1994;22:171–176.

294. Cartland JP, Crues JV III, Stauffer A, et al. MR imaging in the evaluation of SLAP injuries of the shoulder: findings in 10 patients. *AJR Am J Roentgenol* 1992;159:787–792.

295. Rames RD, Karzel RP. Injuries to the glenoid labrum, including SLAP lesions. *Orthop Clin North Am* 1993;24:45–53.

296. Hodler J, Kursumoglu-Brahme S, Flannigan B, et al. Injuries of the superior portion of the glenoid labrum involving the insertion of the biceps tendon: MR imaging findings in nine cases. *AJR Am J Roentgenol* 1992;159:565–568.

297. Hunter JC, Blatz DJ, Escobedo EM. SLAP lesions of the glenoid labrum: CT arthrographic and arthroscopic correlation. *Radiology* 1992;184:513–518.

298. Smith AM, McCauley TR, Jokl D. SLAP lesions of the glenoid labrum diagnosed with MR imaging. *Skeletal Radiol* 1993;22:507–510.

299. Snyder SJ, Karzel RP, Del Pizzo W, et al. SLAP lesions of the shoulder. *Arthroscopy* 1990;6:274–279.

300. Snyder SJ, Bonas MP, Karzel RP. Analysis of 140 injuries to the superior glenoid labrum. *J Shoulder Elbow Surg* 1995;4:243–248.

301. Maffett MW, Gartsman GM, Moseley B. Superior labral-biceps tendon complex lesions of the shoulder. *Am J Sports Med* 1995;23:93–98.

302. Morgan CD, Burkhart SS, Palmeri M, et al. Type II SLAP lesions: three subtypes and their relationship to superior instability and rotator cuff tears. *Arthroscopy* 1998;14:553–565.

303. Higgins LD, Warner JJ. Superior labral lesions: anatomy, pathology and treatment. *Clin Orthop* 2001;390:73–82.

304. Monu JUV, Pope TL, Chabon SJ, et al. MR diagnosis of superior labral anterior posterior (SLAP) injuries of the glenoid labrum: value of routine imaging without intra-articular injection of contrast material. *AJR Am J Roentgenol* 1994;163:1425–1429.

305. Tuite MJ, Cirillo RL, DeSmet AA, et al. Superior labrum anterior-posterior (SLAP) tears: evaluation of three MR signs on T2-weighted sequences. *Radiology* 2003;215:841–845.

306. Smith DK, Chopp TM, Aufdemorte TB, et al. Sublabral recess of the superior glenoid labrum: study of cadavers with conventional nonenhanced MR imaging, MR arthrography, anatomic dissection, and limited histologic examination. *Radiology* 1996;201:251–256.

307. Tung GA, Hou DD. MR arthrography of the posterior labrocapsular complex; relationship with glenohumeral joint alignment and clinical posterior instability. *AJR Am J Roentgenol* 2003;180:369–375.

308. Chan KK, Muldoon KA, Yeh L-R, et al. Superior labral anteroposterior lesions: MR arthrography with arm traction. *AJR Am J Roentgenol* 1999;173:1117–1122.

309. Waldt S, Burkart A, Lange P, et al. Diagnostic performance of MR arthrography in assessment of superior labral anterior posterior lesions of the shoulder. *AJR Am J Roentgenol* 2004;182:1271–1278.

310. Wagner SC, Schweitzer ME, Morrison WB, et al. Shoulder instability: accuracy of MR imaging performed after surgery in depicting recurrent injury—initial findings. *Radiology* 2002;222:196–213.

311. Bankart ABS. The pathology and treatment of recurrent dislocation of the shoulder. *Br J Surg* 1938;26:23–39.

312. Spritzer CE, Collins AJ, Cooperman A, et al. Assessment of instability of the long head of the biceps tendon by MRI. *Skeletal Radiol* 2001;30:199–207.

313. Tuckman GA. Abnormalities of the long head of the biceps tendon of the shoulder: MR image findings. *AJR Am J Roentgenol* 1994;163:1183–1188.

314. Cone RO, Danzig L, Resnick D et al, Radiographic, anatomic and pathologic study. The bicipital groove. *AJR Am J Roentgenol* 1983;141:781–788.

315. Falchok FS, Zlatkin MB, Erbacher GE, et al. Rupture of the biceps tendon: evaluation with MR imaging. *Radiology* 1994;190:659–663.

316. Chan TW, Dalinka MK, Kneeland BJ, et al. Biceps tendon dislocation: evaluation with MR imaging. *Radiology* 1991;179:649–652.

317. Pfirrmann CWA, Zanette M, Weishaupt D, et al. Subscapularis tendon tears: detection and grading at MR arthrography. *Radiology* 1999;213:709–714.

318. Tung GA, Yoo DC, Levine SM, et al. Subscapularis tendon tear: primary and associated signs on MRI. *J Comput Assist Tomogr* 2001;25(3):417–424.

319. Li XX, Schweitzer ME, Bifano JA, et al. MR evaluation of the subscapularis tears. *J Comput Assist Tomogr* 1999;23:713–717.

320. Carrino JA, Chandmanni JP, Mitchell DB, et al. Pectoralis major muscle and tendon tears: diagnosis and grading using magnetic resonance imaging. *Skeletal Radiol* 2000;29:305–313.

321. Wolf SW, Wickiewicz TL, Cavanaugh JT. Ruptures of the pectoralis muscle: anatomic and clinical analysis. *Am J Sports Med* 1992;20:587–592.

322. Fritz RC, Helms CA, Steinbach LS. Suprascapular nerve entrapment: evaluation with MR imaging. *Radiology* 1992;182:437–444.

323. Linker CS, Helms CA, Fritz RC. Quadrilateral space syndrome: findings at MR imaging. *Radiology* 1993;188:675–676.

324. Sjöström L. Suprascapular nerve entrapment in an arthrodesed shoulder. *J Bone Joint Surg Br* 1992;74B:470–471.

325. Warner JJP, Krushell RJ, Masquelet A, et al. Anatomy and relationship of the suprascapular nerve: anatomic constraints of mobilization of the supraspinatus and infraspinatus muscles in management of massive rotator cuff tears. *J Bone Joint Surg* 1992;24A:36–45.

326. Green JR, Freehill MG, Buss DD. III Diagnosis and treatment of ganglion cysts about the shoulder. *Tech Shoulder Elbow Surg* 2001;2(2):100–105.

327. Tung GA, Entzian D, Stern JB, et al. MR imaging and MR arthrography of paraglenoid labral cysts. *AJR Am J Roentgenol* 2000;174:1707–1715.

328. Martin SD, Warren RF, Martin TR, et al. Supra scapular neuropathy: results of non-operative treatment. *J Bone Joint Surg* 1997;79A:1159–1165.

329. Hodler J, Loredo RA, Longo C, et al. Assessment of articular cartilage thickness of the humeral head: MR—anatomic correlation in cadavers. *AJR Am J Roentgenol* 1995;165:615–620.

330. Spritzer CE, Dalinka MK, Kressel HY, et al. Magnetic resonance imaging of pigmented villonodular synovitis: a report of two cases. *AJR Am J Roentgenol* 1986;147:67–71.

331. Yeh LR, Kwak S, Kun Y-S, et al. Evaluation of articular cartilage thickness of the humeral head and glenoid fossa by MR arthrography: anatomic correlation in cadavers. *Skeletal Radiol* 1998;27:500–504.

332. Zlatkin MB, Dalinka MK. Crystal deposition diseases: current concepts. *Postgrad Radiol* 1988;8:88–98.

333. Burk DL, Karasick D, Mitchell DG, et al. MR imaging of the shoulder: correlation with plain radiography. *AJR Am J Roentgenol* 1990;154:549–553.

334. Burk LD, Torres JL, Marone PJ, et al. MR imaging of shoulder improves in professional baseball players. *J Magn Reson Imaging* 1991;1:385–389.

335. McCarty DJ, Halverson PB, Carrera GF, et al. "Milwaukee Shoulder"–association of microspheroids containing hydroxyapatite crystals, active collagenase, and neutral protease with rotator cuff defects. I. Clinical Aspects. *Arthritis Rheum* 1981;24:464–472.

336. Beltran J, Simon DC, Katz W, et al. Increased MR signal intensity in skeletal muscle adjacent to malignant tumors: pathology correlation and clinical relevance. *Radiology* 1987;162:251–255.

337. Mitchell DG, Kundel JL, Steinberg ME, et al. Avascular necrosis of the hip: comparison of and scintigraphy. *AJR Am J Roentgenol* 1996;147:67–71.

338. Blackson MR, Beuovenia J. Neoplasms of the scapula. *AJR Am J Roentgenol* 2000;174:1729–1735.

339. Sundaram M, McDonald DJ. The solitary tumor or tumor like lesion of bone. *Top Magn Reson Imaging* 1989;1(4):17–29.

340. Unni KK. Dahlin's bone tumors. *General aspects and data on 11,087 cases*, 5th ed. Philadelphia, PA: Lippincott-Raven, 1996.

341. O'Connor EE, Dixon LB, Peabody T, et al. MRI of cystic and soft tissue masses of the shoulder. *AJR Am J Roentgenol* 2004;183:39–47.

342. Sundaram M, McGuire MH, Fletcher J, et al. Magnetic resonance imaging of lesions of synovial origin. *Skeletal Radiol* 1986;15:110–116.

343. Weiss SW, Goldblum JP. *Enzinger and Weiss's soft tissue tumors*, 4th ed. St. Louis, MO: Mosby, 2001.

344. Czervionki LF, Daniels DL, Ho PSP, et al. Cervical neural foramina: correlative anatomic and MR imaging studies. *Radiology* 198;169:753–759.

345. Iyer RB, Fenstermacher MJ, Libshitz HI. MR imaging of the treated brachial plexus. *AJR Am J Roentgenol* 1996;167:225–229.

346. Lin J, Mantel W. Cross sectional imaging of peripheral nerve sheath tumors: characteristic signs on CT, MR imaging and sonography. *AJR Am J Roentgenol* 2001;176:75–82.

347. Tsairis P, Dyck P, Mukler DW. Natural history of brachial plexus neuropathy: report of 99 patients. *Arch Neurol* 1972;27:109–117.

348. Helms CA, Martinez S, Speer KP. Acute brachial neuritis (Parsonage-Turner Syndrome): MR imaging appearance—report of 3 cases. *Radiology* 1999;207:255–259.

Elbow and Forearm

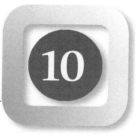

10

Thomas H. Berquist   *Laura W. Bancroft*

Magnetic resonance imaging (MRI) of the elbow and forearm can clearly define normal bone and soft tissue anatomy and pathology (1–4). Clinical information (symptomatic region, the relationship of symptoms to flexion, extension, pronation, and supination) and the type of pathology suspected are important in planning the MRI examination. To solve a given clinical problem, the patient must be comfortable, properly positioned, and the best image planes and pulse sequences selected to optimize lesion identification and characterization.

TECHNIQUE

Patient Positioning and Coil Selection

Patient positioning is as important with MRI as with other radiographic techniques (see Chapter 3). The types of coils available, gantry limitations, patient size, and clinical status may lead to suboptimal examinations, particularly in the upper extremity. The confining nature of the most high field strength MR gantries, excluding open and extremity systems, reduces positioning options, especially for larger patients (1–5). Patients are usually most comfortable when supine with the elbow extended, forearm supinated, and arm at their side (see Fig. 10-1). A dedicated circumferential elbow coil can be used in this position (see Fig. 10-2A). The larger phased array coil is preferred for examination of larger areas such as the forearm or forearm and elbow (see Fig. 10-2B).

Different positions and coils may be required with larger patients (2,3,5,6). With larger patients, the elbow

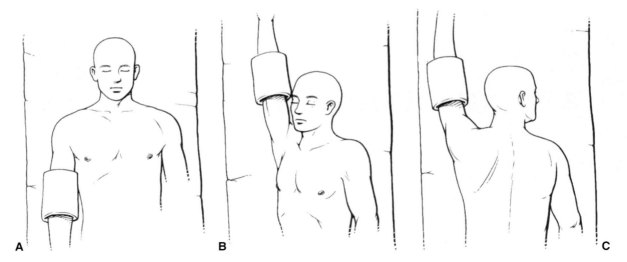

Figure 10-1 Illustration of positions for imaging the elbow. Positioning the arm **(A)** at the side is most comfortable for the patient. When the arm is positioned **(B,C)** above the head, the patients have more difficulty tolerating the examination. The patient is rotated in **B,** which is often necessary with larger patients or when elbow flexion is needed to evaluate the biceps tendon.

may have to be positioned with the arm above the head and the elbow extended as much as possible (Superman position) and the patient in a rotated or prone position (Fig. 10-1) (1–3,5). In this setting, the prone position with the arm above the head is most often selected (1,7–9). Unfortunately, patient discomfort can be significant when the arm is above the head. As a result, images may be degraded by motion artifact. In our initial review of 200 upper extremity cases, we found image degradation due to motion in 25%. Motion artifact is usually not a problem when the patient is supine with the arm at the side (1,2). These positioning approaches can be used with children and adults.

The site of pain or suspected pathology can be marked with a vitamin E capsule. However, care should be taken

not to compress or distort the underlying soft tissues. Marking the symptomatic site is particularly useful when the study is normal (3). Oral sedation may be required in children under 5 years of age (see Chapter 3) (10).

In certain situations, such as biceps insertion pathology, positioning the patient with the elbow flexed displays anatomy to better advantage (see Fig. 10-3). This may be impossible with large patients. Smaller patients can be rotated into the oblique position with the elbow flexed at the side. Axial examinations during pronation and supination are also useful for evaluating the biceps tendon and subtle abnormalities in the radioulnar joint. Both axial and sagittal images should be obtained. When motion studies are required, we have used gradient echo (GRE) sequences (see below) and cine studies. Quick et al. (11) used fast imaging

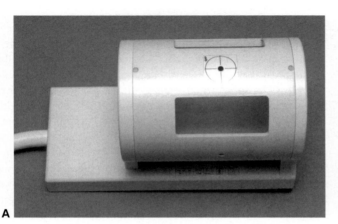
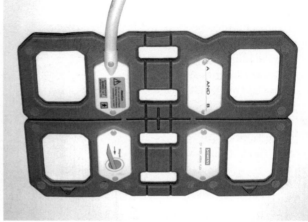

Figure 10-2 Photographs of the elbow **(A)** and larger phased-array **(B)** coils.

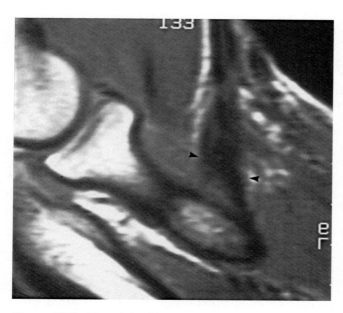

Figure 10-3 Normal distal biceps tendon. Sagittal T1-weighted image with the elbow flexed demonstrates the biceps tendon as it expands (*arrowheads*) near its attachment on the tuberosity of the radius.

steady state precession (FISP) sequence to perform motion studies of the elbow and other joints. True FISP is a steady state precession GRE sequence. The parameters used in this study include repetition time/echo time (TR/TE) of 2.2/1.1 ms, flip angle (FA) 50°, field of view (FOV) 12 to 27 cm, section thickness of 6 mm, and a 256 × 135 matrix (11).

Giuffre and Moss (12) used the flexed abducted supinated position to evaluate the biceps tendon. The elbow is flexed with the arm above the head and the forearm positioned with the thumb up (see Fig. 10-4). This approach improves the ability to include the entire biceps tendon in the image

plane enhancing the ability to differentiate partial from complete tears and other subtle pathology. This position may be difficult to maintain, resulting in motion artifact (1,2).

Comparison of both extremities is useful in patients with subtle pathology. This doubles the examination time with conventional coils. Dual coils allow simultaneous examinations of both upper extremities. This will reduce image time significantly without reduction in image quality (13–15).

Recently, Yoshioka et al. (16) used microscopic coils to evaluate the elbow. Their work is preliminary. Conventional pulse sequences, FOV of 5 to 7 cm, image matrix of 140 to 224 × 512, 2 to 6 acquisitions, and a 14 × 17 cm flex coil with a 23 mm microscopic coil were used together to evaluate the elbow. Signal to noise ratios and spatial resolution were improved compared to conventional coil techniques (16).

Other general parameters for elbow imaging include a small FOV (10 to12 cm); 256 × 192, 256 × 256, 512 × 512 matrixes; and 1 to 2 acquisitions. Section thickness varies with the area of interest and volume of tissue, but it is typically 4 mm or less in the elbow (Table 10-1). A larger FOV is required to examine the forearm or the elbow and forearm together.

Pulse Sequences and Image Planes

Image planes for the elbow and forearm include axial, sagittal, coronal, oblique, and reformatting of thin-section GRE images (1–3,5,17). The axial image plane is useful for neurovascular, tendon, and muscle anatomy. The sagittal plane is useful as a second plane for biceps and triceps tears or to define the extent of a lesion identified on axial images. The coronal plane is useful for evaluating the articular surfaces and the collateral ligaments (2,3). Some authors suggest oblique coronal (parallel to the humeral shaft with the elbow slightly flexed) image planes for evaluating the collateral ligaments (17,18). Reformatting thin (1 mm) GRE image blocks or three-dimensional imaging also provides the flexibility to align complex anatomic structures. Soft tissue contrast is reduced with these sequences compared to conventional or fast spin-echo (FSE) sequences (2,3,5,19).

We begin most examinations with a coronal scout image (Table 10-1) which takes 26 seconds to perform (see Fig. 10-5). Three to five 1-cm-thick images are obtained using a large FOV (32 to 40 cm).

Axial images are obtained using T1-weighted and either FSE T2-weighted or fast STIR sequences. The section thickness is typically 4 mm. Image planes are matched with the T1- and T2-weighted sequences to allow comparison of sections. Additional T2-weighted FSE images are obtained in the coronal and sagittal planes (Table 10-1). We also obtain dual echo steady state (DESS) images in the coronal plane using 1-mm sections to better evaluate the articular cartilage and collateral ligaments.

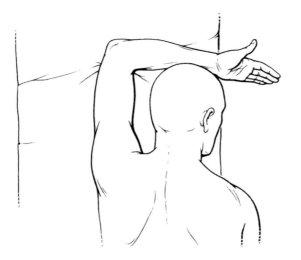

Figure 10-4 Illustration of the flexed abducted supinated view for evaluation of the biceps tendon. The thumb is up.

TABLE 10-1
ROUTINE EXAMINATION MRI OF THE ELBOW AND FOREARM

	Pulse Sequence	Slice Thickness	FOV	Matrix	Excitations (NEX)	Image Time
Scout (coronal)	15/5, FA 40	1 cm/skip 0.5 mm	32–40	256 × 128	1	26 s
Axial T1-weighted	SE 530/17	4 mm	8–12	512 × 512	1	4 min 35 s
Axial STIR	7,090/101, TI 160	4 mm/skip 0.04 mm	8–12	256 × 256	2	4 min 38 s
Or						
Axial T-2 weighted FSE with FS	4,000/102, ETL 8	4 mm/skip 0.04 mm	8–12	256 × 256	2	3 min 18 s
Coronal T2-weighted FSE with FS	4,000/102, ETL 8	4 mm/skip 0.04 mm	8–12	256 × 256	2	3 min 18 s
Coronal DESS	23.87/6.73	1 mm/22/slab	12–14	256 × 256	1	4 min 36 s
MR arthrography						
Axial T1-weighted with FS	500/12	4 mm/skip 0.5 mm	10–14	256 × 256	1	3 min 16 s
Sagittal T1-weighted with FS	500/12	4 mm/skip 0.5 mm	10–14	256 × 256	1	3 min 16 s
Coronal T1-weighted with FS	500/12	4 mm/skip 0.5 mm	10–14	256 × 256	1	3 min 16 s
Coronal PD FSE	2,000/19	4 mm/skip 0.5 mm	10–14	256 × 256	1	3 min 30 s
Coronal T2 FSE with FS	4,140/92	4 mm/skip 0.5 mm	10–14	256 × 256	1	3 min 20 s

SE, spin echo; FA, flip angle; FSE, fast spin echo; FS, fat suppression; DESS, dual echo steady state; PD, proton density

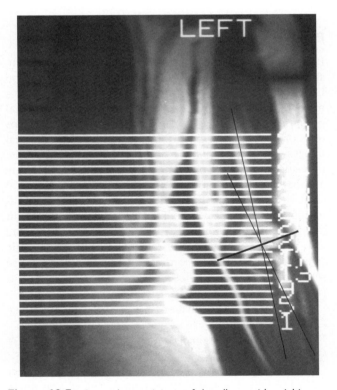

Figure 10-5 Coronal scout image of the elbow with axial image planes selected. The left side of the trunk is also seen due to the large (40 cm) field of view. The axis of the humerus and forearm (*dark lines*) must be considered to obtain true axial images. The normal carrying angle of the elbow is 3° to 29°. Therefore, axial images of the forearm need to be angled (*black transverse line*).

Intravenous gadolinium is commonly given to improve evaluation of synovial, osseous, and soft tissue lesions. Fat-suppressed postcontrast T1-weighted images are obtained in the two most appropriate image planes.

GRE sequences provide less soft tissue contrast, but can be useful for motion studies or reformatting to improve anatomic alignment of structures. Parameters include 400 to 450 TR, 20 TE, FA 45°, and 1-mm sections with a 256 × 256 matrix and two acquisitions (1,3,5). Motion studies may include axial images in differing degrees of pronation and supination or sagittal images in different degrees of flexion and extension. The latter are more difficult to perform in closed high field strength magnets.

We have not performed elbow arthrography commonly in our practice. However, this technique is more optimal for loose bodies when there is no joint effusion, capsular and ligament tears and osteochondral lesions (3,20,21). The elbow can be entered laterally (radio-capitellar joint) or posteriorly in the olecranon fossa. We inject 4 to 5 ccs of diluted gadolinium (1 mmol solution). Gadolinium is mixed with a solution of 50% Marcaine and 50% iodinated contrast. This assists with confirming needle position and confirming that pain, if present, is intraarticular. Following injection, fat-suppressed T1-weighted images are obtained in the axial, coronal, and sagittal planes. In addition, we obtain T2-weighted fat-suppressed FSE images in the coronal plane to better evaluate the capsule and collateral ligaments.

ANATOMY

Anatomy of the elbow and forearm is complex but effectively demonstrated by MRI (see Figs.10-6 to 10-8) (2,3,22–24).

Articular Structures

The elbow articulations are formed by three osseous structures. The lower end of the humerus, consisting of the capitellum and the trochlea, articulates with the radial head and ulna, respectively (Fig. 10-7). The radial head also articulates with the adjacent radial notch of the ulna (Fig. 10-6C) (24–26). This allows the radial head to rotate, providing supination and pronation of the forearm. The trochlear notch of the olecranon surrounds almost 180° of the trochlea, making the elbow one of the most inherently stable joints in humans (27,28). The distal articular surface of the humerus is tilted 30° anteriorly and there is a posterior tilt of the trochlear notch, yielding a resistance to posterior subluxation of the elbow in both flexion and extension (28). The ulnohumeral articulation is the most important stabilizer of the elbow under varus stress, providing 55% of the resistance to varus stress when the elbow is fully extended and 75% of the resistance when the elbow is flexed 90°. The remainder of the stabilization is provided by the capsuloligamentous structures (28). All articular surfaces are covered with hyaline cartilage; this cartilage is best appreciated on DESS or FSE proton-density images (2,19,29).

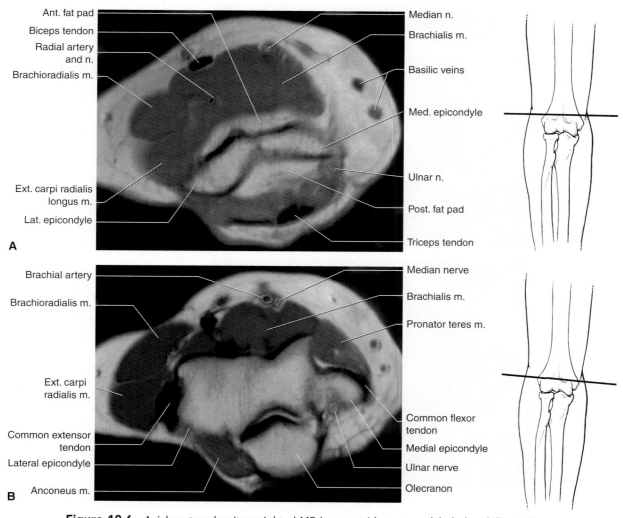

Figure 10-6 Axial proton density-weighted MR images with anatomy labeled and illustration demonstrating the level of section. **A:** Axial image through the supracondylar region. **B:** Axial image through the medial and lateral epicondyle. **C:** Axial image through the radial head. **D:** Axial image at a level just distal to the radial head. **E:** Axial image at the level of the radial tuberosity. **F:** Axial image below the tuberosity level. **G:** Axial image of the proximal forearm.

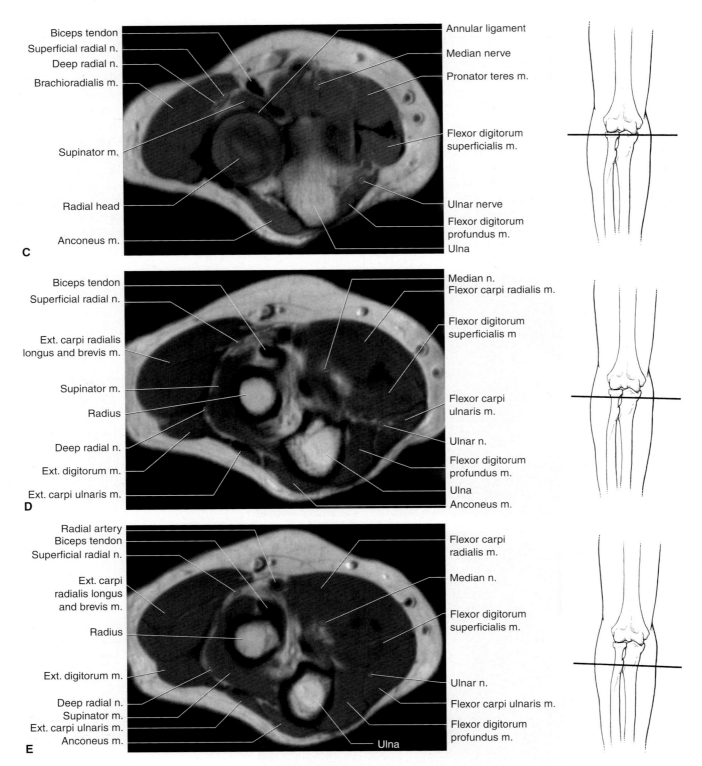

Biceps tendon
Superficial radial n.
Deep radial n.
Brachioradialis m.

Supinator m.

Radial head

Anconeus m.

C

Annular ligament
Median nerve
Pronator teres m.

Flexor digitorum
superficialis m.

Ulnar nerve
Flexor digitorum
profundus m.
Ulna

Biceps tendon
Superficial radial n.

Ext. carpi radialis
longus and brevis m.

Supinator m.
Radius

Deep radial n.
Ext. digitorum m.
Ext. carpi ulnaris m.
D

Median n.
Flexor carpi radialis m.

Flexor digitorum
superficialis m

Flexor carpi
ulnaris m.

Ulnar n.
Flexor digitorum
profundus m.
Ulna
Anconeus m.

Radial artery
Biceps tendon
Superficial radial n.

Ext. carpi
radialis longus
and brevis m.

Radius

Ext. digitorum m.

Deep radial n.
Supinator m.
Ext. carpi ulnaris m.
Anconeus m.
E

Flexor carpi
radialis m.

Median n.

Flexor digitorum
superficialis m.

Ulnar n.
Flexor carpi ulnaris m.

Flexor digitorum
profundus m.
Ulna

Figure 10-6 (continued)

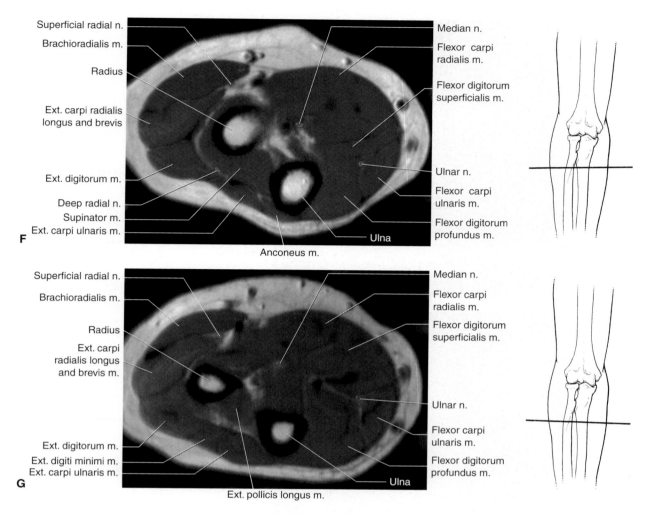

F — Superficial radial n., Brachioradialis m., Radius, Ext. carpi radialis longus and brevis, Ext. digitorum m., Deep radial n., Supinator m., Ext. carpi ulnaris m., Median n., Flexor carpi radialis m., Flexor digitorum superficialis m., Ulnar n., Flexor carpi ulnaris m., Flexor digitorum profundus m., Ulna, Anconeus m.

G — Superficial radial n., Brachioradialis m., Radius, Ext. carpi radialis longus and brevis m., Ext. digitorum m., Ext. digiti minimi m., Ext. carpi ulnaris m., Ext. pollicis longus m., Median n., Flexor carpi radialis m., Flexor digitorum superficialis m., Ulnar n., Flexor carpi ulnaris m., Flexor digitorum profundus m., Ulna

Figure 10-6   (*continued*)

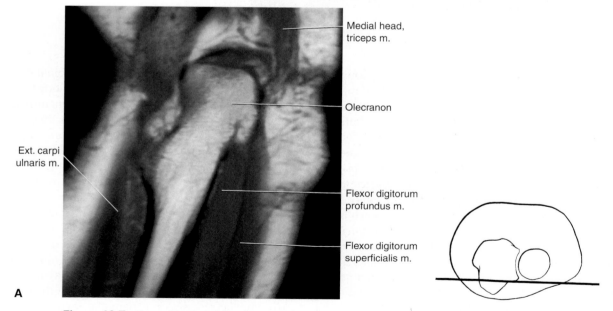

Medial head, triceps m., Olecranon, Ext. carpi ulnaris m., Flexor digitorum profundus m., Flexor digitorum superficialis m.

A

Figure 10-7   Coronal image of the elbow and forearm with anatomy labeled and illustration demonstrating the section level. **A:** Coronal image through the posterior elbow and forearm. **B:** Coronal image through the mid elbow and forearm. **C:** Coronal image through the anterior elbow and forearm.

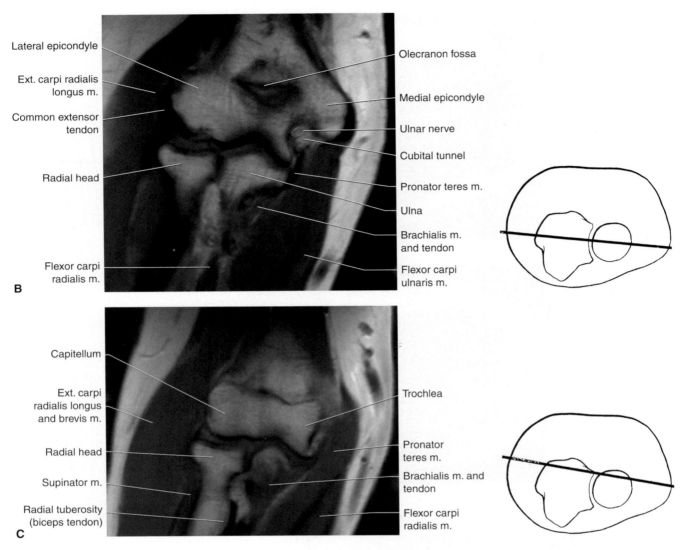

Figure 10-7 (continued)

The articular capsule of the elbow is thin anteriorly and posteriorly with additional support provided anteriorly by the brachialis muscle and posteriorly by the triceps muscle (see Fig. 10-9). The anterior capsule attaches to the humerus just above the radial and coronoid fossa and extends beyond the coronoid process of the ulna to the anterior portion of the annular ligament (Fig. 10-9). The posterior capsule is closely related to the triceps tendon and attaches to the humerus above the olecranon fossa, attaching inferiorly to the upper and lateral margins of the trochlear notch of the ulna, the roughened area on the lateral side of the ulna, and the annular ligament (Fig. 10-9). Medially and laterally, the capsule blends with the medial and lateral collateral ligaments (see Figs. 10-9 and 10-10). The capsule is not usually clearly demonstrated on MRI unless there is an effusion or MR arthrography has been used. In this setting, it is often best appreciated on axial and sagittal images (Figs. 10-6 and 10-9).

It may be difficult to separate the capsule from the brachialis muscle anteriorly and triceps tendon posteriorly (24,30).

Five main synovial recesses can be distinguished within the elbow joint on MRI, especially when there is a joint effusion or when MR arthrography is performed (23).

The olecranon recess is the largest of the five, and is subdivided into the superior, medial, and lateral olecranon recesses. The anterior humeral recess is divided into the coronoid and radial fossae. The annular recess surrounds the radial neck. The ulnar collateral ligament (UCL) and radial collateral ligament (RCL) recesses are deep in the respective UCL and RCL. Synovial folds of various sizes and shapes normally project into the joint space and should not be mistaken for intraarticular loose bodies (23). These synovial folds usually occur at the junction of two synovial recesses or a triangular meniscus-like structure at the joint line margin (23).

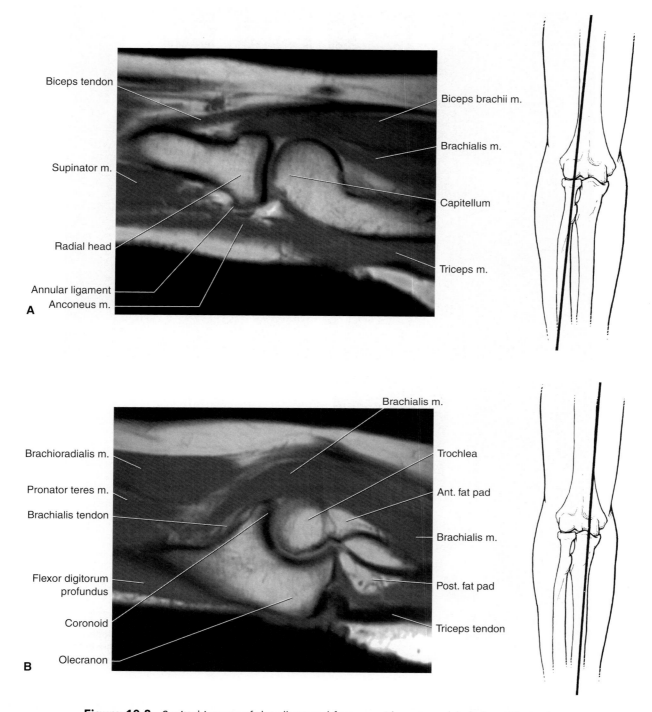

Figure 10-8 Sagittal images of the elbow and forearm with anatomy labeled and illustration demonstrating the section level. **A:** Sagittal image through the lateral radiocapitellar joint. **B:** Sagittal image through the ulnar-trochlear articulation.

Ligaments

Supplementary support for the elbow is provided medially and laterally by the radial and ulnar collateral ligament complexes (see Fig. 10-10 and 10-11) (24,30). These ligaments can be identified on the coronal, posterior coronal oblique, and axial MRIs (Fig. 10-10) (2,17,23). Varus and valgus injuries to the elbow can result in disruption of either the radial or ulnar collateral ligaments and capsule (2,30–33). Therefore, these structures need to be further

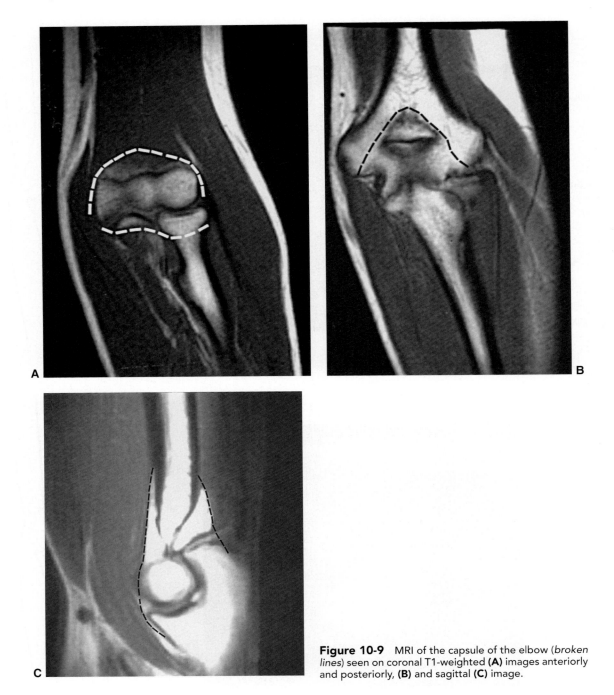

Figure 10-9 MRI of the capsule of the elbow (*broken lines*) seen on coronal T1-weighted **(A)** images anteriorly and posteriorly, **(B)** and sagittal **(C)** image.

defined (Fig. 10-11). The ulnar (medial) collateral ligament is much stronger than the radial (lateral) collateral ligament (24). The UCL is comprised of three bands that are in continuity with each other. The anterior band is the dominant structure and the primary constraint resisting valgus stress on the elbow (24,31,34). It courses anteriorly from the anteroinferior surface of the epicondyle to attach the medial edge of the coronoid process (Fig. 10-11A). The posterior band is smaller and has a fan-like configuration (21). It extends from behind the medial epicondyle and courses slightly posteriorly to attach onto the medial aspect of the

olecranon (Fig. 10-11A). The transverse band is clinically less significant, small, or sometimes absent, and is often difficult to identify on MRI (2,3,21).

The RCL complex is composed of the lateral ulnar collateral ligament, radial collateral ligament, and annular ligament (Fig. 10-11B). The lateral UCL (LUCL) originates from the lateral epicondyle, extends distally along the posterior radial head, blends with some fibers of the annular ligament, then courses obliquely and medially to attach onto the proximal supinator crest of the ulna (17). The LUCL is the primary stabilizer against varus stress, and its

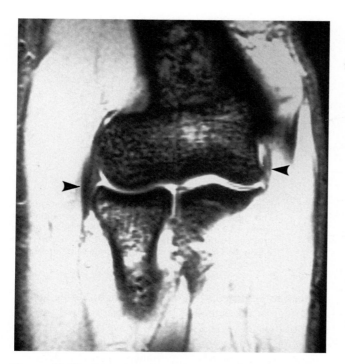

Figure 10-10 Coronal gradient-echo image of the elbow demonstrates the radial and ulnar collateral ligaments (*arrowheads*).

disruption can lead to posterolateral rotatory instability of the elbow (35). The radial collateral ligament arises from the anterior inferior aspect of the lateral epicondyle, deep to the common extensor tendon. It extends distally to insert onto the annular ligament and fibers of the supinator muscle (Fig. 10-11B). The annular ligament encircles the proximal radial neck and attaches anteriorly and posteriorly onto the radial notch of the ulna (Fig. 10-11B). There is an additional ligament, the quadrate ligament, that extends between the radial neck and ulna (24,34).

Bursae

There are several important superficial and deep bursae about the elbow that should be emphasized because of the potential for confusion with cysts or other pathology on MRI. Superficial bursae include the olecranon, medial, and lateral epicondylar bursae. There are three potential olecranon bursae locations. The most common is the subcutaneous olecranon bursa. There are also intratendinous and subtendinous bursae in the olecranon region (see Fig. 10-12) (Table 10-2) (24,30). The subtendinous bursa (bicipitoradialis) is best seen on axial and sagittal MR images and should not be confused with an elbow effusion. An inflamed bursa

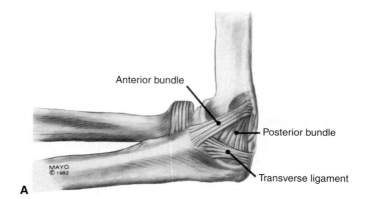

A

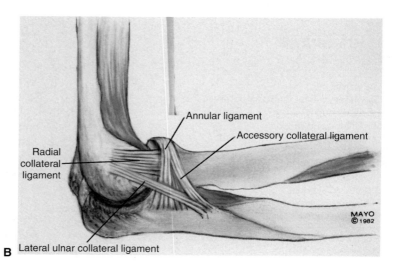

B

Figure 10-11 Lateral illustrations of the ligaments of the elbow from the medial (**A**) and lateral (**B**) sides. (From Morrey BF. *The elbow and its disorders*, 2nd ed. Philadelphia: WB Saunders, 1993.)

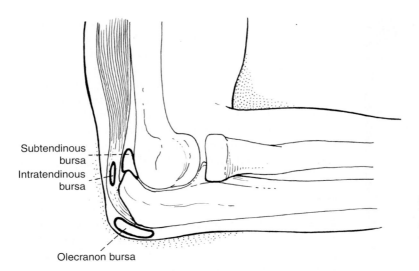

Subtendinous bursa

Intratendinous bursa

Olecranon bursa

Figure 10-12 Illustration of the olecranon bursae. The superficial subcutaneous bursa is most commonly seen. The intratendinous and subtendinous bursae are less frequently identified. (From Morrey BF. *The elbow and its disorders*, 2nd ed. Philadelphia, PA: WB Saunders, 1993.)

can be differentiated from a simple effusion by the lack of fluid in the anterior compartment of the elbow. The other two superficial bursae, the medial epicondylar and lateral epicondylar, should not be confused with disruptions or tears in the medial and lateral collateral ligaments. Figure 10-13 demonstrates the location of the other superficial and deep bursa in the elbow region. The relationship of these bursae to branches of the radial and ulnar nerves (Fig. 10-13) is important (24,30). These bursae are normally not identified, but when inflamed and fluid-filled (due to trauma, infection, synovitis, or gout), they can be demonstrated on T2-weighted or GRE images (5). In this setting, the bursae will appear as homogeneous, high intensity structures with clearly defined margins (1,2).

Muscles of the Elbow and Forearm

The muscular anatomy of the elbow and forearm is complex (Tables 10-3 and 10-4) (24,30,36). Generally, there are four basic movements in the elbow and forearm. The elbow is limited to flexion and extension. Pronation and supination

TABLE 10-2
ELBOW BURSAE

Superficial
Olecranon (subcutaneous, intratendinous, subtendinous)
Medial epicondylar
Lateral epicondylar
Deep
Radiohumeral bursa
Supinator bursa
Bicipitoradial bursa
Subextensor carpi radialis brevis bursa
Ulnar nerve bursa

From Morrey BF. *The elbow and its disorders*, 3rd ed. Philadelphia, PA: WB Saunders, 2000.

occurs between the radius and ulna. It should be kept in mind that in the extended position, the normal carrying angle of the elbow ranges from 3° to 29° (Fig. 10-5). When discussing the muscles of the elbow and forearm, it is simplest to discuss them based upon their function (Tables 10-3 and 10-4) (24,26,30).

There are two major categories as described above, namely flexors and extensors, and pronators and supinators. The chief flexors of the elbow are the biceps, brachialis, and brachioradialis (see Figs. 10-6, 10-8, and 10-14) (Table 10-3). The biceps brachii crosses the elbow anteriorly to insert onto the radial tubercle and serves as a supinator and flexor (Figs. 10-3, 10-6, and 10-14) (24). The brachialis is a large muscle that arises from the anterior humerus and passes anterior to the elbow before inserting onto the proximal ulna near the coronoid process (Figs. 10-6, 10-7, and 10-14). The brachioradialis arises from the radial side of the distal humerus (Fig. 10-14), crosses the lateral epicondyle, and extends distally to insert just proximal to the metaphysis of the radius (Figs. 10-6 through 10-8). In its activity as a flexor, the brachioradialis is aided by the adjacent muscles of the extensor group, especially the extensor carpi radialis longus (3,24,30). A fourth and less important flexor of the elbow is the pronator teres, which functions optimally only when the forearm is pronated. The pronator teres arises from the supracondylar portion of the humerus, extends obliquely across the medial aspect of the elbow, and inserts onto the upper third of the radius (Figs. 10-6, 10-7, and 10-14) (24,30).

Extension of the elbow (Table 10-3) is accomplished primarily by the triceps, especially the medial head, and the anconeus (see Figs. 10-6, 10-8, and 10-15) (24,25). The triceps (Fig. 10-15) takes its origin (three heads) from the infraglenoid tubercle of the scapula, posterior humerus above the radial groove, and the lower posterior humerus (24,30,37). It inserts onto the olecranon. The anconeus (Figs. 10-6 and 10-15) arises from the posterior lateral epicondyle and extends distally and medially to insert onto the lateral ulna (Fig. 10-15).

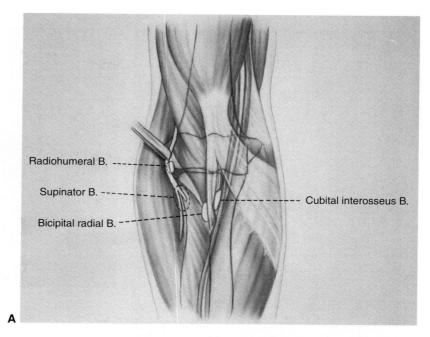

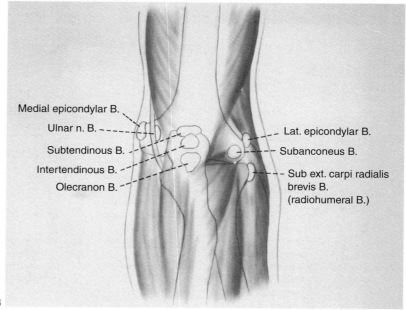

Figure 10-13 Illustrations of the bursae of the elbow as seen **(A)** anteriorly and **(B)** posteriorly. Note the relationship of the bursae to the ulnar nerve and neural branches anteriorly. T2-weighted sagittal. **(C)** and axial **(D)** images in a patient with olecranon bursitis demonstrate fluid distending the olecranon bursa (*arrows*). (From Morrey BF. *The elbow and its disorders*, 2nd ed. Philadelphia, PA: WB Saunders, 1993, with permission.)

The main pronators of the radius and ulna are the pronator teres proximally and the pronator quadratus distally (Tables 10-3 and 10-4) (see Fig. 10-16). The pronator teres (Figs. 10-6, 10-8, and 10-16) originates from the medial supracondylar ridge and coronoid of the ulna. It passes distally and laterally to insert onto the lateral aspect of the midradius (24,25). The origins and insertions of the pronator quadratus are discussed in Chapter 11.

Supination is accomplished by the supinator and biceps brachii muscles, with some supination resulting from contraction of the extensor pollicis longus, abductor pollicis longus, and, to a lesser extent, the extensor carpi radialis longus and brachioradialis (see Fig. 10-17) (24,30). The supinator (Figs. 10-6 and 10-17) originates from the lateral epicondyle, lateral collateral ligament complex, and adjacent ulna. The muscle passes distally to insert onto the upper lateral radius (24,25). The muscles responsible for pronation are almost exclusively innervated by the median nerve, while those responsible for supination are innervated by the musculocutaneous and radial nerves (Table 10-3) (24).

The majority of the forearm muscles arise from the humerus and cross the elbow prior to inserting distally (31,32,38). The flexor group arises from the medial humerus and/or ulna. This muscle group is innervated by both the median and ulnar nerves, but the median nerve is the major contributor (Table 10-4). The extensors arise from

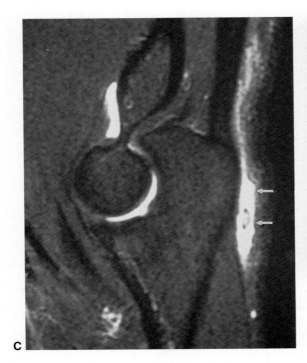

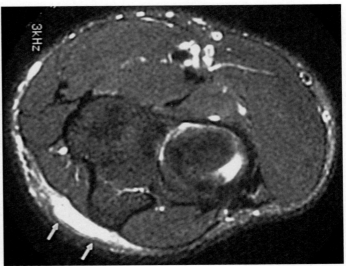

Figure 10-13 *(continued)*

TABLE 10-3
MUSCLES OF THE ELBOW

Muscle	Origin	Insertion	Action	Blood Supply	Innervation
Biceps brachii	Two heads 1) Supraglenoid tubercle 2) Coracoid	1) Radial tuberosity (bursa separates tendon from tuberosity) 2) Aponeurosis to forearm flexors	Elbow flexor supinator	Brachial branches	Musculocutaneous C5–C6
Brachialis	Low 2/3 anterior humerus	Coronoid and ulnar tuberosity	Elbow flexor	Brachial branches	Musculocutaneous C5–C6
Brachioradialis	Supracondylar ridge lateral humerus	Distal lateral radius	Elbow flexor	Radial and radial recurrent arteries	Radial C5–C6
Pronator teres	Two heads 1) Medial supracondylar ridge and interosseous membrane 2) Coronoid of ulna	Midlateral radius	Pronation accessory elbow flexor	Ulnar and recurrent ulnar arteries	Median C5–C7
Triceps brachii	Three heads 1) Infraglenoid tubercle 2) Posterior humerus above radial groove 3) Lower 2/3	Olecranon	Elbow extensor	Profunda brachii	Radial
Anconeus	Posterolateral epicondyle	Lateral olecranon and proximal ulna	Elbow extensor	Recurrent radial artery	Radial
Supinator	Lateral epicondyle, radial ligament, annular ligament, ulna	Upper lateral radius	Supination	Radial artery	Median

From Berquist TH. *MRI of the musculoskeletal system*, 4th ed. Philadelphia, PA: Lippincott Williams & Wilkins, 2001; Rosse C, Rosse PC. *Hollinshead's textbook of anatomy*. Philadelphia, PA: Lippincott–Raven, 1997; and Morrey BF. *The elbow and its disorders*, 3rd ed. Philadelphia, PA: WB Saunders, 2000.

TABLE 10-4
MUSCLES OF THE FOREARM

Muscles	Origin	Insertion	Action	Innervation
Flexors				
Superficial group				
Pronator teres	Two heads 1) Medial supracondylar ridge and interosseous membrane 2) Coronoid of ulna	Midlateral radius	Pronator, elbow flexor	Median C5–C7
Flexor carpi radialis	Common flexor tendon (medial epicondyle)	Second metacarpal base	Wrist flexor	Median
Palmaris longus	Common flexor tendon (medial epicondyle)	Palmar aponeurosis	Wrist flexor	Median
Flexor carpi ulnaris	Two heads 1) Common flexor tendon 2) Upper radius and distal to tubercle	Hamate hook and 5th metacarpal base	Wrist flexor	Ulnar nerve
Intermediate group				
Flexor digitorum superficialis	Two heads 1) Common flexor tendon 2) Upper radius and distal to tubercle	Base 2–5 middle phalanx	Flexion proximal interphalangeal joints	Median
Deep group				
Flexor digitorum profundus	Anterior 2/3 ulna and interosseous membrane	Distal phalanges 2–5	Flexion of fingers	Median and ulnar
Flexor pollicis longus	Middle 1/3 radius and interosseous membrane	Distal phalanx thumb	Thumb flexor	Median
Pronator quadratus	Distal 1/4 anterior ulna	Distal 1/4 anterior radius	Pronation	Median
Extensors				
Superficial group				
Brachioradialis	Low 2/3 anterior humerus	Coronoid and ulnar tuberosity	Elbow flexor	Radial C5–C6
Extensor carpi radialis longus	Low 1/3 supracondylar ridge humerus	Radial dorsal base 2nd metacarpal	Extend wrist	Radial
Extensor carpi radialis brevis	Common extensor tendon lateral epicondyle	Base 3rd metacarpal	Extend wrist	Radial
Extensor digitorum	Common extensor tendon lateral epicondyle	Distal 2–5 phalanges	Common extensor fingers	Radial
Extensor digiti minimi	Extensor digitorum	Distal small finger	Extensor 5th finger	Radial
Extensor carpi ulnaris	Two heads 1) common extensor tendon 2) posterior ulnar border	Medial side base 5th metacarpal	Wrist extensor, ulnar abduction	Radial
Deep group				
Abductor pollicis longus	Posterior ulna, interosseous membrane, middle posterior radius	Lateral base 1st metacarpal	Long abduction thumb	Radial
Extensor pollicis brevis	Midposterior radius	Base proximal phalanx of thumb	Extensor thumb	Radial
Extensor pollicis longus	Mid 1/3 posterior radius	Base distal phalanx of thumb	Extends phalanges of thumb	Radial
Extensor indicis	Posterior radius and interosseous membrane	Proximal phalanx index finger	Extensor index finger	Radial

From Berquist TH. *MRI of the musculoskeletal system*, 4th ed. Philadelphia, PA: Lippincott Williams & Wilkins, 2001; Rosse C, Rosse PC. *Hollinshead's textbook of anatomy*. Philadelphia, PA: Lippincott–Raven, 1997; and Morrey BF. *The elbow and its disorders*, 3rd ed. Philadelphia, PA: WB Saunders, 2000.

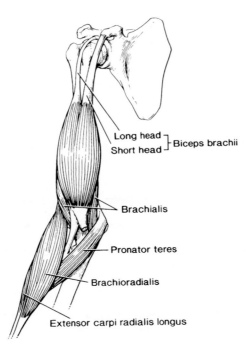

Figure 10-14   Illustration of the superficial flexor muscles of the elbow.

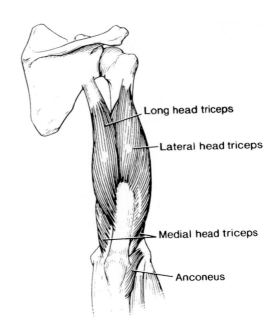

Figure 10-15   Illustration of the extensors of the elbow.

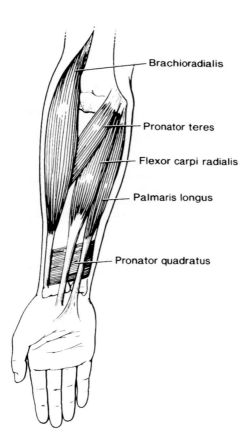

Figure 10-16   Illustration of the pronators of the forearm.

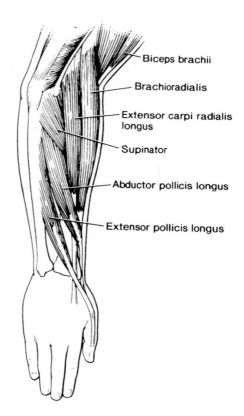

Figure 10-17   Illustration of the supinators of the forearm.

the lateral aspect of the humerus and radius and are supplied predominantly by the radial nerve (Table 10-4) (24).

The flexor group is divided into three layers—superficial, intermediate, and deep (24). The superficial layer originates predominantly from the common flexor tendon at the medial epicondyle (see Fig. 10-18). Muscles in the superficial group include the pronator teres, flexor carpi radialis, palmaris longus, and flexor carpi ulnaris (Fig. 10-18) (Table 10-4). The two heads of the pronator teres originate from the common flexor tendon and the coronoid process of the elbow. The pronator teres extends under the brachialis and inserts onto the lateral aspect of the midradius. The flexor carpi radialis also originates from the common flexor tendon at the medial epicondyle and extends distally, crosses the flexor retinaculum along the groove of the trapezium, and inserts onto the second metacarpal base. Along its course, the flexor carpi radialis covers part of the flexor digitorum superficialis (Fig. 10-6). The palmaris longus arises from the common flexor tendon medially and extends for only about one third the length of the forearm. Distally the tendinous portion crosses the wrist superficial to the flexor retinaculum (Fig. 10-18) and continues to become a part of the palmar aponeurosis in the hand. The flexor carpi ulnaris (the last of the superficial group) also has two heads, the first arising from the common flexor tendon, the second

from the olecranon and posterior upper two thirds of the ulna (Fig. 10-18). This muscle covers the ulnar nerve and vessels along much of its course in the forearm (Fig. 10-6) and crosses the wrist through the pisohamate and pisometacarpal ligaments to insert onto the hamate hook and fifth metacarpal base (24,25).

The flexor digitorum superficialis (sublimis) forms the intermediate layer of the flexor group (see Fig. 10-19). This muscle also arises from the medial common flexor tendon; a second head originates from the upper radius, distal to the tubercle. This large, flat muscle covers the median nerve and ulnar nerve and artery as it courses distally in the forearm (Figs. 10-6 and 10-19) (24,26). Prior to transversing the flexor retinaculum, the flexor digitorum superficialis gives off four tendons. After passing through the flexor retinaculum and carpal tunnel, these four tendons have common sheaths with the flexor digitorum profundus and split distally to insert onto either side of the bases of the second through fifth middle phalanges (24,25).

The deep flexor group includes the flexor digitorum profundus, flexor pollicis longus, and pronator quadratus (see Fig. 10-20) (Table 10-4). The flexor digitorum profundus arises from the anterior two thirds of the ulna in its midportion and the interosseous membrane. This muscle also divides into four tendons that join the flexor digitorum

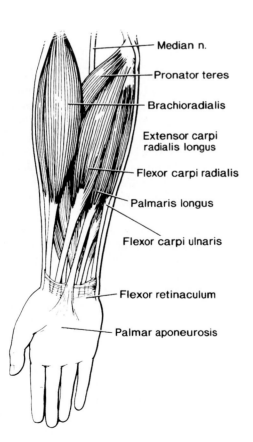

Figure 10-18 Illustration of the superficial flexor and extensor muscles of the forearm.

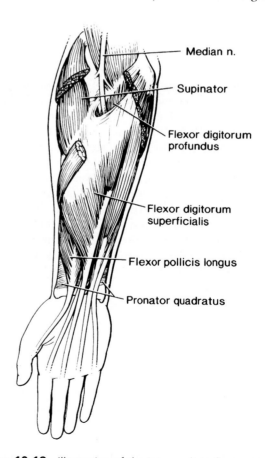

Figure 10-19 Illustration of the intermediate flexor compartment of the forearm.

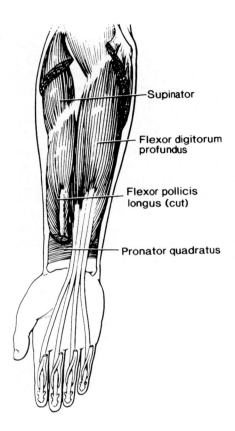

Figure 10-20 Illustration of deep flexors of the forearm.

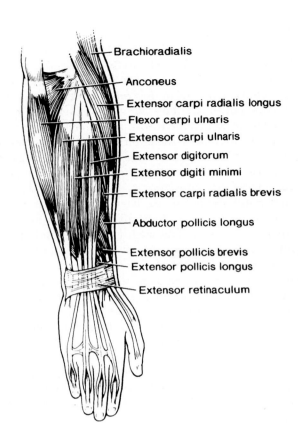

Figure 10-21 Illustration of extensor muscles of the forearm.

superficialis in a common tendon sheath as they pass beneath the flexor retinaculum and carpal tunnel. The tendons insert onto the bases of the distal second through fifth phalanges (25,26,39). The flexor pollicis longus arises from the middle one third of the radius and interosseous membrane and has an independent tendon sheath distally as it passes through the carpal tunnel. Thus, it is located more radially and separate from the flexor digitorum profundus and flexor digitorum superficialis tendons (Fig. 10-20). Upon leaving the carpal tunnel, the flexor pollicis longus passes through the thenar muscle region to insert onto the distal phalanx of the thumb. The third and final muscle of the deep group is the pronator quadratus, which is a flat, quadrangular muscle lying behind the flexor digitorum longus and flexor pollicis longus. This muscle arises from the distal ulna to insert onto the distal radius in a near-transverse direction (Fig. 10-20) (24–26,30).

Extensors

The extensor muscles of the forearm are actually flexors of the elbow, as noted above. All of the extensor muscles are innervated by the radial nerve (24). The extensor muscles, like the flexors, are divided into superficial and deep compartments. The superficial group includes the brachioradialis, extensor carpi radialis longus, extensor

digitorum, extensor digiti minimi, and extensor carpi ulnaris (see Fig. 10-21) (24,25). The brachioradialis, as described above, has a long origin above the supracondylar ridge, where it lies between the brachialis and triceps muscles. The radial nerve lies between it and the brachialis (Fig. 10-6). Superiorly, the brachioradialis partially covers the extensor carpi radialis longus as it passes distally to insert onto the lateral side of the distal radius. The extensor carpi radialis longus arises from the lower third of the anterior supracondylar ridge and is covered superiorly by the brachialis. The extensor carpi radialis longus overlaps the extensor carpi radialis brevis and gives rise to a flat tendon at the level of the mid forearm. It then accompanies its companion, the extensor carpi radialis brevis, distally. The extensor carpi radialis longus extends along the posterior radial surface deep to the abductor pollicis longus and extensor pollicis longus, passes under the extensor retinaculum (where it shares a common tendon sheath with the extensor carpi radialis brevis), and inserts onto the radial dorsal aspect of the base of the second metacarpal (Figs. 10-6 through 10-8). At this location, there may be a small bursa between the second metacarpal base and the tendon. This bursa is usually not visible on MRI unless it is inflamed and distended with fluid. The extensor carpi radialis brevis is the most lateral of the extensor muscles and arises from the common extensor tendon at the lateral epicondyle, and also has a small head that arises from the radial collateral ligament. This muscle is largely covered by the extensor carpi radialis longus in its proximal portion (Figs. 10-6 and 10-21). The extensor digitorum is located adjacent to it on the ulnar side. In the distal forearm, the muscle is separated from the extensor digitorum by the abductor pollicis longus and extensor pollicis brevis (Figs. 10-6 and 10-21). At the wrist, the tendon of the extensor carpi radialis brevis lies immediately adjacent to the ulnar side of the extensor carpi radialis longus, and both tendons share a common sheath as they pass under the extensor retinaculum. The extensor carpi radialis longus inserts onto the base of the third metacarpal. Its chief function is to extend the wrist, but it also assists in elbow flexion. The extensor digitorum (extensor digitorum communis) is the common extensor of the fingers. This muscle occupies the central portion of the dorsal forearm. It originates from the common extensor tendon and shares an origin with the belly of the extensor digiti minimi. Distally, three to four tendons are present with a common sheath within the extensor retinaculum. The sheath is shared with the extensor digiti indicis. The tendons pass under the extensor retinaculum and receive slips from the lumbricals and interosseous muscles in the hand, thereafter dividing into central and lateral bands (see Chapter 11). The central bands insert onto the middle and lateral bands on the sides of the distal phalanges. The primary function of the extensor digitorum is to serve as an extender and abductor of the fingers. The extensor digiti minimi arises largely from a septum adjacent to the extensor digitorum and occupies a superficial position on the dorsal forearm between the extensor digitorum and extensor carpi ulnaris. The slender tendon of this muscle continues in a separate compartment under the extensor retinaculum to insert onto the dorsal aspect of the small finger in a similar fashion to the extensor digitorum. The extensor carpi ulnaris is the most medial of the superficial muscles. It has two heads, the first arising from the lateral epicondyle via the common extensor tendon, and the second from the posterior border of the ulna. The tendon of this muscle passes through a special compartment in the extensor retinaculum and also through the ulnar groove. The insertion is the medial side of the base of the fifth metacarpal. Its primary functions are wrist extension and ulnar abduction (24–26,30).

Deep Extensors

The deep extensors of the forearm include the abductor pollicis longus, extensor pollicis brevis, extensor pollicis longus, and extensor indicis (see Fig. 10-22). The supinator is included in this group because of its position in the deep compartment (Fig. 10-6). The abductor pollicis longus is the long abductor of the thumb and arises from the posterior ulna distal to the supinator, the interosseous membrane, and the middle third of the posterior radius. This muscle passes obliquely to emerge between the extensor

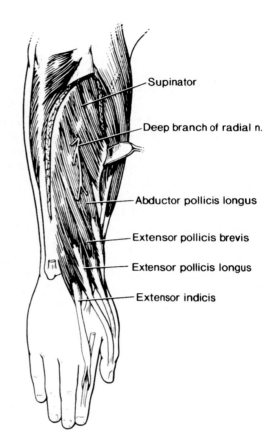

Figure 10-22 Illustration of the deep extensor muscles of the forearm.

carpi radialis brevis and extensor digitorum with the extensor pollicis brevis medial and inferior to it (Figs. 10-6 and 10-22). The abductor pollicis longus and extensor pollicis brevis pass superficial to the radial extensor tendons and both share a common sheath at the wrist. At this level, it lies superior to the radial artery and passes to the dorsum of the hand where it inserts onto the base of the first metacarpal on its lateral side (see Chapter 11). The abductor pollicis longus serves as a radial abductor of the wrist and also a radial extender of the thumb. The extensor pollicis brevis is the short extensor of the thumb and arises from the midportion of the posterior radius distal to the abductor pollicis longus and also from the interosseous membrane. It passes between the extensor digitorum and abductor pollicis longus and crosses the wrist superficial to the radial extensors. This tendon forms the anterior boundary of the anatomic snuff box. The radial artery is deep to this tendon and the tendon of the abductor pollicis longus. The extensor pollicis brevis inserts onto the base of the proximal phalanx of the thumb, where it serves as an extensor of the thumb and radial abductor of the wrist. The extensor pollicis longus arises from the middle posterior third of the radius and interosseous membrane, is in contact with the abductor pollicis longus, and partially overlaps the extensor pollicis brevis superiorly. At the wrist, it lies on the radial side of the extensor digitorum. The tendon runs obliquely across the wrist in a separate compartment under the extensor retinaculum and in a groove just medial to the radial tubercle. It emerges to form the dorsal margin of the anatomic snuff box. Its tendon covers or is dorsal to the extensor pollicis brevis and inserts onto the base of the distal phalanx of the thumb. This muscle serves as an extensor of both phalanges of the thumb. The final muscle of the deep compartment is the extensor indicis (extensor indicis proprius), which is the extensor of the index finger. It arises distal to the extensor pollicis longus on the posterior radius and interosseous membrane, and is largely covered by the superficial muscle group along its course. The tendon passes deep to the extensor digiti minimi and deep to the extensor digitorum, with which it shares a common sheath in the dorsum of the hand. Along the dorsal aspect of the hand, the extensor indicis lies on the ulnar side of the extensor digitorum and inserts with an expansion onto the dorsal aspect of the proximal phalanx (3,24,25).

Neurovascular Anatomy

Knowledge of the neurovascular anatomy and the relationship of the neurovascular structures to the various muscles and compartments of the elbow and forearm is critical for evaluating MRIs (see Fig. 10-23) (40). Soft tissue masses and traumatic conditions, including nerve compression syndromes involving these structures, can cause significant clinical symptoms (2,24,26,41). Therefore, it is important that the relationship of the arteries, veins, and nerves to the various compartments and muscle groups is appreciated. Following the nerves and vessels is most easily accomplished with contiguous axial images (Fig. 10-6), especially when viewed in cine mode. Because of the variation in the course of these structures, they are rarely included in their entirety in the coronal or sagittal planes. Three-dimensional volume imaging and angiographic techniques will provide excellent visualization of the major vascular structures; however, following the course of nerves and identifying lesions in or adjacent to them will likely still be most easily accomplished on axial images (3,26,29).

At the level of the distal humerus (Fig. 10-6A), the brachial artery is located anteromedially adjacent to its accompanying vein. The median nerve usually lies along the medial aspect at the junction of the biceps and brachialis muscles. The ulnar nerve is positioned more posteriorly along the medial aspect of the triceps (Figs. 10-6 and 10-23). At this same level, the radial nerve is most commonly seen between the brachialis muscle and brachioradialis just anterior to the lateral aspect of the supracondylar portion of the humerus. Near the elbow, the

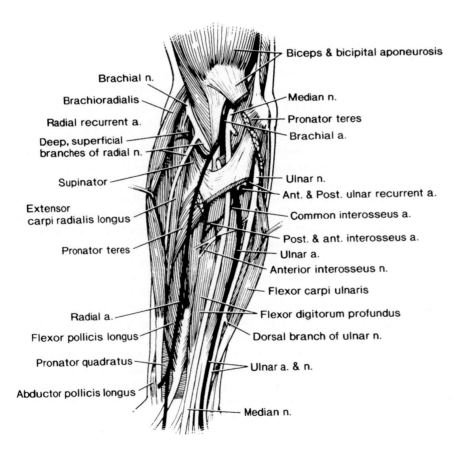

Figure 10-23 Illustrations of the neurovascular anatomy of the elbow and forearm.

radial nerve courses anteriorly along the margin of the brachialis muscle and medial to the brachioradialis (Fig. 10-23) to a point just above the supinator, where it divides into the deep and superficial branches. Once this division has occurred, the nerve is more difficult to follow into the forearm on MRI (Fig. 10-6). However, at this point, the superficial branch of the nerve lies anterior to the extensor carpi radialis longus and the deep branch is generally seen either within or between the supinator and extensor digitorum, posterior to the radius (Figs. 10-6 and 10-23). The median nerve courses along the anterior aspect of the antecubital fossa, passes beneath the flexor digitorum superficialis, and lies between this muscle and the flexor digitorum profundus as it passes distally into the forearm (Figs. 10-19 and 10-23). The median nerve is a larger structure and usually can be easily identified on axial MRI (Fig. 10-6). The ulnar nerve passes posterior to the medial epicondyle and is clearly identified on most images at this level (Fig. 10-6). More distally, the ulnar nerve is usually located between the flexor digitorum profundus and the flexor carpi ulnaris (Figs. 10-6 and 10-23) (24,30).

The major vessels in the elbow and forearm are more easily identified than the smaller, low signal intensity nerves. The brachial artery courses with the median nerve in the antecubital fossa prior to dividing into the radial and ulnar arteries. The radial artery lies superficial to the flexor pollicis longus as it extends into the forearm. The ulnar artery usually accompanies the median nerve along its course superficial to the flexor digitorum profundus. Figure 10-23 demonstrates the major neurovascular anatomy of the forearm and elbow (24,41). Figure 10-24 depicts the normal MR angiogram of the elbow and proximal forearm.

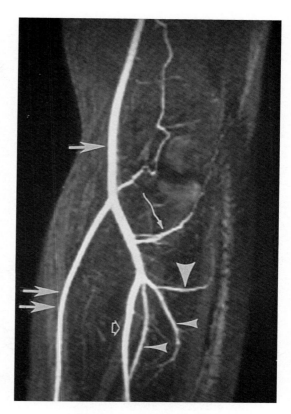

Figure 10-24 Normal MR angiogram of the elbow and proximal forearm. The distal brachial artery (*large arrow*), proximal radial, (*large double arrows*) and ulnar (*open arrow*) arteries are illustrated. The proximal portions of the anterior and posterior ulnar recurrent arteries (*curved arrow*), anterior and posterior interosseous arteries (*small arrowheads*), and posterior interosseous recurrent artery (*large arrowhead*) are well-visualized.

PITFALLS

Pitfalls when interpreting MRIs of the elbow and forearm are usually related to normal anatomic variants, technical errors, improper coil selection, patient motion or flow, and other imaging artifacts (1,2,38,42–44).

The list of normal anatomic variants involving the elbow and forearm is potentially long. A frequent osseous variant is the supracondylar process. This hook-like, bony projection is a vestigial remnant that is also seen in birds, and is usually noted 1 to 2 inches above the medial epicondyle in humans. This structure is almost always asymptomatic. However, a ligamentous structure (ligament of Struthers) can extend from the supracondylar process to the medial epicondyle and compress the median nerve or brachial artery (24,45–48). Identification of the supracondylar process is easily accomplished with routine radiography. However, the relationship of the ligament of Struthers to the neurovascular structures may be most easily viewed with coronal and axial MRI (2). Rosenberg et al.

(38,43,49,50) described a pseudodefect at the junction of the capitellum and lateral epicondyle (see Fig. 10-25) that should not be confused with osteochondritis dissecans or an osteochondral fracture. This pseudodefect is due to a normal osseous groove in this region that can give the appearance of an osteochondral abnormality on axial and coronal T2-weighted or GRE MRI. The pseudodefect deepens as the images proceed more laterally. Occasionally, one or more fine, low signal lines extend from the pseudodefect into the marrow; these should not be mistaken for fractures (38,43,49,50). Similarly, there is normally a transverse ridge in the trochlear notch that is not covered with hyaline cartilage. This finding is most easily appreciated on sagittal images and should not be mistaken for a cartilage lesion (51).

A small, normal groove in the olecranon, subjacent to the trochlea (Fig. 10-25), should not be mistaken for a cartilaginous defect (50,52,53). In most individuals, the trochlear groove is traversed by a cartilage-free bony ridge (2 to 3 mm in height) at the junction of the olecranon and the coronoid process (38).

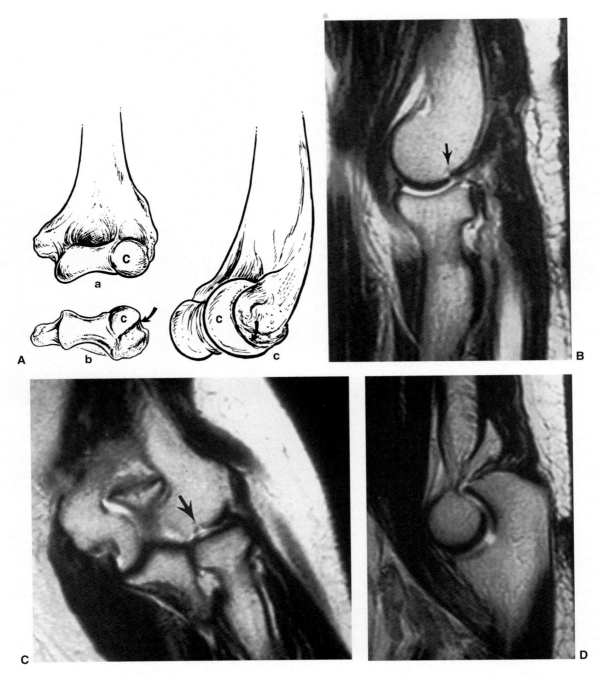

Figure 10-25 Normal variants: capitellar pseudodefect and trochlear groove. Illustration of the distal humerus **(A)** seen from anterior (a), inferior (b), and oblique (c) views. The capitellum (c) is separated from the lateral epicondyle by a groove *(curved arrow)* that may appear as an osteochondral defect on MR images. (From Rosenberg ZS, Beltran J, Cheung YY, et al. Pseudodefect of the capitellum: potential pitfall in MRI. *Radiology* 1994; 191:1821–1823.) Sagittal T1-weighted **(B)** and coronal T2-weighted **(C)** images demonstrate a focal cortical concavity *(arrow)* at the level of the pseudodefect. **D:** Sagittal T2-weighted image depicts the small normal groove in the olecranon subjacent to the trochlea, which should not be mistaken for a cartilaginous defect.

Soft tissue anomalies, including combination of muscle bellies, accessory origins or absence of one of the heads when multiple origins are present, and total absence (palmaris longus 12.9%) are not unusual. These changes are not usually clinically significant (24). Certain anomalous muscles can be significant. The anconeus epitrochlearis is present in place of

the cubital tunnel retinaculum in up to 11% of patients. This can result in ulnar nerve compression (see Fig. 10-26) (30). Readers are referred to anatomic references for a more complete discussion of normal anatomic variants (24,25,30).

Other errors in interpretation of MR images are due to improper choice of pulse sequences, image planes, coils, and

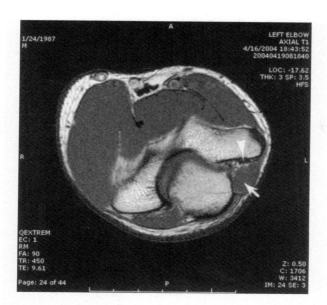

Figure 10-26 Axial T1-weighted image of the elbow demonstrates an anconeus epitrochlearis (*arrow*) compressing the ulnar nerve (*arrowhead*).

patient position (see Chapter 3). Many mistakes can be avoided by careful review of clinical history and physical findings.

Image artifacts have been more fully discussed in Chapters 1 and 3. Most artifacts in the upper extremity are due to motion and/or flow artifacts (1,54–57). Flow artifacts may also create problems in image interpretation. Flow artifact suppression techniques (see Chapter 3) can reduce artifacts; however, it is still useful to change the phase encoding direction to prevent artifacts from degrading important areas on the image (see Fig. 10-27) (1,2,58).

Pitfalls may also be avoided by comparing radiographs and other imaging modalities with MRI. Metal artifact can cause significant signal intensity distortion. Knowledge of the type of implant is useful to select the proper pulse sequence parameters to reduce the artifact or confirm that MRI would not be useful (2,3). Titanium implants cause less artifact due to reduced ferromagnetic content.

Heterotopic calcification or ossification is common about the elbow, especially at the flexor and extensor tendon attachments. Signal intensity may vary depending upon the

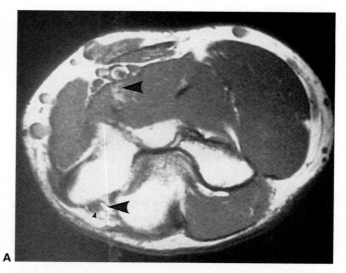

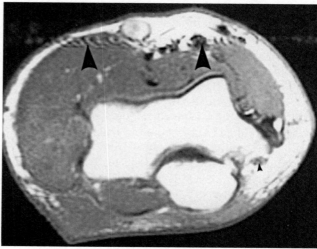

Figure 10-27 Flow artifact. Axial images of the elbow showing flow artifact in the (**A**) vertical *y* axis and (**B**) transverse or *x* axis. The ulnar nerve region (*small arrowhead*) is distorted by flow artifact (*large arrowheads*) in **A**, which could interfere with diagnosis of pathology in this region.

presence of marrow in ossifications. Calcifications are low signal intensity on all pulse sequences (59).

The presence of joint effusion on radiographs after trauma has been considered synonymous with occult fracture. However, in children this may not be the case (60–62). Donnelly et al. (60,61) reported fractures in 17% of children on follow-up when initially presenting with joint effusion. When the effusion persisted, the incidence of fracture was 78% (60).

APPLICATIONS

The most common clinical indications for MR of the elbow and forearm are trauma, neoplasms and other mass lesions, avascular necrosis (AVN, osteonecrosis), infection, nerve compression syndromes, and arthropathies. MRI is also an excellent technique in patients with complex symptoms who have had normal conventional studies including computed tomography (CT), ultrasonography, and arthrography (1,3,4,49,63–65).

TRAUMA

Fractures

Elbow fractures and other injuries are common in infants, children, and adolescent and adult throwing athletes (5,66–72). In children, supracondylar humeral fractures account for 50% to 60% of all fractures (71). This fracture is most common prior to age 10 (84%), with a peak incidence at 7 years of age. Supracondylar fracture also has the highest complication rate (30). Physeal fractures are also common in children and adolescents (73,74). Fractures of the lateral humeral condyle are most common. These are usually Salter-Harris type IV injuries (5,71). In adults, the radial head is most often fractured. However, avulsion fractures and ulnar stress fractures are also common in throwing athletes (39,70,73).

Routine radiographs, radionuclide studies, and conventional tomography or CT are generally sufficient for the detection and classification of skeletal injuries. However, it is not uncommon to detect subtle skeletal injuries with MRI that were overlooked or not identifiable with conventional techniques (see Figs. 10-28 through 10-30) (1,2). Beltran et al. (7) reported MRI changed the radiographic diagnosis in 50% and management in 36% of pediatric fractures. Griffith et al. (10) compared radiographic features with MRI in 50 children (32 males and 18 females, mean age 7.3 years) after trauma. Radiographs were normal in 14%, demonstrated effusion in 17% (Fig. 10-28), and a fracture was suggested in 52%. MRI demonstrated a joint effusion in 96% and fractures in 74%. Physeal fractures were evident in 20% (Fig. 10-29), bone bruises in 90%, ligament injuries in 14%, and muscle injuries in 38% (10).

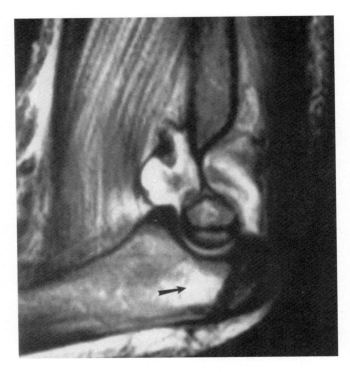

Figure 10-28 Ten-year-old male with acute elbow trauma. Sagittal STIR image demonstrates a large effusion, edema in the brachialis, and an ulnar bone bruise (*arrow*). (From Griffith JF, Roebuck DJ, Cheng JCY, et al. Acute trauma in children: spectrum of injury revealed by MRI not apparent on radiographs. *AJR* 2001; 176:53–60.)

Occult fractures in the marrow and physeal fractures can be identified early with MRI (7,60,75,76). Cortical changes are most obvious on T2-weighted or STIR sequences. Fractures have high signal intensity compared with the low signal intensity of cortical bone. Marrow fat is suppressed with the use of these sequences, so a stellate area of high or low signal intensity may be noted. The former occurs with edema and blood at the fracture site (1,2,76). When signal intensity is decreased on T2-weighted sequences, it usually is due to trabecular compression. Marrow edema or bone bruises are low signal intensity on T1-weighted images (Fig. 10-30). The fracture line may be less conspicuous compared to T2-weighted sequences, but if visible, it is low signal intensity. MRI also can be useful in monitoring the healing process and for differentiating between fibrous union and nonunion. In patients with fibrous union, the signal intensity is decreased on both T1- and T2-weighted sequences. If nonunion is present, the signal intensity is increased due to fluid between the fracture fragments (see Fig. 10-31) (1,2).

MRI may be particularly useful for evaluating physeal injuries in patients with incomplete ossification of the epiphyses (5,7,10,71,74,77). Radiographs may be difficult to interpret because epiphyses may be poorly ossified until age 12 or beyond (7). Early detection and treatment of elbow injuries, specifically distal humeral fractures (see Fig. 10-32),

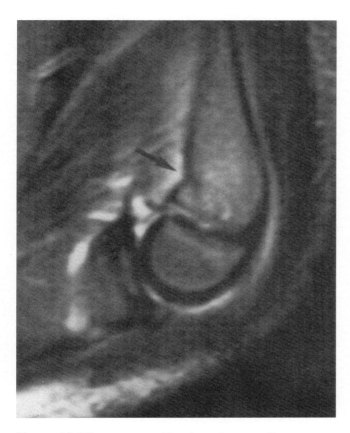

Figure 10-29 Nine-year-old male with acute elbow trauma. Sagittal T2-weighted image shows a supracondylar fracture (*arrow*). (From Griffith JF, Roebuck DJ, Cheng JCY, et al. Acute elbow trauma in children: spectrum of injuries revealed by MRI not apparent on radiographs. *AJR* 2001;176:53–60.)

are important, since these fractures are frequently unstable and require surgical intervention to prevent residual deformity (cubitus valgus, ulnar nerve palsy) (7,30). Complications from physeal injuries include angular deformity due to tethering in eccentric physeal injury, cupping of the metaphysis and shortening of the bones in central physeal injuries, and interference of longitudinal growth due to premature partial closure of the physis by bridging osseous bars (see Fig. 10-33) (18). These complications are more severe in younger children. Thin section T2 or T2* GRE sequences with reformatting are effective for evaluation of premature closure and other growth plate complications (18,78).

The majority of physeal injuries in the elbow occur between 4 and 8 years, when epiphyses are not well-ossified (7,30,79). Fractures of the lateral condyle (Fig. 10-32) are most common, accounting for more than 54% of fractures (7). "Little Leaguer's elbow" is avulsion and fragmentation of the medial humeral epicondyle due to repeated valgus stress from the flexor and pronator muscles across the growth plate (Fig. 10-31). This injury typically occurs in 9 to 12-year-old baseball pitchers prior to fusion of the secondary ossification center of the medial humeral epicondyle. The physeal plate is the weakest link of the attachment of the flexor–pronator muscle group to the bone (53,80). T2- or T2*-weighted sequences are best for evaluation. Because of the age group and need to minimize examination time, we prefer coronal T1-weighted and T2* GRE sequences, which provide excellent detail with reduced examination time compared to conventional SE sequences. FSE sequences with fat suppression could also be used (1,2).

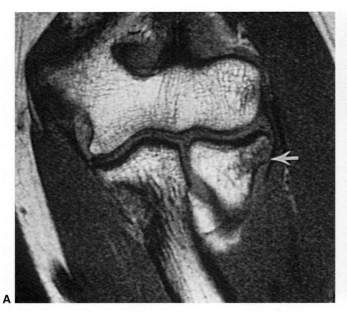

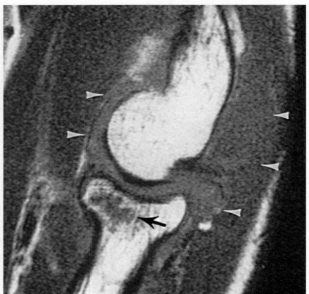

A   B

Figure 10-30 Occult radial head fracture. Coronal **(A)** and sagittal T1-weighted images **(B)** through the radiocapitellar joint demonstrate the radiographically occult marrow edema and transverse fracture (*arrow*) as a hypointense line on the coronal image (*arrow*). Note the intermediate intensity joint effusion (*arrowheads*).

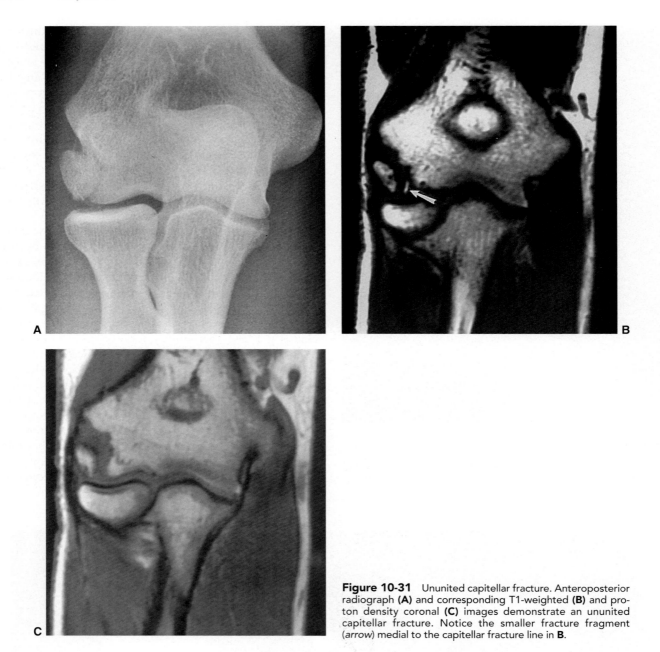

Figure 10-31 Ununited capitellar fracture. Anteroposterior radiograph **(A)** and corresponding T1-weighted **(B)** and proton density coronal **(C)** images demonstrate an ununited capitellar fracture. Notice the smaller fracture fragment (*arrow*) medial to the capitellar fracture line in **B**.

Osseous injuries in adults and throwing athletes go beyond the common radial head fracture to include avulsion fractures and stress fractures (5,39,81). Repetitive valgus stress creates the potential for medial osseous and ligament injury (see Fig. 10-34). Throwing athletes, especially baseball pitchers, typically present with medial or posteromedial elbow pain. In this setting, the differential diagnostic considerations include ulnar collateral ligament tears, muscle injury, medial epicondyle avulsion (adolescents), osteoarthritis, and avulsion of the coronoid tubercle (5,39,51,66,73). Stress injuries with ulnar marrow edema have also been reported in baseball pitchers. These injuries have marrow edema in the proximal ulna that is low signal

intensity on T1- and high signal intensity on T2-weighted or STIR images (see Fig. 10-35). Salvo et al. (39) found coronal GRE images most useful for detection of coronoid (sublime) tubercle avulsions (see Figs. 10-34 and 10-36). Though less common than ligament injury, this avulsion should be considered in throwing athletes (5,39). Because of the differential diagnoses listed above, MR arthrography may be required to completely evaluate throwing athletes with medial elbow pain.

Osteochondral fractures or impaction can be easily defined with MRI (see Fig. 10-37). At least two image planes should be used so the size of the defect and its position can be clearly defined. Defects in the capsule are

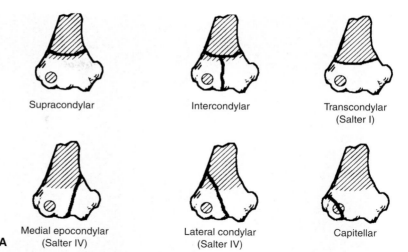

Supracondylar

Intercondylar

Transcondylar
(Salter I)

Medial epocondylar
(Salter IV)

Lateral condylar
(Salter IV)

Capitellar

A

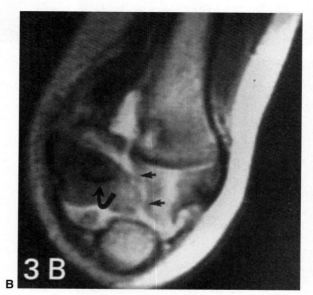

Figure 10-32 Distal humeral fractures. **A:** Illustrations of distal humeral fractures with Salter-Harris classification in parentheses when present. **B:** Coronal T2-weighted image shows a lateral condylar fracture (*straight arrows*) through the metaphysis and epiphysis. Note the ossification center of the capitellum (*curved arrow*). (From Beltran J, Rosenberg ZS, Kawelblum M, et al. Pediatric elbow fractures: MRI evaluation. *Skel Radiol* 1994; 23:277–281.)

B

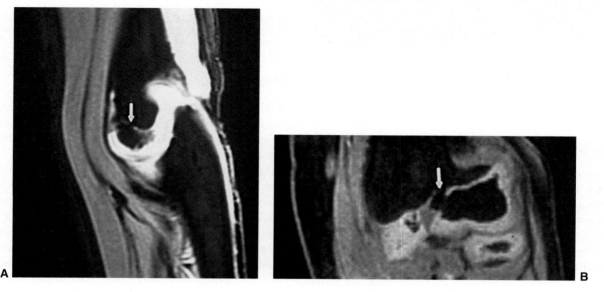

A

B

Figure 10-33 Capitellar physeal osseous bridge. Sagittal **(A)** and reformatted coronal three-dimensional GRE **(B)** images through the medial capitellum demonstrate a hypointense osseous bridge (*arrow*) connecting the distal humerus to the epiphysis. Osseous bridges are usually post-traumatic in origin and can potentially inhibit longitudinal growth.

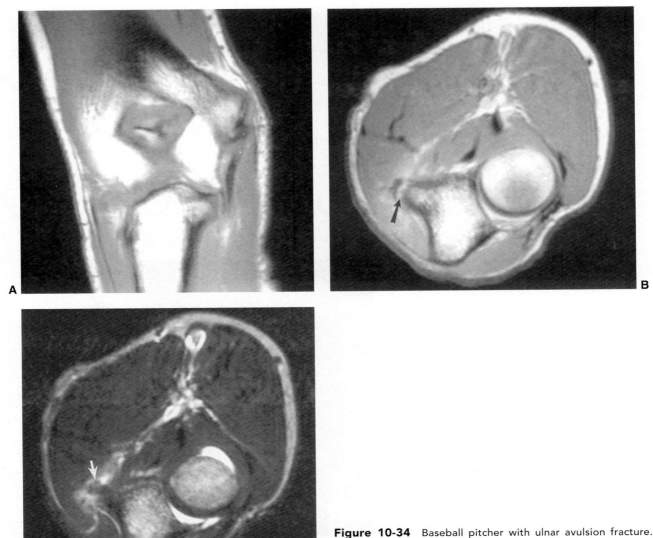

Figure 10-34 Baseball pitcher with ulnar avulsion fracture. Coronal **(A)** and axial **(B)** T1-weighted images demonstrate an ulnar avulsion (*arrow*) with increased signal intensity in the ulnar collateral ligament. Axial T2-weighted image **(C)** shows the fragment (*arrow*) and increased signal intensity in the adjacent soft tissues.

usually easily defined. In certain cases, MR arthrography may be necessary to better define subtle articular and soft tissue injuries (17,23).

Dislocations

Elbow dislocations are second only to the shoulder in frequency. In children, it is the most common dislocation. Simple posterior dislocations of the elbow usually result in complete disruption of all of the capsuloligamentous structures, with variable adjacent muscular injury (62,82). Persistent instability after a closed reduction of a simple dislocation may be due to soft-tissue interposition or entrapment of an intraarticular chondral or osteochondral fragment (62). MRI and MR arthrography may be useful in these circumstances for further evaluation.

Osteochondroses

Osteochondral lesions in the elbow typically involve the capitellum and may be secondary to acute trauma, osteochondrosis (Panner disease), osteochondritis dissecans (OCD), or AVN. The trochlea is rarely involved (83). The etiology is unclear. However, a tenuous blood supply and repetitive trauma due to lateral impaction forces is the leading theory (3,84,85). Both Panner disease (self limited) and osteochondritis dissecans (OCD) (progressive) may represent stages of the same process (86–88). Panner disease, an osteochondrosis, is characterized by irregularity and fragmentation of the entire capitellum, and is not associated with loose body formation (71,77,86,87). The condition is frequently seen in young males (age 4 to 12) during ossification of the capitellar epiphysis. Patients present with dull

OCD is a lesion of bone and cartilage due to chronic lateral impaction that commonly involves the central or anterolateral surface of the capitellum in older patients (age 12 to 20) (77,89). Lesions typically occur in boys, are more common on the dominant side, but can be bilateral in 15% to 20% of patients (80). Up to 67% of patients are involved in competitive sports (baseball, gymnastics) (89). Lesions may progress to fragmentation and destruction of the articular cartilage and bone (5,87,90). Imaging of OCD should begin with routine radiography. In certain cases, radionuclide scans are important for early detection. However, if one considers the importance of classifying this lesion and evaluating unossified cartilage, it becomes apparent that MRI or MR arthrography are ideally suited to evaluate these patients (see Fig. 10-38). Because treatment is dictated by the imaging appearance of these lesions, it is important to accurately define the bone and cartilage changes. Care should be taken not to mistake the capitellar pseudodefect, a normal variant, for OCD (50). Type I lesions are undisplaced fragments with intact articular cartilage. Type II lesions have defects in the articular cartilage and may be partially displaced. Type III lesions are completely detached (87,88). Operative or arthroscopic repair is indicated for type II and type III lesions (30,88,91).

Prior to MRI, arthrography was frequently required to evaluate the articular cartilage in patients with OCD. However, T2-weighted or GRE sequences in two image planes provide excellent visualization of the size and position of the osseous or cartilaginous lesion and the articular

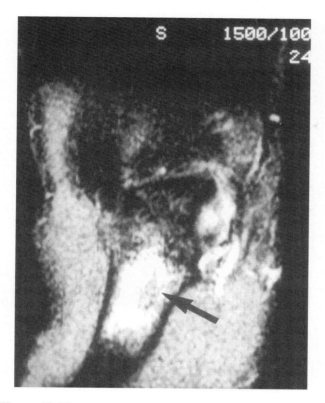

Figure 10-35 Baseball pitcher with proximal ulnar stress injury. T2-weighted coronal image demonstrates increased signal intensity in the marrow (*arrow*). (From Schickendantz MS, Ho CP, Koh J. Stress injury of the proximal ulna in professional baseball players. *Am J Sports Med* 2002; 30:737–741.)

pain in the elbow. Symptoms frequently increase with exercise. Local swelling and reduced elbow extension are common findings. Younger patients generally have more favorable prognoses, with remodeling and complete healing with conservative therapy (80,87).

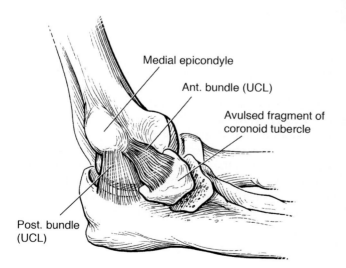

Medial epicondyle

Ant. bundle (UCL)

Avulsed fragment of coronoid tubercle

Post. bundle (UCL)

Figure 10-36   Illustration of avulsion injury of the coronoid (sublime) tubercle.

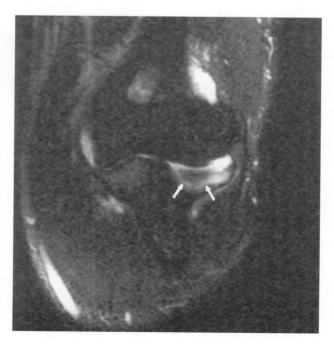

Figure 10-37   Coronal STIR image demonstrating an effusion and ulnar impaction fracture (*arrows*).

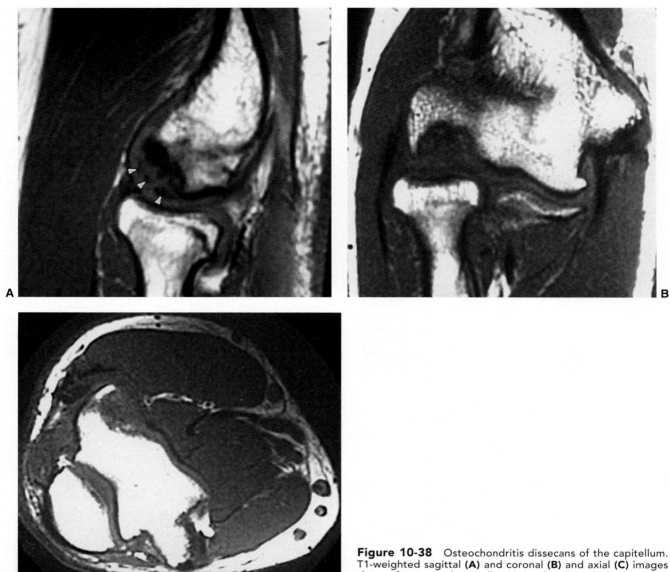

Figure 10-38 Osteochondritis dissecans of the capitellum. T1-weighted sagittal **(A)** and coronal **(B)** and axial **(C)** images show a fragmented capitellum (*arrowheads*) with displacement of several of the smaller fragments.

cartilage. In general, sagittal and coronal images are most useful. MR arthrography is useful in selected cases (2).

Osteonecrosis or AVN occurs less frequently in the elbow than other anatomic sites. However, patients with systemic disease or on steroid therapy can develop osteonecrosis in this region. The MRI features of osteonecrosis in the elbow are similar to the changes described in the hip. On T1-weighted images, the area of necrosis is usually isointense with normal marrow and it is surrounded by a low-intensity margin (see Fig. 10-39). During the early stages, the low-intensity margin is due to hyperemia. On T2-weighted images, high signal intensity is noted in this hyperemic region. When new bone formation occurs around the region of infarction, the signal intensity is reduced on both T1- and T2-weighted sequences. Variable signal intensity at the necrotic margin is due to mixed resorption and new bone deposition. Articular cartilage (intermediate signal intensity) can be clearly defined on either T1- or T2-weighted sequences. However, subtle fissures or linear defects may be more easily identified on proton-density fat-suppressed DESS or GRE sequences. Early experience with MRI in the hip and wrist suggests that the technique is also useful for following patients with low-grade lesions who are considered for conservative therapy. Return of normal signal intensity has been correlated with improvement in patient symptoms (1,2).

Tendon Injuries

Tendon injuries are more common in the upper extremity than the lower extremity (4). Isolated ruptures of tendons

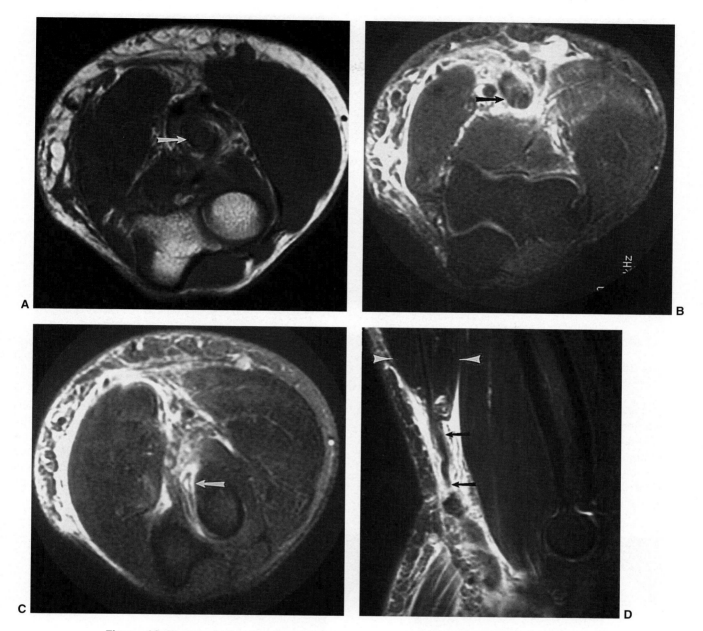

Figure 10-45 Distal biceps tendon rupture. Axial T1-weighted **(A)** and T2-weighted **(B)** images display a markedly thickened distal biceps containing increased T2-weighted signal (*arrow*) proximal to the point of rupture. Increased T2-weighted fluid (hemorrhage) surrounds the tendon and extends throughout the deep fascial planes and the subcutaneous soft tissues. **C:** Axial T2-weighted image near the radial tuberosity demonstrates some frayed tendinous remnants (*arrow*) at the site of rupture. **D:** Sagittal FSE T2-weighted fat-saturated image displays the retracted biceps muscle (*arrowheads*) and the undulating ruptured biceps tendon (*arrows*).

neuropraxia is commonly seen in conjunction with medial tennis elbow (3,95). Posterior tennis elbow is related to tendinosis at the triceps attachment. This condition is seen in baseball pitchers and javelin throwers. Olecranon synovitis and loose bodies are commonly associated findings (95). It is not unusual to have symptoms in multiple sites (95,97).

The lack of inflammatory cells in tennis elbow has created a new description of epicondylitis or tendinitis. The more appropriate term is angiofibroblastic tendinosis (3,91,95). Kraushaar and Nirschl (91) described four stages. Stage 1 is inflammatory and resolves. In stage 2, tendinosis and angiofibroblastic degeneration occur (see Fig. 10-53). Stage 3 includes tendinosis with rupture, and

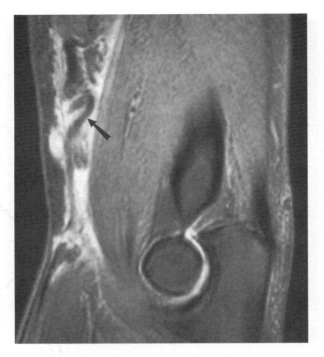

Figure 10-46 Sagittal T2-weighted image shows a ruptured, retracted biceps tendon (*arrow*).

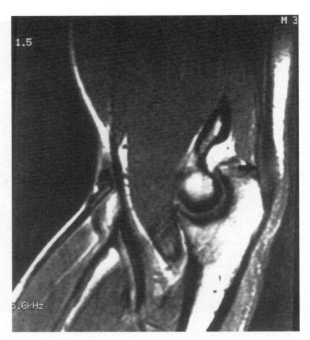

Figure 10-48 Sagittal T1-weighted image demonstrates thickening and increased signal intensity in the distal triceps tendon (*arrow*).

stage 4 is a combination of stages 2 and 3 plus scarring and calcification (91).

MRI demonstrates thickening and intermediate signal in the common extensor origin in tendinopathy (stages 1 and 2). Partial tears are depicted by thinning or partial disruption of the tendon, and increased T2-weighted signal within and adjacent to the tendon origin (see Fig. 10-54).

Complete rupture of the tendons will lead to a tendinous gap containing fluid signal, and distal retraction of the involved muscle(s) (see Fig. 10-55). Dystrophic calcifications (stage 4) can arise adjacent to the lateral epicondyle and are best demonstrated on GRE images (53). Coronal and axial images using fat-suppressed T2-weighted FSE sequences are most useful for evaluating the extent of injury (2,3,79).

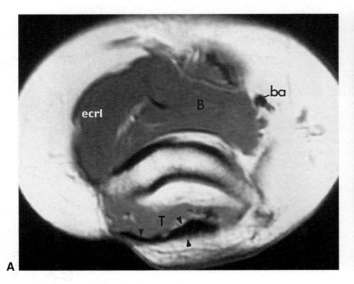

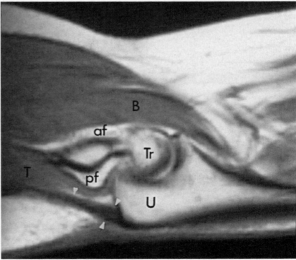

Figure 10-47 Normal triceps tendon. **A:** Axial T1-weighted image just above the elbow demonstrates the normal variation in thickness (*arrowheads*) of the triceps tendon. **B:** Sagittal T1-weighted image demonstrates the triceps tendon (*arrowheads*). *T*, triceps muscle; *ba*, brachial artery; *B*, brachialis; *ecrl*, extensor carpi radialis longus; *Tr*, trochlea; *af*, anterior fat pad; *pf*, posterior fat pad.

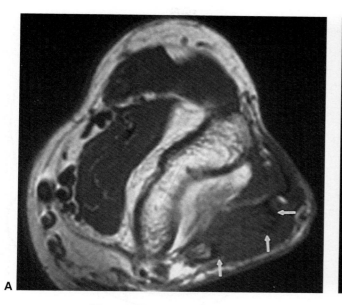
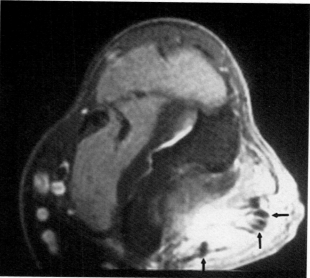

Figure 10-49 High-grade partial tear of the triceps tendon. Axial T1-weighted **(A)** and T2-weighted **(B)** images proximal to the olecranon process demonstrate absence of the majority of the midportion of the triceps tendon and fluid within the posterior soft tissues. Note the several remaining hypointense tendinous fibers (*arrows*).

Injuries to the common flexor tendon origin (medial tennis elbow) are less common than injuries to the common extensor tendon origin (30,95). Common flexor tendon injury (see Fig. 10-56) occurs at the origins of the flexors and pronator teres (19,30,65,80,93). This syndrome occurs in

1% to 3% of adults 35 to 55 years of age, and is often seen in golfers, high-performance throwers, swimmers, racquetball and squash players, and bowlers (3,79). Tears in the flexor/pronator muscle group are more common than extensor muscle tears even though symptoms are far more

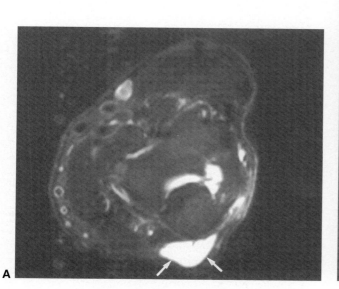
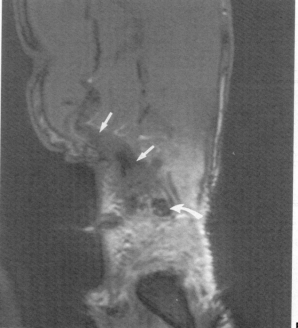

Figure 10-50 Triceps avulsion with retraction. **A:** Axial T2-weighted image demonstrates a fluid collection (*arrows*) adjacent to the olecranon. **B:** Coronal fat-suppressed T2-weighted image shows retraction of the tendon (*arrows*) and an avulsed osseous fragment (*curved arrow*).

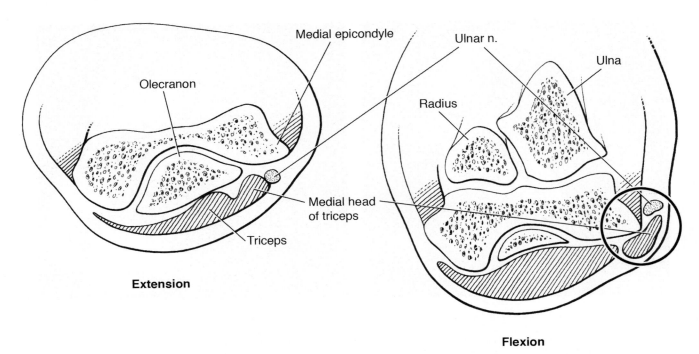

Figure 10-51 Snapping triceps tendon. Illustration of the change of position of the medial head of the triceps and ulnar nerve in flexion and extension.

common laterally (3,79,95). MR arthrography has been advocated by many in the literature for the detection of partial tears (30). The diagnosis of partial tears is critical to throwing athletes, because these patients will likely undergo surgery (30). Inflammation medially may result in ulnar nerve compression (Fig. 10-56) (95). In advanced cases, surgical intervention with ulnar nerve transfer may be indicated (21). In this setting, MRI may be useful to evaluate the position of the ulnar nerve in relation to the medial epicondyle and adjacent soft tissues. Increased signal within the extensor muscles, including the anconeus, can also been seen in patients with lateral epicondylitis (65). In patients with medial elbow symptoms, the ulnar collateral ligament

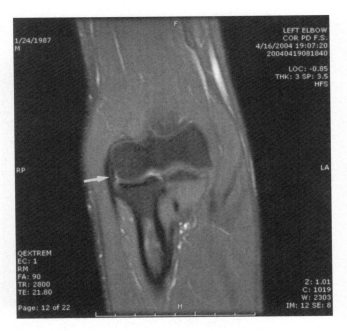

Figure 10-52 Normal ulnar nerve. Axial T1-weighted image demonstrates the low intensity ulnar nerve (*un*) surrounded by fat as it passes behind the medial epicondyle (*M*). *L*, lateral epicondyle; *B*, brachialis; *ecrl*, extensor carpi radialis longus.

Figure 10-53 Common extensor tendinosis. Coronal T2-weighted image demonstrates thickening with increased signal in the substance of the tendons (*arrow*).

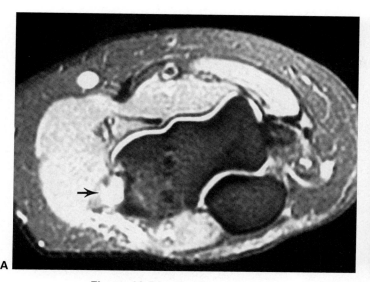
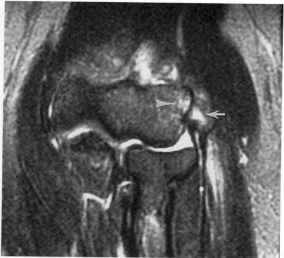

Figure 10-54 Partial tear of the common extensor origin. Axial **(A)** and coronal T2-weighted **(B)** images through the common extensor origin display hyperintense signal at the site of partial tendinous tear (*arrow*) and marrow edema within the lateral epicondyle (*arrowhead*).

should also be evaluated. Avulsion of the medial epicondyle may occur in skeletally immature individuals (3,79,95).

MRI in the axial and coronal planes is most useful to evaluate changes in tendons and osseous edema of the epicondyles. T2-weighted, FSE T2-weighted fat-suppressed or GRE sequences are most useful. Comparison with routine radiographs is essential to avoid confusion caused by tendon calcification. In fact, we generally reserve MRI for

patients who do not respond to normal therapy or to exclude other pathology (1).

Several associated conditions must be considered when evaluating patients with epicondylar symptoms. Ulnar nerve compression was noted earlier with medial tennis elbow. Radial nerve entrapment in the lateral tunnel may occur with lateral tennis elbow. Posterior interosseous nerve entrapment may also present with lateral elbow pain

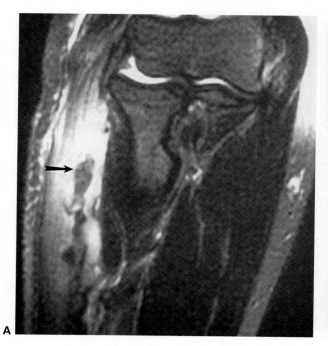
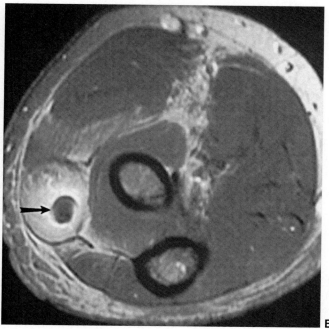

Figure 10-55 Complete rupture of the extensor carpi radialis brevis tendon, secondary to chronic "tennis elbow." Coronal T2-weighted **(A)** and axial proton density fat-suppressed **(B)** images demonstrate complete rupture of the extensor carpi radialis brevis tendon (*arrow*), with distal retraction of the tendinous remnant and associated hemorrhage.

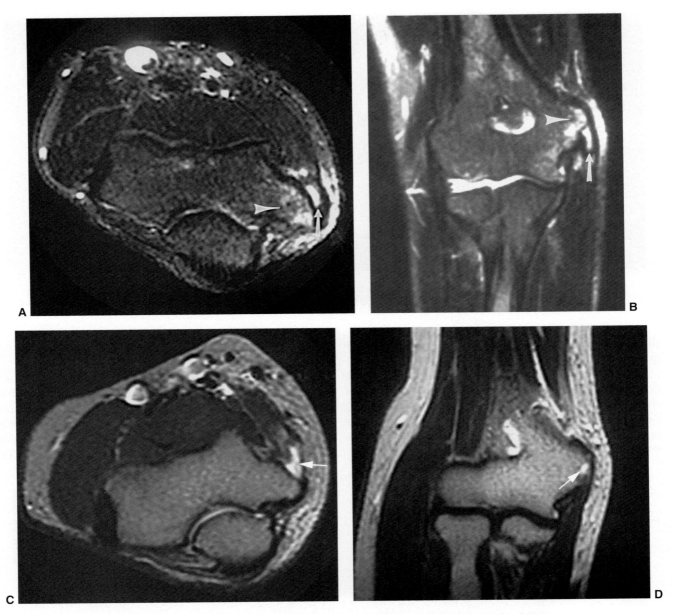

Figure 10-56   Partial tear of the common flexor origin. Axial **(A)** and coronal T2-weighted **(B)** images through the common flexor origin demonstrate hyperintense signal at the site of partial tendinous tear (*arrow*), hyperintense hemorrhage within the proximal flexor muscles, and marrow edema within the medial epicondyle (*arrowhead*). Axial **(C)** and sagittal T2-weighted **(D)** images in a different patient show similar findings (*arrow*), except there is the absence of epicondylar marrow changes.

(48,95). These conditions will be more completely discussed in the section on nerve compression syndromes.

Treatment is designed to control pain and avoid stress overload to the elbow. Stage 1 disease is treated with rest and antiinflammatory medications. Patients with stage 2 disease are also successfully treated with this regimen if less than 50% of the tendon is involved. Surgery may be considered for more advanced stage 2 and stages 3 and 4 disease (95). Lateral epicondylar exostoses, tendon calcification, chondromalacia, loose bodies, and pain at rest suggest refractory process that may require operative intervention (95).

Muscle Injuries

Muscle injuries in the upper extremity, excluding those related to medial or lateral tennis elbow, are much less common than in the lower extremity (30,96,109,110). Muscle strain is a stretch-induced injury that occurs most commonly in eccentric overload (i.e., when a muscle increases in length while it is contracting) and pathologically is a microtraumatic disruption of the muscle fibers near the myotendinous junction (80,111). Muscle strain appears as increased T2-weighted signal at the myotendinous junction without

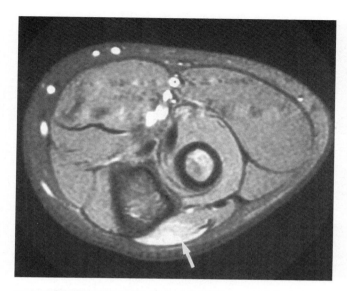

Figure 10-57 Anconeus muscle strain. Axial T2-weighted distal to the elbow joint demonstrates increased signal in the anconeus muscle (*arrow*) in a patient who had performed repetitive extension and flexion exercises of the elbow.

evidence of tear or hematoma formation (see Fig. 10-57). Partial muscle tears are macroscopic tears that can be associated with hemorrhage and edema. Complete muscle disruption is less common and is evidenced by discontinuity of the muscle on MRI. MRI in two planes is an excellent technique for determining the extent of injury (see Fig. 10-58). T2-weighted or STIR sequences are most useful (1,96). Other subtle muscle changes can also be appreciated on MRI (2,111).

Ligament Injuries

The radial and ulnar collateral ligament complexes (Fig. 10-11) are important for elbow stability (4,30,81). The UCL complex is most important for elbow stability (30,32, 71,74). This ligamentous complex is composed of an anterior band (primary stabilizer), and the thinner posterior and transverse bands (see Fig. 10-59). The UCL complex is frequently injured due to excessive valgus stress in individuals such as baseball pitchers and javelin throwers (Fig. 10-60) (39,73,79). Maximum stress occurs during cocking and the acceleration phases of throwing. Because of the valgus mechanism for injury, the radiocapitellar joint is also often injured due to compressive forces. Excessive valgus stress to the elbow may leave the UCL intact and lead to an avulsion fracture of the sublime (coronoid tubercle) tubercle of the ulna, at the attachment of the anterior band of the UCL (Figs. 10-34 and 10-36) (112).

The anterior bundle of the UCL is best depicted on MRI in the coronal plane aligned with the humeral shaft with the elbow flexed (Fig. 10-59) (17). The anterior band is taut when the elbow is extended, whereas the posterior band is taut when the elbow is flexed (30,32).

The transverse band is clinically less significant, small, or sometimes absent, and is often difficult to identify on MRI (21).

Routine radiographs may be useful. Heterotopic calcification or ossification may be present radiographically. In this setting, 76% of patients demonstrate partial or complete UCL tears at surgery (59). These findings may be difficult to appreciate on MRI, stressing the importance of radiographs for comparison. Over time, there may also be cartilage loss and medial trochlear osteophyte formation leading to posteromedial impingement and ulnar nerve involvement (59,79,113,114).

Stress views with comparison of both elbows can also be performed. If the medial joint space opens more than 0.5 mm on the involved side compared to the uninjured elbow, a ligament tear is almost certainly present (33).

Coronal or oblique coronal and axial T2-weighted, STIR, or GRE images are most useful in the evaluation of ligamentous injuries (see Figs. 10-60 through 10-62). Carrino et al. (20) found FSE proton density and T2-weighted images most useful for detection of UCL injuries. Acute ruptures are not a diagnostic dilemma, and are seen as discontinuity and abnormal course of a ligament. Partial tears are more difficult to diagnose; undersurface tears are more accurately assessed with MR arthrography (17,21,51). Most acute injuries occur at or near the humeral attachment, and demonstrate increased signal intensity on the second echo (T2-weighted) compared to the first echo (proton density) (1,2,115). Chronic or degenerative changes are less likely to have increased signal intensity of T2-weighted compared to proton density sequences (2).

In the asymptomatic immature elbow before epiphyseal fusion, increased T1-weighted and T2-weighted signal is seen at the origin and insertion of the UCL, as well as the ulnar periosteum (39,73,112). In the symptomatic immature elbow, segmentation and subchondral bone resorption of the ossification center can be seen with or without an associated capsular tear (44,50).

Several studies have compared UCL evaluation with conventional MRI and MR arthrography (15,20,21,37,51,67). Hill et al. (80) used coronal GRE sequences (68/18, 20° FA, 28.9-mm sections, 256 ×192 matrix, 1.5 acquisitions, FOV 10 cm) for evaluating the UCL. Carrino et al. (20) used FSE proton density and T2-weighted sequences and found conventional MRI demonstrated 57% sensitivity and 100% specificity. MR arthrography demonstrated sensitivity of 86% for partial tears and 95% for complete tears. Specificity for MR arthrography was also 100%.

Table 10-5 summarizes other conditions that should be considered in patients with medial elbow pain (Fig. 10-62). In patients with prior UCL repair, it is important to evaluate the ligament and nerve, as ulnar neuropathy is a potential complication of ligament repair (31,59,114).

Injury to the RCL complex (Fig. 10-58) is less common and usually is the result of varus stress (55,115). The RCL is less crucial to elbow stability and is best demonstrated in

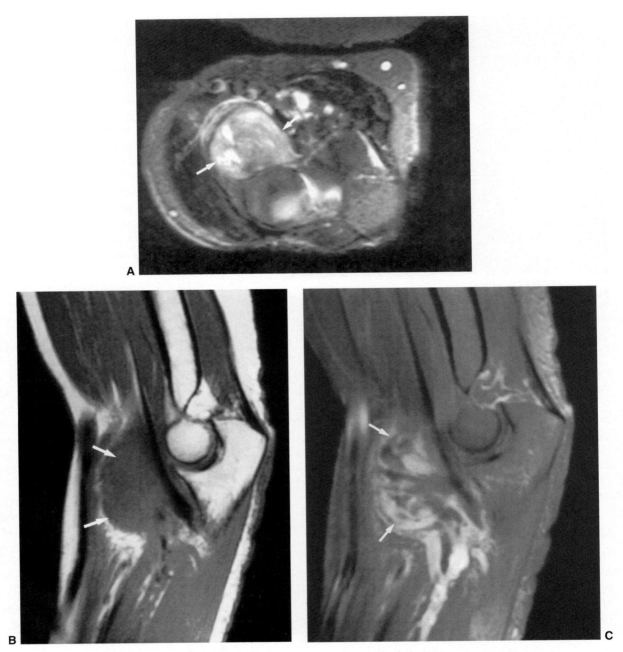

Figure 10-58 Brachialis tear. Axial T2-weighted **(A)** image demonstrates an inhomogeneous antecubital mass (*arrows*). Sagittal T1-weighted **(B)** and contrast-enhanced fat-suppressed T1-weighted **(C)** images show the extent of the mass (*arrows*) with irregular enhancement.

the coronal plane aligned along the humeral shaft with the elbow in 20° to 30° of flexion (17). The annular ligament is somewhat thin and best seen on axial MRI (Fig. 10-6) (73,90,116). As noted earlier (see Pitfalls section), the appearance of the ligaments varies with age and epiphyseal ossification (44).

Radial collateral ligament injuries are less common than medial ligament injury. The mechanism is usually acute varus stress or subluxation/dislocation. Overly aggressive surgical procedures such as common extensor tendon release or radial head resection can also lead to RCL injury (51,79). Since the RCL attaches to and is associated with the annular ligament, both structures should be carefully evaluated. The same MRI approaches described with UCL imaging can be employed for RCL evaluation (see Figs. 10-63 and 10-64).

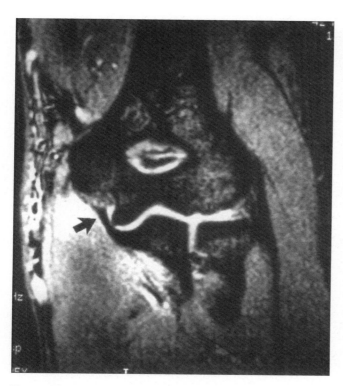

Figure 10-59 Coronal STIR image demonstrating a normal ulnar collateral ligament (*arrow*).

TABLE 10-5

MEDIAL ELBOW PAIN IN THROWING ATHLETES

Medial tendon overuse
Flexor–pronator muscle tears
Ulnar collateral ligament tears
Avulsion of the coronoid tubercle
Posteromedial impingement
Ulnar neuropathy
Ulnar nerve subluxation
Medial antebrachial cutaneous nerve injury

From references 3, 39, 73, 74, and 113.

Synovial Fold Syndrome

Plicae are synovial folds that are remnants of embryonic development (24). Thickened folds may become symptomatic. Plica syndrome in the knee is well-recognized (2). However, this condition in the elbow has not been given much attention in the literature until recently.

The elbow develops as three cavities that merge. Plicae are synovial remnants of this developmental process. They are usually not symptomatic (30). Awaya et al. (117) described elbow plica. Plicae may occur anteriorly or posteriorly (see Fig. 10-65). In cadavers, plicae were uniformly

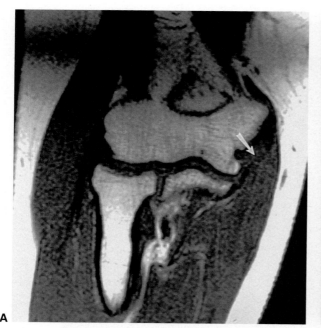

A

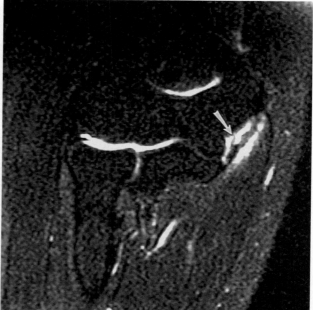

B

Figure 10-60 Partial tear of the anterior band of the ulnar collateral ligament. Coronal T1-weighted **(A)** and T2-weighted **(B)** images demonstrate increased signal within the midsubstance of the anterior band of the ulnar collateral ligament and partial tear (*arrow*), better seen on the T2-weighted image. Fluid extends deep and superficial to the injured ligament.

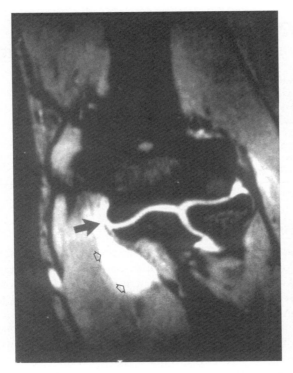

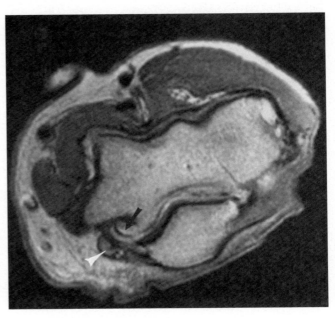

Figure 10-61   Coronal STIR image shows a complete ulnar collateral ligament tear (*arrow*) with a large fluid collection (*open arrows*).

Figure 10-62   Axial proton density image demonstrates osteophyte formation (*arrow*) displacing the ulnar nerve (*arrowhead*).

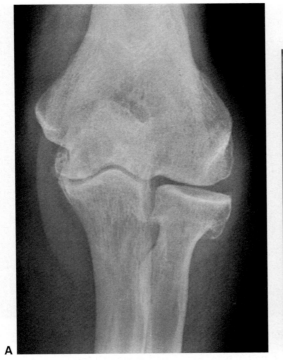

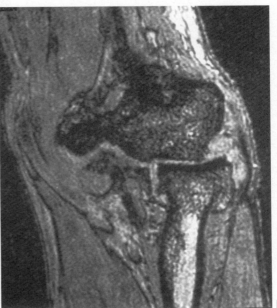

A

B

Figure 10-63   Rupture of the entire radial collateral ligament complex. **A:** Anteroposterior radiograph depicts widening of the radiocapitellar joint and degenerative change of the ulnohumeral and proximal radioulnar joints. **B:** Coronal gradient-echo image demonstrates a radial collateral ligament complex tear.

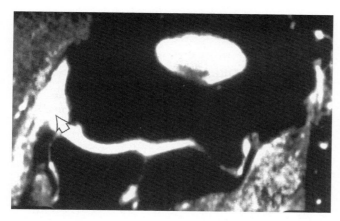

Figure 10-64 Coronal fat-suppressed T2-weighted image demonstrates a complete radial collateral ligament tear (*open arrow*).

thin (2 mm). Review of 153 cases with nonlocking elbows demonstrated plicae in the posterior superior olecranon recess in 48.4% of cases. Symptomatic patients with locking or limited extension demonstrated thickening of the posterior plicae.

Sagittal T2-weighted images (Fig. 10-65B) may be adequate for detection in the presence of a joint effusion. MR arthrography is a more optimal imaging approach to define plicae in the elbow.

BONE AND SOFT TISSUE NEOPLASMS

A large number of patients are referred for evaluation of the elbow and forearm because of suspected soft tissue masses or to exclude postoperative residual or recurrent neoplasms (2,64). Although MRI is generally requested, CT is still valuable for certain cortical lesions, lesions with subtle soft tissue calcification, and for patients who are difficult to examine with MRI due to size or claustrophobia.

Bone Tumors

MRI examinations for suspected musculoskeletal neoplasm in the elbow region usually begin with a coronal scout image. Axial T2- weighted spin-echo or FSE with fat-suppression sequences are used to evaluate the extent of cortical and soft tissue involvement. If the nature of the lesion is obvious, a sagittal or coronal T1-weighted image is obtained, with care being taken to select an image plane that includes the entire osseous or soft tissue region in the image slices. This usually requires an oblique adjustment in the sagittal or coronal images. Postgadolinium fat-suppressed T1-weighted images are added in most cases. Slice thicknesses can be varied depending upon the size of the lesion. We typically use 4- to 5-mm sections. As noted above, the coil selected should include the region of interest plus potential skip areas. Chapter 12 will discuss technical aspects more completely.

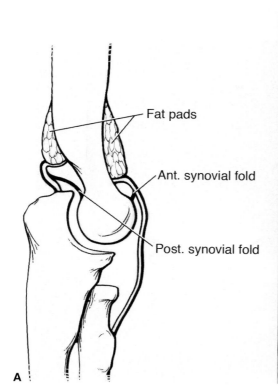

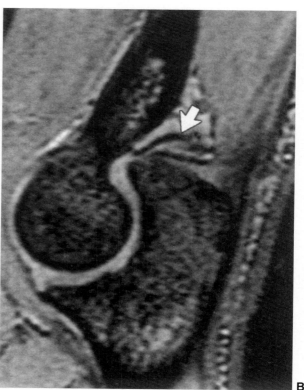

Fat pads

Ant. synovial fold

Post. synovial fold

A

B

Figure 10-65 **A:** Illustration of the anterior and posterior synovial folds. **B:** Sagittal spoiled gradient-echo steady state with fat suppression demonstrates a posterior synovial fold (*arrow*). (**B** from Awaya H, Schweitzer ME, Feng SA, et al. Elbow synovial fold syndrome. *AJR Am J Roentgenol* 2001;177:1377–1381.)

Osseous neoplasms in the elbow are rare and are not commonly evaluated with MRI (see Fig. 10-66 and 10-67) (Table 10-6) (64,118). For example, only 2.3% of benign and 1.6% of malignant primary bone lesions listed in Table 10-6 involved the elbow region (119,120). Routine radiographs usually are sufficient for detection of skeletal neoplasms. Characterization of the lesion also is usually possible with radiographs, so that only indeterminate or obviously malignant lesions require staging with MRI. When an MR examination is required, it is usually to determine the extent of bone and soft tissue involvement. This is accomplished most easily with the use of a dedicated elbow coil. The larger phased array coil allows a larger FOV, so that skip areas in the humerus or forearm are not overlooked when a lesion in the elbow is being studied (1,2).

Soft Tissue Tumors

Table 10-7 summarizes common benign and malignant soft tissue tumors about the elbow. Benign soft tissue tumors usually are well marginated, have homogeneous signal intensity, and do not encase neurovascular structures or invade bone (64,121). Edema is common with malignant lesions but also occurs with benign tumors (2,45,64). Though histology may be difficult to predict using signal intensity and morphological features, the appearance of certain lesions can be accurately defined with the use of the previously described criteria and the increased experience with MR (64).

TABLE 10-6

SKELETAL NEOPLASMS OF THE ELBOW AND UPPER FOREARM

	No. of Elbow and Forearms/Total
Benign	
Osteoid osteoma	22/331
Osteochondroma	12/872
Giant cell tumor	12/568
Chondroma	1/290
Chondromyxoid fibroma	2/45
TOTAL	49/2106
Malignant	
Lymphoma	28/694
Osteosarcoma	14/1649
Ewing sarcoma	15/512
Myeloma	15/814
Chondrosarcoma	6/895
Fibrosarcoma	3/255
TOTAL	81/4819

From Unni KK. Dahlin's Bone Tumors: General aspects and data on 11,087 cases. 5th ed. Philadelphia, PA: Lippincott-Raven, 1996.

Lipomas are common benign soft tissue lesions that maintain a homogeneous signal intensity equivalent to subcutaneous fat on both T1- and T2-weighted sequences (see Fig. 10-68). The lesions are well marginated but may contain fibrous septations (64,122). Liposarcoma should

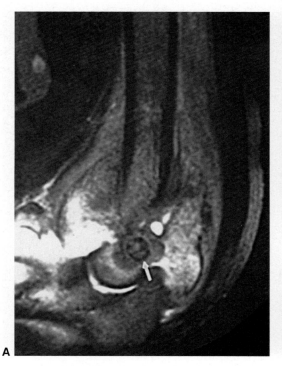
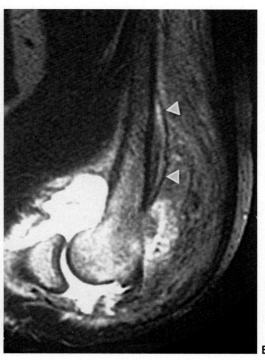

Figure 10-66 Osteoid osteoma. Sagittal FSE T2-weighted fat-saturated images **(A,B)** display a rounded hypointense (partially calcified) nidus in the capitellum (*arrow*), with secondary humeral edema, periosteal reaction (*arrowheads*), large joint effusion, and synovitis.

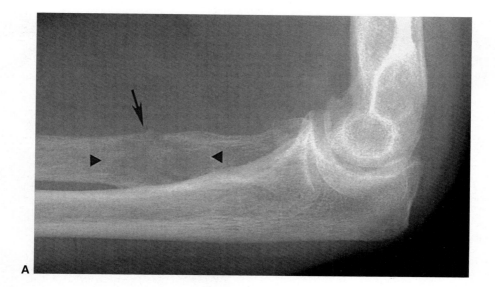

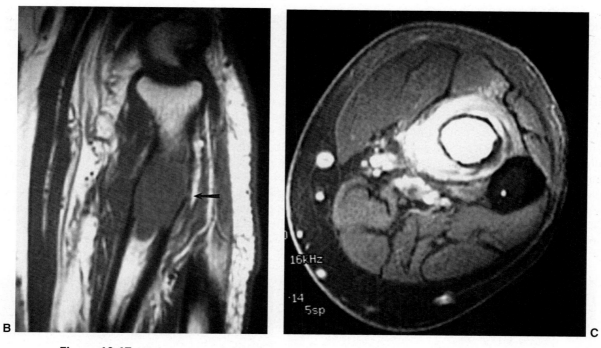

Figure 10-67 Plasmacytoma of the proximal radius. **A:** Lateral radiograph of the elbow demonstrates a pathologic fracture (*arrow*) through a permeative lesion (*arrowheads*) in a 70-year-old patient without a history of a primary tumor. **B:** Sagittal T1-weighted image through the radius demonstrates a marrow-replacing, expansile lesion with associated cortical fracture (*arrow*). **C:** Proton-density fat-saturated axial image shows markedly hyperintense intramedullary and periosteal tumor signal in this plasmacytoma.

be considered when areas of nodularity, inhomogeneity, or irregular margins are noted in a fatty tumor (64).

Lipoma arborescens is a rare subsynovial proliferation of fatty tissue. Most patients have chronic arthropathy. Therefore, many consider the lesion a response to inflammation. The knee is the most common location, though lesions have also been reported in the elbow and bicipital bursa (123,124). T1- and T2-weighted sequences

are adequate for diagnosis. In fact, contrast should not be given, as this lesion does enhance, giving it a more aggressive appearance (124).

Benign cysts (see Fig. 10-69) have high signal intensity on T2-weighted sequences and homogeneous low signal intensity on T1-weighted images. These lesions are very distinct and well marginated, but when complicated by hemorrhage or infection, the signal intensity of these

TABLE 10-7

SOFT TISSUE NEOPLASMS OF THE ELBOW AND FOREARM

Benign
Nodular fasciitis
Lipoma
Benign peripheral nerve sheath tumors
Myxoma
Hemangioma

Malignant
Malignant fibrous histiocytoma
Liposarcoma
Fibrosarcoma
Malignant peripheral nerve sheath tumors
Synovial sarcoma

From Weiss SW, Goldblum JR. *Enzinger and weiss soft tissue tumors*, 4th ed. St. Louis, MO: Mosby, 2001.

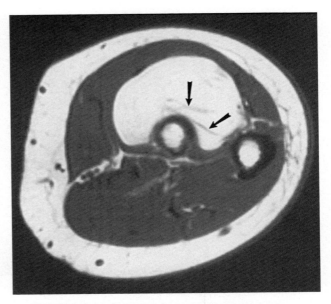

Figure 10-68 Lipoma. Axial image of a benign lipoma depicts a homogeneous tumor with the same signal intensity as subcutaneous fat, except for a few thin, fibrous septae (*arrows*).

complicated cysts may be lower on T2- and higher on T1-weighted sequences (1,2,116).

Other than lipomas, most benign lesions are well marginated, homogeneous, and have a high signal intensity on T2-weighted sequences and a low signal intensity on T1-weighted sequences. The exception to this general rule occurs with two lesions: hemangiomas and desmoid tumors (1,2). Hemangiomas and other vascular malformations often are irregular, have mixed signal intensity, and may be extensive. Intramuscular vascular malformations can be associated with fatty replacement of the involved muscle, which may be attributed to a vascular steal phenomenon. The numerous vessels are usually obvious as signal flow voids, and when MRI data are combined with clinical data, the diagnosis usually is obvious. Differentiation of veins, arteries, and dilated lymphatic vessels is not always possible. MR angiography may be helpful in identifying the feeding arteries and draining veins in arteriovenous malformations (1,2,125).

Desmoid tumors are aggressive, often hypocellular fibrous lesions. The margins are frequently irregular (80% in the Mayo Clinic experience), and the masses have inhomogeneous signal intensity. Lesions usually contain areas of low signal intensity even on T2-weighted sequences due to fibrous tissue (see Fig. 10-70). Resection of these lesions often requires extensive surgery and recurrence is common (see Chapter 12) (1,2).

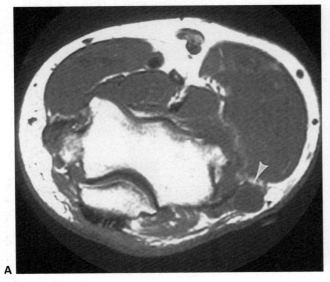
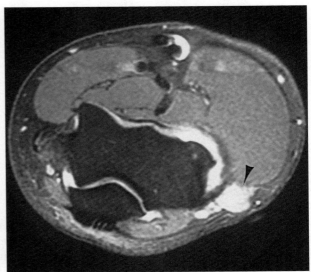

Figure 10-69 Ganglion. **(A)** Axial T1-weighted and **(B)** T2-weighed images demonstrate a well defined, high signal intensity ganglion cyst (*arrowheads*) superficial to the lateral humeral epicondyle.

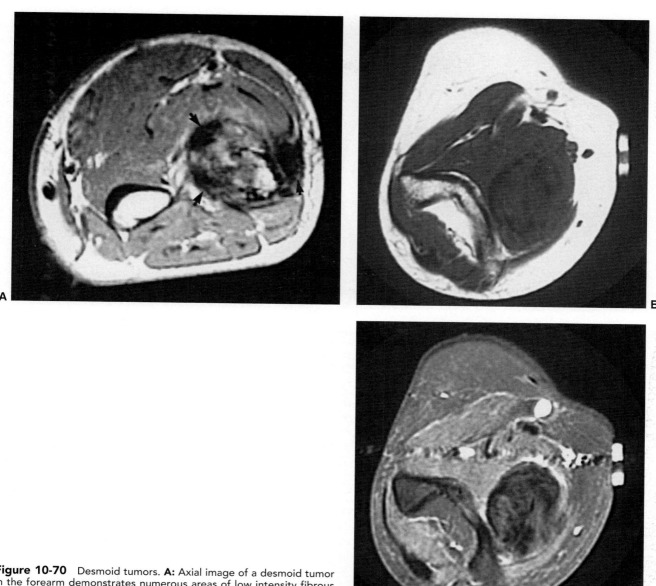

Figure 10-70 Desmoid tumors. **A:** Axial image of a desmoid tumor in the forearm demonstrates numerous areas of low intensity fibrous tissue (*arrows*). Axial T1-weighted **(B)** and T2-weighted **(C)** images in a different patient demonstrate the predominantly low signal intensity throughout this desmoplastic fibroma near the antecubital fossa.

Neural tumors and neural sheath tumors may also be seen in the elbow region (121,126). A complete discussion of these lesions can be found in Chapter 12.

Malignant soft tissue tumors are uncommon in the elbow. Most malignant soft tissue neoplasms are irregular, at least at some point along their margins. Irregular margins also may be due to local inflammation rather than malignant extension. Beltran et al. (45) described increased signal intensity around masses on T2-weighted sequences. This finding was more common with malignant lesions but also was seen in some patients with infection and hemorrhage. The sensitivity of this finding in predicting malignancy was 80%, specificity 50%, and accuracy 64%. Some malignant lesions are well marginated. Therefore, inhomogeneous signal intensity, which is noted in most malignancies, may be a more useful sign for distinguishing benign from malignant disorders. Generally, the signal intensity is inhomogeneous on both T1- and T2-weighted sequences (see Fig. 10-71). Neurovascular encasement and bone involvement also occur more frequently with malignant lesions (64).

The above image criteria are less useful in patients who have recently undergone surgery or a diagnostic needle biopsy. Inflammatory changes and hemorrhage from the procedure can create inhomogeneity in the signal intensity, which makes classification of lesions difficult (1,64).

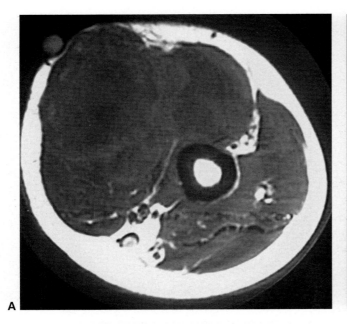

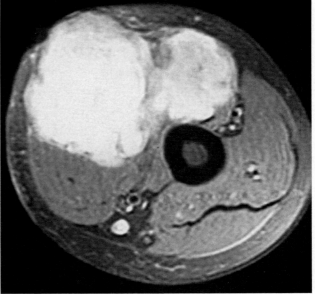

Figure 10-71 Malignant fibrous histiocytoma. Axial T1-weighted **(A)** and T2-weighted **(B)** images of an anterior compartment malignant fibrous histiocytoma display several characteristics worrisome for malignancy. The mass is large, inhomogeneous on both T1- and T2-weighted sequences, and crosses the fascial planes into the brachialis muscle, biceps muscle, and subcutaneous fat.

A more complete discussion of musculoskeletal neoplasms, postoperative changes, metastasis, and MR specificity is discussed in Chapter 12.

INFECTION

Musculoskeletal infections may present with an acute, rapidly progressing course or be insidious. Determination of the extent of involvement is important in planning proper medical or surgical management. Routine radiographs and

CT are useful for these purposes (46,127,128). Radioisotope studies are particularly sensitive in the early stages of infection. The anatomic extent, however, may be inaccurate, especially in the articular regions, and differentiation of cellulitis or soft tissue infection from bone involvement is not always possible (2,129).

Hematogenous skeletal infections typically begin in medullary bone. The resulting hyperemia and inflammation causes alterations in the signal intensity of medullary bone on MRIs (see Fig. 10-72). Osteomyelitis can also result from the direct inoculation of an infectious agent into the bone

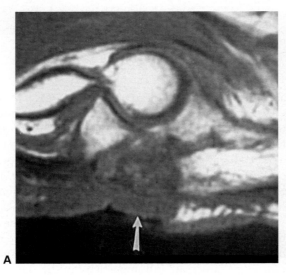

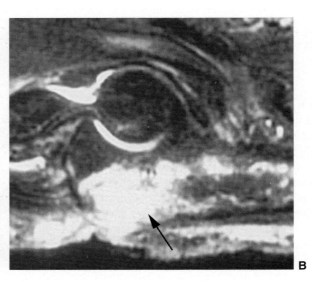

Figure 10-72 Sagittal T1- **(A)** and T2-weighted **(B)** images demonstrate abnormal signal intensity in the ulna (*arrows*) due to osteomyelitis.

from a puncture wound or surgical procedures and from contiguous spread from an adjacent soft tissue infection or septic arthritis. The excellent tissue contrast and multiplanar imaging provided by MRI may allow earlier and more accurate assessment than is possible with current imaging techniques. Therefore, acute osteomyelitis may be evident on MRI when radiographic findings are negative (2,127,130,131).

MRI evaluation for diagnosing osteomyelitis is fully discussed in Chapter 13. Generally, a combination of T1-weighted, STIR or FSE T2-weighted fat-suppressed, and enhanced T1-weighted fat-suppressed images is the most sensitive technique for the detection of osteomyelitis. Short TR/TE SE sequences (SE 500/10–20) can be performed quickly and provide high spatial resolution. Infection is seen as an area of decreased marrow signal intensity compared with the high signal intensity of normal fatty marrow. Changes in cortical bone (osteitis), periosteum (periostitis), and muscle are often less obvious. Osteomyelitis is evident on STIR or FSE T2-weighted fat-suppressed images as foci of high signal intensity. Enhancement of the marrow on T1-weighted enhanced fat-suppressed images is also a feature of osteomyelitis. The presence of associated cortical destruction, sinus tracts, low intensity sequestra, cloaca, and adjacent soft tissue inflammatory signal changes can also be evaluated with MR.

Infectious arthritis generally is monoarticular and, like osteomyelitis, usually involves the lower extremities. Joint-space changes and soft-tissue swelling may be noted on radiographs, but early bone changes are not appreciated for 1 to 2 weeks in a pyogenic infection, and may take months to develop with more indolent infections such as

tuberculous or atypical mycobacteria (2,132). Septic arthritis, if left untreated, can lead to secondary osteomyelitis of the adjacent bones (see Fig. 10-73). Isotope studies with the use of ^{99m}Tc are sensitive in detecting early changes, but are nonspecific. ^{67}Ga and ^{111}In leukocyte scans are more specific in this regard (2,129,133).

The role of MRI in joint space infection continues to evolve. Early bone and soft tissue changes and effusions are easily detected (133,134). Findings, however, are nonspecific and could be noted with other arthropathies (135,136). Characterization of the type of fluid present in the joint may be useful. Infected fluid and blood in the joint may have an intermediate signal intensity, or fluid may be inhomogeneous on T2-weighted images (Fig. 10-73). Normal synovial fluid has a uniformly high signal intensity on T2-weighted sequences. Fluid signal intensity is not usually very useful and does not obviate joint aspiration to identify the offending organism. In addition, effusions and capsular distention may be evident with any of the inflammatory arthropathies.

ARTHROPATHIES

MRI is not required for the diagnosis of osteoarthritis. However, since it is such a common disorder, osteoarthritis is concomitantly imaged in patients with other diagnostic dilemmas. The hallmark characteristics of osteoarthritis (osteophytes, joint space narrowing, chondromalacia, loose bodies, etc.) are exquisitely outlined by multiplanar MRI (see Fig. 10-74) (3,137,138). Cartilage is optimally imaged using DESS sequences or with MR arthrography (17,21,51).

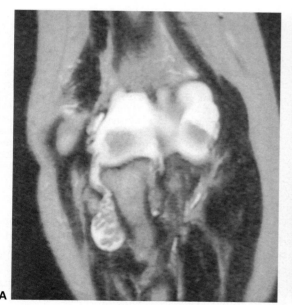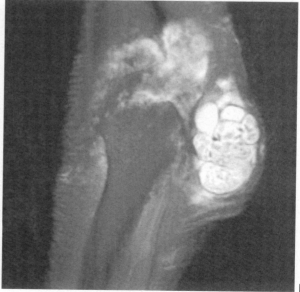

Figure 10-73 Coronal T2-weighted images **(A,B)** demonstrate joint distention with multiple low intensity rice bodies due to atypical mycobacterial infection.

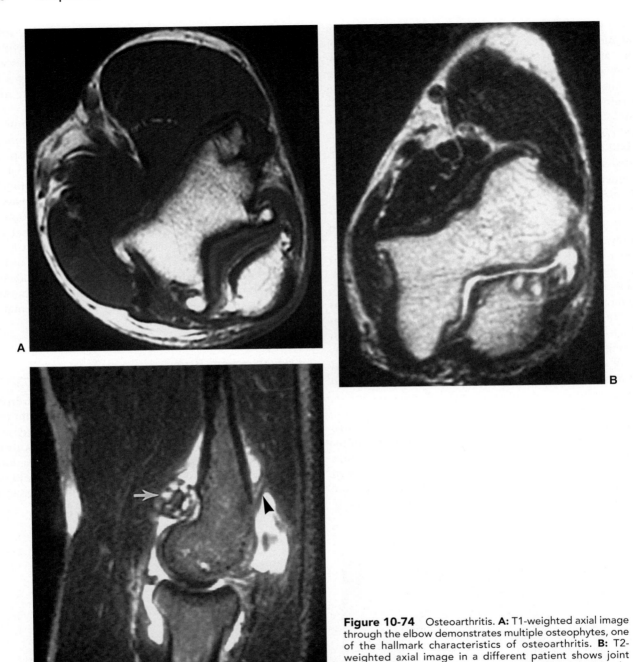

Figure 10-74 Osteoarthritis. **A:** T1-weighted axial image through the elbow demonstrates multiple osteophytes, one of the hallmark characteristics of osteoarthritis. **B:** T2-weighted axial image in a different patient shows joint space narrowing due to extensive chondromalacia, subchondral cysts in the olecranon, osteophytes, and a small joint effusion. **C:** A large joint effusion outlines an osteochondral loose body (*arrow*) in this T2-weighted sagittal image. There is also thickened posterior synovial fold (*arrowhead*).

When the elbow is affected by rheumatoid arthritis, the wrist and hand are invariably involved (62). MRI provides a method for early detection of synovial inflammation and bone erosions. Response to therapy (active synovial inflammation and new erosions) can also be monitored with contrast-enhanced MRI. Joint effusions are easily appreciated on T2-weighted images. However, the presence of a joint effusion is a nonspecific finding (3,139).

Gout may also involve the elbow. The olecranon bursa is involved more commonly than the joint. Fluid in the bursa may be due to bursitis, but gout should always be considered (3).

Certain MRI features are not useful for specific classification of inflammatory or infectious arthropathies. Changes demonstrated with pigmented villonodular synovitis (PVNS) and hemophilic arthropathy (see Fig. 10-75) are exceptions to the rule. The lipid-laden macrophages and hemosiderin deposition seen in PVNS create fairly specific MRI changes of nodular low signal intensity on both T1-weighted and T2-weighted images (135).

Patients with hemophilia may have recurrent intraarticular bleeds leading to aggressive articular and periarticular abnormalities (2,3,139). Recurrent bleeds can be prevented or reduced by prophylaxis with factor VIII or IX therapy. MRI can identify early changes such as joint effusion or hemarthrosis. Chronologically, these changes are followed by hemosiderin deposition and synovial hypertrophy, then cartilage loss, subchondral cysts, and bone erosions (139). The extent of changes seen on MRI correlates with the number of intraarticular bleeding episodes. Joints with fewer

than three bleeds have minimal changes, while joints with four or more bleeds demonstrate more advanced changes (139). T1- and T2-weighted images are useful for detection of most changes. Fat-suppressed proton density or DESS sequences are most useful for evaluation of articular cartilage. As seen on radiographs, epiphyseal overgrowth, early growth plate closure, and destructive changes can be depicted on MRI (see Fig. 10-76).

Synovial chondromatosis is rare in the elbow. The hip and knee are more commonly affected (19). Patients present with pain, swelling, and decreased range of motion or locking. In the presence of an effusion, T2-weighted images may be adequate for diagnosis. In the early stages of synovial nodularity, MR arthrography is more accurate (17).

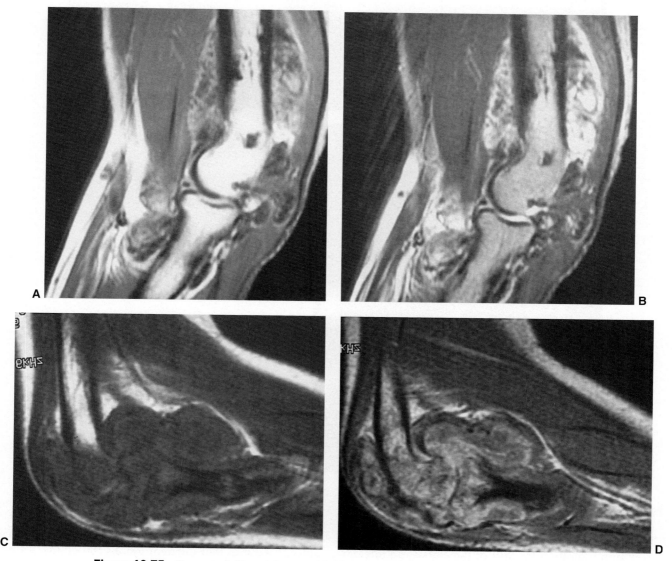

Figure 10-75 Pigmented villonodular synovitis (PVNS). Sagittal T1-weighted **(A)** and T2-weighted **(B)** images demonstrate extensive synovitis with multiple areas of low signal intensity due to PVNS. Sagittal T1-weighted **(C)** and T2-weighted **(D)** images in a different patient demonstrate an extensive synovial soft tissue mass, which is hypointense on the T1-weighted image and has mixed intermediate/hypointense signal intensity on the T2-weighted image. The process is resulting in marked osseous destruction.

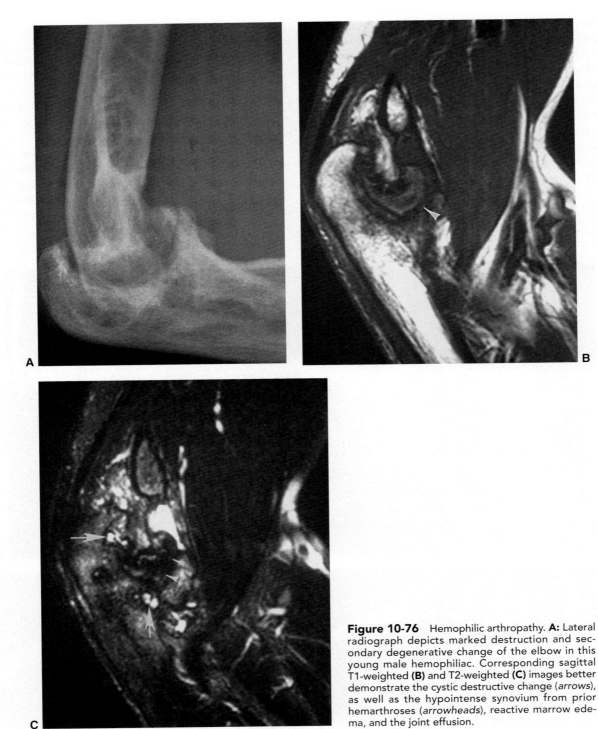

Figure 10-76 Hemophilic arthropathy. **A:** Lateral radiograph depicts marked destruction and secondary degenerative change of the elbow in this young male hemophiliac. Corresponding sagittal T1-weighted **(B)** and T2-weighted **(C)** images better demonstrate the cystic destructive change (*arrows*), as well as the hypointense synovium from prior hemarthroses (*arrowheads*), reactive marrow edema, and the joint effusion.

NERVE ENTRAPMENT SYNDROMES

Chronic pain with or without localized neurologic disease is a common indication for MRI of the elbow and forearm (140,141). Generally, patients are referred to exclude soft tissue masses or primary peripheral nerve tumors. There is no question that MRI is ideally suited for detection of these lesions (1,2,49,63). However, subtle changes along the nerves of the elbow and forearm may also be evaluated with MRI (Fig. 10-23). This requires careful evaluation of the nerves and adjacent anatomy.

Nerve compression or entrapment syndromes have been categorized into four different lesions (30,41,48). A first-degree lesion (neuropractic) shows conduction defects, but there are no structural changes in the nerve. This type of lesion may be due to blunt trauma, ischemia, or compression, and functional return can be expected with proper treatment. Second-degree lesions (axonometric) have disruption of the sheath and nerve fibers, but connective tissue is intact and regeneration can occur. More advanced third-degree and fourth-degree lesions (neurometric) usually result in complete motor and sensory loss and typically occur when compression has been present for more than 1.5 years (48). Third- and fourth-degree injuries are more common in regions where motion or friction occur in addition to compression (41,48).

Clinical diagnosis may be relatively easy with physical examination and electromyographic data. However, in some cases, findings are not straightforward. For example, multiple nerves may be involved by the same or different processes, or nerve compression may occur at multiple levels (48,90). Clinical and anatomic knowledge of the nerve and perineural anatomy is critical for planning the MR examination when imaging is required (2,3).

The causes of nerve compression are numerous and vary to some degree with the nerve involved and the location (3,52).

Ulnar Nerve

In the arm, the ulnar nerve typically passes from anterior to posterior through the arcade of Struthers about 8 cm above the medial epicondyle (see Fig. 10-77) (24,41,48). The ulnar nerve passes posteriorly to the medial epicondyle at the elbow. It is easily identified on axial images (see Fig. 10-78 and 10-79). The nerve passes form posterior to the medial epicondyle into the anterior compartment a few centimeters distal to the epicondyle and cubital tunnel (Fig. 10-78) (44,93,95). In the cubital tunnel (Fig. 10-78), the nerve passes between the medial epicondyle and the olecranon deep to the cubital tunnel retinaculum and arcuate ligament. In the region, the nerve also lies between the humeral origins of the flexor carpi ulnaris (24,52,140).

Ulnar nerve compression can be due to multiple factors (see Figs. 10-79 and 10-80) (Table 10-8). Patients present with medial elbow pain, parasthesias in the fourth and fifth fingers, and varying degrees of sensory

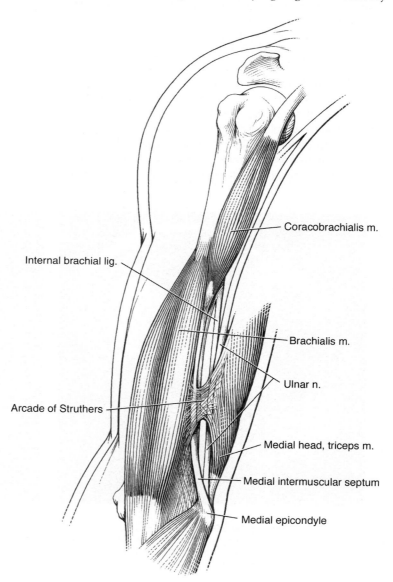

Coracobrachialis m.

Internal brachial lig.

Brachialis m.

Ulnar n.

Arcade of Struthers

Medial head, triceps m.

Medial intermuscular septum

Medial epicondyle

Figure 10-77 Illustration of the ulnar nerve in the arm and the arcade of Struthers.

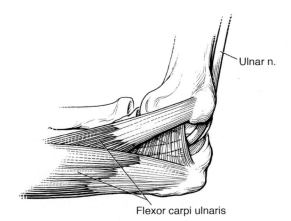

Ulnar n.

Flexor carpi ulnaris

Figure 10-78 Illustration of the cubital tunnel and ulnar nerve.

and motor loss (3,48,52). Symptoms are often aggravated by elbow flexion (48,52). Proximal ulnar nerve injury may occur at the cervical spine, thoracic outlet, or in the arm at the arcade of Struthers (3,24,29,48,52).

The ulnar nerve is most frequently injured at the elbow as it passes through the cubital tunnel (3,52). Cubital tunnel syndrome or spontaneous nerve compression neuritis is seen second to carpal tunnel syndrome in frequency (48,52).

Anatomic variations may cause ulnar nerve compression at the cubital tunnel. Thickening of the retinaculum, UCL thickening, and osteophyte formation may cause nerve compression, especially during flexion. In 11% of patients, an anomalous muscle, anconeus epitrochlearis, replaces the retinaculum, resulting in nerve compression

TABLE 10-8

ULNAR NERVE COMPRESSION SYNDROME

Etiology

Fibrous adhesions
Muscle anomalies (anconeus epitrochlearis)
Absent cubital retinaculum
Thickened cubital retinaculum
Thickened ulnar collateral ligament
Vascular anomalies
Bursal enlargement
Ganglia
Musculotendinous inflammation
Bone and soft tissue trauma
Neoplasms
Inflammatory arthropathies
Hypermobility
Snapping medial triceps
Osteophytes
Loose bodies
Iatrogenic

From references 3, 48, 49, 52, 63, and 140.

(Fig. 10-26). In 10% of patients, the cubital tunnel retinaculum is absent, allowing for dislocation of the ulnar nerve over the medial epicondyle, resulting in friction neuritis (3,48,90).

Treatment is conservative in most cases, with rest, reduced flexion, and, in some cases, steroid injections (3,48). When conservative treatment fails, surgical intervention may be

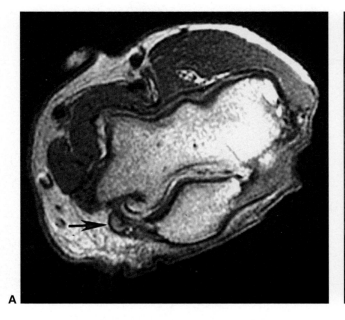

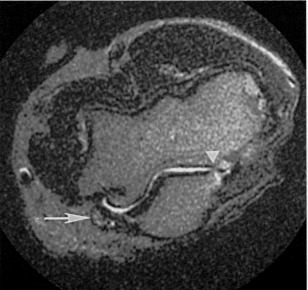

Figure 10-79 Ulnar neuritis due to osteophytic impingement in the cubital tunnel. Axial T1-weighted **(A)** and T2-weighted **(B)** images through the level of the cubital tunnel demonstrate a degenerative osteophyte medially displacing an enlarged ulnar nerve (*arrow*), which is increased in signal intensity. Note the degenerative change of the lateral ulnohumeral joint (*arrowhead*).

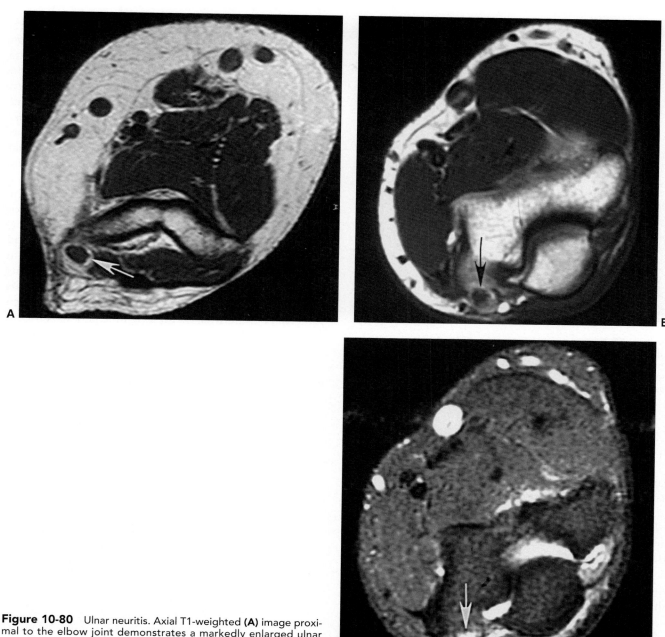

Figure 10-80 Ulnar neuritis. Axial T1-weighted **(A)** image proximal to the elbow joint demonstrates a markedly enlarged ulnar nerve (*arrow*). Axial T1-weighted **(B)** and T2-weighted **(C)** images at the level of the elbow joint in a different patient display thickening and increased T2-weighted signal in the inflamed nerve (*arrow*).

required—procedures such as osteophyte removal, retinacular release, and anterior transposition of the ulnar nerve (see Fig. 10-81) (3,48). Some surgeons perform epicondylectomy, but this is infrequently used at our institution (48).

Median Nerve

In the arm, the median nerve lies on the brachialis beneath the brachial fascia. The brachial artery and vein and the biceps tendon course along the nerve (24). The nerve passes distally to lie deep to the humeral head of the pronator teres.

It then courses between the deep humeral and ulnar heads of the pronator (48). The anterior interosseous branch arises deep to the pronator teres near the bifurcation of the radial and ulnar arteries. The median nerve then passes deep to the tendinous arch of the flexor superficialis. The lacertus fibrosis extends from the biceps tendon obliquely over the flexor and pronator muscles (24,48).

Median nerve compression can occur at the supracondylar process and ligament of Struthers, palmaris longus, the flexor carpi radialis brevis (a variant of the lacertus fibrosis), and by vascular tethering of the nerve

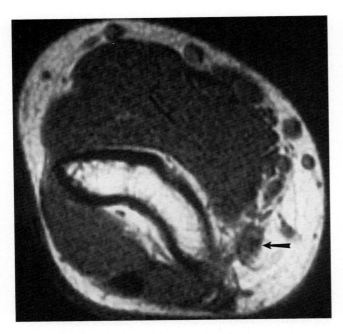

Figure 10-81 Ulnar nerve transposition. Axial T1-weighted image proximal to the elbow joint demonstrates postsurgical change of the posteromedial elbow. The ulnar nerve is now positioned anteromedial to the distal humerus and is surrounded by low intensity fibrous tissue (*arrow*).

(48). Fractures of the humerus and elbow dislocation commonly injure the median nerve (3,48).

Median nerve compression at the level of the supracondylar process accounts for about 1% of median nerve compression syndromes. The ulnar nerve is rarely associated (48).

Pronator syndrome is the most common cause of median nerve compression (3,142). Patients present with anterior elbow pain and may have numbness or tingling in the distribution of the median nerve (24,48). Repetitive activities such as weight training or manual labor provoke the symptoms. The condition is more common in females than males (48).

The median nerve is compressed between the two heads of the pronator teres, fibrous arch of the flexor digitorum superficialis or lacertus fibrosis (3,48). Cubital bursitis or partial biceps tendon tears can also compress the median nerve (Figs. 10-44 and 10-45) (3). Conservative therapy with rest and immobilization or activity reduction is the first approach. Surgery with muscle or lacertus fibrosis release are reserved for cases that don't respond to conservative regimens (48).

The motor branch of the median nerve (anterior interosseous nerve) may also be compressed by soft tissue masses, fibrous bands, accessory muscles, or enlarged bursae. Patients present with weakness in pinch and motor symptoms. Surgery is reserved for patients who do not respond to conservative therapy for 6 to 8 weeks (48,143). If MRI demonstrates a soft tissue mass or enlarged bursa, operative intervention is indicated.

Radial Nerve

The radial nerve takes an anterior course about 10 cm proximal to the lateral epicondyle (24,48,144). At the radiocapitellar joint, it divides into the superficial and posterior interosseous branches (see Fig. 10-82) (24). At the elbow, the posterior interosseous nerve courses between the two heads of the supinator muscle. The proximal edge of the supinator forms an arch for the nerve, termed the arcade of Frohse (24,48,144). The superficial branch passes anterior to the supinator and deep to the brachioradialis. The posterior interosseous nerve takes a dorsoradial course in the forearm. It passes through the supinator with small branches that innervate the extensor muscle groups and abductor pollicis longus (24,48,144).

The radial nerve or its major branches (superficial and posterior interosseous) is vulnerable to compression from the level of the lateral head of the triceps muscle to the distal forearm. Radial nerve injury proximal to the elbow occurs with humeral shaft fractures and poor technique when patients are using crutches for long time periods. Pressure from cast immobilization may also cause radial nerve compression in the arm (3,48).

Thickening of the arcade of Froshe can lead to posterior interosseous nerve syndrome. The nerve may also be

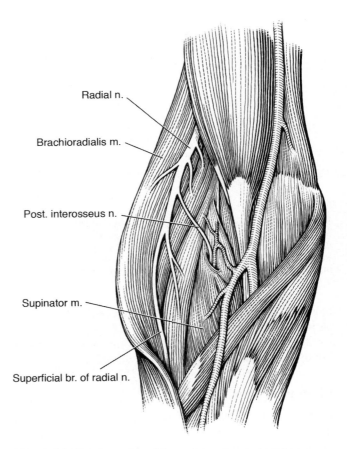

Figure 10-82 Illustration of the radial and posterior interosseous nerves.

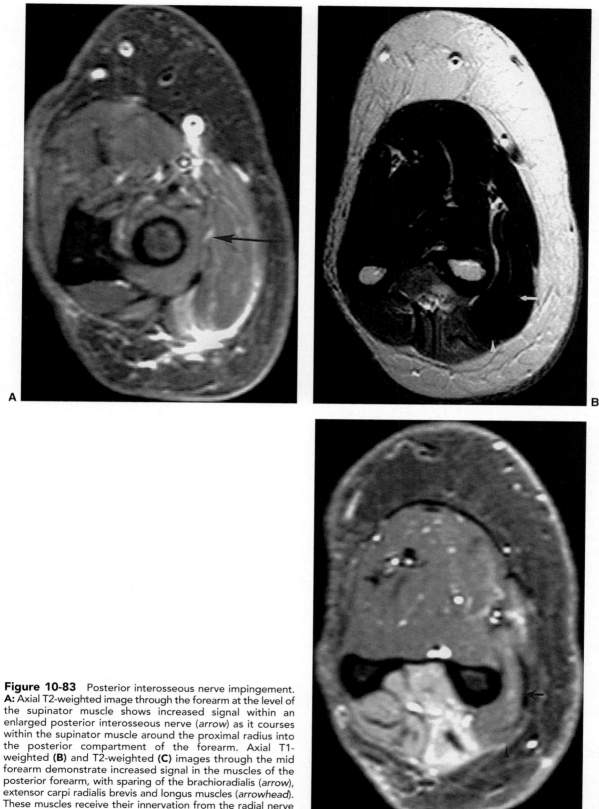

Figure 10-83 Posterior interosseous nerve impingement. **A:** Axial T2-weighted image through the forearm at the level of the supinator muscle shows increased signal within an enlarged posterior interosseous nerve (*arrow*) as it courses within the supinator muscle around the proximal radius into the posterior compartment of the forearm. Axial T1-weighted **(B)** and T2-weighted **(C)** images through the mid forearm demonstrate increased signal in the muscles of the posterior forearm, with sparing of the brachioradialis (*arrow*), extensor carpi radialis brevis and longus muscles (*arrowhead*). These muscles receive their innervation from the radial nerve proximal to the posterior interosseous nerve.

TABLE 10-9
RADIAL NERVE COMPRESSION SYNDROME

Humeral shaft fractures
Fracture/dislocation proximal radius
Cast immobilization
Poor crutch technique
High radial nerve bifurcation
Thickened arcade of Froshe
Radiocapitellar pannus
Vascular anomalies
Muscle anomalies
Inflamed bursae
Soft tissue masses
Synovial chondromatosis

From references 3, 48, 143, and 144.

compressed proximal to the lateral epicondyle by the lateral intermuscular septum. This occurs when the bifurcation (division into superficial and posterior interosseous branches) occurs more proximally (48). More distally, nerve compression may result from radiocapitellar synovitis with pannus formation, the radial recurrent artery, or the extensor carpi radialis brevis. There are multiple other causes, as well (Table 10-9) (3,48).

Patients present with pain and motor or sensory deficits. The posterior interosseous nerve is the motor branch and the superficial radial nerve the sensory branch. Uncommonly, both nerves can be effected (48,144). Pain may mimic lateral tennis elbow. In this setting, imaging is particularly useful to define the nature of the symptoms (2,3,48).

T1- and T2-weighted axial MRI is useful to follow the course of the nerves and define adjacent pathology. Muscles affected by the nerve distribution are high signal intensity on T2-weighted or STIR sequences (see Fig. 10-83). If not treated appropriately, fatty infiltration and atrophy of the involved muscles occurs over time. Contrast-enhanced images are useful in selected cases to detect neural ischemia and characterize soft tissue masses (2,3).

Treatment of radial nerve compression syndromes is conservative initially. For patients who do not respond to conservative measures, surgery should be performed within 4 months to avoid irreversible nerve damage (48).

MRI applications for the elbow and forearm will continue to expand. Chapter 15 discusses evolving MR applications in the musculoskeletal system.

REFERENCES

1. Berquist TH. MR imaging of the elbow and wrist. *Top Magn Reson Imaging* 1989;1:15–27.
2. Berquist TH. *MRI of the musculoskeletal system*, 4th ed. Philadelphia, PA: Lippincott Williams & Wilkins, 2001.
3. Major N. Magnetic resonance imaging of the elbow. *Curr Probl Diagn Radiol* 2000;1:27–40.
4. Murphy BJ. MR imaging of the elbow. *Radiology* 1992;184: 525–529.
5. Sofka CM, Potter HG. Imaging of elbow injuries in children and adults. *Radiol Clin North Am* 2002;40:251–265.
6. Narayama PA, Brey WW, Kulkarni MV, et al. Compensation for surface coil sensitivity variation in magnetic resonance imaging. *Magn Reson Imaging* 1988;6:271–274.
7. Beltran J, Rosenberg ZS, Kawelblum M, et al. Pediatric elbow fractures: MRI evaluation. *Skeletal Radiol* 1994;23:277–281.
8. Falchook FS, Zlatkin MB, Erbacher GE, et al. Rupture of the distal biceps tendon: evaluation with MR imaging. *Radiology* 1994;190: 659–663.
9. Fitzgerald SW, Curry DR, Erickson SJ, et al. Distal biceps tendon injury: MR imaging diagnosis. *Radiology* 1994;191:203–206.
10. Griffith JF, Roebuck DJ, Cheng JC, et al. Acute elbow trauma in children: spectrum of injury revealed by MR imaging not apparent on radiographs. *AJR Am J Roentgenol* 2001;176:53–60.
11. Quick HH, ladd ME, Hoevel M, et al. Real-time MRI of joint involvement with true FISP. *J Magn Reson Imaging* 2002;15: 710–715.
12. Giuffre BM, Moss MJ. Optimal positioning for MRI of the distal biceps brachii tendon: flexed abducted supinated view. *AJR Am J Roentgenol* 2004;182:944–946.
13. Hardy CJ, Katzberg RW, Frey RL, et al. Switched surface coil system for bilateral MR imaging. *Radiology* 1988;167:835–838.
14. Wright SM, Wright RM. Bilateral MR imaging with switched mutually coupled receiver coils. *Radiology* 1989;170:249–255.
15. Zou KH, Carrino JA. Comparison of accuracy and inter-reader agreement in side by side versus independent evaluation of MR imaging of the medial collateral ligament of the elbow. *Acad Radiol* 2002;9:520–525.
16. Yoshioka H, Ueno T, Tanaka T, et al. High resolution MR imaging of the elbow using a microscopy surface coil and a clinical 1.5T MR machine: preliminary results. *Skeletal Radiol* 2004;33: 265–271.
17. Cotten A, Jacobson J, Brossmann J, et al. Collateral ligaments of the elbow: conventional MR imaging and MR arthrography with coronal oblique plane and elbow flexion. *Radiology* 1997;204: 806–812.
18. Craig JG, Cramer KE, Cody DD, et al. Premature partial closure and other deformities of the growth plate: MR imaging and three-dimensional modeling. *Radiology* 1999;210:835–843.
19. Holtz P, Erickson SJ, Holmquist K. MR imaging of the elbow: technical considerations. *Semin Musculoskelet Radiol* 1998;2: 121–131.
20. Carrino JA, Morrison WB, Zou KH, et al. Non-contrast MR imaging and MR arthrography of the ulnar collateral ligament of the elbow: prospective evaluation of two-dimensional pulse sequences for detection of complete tears. *Skeletal Radiol* 2001; 30:625–632.
21. Nakanishi K, Masatomi T, Ochi T, et al. MR arthrography of the elbow: evaluation of the ulnar collateral ligament of the elbow. *Skeletal Radiol* 1996;25:629–634.
22. Boles CA, Kannam S, Cardwell AB. The forearm: anatomy of muscle compartments and nerves. *AJR Am J Roentgenol* 2000;174: 151–159.
23. Cotton A, Boutin RD, Resnick D. Normal anatomy of the elbow on conventional MR imaging and MR arthrography. *Semin Musculoskelet Radiol* 1998;2:133–140.
24. Rosse C, Rosse PC. *Hollinshead's textbook of anatomy*. Philadelphia, PA: Lippincott–Raven Publishers, 1997.
25. Anzel SH, Covey KW, Weiner AD, et al. Disruption of muscles and tendons: analysis of 1,014 cases. *Surgery* 1959;45:406–414.
26. Carter BL, Morehead J, Walpert SM, et al. *Cross-sectional anatomy: computed tomography and ultrasound correlation*. New York: Appleton-Century-Crofts, 1977.
27. Gaary EA, Potter HG, Altchek DW. Medial elbow pain in the throwing athlete: MR imaging evaluation. *AJR Am J Roentgenol* 1997;168:795–800.
28. Ring D, Jupiter JB. Current concepts review: fracture-dislocation of the elbow. *J Bone Joint Surg* 1998;80A:566–580.
29. Middleton WD, Lawson TL. *Anatomy and MRI of the joints*. New York: Raven Press, 1989.
30. Morrey BF. *The elbow and its disorders*, 3rd ed. Philadelphia, PA: WB Saunders, 2000.
31. Conway JE, Jobe FE, Glousman RE, et al. Medical instability of the elbow in throwing athletes. *J Bone Joint Surg* 1992;74A:67–83.

32. Mirowitz SA, London SL. Ulnar collateral ligament injury in baseball pitchers: MR imaging evaluation. *Radiology* 1992;185: 573–576.

33. Rijke AM, Goitz HT, McCue FC, et al. Stress radiography of the medial elbow ligaments. *Radiology* 1994;191:213–216.

34. Munshi M, Pretterkieber ML, Chung CB, et al. Anterior bundle of ulnar collateral ligament: evaluation of anatomic relationships by using MR imaging, MR arthrography and gross anatomic analysis. *Radiology* 2004;231:203–797.

35. Cohen MS, Hastings H. Rotatory instability of the elbow. *J Bone Joint Surg Am* 1997;79A:225–232.

36. Ho CP. Sports and occupational injuries of the elbow: MR imaging findings. *AJR Am J Roentgenol* 1995;164:1465–1471.

37. Hill NB, Bucchier JS, Shon F, et al. Magnetic resonance imaging of injury to the medial collateral ligament of the elbow. *J Shoulder Elbow Surg* 2000;9:418–422.

38. Rosenberg ZS, Beltran J, Cheung Y, et al. MR imaging of the elbow: normal variant and potential pitfalls of the trochlear groove and cubital tunnel. *AJR Am J Roentgenol* 1995;164: 415–418.

39. Salvo JP, Rizio L, Zvijac JE, et al. Avulsion fracture of the ulnar sublime tubercle in overhead throwing athletes. *Am J Sports Med* 2002;30:426–431.

40. Yamaguchi K, Sweet F, Bindra R, et al. The extraosseous and intraosseous arterial anatomy of the adult elbow. *J Bone Joint Surg Am* 1997;79A:1653–1661.

41. Sutherland S. *Nerves and nerve injuries.* Baltimore, MD: Lippincott Williams & Wilkins, 1978.

42. Pusey E, Lofkin RB, Brown RK, et al. Magnetic resonance imaging artifacts: mechanism and clinical significance. *RadioGraphics* 1986;6(5):891–911.

43. Rosenberg ZS, Beltran J, Cheung YY. Pseudo defect of the capitellum: potential MR imaging pitfall. *Radiology* 1994;191:821–823.

44. Sugimoto H, Ohsawa T. Ulnar collateral ligament in the growing elbow: MR imaging of normal development and throwing injuries. *Radiology* 1994;192:417–422.

45. Beltran J, Simon DC, Katz W, et al. Increased MR signal intensity in skeletal muscle adjacent to malignant tumors. *Radiology* 1987;162:251–255.

46. Beltran J, Rosenberg ZS. Nerve entrapment. *Semin Musculoskelet Radiol* 1998;2:175–184.

47. Pecina M, Boric I, Anticeric D. Intraoperatively proven anomalous Struther's ligament diagnosed by MRI. *Skeletal Radiol* 2002;31:532–535.

48. Spinner RJ, Spinner M. Nerve entrapment syndromes. In: Morrey BF, ed. *The elbow and its disorders,* 3rd Ed. Philadelphia, PA: WB Saunders, 2000:839–862.

49. Rosenberg ZS, Beltran J, Cheung YY, et al. The elbow: MR features of nerve disorders. *Radiology* 1993;188:235–240.

50. Rosenberg ZS, Bencardino J, Beltran J. MRI of normal variants and interpretation pitfalls of the elbow. *Semin Musculoskelet Radiol* 1998;2:141–153.

51. Grainger AJ, Elliott JM, Campbell RSD, et al. Direct MR arthrography: a review of current uses. *Clin Radiol* 2000;55:163–176.

52. O'Driscoll SW, Horii E, Carmichael S, et al. The cubital tunnel and ulnar neuropathy. *J Bone Joint Surg Br* 1991;73A:613–617.

53. Patten RM. Overuse syndromes and injuries involving the elbow: MR imaging findings. *AJR Am J Roentgenol* 1995;164:1205–1211.

54. Axel L. Blood flow effects in magnetic resonance imaging. *AJR Am J Roentgenol* 1984;143:1157–1166.

55. Bradley WG, Waluch V Jr. Blood flow: magnetic resonance imaging. *Radiology* 1985;154:443–450.

56. Bradley WG Jr, Waluch V, Lai KS, et al. Appearance of rapidly flowing blood on magnetic resonance images. *AJR Am J Roentgenol* 1984;143:1167–1174.

57. Bradley WG Jr. Flow phenomena in MR imaging. *AJR Am J Roentgenol* 1988;150:983–994.

58. Felmlee JP, Ehman RL. Spatial presaturation: a method for suppressing flow artifacts and improving depiction of vascular anatomy in MR imaging. *J Comput Assist Tomogr* 1987;11:369–377.

59. Mulligan SA, Schwartz ML, Broussard MF, et al. Heterotopic calcification and tears of the ulnar collateral ligament. Radiographic and MR imaging findings. *AJR Am J Roentgenol* 2000;175: 1099–1102.

60. Donnelly LF, Klostermeier TT, Klosterman LA. Traumatic elbow effusions in pediatric patients: are occult fractures the rule? *AJR Am J Roentgenol* 1998;171:243–245.

61. Donnelly LF. Traumatic elbow effusion in children are not synonymous with occult fractures even with evaluation with MR imaging. *AJR Am J Roentgenol* 2002;179:531–532.

62. Major N, Crawford ST. Elbow effusion in trauma in adults and children: is there occult fracture? *AJR Am J Roentgenol* 2002;178: 413–418.

63. Beltran J, Rosenberg ZS. Diagnosis of compression and entrapment neuropathies of the upper extremity: value of MR imaging. *AJR Am J Roentgenol* 1994;163:525–531.

64. Berquist TH. Magnetic resonance imaging of musculoskeletal neoplasms. *Clin Orthop* 1989;244:101–118.

65. Coel M, Yamada CY, Ko J. MR imaging of patients with lateral epicondylitis of the elbow (tennis elbow): importance of increased signal of the anconeus muscle. *AJR Am J Roentgenol* 1993;161:1019–1021.

66. Burn PR, Hunt JL, King CM, et al. MR imaging of acute trauma to the elbow. *AJR Am J Roentgenol* 2002;179:1076.

67. Carrino JA, Morrison WB, Zou KH, et al. Lateral ulnar collateral ligament of the elbow: opimization of evaluation with two-dimensional MR imaging. *Radiology* 2001;218:118–125.

68. Raupp P, Haas D, Lovasz G. Epiphyseal separation of the distal humerus. *J Perinat Med* 2000;30:528–530.

69. Sawant MR, Narayaman S, O'Neill K, et al. Distal humeral epiphysis fracture separation in neonates-diagnosis using MRI scan. *Injury* 2002;33:179–181.

70. Schickendantz MS, Ho CP, Koh J, et al. Stress injury of the proximal ulna in baseball players. *Am J Sports Med* 2002;30: 737–741.

71. Thornton R, Riley GM, Steinbach LS. Magnetic resonance imaging of sports injuries of the elbow. *Top Magn Reson Imaging* 2003;14:69–86.

72. Costa M, Owen-Johnstone S, Tucker J, et al. The value of MRI in the assessment of elbow injuries in a neonate. *J Bone Joint Surg Br* 2001;83B:544–546.

73. Akagi M, Ito T, Ikeda N, et al. Total avulsion fracture of the coronoid tubercle caused by baseball pitching. A case report. *Am J Sports Med* 2000;28:580–582.

74. Sofka CM, Pavlov H. Sports injury update: imaging features. *Curr Probl Diagn Radiol* 2001;30:174–187.

75. Lee JK, Yao L. Stress fractures: MR imaging. *Radiology* 1988;169:217–220.

76. Yao L, Lee JK. Occult intraosseous fracture: detection with MR imaging. *Radiology* 1988;167:749–751.

77. Anderson SE, Otsuka NY, Steinbach LS. MR imaging of pediatric elbow trauma. *Semin Musculoskelet Radiol* 1998;2:185–198.

78. Skaggs DL, Cluck MW, Mostofi A, et al. Lateral entry pin fixation in management of supracondylar fractures in children. *J Bone Joint Surg Am* 2004;86A:702–707.

79. Chung CB, Kim HJ. Sports injuries of the elbow. *Magn Reson Imaging Clin N Am* 2003;11:239–253.

80. Herzog RJ. Magnetic resonance imaging of the elbow. *Magn Reson Q* 1993;9:188–210.

81. Schwartz ML. Collateral ligaments. *Semin Musculoskelet Radiol* 1998;2:155–161.

82. Potter HG, Weiland AJ, Schatz JA, et al. Posterolateral rotatory instability of the elbow: usefulness of MR imaging in diagnosis. *Radiology* 1997;204:185–189.

83. Patel N, Weiner SD. Osteochondritis dissecans involving the trochlea: report of two patients and review of the literature. *J Pediatr Orthop* 2002;24:48–51.

84. Le TB, Mont MA, Jones LC, et al. Atraumatic osteonecrosis of the adult elbow. *Clin Orthop Relat Res* 2000;373:141–145.

85. Sonin AH, Fitzgerald SW. MR imaging of sports injuries in the adult elbow: a tailored approach. *AJR Am J Roentgenol* 1996;167:3 25–331.

86. Bowen RE, Otsuka NY, Yorn T, et al. Osteochondral lesions of the capitellum in pediatric patients. Role of magnetic resonance imaging. *J Pediatr Orthop* 2001;21:298–301.

87. Shaughnessy WJ. Osteochondritis dissecans. In: Morrey BF, ed. *The elbow and its disorders,* 3rd Ed. Philadelphia, PA: WB Saunders, 2000:255–260.

88. Woodward AH, Bianco AJ. Osteochondritis dissecans of the elbow. *Clin Orthop* 1975;110:35–44.

89. Krijnen MR, Lim L, Williams WJ. Arthroscopic treatment of osteochondritis dissecans of the capitellum: report of five male athletes. *J Arthro Related Surg* 2003;19:210–214.

90. Herrmann DN, Preston DC, McIntesh KA, et al. Localization of ulnar neuropathy with conduction block across the elbow. *Muscle Nerve* 2001;24:698–670.

91. Kraushaar BS, Nirschl RL. Tendinosis of the elbow (tennis elbow). *J Bone Joint Surg Am* 1999;81A:259–278.

92. Williams BD, Schweitzer ME, Weisharpt D, et al. Partial tears of the distal biceps tendon: MR appearance and associated findings. *Skeletal Radiol* 2001;30:560–564.

93. Sonin A. Tendon disorders. *Semin Musculoskelet Radiol* 1998;2:163–173.

94. Miller TT, Adler RS. Sonography of tears of the distal biceps tendon. *AJR Am J Roentgenol* 2000;175:1081–1086.

95. Nirschl RP. Muscle and tendon trauma: tennis elbow. In: Morrey BF, ed. The elbow and its disorders, 3rd ed. Philadelphia, PA: WB Saunders, 2000:523–535.

96. Berquist TH. *Imaging of orthopedic trauma*, 2nd ed. New York: Raven Press, 1992.

97. Pasternack I, Touvinen E-M, Lohman M, et al. MR findings in humeral epicondylitis. *Acta Radiol* 2001;42:434–440.

98. Liessi G, Cesari S, Spalviero B, et al. The US, CT and MR findings of cubital bursitis: a report of five cases. *Skeletal Radiol* 1996;25:471–475.

99. Skaf AY, Boutin RD, Dantas RWM, et al. Bicipitoradial bursitis: MR imaging findings in eight patients and anatomic data from contrast material opacification of bursae followed by routine radiography and MR imaging in cadavers. *Radiology* 1999;212:111–116.

100. Yamamoto T, Mizuno K, Soejima T, et al. Bicipital radial bursitis. CT and MR appearance. *Comput Med Imaging Graph* 2001;25:531–533.

101. Tiger E, Mayer DP, Glazer R. Complete avulsion of the triceps tendon: MRI diagnosis. *Comput Med Imaging Graph* 1993;17:51–54.

102. Farrar EL III, Lippert FG III. Avulsion of the triceps tendon. *Clin Orthop* 1981;161:242–246.

103. Spinner RJ, Hayden FR, Hipps CT, et al. Imaging the snapping triceps tendon. *AJR Am J Roentgenol* 1996;167:1550–1551.

104. Yiannoakopoulos CK. Imaging of snapping triceps syndrome. *Radiology* 2002;225:607–608.

105. Dreyfuss U, Kessler I. Snapping elbow due to dislocation of the medial head of the triceps. *J Bone Joint Surg Br* 1978;60B:56–57.

106. Miller TT, Shapiro MA, Schultz E, et al. Comparison of sonography and MRI for diagnosing epicondylitis. *J Clin Ultrasound* 2002;30:193–202.

107. Potter HG, Hannafin JA, Morwessel RM, et al. Lateral epicondylitis: correlation of MR imaging, surgical, and histopathologic findings. *Radiology* 1995;196:43–46.

108. Mackay D, Rangan A, Hide G, et al. The objective diagnosis of early tennis elbow by magnetic resonance imaging. *Occup Med (Lond)* 2003;53:309–312.

109. Van den Berghe GR, Queenan JF, Murphy DA. Isolated rupture of the brachialis. *J Bone Joint Surg Am* 2001;83A:1074–1075.

110. Shellock FG, Fukunaga T, Mink JH, et al. Acute effects of exercise on MR imaging of skeletal muscle: concentric vs eccentric actions. *AJR Am J Roentgenol* 1991;156:765–768.

111. Fleckstein JL, Bertocci LA, Nunnally RL, et al. Exercise enhanced MR imaging of variations in forearm muscle anatomy and sue: importance in MR spectroscopy. *AJR Am J Roentgenol* 1989;153:693–698.

112. Glajchen N, Schwartz ML, Andrews JR, et al. Avulsion fracture of the sublime tubercle of the ulna: a newly recognized injury in the throwing athlete. *AJR Am J Roentgenol* 1998;170:627–628.

113. David TS. Medial elbow pain in the throwing athlete. *Orthopedics* 2003;26:94–103.

114. Potter HG. Imaging of post-traumatic and soft tissue dysfunction of the elbow. *Clin Orthop Relat Res* 2000;370:9–18.

115. Sonin AH, Tutton SM, Fitzgerald SW, et al. MR imaging of the adult elbow. *RadioGraphics* 1996;16:1323–1336.

116. Feldman MD. Arthroscopic excision of a ganglion cyst from the elbow. *J Arthro Related Surg* 2000;16:661–664.

117. Awaya H, Schweitzer ME, Feng SA, et al. Elbow synovial fold syndrome: MR imaging findings. *AJR Am J Roentgenol* 2001;177:1377–1381.

118. Unger E, Moldofsky P, Gateby R, et al. Diagnosis of osteomyelitis by MR imaging. *AJR Am J Roentgenol* 1988;150:605–610.

119. Dzupa V, Bartonicek J, Sprindrich J, et al. Osteoid osteoma of the olecranon process of the ulna in subchondral location. *Arch Orthop Trauma Surg* 2001;121:117–118.

120. Unni KK. *Dahlin's bone tumors: general aspects and data on 11,087 cases*, 5th ed. Philadelphia, PA: Lippincott–Raven, 1996.

121. Weiss SW, Goldblum JR. *Enzinger and Weiss soft tissue tumors*, 4th ed. St Louis, MO: Mosby, 2001.

122. Dooms GC, Hricak H, Sollitto RA, et al. Lipomatous tumors and tumors with fatty component: MR imaging potential and comparison of MR and CT results. *Radiology* 1985;157:479–483.

123. Dinauer P, Bojescul JA, Kaplan KJ, et al. Bilateral lipoma arborescens of the bicipitoradial bursa. *Skeletal Radiol* 2002;31:661–665.

124. Doyle AJ, Miller MV, French JG. Lipoma arborescens in the bicipital bursa of the elbow: MRI findings in two cases. *Skeletal Radiol* 2002;31:656–660.

125. Cohen JM, Weinreb JC, Redman HC. Arteriovenous malformations of the extremities. MR imaging. *Radiology* 1986;158:475–479.

126. Anderson SE, Johnston JO, Zalaudek CJ, et al. Peripheral nerve ectopic meningioma of the elbow. *Skeletal Radiol* 2001;30:639–642.

127. Rosen BR, Flemings DM, Kushner DC, et al. Hematologic bone marrow disorders: quantitative chemical shift MR imaging. *Radiology* 1988;169:799–804.

128. Wing VW, Jeffrey RB, Federle MP, et al. Chronic osteomyelitis examined by CT. *Radiology* 1985;154:171–174.

129. Lewin JS, Rosenfield NS, Hoffner PB, et al. Acute osteomyelitis in children: combined Tc-99m and Ga-67 imaging. *Radiology* 1986;158:795–804.

130. Tang JSH, Gold RH, Bassett LW, et al. Musculoskeletal infection of the extremities: evaluation with MR imaging. *Radiology* 1988;166:205–209.

131. Vogler JB III, Murphy WA. Bone marrow imaging. *Radiology* 1988;168:679–693.

132. Crum NF. Tuberculosis presenting as epitrochlear lymphadenitis. *Scand J Infect Dis* 2003;35:888–890.

133. Beltran J, Noto AM, Herman LJ, et al. Joint effusions: MR imaging. *Radiology* 1986;158:133–137.

134. Beltran J, Caudell JL, Herman LA, et al. Rheumatoid arthritis: MR imaging manifestations. *Radiology* 1987;165:153–157.

135. Spritzer CE, Dalinka MK, Kressel HY. Magnetic resonance imaging of pigmented villonodular synovitis: a report of two cases. *Skeletal Radiol* 1987;16:316–319.

136. Yulish BS, Lieberman JM, Newman AJ, et al. Juvenile rheumatoid arthritis: assessment with MR imaging. *Radiology* 1987;165:149–152.

137. Quinn SF, Haberman JJ, Fitzgerald SW, et al. Evaluation of loose bodies of the elbow with MR imaging. *J Magn Reson Imaging* 1994;4:169–172.

138. Jazrawi LM, Ong B, Jazwari AJ, et al. Synovial chondromatosis of the elbow. *Am J Orthop* 2001;30:223–224.

139. Funk MB, Schmidt H, Becker S, et al. Modified magnetic resonance imaging score compared with orthopedic and radiologic scores for hemophilic arthropathy. *Hemophilia* 2002;8:98–103.

140. Martinoli C, Bianchi S, Gandolfo G, et al. US of nerve intrapment in osseofibous tunnels of the upper and lower limbs. *RadioGraphics* 2000;20:S199–S217.

141. Sullivan PP, Berquist TH. Magnetic resonance imaging of the hand, wrist and forearm: utility in patients with pain and dysfunction as a result of trauma. *Mayo Clin Proc* 1991;66:1217–1221.

142. Kopell HP, Thompson WAL. The pronator syndrome. *N Engl J Med* 1958;259:713–715.

143. Yanagisawa H, Okada K, Sashi R. Posterior interosseous nerve palsy caused by synovial chondromatosis of the elbow joint. *Clin Radiol* 2001;56:510–514.

144. Chien AJ, Jamador DA, Jacobson JA, et al. Sonography and MR imaging of posterior interosseous nerve syndrome with surgical correlation. *AJR Am J Roentgenol* 2003;181:219–221.

Hand and Wrist

Thomas H. Berquist

Imaging of the hand and wrist can be difficult due to the complex bone and soft tissue anatomy. Optimization of the numerous imaging techniques and approaches is essential in today's cost-conscious environment (1–6). Routine radiographs or computed radiography (CR) and fluoroscopically positioned spot films are usually adequate for identification of fractures and other osseous pathology. Subtle changes may require radionuclide studies followed by computed (CT) or conventional tomography to define clearly the nature of bone lesions. Invasive techniques such as arthrography and tenography have been used to identify ligament and tendon injuries (7). Ultrasonography has been used to evaluate tendons, and CT is the technique of choice for evaluating subluxations of the distal radioulnar joint (8,9). The role of magnetic resonance imaging (MRI) in the hand and wrist has continued to expand with new pulse sequences, coil technology, and higher field strength magnets [3 Tesla (T) and 8 T]. MR arthrography and MR angiography have contributed to the increased utilization of MRI for evaluation of hand and wrist disorders (10–15).

Recent studies have demonstrated the clinical impact of MRI. Hobby et al. (5) demonstrated that MR studies changed the clinical diagnosis in 55%, modified the treatment plan in 45%, and improved the physicians understanding of the disease process in 67%.

TECHNIQUE

Multiple factors must be considered to optimize MR examinations. Considerations include the presence of metal or electrical devices, the area of interest (small vs. large), patient size, patient condition, the need for sedation, and whether intravenous or intraarticular contrast may be required (16,17).

Patient Positioning/Coil Selection

MRI examinations of the hand and wrist can be difficult to perform due to limitations in positioning and the demanding anatomic detail required for lesion detection

(16,18,19). Patient comfort is an essential part of the examination. If the position is difficult to tolerate, motion artifact and image degradation will occur. In our initial review of upper extremity MRI studies, we noted motion artifacts or incomplete studies due to patient discomfort in 25% of cases (18).

Positioning depends upon patient size, information required (i.e., motion studies), software, and coil availability. When possible, we position the patient with the arm at the side and the hand and wrist in the optimal or most comfortable position (pronation, supination, or thumb up) (see Fig. 11-1). The wrist can also be placed over the abdomen with the arm flexed. However, the coil must be separated from the abdominal wall to prevent respiratory motion artifact. Larger patients and children may be positioned in the prone or lateral decubitus position with the arm above the head (see Fig. 11-2). In this setting, shoulder discomfort frequently leads to motion artifact and reduced image quality (18–20).

Once the hand and wrist are positioned they should be supported with pads or bolsters to reduce motion and enhance comfort. The exception to this approach is when motion studies are required. In this case, motion control devices can be used to optimize position changes (7,21).

Uniform signal intensity is most easily obtained using new flat or circumferential coil systems (see Fig. 11-3) (19,22–26). The small, flat coils (3 and 5 inch) are also adequate for hand and wrist imaging. Flat coils allow more flexibility for positioning and motion studies (16). Dual coils allow simultaneous evaluation of both hands and wrists when pathology is bilateral or comparison is required (23).

Recently, Yoshioka et al. (26) used 23-mm flat circular microscopy coils to achieve improved spatial resolution and signal-to-noise ratios compared to conventional 5-inch coils.

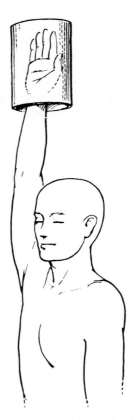

Figure 11-2 Patient positioned for evaluation of the hand and wrist using a circumferential (volume) coil. The arm is above the head. This position is not easily tolerated, and motion artifacts are likely to occur. Shoulder discomfort frequently develops early in the examination.

Optimal image quality for hand and wrist imaging requires a small field of view (FOV) (see Fig. 11-4) (19,27,28). We typically use an 8- to 12-cm FOV for examinations with both flat and volume coils. The image matrix should be 256 to 512 with 1- to 3-mm sections (Table 11-1). Smaller sections (0.6 to 1.0 mm) are used for volume acquisitions and three-dimensional imaging (16,29). In general, one acquisition is adequate, though for improved image quality we occasionally use two acquisitions.

Most imaging of the hand and wrist is performed at 1.5 T. However, experience with 3 T magnets is increasing. The primary advantage of extremity imaging at 3 T is increased signal-to-noise ratio (SNR). SNR increases linearly with field strength; hence, the SNR at 3 T is twice that of standard systems at 1.5 T. This allows significant improvement in spatial resolution without increasing image time. More detailed anatomic information may be provided for small structures including the ligaments, articular cartilage and triangular fibrocartilage complex (TFCC).

We have used custom designed transmit/receive coils (Fig. 11-3D) with 6-cm internal diameter for fingers and 10-cm diameter for wrists. This results in even greater SNR compared to phased array coils. Though experience is early, imaging of the hand and wrist at 3 T may offer advantages over 1.5 T.

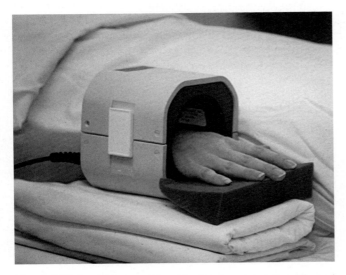

Figure 11-1 Patient positioned with the arm at the side and supported for comfort.

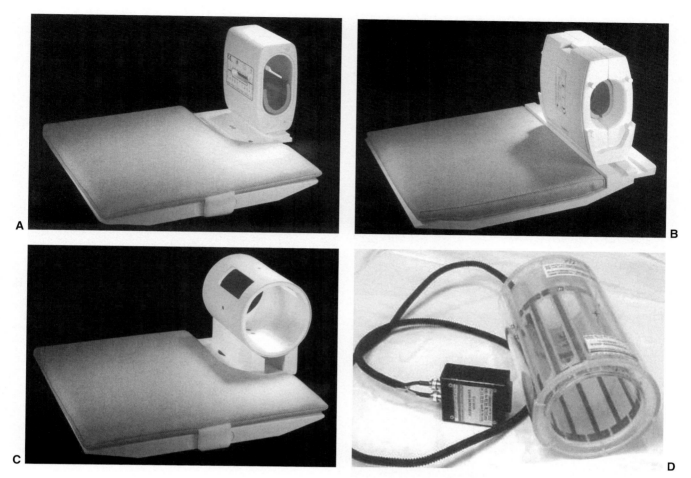

Figure 11-3 Coils for hand and wrist imaging. **A:** Quadrature or phased array configuration can be positioned either vertically or horizontally. **B:** Four-channel phased array coil for the wrist that can be used with less than 6-cm field of view. Coil can be positioned similar to **A**. **C:** Small extremity quadrature phased array coil. **A–C** can be used with GE or Siemens systems. (Courtesy of MRI Devices Corp., Waukesha, Wisconsin.) **D:** Birdcage 10-cm coil for hand and wrist imaging at 3 T. Coil designed by Joel Felmlee, PhD. With postdoctoral fellow Armen Kocharian, PhD, Mayo Clinic, Rochester, MN.

TABLE 11-1

MR TECHNIQUES FOR HAND AND WRIST IMAGING

Procedure	Plane	Sequences	Sections/Skip	FOV	Matrix	Acquisitions NEX
Screening						
Wrist	Axial	T1 400–500/10–20	3 mm/0.5	8 cm	512 × 224	1
	Axial	FSE PD 2,400–2,500/20–30	3 mm/0.5	8 cm	256 × 224	1
	Coronal	T1 400–500/10–20	3 mm/0.5	8 cm	512 × 224	1
	Axial	FSE T2 3,500–3,600/70–90	3 mm/0.5	8 cm	256 × 192	1
	Coronal	DESS 24/7, FA 25°	3 mm/0.5	8 cm	256 × 192	1
Hand/finger[a]	Coronal	T1 400–500/10–20	1–3 mm/0.5	6 cm	512 × 224	1
	Axial	T1 400–500/10–20	3 mm/0.5	6 cm	512 × 224	1
	Sagittal[a]	FSE T2 3,500–4,000/70–90	1–3 mm/0.5	6 cm	256 × 192	1
	Sagittal[a]	T1 400–500/10-20	1–3 mm/0.5	6 cm	512 × 224	1
Wrist arthrogram	Coronal	T1 FS 600/18	3 mm/0.5	8 cm	256 × 256	2
	Sagittal	T1 FS 600/18	3 mm/0.5	8 cm	256 × 256	2
	Axial	T1 FS 600/18	3 mm/0.5	8 cm	256 × 256	2
	Coronal	3D GRE 45/9, 30°	1 mm/60/0.5	8 cm	256 × 192	1
Angiogram	Coronal	21/6, 30° or 3.8/1.4, 30°	1 mm/40	8 cm	512 × 256	1

FSE, fast spin echo; PD, proton density; FS, fat suppression; GRE, gradient echo; FOV, field of view; FA, flip angle
[a]flexion and extension

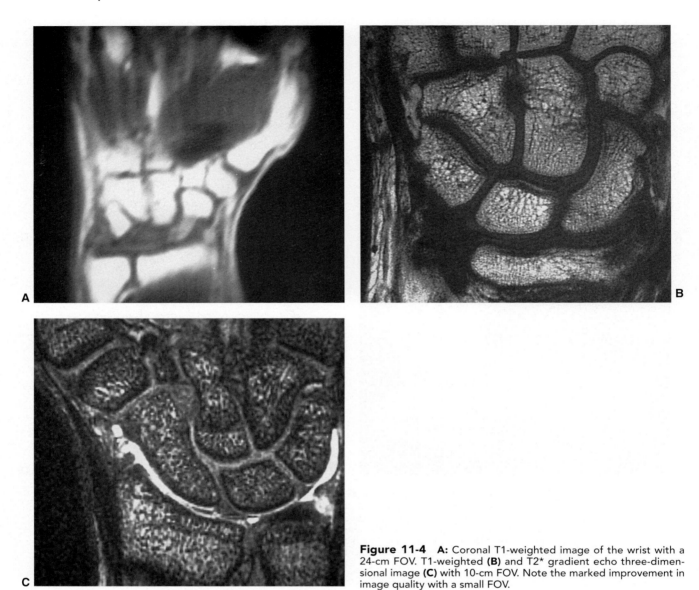

Figure 11-4   A: Coronal T1-weighted image of the wrist with a 24-cm FOV. T1-weighted **(B)** and T2* gradient echo three-dimensional image **(C)** with 10-cm FOV. Note the marked improvement in image quality with a small FOV.

Pulse Sequences/Image Planes

Once the patient has been positioned, the proper pulse sequences and image planes must be selected to demonstrate the anatomy and characterize the lesion (Table 11-1). An effective screening examination can be accomplished by the beginning with either a coronal or sagittal scout (SE 500-400/10-20). This should include the full area of the hand and wrist to be examined. The sequences and image planes vary with clinical indication. One can begin with a standard screening examination and add additional sequences or gadolinium when indicated. T1- and T2-weighted sequences are performed. We use conventional spin-echo T1-weighted sequences and fast spin-echo (FSE) T2-weighted sequences with fat suppression in most cases (Table 11-1). Conventional short TI inversion recovery (STIR) sequences have

been replaced with FSE inversion recovery sequences. Fluid and pathologic tissues have high signal intensity in comparison to suppressed marrow and fat signal.

Gradient-echo (GRE) sequences can be performed using two- or three-dimensional techniques. We use the latter with sixty 0.6- to 1.0-mm sections to allow reformatting in any image plane. Ligament, capsular, and articular anatomy are well defined using this approach (19,29). We are also routinely performing a coronal dual echo steady state (DESS) sequence to evaluate articular cartilage (see Fig. 11-5). Multiple (about 100) 1.0-mm sections can be performed in 6 minutes, 26 seconds. Our screening examination includes all three image planes (axial, coronal, and sagittal). For certain anatomy, oblique planes are useful (Table 11-2). This is particularly true for the carpal bones (see Fig. 11-6) and individual digits of the hand.

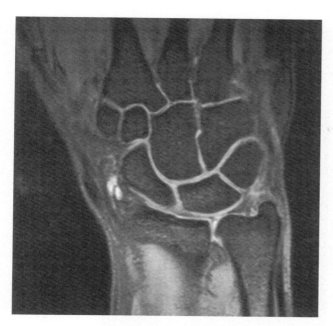

Figure 11-5 Coronal DESS image demonstrating high signal intensity of articular cartilage and low signal intensity marrow.

Magnetic Resonance Arthrography

Wrist and hand arthrograms are performed using either indirect (intravenous) or intraarticular injections.

Indirect arthrography has several advantages in that it is minimally invasive, enhances joint fluid (giving an arthrographic effect), and does not require additional time for intraarticular monitoring and injection. Passive or active exercise is performed prior to imaging to enhance fluid distribution. Using this approach, Schweitzer et al. (30) reported 100% accuracy for triangular fibrocartilage tears and 96% for scapholunate ligament tears.

Disadvantages of indirect arthrography include lack of fluid control (cannot measure joint volume), inability to

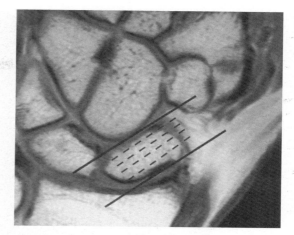

Figure 11-6 Coronal T1-weighted image demonstrating selection of oblique sagittal images to evaluate the scaphoid.

aspirate fluid, inability to perform diagnostic injections, and inability to do isolated compartment studies (19,30). The last may make subtle lesions more difficult to detect.

Patients should be preselected so schedules can be adjusted. Ultrasound, palpation, or fluoroscopy can be used for needle position and injection (19,31). We prefer fluoroscopic monitoring of injections. The radiocarpal, intercarpal, and distal radioulnar joint may all need to be injected. We begin with the most symptomatic region or area of suspected pathology.

The patient can be seated next to the fluoroscopic table or lying supine with the arm extended and hand resting palm down. The wrist is prepared using sterile technique. The entry site is injected with local anesthetic (1% lidocaine) using a 25-gauge needle. The radiocarpal joint is entered dorsally with the wrist slightly flexed (see Fig. 11-7). The extensor tendon and area of the scapholunate ligament should be avoided. The needles should be angled proximally (Fig. 11-7) to avoid the dorsal lip of the radius. Injection of the intercarpal or distal radioulnar joint is performed with the hand flat and palm down (see Fig. 11-8). It is necessary that fluid be aspirated and studied prior to injection. Three to four mL of diluted gadolinium (0.2 mL in 20 mL of 50% iodinated contrast and 50% lidocaine or marcaine) is injected using fluoroscopic guidance.

When the injection is completed, the patient is transferred to the MR gantry. A phased array wrist coil is used. The patient is positioned as described above. For conventional arthrography, the standard wrist or hand coils are used. When motion studies are required, a positioning device can be used with a noncircumferential coil (19,21). Conventional sequences and image planes are described in Table 11-1. GRE sequences are used for motion studies.

Sahin et al. (32) used three-dimensional spoiled GRE sequences after intraarticular contrast to create virtual arthroscopic images of the triangular fibrocartilage. Image data was

TABLE 11-2

MRI OF THE HAND AND WRIST: IMAGE PLANES

Anatomic Structure	Image Plane
Distal radius and ulna	Axial and coronal
	Sagittal for fragment alignment
Distal radioulnar joint	Coronal, axial (neutral, pronation, supination)
Soft tissue proximal wrist	Axial and sagittal
Carpal tunnel	Axial
Carpal bones—scaphoid	Axial and coronal, add oblique sagittal
Metacarpal/phalanges	Axial and oblique sagittal
Tendons	Axial and sagittal
Ligaments	Axial, coronal, and oblique reformats

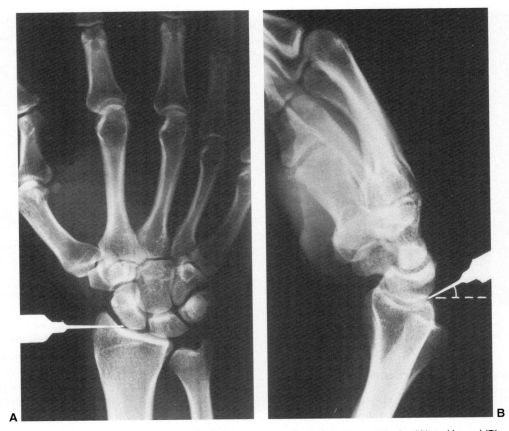

Figure 11-7 Injection site for the radiocarpal joint seen from the posteroanterior **(A)** and lateral **(B)** views. Flexing the wrist slightly facilitates needle placement. The needle is angled proximally. The region of the scapholunate ligament should be avoided.

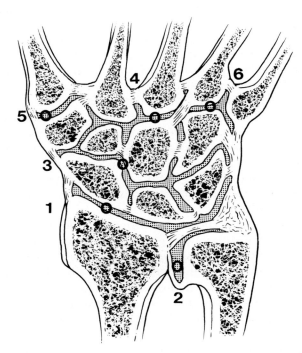

Figure 11-8 Injection sites for the radiocarpal (*1*), distal radioulnar joint (*2*), and intercarpal joint (*3*). The common carpometacarpal joint (*4*), first carpometacarpal joint (*5*), and outer carpometacarpal (*6*) joints are rarely injected.

transferred to a computer and using navigator software the images were recreated. Preliminary results were promising.

MR Angiography

Contrast enhanced MR angiography has improved significantly in recent years. Major and digital vessels can easily be demonstrated. Aneurysms, pseudoaneurysms, and vasculitis can be clearly demonstrated (see Fig. 11-9) (10,33–35). Osseous ischemic changes and vascular tumors are also more readily evaluated (12,36,37).

ANATOMY

The osseous and soft tissue anatomy of the hand and wrist is complex. Therefore, in the past, numerous imaging techniques have been required for thorough evaluation. MRI is an additional technique that can provide valuable information regarding subtle soft tissue and bone pathology (7,16,18,19,22,29,38–47).

Osseous Anatomy

There are eight carpal bones in the wrist and five metacarpals and 14 phalanges in the hand (see Fig. 11-10).

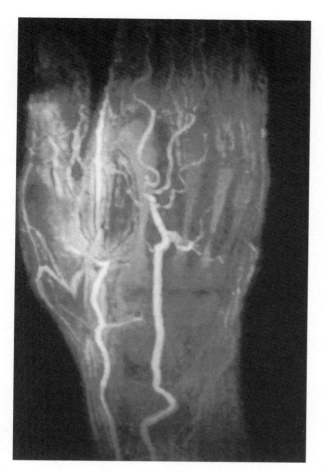

Figure 11-9 MR angiogram of the hand and wrist in a patient with vasculitis. There are multiple occlusions and vascular irregularities.

Bones of the wrist form three major articular groups composed of the distal radioulnar joint, the radiocarpal joint, and the midcarpal articulation. The distal radial metaphysis and epiphysis is a largely cancellous bone with only a thin cortical shell which makes this region ideally suited for MR imaging (48,49). The distal radius is elongated on its radial side, forming the radial styloid (Fig. 11-10). Distally, the radius has two articular fossae for the scaphoid and lunate, respectively. The distal articular surface normally angles 24° toward the ulna in the frontal plane and 12° to 15° volarly in the lateral or sagittal plane (see Fig. 11-11). There is a notch in the ulnar side of the radius termed the sigmoid notch that articulates with the distal ulna (see Fig. 11-12). Of importance, on the dorsal surface of the radius are the sulci and palpable dorsal protuberance termed Lister tubercle (Fig. 11-12). These osseous changes assist in forming the dorsal compartments for the extensor tendons of the wrist (see Figs. 11-12 and 11-13) (48,49). The cortex in the distal ulna is somewhat thicker than the radius and it also has a spikelike projection on the most medial aspect termed the ulnar styloid. There is a groove in the dorsal ulna for the sixth dorsal compartment (extensor carpi ulnaris [ECU]) (Fig. 11-13)

(38,48,50). The head of the ulna articulates with the distal radius via the sigmoid notch and the lunate and triquetrum distally. It is separated from the latter two structures by a TFCC. This will be discussed more completely below. The carpal bones are composed of three anatomic groups (Fig. 11-10). The proximal row consists of the scaphoid, lunate, triquetrum, and overlapping pisiform. The proximal surfaces of these bones should form a smooth, unbroken arch in the coronal plane. In the sagittal plane, the angle formed by the scaphoid and lunate should be between 30° and 60°. A second osseous anatomic group, or the distal carpal row, consists of the trapezoid, capitate, and hamate. The third compartment is composed of the trapezium and five metacarpals (19,38,48,50).

Certain key features of carpal anatomy deserve mention. The scaphoid is the largest carpal bone in the proximal row and serves as a link between the proximal and distal rows (see Figs. 11-4 through 11-6). The scaphoid articulates with the radius, lunate medially, capitate distomedially and the trapezium and trapezoid distally. The scaphoid ridge is located on the mid surface and accepts 80% of the vascular supply to the scaphoid (19,48,50).

The lunate has four articular facets for the radius proximally, the scaphoid laterally, the triquetrum medially, and the capitate distally. Viegas et al. (51) described the lunate as type 1 or 2 based upon the presence of a hamate articular surface. Type 1 (34.5%) has no hamate facet and type 2 (65.5%) has a hamate articular facet (Fig. 11-14) (51,52).

The capitate is the largest carpal bone (see Figs. 11-15E, 11-16A, and 11-17B) and plays an important role in the transverse carpal arch. In about 85% of patients, there is a small facet that articulates with the fourth metacarpal base (19,48,53).

The hamate has a prominent palmar projection (hook) (Fig. 11-15E) that forms the medial boundary of the carpal tunnel. This serves as the attachment for the flexor retinaculum.

The trapezium also has four articular facets. On the palmar surface there is a groove for the flexor carpi radialis tendon and a prominent ridge (trapezial ridge) for attachment of the flexor retinaculum and scaphotrapezial and anterior oblique ligaments (Figs. 11-10 and 11-16A) (12,48).

The proximal and middle phalanges of the fingers are similar in structure with proximal and distal flaring. The osseous composition of these structures is primarily cancellous. There are two phalanges on the thumb as it lacks a middle phalanx. The remaining digits have three phalanges (Fig. 11-10) (38,48,50).

There are numerous osseous variants (54–56). Identification of these structures, especially ossicles, may be difficult on MRIs unless their location is clearly understood or routine radiographs are available for comparison (56). Coalitions may occur between the lunate and triquetrum and capitate and hamate. These may be fibrous, cartilaginous, or osseous (54,56). A more complete discussion of

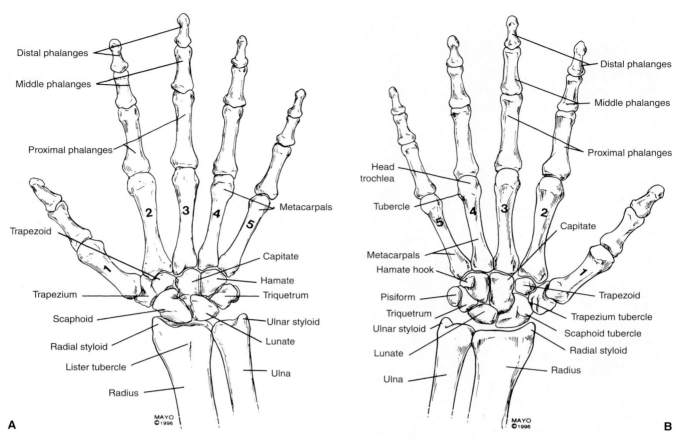

Figure 11-10 Osseous structures of the hand and wrist seen dorsally **(A)** and from the palmar surface **(B)**. (From Berger RA. General anatomy. In: Cooney WP III, Linscheid RL, and Dobyns JH, eds. *The wrist: diagnosis and operative treatment.* St. Louis: Mosby; 1998:32–60.)

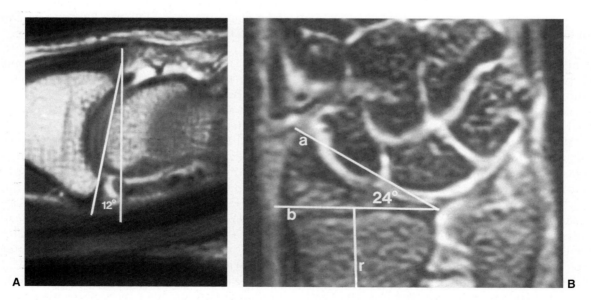

Figure 11-11 **A:** Sagittal MR arthrogram demonstrating the normal 12° palmar tilt of the distal radius. **B:** Coronal MRI demonstrating the normal radial inclination angle of 24°. The angle is formed by a line from the styloid tip to the articular margin (a) and a line (b) perpendicular to the radial shaft (r) at the level of the ulnar articular margin.

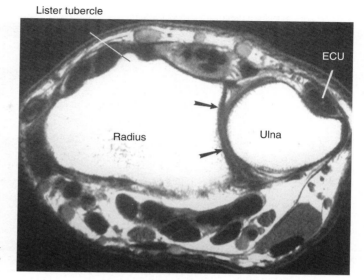

Figure 11-12 Axial T1-weighted image of the wrist demonstrating Lister tubercle, the sigmoid notch (*arrows*), and the groove in the dorsal ulna for the ECU.

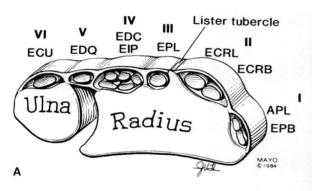

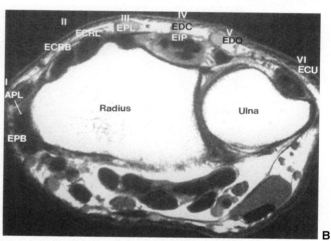

Figure 11-13 Illustration **(A)** and axial MRI **(B)** demonstrating the six dorsal compartments of the wrist. *I,* abductor pollicis longus (APL), extensor pollicis brevis (EPB); *II,* extensor carpi radialis longus (ECRL) and brevis (ECRB); *III,* extensor pollicis longus (EPL); *IV,* extensor digitorum communis (EDC) and extensor indicis proprius (EIP), *V,* extensor digiti quinti (EDQ); *VI,* extensor carpi ulnaris (ECU).

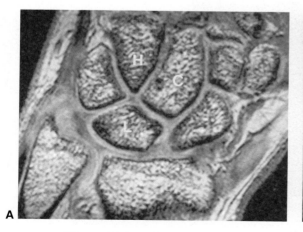

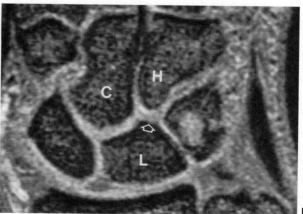

Figure 11-14 **A:** Coronal gradient-echo image demonstrating a type I (single facet) lunate articulating with the capitate. **B:** Coronal gradient-echo image of the lunate with a second small facet (*open arrow,* type II) articulating with the hamate. *C,* capitate; *H,* hamate; *L,* lunate.

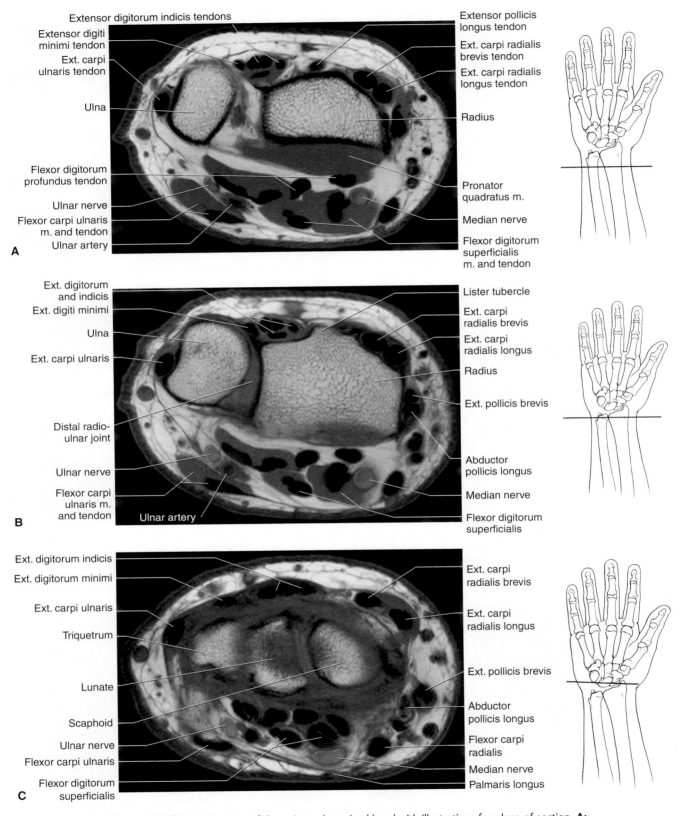

Figure 11-15 Axial images of the wrist and proximal hand with illustrations for plane of section. **A:** Axial images of distal forearm. **B:** Axial image through the distal radioulnar joint. **C:** Axial image through radiocarpal joint. **D:** Axial image through pisotriquetral joint and Guyon's canal. **E:** Axial image through the distal carpal row and hamate hook. **F:** Axial image through the thenar region. **G:** Axial image through the metacarpals. **H:** Axial image through the base of the proximal phalanx.

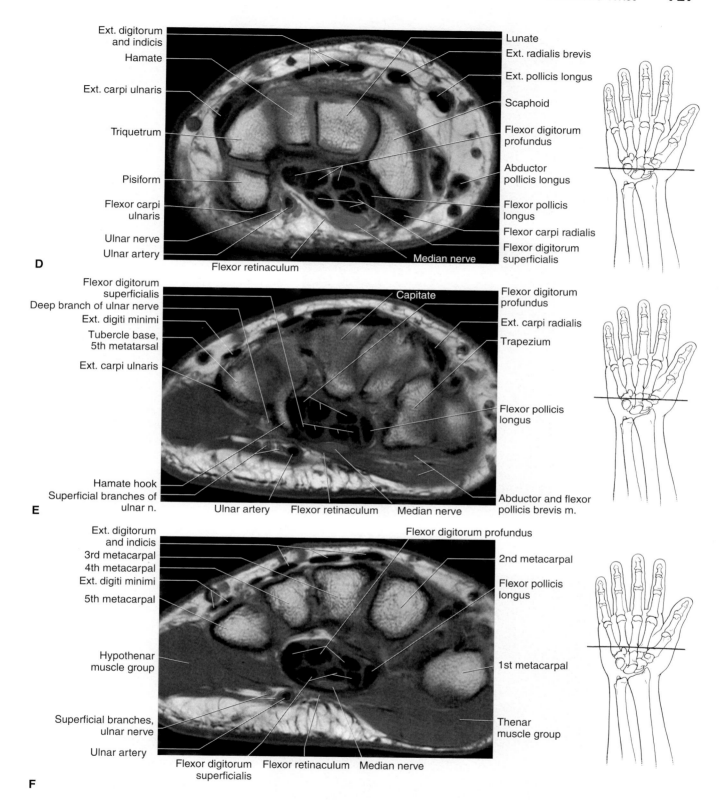

D

E

F

Figure 11-15 (*continued*)

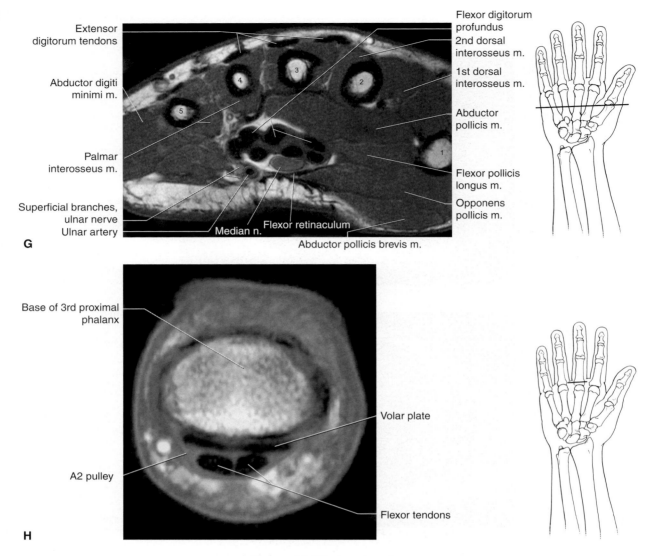

G

Extensor digitorum tendons

Abductor digiti minimi m.

Palmar interosseus m.

Superficial branches, ulnar nerve
Ulnar artery

Median n.

Flexor retinaculum

Abductor pollicis brevis m.

Flexor digitorum profundus
2nd dorsal interosseus m.
1st dorsal interosseus m.
Abductor pollicis m.
Flexor pollicis longus m.
Opponens pollicis m.

H

Base of 3rd proximal phalanx

A2 pulley

Volar plate

Flexor tendons

Figure 11-15 (*continued*)

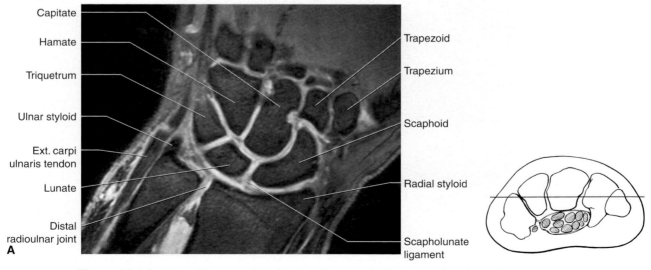

A

Capitate

Hamate

Triquetrum

Ulnar styloid

Ext. carpi ulnaris tendon

Lunate

Distal radioulnar joint

Trapezoid

Trapezium

Scaphoid

Radial styloid

Scapholunate ligament

Figure 11-16 Coronal images of the hand and wrist with illustrations for plane of section. **A:** DESS image of the wrist. **B:** DESS image through the triangular fibrocartilage. **C:** Proton density-weighted image through the carpal bones and thenar muscles. **D:** Proton density-weighted image through the flexor tendons. **E:** T1-weighted image through the proximal interphalangeal joint.

730

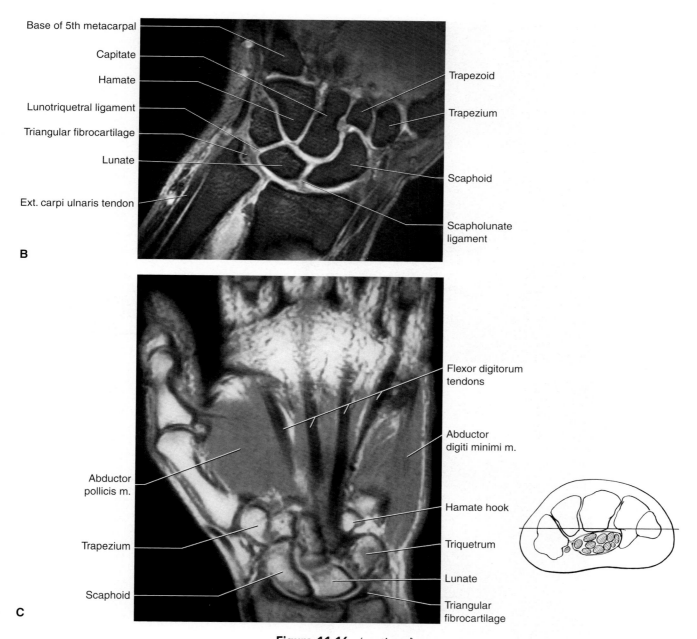

Base of 5th metacarpal

Capitate

Hamate

Lunotriquetral ligament

Triangular fibrocartilage

Lunate

Ext. carpi ulnaris tendon

B

Trapezoid

Trapezium

Scaphoid

Scapholunate ligament

Flexor digitorum tendons

Abductor digiti minimi m.

Abductor pollicis m.

Hamate hook

Trapezium

Triquetrum

Scaphoid

Lunate

C

Triangular fibrocartilage

Figure 11-16   (*continued*)

osseous variants is included in the Pitfalls section of this chapter.

Ligamentous and Articular Anatomy

The ligamentous anatomy of the wrist is complex due to the stabilization required for the numerous carpal bones and extensive motion (Figs. 11-15 through 11-17). The orientation of the ligaments about the wrist is also complex, making it difficult to include all of the dorsal or volar ligaments in any one orthagonal MR image plane (29,42–45, 48,49,57–60). MR images must be obtained using thin sections (≤1 to 2 mm), a small FOV (≤10 cm) and 256 × 256

or 256 × 192 matrix. Three-dimensional Fourier techniques are preferred for thinner contiguous sections, and reformatting can be accomplished. Volar, dorsal, and interosseous ligaments can be defined most consistently with these techniques or MR arthrography (29,42–45,61).

The distal radioulnar joint is primarily stabilized by the TFCC. This complex consists of several components that blend with one another and include the triangular fibrocartilage, the ulnocarpal meniscus, the ulnar collateral ligament (UCL), and the palmar and dorsal distal radioulnar ligaments (see Figs. 11-15B, 11-16B, and 11-18). The articular disc is composed of fibrocartilage. The disc attaches to the ulnar margin of the radius with a broader

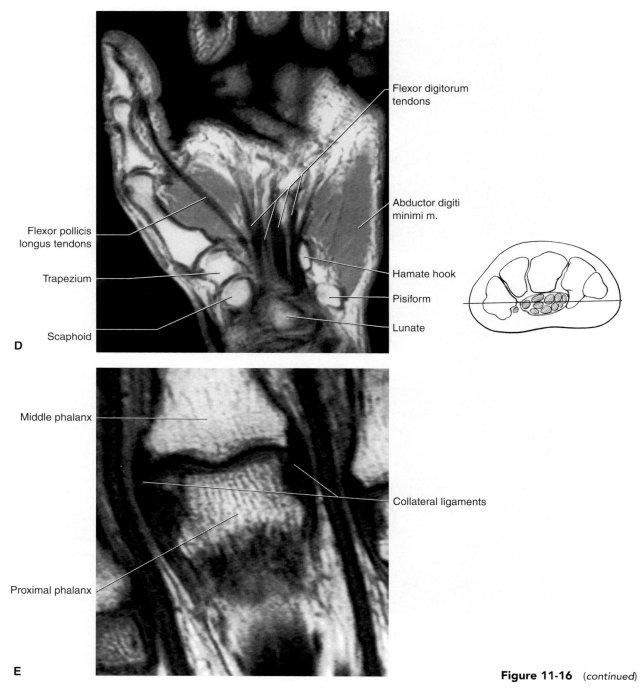

Flexor digitorum
tendons

Abductor digiti
minimi m.

Flexor pollicis
longus tendons

Trapezium

Hamate hook

Scaphoid

Pisiform

Lunate

D

Middle phalanx

Proximal phalanx

Collateral ligaments

E

Figure 11-16 *(continued)*

ulnar portion attaching to the ulnar styloid, ulnar fovea and deep lamina of the antebrachial fascia. The deep lamina is separated from the superficial lamina by the ECU tendon and its sheath (48,57). The triangular fibrocartilage (TFC) is most easily identified on coronal images (Fig. 11-16) with the dorsal and volar ligaments most easily seen on axial or three-dimensional images (29,42–45, 62,63). The TFC is normally of low signal intensity on MR images. However, degeneration, especially on the ulnar aspect, is common on patients over 50 years of age creating areas of increased signal intensity (64–66). Additional support of the distal

radioulnar joint is provided by the interosseous membrane between the radius and ulna, the ECU tendon and the concavity of the sigmoid notch of the radius (Figs. 11-18 and 11-12) (19,48,57).

Wrist stability is provided by the palmar and dorsal ligaments (see Fig. 11-19) (29,45,57,63).

Palmar Ligaments

The palmar ligaments consist of two concentric arches originating 1 to 2 mm from the volar margin of the radius

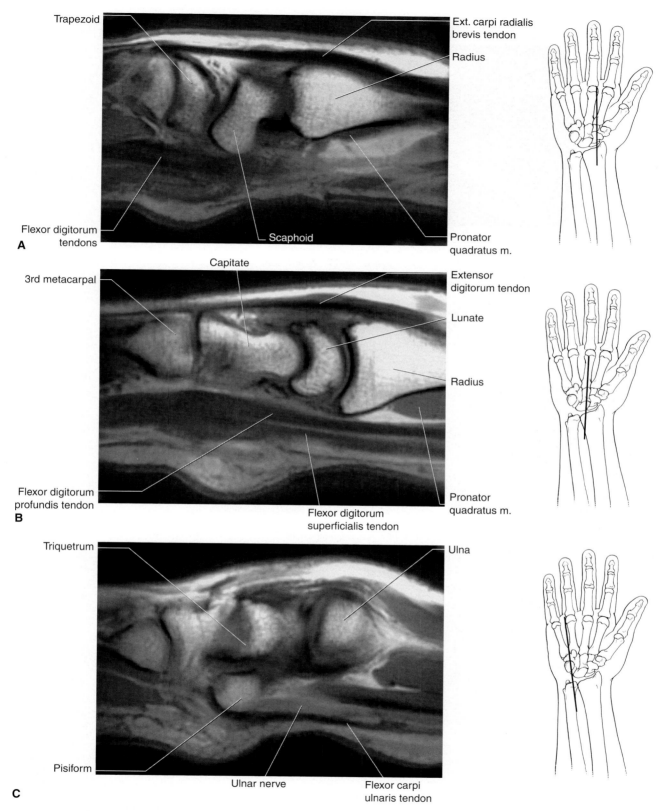

Figure 11-17 Sagittal images of the hand and wrist with illustrations for plane of section. **A:** T1-weighted image through the scaphoid. **B:** T1-weighted image through the lunocapitate region. **C:** T1-weighted image through the pisiform. **D:** T1-weighted image through the finger with pulley systems labeled.

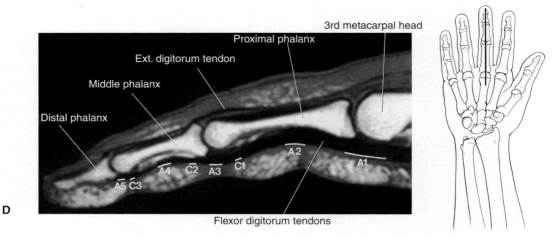

3rd metacarpal head

Proximal phalanx

Ext. digitorum tendon

Middle phalanx

Distal phalanx

A2

A4 C2 A3 C1 A1

A5 C3

D

Flexor digitorum tendons

Figure 11-17 (*continued*)

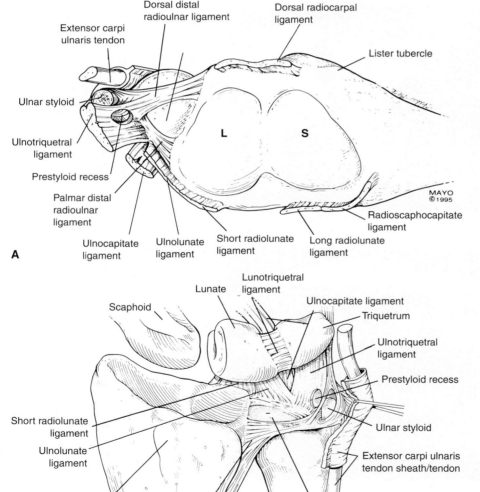

Dorsal distal radioulnar ligament

Extensor carpi ulnaris tendon

Dorsal radiocarpal ligament

Lister tubercle

Ulnar styloid

Ulnotriquetral ligament

Prestyloid recess

Palmar distal radioulnar ligament

L   S

MAYO ©1995

Radioscaphocapitate ligament

Ulnocapitate ligament

Ulnolunate ligament

Short radiolunate ligament

Long radiolunate ligament

A

Lunotriquetral ligament

Lunate

Scaphoid

Ulnocapitate ligament

Triquetrum

Ulnotriquetral ligament

Prestyloid recess

Short radiolunate ligament

Ulnolunate ligament

Ulnar styloid

Extensor carpi ulnaris tendon sheath/tendon

Lister tubercle

MAYO ©1995

Dorsal distal radioulnar ligament

Triangular disk

B

Figure 11-18 **A:** Distal radius including the scaphoid *(S)* and lunate *(L)* fossae and the TFCC. **B:** Ulnocarpal ligament complex and TFCC seen dorsally. (From Berger RA. Ligament anatomy. In: Cooney WP III, Linscheid RL, Dobyns JH, eds. *The wrist: diagnosis and operative treatment.* St. Louis: Mosby; 1998: 73–105.)

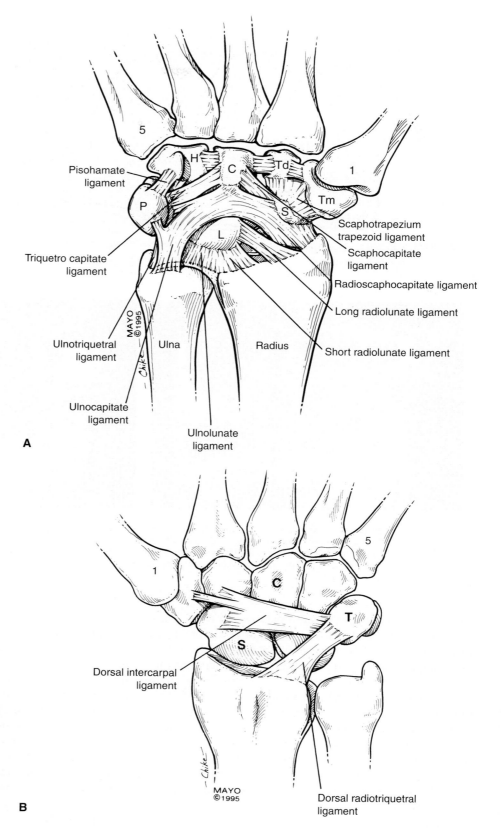

Figure 11-19 Palmar **(A)** and dorsal **(B)** carpal ligaments. *1*, first metacarpal; *5*, fifth metacarpal; *Tm*, trapezium; *Td*, trapezoid; *C*, capitate; *H*, hamate; *P*, pisiform; *L*, lunate; *S*, scaphoid; *T*, triquetrum. (From Berger RA. Ligament Anatomy. In: Cooney WP III, Linscheid RL, Dobyns JH, eds. *The wrist: diagnosis and operative treatment*. St. Louis: Mosby; 1998: 73–105.)

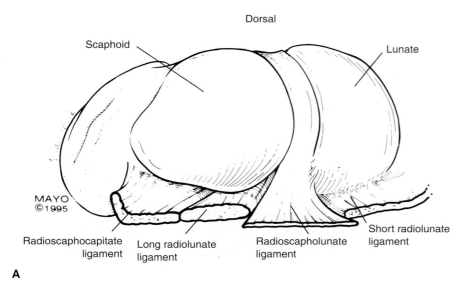

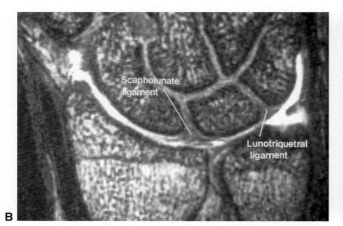

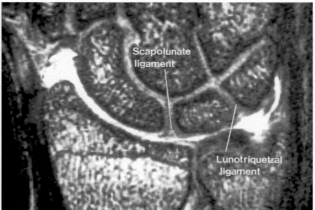

Figure 11-20   A: Scapholunate ligament from proximally and a slightly radial perspective. (From Berger RA. Ligament anatomy. In: Cooney WP III, Linscheid RL, Dobyns JH, eds. *The wrist: diagnosis and operative treatment.* St. Louis: Mosby; 1998:73–105.) **B,C:** Coronal gradient echo MR arthrogram images at different levels demonstrating variation in thickness of the scapholunate and lunotriquetral ligaments.

and inserting into the proximal carpal row and TFCC (Figs. 11-18 and 11-19) (50,57). The radioscaphocapitate ligament (Fig. 11-19A) is most lateral, extending from the radial styloid to the scaphoid waist and capitate. At the capitate it joins the ulnocapitate ligament to form the arcuate ligament. The long radiolunate ligament lies medial to the radioscaphocapitate ligament (Fig. 11-19A). The radioscapholunate ligament (ligament of Testut) extends vertically between the short and long radiolunate ligaments to insert on the lunate and medial scaphoid. The short radiolunate ligament extends from the medial radius to the lunate forming the floor of the radiolunate space (48,57,58).

The palmar midcarpal ligaments include the scaphotrapezium trapezoid, scaphocapitate, triquetrocapitate, triquetrohamate, and pisohamate ligaments (Fig. 11-19A). These ligaments are contiguous, with the radiocarpal and ulnocarpal ligaments joining to form the nearly contiguous palmar capsule (48,57).

The ulnocarpal ligaments (ulnolunate, ulnocapitate and lunotriquetral) (Figs. 11-18 and 11-19A) originate primarily from the palmar radiolunate ligament and the triangular fibrocartilage (57,58).

Smith (45) was able to define six of the eight palmar ligaments—*1,* radioscaphocapitate; *2,* radiolunotriquetral; *3,* radiolunate; *4,* ulnolunate; *5,* ulnotriquetral; and *6,* triquetroscaphoid—in 95% of wrists. The radioscaphoid and radioscapholunate were demonstrated in 66% and 26%, respectively. Three-dimensional techniques were used.

Dorsal Ligaments

The dorsal radiocarpal ligament is a broad band extending from Lister tubercle obliquely to insert on the lunate and triquetrum. This is the floor of the fourth through sixth extensor compartments (Fig. 11-19B). The dorsal intercarpal ligament (Fig. 11-19B) extends from the triquetrum to insert with three slips onto the scaphoid, trapezium, and trapezoid (57).

Interosseous Ligaments

The scapholunate and lunotriquetral ligaments are C-shaped (see Fig. 11-20), extending from dorsal to proximal to palmar surfaces of the joints (57,59,60). The scapholunate ligament is thicker dorsally (59,60). Both the dorsal and palmar portions of the lunotriquetral ligament are thicker than the proximal portion.

The scapholunate ligament is low signal intensity in 63% and has areas of intermediate signal intensity in 37% of patients. The ligament may be triangular (90%) or linear (10%) in its configuration (see Fig. 11-21) (44). Signal intensity was low and uniform (type 1) in 49% of wrists. Areas of intermediate signal intensity were noted in 51%. Type 2 increased signal in the ligament occurred in 14%, type 3 increased signal distally in 16% and increased signal proximally (type 4) in 2%. Intermediate signal intensity extended through the ligament (type 5) in 19% of patients (Fig. 11-21) (44).

Similarly, the lunotriquetral ligament may also have a linear or triangular configuration with variations in signal intensity in asymptomatic individuals (42,48). The lunotriquetral ligament is triangular in 63% and more linear in 37% of patients. An amorphous appearance was noted in a few patients by Smith and Snearly (see Fig. 11-22) (42). Signal intensity is not always uniformly low, similar to variations described in the scapholunate ligament (Fig. 11-22) (42,44).

The interosseous ligaments in the second carpal row consist of dorsal and palmar transverse interosseous bands (see Fig. 11-23). The trapeziocapitate and capitohamate interosseous ligaments have deep ligaments between the articulating surfaces (48,57).

Ligamentous anatomy of the metatarsophalangeal and interphalangeal joints is similar with collateral and volar ligaments incorporated into the joint capsule (Figs. 11-16E and 11-24) (19,67). These ligaments are tight in extension and relax with flexion of the joints. The collateral ligaments are seen on axial and coronal MRI (Figs. 11-15 and 11-16). The palmar plate is clearly seen on axial and sagittal images (67).

Muscular Anatomy

Many of the muscles and tendons that cross the wrist originate at the elbow and forearm. These myotendinous

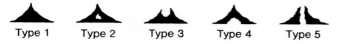

Figure 11-21 Signal intensity patterns in the scapholunate ligament described by Smith (44). *Type I,* uniform low signal intensity; *type II,* central intermediate signal intensity; *type III,* distal intermediate signal intensity; *type IV,* proximal intermediate signal intensity; *type V,* intermediate signal intensity extending through the ligament.

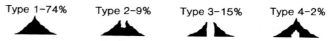

Figure 11-22 Signal intensity variations in the lunotriquetral ligament described by Smith and Snearly (42). *Type I,* homogenous low signal intensity; *type II,* distal intermediate signal intensity; *type III,* intermediate signal intensity extending through the ligament; *type IV,* proximal intermediate signal intensity.

units were previously discussed in Chapter 10. The muscles of the forearm, which are largely responsible for flexion and extension of the wrist, have been thoroughly discussed in Chapter 10. Therefore, except for essential anatomy, they will not be reviewed here (68). This section will primarily deal with those muscles directly related to bones of the hand and wrist with regard to their origins and insertions (Table 11-3).

The chief flexors of the wrist are the flexor carpi radialis and flexor carpi ulnaris. The palmaris longus is a minor flexor of the wrist (see Fig. 11-25) (38,48). Extension of the wrist is largely due to the extensor carpi radialis longus and brevis and the ECU (Fig. 11-25). During radial deviation of the wrist, primary muscles involved are the abductor pollicis longus and extensor pollicis brevis. Ulnar deviation of the wrist is accomplished primarily by the ECU (38,48,70).

There are typically four lumbrical muscles that arise from the flexor digitorum profundus tendons and extend along the radial aspects of the second through fifth metacarpals to insert in the extensor aponeurosis of the proximal phalanx on the radial side. The muscles can be identified in the axial and coronal planes (Figs. 11-15 and 11-16). The lumbricals are seen as tissue of muscle signal intensity between the flexor digitorum profundus tendons proximally and along the radial aspect of the metacarpals adjacent to the interosseous muscles more distally (38,48). Insertions are not usually clearly defined on MRI. The flexor pollicis longus has been discussed in Chapter 10; however, its function is important in the hand and wrist, so certain aspects of its anatomy needs to be repeated. As noted in Table 11-3, the muscle originates from the anterior aspect of the middle third of the radius (48,71). The tendon passes through the radial side of the carpal tunnel (Figs. 11-15) radial to the superficial and deep flexor tendons (Figs. 11-15, 11-16, and 11-25). A synovial sheath of the flexor pollicis longus tendon begins just proximal to the flexor retinaculum and extends distally to near the insertion of the tendon on the distal phalanx of the thumb (Table 11-3) (38,48).

The interosseous muscles form the deepest layer of the muscles in the hand and are divided into palmar and dorsal groups (Fig. 11-15). The palmar group consists of three muscles that take their origin on the radial aspect of the fifth and fourth metacarpals and the ulnar aspect of the second metacarpal. The muscles pass distally between the metacarpophalangeal joints to insert on the extensor aponeurosis. The dorsal interossei originate from adjacent metacarpals, the first from the first and second metacarpals,

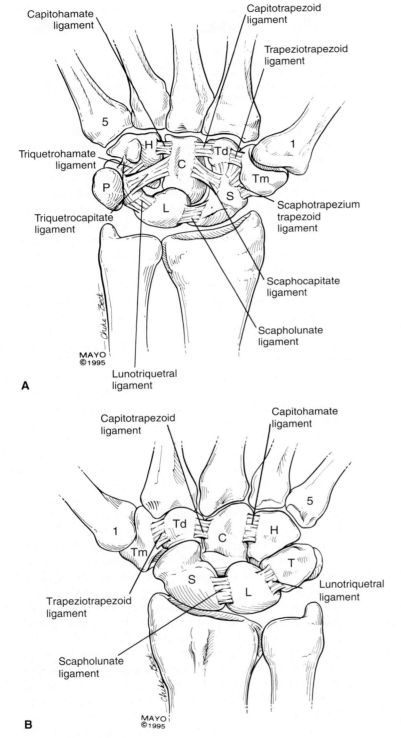

Capitohamate ligament

Capitotrapezoid ligament

Trapeziotrapezoid ligament

Triquetrohamate ligament

Triquetrocapitate ligament

Scaphotrapezium trapezoid ligament

Scaphocapitate ligament

Scapholunate ligament

Lunotriquetral ligament

A

Capitotrapezoid ligament

Capitohamate ligament

Trapeziotrapezoid ligament

Lunotriquetral ligament

Scapholunate ligament

B

Figure 11-23 Palmar **(A)** and dorsal **(B)** intercarpal ligaments. (From Berger RA. Ligament anatomy. In: Cooney WP III, Linscheid RL, Dobyns JH, eds. *The wrist: diagnosis and operative treatment.* St. Louis: Mosby; 1998:73–105.)

the second from the second and third, the third from the third and fourth, and the fourth from the fourth and fifth metacarpal diaphyses. The muscles pass dorsally and distally to insert with a palmar and dorsal slip into the bases of the proximal phalanges. The interosseous muscles, both palmar and dorsal, are innervated by the deep branch of the ulnar nerve. The interosseous muscles aid in abduction and adduction of the fingers of the hand (Table 11-3) (48).

The thenar eminence or muscle group is comprised of the abductor pollicis brevis and superficial head of the flexor pollicis brevis that overlie the opponens pollicis (Fig. 11-15). The abductor pollicis brevis arises from the flexor

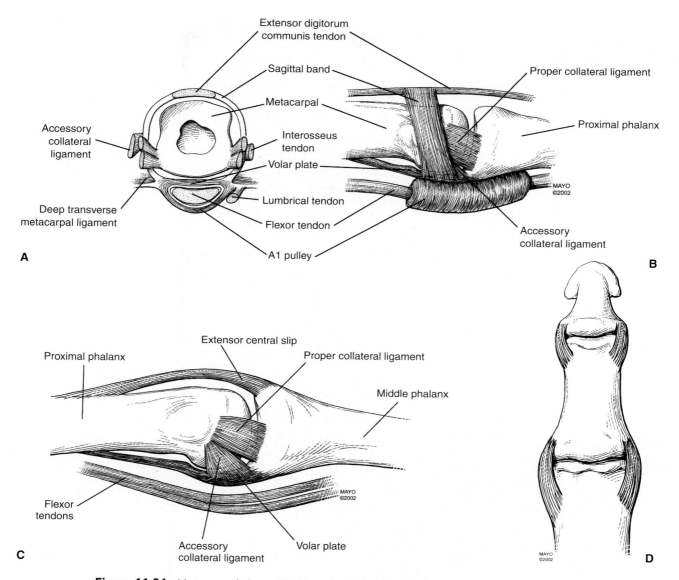

Figure 11-24 Metacarpophalangeal **(A,B)** and interphalangeal **(C,D)** joint anatomy.

retinaculum and has deeper origins from the trapezium and trapezoid. This somewhat triangular muscle extends distally to insert in the radial aspect of the proximal phalanx of the thumb. It serves as the primary abductor of the thumb. The flexor pollicis brevis has two heads, one superficial and the other deep. The superficial head arises from the trapezium and flexor retinaculum and the deep head from the trapezoid. The muscle extends distally to form a tendon that inserts on the radial flexor side of the base of the proximal phalanx of the thumb. The primary function is flexion and rotation of the thumb. The opponens pollicis is partially covered by the abductors and flexors of the thumb and arises from the flexor retinaculum and trapezium to insert on the radial surface of the diaphysis of the first metacarpal. The adductor pollicis arises with both oblique and transverse heads. The transverse head arises

from the ulnar surface of the third metacarpal diaphysis and the oblique head from the base of the third metacarpal and flexor aspects of the trapezium, trapezoid, and capitate. The triangular muscle extends to insert at the base of the proximal phalanx of the thumb. This muscle serves to adduct the metacarpal and flex the metacarpophalangeal joint of the thumb (Table 11-3) (38,48).

The hypothenar muscle group consists of one superficial and three deep muscles. The superficial muscle is the palmaris brevis that arises from the ulnar side of the palmar aponeurosis and extends medially to attach into the skin along the medial border of the palm. This muscle is superficial to the ulnar nerve and artery (48). The deep muscles include the abductor digiti minimi, flexor digiti minimi brevis, and opponens digiti minimi (Figs. 11-15 and 11-16). The abductor digiti minimi is the most superficial of the

TABLE 11-3
MUSCLES OF THE HAND

Muscles	Origin	Insertion	Action	Innervation
Lumbricals (4)	Tendons of flexor digitorum profundus	Extensor aponeurosis	Extensors of interphalangeal joints	Radial or 1st and 2nd lumbricals-median nerve, 3rd and 4th ulnar nerve
Flexor pollicis longus	Anterior middle one-third radius and interosseous membrane	Distal phalanx thumb	Flexor of thumb	Median nerve (anterior interosseous branch)
Interossei palmar (3)	2,4,5 metacarpal diaphysis	Extensor aponeurosis	Abduction and adduction of fingers	Deep branch of ulnar nerve
Dorsal (4)	1st to 5th metacarpal diaphyses	Proximal phalanges		
Abductor pollicis brevis	Flexor retinaculum, trapezium	Radial side proximal phalanx thumb	Abductor of thumb	Median nerve
Flexor pollicis brevis	Flexor retinaculum, trapezium, and trapezoid	Radial flexor aspect proximal phalanx thumb	Flexes and rotates thumb	Median nerve
Opponens pollicis	Flexor retinaculum, trapezium	Radial diaphysis 1st metacarpal	Stabilize and opposition of thumb	Median nerve
Adductor pollicis	3rd metacarpal, trapezium, trapezoid, capitate	Base proximal phalanx thumb		Median nerve
Palmaris brevis	Palmar aponeurosis (ulnar side)	Medial skin palm	Draws skin laterally	Deep branch ulnar nerve
Abductor digiti minimi	Pisiform	Ulnar base 5th proximal phalanx	Abductor 5th finger	Deep branch ulnar nerve
Flexor digiti minimi brevis	Hamate hook, flexor retinaculum	Ulnar base 5th proximal phalanx	Flexor 5th metacarpophalangeal (MCP) joint	Deep branch ulnar nerve
Opponens digiti minimi	Flexor retinaculum, distal hamate hook	5th metacarpal diaphysis	Draws 5th metacarpal anteriorly	Deep branch ulnar nerve

From Berquist TH. Magnetic resonance imaging of the elbow and wrists. *Top Magn Reson Imaging* 1989;1:15–27; Rosse C, Rosse PC. *Hollinshead's textbook of anatomy*. Philadelphia, PA: Lippincott–Raven, 1997 and Bishop AT, Gabel G, Carmichael SW. Flexor carpi radialis tendinitis. Part I: operative anatomy. *J Bone Joint Surg Am* 1994;76A:1009–1014.

three deep muscles. It arises from the distal surface of the pisiform and passes distally along the medial aspect of the hand to insert along the ulnar side of the base of the fifth proximal phalanx. This muscle abducts the little finger at the metacarpophalangeal joint. It acts along with the dorsal interosseous muscle to assist in abduction or spreading of the fingers. The flexor digiti minimi brevis arises more distally than the abductor digiti minimi and takes its origin from the hook of the hamate and flexor retinaculum. This muscle passes more obliquely and medially and inserts in the same position as the abductor. The main function of this muscle is as flexor of the fifth metacarpophalangeal joint. The third and final muscle of the deep hypothenar group is the opponens digiti minimi. This muscle is the deepest and arises deep to the abductor and flexor from the flexor retinaculum and distal hook of the hamate, taking an oblique course to insert along the ulnar aspect of the fifth metacarpal diaphysis. This muscle draws the fifth

metacarpal anteriorly. All of the hypothenar muscle group is innervated by the deep branch of the ulnar nerve (Table 11-3) (38,48).

Numerous muscular variations have been described (72,73).

The accessory abduction digit minimi has been reported in up to 24% of patients. The extensor digitorum manus muscle is reported in 1% to 3% of the general population. The origin of the lumbrical muscles (Table 11-3) may vary, with the origin arising in the carpal tunnel in 22% of patients. The palmaris longus is typically seen only as a tendon at the level of the wrist. In up to 13% of patients, the muscle may be absent. There are numerous other variations, including palmaris longus inversus (muscle distally, tendon proximally), nontendinous variation (muscle from origin to insertion), central tendon with muscle tissue proximally and distally, and a bifid variant with two tendinous insertions distally

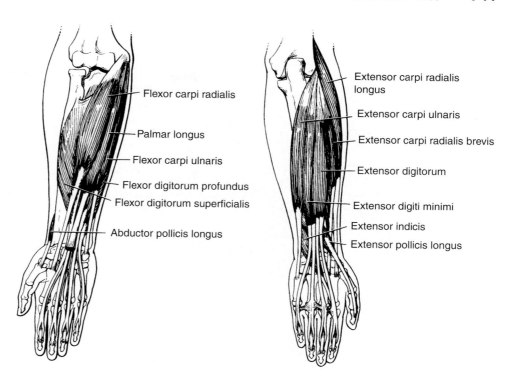

Flexor carpi radialis

Palmar longus

Flexor carpi ulnaris

Flexor digitorum profundus

Flexor digitorum superficialis

Abductor pollicis longus

Extensor carpi radialis longus

Extensor carpi ulnaris

Extensor carpi radialis brevis

Extensor digitorum

Extensor digiti minimi

Extensor indicis

Extensor pollicis longus

Figure 11-25 Flexor and extensor muscle groups.

(48,73). A more complete discussion of muscle variants and clinical implications is included it the Pitfalls section of this chapter.

Neurovascular Anatomy

The neurovascular anatomy of the hand and wrist is complex (see Fig. 11-26). Because there are numerous causes of nerve compression in this region, it is especially essential to understand the anatomy and relationship of these structures in the hand and wrist (Figs. 11-26 and 11-27) (46–48,74–79). MR evaluation of neurovascular anatomy is most easily accomplished by following these structures from proximal to distal on axial images (see Figs. 11-15 and 11-27). On the ulnar side of the distal forearm proximal to the carpal tunnel, the ulnar artery, nerve, and the accompanying veins lie deep to the flexor carpi ulnaris (Fig. 11-15) (46,48). The nerve is generally medial to the artery at this level. At the level of the pisiform, these structures pass along the lateral or radial side of the pisiform, passing deep to the volar carpal ligament and then distally into the palm of the hand anterior to the flexor retinaculum but deep to the palmaris brevis muscle (Fig. 11-27B) (74). At the level of the pisiform, the ulnar nerve typically divides into superficial and deep branches (Fig. 11-27B). Also, at the pisiform level, the nerve and accompanying vascular structures lie between the volar carpal ligament and flexor retinaculum in a space commonly known as Guyon canal (46,48). Lesions proximal to or within the canal can produce both sensory and motor abnormalities in the ulnar nerve distribution (46,48).

The two flexor digitorum muscles (superficial and profundus) are lateral to the ulnar nerve and vessels at the level of the wrist (Fig. 11-27). The tendon of the palmaris longus lies superficially. These structures are most easily identified on axial MR images (Figs. 11-15 and 11-27). The midline volar structures of the wrist, as they enter the carpal tunnel, tend to form three layers. The most superficial or anterior layer is formed by the flexor digitorum superficialis. The middle layer is formed by the superficial flexor of the index and middle fingers, and the most posterior or deepest layer is formed by the flexor digitorum profundus tendons. All tendons have a common sheath just before they pass under the flexor retinaculum. The palmaris longus tendon is the most superficial and midline structure at the wrist level (Figs. 11-15 and 11-27) (38,48).

The median nerve lies deep to the flexor digitorum superficialis through much of the forearm (Figs. 11-15 and 11-27). Just proximal to the wrist, it emerges on the radial side of the superficial flexor and passes forward and medially to lie in front of the flexor tendons in the carpal tunnel (Figs. 11-15 and 11-27). At the distal margin of the flexor retinaculum, the median nerve divides into five or six branches. These small branches are difficult to identify, even when thin axial MR sections are obtained (19,47,80).

The muscle planes and fascial compartments of the palm basically divide the palm into three compartments—the thenar, hypothenar, and central compartments (Figs. 11-15 and 11-26). These compartments, along with the tendon sheaths of the flexor tendons, are anatomically important in the spread of inflammatory and infectious diseases (48).

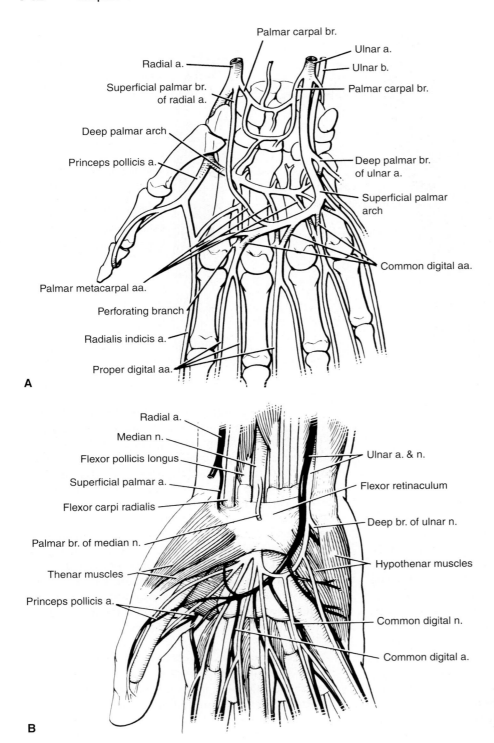

Palmar carpal br.

Radial a.

Superficial palmar br.
of radial a.

Deep palmar arch

Princeps pollicis a.

Palmar metacarpal aa.

Perforating branch

Radialis indicis a.

Proper digital aa.

A

Ulnar a.

Ulnar b.

Palmar carpal br.

Deep palmar br.
of ulnar a.

Superficial palmar
arch

Common digital aa.

Radial a.

Median n.

Flexor pollicis longus

Superficial palmar a.

Flexor carpi radialis

Palmar br. of median n.

Thenar muscles

Princeps pollicis a.

B

Ulnar a. & n.

Flexor retinaculum

Deep br. of ulnar n.

Hypothenar muscles

Common digital n.

Common digital a.

Figure 11-26 Vascular (**A**) and neurovascular (**B**) anatomy of the hand and wrist.

PITFALLS

Pitfalls of MRI of the hand and wrist may be due to anatomic variants, improper techniques, and software and hardware artifacts. Patient motion, flow artifacts, and other technical errors can lead to suboptimal images (see Fig. 11-28).

Flow artifacts vary with different pulse sequences, and they are more common in the peripheral extremities (see Fig. 11-29). When flow artifacts enter the area of interest, lesions—especially small lesions—can be overlooked. In this setting, images can be repeated with change in the phase direction that will direct the artifact out of the area of interest. Flow-suppression techniques are also useful for reducing artifacts (19).

The magic angle phenomenon may cause increased signal intensity in tendons or ligaments oriented 45° to 65° to

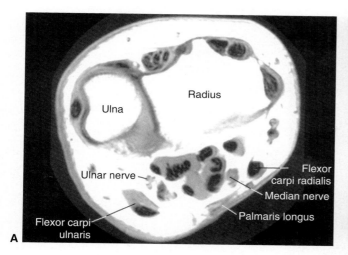

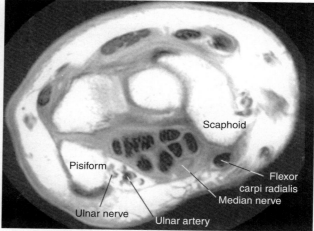

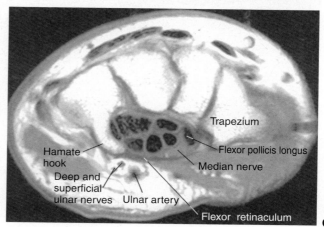

Figure 11-27 Axial MRI demonstrating the relationships of the ulnar and median nerves at the level of the distal radioulnar joint (**A**), pisiform (**B**), and hamate hook (**C**).

the magnetic field (**B₀**) (81). The direction of **B₀** varies with the type of magnet. It is aligned with the bore in closed high field systems, vertical in open systems, and left to right in small extremity units. Proper positioning or use of radial or ulnar deviation of the wrist may reduce this phenomenon (see Fig. 11-30).

Magic angle occurs with short TE spin-echo and many GRE sequences, but it is not a problem with long TE or T2-weighted sequences (2,19,81). Abnormal signal intensity not related to magic angle phenomenon has been described in the ECU tendon (82). However, pathology is unlikely in the absence of tendon enlargement or fluid in the tendon sheath (2,19).

Anatomic variants may involve osseous or soft tissue structures (83–87).

Osseous Variants

The carpal bones generally develop from a single ossification center. Therefore, anomalous conditions such as bipartate and tripartate carpal bones are not common (54,55). Unfortunately, when bipartate and tripartate carpal bones do occur, they involve the most commonly fractured carpal bone, the scaphoid (48,54). The most

common appearance is two separate ossicles separated at the waist, a common site of scaphoid fractures. The capitate and hook of the hamate may also develop from multiple ossification centers. When this occurs, differentiation from fracture may be difficult with MRI (55). Hypoplastic hamate hooks have been described in females (55,88).

Osseous coalitions may be fibrous, cartilaginous, or osseous. Lunotriquetral coalitions are most common, but capitohamate coalitions also occur (see Fig. 11-31) (54–56). Coalitions are more common in females and African-Americans, occurring in up to 6% of the black population (48,54). Minaar classified lunotriquetral coalitions. Type I coalitions (see Fig. 11-32A) are fibrous or cartilaginous and may be painful. Type II coalitions are incomplete osseous coalitions with a distal notch (see Fig. 11-32B), and type III show complete osseous fusion (see Fig. 11-32C). Type IV coalitions (see Fig. 11-32D) are complete osseous fusions with other carpal anomalies (48,56).

As noted in the anatomy section, the lunate may have one distal facet (type 1) or two facets, one for articulation with the hamate (type 2) (Fig. 11-14). The type 2 lunate is more common (50% to 65%) and is associated with cartilage damage on the proximal pole of the hamate

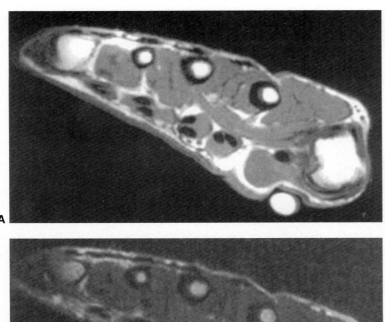

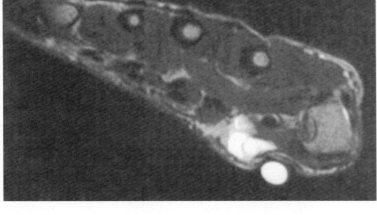

Figure 11-28 Axial T1- **(A)** and T2-weighted **(B)** images. The large vitamin E capsule compresses and distorts the underlying anatomy and ganglion cyst (*arrow*).

(56). Pfirrmann et al. (89) found no correlation with interosseous and triangular fibrocartilage tears.

Irregularity of the palmar aspect of the lunate may be seen on sagittal T1-weighted MRI. This is due to nutrient vessels and ligament attachments (see Fig. 11-33) (54,90).

There are numerous ossicles in the hand and wrist (see Fig. 11-34). Common ossicles and their locations may be most easily appreciated on radiographs. They should not be confused with loose bodies or fractures. The lunula (Table 11-4) is an ossification center that lies between the

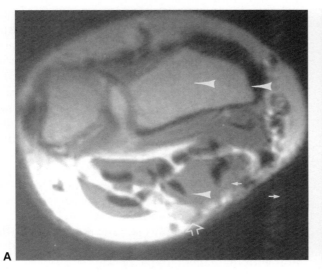

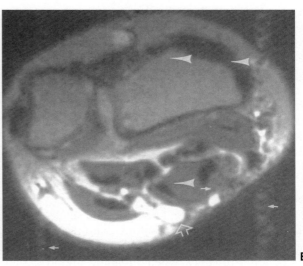

Figure 11-29 Proton density **(A)** and T2-weighted **(B)** images. Flow artifacts (*small arrows*) and small ganglion cyst (*open arrow*). Swapping the phase direction (*arrowheads*) can move the artifact out of the area of interest.

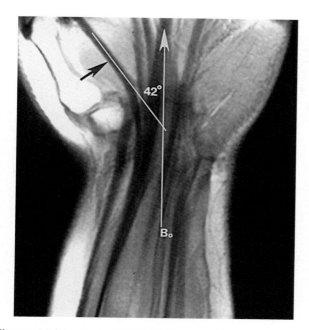

Figure 11-30 Coronal SE 500/10 image of the flexor tendons. Most tendons are oriented in the plane of this closed high field magnet (B₀). The flexor pollicis longus is oriented 42° to B₀. Magic angle phenomenon could come into play depending upon the degree of radial or ulnar deviation of the wrist.

triangular fibrocartilage and the triquetrum. In some cases, it may fuse to the ulnar styloid (see Figs. 11-34 and 11-35) (54). The os styloideum, also known as a carpal boss, lies dorsal to the second and third metacarpal bases.

TABLE 11-4

COMMON OSSICLES OF THE HAND AND WRIST

Ossicle	Location
Lunula	Between triangular fibrocartilage complex and triquetrum, may fuse to ulnar styloid
Os styloideum	Dorsal to 2nd and 3rd metacarpal bases
Os triangulare	Distal to fovea
Trapezium secondarium	Superomedial aspect of trapezium
Epilunate	Dorsal to lunate
Os hamuli	Adjacent to hamate hook
Os Gruber	Between capitate, hamate, and 3rd and 4th metacarpal bases

From references 54–56, 88, and 90.

This ossicle may be congenital or degenerative and may mimic a ganglion cyst clinically (54,56). The os triangulare (Table 11-4) is congenital and lies in the ulnar fovea. The trapezium secondarium lies at the superomedial border of the trapezium (Fig. 11-35) (54,56). The epilunate lies dorsal to the lunate and because of its location is easily mistaken for a loose body (82). The os hamuli lies at the tip of the hamate hook, and the os Gruber lies between the capitate, hamate, and third and fourth metacarpal bases (54,56).

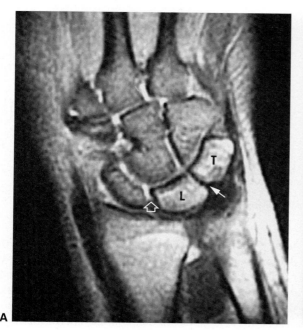
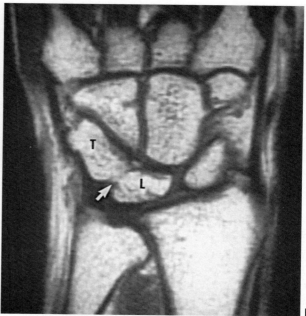

Figure 11-31 Lunotriquetral coalitions. **A:** Coronal T2-weighted image demonstrates a fibrous (type I) coalition. Note the low signal intensity and decreased joint space (*arrow*). The space is normal between the scaphoid and lunate and there is fluid in the joint space (*open arrow*). **B:** Coronal T1-weighted image demonstrating an osseous coalition with a proximal notch (*arrow*). *T*, triquetrum; *L*, lunate.

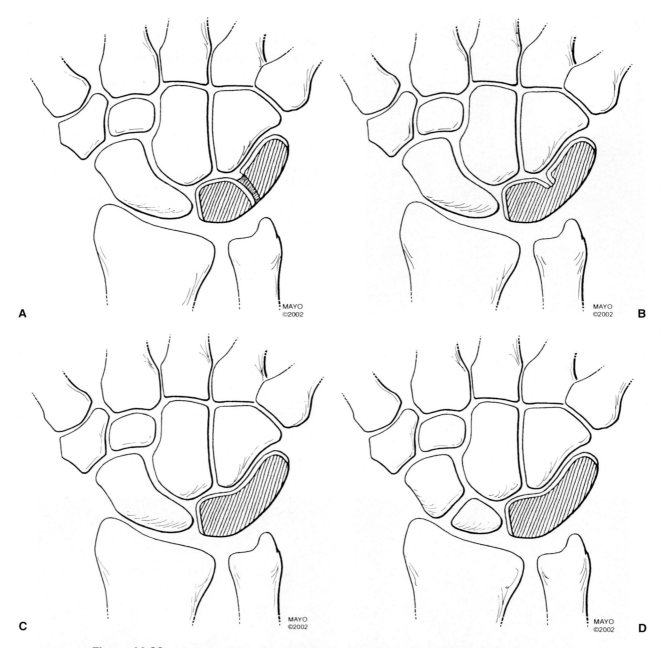

Figure 11-32 Lunotriquetral coalitions. **A:** Type I, fibrous or cartilagenous. **B:** Type II, incomplete osseous coalition with a distal notch. **C:** Type III, complete osseous fusion. **D:** Type IV, complete osseous fusion with other carpal anomalies, in this case a bipartate scaphoid. (From Berquist TH. *MRI of the hand and wrist.* Philadelphia, PA: Lippincott Williams & Wilkins, 2003.)

Soft Tissue Variants

Soft tissue variants are common. Neurovascular variations in the dorsal and palmar arches may be noted in up to one third of patients (48). Fortunately, this is not usually a significant problem when interpreting MRIs. Anomalous muscles may cause problems clinically as patients present with soft tissue masses or asymmetry when compared with the opposite extremity (Table 11-5) (91,92). The exact variation may not be apparent on MRI. However, the demonstration of a muscle density structure

is obvious on MRI. Thus, a neoplasm can be excluded. Anomalous muscles have also been described in Guyon canal in 25% of patients. Anomalies are bilateral in 67%. Anomalous muscles can result in nerve compression syndrome (47,73).

The accessory abductor digiti minimi is a common variant reported in 24% of the general population (see Fig. 11-36). This muscle may originate from the palmar carpal ligament, palmaris longus, or forearm fascia. It inserts on the medial aspect of the fifth proximal phalanx. Ulnar and median

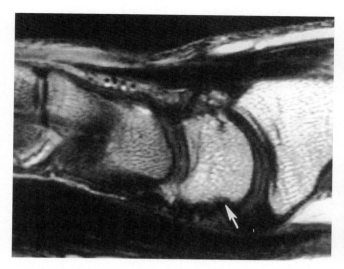

Figure 11-33 Sagittal T1-weighted image demonstrating volar irregularity of the lunate (*arrow*) due to normal ligament attachments.

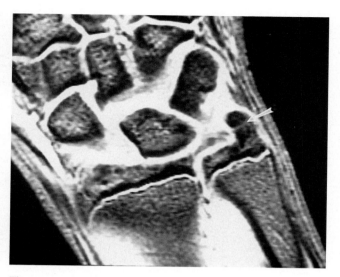

Figure 11-34 Coronal gradient-echo image demonstrating an elongated ulnar styloid with faint signal intensity increase (*arrow*) due to a partially fused lunula.

nerve symptoms have been associated with this anomaly (Fig. 11-36B) (48,73).

The extensor digitorum brevis manus muscle occurs in 1% to 3% of patients. This muscle arises from the distal radius or radiocarpal ligament and inserts on the distal second metacarpal (see Fig. 11-37) (73,82,83,94). This muscle is generally not symptomatic, but it may mimic a ganglion cyst (83).

In 22% of patients, the lumbrical muscles may have a more proximal origin in the carpal tunnel. Nerve compression may occur with finger flexion (83).

The palmaris longus typically takes its origin from the medial epicondyle. There are numerous variants (see Fig. 11-38), and in 13% of the population the muscle is absent (73,95).

Variations in the flexor tendon sheaths are more significant. Anomalies may lead to changes in patterns of spread of infection. Also, confusion of tenosynovitis with a ganglion can occur. Most often, the common flexor tendon sheath ends in the midpalm (71.4% of the population). The digital sheaths in the fingers do not usually communicate with the common flexor tendon sheath (48).

As noted above (Figs. 11-20 through 11-22), variations in shape and signal intensity of the ligaments and TFC complex may also cause confusion (96,97). The ulnar aspect of the TFC is rich in vascular tissue that can result in increased signal intensity (see Fig. 11-39). These changes should not be confused with a tear (73,82). Variations in signal intensity, as with arthrography, need to be correlated with clinical symptoms. In some cases, arthrography with diagnostic injection may be necessary to confirm MR findings and localize the patient's symptoms. Also, similar to the meniscus in the knee, signal

TABLE 11-5
MUSCLE VARIANTS OF THE HAND AND WRIST

Muscle	Incidence	Clinical Significance
Accessory abductor digiti minimi	24%	Usually none, may compress ulnar or median nerve
Extensor digitorum brevus manus muscle	1%–3%	None, may mimic a ganglion
Lumbrical origin anomaly	22%	Mimics carpal tunnel pathology
Palmaris longus	13% absent multiple variants	May mimic soft tissue mass or muscle tear, nerve compression
Accessory flexor digitorum superficialis	?	Mimics soft tissue mass
Flexor digiti minimi (anomalous origin)	?	Ulnar nerve compression

From references 73, 82, 83, and 93.

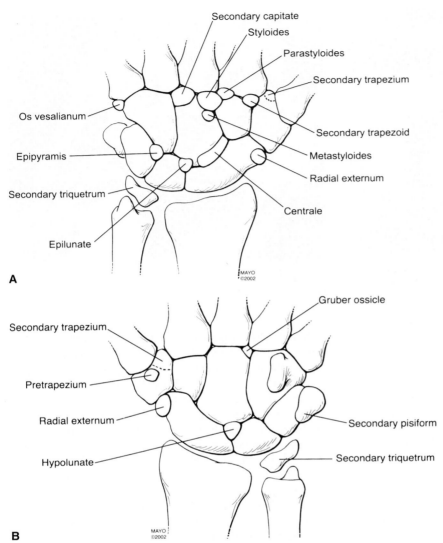

A

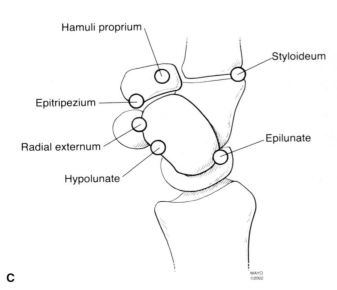

B

C

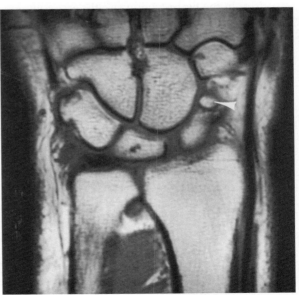

D

Figure 11-35 Ossicles of the wrist seen from dorsal **(A)**, volar **(B),** and sagittal **(C).** Coronal T1-weighted image **(D)** demonstrates an os centrale (*arrowhead*). (From Berquist TH. *MRI of the hand and wrist*. Philadelphia, PA: Lippincott Williams & Wilkins, 2003.)

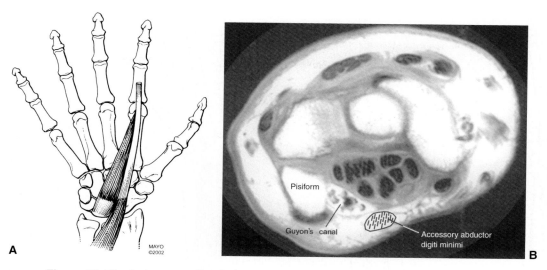

Figure 11-36 **A:** Accessory abductor digiti minimi. **B:** Axial MR image demonstrating the relationships of the muscle to Guyon's canal. Normally, there is no muscle in this region.

changes in the TFC have also been described with aging (98,99).

Variations in the median nerve may also cause confusion. The normal median nerve is elliptical on axial MR images with variable signal intensity (19,79,98). Signal intensity is increased with changes in nerve configuration on T2-weighted sequences when the nerve is abnormal (19,82).

A bifid median nerve has been described in 2.8% of the population. A persistent median artery may be present between the nerve segments (100).

CLINICAL APPLICATIONS

Clinical applications for MRI of the hand and wrist have expanded dramatically due to improve surface coil technology, new pulse sequences, and increased utilization of MR arthrography and MR angiography (10,28,101–106). Major applications for MRI in our practice include trauma, neoplasms, infection, avascular necrosis (AVN), nerve compression syndromes, and arthropathies. MRI may also be of value in imaging other conditions in the hand and wrist. However, experience is still evolving in these areas (26,37,107–109).

TRAUMA

Osseous Injuries

MRI techniques are useful to evaluate acute and chronic musculoskeletal injuries to the hand and wrist fully

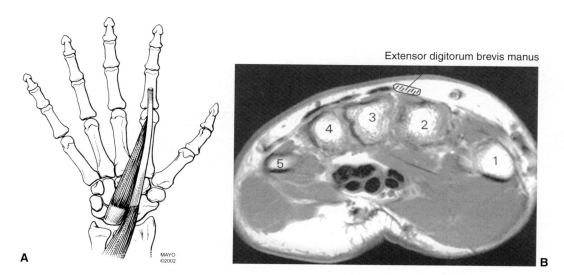

Figure 11-37 **A:** Extensor digitorum manus. **B:** Axial MR image demonstrating the location at the level of the metacarpal bases. The muscle is radial to the extensor tendons and between the second and third metacarpals.

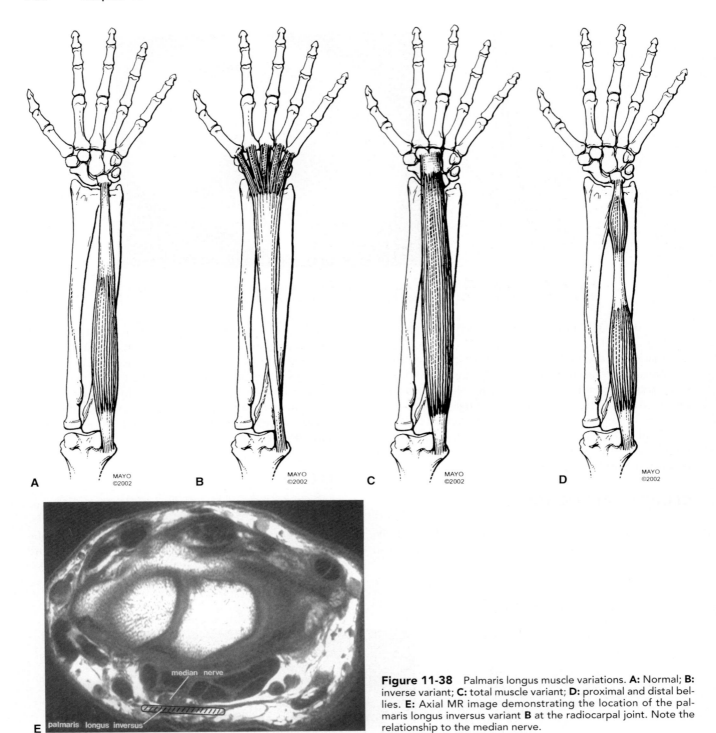

Figure 11-38 Palmaris longus muscle variations. **A:** Normal; **B:** inverse variant; **C:** total muscle variant; **D:** proximal and distal bellies. **E:** Axial MR image demonstrating the location of the palmaris longus inversus variant **B** at the radiocarpal joint. Note the relationship to the median nerve.

(19,22,43,108,110–113). Most acute skeletal injuries are adequately diagnosed with routine radiography. CT and isotope studies are valuable supplemental radiographic techniques (7,114–117).

MRI is useful for early diagnosis of subtle injuries and to evaluate the extent of osseous, physeal, and soft tissue injury in more complex cases (19,118–122). Osseous injuries include incomplete fractures, complete fractures, physeal fractures, stress fractures, and bone bruises (19,118,120,123,124).

Early diagnosis of fractures, especially of the scaphoid, is essential to reduce complications. MRI should be considered when radiographs or computed radiography (CR) images are normal, but fracture is suspected clinically. Up

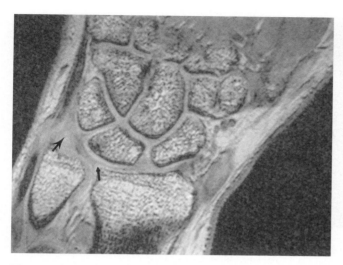

Figure 11-39 Coronal gradient-echo image demonstrating normal increased signal at the ulnar attachment (*large arrow*) and radial cartilage attachment (*small arrow*) of the triangular fibrocartilage.

to 35% of fractures detected on MRI cannot be identified on radiographs (124).

Fractures of the distal radius and ulna are common (see Fig. 11-40). MRI may be particularly useful in children. Forty percent of physeal injuries in children involve the distal radius and 5% the ulna (125). Physeal fractures and soft tissue injuries are included in the spectrum of gymnast's wrist (126–128). High loads applied to the wrist during gymnastics commonly result in injury, especially between the ages of 12 and 14 years (126). Radiographs may demonstrate irregularity and cystic changes in the physis. Ulnar positive variance has also been described with this condition (126,128).

TABLE 11-6

CARPAL FRACTURES: IMAGE PLANES

Osseous Structure	Image Planes
Scaphoid	Coronal, oblique sagittal
Lunate	Coronal and sagittal
Triquetrum	Coronal, axial, oblique sagittal
Pisiform	Axial and sagittal
Trapezium	Coronal and axial
Trapezoid	Coronal and axial
Capitate	Coronal and sagittal
Hamate	Coronal and axial

Carpal fractures are rare in children, but common in adults (125,129). The scaphoid is the most commonly fractured carpal bone in adults and children. However, in children scaphoid fractures account for only 2.9% of hand and wrist fractures. In adults, fractures most commonly involve the waist, while in children the distal third is the most common fracture site (125,129). Fractures of the triquetrum are the second most common carpal fracture followed by the capitate and lunate (7,125).

MRI is sensitive and specific for early detection of fractures, including bone bruises (130). Imaging approaches vary depending upon the site of injury. Specifically, different image planes may be required to fully evaluate each carpal bone (Table 11-6). Both T1- and T2-weighted sequences are obtained. In some cases, STIR or fast inversion recovery are added to the examination. Marrow edema is low signal intensity on T1- and high signal intensity on T2-weighted or STIR sequences. Signal intensity is low along the fracture line on both T1- and T2-weighted

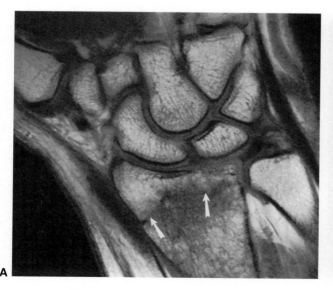

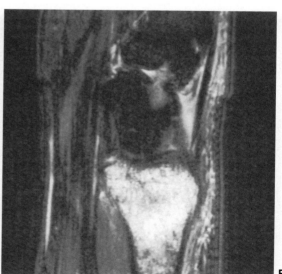

Figure 11-40 Distal radial fracture. Coronal T1- **(A)** and sagittal T2-weighted **(B)** images demonstrate an undisplaced distal radial fracture (*arrows*) with marrow edema.

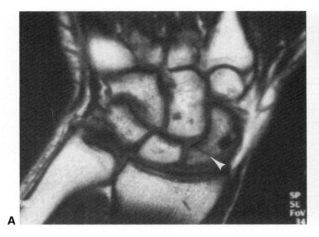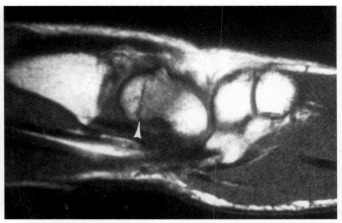

Figure 11-41 Scaphoid fracture. Coronal **(A)** and sagittal **(B)** T1-weighted images demonstrate an undisplaced fracture (*arrowhead*). There is associated low signal intensity due to edema.

sequences with trabecular compression or impaction (see Figs. 11-41 and 11-42). Increased signal intensity is seen in the fracture line on T2-weighted sequences when fragments are not impacted (16,19). Image planes are especially important for the scaphoid (see Fig. 11-43). Sagittal image planes aligned with the scaphoid are important to exclude "hump back" deformity (7).

Metacarpal and phalangeal fractures are usually easily identified on radiographs; therefore, MRI is rarely indicated (see Fig. 11-44).

Fracture Complications

Complications of osseous trauma vary with age and location. In children, physeal injuries can result in deformity due to premature closure or overgrowth of the growth plate. Other complications include delayed union, nonunion, malunion, AVN, soft tissue injuries, and infection (7,16).

Physeal injuries may result in fibrous or osseous bars leading to joint asymmetry. Thin section T2* or three-dimensional GRE sequences through and perpendicular to the physis are useful for operative planning (131,132).

In a similar fashion, T1- and T2-weighted sequences can be used to confirm fibrous union or nonunion (see Fig. 11-45). Fibrous union is low signal intensity on both sequences, while there is high signal intensity in the fracture line with low signal intensity bone margins with nonunion. Gadolinium-enhanced fat-suppressed T1-weighted images are useful to evaluate flow and healing (124,133).

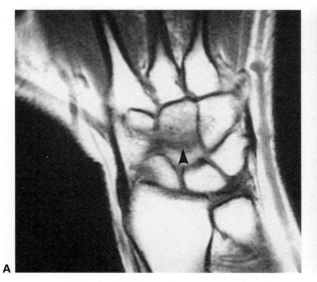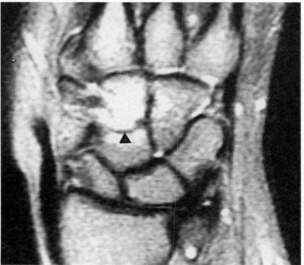

Figure 11-42 Coronal T1- **(A)** and T2-weighted **(B)** images of a capitate fracture. The fracture line is low signal intensity on both sequences. Edema is more obvious on the T2-weighted sequence.

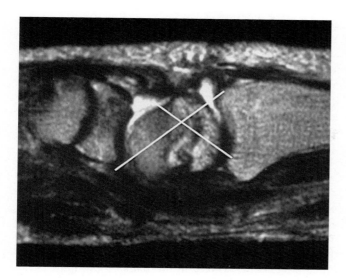

Figure 11-43 Sagittal T2-weighted image of a scaphoid fracture with "hump back" (*lines*) deformity. Compare to Fig. 11-41B, where there is no displacement.

Avascular necrosis occurs in up to 30% of proximal scaphoid fracture. This complication may also be seen in capitate and lunate fractures (134). In the acute setting, changes in signal intensity may be detected in both the proximal and distal fragments (see Fig. 11-46). Therefore, AVN may be suspected when, in fact, we are only seeing acute posttraumatic changes or edema. Abnormal signal intensity that develops or persists more than 6 weeks is more accurate for diagnosis of AVN (16,19,135). A more complete discussion of AVN of the scaphoid and lunate will follow in a later section of this chapter.

Soft Tissue Injuries

Soft tissue injuries may occur alone or in association with osseous injuries (see Fig. 11-47). Injuries are commonly related to repetitive microtrauma with secondary degeneration (overuse syndromes) (19,27,70,136). Routine radiographs are useful as a screening tool, as bone and soft tissue changes may suggest that additional imaging may be

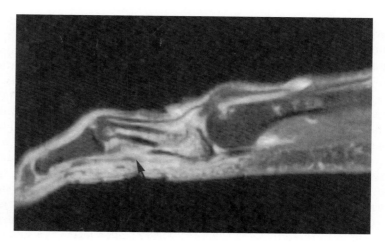

Figure 11-44 Sagittal fast spin-echo T2-weighted image of the middle finger demonstrates an angulated fracture of the proximal phalanx with rupture of the A2 pulley (*arrow*).

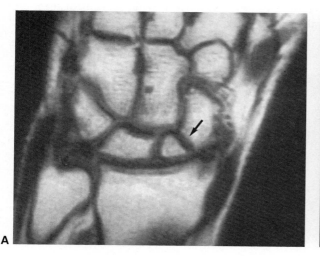

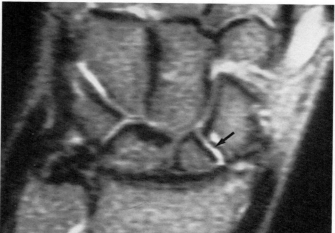

A **B**

Figure 11-45 Scaphoid nonunion. Coronal T1- **(A)** and T2-weighted **(B)** sequences demonstrate fluid in the fracture line with sclerotic margins along the fracture fragments **B**. Signal intensity in the proximal fragment is normal, excluding AVN.

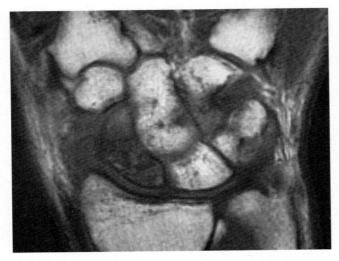

Figure 11-46 Coronal T1-weighted image of an acute scaphoid fracture. There is edema involving the entire scaphoid in the acute setting. Therefore, it is too early to evaluate potential AVN.

required. Depending on radiographic and clinical findings, ultrasound, CT, MRI, conventional arthrography, MR arthrography, or MR angiography may be selected (19,83, 137–139).

Triangular Fibrocartilage Complex (TFCC)

The TFCC includes the disc, supporting ligaments, and ECU tendon and its sheath (Fig. 11-18) (136,140–144). Patients with TFCC injuries present with ulnar-sided wrist pain. Associated ulnar styloid fractures and lunotriquetral ligament tears (70%) are common (142,144–147). Traumatic tears are more common in younger patients and usually occur near the radial attachment. Ulnar minus variance is common in these patients (27,145). Degenerative tears occur more commonly in the vascular zone near the ulnar attachment. These tears are more likely to heal without surgical intervention. Degenerative tears may be associated

with ulnar positive variance and ulnar lunate impaction syndrome (140,148,149).

The Palmer classification is commonly used to define the type of TFCC injury and associated findings (147). Type I tears are traumatic and type II tears are degenerative (146,147) (see Fig. 11-48). Type IA and IB lesions are the most common traumatic lesions. Degenerative lesions lead to internal derangement with progression to perforation (type IIC) and associated arthropathy (type IIE) (see Fig. 11-49) (65,66,146).

Ulnar length, radioulnar arthrosis, old radial fractures with shortening, ulnolunate arthrosis, and changes in the length or configuration of the ulnar styloid may be evident on radiographs. These findings may assist with classifying the type of TFCC injury (19,146,149). Arthrography is still a useful tool for evaluation of the TFCC and lunotriquetral ligament. Keep in mind that asymptomatic perforations in the TFCC may be evident in up to 27% of older individuals (16,19).

Both conventional MRI and MR arthrography have been correlated with arthroscopic and surgical findings for evaluating the TFCC (97,150–152). Conventional MRI techniques have included spin echo T1- and T2-weighted sequences, T2* GRE, FSE T2-weighted sequences, and high resolution three-dimensional GRE techniques (19,142). Results have varied with pulse sequence and location of the TFCC tear. Sensitivity for central defects is 91%, radial defects 86% to 100%, and ulnar defects 25% to 50% (144). Haims et al. (141) evaluated ulnar attachment tears. They compared indirect MR arthrography and MRI with surgical findings. MRI had a sensitivity of 17%, specificity of 79%, and accuracy of 64%. Using high signal intensity on T2-weighted sequences as a marker, the sensitivity was 42%, specificity 63%, and accuracy 55%. These findings suggest conventional MRI is suboptimal for peripheral tears (see Fig. 11-50) (141,144). This finding is significant in that peripheral tears can be repaired (good vascularity), whereas central tears typically are debrided (141).

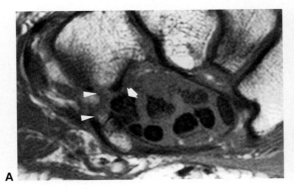
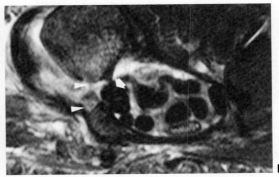

Figure 11-47 Axial T1-weighted **(A)** and STIR **(B)** images demonstrate a fracture of the hamate hook with separation of the fragments and interposition of a flexor tendon (*arrow*) between the fragments.

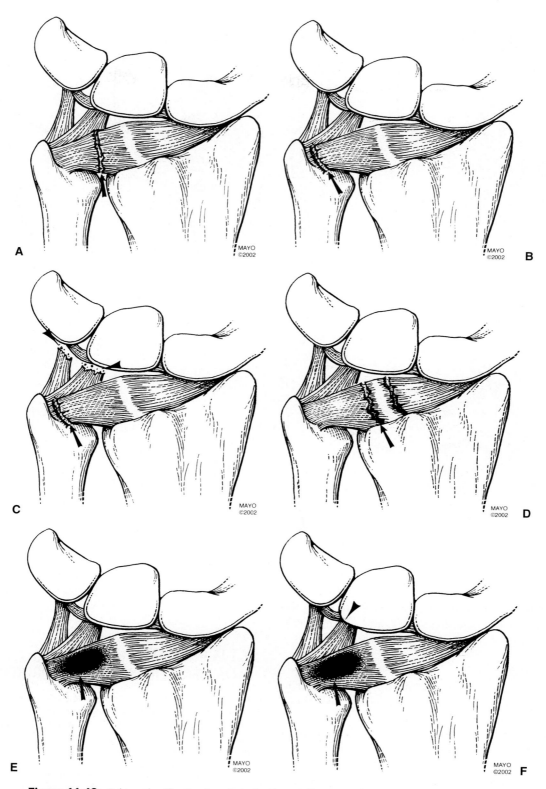

Figure 11-48 Palmer classification for triangular fibrocartilage complex (TFC) tears. **A:** Type IA, central perforation (*arrow*). **B:** Type IB, ulnar avulsion (*arrow*) with or without distal ulnar fracture. **C:** Type IC, distal avulsion (*arrow*) with peripheral volar attachment tears of the ulnolunate and ulnotriquetral ligaments (*arrowheads*). **D:** Type ID, radial avulsion (*arrow*) in the sigmoid notch with or without radial fracture. **E:** Type IIA, degenerative TFC complex wear (*arrow*). **F:** Type IIB, degenerative TFC wear (*arrow*) with lunate or ulnar chondromalacia (*arrowhead*). **G:** Type IIC, TFC perforation (*arrow*) with lunate or ulnar chondromalacia (*arrowhead*). **H:** Type IID, TFC perforation (*arrow*) with lunate or ulnar chondromalacia (*arrowhead*) and lunotriquetral ligament tear (*curved arrow*). **I:** Type IIE, TFC perforation (*arrow*) with complex ligament tears (*curved arrows*) and ulnocarpal arthrosis (*arrowheads*).

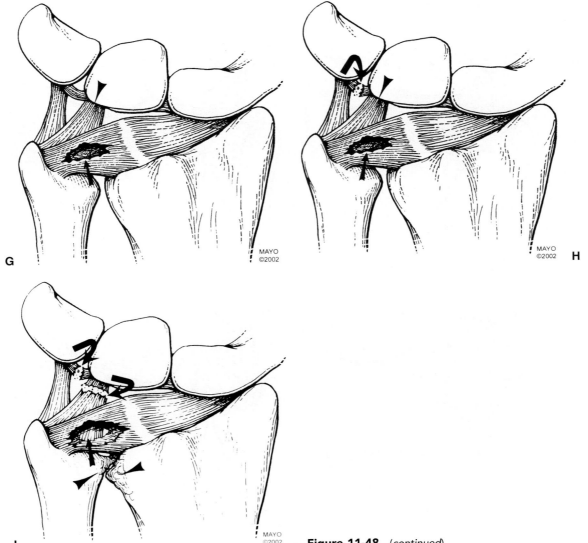

Figure 11-48 (continued)

When MR arthrography was compared to MRI, the sensitivity was 100%, specificity 90%, and accuracy 97% (Fig. 11-49) (151).

Impaction Syndromes

There are multiple impaction syndromes that result in ulnar-sided wrist pain. Certain syndromes are associated with TFCC defects (Table 11-7) (140,149,153).

Ulnar impaction syndrome (ulnar lunate abutment or impaction syndrome) is the most common of these disorders (140). Patients have ulnar positive variance and chronic wrist pain that increases with activity and is relieved by rest. Radiographs demonstrate ulnar positive variance with sclerosis and/or cystic changes in the lunate and triquetrum (see Fig. 11-51) (140,153). Degenerative TFCC tears (Palmer type II) are common (143,147). Coronal MR images (see Fig. 11-52) more clearly demonstrate the triangular fibrocartilage tear and articular changes.

TABLE 11-7
ULNAR-SIDED IMPACTION SYNDROMES

Ulnar impaction syndrome—chronic impaction of ulnar head, trangular fibrocartilage, and adjacent lunate and triquetrum.

Ulnar carpal impaction syndrome—due to ulnar styloid nonunion, ununited fragment acts as loose body.

Ulnar styloid impaction syndrome—chronic impaction due to long styloid abutting triquetrum.

Ulnar impingement syndrome—shortened ulna impinges on radius.

Hamatolunate impaction syndrome—due to type II lunate, arthrosis, and impingement with wrist in ulnar deviation.

From Cerezal L, del Pinal F, Abascal F, et al. Imaging findings in ulnar sided wrist impaction syndromes. *Radiographics* 2002;22:105–121; and Imaeda T, Nakamura R, Shionoya K, et al. Ulnar impactions syndrome: MR image findings. *Radiology* 1996;201:202–208.

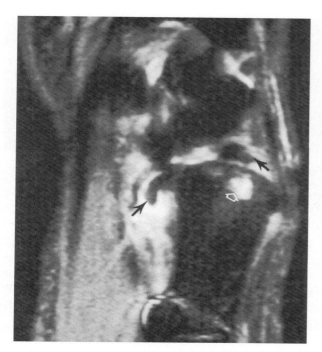

Figure 11-49 Degenerative triangular fibrocartilage tear with separation of the fragments (*arrows*) and an ulnar geode (*open arrow*) seen on a sagittal MR arthrogram image.

Focal signal refers to signal abnormality in the lunate in 87%, triquetrum 43%, and radial aspect of the ulna in 10% of the patients with ulnar impaction syndrome (153).

Ulnar carpal impactions syndrome (Table 11-7) is due to an ununited ulnar styloid fracture. The fragment may act as a loose body, causing arthrosis or impinging on the ECU

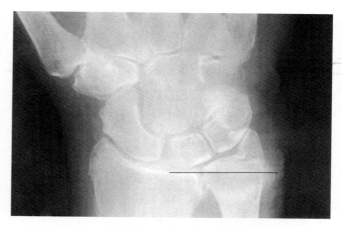

Figure 11-51 Posteroanterior radiograph demonstrates ulnar positive variance (*line*) with an elongated ulnar styloid. There is subchondral sclerosis in the lunate and triquetrum secondary to ulnar lunate impaction syndrome.

tendon. There may also be associated TFCC tears (140,153). Radiographs are usually adequate for diagnosis. However, MRI will confirm the nonunion and demonstrate cartilage and ECU changes more clearly (19,140).

Ulnar styloid impaction syndrome is due to an elongated styloid that causes chronic triquetral impaction (Fig. 11-7) (140). Ulnar impaction syndrome is due to a shortened ulna impinging on the radius. Hamate–lunate impaction is associated with a type 2 lunate (Fig. 11-14) that is present in up to 50% to 65% of patients. Up to 25% of patients develop hamate chondromalacia and arthrosis (140,149). Changes are easily appreciated on coronal T1- and T2-weighted or DESS sequences (19).

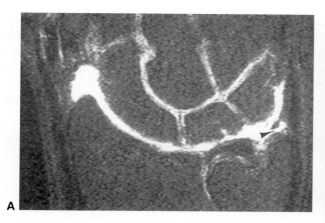

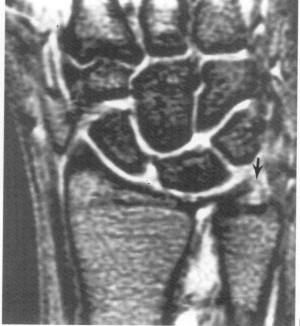

Figure 11-50 Ulnar attachment tears. **A:** Coronal gradient-echo image demonstrating a peripheral tear with high signal intensity fluid (*arrowhead*). **B:** Coronal gradient-echo image with increased signal intensity peripherally (*arrow*) but no tear.

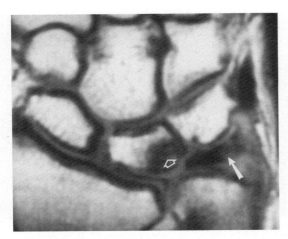

Figure 11-52 Coronal T1-weighted image demonstrates a triangular fibrocartilage tear (*arrow*) and abnormal signal intensity in the lunate (*open arrow*) due to ulnar lunate impaction syndrome.

Treatment of impaction disorders may involve arthroscopic or open approaches. Ulnar shortening may be required in patients with ulnar positive variance (140,153).

Ligament Tears/Instability

The intracapsular ligaments are divided into extrinsic and intrinsic (interosseous) groups. The scapholunate and lunotriquetral ligaments are the most important intrinsic ligaments (154).

Carpal instability can be seen following fracture malalignment, ligament tears, or inflammatory arthropathies (19,150,154). Disruption of the radioulnar ligaments and TFCC can result in ulnar translocation of the wrist and subluxation or dislocation of the distal radioulnar joint (154).

Carpal instability may be static (malalignment visible on radiographs) or dynamic where malalignment is demonstrated on physical examination or motion/stress views (18,154). Several carpal collapse patterns have been described based upon radiographic features. Dorsal intercalated segment instability (DISI) is the most common. There is an increased scapholunate angle (normal, 45°) on lateral radiographs with the lunate tilted dorsally and the scaphoid more plantar-flexed (see Fig. 11-53). The DISI pattern is associated with scapholunate and palmar extrinsic ligament disruptions (155). The scapholunate angle is reduced with volar intercalated segment instability (VISI). The lunate is in palmar flexion with associated capitate shift (see Fig. 11-54). The VISI pattern is seen with lunotriquetral and dorsal extrinsic ligament tears and in patients with rheumatoid arthritis (2,16,156). Scapholunate advanced collapse is seen with posttraumatic arthropathies. Detection of these patterns is usually obvious on anteroposterior and lateral radiographs or motion studies. MRI is not commonly required and may be confusing. Wrist positioning is artificial, and slight radial or ulnar deviation or standard MR positioning tends to exaggerate the scapholunate angle (19,154).

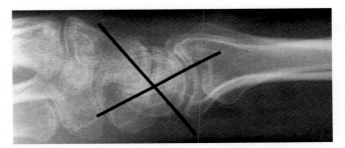

Figure 11-53 Lateral radiograph demonstrating dorsal intercalated segment instability deformity. The lunate is tilted dorsally and the scapholunate angle (*lines*) is increased. The capitate is shifted dorsally.

Similarly, ligament tears may also involve the metacarpophalangeal and interphalangeal joints. Imaging of ligament injuries in the hand and wrist should begin with radiographs (standard views and motion studies) (7). MRI or MR arthrography can be selected, depending on radiographic and clinical features.

Distal Radioulnar Joint

Distal radioulnar joint instability may follow trauma, radial shortening, or inflammatory arthropathies (18,157). CT or MRI can be performed to evaluate instability or subluxation. Axial images are obtained in neutral, pronation, and supination (16,136,158). Intraarticular contrast is not required unless the TFCC or other ligaments need to be evaluated. Noncontrast MR images can be obtained using T2-weighted or T2* GRE images. All positions should be reviewed. The ulna may look slightly dorsally subluxed in normal patients when the hand is positioned palm-down (see Figs. 11-55 and 11-56) (19,136).

Scapholunate Ligament Tears

The appearance of the scapholunate ligament varies with the portion included in the image plane. The ligament is C-shaped, extending from dorsal to proximal to palmar (Fig. 11-20). Thus, the distal joint is open and fills with contrast on conventional or MR arthrography. Contrast should

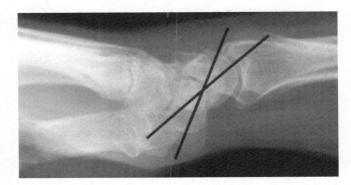

Figure 11-54 Volar intercalated segment instability deformity with the lunate tilted volarly and the scapholunate angle (*lines*) decreased.

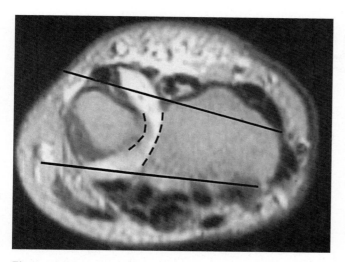

Figure 11-55 Axial T2-weighted image demonstrating a large effusion in the distal radioulnar joint. The radioulnar relationship is normal. *Broken lines* mark the articular surfaces. The ulna is completely within the radial lines, indicating normal position.

not extend through the joint space proximally. On coronal images, the ligament appears to have a trapezoid configuration on palmar sections, triangular in the proximal region, and band-like dorsally (see Fig. 11-57) (61,62).

Conventional and MR arthrography and MRI have been used to evaluate the SL ligament (16,48,62,136,148). MRI can be performed using FSE T2-weighted or T2* GRE sequences. Three-dimensional GRE sequences may be superior to assess fully the segments of the ligament (19,44, 61,62). Variations in signal intensity may be evident in addition to changes in shape in different sections. Higher signal intensity in the volar portion may be due to loose collagen fibers and vascular tissue (44,62). Smith (44) described several SL ligament appearances in normal individuals. Signal intensity was low and uniform in type I (49%), there was central intermediate signal in type II (14%), and signal increased proximally in type III and distally in type IV (18%). Intermediate signal extended through the ligament in a linear fashion in type V (19%) (see Figs. 11-21 and 11-58).

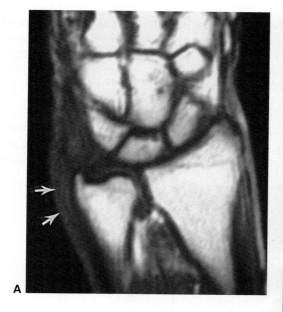

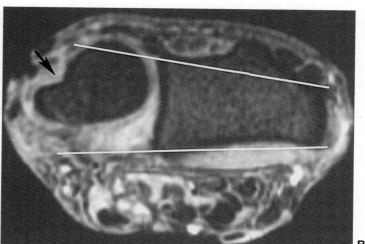

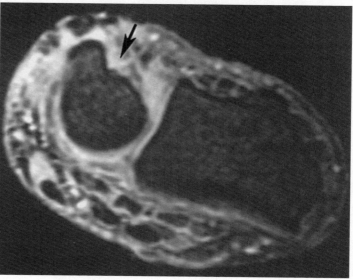

Figure 11-56 Subluxation of the distal radioulnar joint with extensor carpi ulnaris (ECU) tendon dislocation. Coronal T1-weighted image **(A)** shows swelling along the ulnar styloid (*arrows*). Axial fat-suppressed fast spin-echo T2-weighted images **(B,C)** show dorsal subluxation (*lines* in **B**). The ECU tendon is absent (*arrow*) from the sixth dorsal compartment in **B,C**.

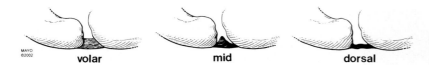

Figure 11-57 Scapholunate ligament seen in the coronal plane in volar, mid (proximal), and dorsal sections.

Scapholunate ligament tears are seen as high signal intensity extending through a portion or the entire ligament on T2-weighted sequences. Fragmentation, absence of the ligament, and widening of the SL space may also be evident (16,61). Though controversial, Berger et al. (60) demonstrated that tears of the proximal ligament were less likely to lead to instability. Dorsal SL ligament tears are more likely to result in instability. Conventional MRI studies demonstrate sensitivities ranging from 50% to 93%, specificities of 86% to 100%, and accuracies of 77% to 87% (19,107,156).

Magnetic resonance arthrography is more accurate (see Fig. 11-59). Radiocarpal injections are usually adequate. Intercarpal injections may be required to exclude partial tears in the distal surface. Fat-suppressed T1-weighted and three-dimensional GRE images are performed after injection (Table 11-1). Scheck et al. (61) reported accurate detection of SL ligament tears in 94% of MR arthrograms. Sensitivities and specificities were 52% and 34% for conventional MRI, compared to 09% and 87% for MR arthrography.

Lunotriquetral Ligament Tears

The configuration of the lunotriquetral (LT) ligament is similar to the SL ligament. Similar to the SL ligament, there are membranous and triangular portions (Fig. 11-20)

(19,42,62). Smith and Snearly (42) described variations in the LT ligament. The ligament was triangular in 63% and linear in 37% of patients (see Fig. 11-60). The ligament was uniformly low signal intensity (type I) in 74%, had intermediate signal distally (type II) in 9%, demonstrated a linear cleft (type III) in 15%, and proximal intermediate signal intensity (type IV) in 2% (Fig. 11-22). Variations in signal intensity were also described at the bony attachments (Fig. 11-60B) (42).

Asymptomatic perforation of the LT ligament occurs in 13% of the general population over age 40. Also, there is a high incidence of LT ligament tears with TFCC tears (see Fig. 11-61). Therefore, we may inject the DRUJ first when performing conventional or MR arthrography. Lunotriquetral ligament tears may be partial, which may require injecting two compartments (16). MRI sequences can be the same as those described with SL ligament tears. Conventional MRI is less accurate for LT ligament tears compared to SL data. Sensitivity ranges from 40% to 56% and specificity 45% to 100% (19).

Extrinsic Ligament Tears

Evaluation of the dorsal and palmar ligaments is more difficult (Fig. 11-23) (1,19,159). Multiple image planes or three-dimension approaches following arthrography are probably

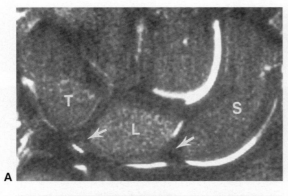

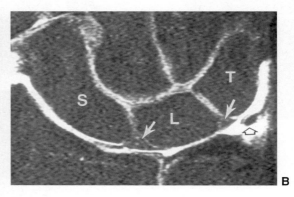

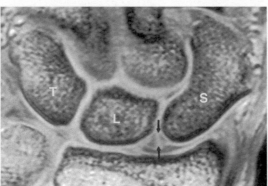

Figure 11-58 Scapholunate ligament appearance seen on MRI (Fig. 11-21). **A:** Coronal MR arthrogram image demonstrating low signal intensity scapholunate and lunotriquetral ligaments (*arrows*) (type I). **B:** Coronal MR arthrogram showing triangular scapholunate and lunotriquetral ligaments with central intermediate signal intensity (*arrows*) (type II). **C:** Coronal gradient-echo image demonstrating linear increased signal through the ligament (*arrows*) (type V). *S*, scaphoid; *L*, lunate; *T*, triquetrum.

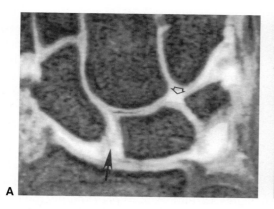 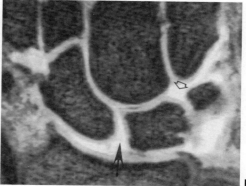

Figure 11-59 Scapholunate ligament tear. Coronal radiocarpal MR arthrogram images **(A,B)** demonstrate subtle widening of the scapholunate space compared to the lunotriquetral joint. There is contrast in the intercarpal joint (*open arrow*), with increased signal intensity in the scapholunate ligament (*arrow*).

best. However, there are limited data on the accuracy of MRI in this regard.

Metacarpophalangeal/Interphalangeal Ligament Tears

Injuries to the ligaments of the hand may be isolated or associated with fractures and other soft tissue injuries (160,161). One of the most common injuries is the UCL of the thumb. The injury was initially termed "gamekeeper thumb" because it occurred in Scottishgame keepers due to

the method used to kill rabbits (162). Today, the injury is common in skiers, accounting for 6% to 9.5% of all skiing injuries (124,160,161).

The fibrocartilagenous palmar plate is thin proximally and thickens distally. The sesamoids are located at the insertions of the flexor pollicis brevis and adductor brevis (48,161). The UCL arises from the medial tubercle of the metacarpal condyle and takes an oblique course to insert on the base of the proximal phalanx near the volar plate. The

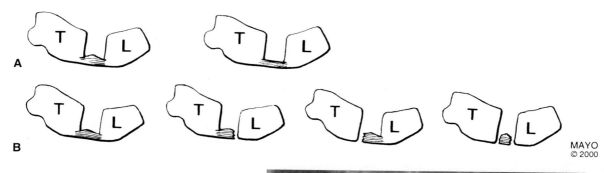

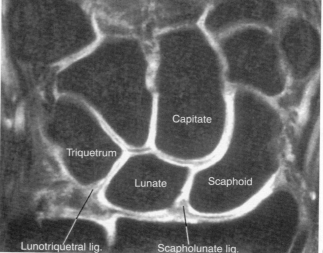

Figure 11-60 Signal intensity variations in the lunotriquetral ligament (Fig. 11-22). **A:** The ligament may be triangular (63%) or linear (37%). **B:** Signal intensity may vary at the bone attachments. *(1)* normal, *(2)* cleft at lunate attachment, *(3)* cleft at triquetral attachment, *(4)* cleft at both attachments. **C:** MR arthrogram demonstrating the scapholunate and lunotriquetral ligaments. *L,* lunate; *T,* triquetrum.

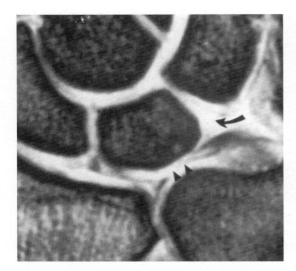

Figure 11-61 Coronal gradient-echo image demonstrating a lunotriquetral ligament tear (*curved arrow*) and a triangular fibrocartilage tear (*arrowheads*) with ulnar positive variance and lunate chondromalacia. (From Oneson SR, Timins ME, Scales LM, et al. MR diagnosis of triangular fibrocartilage pathology with arthroscopic correlation. *AJR Am J Roentgenol* 1997;168:1513–1518.)

adductor brevis has three insertions, including the ulnar sesamoid and palmar plate, the lateral tubercle of the proximal phalanx, and the dorsal expansion (161). The insertion confluent with the dorsal expansion hood and superficial to the UCL is termed the adductor aponeurosis (48,162).

Ulnar collateral ligament injuries occur with forced abduction of the thumb. Tears occur most commonly near the phalangeal insertion (distally) (124,160,162). When the ligament is displaced so that it lies superficial to the adductor aponeurosis, it is termed a Stener lesion (see Fig. 11-62) (160,162). This is important to identify, as it requires surgical repair (162).

Diagnosis is accomplished with stress views of both thumbs for comparison. Anesthetic injection is required in

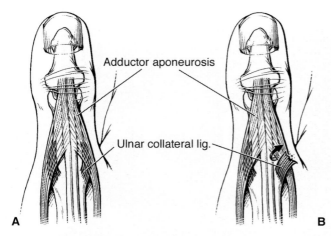

Figure 11-62 Stener lesion. **A:** Normal anatomy of the UCL and adductor aponeurosis. Following forced abduction of the thumb a tear may occur in the UCL. When the proximal fragment is displaced superficial to the aponeurosis **(B)** it is termed a Stener lesion.

the acute setting to perform an adequate examination (7). Conventional arthrography can be performed in this setting by injecting contrast with the anesthetic. In many institutions, MRI or MR arthrography has replaced more conventional imaging approaches (124,160,162,163). Conventional arthrography demonstrates 83% of tears but only 61% of Stener lesions. MRI demonstrated 90% and MR arthrography 100% of displaced tears (Stener lesions) (see Fig. 11-63) (162).

Tendon Injuries

Certain key aspects of tendon anatomy and surgical landmarks are important to plan and interpret MRI examinations. The flexor tendons begin in the distal third of the forearm. At the wrist, the flexor pollicis longus passes the transverse flexor retinaculum and is enclosed in its own tendon sheath (radial bursa) (see Fig. 11-64). The flexor digitorum profundus and superficialis tendons lie dorsal and medial to the median nerve and are enclosed in a common tendon sheath (ulnar bursa) (Fig. 11-64; Fig. 11-15). The relationships of the flexor tendons to the MCP and interphalangeal (IP) joints are also important. At the MCP joint, the flexor tendon lies just palmar to the volar plate in the A1 pulley (see Fig. 11-65). It has a similar position at the proximal interphalangeal joint in the A3 pulley (Fig. 11-65). Zones have been described for surgical planning. Figure 11-64 demonstrates the flexor tendon zones. It is useful to use these surgical zones when describing tendon injuries (16,48,101).

The extensor tendons are stabilized in six dorsal compartments of the wrist (see Fig. 11-66). At the level of the extensor retinaculum, the tendons are enclosed in tendon sheaths. Just proximal to the MCP joints, the extensor digitorum communis tendons are joined together by the junctura tendinum (Fig. 11-66). The relationship of the extensor tendons to the MCP and interphalangeal joints is summarized in Figs. 11-15 and 11-66B. As with the flexor tendons, zones are established for surgical planning (see Fig. 11-67) (15,16,48,101).

Injuries to the tendons of the hand and wrist occur commonly (Table 11-8) (15,19,70,101,164,165). Inflammation of the tendon (tendinitis), tendon sheath (tenosynovitis), or perivascular bundle (peritendinitis) may occur alone or in combination. Tendinosis is a degenerative process seen in overuse and aging that results in mucoid degeneration, vascular ingrowth, and cartilage metaplasia. Tendon ruptures may be partial or complete (15,101,166–169).

Patients with tendon injuries present with pain and diminished function involving the affected tendon or tendons. Routine radiography is still an important screening tool and may demonstrate subtle avulsion fractures or other changes that may suggest the diagnosis (19). Prior to MRI, clinical diagnosis, ultrasound, or tenography were used to evaluate tendon disorders of the hand and wrist.

Conventional MRI or, rarely, MR tenography is commonly used today. Normal tendons have low signal intensity on all pulse sequences. There is normally minimal

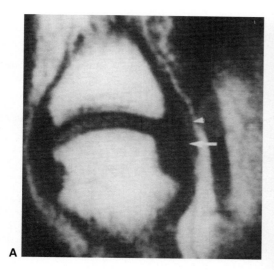

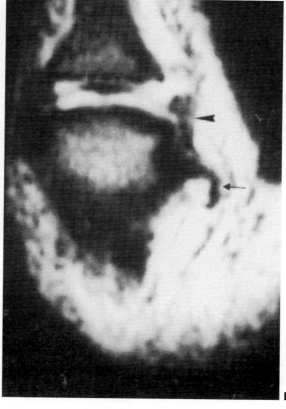

Figure 11-63 MRI in gamekeeper thumb. **A:** Coronal SE 600/20 image demonstrating a normal UCL (*arrow*) and adductor pollicis aponeurosis (*arrowhead*). **B:** Coronal SE 2,000/80 image demonstrating a Stener lesion with proximally retracted and torn UCL (*arrow*) in respect to the adductor aponeurosis (*arrowhead*). (From Harper MT, Chandnani VP, Spaeth J, et al. Gamekeeper thumb: diagnosis of UCL injury using magnetic resonance imaging, magnetic resonance arthrography and stress radiography. *J Magn Reson Imaging* 1996;6:322–328.)

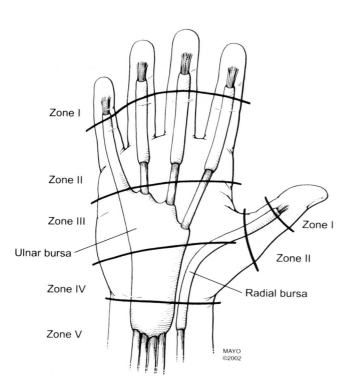

Figure 11-64 Flexor tendon sheaths and zones of injury in the hand and wrist. (From Berquist TH. *MRI of the hand and wrist.* Philadelphia, PA: Lippincott Williams & Wilkins, 2003.)

fluid in the tendon sheath. When fluid completely surrounds the tendon, inflammation is more likely. Inflammatory changes in the tendon or sheath are most easily demonstrated on T2-weighted sequences (Table 11-8) (see Fig. 11-68) (2,16,150). Tendon inflammation and partial tears show increased signal intensity and thickening in the area of involvement on T2-weighted sequences (see Fig. 11-69). Signal intensity increases on T2-weighted compared to proton density sequences. In general, signal intensity is intermediate on both sequences with tendonosis. The tendon ends are separated and may be retracted with complete tears (16,170).

Tendon/Pulley System Ruptures

Tendon ruptures may occur with acute trauma or degeneration. Ruptures may also result from fracture malunion or nonunion and inflammatory arthropathies (19,168,169). Patients with rheumatoid arthritis develop tenosynovitis in 64% of cases. Chronic inflammation frequently leads to partial or complete tendon tears (168). Tendon tears in the fingers and hand are often associated with skin wounds or lacerations (167,171).

The pulley system (Fig. 11-65C) is critical for flexor tendon function. These structures keep the tendon in position along the phalanges during finger flexion (172). Rupture of the pulley system occurs with forced extension when the finger is flexed (see Fig. 11-70). Pulley system rupture is associated with activities such as rock climbing (173).

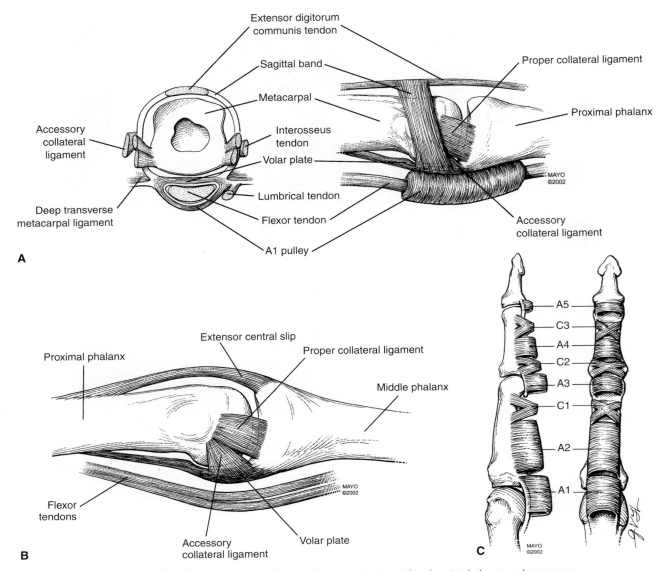

Figure 11-65 **A:** Flexor and extensor tendons seen in the axial and sagittal planes at the metacarpophalangeal joint. **B:** Illustration of the flexor and extensor tendons at the interphalangeal joint.
C: Five annular (A) and three C-shaped (C) pulleys to maintain flexor tendon position.

Injury to the pulley system may result in "bowstring" deformity of the involved tendons (see Fig. 11-71) (172–174).

Tendon injuries can be evaluated with dynamic ultrasound or MRI. Image planes used most commonly are
axial and sagittal for the fingers, axial and coronal for the
hand, and axial and coronal or sagittal for the wrist
(19,168,171). Sagittal images in flexion and extension
may be required to evaluate the pulley system fully (Fig.
11-71) (19,166). FSE T2-weighted sequences with fat
suppression, 2- to 3-mm-thick sections, 8 cm FOV, 1
acquisition, and a 256 × 256 matrix are used. Volume
three-dimensional GRE sequences can be obtained in the
coronal plane for the wrist.

Flexor tendon injuries are more common than extensor
tendon disorders. Tendon injuries are treated differently,
depending upon the degree of displacement. Therefore, it
is important to demonstrate both ends in complete tears.
Retraction of the flexor tendon back into the hand results
in loss of vascular supply to the tendon ends. The vascular
supply is preserved if the tendon is retracted to the proximal interphalangeal joint level. Therefore, it is important
to repair tendons retracted into the hand early. Delay is less
critical with mild retraction (see Fig. 11-72) (166,171).

Tendon Subluxation/Dislocation

Subluxation or dislocation of the tendons in the hand and
wrist may occur with trauma, previous fracture with deformity, or inflammatory arthropathies. Patients may have subtle symptoms or present with pain, swelling, and reduced
function (7,16).

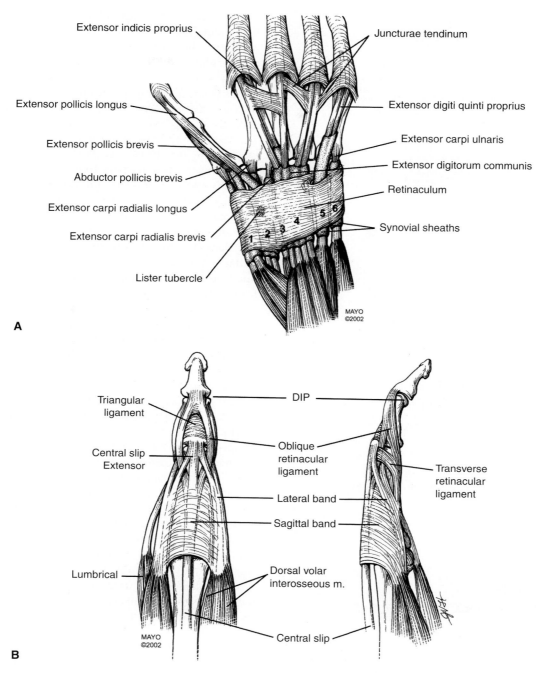

Figure 11-66 A: Extensor tendons, tendon sheaths, and six dorsal compartments. **B:** Extensor tendons in the fingers, seen dorsally and laterally.

Imaging should include radiographic screening to evaluate osseous structures, joint deformity, and areas of soft tissue swelling. Ultrasound or MRI can be used to evaluate tendon position. Flexion, extension, pronation, and supination may be required to detect subtle abnormalities, especially in the wrist (see Fig. 11-73).

Inflammatory Disorders
Inflammatory disorders involving the tendons are common (16,69,175). Tendinitis or tenosynovitis of the first

dorsal compartment (de Quervain tenosynovitis) occurs most commonly (2,176). The ECU tendon is the second most common location for tenosynovitis, followed by the extensor carpi radialis, flexor carpi radialis, flexor carpi ulnaris, and extensor pollicis longus (third dorsal compartment) (87,177,178).

De Quervain stenosing tenosynovitis involves the first dorsal compartment (see Fig. 11-74). Patients present with pain and restriction of the extensor pollicis brevis and abductor pollicis longus (176). This condition is most

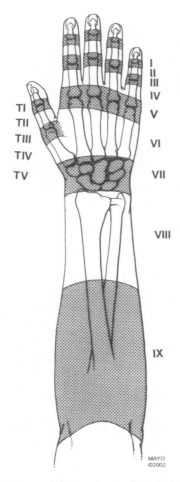

Figure 11-67 Zones for extensor tendon injuries.

TABLE 11-8
TENDON DISORDERS: MRI FEATURES

Condition	MRI Features
Tendinosis	Intermediate increased signal intensity, proton density and T2-weighted sequences, tendon thickening
Tendinitis	Intermediate signal intensity, proton density with high signal intensity on T2-weighted sequence, tendon thickening
Tenosynovitis	Increased signal intensity surrounding tendon, T2-weighted sequences, tendon signal intensity normal
Partial tear	Increased signal intensity and thickening on T2-weighted sequences
Complete tear	Increased signal intensity on T2-weighted sequences with segments separated, with or without retraction

common between the ages of 30 and 50 years. Up to 77% of patients are women involved in nursing, secretarial work, or other occupations resulting in overuse (pinch, grasp, radial and ulnar deviation of the wrist) symptoms. The incidence of de Quervain is also increased during pregnancy (176). Clinical symptoms may mimic a scaphoid fracture, flexor carpi radialis tendonitis, degenerative arthritis, or intersection syndrome (squeaker wrist) (7). The last is an overuse syndrome slightly proximal to de Quervain tendonitis (Fig. 11-74A). A bursa forms between the extensor carpi radialis longus and brevis and the abductor pollicis longus and extensor pollicis brevis. Patients usually are involved in racquet sports and present with pain, weak grip, and crepitation (squeaker wrist).

Radiographs in patients with de Quervain tenosynovitis may demonstrate soft tissue swelling and osteopenia of the radial styloid, focal periosteal reaction, or bone erosion due to thickened inflamed synovium (19,176). Multiple features have been described on MR images. Thickening of the extensor pollicis brevis and abductor pollicis longus tendons is the most consistent finding. Peritendinous fluid and marrow edema may be seen on T2-weighted images (Fig. 11-74). A septum dividing the first dorsal compartment is evident in 30% of patients with de Quervain tenosynovitis (176).

MRI features are similar with tendinitis and tenosynovitis involving other tendons. Inflammatory changes in the ECU may result in recurrent subluxation. Therefore, axial images should be obtained in neutral, pronation, and supination, or cine motion studies should be considered to exclude subluxation (Fig. 11-73) (19).

Patients with extensor indicis proprius syndrome present with pain in the forearm and wrist with flexion of the wrist and fingers together (87). MR images demonstrate thickening of the fourth dorsal compartment and hypertrophy of the muscle. Findings are easily appreciated on axial T1- and T2-weighted images (87).

Generalized inflammatory changes in the tendons or tendon sheaths are unusual except in rheumatoid arthritis, infection, and gymnast's wrist (128,178,179).

Miscellaneous Conditions

The previous sections have discussed osseous, ligament, tendon, and TFCC injuries. Other soft tissue injuries may include the neurovascular tissues. Injuries to the digital arteries can occur with lacerations. Occlusion and aneurysm formation in the ulnar artery does occur in the region of the hamate hook. Chronic trauma to this region is reported in handball players, jackhammer operators, tennis players, and golfers (180).

Anatomically, the ulnar artery divides into deep and superficial branches in Guyon canal. The arteries are bounded by the pisiform and hamate hook laterally, the transverse carpal ligament dorsally, and the volar carpal ligament superficially. The superficial branch of the ulnar artery penetrates the palmar aponeurosis to form

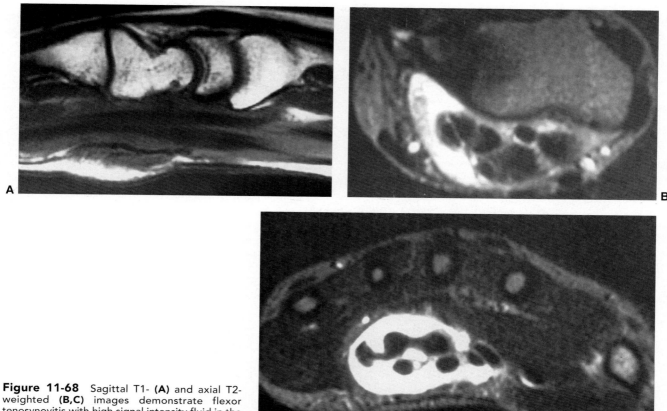

Figure 11-68 Sagittal T1- **(A)** and axial T2-weighted **(B,C)** images demonstrate flexor tenosynovitis with high signal intensity fluid in the tendon sheaths and normal low signal intensity tendons in a gymnast with overuse syndrome.

the superficial palmar arch. At this point, the artery is unprotected and the hamate hook serves as an anvil to which chronic trauma can damage the vessel (48,180).

Angiography has been the gold standard for imaging the arteries of the hand and wrist (33,35). Thrombi, neural damage, and aneurysms have been identified with ulnar artery injury (hypothenar hammer syndrome) (see Fig. 11-75).

Improvements in MR angiography using intravenous gadolinium and other techniques now provide excellent image quality for evaluation of vascular structures (19,33,35,181).

Other arteries can also be injured, most frequently by lacerations or open wounds (33,181). An exception is frostbite injuries that result from microvascular occlusion

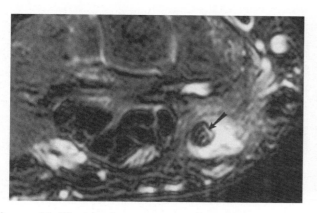

Figure 11-69 Partial tear in the flexor carpi radialis. T2-weighted image shows thickening of the tendon with increased signal intensity (*arrow*). There is fluid surrounding the tendon.

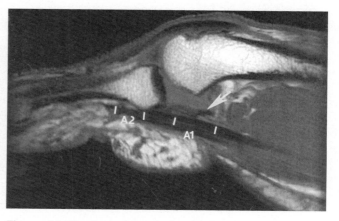

Figure 11-70 Sagittal T1-weighted image demonstrates volar subluxation with disruption of the volar plate (*arrow*) and tendon displacement due to A1 pulley rupture (Fig. 11-65C). The A2 pulley and tendon position are normal.

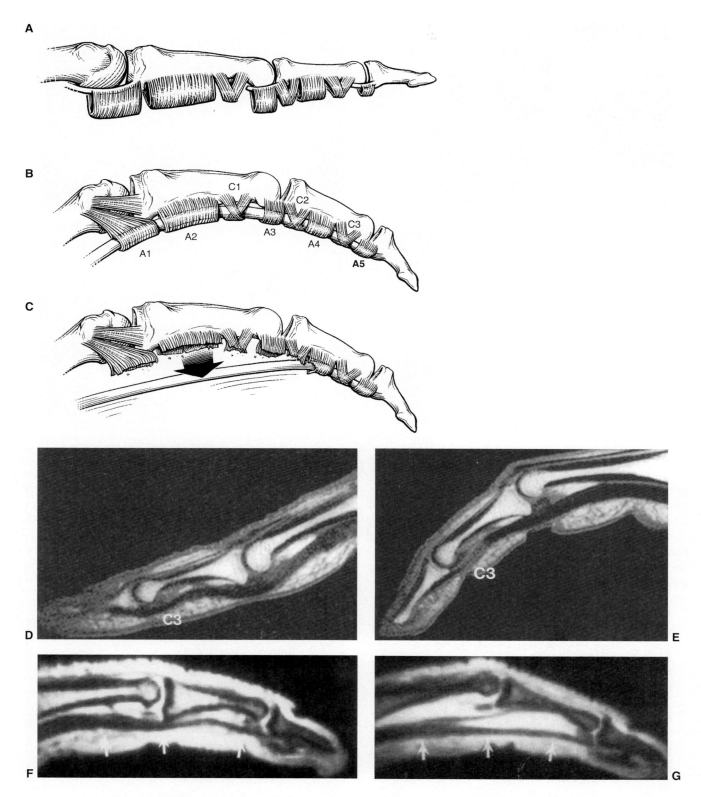

Figure 11-71 Pulley system rupture. Illustration of the pulley system with the finger extended **(A)**, flexed **(B)**, and bow-string appearance with pulley rupture **(C)**. Sagittal T1-weighted images in the extended **(D)** and flexed **(E)** positions, demonstrating an intact pulley system with normal relationship of the flexor tendons to the phalanges. T1-weighted extended **(F)** and flexed **(G)** images in a patient with pulley system rupture. The flexor tendon is separated from the phalanx in extension *(arrows)* and there is obvious bow-stringing with flexion *(arrows* in **G**). **(F,G** from Bowers WH, Kuzma AR, Byrum DK. Closed traumatic rupture of the finger pulleys. *J Hand Surg* 1994;19A: 782–787.)

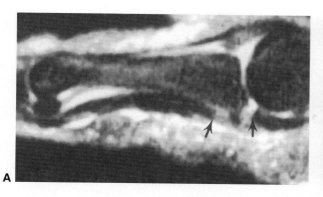
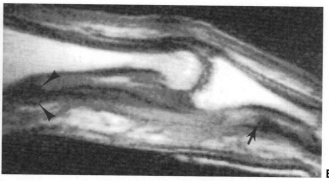

Figure 11-72 Flexor tendon ruptures. **A:** Sagittal T2-weighted fast spin-echo image demonstrates mild retraction (*arrows*). **B:** Sagittal T1-weighted image shows the distal segment (*arrow*) with retraction of the proximal fragment to the base of the proximal phalanx (*arrowheads*).

and intracellular ice crystal formation. MR angiography can demonstrate the extent of vascular and soft tissue involvement (181,182).

MUSCULOSKELETAL NEOPLASMS

Tumors in the hand and wrist are uncommon compared to the lower extremities and axial skeleton. Benign tumors occur more frequently than malignant tumors (16,19,74, 183–189). Generally, routine radiographs are most useful for determining the nature of skeletal lesions; that is, whether a lesion is potentially benign or malignant. Table 11-9 lists the most common benign (tumor or tumor-like) and malignant osseous neoplasms in the hand and wrist. The most common benign tumors in the hand and wrist, as noted in Table 11-9 (in order of decreasing frequency), are enchondromas (see Fig. 11-76), giant cell

tumors (see Fig. 11-77), osteoid osteoma, chondromyxoid fibromas, and aneurysmal bone cysts (190). These lesions can usually be accurately diagnosed with routine radiographs. Therefore, MRI is not often indicated. Certain lesions, such as osteoid osteoma, are often more easily characterized with CT (191). MRI is reserved for equivocal cases or to plan operative approaches.

Malignant lesions of bone in the hand and wrist are even less common than benign lesions (Table 11-9) (188,192,195). Malignant vascular tumors are most common (193). As in other areas of the extremities, if a malignant lesion is suspected, MRI is superior to CT for demonstrating the extent of medullary bone, soft tissue, and neurovascular involvement. Most frequently, both T1- and T2-weighted sequences are needed to characterize lesions. T2-weighted sequences are best suited for soft tissue characterization and T1-weighted sequences for distinction between marrow and tumor (see Fig. 11-78)

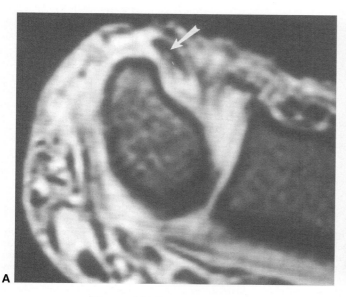
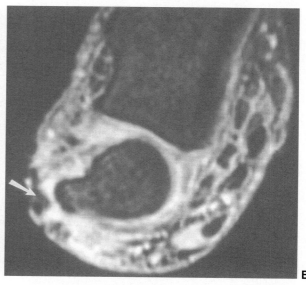

Figure 11-73 Extensor carpi ulnaris dislocation. Axial gradient-echo images at the level of the distal radioulnar joint in different positions show subluxation **(A)** progressing to dislocation **(B)**.

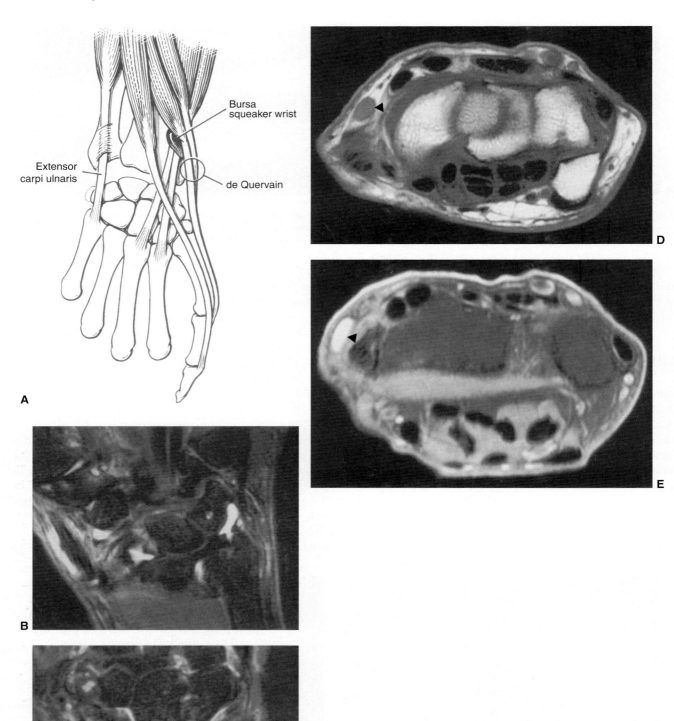

Figure 11-74   A: Illustration of the location of de Quervain tenosynovitis and a bursa that can form proximal to this resulting in intersection syndrome (squeaker wrist). Coronal T2-weighted fast spin-echo images **(B,C)** show inflammatory changes along the radial styloid and marrow edema (*arrow*). Axial T1- **(D)** and fat-suppressed fast spin-echo T2-weighted **(E)** images demonstrate a localized fluid collection (*arrowhead*) in the first extensor compartment due to de Quervain tenosynovitis.

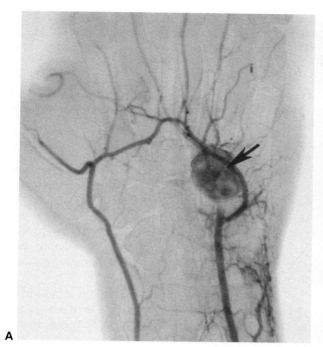

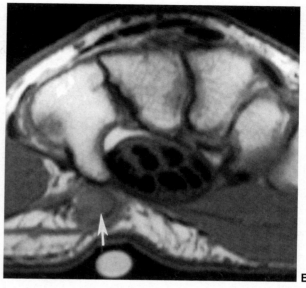

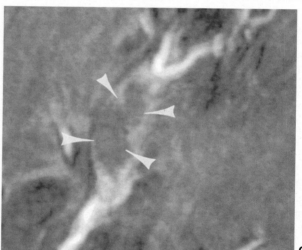

Figure 11-75 Posttraumatic ulnar artery aneurysm. **A:** Angiogram shows a large ulnar artery aneurysm (*arrow*). Axial T1-weighted image **(B)** demonstrates a soft tissue mass (*arrow*) at the hook of the hamate. Coronal MR angiogram **(C)** shows a thrombosed (*arrowheads*) ulnar artery aneurysm.

(16,19). Short TI inversion recovery sequences are useful for detection of subtle marrow or soft tissue lesions. Gadolinium does not routinely improve histologic accuracy of MRI, but it has become a routine approach when imaging bone or soft tissue tumors.

The role of MRI in evaluation of soft tissue neoplasm differs significantly from osseous neoplasms (16, 196–200). Routine radiographs, except for lipomas and calcifications, are not usually able to identify soft tissue lesions (see Fig. 11-79). Secondary bone erosion can occur with giant cell tumors of the tendon sheath and epidermoids (189,193). Soft tissue contrast with MRI in the peripheral extremities is superior to CT. The ability to image in multiple planes with the variable pulse sequences and the superior soft tissue contrast of MRI make identification and characterization of soft tissues in the hand and wrist much easier to accomplish (16,19). Also, compared to skeletal lesions, characterization of lesions, especially benign soft tissue tumors, is more easily

accomplished (see Chapter 12) (18). New angiographic techniques are also available that allow better definition of vascular lesions (33,181).

Certain lesions in the hand and wrist deserve further discussion (Table 11-10) (201,202). Epidermoids, glomus tumors, ganglia, giant cell tumors of the tendon sheath, and mucoid cysts, and lipomas occur commonly in the hand and wrist (12,36,183,197,202–204).

Ganglion Cysts

Ganglion cysts are the most common soft tissue masses in the hand and wrist. Ganglion cysts are synovial outpouchings that occur most commonly along the dorsal aspects of the hand and wrist (36,143,164,204,206). Ganglia are well marginated but vary in size. In some cases, they appear as elongations of the tendon sheath. Most often they have high signal intensity on T2-weighted sequences and are near muscle intensity on T1-weighted sequences (see Fig. 11-80). Slight shortening of T1- and T2-relation times can occur

TABLE 11-9

BONE TUMORS AND TUMORLIKE CONDITIONS OF THE HAND AND WRIST (11,087 TUMORS)

Benign	No. of Cases	No. of (%) Tumors in Hand and Wrist
Enchondromas	290	130 (45%)
Giant cell tumors	568	84 (15%)
Osteoid osteoma	331	29 (9%)
Aneurysmal bone cysts	289	16 (6%)
Osteochondroma	827	30 (4%)
Osteoblastoma	87	3 (3%)
Chondromyxoid fibroma	45	3 (3%)
Fibrous defects	125	3 (2%)
Chondroblastoma	119	1 (0.7%)
Benign vascular tumors	108	0 (0%)
Malignant		
Hemangioendothelioma	80	7 (9%)
Fibrosarcoma	255	5 (2%)
Chondrosarcoma	895	17 (2%)
Malignant fibrous histiocytoma	83	2 (2%)
Ewing sarcoma	512	6 (1%)
Lymphoma	694	6 (0.8%)
Osteosarcoma	1,649	17 (0.1%)
Metastasis	3,000	2 (0.1%)

From references 181,188, and 192–194.

with viscous or proteinaceous debris so that signal intensity is slightly reduced on T2-weighted and slightly increased on T1-weighted sequences (16). Ganglia are commonly associated with internal derangements of the wrist (207).

Giant Cell Tumors

Giant cell tumors of the tendon sheath are the second most common soft tissue mass in the hand. Most patients are in their third or fourth decades and, like ganglion cysts, there is a slight female predominance (202,208). In the hand and wrist, most patients present with a slowly growing subcutaneous mass. The lesion is most often palmar and involves the first three fingers most frequently. Lesions may be painful and, though unusual, multiple lesions may occur (208). Malignant giant cell tumors of the tendon sheath have been reported, but they are rare (202,208).

Radiographs demonstrate swelling or a focal mass. Erosion of the adjacent osseous structures occurs in 15% of cases (see Fig. 11-81) (208). On MR images, the lesion is muscle intensity on T1-weighted sequences. Lesions may be high or low signal intensity and inhomogeneous on T2-weighted sequences. Areas of low signal intensity due to hemosiderin are typical of this lesion (16). Nonuniform enhancement is common on postcontrast fat-suppressed T1-weighted images (Fig. 11-81E). Fibroma of the tendon

sheath can have a similar appearance (16,208,209). However, they are low signal intensity on all pulse sequences and there is little or no enhancement after intravenous gadolinium.

After resection, these lesions recur in about 50% of cases (see Fig. 11-82). Therefore, a postoperative baseline study is important to improve the ability to detect recurrent lesions (19).

Hemangiomas

Hemangiomas account for 7% of benign soft tissue tumors (202,210). Twelve percent of these lesions occur in the hand and wrist. Hemangiomas represent a spectrum of benign vascular lesions that may also contain fat, fibrous tissue, or bone (9,210). Hemangiomas may be cavernous (large vessels) or capillary (small vessels) or mixed. Nonvascular components are more common in cavernous hemangiomas (183).

Radiographs may demonstrate swelling, a focal mass, or phleboliths (see Fig. 11-79). Phleboliths are most characteristic of cavernous hemangiomas (183). MR features are frequently definitive with intermixed fat signal on T1-weighted sequences and serpiginous high signal intensity vascular structures on T2-weighted sequences. Phleboliths are demonstrated as round areas of low signal intensity (16,183,210).

Resection is not normally indicated unless the lesion interferes with growth, is bleeding, or diminishes function (9). When surgery is suggested, conventional or MR angiography should be performed to define clearly the extent of the lesion (see Fig. 11-83) (9,184,201).

Lipomas

Lipomas account for 6% of benign tumors in the hand and wrist (211). Lipomas are composed of adipose tissue and occur most commonly in patients over 50 years of age. Lesions may be superficial or deep. The former may be difficult to separate from subcutaneous fat. Multiple lesions occur in 5% to 7% of patients (16,211).

Radiographs may demonstrate a fat density mass. On MR images the mass has fat signal intensity on T1- and T2-weighted sequences. Well-defined septae and a lobulated appearance are common findings (16,211). Intramuscular lipomas may infiltrate between muscle fibers resulting in more irregular margins compared to the usually well-defined margins of a benign lipoma (16).

Fatty tissue may be seen along or around tendons of the hand and wrist (see Fig. 11-84). Neurofibrolipomas frequently involve the median nerve (80%) (see Fig. 11-85). Patients usually present during early adulthood with a slowly growing palmar mass. Patients may have pain and carpal tunnel syndrome. Up to 66% have macrodactyly (2,212,213).

Macrodystrophia lipomatosis is a rare localized form of gigantism present at birth. The condition is due to mesenchymal overgrowth and typically involves the second and

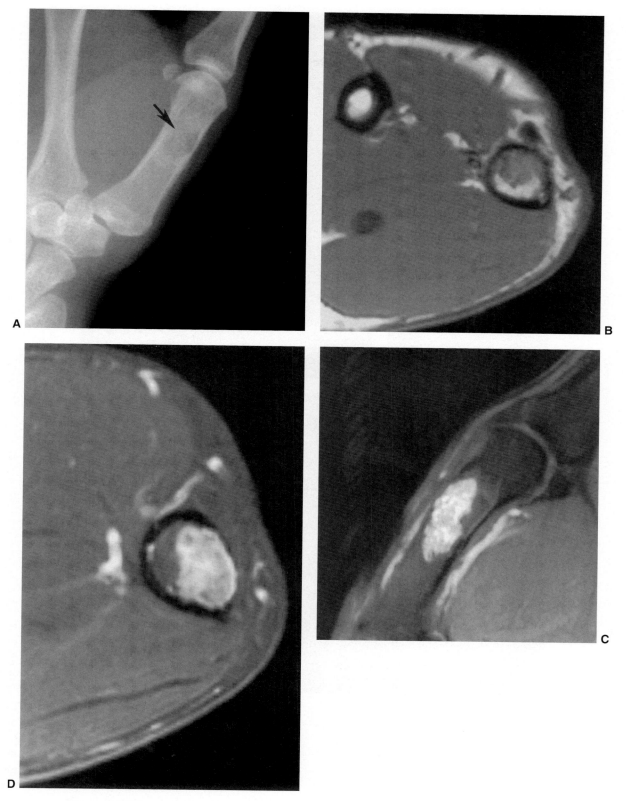

Figure 11-76   Enchondroma. **A:** Radiograph demonstrates a lytic lesion (*arrow*) in the thumb. Axial T1- **(B)** and T2-weighted axial **(C)** and sagittal **(D)** images demonstrate the enchondroma.

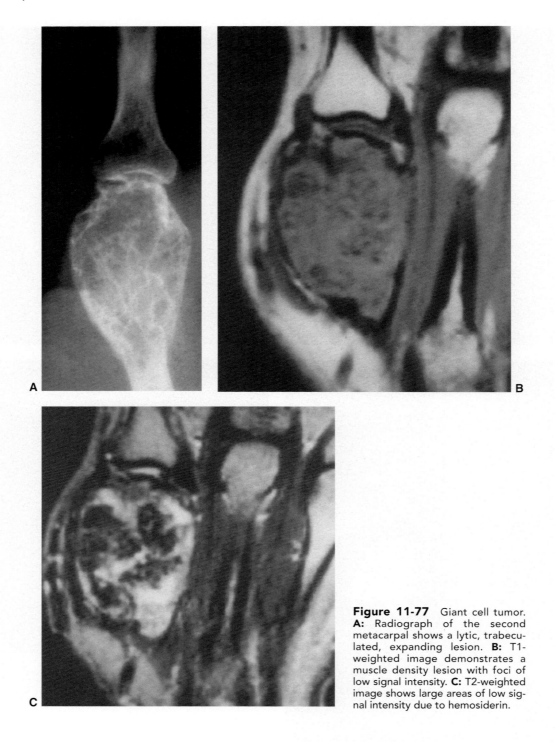

Figure 11-77 Giant cell tumor. **A:** Radiograph of the second metacarpal shows a lytic, trabeculated, expanding lesion. **B:** T1-weighted image demonstrates a muscle density lesion with foci of low signal intensity. **C:** T2-weighted image shows large areas of low signal intensity due to hemosiderin.

third digits of the hand or foot. Considerable fatty tissue is present in the involved fingers or toes. Median nerve involvement (fibrolipoma) is not uncommon (214).

Glomus Tumors
Glomus bodies are arteriovenous anastomoses for thermoregulation. Glomus bodies are present in the dermis throughout the body, but they are most evident in the digits of the hands and feet (83,184,201,204).

Glomus tumors are small (<1 cm) hamartomas of the neuromyoarterial apparatus. Most are localized in the fingertips (75%), usually beneath the nail beds. Though they account for only 1.2% to 5% of hand tumors, 52% of glomus tumors are found in the hand (12,184,204). Patients are usually 30 to 50 years of age and present with local pain that may fluctuate with temperature changes. Up to 65% are subungual, which makes clinical diagnosis more difficult. Lesions are multiple in 2.3% of cases (12,19,205).

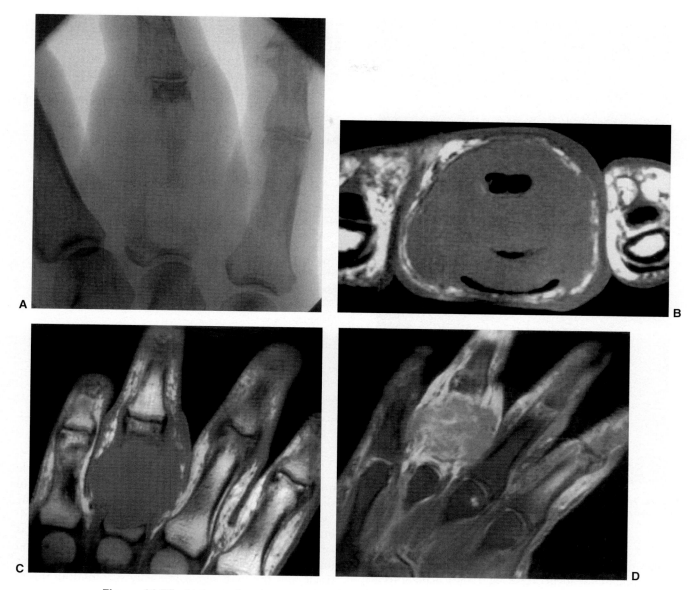

Figure 11-78 Malignant lymphoma. **A:** Radiograph demonstrates marked swelling and destruction of the third proximal phalanx. Axial **(B)** and coronal **(C)** T1-weighted and coronal contrast-enhanced **(D)** images demonstrate the extent of bone and soft tissue involvement and nonuniform enhancement.

Radiographs demonstrate focal bone erosion in up to 60% of cases (205,215). Lesions are low signal intensity on T1-weighted sequences and have homogeneous high signal intensity on T2-weighted or STIR sequences. Lesions demonstrate intense uniform enhancement on postcontrast images (see Fig. 11-86) (215). MR angiography is also useful using gadolinium and three-dimensional GRE sequences (12).

Treatment is surgical resection. Recurrences (see Fig. 11-87) are reported in 5% to 50% of cases (12,184,204,205). Therefore, baseline postoperative MRI is useful for patient management (19).

Mucoid Cyst

Mucoid cysts have been termed epidermoid cysts, dorsal cysts, synovial cysts, and myomyxomatous cysts. Lesions are most common in older patients (mean age 63 years). There is frequently a history of trauma (204). Lesions are most commonly located dorsally between the nail bed and the distal interphalangeal joint. Drape et al. (197) categorized cysts into three types: cysts in the proximal nail fold (48%), multiple flat cysts proximal to the nail fold (22%), and subungual (30%).

Cysts proximal to the nail fold can be diagnosed clinically. There is frequently associated osteoarthritis. On MRI, a pedicle can be defined leading to the joint. This is important to define, as recurrence is common if the pedicle is not resected (197). Multiple flat cysts and subungual cysts are difficult to diagnose clinically (197,204).

Radiographs demonstrate bone erosion less commonly (14%) than glomus tumors (60%) (197,204). MR

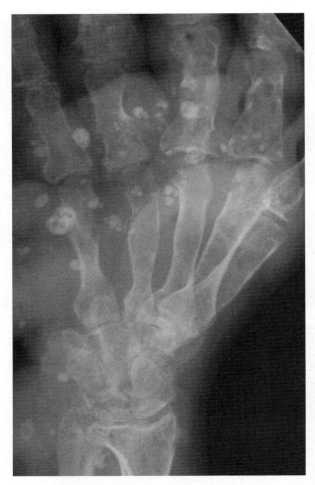

Figure 11-79 Oblique view of the hand and wrist with multiple phleboliths and enchondromas due to Maffucci syndrome.

TABLE 11-10
SOFT TISSUE TUMORS AND TUMORLIKE CONDITIONS IN THE HAND AND WRIST

Lesions	No. of Total Cases	No. in Hand and Wrist/% total
Benign		
Ganglion cyst	—	—
Glomus tumors	52	27 (52%)
Giant cell tumor tendon sheath	410	180 (44%)
Hemangioma	443	53 (12%)
Neurofibroma	85	10 (12%)
Nodular fasciitis	19	2 (11%)
Periosteal pseudotumor	182	20 (11%)
Lipoma	402	24 (6%)
Myxoma	49	1 (2%)
Malignant		
Synovial sarcoma	229	19 (8%)
Malignant nerve sheath tumor	94	4 (4.2%)
Fibrosarcoma	311	13 (4%)
Rhabdomyosarcoma	91	3 (3.2%)
Malignant fibrous histiocytoma	381	7 (2%)
Leiomyosarcoma	70	1 (1.4%)
Liposarcoma	307	1 (0.3%)

From references 12, 83, 183, 184, 197, 202, 203, and 205.

images reveal a well-defined high signal intensity lesion on T2-weighted sequences (see Fig. 11-88). Septations may be evident in 39% of cases (197).

Epidermoids

Epidermoids are usually posttraumatic. They occur in the distal phalangeal region varying in size from 1 to 20 mm. Pain is a common presenting symptom. Radiographs may demonstrate a well-defined soft tissue lucency. Bone erosion can occur. On MRI, lesions have low intensity on T1- and inhomogeneous high signal intensity on T2-weighted sequences (197,204).

Benign Neural Lesions

Benign nerve sheath tumors (BNST) (neurofibroma and schwannoma) and mucoid cysts in the nerve occur in the hand and wrist (2,28,216). Fibrolipoma of the median nerve was described above. Patients with BNSTs present with a soft tissue mass and/or signs of nerve compression (19,204). Schwannomas are fusiform and most commonly involve the ulnar nerve (2).

Benign nerve sheath tumors are isointense with muscle on T1-weighted sequences (see Fig. 11-89). Two useful signs have been described on T2-weighted sequences. The "split fat" sign is seen as a peripheral rim of fat surrounding the lesion. The target sign (seen with neurofibromas) is a low signal intensity center with peripheral high signal intensity. The central low signal intensity is due to fibrous tissue and the high signal intensity surrounding this is myxomatous tissue (2,16).

Intraneural mucoid cysts occur in elderly patients and are most common in the digital and ulnar nerves. Lesions are low signal intensity on T1- and high signal intensity on T2-weighted sequences (156).

Malignant Soft Tissue Tumors

Malignant soft tissue tumors in the hand and wrist are uncommon. Only 4% of lesions listed in Table 11-10 involve the hand (83,184,202). Of the malignant lesions, epitheliod sarcomas involve the hand and wrist in 32% of cases (184,201,202). MR features are not histologically specific. However, malignant lesions tend to be poorly marginated with inhomogeneous signal intensity on T2-weighted sequences. Lesions show irregular enhancement after intravenous gadolinium (16).

More detailed information regarding musculoskeletal tumors is available in Chapter 12.

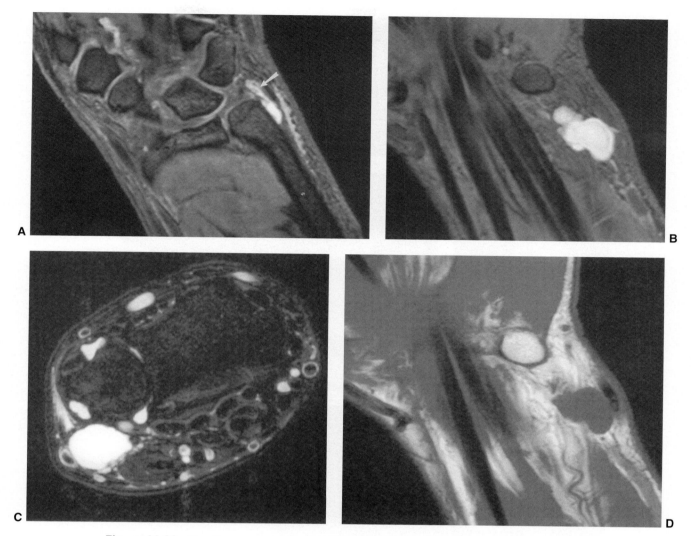

Figure 11-80 Ganglion cyst extending from the TFCC. Coronal **(A,B)** and axial **(C)** T2-weighted images demonstrate a sharply marginated lobulated cyst extending from the TFCC volarly (*arrow*). Coronal T1-weighted image **(D)** shows uniform low signal intensity.

INFECTION

Chapter 13 covers musculoskeletal infections. Therefore, we will focus on infections more prone to involve the hand and wrist. Infections in the hand and wrist may involve the soft tissues (muscle, subcutaneous, cutaneous, tendon sheaths, fascia, and nail beds), bones, and joints. Onset may be acute or more insidious, depending on the organism and clinical setting (8,16,72,217,218).

Typical mechanisms of implantation, such as hematogenous, spread from contiguous source, direct implantation (puncture wound, abrasion, or bite), and surgical procedures also apply to the hand and wrist (219–223). Certain soft tissue infections are specific to the hand. These include subcutaneous abscess of the nail fold (paronychia) and pulp infections of the distal finger (felon) (19,217).

To avoid redundancy, we will focus on infections resulting from direct implantation and surgical interventions. Soft tissue infections are common after direct implantation. Cellulitis is limited to the skin and subcutaneous tissues. Staphylococcal and streptococcal organisms are most commonly involved (16,72,224). Deep fascial infections, such as necrotizing fasciitis, do not commonly occur in the hand and wrist.

Soft tissue abscesses are well-defined fluid collections that may be superficial or deep (see Fig. 11-90). Wall thickness varies, depending on the organism (225).

Infections involving the tendon sheaths are common in the hand and wrist. Infectious tenosynovitis may be caused by multiple organisms including tuberculosis, atypical mycobacteria, and fungi (72,175,226–230). The tendon sheaths of the hand and wrist are the most common site for

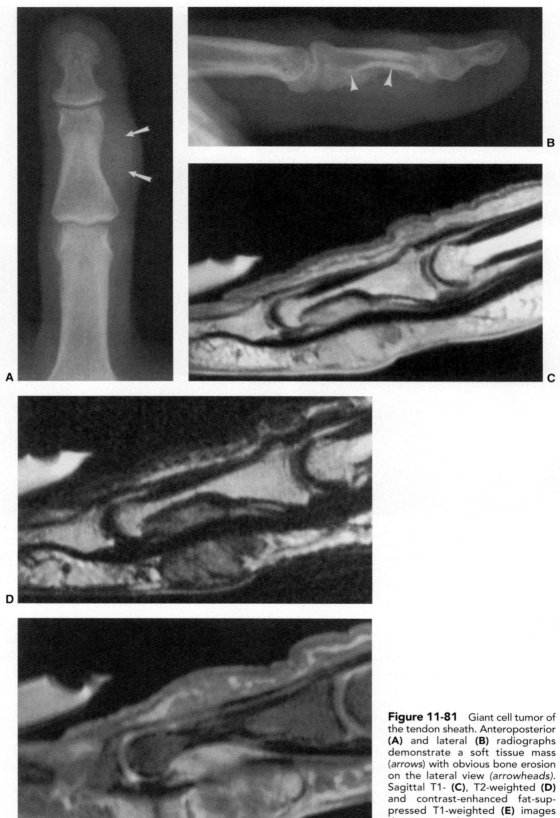

Figure 11-81 Giant cell tumor of the tendon sheath. Anteroposterior **(A)** and lateral **(B)** radiographs demonstrate a soft tissue mass *(arrows)* with obvious bone erosion on the lateral view *(arrowheads)*. Sagittal T1- **(C)**, T2-weighted **(D)** and contrast-enhanced fat-suppressed T1-weighted **(E)** images demonstrate low signal intensity on T2 in **D** and nonuniform contrast enhancement in **E**.

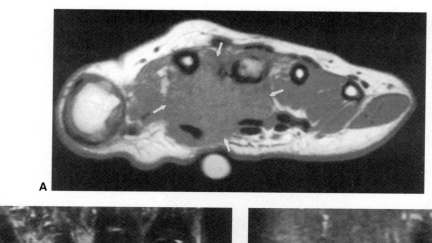

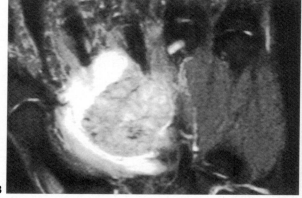

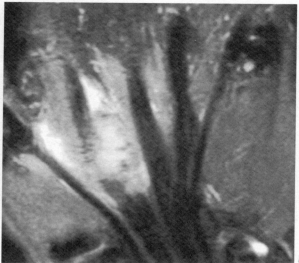

Figure 11-82 Recurrent giant cell tumor of the tendon sheath. Axial T1-weighted image **(A)** demonstrates a large soft tissue mass (*arrows*) displacing the tendons. Coronal contrast-enhanced images **(B,C)** demonstrate displacement and encasement of the flexor tendons.

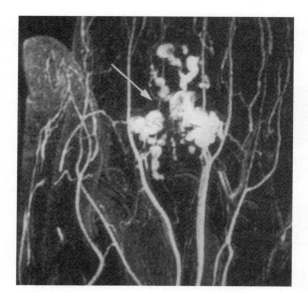

Figure 11-83 Hemangioma. Contrast-enhanced angiogram shows the common and proper digital arteries to the second, third, and fourth digits. The hemangioma fills at the base of the third digit (*thin arrow*). (From Connell DA, Koulouris G, Thorn DA, et al. Contrast enhanced MR angiography of the hand. *Radiographics* 2002; 22:583–599.)

atypical mycobacteria infections (16,231). Musculoskeletal infections occur in up to 15% of patients with tuberculosis (231). Patients with mycobacterial infections present with indolent soft tissue swelling that most often involves the tendon sheaths. Carpal tunnel syndrome may be associated with these infections (232,233). When the extensor tendons are involved, the extensor pollicis is most commonly affected (232). In advanced cases, bone and joint involvement may also be evident (19).

Infection following surgical intervention may affect the osseous, articular, or soft tissue structures, depending on the type of procedure. Image quality may be suboptimal due to metal fixation devices or joint implants. Silicone implants do not cause image distortion (16).

Radiographic or CR images are still a useful screening tool. CT is useful for cortical and osseous changes. MRI is more effective for evaluating the extent of bone and soft tissue involvement. T1- and T2-weighted sequences are usually adequate to define the area of involvement (see Fig. 11-91). Postcontrast fat-suppressed T1-weighted images provide additional information regarding tendon sheath or synovial inflammation as well as bone involvement (16, 221,233,234).

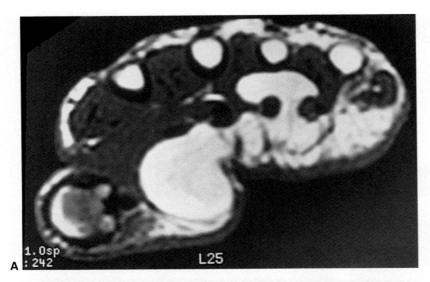

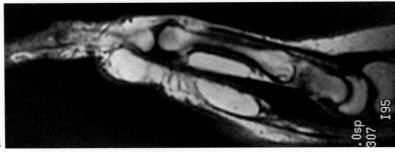

Figure 11-84 Axial **(A)** and sagittal **(B)** T1-weighted images of a benign lipoma extending around the flexor tendons.

ARTHROPATHIES

Routine radiographs have been valuable in staging and monitoring bone and joint changes in patients with inflammatory arthropathies (19,235–237). However, early soft tissue and cartilaginous changes are difficult to detect with conventional techniques. High field surface coil techniques are particularly useful for early detection of subtle changes in the synovium, articular cartilage, and bone before they are evident radiographically (25,28,168,238–243). Synovial changes can be seen on T2-weighted sequences (16). Inflamed synovium has high signal intensity and there is

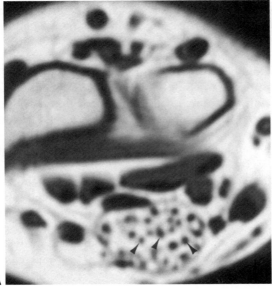

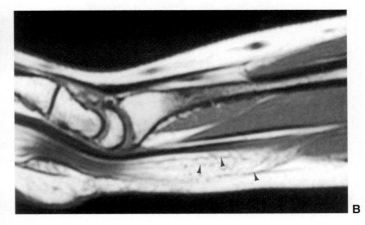

Figure 11-85 Axial **(A)** and sagittal **(B)** T1-weighted images of a fibrolipomatous lesion of the median nerve. Note the low intensity neural and fibrous strands within the fatty tissue (*arrowheads*).

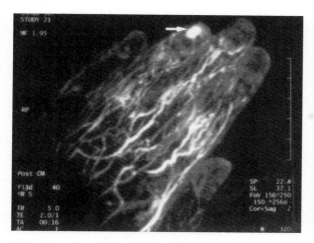

Figure 11-86 MR angiogram demonstrating a small glomus tumor in the ulnar side of the fourth distal tuft. (From Boudghene FP, Gouny P, Tassart M, et al. Subungual glomus tumor. Combined use of MRI and three-dimensional contrast angiography. *J Magn Reson Imaging* 1998;8:1326–1328.)

almost always an associated effusion. Intravenous gadolinium is particularly useful for detection of early synovitis and cartilage loss (11,142,244). Fat-suppressed T1-weighted sequences after contrast identify synovial and erosive changes more clearly (see Fig. 11-92) (99). More chronic synovial proliferation (fronds) appears as low signal intensity nodules or strands contrasted to the high signal intensity of fluid.

More recently, three-dimensional SPGR (102/64, FA 60°) sequences have been used after contrast injection to better evaluate synovial and articular changes. A bolus injection technique can be used to evaluate synovial enhancement more effectively. Images are obtained every 30 seconds after injection (98,245).

MRI has been most commonly used for early detection, and monitoring treatment response and remission in patients with rheumatoid arthritis (2,179,244–248). McQueen et al. (249) demonstrated erosions in 45% of patients with rheumatoid arthritis of less than 4 months

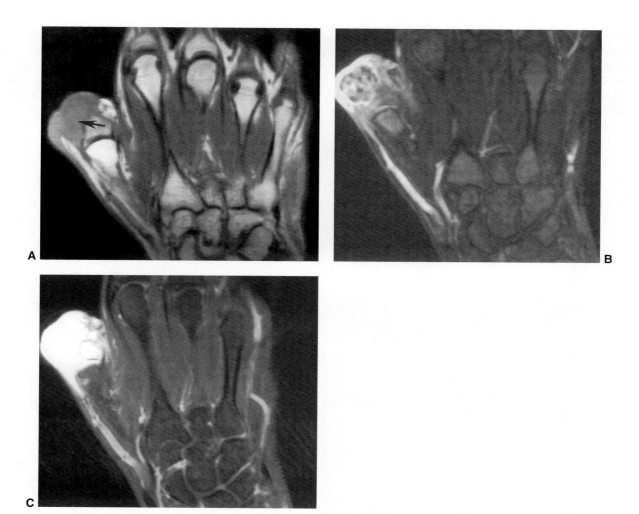

Figure 11-87 Recurrent glomus tumor. T1-weighted coronal image **(A)** demonstrates an intermediate signal intensity soft tissue mass (*arrow*). MR angiogram images **(B,C)** demonstrate dramatic enhancement.

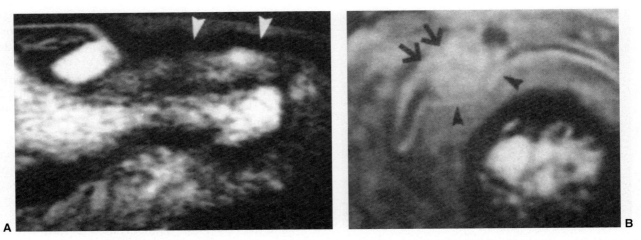

Figure 11-88 Mucoid cyst. **A:** Sagittal T2-weighted image demonstrates a well-defined high signal intensity 4-mm cyst in the proximal nail fold with distal nail atrophy (*arrowheads*). **B:** Axial three-dimensional gradient-echo image shows the slightly hyperintense cyst deep to the lateral groove with compression of the proximal (*arrows*) and distal nail matrix (*arrowheads*). The cyst healed after injection of sclerosing solution. (From Drape J-L, Idy-Petetti I, Goettman S, et al. MR imaging of digital mucoid cysts. *Radiology* 1996;200:531–536.)

duration. Radiographs demonstrated erosions in 15%. The capitate and ulnar side of the radiocarpal joint were involved early. Erosions were evident in 74% of patients on MRI at one year.

MRI can also provide valuable information regarding disease activity and response to therapy (see Fig. 11-93). The dynamic technique described above can be used to monitor the synovial volume and extent of inflammation (245,247). Patients with active disease demonstrate more rapid synovial enhancement and increased pannus volume (245). Patients with inactive disease show decreased synovial enhancement, decreased edema and no new erosions (245,247).

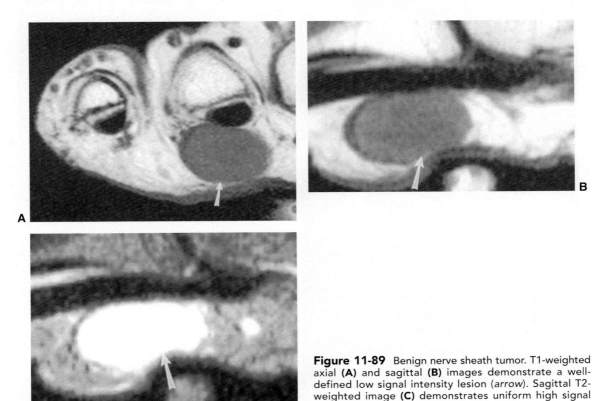

Figure 11-89 Benign nerve sheath tumor. T1-weighted axial **(A)** and sagittal **(B)** images demonstrate a well-defined low signal intensity lesion (*arrow*). Sagittal T2-weighted image **(C)** demonstrates uniform high signal intensity (*arrow*).

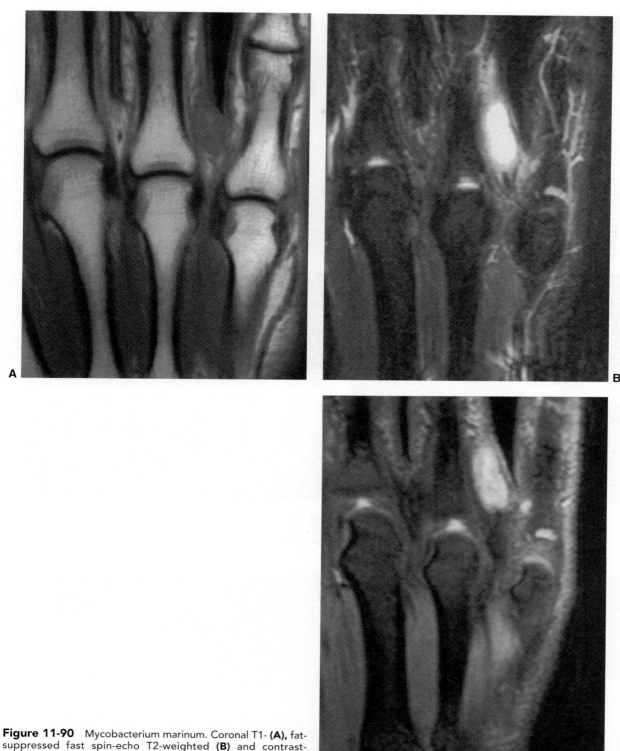

Figure 11-90 Mycobacterium marinum. Coronal T1- **(A)**, fat-suppressed fast spin-echo T2-weighted **(B)** and contrast-enhanced **(C)** images demonstrate a focal soft tissue infection at the base of the fourth proximal phalanx.

MRI is not commonly required to evaluate patients with gout. Clinical, laboratory data, and, after 6 to 8 years, radiographs are generally adequate for diagnosis and management. MRI can detect changes earlier and also detect associated complications of AVN of the capitate and lunate (250). MR studies should include T1- and T2-weighted images along with contrast-enhanced fat-suppressed T1-weighted images. Signal intensity may be increased or

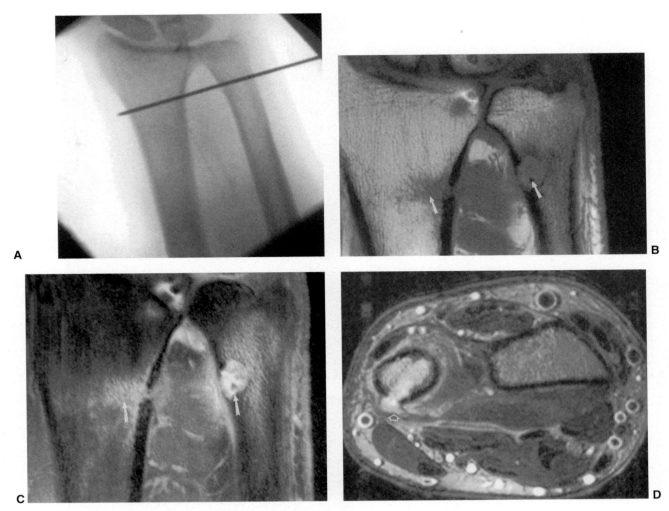

Figure 11-91 Pin tract infection. **A:** Radiograph demonstrates a K-wire through the distal radius and ulna. Coronal T1- **(B)** and T2-weighted **(C)** images show signal abnormality in the region of the previous K-wire (*arrows*). Axial T2-weighted **(D)** image shows a focal abscess (*open arrow*).

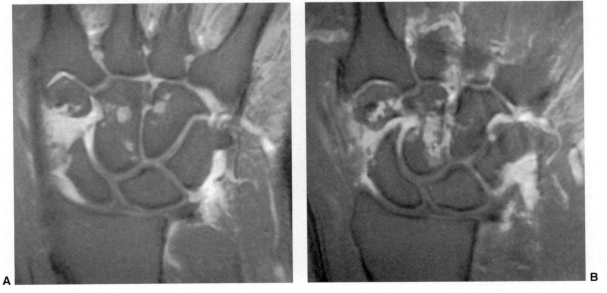

Figure 11-92 Contrast-enhanced fat-suppressed T1-weighted images **(A,B)** show synovial enhancement and multiple erosions, most obvious in the capitate and hamate.

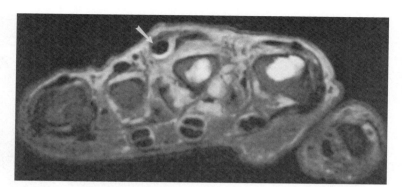

Figure 11-93 Axial image at the level of the metacarpophalangeal joints demonstrates large osseous erosions and subluxation of the extensor tendon (*arrow*) with tenosynovitis.

decreased depending on the extent of calcification and fibrosis in this chronic process. Contrast enhancement in tophi is typically uniform (251).

Pigmented villonodular synovitis (PVNS) is a monoarticular synovial proliferative disorder that typically affects large joints in adults (30 to 50 years old) (252–254). The knee is most commonly involved. Patients present with pain and swelling in the involved joint. Synovial histology is similar to giant cell tumor of the tendon sheath (252,255).

Though the condition is uncommon in the hand and wrist, the image features are characteristic. Hemosiderin deposition and fibrosis result in areas of low signal intensity on both T1- and T2-weighted sequences (see Fig. 11-94). Contrast enhancement is not uniform.

Following resection, recurrence occurs in up to 50% of patients. Therefore, baseline MR examinations should be performed several weeks after resection to optimize evaluations for recurrence (252,255).

On patients with interposition or silicone implant arthroplasty, MRI is useful to evaluate infection, loosening, and silicone synovitis (see Fig. 11-95). T1- and T2-weighted sequences provide useful data on bone loss and

implant fragmentation. Contrast-enhanced fat-suppressed T1-weighted images are useful for evaluating silicone synovitis (19,227,256).

AVASCULAR NECROSIS

There are numerous causes of osteonecrosis. In the hand and wrist, changes most often effect the scaphoid (post fracture), lunate, capitate, and, less commonly, the other carpal bones, metacarpal heads, phalanges, and accessory ossicles (2,19,257,258).

Scaphoid

The vascular entry for the scaphoid places the proximal 33% to 50% at risk for AVN. The major vascular supply to the distal third of the scaphoid is from dorsal, distal, and palmar branches of the radial artery (129). There is a single central vessel to the proximal pole. Interosseous branches progress primarily distal to proximal (134,258).

Scaphoid fractures may involve the proximal pole, waist, distal scaphoid, or scaphoid tubercle (see Fig. 11-96). In

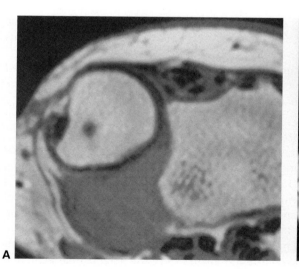

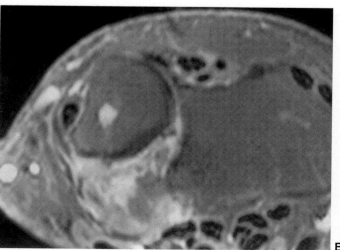

Figure 11-94 Pigmented villonodular synovitis of the distal radioulnar joint. Axial T1- **(A)** and contrast-enhanced **(B)** images demonstrate an irregularly enhancing lesion with dorsal ulnar subluxation.

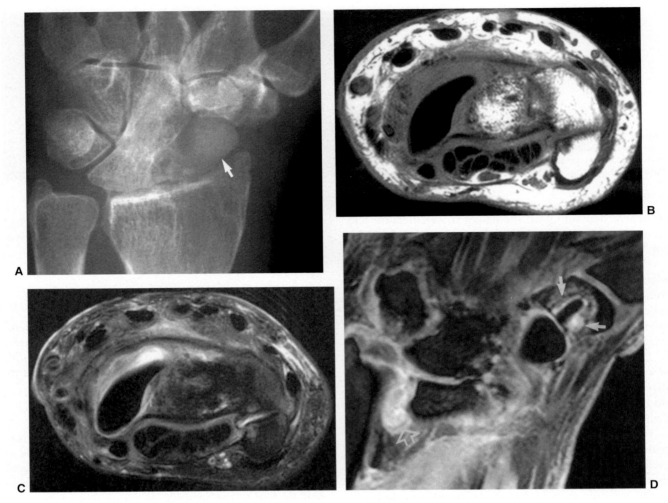

Figure 11-95 Silicone synovitis with staphylococcal infection. **A:** Posteroanterior radiograph shows the silicone implant (*arrow*) and lunocapitate fusion. Axial T1- **(B)** and T2-weighted fast spin-echo **(C)** images demonstrate fluid around the implant. Note there is no adjacent artifact. Coronal STIR image **(D)** shows increased signal intensity about the stem in the trapezium (*arrows*) and fluid in the distal radioulnar joint (*open arrow*).

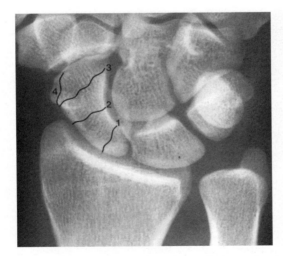

Figure 11-96 Posteroanterior radiograph demonstrating the location of scaphoid fractures. *(1)* proximal pole (10%); *(2)* waist (80%); *(3)* distal; and *(4)* tuberosity.

adults, 80% of fractures involve the waist. Fractures of the waist and proximal pole lead to AVN in 30% of patients (14,134,258).

Scaphoid fractures that are not displaced can be treated with cast immobilization. Displaced fractures require internal fixation using a Herbert screw (134,258).

Lunate

The tenuous vascular supply to the lunate results in ANV (Kienbock disease) more commonly than other carpal bones (134,154,259). The dorsal vascular supply is provided by a branch of the radial artery. Branches from the radiocarpal arch and a dorsal branch of the interosseous artery may also contribute to the dorsal lunate vascularity. The palmar vascular supply is from branches of the anterior interosseous artery, recurrent branches from the deep palmar arch, and direct branches from the radial and ulnar arteries. The vascular supply is primarily dorsal to palmar (78). In 8% of

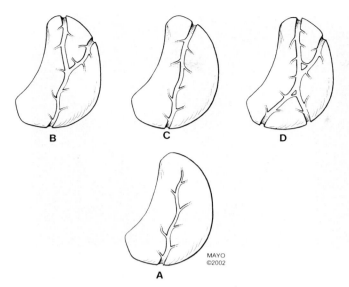

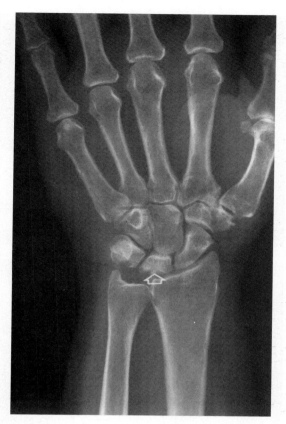

Figure 11-97 Vascular patterns of the lunate. **A:** Single palmar vessel (8%); **B:** *Y* pattern, with single palmar and two dorsal vessels (59%); **C:** *I* pattern with single dorsal and palmar vessels (10%); **D:** *X* pattern with two dorsal and two palmar vessels (23%). (From Berquist TH. *MRI of the hand and wrist.* Philadelphia, PA: Lippincott Williams & Wilkins, 2003.)

patients, the lunate is supplied by only palmar vessels; 59% have two dorsal and a single palmar vessel, 10% have single dorsal and palmar vessels, and 23% have two dorsal and two palmar arteries (see Fig. 11-97) (78,121,134).

The etiology of Kienbock disease is unclear, but trauma, its fixed position in the wrist, vascular supply, connective tissue diseases, gout, and ulnar minus variance have all been implicated (78,154,250,259,260). Seventy percent of patients have ulnar minus variance greater than 1 mm and 95% are involved in manual labor (2). The condition is more common in males and patients are usually in the 20- to 40-year age group (2,19).

Patients with Kienbock disease present with a history of trauma in most cases, wrist pain related to activity and relieved by rest and pain, and tenderness over the dorsal wrist on physical examination. Delay in diagnosis for 1 to 2 years is not uncommon (259,261).

Management may be conservative or surgical depending on the stage of disease (121,259). Lichtman and Degnan (121) described radiographic staging. Stage I lunates are normal radiographically but may have signal intensity abnormalities on MRI. In patients with stage II disease, there is increased density or sclerosis in the lunate without collapse. Stage III (see Fig. 11-98) demonstrates collapse and fragmentation without (IIIA) or with (IIIB) fixed scaphoid rotation and scapholunate dissociation. Stage IV disease includes features of stage III plus radiocarpal arthrosis.

Treatment for early stage disease is cast immobilization. Up to 80% of patients have excellent results following three months of immobilization. More advance disease is treated with radial shortening, ulnar lengthening, revascularization, or resection with silicone implantation (19,121,259).

Figure 11-98 Posteroanterior radiograph shows a Lichtman stage III (sclerosis and collapse) (*open arrow*) AVN with ulnar minus variance.

Capitate/Other Carpal Bones

The vascular supply to the capitate is similar to the scaphoid, placing the proximal third at risk after fracture (14,78,134). Avascular necrosis of the other carpal bones is rare due to their rich vascular supply (78).

Metacarpal Heads/Phalanges

Avascular necrosis of the metacarpal heads and phalanges is rare (262). Osteonecrosis of the metacarpal head may be related to a single vascular supply. In 35% of patients, multiple arterioles supply the metacarpal head (2,105). When AVN occurs in the phalanges, the bases of the second and third proximal phalanges are most commonly involved (16,78,263).

Magnetic Resonance Imaging

MRI is the technique of choice for detection, staging, and follow-up of patients with AVN (16,261,264). Both conventional and contrast-enhanced studies may be required. The MR features are similar regardless of the osseous structure involved. Normal signal intensity on T1- and T2-weighted sequences and uniform enhancement after intravenous contrast indicate normal flow. Low signal intensity on T1- and high signal intensity on T2-weighted sequences can be seen with transient marrow edema, after

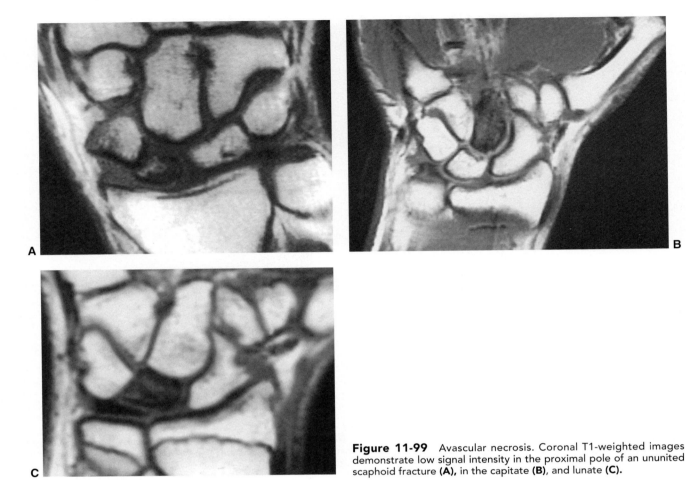

Figure 11-99 Avascular necrosis. Coronal T1-weighted images demonstrate low signal intensity in the proximal pole of an ununited scaphoid fracture **(A)**, in the capitate **(B)**, and lunate **(C)**.

fracture, or with AVN (see Fig. 11-99) (2,19,259,260). In more advanced stages with bone sclerosis, signal intensity is low on T1- and inhomogeneous but low on T2-weighted sequences. Comparison of MR images with radiographs reduces errors in interpretation. Changes with AVN typically involve the entire structure compared to focal defects

seen with arthropathies or ulnar lunate impaction syndrome (Figs. 11-50 and 11-51) (16,260).

Conventional MRI studies are usually adequate for diagnosis. Contrast-enhanced fat-suppressed T1-weighted sequences are more critical to evaluate treatment response after vascularized bone grafts (see Fig. 11-100) (19).

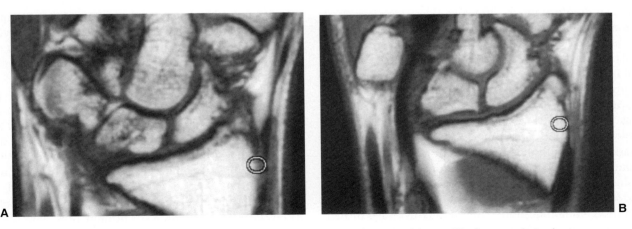

Figure 11-100 Coronal T1-weighted images at 6 months **(A)** and 1 year **(B)** after vascularized grafting. The signal intensity has returned to normal.

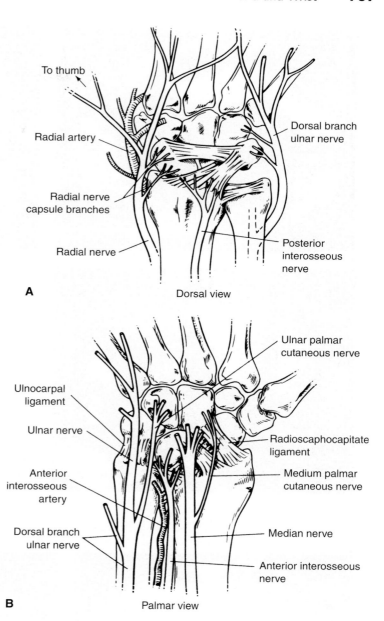

A   Dorsal view

To thumb

Radial artery

Dorsal branch
ulnar nerve

Radial nerve
capsule branches

Radial nerve

Posterior
interosseous
nerve

Ulnar palmar
cutaneous nerve

Ulnocarpal
ligament

Ulnar nerve

Radioscaphocapitate
ligament

Anterior
interosseous
artery

Medium palmar
cutaneous nerve

Dorsal branch
ulnar nerve

Median nerve

Anterior interosseous
nerve

B   Palmar view

Figure 11-101 Dorsal **(A)** and palmar **(B)** illustrations of the nerve supply to the hand and wrist. (From Cooney WP III. Vascular and neurological anatomy of the wrist. In: Cooney WP III, Linscheid RL, Dobyns JH, eds. *The wrist: diagnosis and operative treatment.* St. Louis: Mosby; 1998:106–123.)

NERVE COMPRESSION SYNDROMES

Nerve compression syndromes involving the hand and wrist (see Fig. 11-101) most often involve the median nerve as it passes through the carpal tunnel and the ulnar nerve in the region of Guyon canal (19,85,107,155, 204,265–269). Clinical evaluation and electromyogram (EMG) are often diagnostic. Imaging studies are usually reserved for difficult or atypical cases. CT and ultrasound may be useful in some cases (16,36,270,271). However, MRI is preferred in our practice. Median and ulnar nerve anatomy is easily appreciated using axial T1- and T2-weighted images (see Fig. 11-102). Fat in Guyon canal and the carpal tunnel helps clearly define the lower signal

intensity nerve. Therefore, we do not usually use fat suppression techniques in these situations.

Carpal Tunnel Syndrome

The carpal tunnel is cone shaped, wider proximally (radiocarpal joint) than distally (metacarpal base level). The length of the carpal tunnel is about 3.6 cm (48,88). The carpal tunnel is bordered dorsally by the carpal bones and volarly by the flexor retinaculum. Eight flexor tendons (superficialis and profunda), the flexor pollicis longus tendon, and the median nerve pass through the carpal tunnel (27,73,75,82,85,272,273). The median nerve may lie volar to the flexor tendons, typically the second (Fig. 11-102) or between the flexor pollicis longus and the flexor digitorum superficialis (see Fig. 11-103) (274).

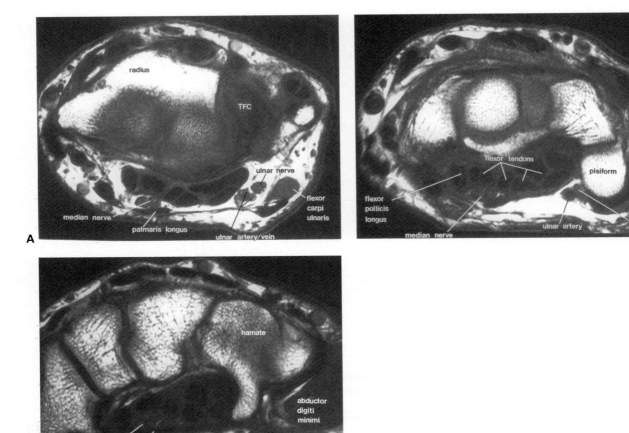

Figure 11-102   Axial T1-weighted images demonstrating the neuroanatomy at the radiocarpal joint **(A)**, pisiform **(B)**, and hamate hook **(C)** levels. *TFC*, triangular fibrocartilage.

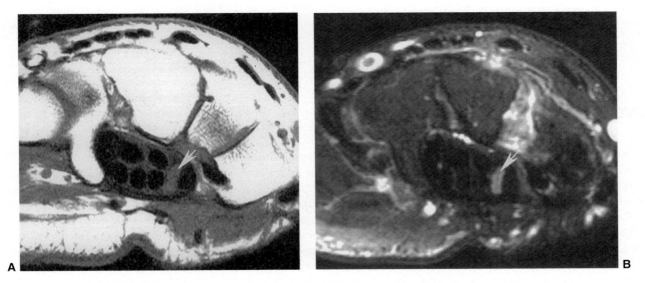

Figure 11-103   Axial T1- **(A)** and T2-weighted **(B)** images demonstrating the median nerve (*arrow*) in a vertically oriented configuration lying between the flexor tendons and flexor pollicis longus.

Carpal tunnel syndrome is the most common nerve compression disorder in the upper extremity. This condition has increased in the workforce dramatically since 1980. The cost for compensation and lost work days is estimated at $20,000 to $200,000 per patient (27,79,137,273,275).

Patients with carpal tunnel syndrome present with chronic discomfort and tingling of the fingers in the median nerve distribution (thumb through radial side of the ring finger) (79,272,273). Nocturnal symptoms are common (47,155). Thenar muscle atrophy may also be present. Most often patients are 30 to 60 years of age, and females outnumber males by up to 5:1. The condition may be bilateral in up to 50% of cases. The condition is generally thought to be due to compression of the median nerve (Table 11-11). Clinical features and nerve conduction studies have been the most common methods of diagnosis.

Positive Tinel and Phalen signs are useful clinically. A positive Tinel sign occurs when tingling is noted in the nerve distribution after percussion over the nerve. Phalen test is performed by constricting or reducing the volume of the carpal tunnel by flexing or extending the wrist for 30 to 60 seconds, during which time the patient's symptoms are reproduced (79,155,272,273).

Though most clinical and imaging studies are designed to demonstrate compression, ischemia has also been proposed as a possible etiology for carpal tunnel syndrome (278). This could explain why the nerve and surrounding structures may appear normal on MR images on patients with clinical and EMG features of carpal tunnel syndrome. Sugimoto et al. (278) studied the median nerve with dynamic gadolinium techniques. Two abnormal patterns were described. Enhancement can occur with edema or there may be lack of enhancement or decreased signal intensity with ischemia. Increased signal patterns reverted to decreased enhancement when the wrist was in marked flexion or extension.

The superior soft tissue contrast obtained with MRI makes the technique ideal for identification of the nerves, vessels, and tendons in the carpal tunnel (Fig. 11-102) (19,79,269,272,273). The median nerve typically lies just deep to the flexor retinaculum and superficial to the flexor tendons (Fig. 11-102) (85). On axial images, the nerve is elliptical with signal intensity that is higher than the adjacent tendons (19,79,269). There are multiple fascicles enclosed in the epineurium (85).

The position and shape of the nerve may vary depending on the position of the wrist. Zeiss et al. (47) studied the position and configuration of the median nerve with the wrist in neutral, flexed, and extended positions. In the neutral position, the median nerve is typically located either anterior to the superficial flexor tendon of the index finger or between this tendon and the flexor pollicis longus tendon. The nerve is more often between the flexor retinaculum and tendon to the index finger during extension. The nerve tends to flatten in the flexed position and again will most often lie anterior to the superficial flexor tendon to the index finger (47).

We prefer thin-slice (3 mm) axial images with a small FOV (8 to 10 cm), 256 × 256 or 256 × 192 matrix, and surface coil technique to evaluate the carpal tunnel. Both T1- and T2-weighted sequences should be performed. Gradient echo sequences are used to study nerve position with flexion–extension motion studies. It may be helpful to evaluate both wrists when symptoms are unilateral. Additional sequences or contrast enhancement may be useful in selected cases. Comparison is especially useful when subtle MR changes are noted in the involved wrist. If the MR of the wrist is normal, one must consider a lesion located more proximally, such as the elbow, thoracic outlet, or cervical spine (79,272).

Patients with carpal tunnel syndrome may demonstrate changes in the median nerve (size, shape, signal intensity, edema, or no flow with enhancement) or contents of the carpal tunnel (75,76,279,280) (Table 11-12). Pathology such as nerve sheath tumors or fibrolipomatous hamartomas of the median nerve are easily detected (Fig. 11-85) (19,79,216).

Changes in size, shape, and signal intensity are easily evaluated on contiguous axial MR images (16,19). The nerve is typically oval in the proximal tunnel (radiocarpal level) becoming flatter at the level of the pisiform and smaller in the distal carpal tunnel (2,47). Swelling is best evaluated at the level of the pisiform (see Fig. 11-104). In

---

TABLE 11-11

NERVE COMPRESSION SYNDROMES ETIOLOGY

Tenosynovitis
Soft tissue tumors (extrinsic and neural)
Ganglion cysts
Osseous deformity (posttraumatic)
Anomalous muscles
Ischemia

From references 79, 155, 273, 276, and 277.

TABLE 11-12

CARPAL TUNNEL SYNDROME FEATURES ON MRI

Median nerve shape: flattening, swelling, deformed
Increased signal intensity median nerve
Bowing of flexor retinaculum
Deep palmar bursitis
Tenosynovitis
Soft tissue masses
Carpal tunnel contents/volume ratios
Carpal tunnel volume/wrist volume ratios

From references 75, 76, 137, 225, 267, 275, and 279.

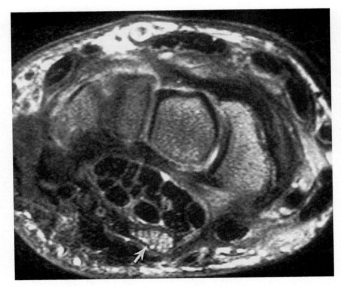

Figure 11-104 Axial T2-weighted image at the pisiform level demonstrating enlargement and increased signal intensity in the median nerve (arrow).

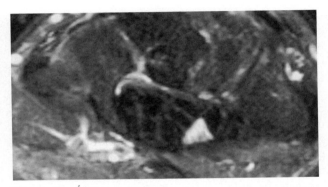

Figure 11-106 Carpal tunnel syndrome in a 40-year-old female. T2-weighted image shows distortion and increased signal intensity in the median nerve.

patients with carpal tunnel syndrome, the nerve is 1.6 to 3.5 times larger compared to the more proximal radiocarpal level (27,274). Enlargement of the nerve is reported in 62% to 95% of patients with documented carpal tunnel syndrome (79,269,274). Flattening of the nerve is optimally evaluated at the level of the hamate hook. Normal patients have a major to minor axis ratio of 2.9 (see Fig. 11-105). Patients with carpal tunnel syndrome have a ratio of 1.8 at the radiocarpal level, compared to 3.8 at the level of the hamate hook (27,79,137).

Bak et al. (137) correlated nerve conduction studies with median nerve size at the radiocarpal, pisiform, and hamate hook levels. The width (major axis) and the thickness (minor axis) were measured and the area calculated at

all three levels. Flattening and swelling ratios were calculated. In this study, there was poor correlation between MRI findings and nerve conduction studies. Others report sensitivities of 27% to 65% and specificities of 70% to 97% for flattening (98,267). Obvious distortion of the nerve is usually associated with significant pathology (see Fig. 11-106) (19,82).

Abnormal signal intensity in the median nerve has also been described in patients with carpal tunnel syndrome (2,19,137). Abnormally high signal intensity has been reported in 52% to 85% of patients. As a solitary finding, abnormal signal intensity on T2-weighted images demonstrated a sensitivity range of 59% to 95% and a specificity range of 51% to 59% (98,269). When increased signal intensity is associated with swelling, flattening, or nerve distortion, the accuracy is increased (16).

Bowing of the flexor retinaculum, nerve flattening, and palmar synovitis have been suggested as the most useful MRI criteria for diagnosis of carpal tunnel syndrome (98). Bowing of the flexor retinaculum is optimally evaluated at the level of the hamate hook (2,27). The flexor retinaculum is normally straight to concave (2,127,137). Bowing is caused by increased pressure or tissue volume in the carpal tunnel. Bowing is expressed in a ratio (see Fig. 11-107). To calculate the ratio, a line is drawn from the hamate hook to the trapezial tubercle (TH). The distance from line TH to the flexor retinaculum (palmar displacement, PD) is divided by the length of line TH. The normal ratio is 0.15 (mean 0.10) compared to 0.14 to 0.26 (mean 0.18) in patients with carpal tunnel syndrome (27,137). The sensitivity of this ratio is 16% to 32% and specificity 91% to 94% (98,267). Overall, bowing of the flexor retinaculum is identified in 73% to 85% of patients with carpal tunnel syndrome (269).

Soft tissue masses and tenosynovitis in the carpal tunnel are obvious on conventional MR images. Tenosynovitis may be related to overuse, inflammatory arthropathies, infections, pigmented villonodular synovitis, sarcoidosis, gout, and amyloidosis (16,19,231,281).

Dynamic studies with contrast enhancement or motion studies have been suggested in selected cases (47,278).

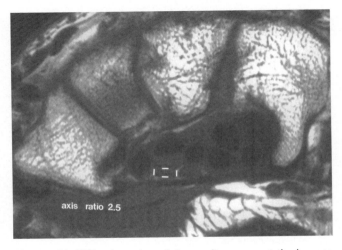

axis ratio 2.5

Figure 11-105 Flattening of the median nerve at the hamate hook level. Axial T1-weighted image with a major (width)/minor (height) ratio of 2.5. Normal is 2.9.

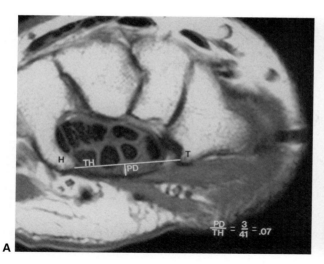
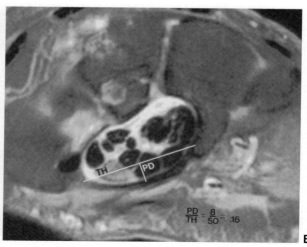

Figure 11-107 Bowing ratio. A line from the attachment on the hamate hook *(H)* to the trapezial tubercle *(T)* termed *TH* is measured. A perpendicular line (PD, palmar displacement) is drawn to the flexor retinaculum. PD/TH results in the bowing ratio. Normal is 0 to 0.15. **A:** Axial T1-weighted image in a normal patient with TH = 41 mm, PD = 3 mm, for a bowing ratio of 0.07. **B:** Axial post-contrast fat-suppressed T1-weighted image in a patient with tenosynovitis and swelling of the median nerve with TH = 50, PD = 8, for a bowing ratio of 0.16.

Gradient echo axial images can be obtained in varying degrees of flexion and extension to evaluate nerve position changes and or deformity caused by adjacent tendons (47,216).

Ischemia has been implicated as a cause of carpal tunnel syndrome (137,278). In this setting, the nerve and structures around the nerve are normal despite electrodiagnostic abnormalities. Sugimoto et al. (278) performed dynamic contrast studies and noted edema or decreased flow to the nerve in these patients. Table 11-12 summarizes MR features of carpal tunnel syndrome.

Many patients with carpal tunnel syndrome are treated conservatively. When conservative methods fail, open or arthroscopic decompression can be performed. A recent study demonstrated that performing tenosynovectomy with decompression did not provide additional benefit (282).

MRI is useful postoperatively to confirm complete release of the flexor retinaculum and detect other complications or causes of recurrent symptoms. Following decompression, axial images demonstrate a defect in the retinaculum with volar displacement of the separated fragments (see Fig. 11-108). Over time, there may be an increase in the carpal tunnel fat and scarring may occur (2). As with other conditions, postoperative baseline MRI is useful. MRI is capable of detecting acute (hemorrhage, hematoma) and late (mass recurrence, scarring around the nerve) complications (see Fig. 11-109) (19).

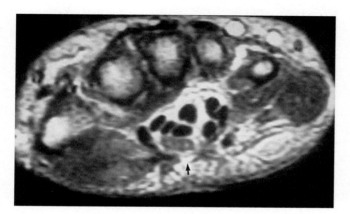

Figure 11-108 Carpal tunnel release. Axial proton density image shows separation of the flexor retinaculum *(arrow)* with palmar displacement of the nerve and tendons. Complete release.

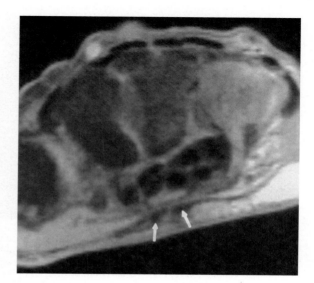

Figure 11-109 Fast spin-echo T2-weighted image demonstrates scarring *(arrows)* without separation of the flexor retinaculum as seen in Fig. 11-108. Incomplete release.

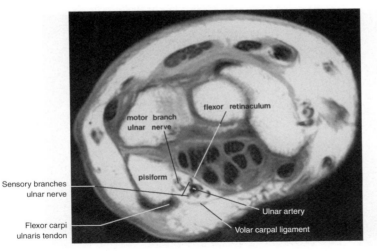

Figure 11-110 Axial MR image at the level of the pisiform, demonstrating the anatomy of Guyon canal.

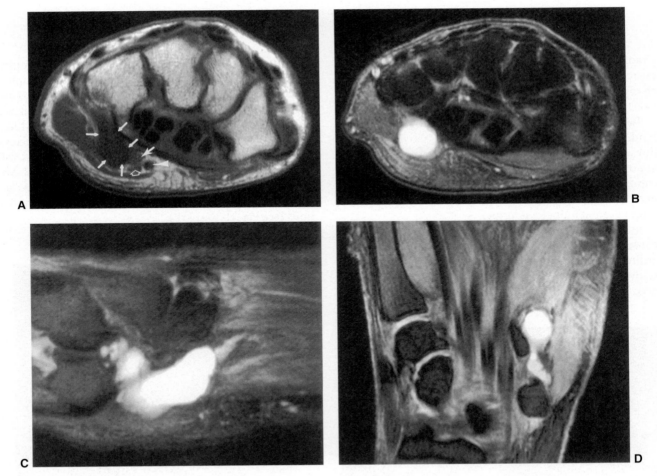

Figure 11-111 Ganglion cyst in Guyon canal compressing the deep branch of the ulnar nerve resulting in motor weakness. **A:** Axial T1-weighted image demonstrates the deep (*arrows*) and superficial (*open arrow*) braches of the ulnar nerve with the artery (*arrowhead*) adjacent. There is a low signal intensity mass (*small white arrows*) compressing the deep branch of the ulnar nerve. Axial **(B)** and sagittal **(C)** T2-weighted and coronal **(D)** DESS images demonstrate the extent and high signal intensity of the cyst.

Ulnar Nerve Compression

Ulnar nerve compression or injury can occur in the elbow region, forearm, or, more commonly, in Guyon canal (see Fig. 11-110) (2,10,16,18,283). Guyon canal begins at the proximal margin of the volar canal ligament and extends to the fibrous arch of the thenar muscles. The canal is bordered by the volar carpal ligament, deep transverse carpal ligament, flexor carpi ulnaris tendon, and the pisiform (48,284). Symptoms vary, depending on the zone involved (283). Zone 1 is the proximal canal before the nerve bifurcates. Injury or compression in this region leads to motor and sensory deficits (type I syndrome). Zone 2 includes the deep branch of the ulnar nerve. Pathology in zone 2 leads to motor deficits. Zone 3 includes the superficial branch of the ulnar nerve that contains primarily sensory fibers. Therefore, patients present with sensory deficits (type III syndrome) (88,284).

Ulnar nerve injury or compression in the wrist may be related to blunt trauma, fractures, arthropathies, anomalous muscles, vascular anomalies, and soft tissue masses (2,16,46,284). Soft tissue masses in Guyon canal are uncommon, but include ganglion cysts (see Fig. 11-111), lipomas, giant cell tumors, posttraumatic neuromas, neurofibromas, intraneural cysts, and other primary nerve lesions (see Fig. 11-112) (2,46,74,284).

Axial MR images can be obtained using the same sequences described above. MRI can clearly define anatomy and pathology. If MR studies are normal, imaging at the elbow or forearm levels should be considered (16,284).

Patients with blunt trauma or overuse syndromes can be treated conservatively. Surgical decompression is required if neural pathology or soft tissue masses are defined (2,19).

Miscellaneous Compression Conditions

Anterior interosseous nerve compression can also occur (78,285). The anterior interosseous nerve is a branch of the median nerve that comes off 2 to 8 cm distal to the medial epicondyle (48,78). The motor nerve supplies the flexor pollicis longus, flexor digitorum profundus of the index finger and middle fingers, and the pronator quadratus (48,286). Compression causes weakness in these muscles but no sensory deficits. Clinically, it is difficult to differentiate anterior interosseous nerve syndrome from tendon rupture (286). Nerve conduction studies may be diagnostic. Increased signal intensity is identified in the muscles on T2-weighted or STIR sequences (see Fig. 11-113) (46,286).

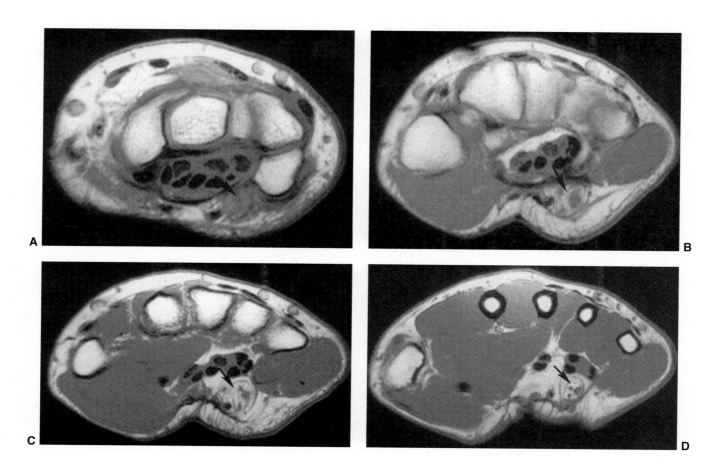

Figure 11-112 Fibrolipoma of the ulnar nerve. Axial T1-weighted images from the level of the pisiform **(A)** and distally **(B–D)** demonstrate a fibrofatty lesion of the ulnar nerve (*arrow*).

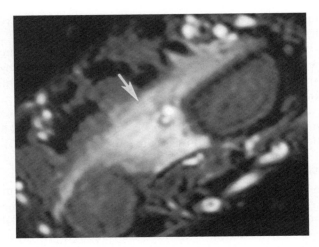

Figure 11-113 Anterior interosseous nerve compression. Axial T2-weighted sequence shows increased signal intensity in the pronator muscle.

Radial nerve branch compression is rare but can be seen with dorsal ganglion cysts of the wrist (19,78).

MISCELLANEOUS CONDITIONS

There are numerous other abnormalities in the musculoskeletal system that may involve the hand and wrist. These include congenital abnormalities, metabolic diseases, hematologic disorders, etc. (16,281,287–290). The exact role of MRI in these conditions is limited at this time (see Chapter 15).

REFERENCES

1. Adler BD, Logan PM, Janzen DL, et al. Extrinsic radiocarpal ligaments: magnetic resonance imaging of normal wrists and scapholunate dissociation. *Can Assoc Radiol J* 1996;47:417–422.
2. Anderson MW, Kaplan PA, Dussault RG, et al. Magnetic resonance imaging of the wrist. *Curr Probl Diagn Radiol* 1998;27:187–229.
3. Disler DG, Recht MP, McCauley TR. MR imaging of articular cartilage. *Skeletal Radiol* 2000;29:367–377.
4. Erickson SJ, Kneeland JB, Middleton WD, et al. MR imaging of the finger: correlation with normal anatomic sections. *AJR Am J Roentgenol* 1989;152:1013–1019.
5. Hobby JL, Dixon AK, Bearcroft PWP, et al. MR imaging of the wrist: effect on clinical diagnosis and patient care. *Radiology* 2001;220:589–593.
6. Louis DS, Buckwalter KA. Magnetic resonance imaging of the collateral ligaments of the thumb. *J Hand Surg Am* 1989;14A:739–741.
7. Berquist TH. *Imaging of orthopedic trauma*, 2nd ed. New York: Raven Press, 1992.
8. Berquist TH, Brown ML, Fitzgerald RH, et al. Magnetic resonance imaging: application in musculoskeletal infection. *Magn Reson Imaging* 1985;3:219–230.
9. Disa JJ, Chung KC, Gillad FE, et al. Efficiency of magnetic resonance angiography in the evaluation of vascular malformations of the hand. *Plast Reconstr Surg* 1997;99:136–144.
10. Bilecen D, Aschwanden M, Heidecker HG, et al. Optimized assessment of hand vascularization on contrast-enhanced MR angiography with subsystolic continuous compression technique. *AJR Am J Roentgenol* 2004;182:180–182.
11. Bonel HM, Schneider P, Seemann MD, et al. MR imaging of the wrist in rheumatoid arthritis using gadobenate dimeglumine. *Skeletal Radiol* 2001;30:15–24.
12. Boudghene FP, Gouny P, Tassat M, et al. Subungual glomus tumor: combined use of MRI and three-dimensional contrast enhanced MR angiography. *J Magn Reson Imaging* 1998;8:1326–1328.
13. Brady TJ, Gebhardt MC, Pykett IL, et al. NMR imaging of forearms in healthy volunteers and patients with giant-cell tumor of bone. *Radiology* 1982;144:549–552.
14. Cristiani G, Cerofolini E, Squarzina PB, et al. Evaluation of ischemic necrosis of the carpal bones by magnetic resonance imaging. *J Hand Surg Br* 1990;15B:249–255.
15. Drape JL, Dubert T, Silbermann O, et al. Acute trauma of the extensor hood of the metacarpophalangeal joint: MR imaging evaluation. *Radiology* 1994;192:469–476.
16. Berquist TH. *MRI of the musculoskeletal system*, 4th ed. Philadelphia, PA: Lippincott Williams & Wilkins, 2001.
17. Shellock FG. *Pocket guide to MR procedures and metal objects: update 1998*. Philadelphia, PA: Lippincott-Raven, 1998.
18. Berquist TH. Magnetic resonance imaging of the elbow and wrists. *Top Magn Reson Imaging* 1989;1:15–27.
19. Berquist TH. *MRI of the hand and wrist*. Philadelphia, PA: Lippincott Williams & Wilkins, 2003.
20. Dalinka MK. MR imaging of the wrist. *AJR Am J Roentgenol* 1995;164:1–9.
21. Tajiri Y, Nakamura K, Matsushita T, et al. A positioning device to allow rotation for cine-MRI of the radioulnar joint. *Clin Radiol* 1999;54:402–405.
22. Baker LL, Hajek PC, Björkengren A, et al. High-resolution magnetic resonance imaging of the wrist: normal anatomy. *Skeletal Radiol* 1987;16:128–132.
23. Hardy CJ, Katzberg RW, Frey RL, et al. Switched surface coil system for bilateral MR imaging. *Radiology* 1988;167:835–838.
24. Middleton WD, Macrander S, Lawson TL, et al. High resolution surface coil magnetic resonance imaging of the joints: anatomic correlation. *Radiographics* 1987;7:645–683.
25. Wong EC, Jesmanowicz A, Hyde JS. High-resolution short echo time MR imaging of the fingers and wrist with a local gradient coil. *Radiology* 1991;181:393–397.
26. Yoshioka H, Ueno T, Tanaka T, et al. High-resolution MR imaging of triangular fibrocartilage complex (TFCC): comparison of microscopy coils and conventional small surface coils. *Skeletal Radiol* 2003;32:575–581.
27. DiMarcangelo MT, Smith PA. Use of magnetic resonance imaging in common wrist disorders. *J Am Osteopath Assoc* 2000;10: 228–231.
28. Weiss KL, Beltran J, Shamam OM, et al. High-field MR surface-coil imaging of the hand and wrist. Part I: normal anatomy. *Radiology* 1986;160:143–146.
29. Smith DK. Dorsal carpal ligaments of the wrist: normal appearance on multiplanar reconstructions of three dimensional fourier transform MR images. *AJR Am J Roentgenol* 1993;161:119–125.
30. Schweitzer ME, Natale P, Winalski CS, et al. Indirect wrist MR arthrography: the effects of passive motion versus active exercise. *Skeletal Radiol* 2000;29:10–14.
31. Beaulieu CF, Ladd AL. MR arthrography of the wrist: scanning room injection of the radiocarpal joint based on clinical landmarks. *AJR Am J Roentgenol* 1998;170:606–608.
32. Sahin G, Ergruvan Dogan B, Demirtas M. Virtual MR arthroscopy of the wrist joint: a new intraarticular perspective. *Skeletal Radiol* 2004;33:9–14.
33. Abouzahr MK, Coppa LM, Boxt LM. Aneurysms of the digital arteries: a case report and review of the literature. *J Hand Surg Am* 1997;22:311–314.
34. Anderson SE, De Monaco D, Buechler U, et al. Imaging features of pseudoaneurysms of the hand in children and adults. *AJR Am J Roentgenol* 2003;180:659–654.
35. Erdoes LS, Brown WC. Ruptured ulnar artery pseudoaneurysm. *Ann Vasc Surg* 1995;9:394–396.
36. Cardinal E, Buckwalter KA, Braunstein EM, et al. Occult dorsal carpal ganglion: comparison of US and MR imaging. *Radiology* 1994;193:259–262.
37. Murhpey MD, Fairbairn KJ, Parman LM, et al. Musculoskeletal angiomatous lesions: radiographic-pathologic correlation. *Radiographics* 1995;15:893–917.
38. Anderson JE. *Grant's atlas of anatomy*, 8th ed. Baltimore, MD: Williams & Wilkins, 1983.

39. Hayman LA, Duncan G, Chiou-Tau FY, et al. Sectional anatomy of the upper limb III: forearm and hand. *J Comput Assist Tomogr* 2001;25:322–325.

40. Hinke DH, Erickson SJ, Chanroy L, et al. Ulnar collateral ligament of the thumb: MR findings in cadavers, volunteers and patients with ligamentous injury (Gamekeeper's Thumb). *AJR Am J Roentgenol* 1994;163:1431–1434.

41. Rominger MB, Bernreuter WK, Kinney PL, et al. MR imaging of anatomy and tears of the wrist ligaments. *Radiographics* 1993;13:1233–1246.

42. Smith DK, Snearly WN. Lunotriquetral interosseous ligament of the wrist: MR appearances in asymptomatic volunteers and arthrographically normal wrists. *Radiology* 1994;191:199–202.

43. Smith DK. Anatomic features of the carpal scaphoid: validation of biometric measurements and symmetry with three-dimensional MR imaging. *Radiology* 1993;187:187–191.

44. Smith DK. Scapholunate interosseous ligament of the wrist: MR appearances in asymptomatic volunteers and arthrographically normal wrists. *Radiology* 1994;192:217–221.

45. Smith DK. Volar carpal ligaments of the wrist: normal appearance on multiplanar reconstructions of three dimensional fourier transform MR images. *AJR Am J Roentgenol* 1993;161:353–357.

46. Zeiss J, Jakab E, Khimji T, et al. The ulnar tunnel of the wrist (Guyon's canal): normal MR anatomy and variants. *AJR Am J Roentgenol* 1992;158:1081–1085.

47. Zeiss J, Skie M, Ebraheim N, et al. Anatomic relations between the median nerve and flexor tendons in the carpal tunnel: MR evaluation in normal volunteers. *AJR Am J Roentgenol* 1989;153:533–536.

48. Rosse C, Rosse PC. *Hollinshead's textbook of anatomy.* Philadelphia, PA: Lippincott-Raven, 1997.

49. Timins ME, Jahnke JP, Krah SE, et al. MR imaging of the major carpal stabilizing ligaments: normal anatomy and clinical examples. *Radiographics* 1995;14:575–587.

50. Berger RA. General anatomy. In: Cooney WP III, Linscheid RL, Dobyns JH, eds. *The wrist: diagnosis and operative treatment.* St. Louis: Mosby, 1998:32–60.

51. Viegas SF, Wagner K, Patterson R, et al. Medial hamate facet of the lunate. *J Hand Surg Am* 1990;15A:564–571.

52. Malik AM, Schweitzer ME, Culp RW, et al. MR imaging of the type II lunate bone. Frequency, extent and associated findings. *AJR Am J Roentgenol* 1999;173:335–338.

53. Viegas SF, Crossley M, Marzke M, et al. The fourth carpometacarpal joint. *J Hand Surg Am* 1990;16A:525–533.

54. O'Rahilly R. A survey of carpal and tarsal anomalies. *J Bone Joint Surg Am* 1953;35A:626–641.

55. Schmidt H, Freyschmidt J. *Koler's/Zimmer's borderlands of normal and early pathologic findings in skeletal radiology,* 4th ed. New York: Thieme Medical Publishers, 1993.

56. Timins ME. Osseous anatomic variants of the wrist. Findings on MR imaging. *AJR Am J Roentgenol* 1999;173:339–344.

57. Berger RA. Ligament anatomy. In: Cooney WP III, Linscheid RL, Dobyns JH, eds. *The wrist: diagnosis and operative treatment.* St. Louis: Mosby, 1998:73–105. in

58. Berger RA, Kauer JMG, Landsmeer JMF. The palmar radiocarpal ligaments. A study of adult and fetal wrists. *J Hand Surg Am* 1991;16A:350–355.

59. Berger RA. The gross and histologic anatomy of the scapholunate interosseous ligament. *J Hand Surg Am* 1996;21A:170–178.

60. Berger RA, Imaedo T, Berglund L, et al. The scapholunate interosseous ligament. In Schind E, ed. *Advances in biomechanics of the hand and wrist.* New York: Plencum Publishers, 1994.

61. Scheck RJ, Kubitzek C, Heisner R, et al. The scapholunate interosseous ligament in MR arthrography of the wrist: correlation with non-enhanced MRI and arthroscopy. *Skeletal Radiol* 1997;26:263–271.

62. Totterman SMS. Scapholunate ligament: normal MR appearance on three-dimensional- gradient-recalled-echo images. *Radiology* 1996;200:237–241.

63. Totterman SMS, Miller R, Wasserman B, et al. Intrinsic and extrinsic carpal ligaments: evaluation by three-dimensional fourier transform MR imaging. *AJR Am J Roentgenol* 1993;160:117–123.

64. Kang HS, Kindynes P, Brahme SK, et al. Triangular fibrocartilage and intercarpal ligaments of the wrist: MR imaging. *Radiology* 1994;181:401–404.

65. Totterman SMS, Miller RJ, McCance SE, et al. Lesions of the triangular fibrocartilage complex: MR findings with a three-dimensional gradient-recalled echo sequence. *Radiology* 1996;199:227–232.

66. Totterman SMS, Miller RJ. Triangular fibrocartilage complex: normal appearance on coronal three-dimensional gradient-recalled echo MR images. *Radiology* 1995;195:521–527.

67. Theumann NH, Pfirrmann CWA, Trudell DJ, et al. MR imaging of the MCP joints of the fingers: conventional MR imaging and MR arthrographic findings in cadavers. *Radiology* 2002;222:431–445.

68. Boles CA, Kannam S, Cardwell AB. The forearm: anatomy of muscle compartments and nerves. *AJR Am J Roentgenol* 2000;174:151–159.

69. Bishop AT, Gabel G, Carmichael SW. Flexor carpi radialis tendinitis. Part I: operative anatomy. *J Bone Joint Surg Am* 1994;76A:1009–1014.

70. Bengston K, Schutt AH, Swee RG, et al. Musician's overuse syndrome: a pilot study of magnetic resonance imaging. *Med Probl Perform Art* 1993;8:77–80.

71. Ham SJ, Konings JG, Wolf RFE, et al. Functional anatomy of the soft tissues of the hand and wrist: in vivo excursion measurement of the flexor pollicis longus-tendon using MRI. *Magn Reson Imaging* 1993;11:163–167.

72. Tang JS, Gold RH, Bassett LW, et al. Musculoskeletal infection of the extremities: evaluation with MR imaging. *Radiology* 1988;166:205–209.

73. Timins ME. Muscular anatomic variants of the wrist and hand. Findings on MR imaging. *AJR Am J Roentgenol* 1999;172:1397–1401.

74. Binkovitz LA, Berquist TH, McLeod RA. Masses of the hand and wrist: detection and characterization using MR imaging. *AJR Am J Roentgenol* 1989;154:223–236.

75. Cobb TK, Dalley BK, Posteraro RH, et al. Anatomy of the flexor retinaculum. *J Hand Surg Am* 1993;18A:91–99.

76. Cobb TK, Carmichael SN, Cooney WP III. Guyon's canal revisited: an anatomic study of the carpal ulnar neurovascular space. *J Hand Surg Am* 1996;21A:861–869.

77. Cobb TK, Bond JR, Cooney WP III, et al. Assessment of the ratio of carpal contents to carpal volume in patients with carpal tunnel syndrome. Preliminary report. *J Hand Surg Am* 1997;22A:635–639.

78. Cooney WP III. Vascular and neurological anatomy of the wrist. In: Cooney WP III, Linscheid RL, Dobyns JH, eds. *The wrist: diagnosis and operative treatment.* St. Louis: Mosby, 1998:106–123.

79. Mesgarzadeh M, Schneck CB, Bonakdapour A, et al. Carpal tunnel: MR imaging. Part II: carpal tunnel syndrome. *Radiology* 1989;171:749–754.

80. Vergel De Dios AM, Bond JR, Shives TC, et al. Aneurysmal bone cyst. A clinicopathologic study of 238 cases. *Cancer* 1992;69:2921–2931.

81. Erickson SJ, Cox IH, Hyde JS, et al. Effect of tendon orientation on MR imaging signal intensity: a manifestation of the "Magic angle" phenomenon. *Radiology* 1991;181:389–392.

82. Timins ME, O'Connell SE, Erickson SJ, et al. MR imaging of the wrist: normal findings that may simulate disease. *Radiographics* 1996;16:987–995.

83. Capelastegui A, Astigarraga E, Fernandez-Canton G, et al. Masses and pseudomasses of the hand and wrist: MR findings in 134 cases. *Skeletal Radiol* 1999;28:498–507.

84. Hunter JC, Escobedo EM, Wilson AJ, et al. MR imaging of clinically suspected scaphoid fractures. *AJR Am J Roentgenol* 1997;168:1287–1293.

85. Ikeda K, Haughton VM, Ho K-C, et al. Correlative MR-anatomic study of the median nerve. *AJR Am J Roentgenol* 1996;167:1233–1236.

86. Oneson SR, Scales LM, Erickson SJ, et al. MR imaging of the painful wrist. *Radiographics* 1996;16:997–1008.

87. Patel MR, Moradia VJ, Bassini L, et al. Extensor indicis proprius syndrome: a case report. *J Hand Surg Am* 1996;21A:914–915.

88. Pierre-Jerome C, Bekkelund SI, Husby G, et al. MRI anatomic variants of the wrists in women. *Surg Radiol Anat* 1996;18:37–41.

89. Pfirrmann CWA, Theuman NH, Chung CB, et al. The hamatolunate facet: characterization and association with cartilage lesions-magnetic resonance arthrography and anatomic correlation in cadaver wrists. *Skeletal Radiol* 2002;31:451–456.

90. Kose N, Ozcelik A, Gunal I. The crowded wrist: a case with accessory carpal bones. *Acta Orthop Scand* 1999;70:96–98.

91. Anderson MW, Benedetti P, Walter J, et al. MR appearance of the extensor digitorum brevis manus muscle: a pseudotumor in the hand. *AJR Am J Roentgenol* 1995;164:1477–1479.

92. Beatty JD, Remedios D, McCullough CJ. An accessory extensor tendon of the thumb as a cause of dorsal wrist pain. *J Hand Surg Br* 2000;25B:110–111.

93. Schuerman AH, Van Gils APG. Reversed palmaris longus muscle on MRI: report of four cases. *Eur Radiol* 2000;10:1242–1244.

94. Fakih RR, Thomas R, Mansour A. The extensor brevis manus. *Bull Hosp Jt Dis* 1997;56:115–116.

95. Polesuk BS, Helms CA. Hypertrophy of the palmaris longus muscle, a pseudotumor of the forearm. MR appearance. Case report and review of the literature. *Radiology* 1998;207:361–362.

96. Golimbu CN, Firooznia H, Melone CP, et al. Tears of the triangular fibrocartilage of the wrist. MR imaging. *Radiology* 1989;173:731–733.

97. Sugimoto H, Shinozaki T, Ohsawa T. Triangular fibrocartilage in asymptomatic subjects: investigation of abnormal MR signal intensity. *Radiology* 1994;191:193–197.

98. Jarvik JG, Kliot M, Maravilla KR. MR nerve imaging of the hand and wrist. *Hand Clin* 2000;16:13–24.

99. Metz VM, Schratter M, Dock WI, et al. Age associated changes of the triangular fibrocartilage of the wrist: evaluation of diagnostic performance of MR imaging. *Radiology* 1992;184:217–220.

100. Propeck T, Quinn TJ, Jacobson JA, et al. Sonography and MR imaging of bifid median nerve and anatomic and histologic correlation. *AJR Am J Roentgenol* 2000;175:1721–1725.

101. Clavero JA, Alomar X, Moukill JM, et al. MR imaging of ligament and tendon injuries in the fingers. *Radiographics* 2002;22:237–256.

102. Clavero JA, Galono P, Farinas O, et al. Extensor mechanisms of the fingers. MR imaging and anatomic correlation. *Radiographics* 2003;23:593–611.

103. Farooki S, Ashman CJ, Yu JS, et al. Invivo high resolution MR imaging of the carpal tunnel at 8 tesla. *Skeletal Radiol* 2002; 31:445–450.

104. Koenig H, Lucas D, Meisser R. The wrist: a preliminary report on high resolution MR imaging. *Radiology* 1986;160:463–467.

105. Weiss KL, Beltran J, Lubbers LM. High-field MR surface coil imaging of the hand and wrist. Part II: pathologic correlations and clinical relevance. *Radiology* 1986;160:147–152.

106. Weiss PC, Akelman E, Lombiase R. Comparison of the findings of triple-injection cine arthrography of the wrist with those of arthroscopy. *J Bone Joint Surg Am* 1996;78A:348–356.

107. Sallomi D, Janzen D, Munk PL, et al. Muscle denervation patterns in the upper limb nerve injuries: MR imaging findings and anatomic bases. *AJR Am J Roentgenol* 1998;171:779–784.

108. Yao L, Lee JK. Occult interosseous fracture: detection with MR imaging. *Radiology* 1988;167:749–751.

109. Yu JS, Brahme SK, Resnick D. MR imaging of the wrist. In: Weisman BN, *Categorical Course in Musculoskeletal Radiology*: RSNA Chicago, IL 1993:87–96.

110. Breitenseher MJ, Metz VM, Gilula LA, et al. Radiographically occult scaphoid fractures: value of MR imaging in detection. *Radiology* 1997;203:245–250.

111. Cerezal L, Abuscal F, Canga A, et al. Usefulness of gadolinium-enhanced MR imaging in the evaluation of the vascularity of scaphoid non-unions. *AJR Am J Roentgenol* 2000;174:141–149.

112. Ehman RL, Berquist TH. Magnetic resonance imaging of musculoskeletal trauma. *Radiol Clin North Am* 1986;24:291–319.

113. Haims AH, Moore AE, Schweitzer ME, et al. MRI in the diagnosis of cartilage injury in the wrist. *AJR Am J Roentgenol* 2004;182:1267–1270.

114. Bain GI, Bennett JD, Richards RS, et al. Longitudinal computed tomography of the scaphoid: a new technique. *Skeletal Radiol* 1995;24:271–273.

115. Chien AJ, Jacobson JA, Martel W, et al. Focal radial styloid abnormalities as manifestation of de Quervain tenosynovitis. *AJR Am J Roentgenol* 2001;177:1383–1386.

116. Munk PL, Lee MJ, Logan PM, et al. Scaphoid bone waist fractures, acute and chronic imaging with different techniques. *AJR Am J Roentgenol* 1997;168:779–786.

117. Fowler C, Sullivan B, Williams LA, et al. A comparison of bone scintigraphy and MRI in the early diagnosis of occult scaphoid waist fracture. *Skeletal Radiol* 1998;27:683–687.

118. Azouz EM, Babyer PS, Mascic AT, et al. MRI of the abnormal pediatric hand and wrist with plain film correlation. *J Comput Assist Tomogr* 1998;22:252–261.

119. Eustace S, Dennison W. Magnetic resonance imaging of acute orthopedic trauma to the upper extremity. *Clin Radiol* 1997;52:338–344.

120. Grampp S, Henk CB, Mostbech GH. Overuse edema in bone marrow of the hand: demonstration with MRI. *J Comput Assist Tomogr* 1998;22:25–27.

121. Lichtman DM, Degnan GG. Staging and its use in determining treatment modalities for Kienbock's disease. *J Hand Surg* 1980;5:272–278.

122. Lee JK, Yao L. Stress fractures: MR imaging. *Radiology* 1988;169:217–220.

123. Alam F, Schweitzer ME, Li X-X, et al. Frequency and spectrum of abnormalities in the bone marrow of the wrist: MR imaging findings. *Skeletal Radiol* 1999;28:312–317.

124. Lohman M, Kivisaari A, Vehmas T, et al. MR imaging of suspected trauma to the wrist bones. *Acta Radiol* 1999;40:615–618.

125. Beatty E, Light TR, Bedsole RJ, et al. Wrist and hand skeletal injuries in children. *Hand Clin* 1990;6:723–728.

126. DiFiori JP, Mandelbaum BR. Wrist pain in a young gymnast: unusual radiographic findings and MRI evidence of growth plate injury. *Med Sci Sport Exerc* 1996;28:1453–1458.

127. DiFiori JP, Puffer JC, Mandelbaum BR, et al. Distal growth plate injury and positive ulnar variance in non-elite gymnasts. *Am J Sports Med* 1997;25:763–768.

128. Gabel GJ. Gymnasts wrist injuries. *Clin Sports Med* 1958;3: 611–621.

129. Cook PA, Yu JS, Wiand W, et al. Suspected scaphoid fractures in skeletally immature patients: applications of MRI. *J Comput Assist Tomogr* 1997;21:511–515.

130. Peh WCG, Gilula LA, Wilson AJ. Detection of occult wrist fractures by magnetic resonance imaging. *Clin Radiol* 1996;51: 285–291.

131. Eckland K, Jaramillo D. Pattens of premature physeal arrest: MR imaging in 111 children. *AJR Am J Roentgenol* 2002;178:967–972.

132. Futami T, Foster BK, Morris LL, et al. Magnetic resonance of growth plate injuries: efficacy and indications for surgical procedures. *Arch Orthop Trauma Surg* 2000;120:390–396.

133. Binkovitz LA, Ehman RL, Cahill DR, et al. Magnetic resonance imaging of the wrist: normal cross sectional imaging and selected abnormal cases. *Radiographics* 1988;8:1171–1202.

134. Cooney WP III. Isolated carpal fractures. In: Cooney WP III, Linscheid RL, Dobyns JH, eds. *The wrist: diagnosis and operative treatment*. St. Louis: Mosby, 1998:474–487.

135. Teisen H, Hjarbaek J. Classification of fresh fractures of the lunate. *J Hand Surg Br* 1988;13B:458–462.

136. Arons MS, Fishbone G, Arons JA. Communicating defects in the triangular fibrocartilage complex without disruption of the triangular fibrocartilage. A report of two cases. *J Hand Surg Am* 1999; 24A:148–151.

137. Bak L, Bak S, Gaster P, et al. MR imaging of the wrist in carpal tunnel syndrome. *Acta Radiol* 1997;38:1050–1052.

138. Gundry CR, Kursunoglu-Brahme S, Schwaighafer B, et al. Is MR better than arthrography for evaluating the ligaments of the wrist. In vitro study. *AJR Am J Roentgenol* 1990;154:337–341.

139. Chiou H-J, Chang C-Y, Chou Y-H, et al. Triangular fibrocartilage of the wrist: presentation of high resolution ultrasonography. *J Ultrasound Med* 1998;17:41–48.

140. Cerezal L, del Pinal F, Abascal F, et al. Imaging findings in ulnar sided wrist impaction syndromes. *Radiographics* 2002;22:105–121.

141. Haims AH, Schweitzer ME, Morrison WB, et al. Limitations of MR imaging in diagnosis of peripheral tears of the triangular fibrocartilage of the wrist. *AJR Am J Roentgenol* 2002;178: 419–422.

142. Nakamura T, Yabe Y, Horiuchi Y. Fat suppression magnetic resonance imaging of the triangular fibrocartilage. Comparison with

spin-echo and gradient echo pulse sequences and histology. *J Hand Surg Br* 1999;24B:22–26.

143. Nishikawa S, Toh S. Ganglion of the triangular fibrocartilage complex. A report of three cases. *J Bone Joint Surg Am* 2003;85A:1560–1563.

144. Oneson SR, Scales LM, Timins ME, et al. MR imaging interpretation of the palmer classification of triangular fibrocartilage complex lesions. *Radiographics* 1996;16:97–107.

145. Oneson SR, Timins ME, Scales LM, et al. MR imaging diagnosis of triangular fibrocartilage pathology with arthroscopic correlation. *AJR Am J Roentgenol* 1997;168:1513–1518.

146. Palmer AK, Werner FW. Triangular fibrocartilage complex of the wrist. Anatomy and function. *J Hand Surg Am* 1981;61A:153–162.

147. Palmer AK. Triangular fibrocartilage complex lesions. A classification. *J Hand Surg Am* 1989;14A:594–605.

148. Schweitzer ME, Brahme SK, Hodler J, et al. Chronic wrist pain: spin-echo and short TI inversion recovery MR imaging and conventional and MR arthrography. *Radiology* 1992;182:205–211.

149. Steinborn M, Schurmann M, Staebler A, et al. MR imaging of ulnocarpal impaction after fracture of the distal radius. *AJR Am J Roentgenol* 2003;181:195–198.

150. Girgis W, Epstein RE. Magnetic resonance imaging of the hand and wrist. *Semin Roentgenol* 2000;35:286–296.

151. Potter HG, Asnis-Ernberg L, Weiland AJ, et al. The utility of high-resolution magnetic resonance imaging in the evaluation of the triangular fibrocartilage complex of the wrist. *J Bone Joint Surg Am* 1997;79A:1675–1684.

152. Zanetti M, Bram J, Hodler J. Triangular fibrocartilage and intercarpal ligament of the wrist: does MR arthrography improve standard MRI? *J Magn Reson Imaging* 1997;7:590–594.

153. Imaeda T, Nakamura R, Shionoya K, et al. Ulnar impactions syndrome: MR image findings. *Radiology* 1996;201:202–208.

154. Gelberman RH, Cooney WP III, Szabo RM. Carpal instability. *J Bone Joint Surg* 2000;82A:578–594.

155. Gelberman RH, Eaton R, Urbaniak JR. Peripheral nerve compression. *J Bone Joint Surg* 1993;75A:1854–1878.

156. Giele H, LeViet D. Intraneural mucoid cysts of the upper limb. *J Hand Surg Br* 1997;22B:805–809.

157. Staron RB, Feldman F, Haramati N, et al. Abnormal geometry of the distal radioulnar joint: MR findings. *Skeletal Radiol* 1994;23:369–372.

158. Nakamura R, Horie E, Imaeda T, et al. Criteria for diagnosing distal radioulnar joint subluxation by computed tomography. *Skeletal Radiol* 1996;25:649–653.

159. Brown RR, Fliszar E, Cotton A, et al. Extrinsic and intrinsic ligaments of the wrist: normal and pathologic anatomy at MR arthrography with three-compartment enhancement. *Radiographics* 1998;18:687–774.

160. Harper MT, Chandnani VP, Spaeth J, et al. Gamekeeper thumb: diagnosis of ulnar collateral ligament injury using magnetic resonance imaging, magnetic resonance arthrography and stress radiography. *J Magn Reson Imaging* 1996;6:322–328.

161. Pfirrmann CWA, Theuman NH, Botte MJ, et al. MR imaging of the metacarpophalangeal joints and fingers II: detection of simulated injuries in cadavers. *Radiology* 2002;222:447–452.

162. Ahn JM, Sartoris DJ, Kang HS, et al. Gamekeeper thumb: comparison of MR arthrography and conventional arthrography and MR imaging in cadavers. *Radiology* 1998;206:737–744.

163. Hergan K, Mittler C, Oser W. Ulnar collateral ligament: differentiation of displaced and nondisplaced tears with US and MR imaging. *Radiology* 1995;194:65–71.

164. Feldman F, Singson RD, Staron RB. Magnetic resonance imaging of peri-articular and ectopic ganglia. *Skeletal Radiol* 1989;18:353–358.

165. Fleckstein JL, Bertocci LA, Nunally RL, et al. Exercise-enhanced MR imaging of variations in forearm muscle anatomy and use: importance in MR spectroscopy. *AJR Am J Roentgenol* 1989;153:693–698.

166. Drape J-L, Silbermann-Hoffman O, Houvet P, et al. Complications of flexor tendon repairs in the hand: MR imaging assessment. *Radiology* 1996;198:219–224.

167. Drape J-L, de Gery ST-C, Chevrot A, et al. Closed ruptures of the flexor digitorum tendons: MRI evaluation. *Skeletal Radiol* 1998;27:617–624.

168. Rubins DJ, Blebea JS, Totterman SMS, et al. Rheumatoid arthritis: evaluation of wrist extensor tendons with clinical examination versus MR imaging—a preliminary report. *Radiology* 1993;187:831–838.

169. Saitoh S, Hata Y, Murakami N, et al. Scaphoid non-union and flexor pollicis longus tendon rupture. *J Hand Surg Am* 1999;24A:1211–1219.

170. Kaplan DA. Anatomy, injuries and treatment of extensor apparatus of the hand and fingers. *Clin Orthop* 1995;18:24–41.

171. Hauger O, Chung CB, Lektrakul N, et al. Pulley system in the fingers: normal anatomy and simulated lesions in cadavers at MR imaging, CT and US with and without contrast material distention of the tendon sheath. *Radiology* 2000;217:201–212.

172. Parellada JA, Balkissoon ARA, Hayes CW, et al. Bowstring injury of the flexor tendon pulley system: MR imaging. *AJR Am J Roentgenol* 1996;167:347–349.

173. Gabl M, Rangger C, Lietz M, et al. Disruption of the finger flexor pulley systems in elite rock climbers. *Am J Sports Med* 1998;26:651–655.

174. Keir PJ, Wells RP. Changes in geometry of the finger flexor tendons in the carpal tunnel with wrist posture and tendon load. An MRI study of normal wrists. *Clin Biomech* 1999;14:635–645.

175. Cauzza E, Stauffer E, Zimmerli S, et al. Mycobacterium marinum. MR imaging and clinical course of a rare soft tissue infection. *Skeletal Radiol* 2004;33:409–412.

176. Glajchen N, Schweitzer M. MRI features in de Quervain's tenosynovitis of the wrist. *Skeletal Radiol* 1996;25:63–65.

177. Gabel G, Bishop AT, Wood MB. Flexor carpi radialis tendinitis. Part II: results of operative treatment. *J Bone Joint Surg Am* 1994;76A:1015–1018.

178. Huang HW, Strauch RJ. Extensor pollicis tenosynovitis: a case report and review of the literature. *J Hand Surg Am* 2000;25A:577–579.

179. Huh Y-M, Suk J-S, Jeong E-K, et al. Role of inflamed synovial volume of the wrist in redefining remission of rheumatoid arthritis with gadolinium-enhanced 3D-SPGR MR imaging. *J Magn Reson Imaging* 1999;10:202–208.

180. Latshaw RF, Weidner WA. Ulnar artery aneurysms: angiographic considerations in 2 cases. *AJR Am J Roentgenol* 1978;131:1093–1095.

181. Connell DA, Koulouris G, Duncan A, et al. Contrast-enhanced MR angiography of the hand. *Radiographics* 2002;22:583–599.

182. Lee VS, Lee HM, Rofsky NM. Magnetic resonance angiography of the hand. *Invest Radiol* 1998;33:687–698.

183. Buetow PC, Kransdorf MJ, Moser RP, et al. Radiologic appearance of intramuscular hemangioma with emphasis on MR appearance. *AJR Am J Roentgenol* 1990;154:563–567.

184. Butler ED, Hamell JP, Seipel RS, et al. Tumors of the hand. A 10 year survey and report of 437 cases. *Am J Surg* 1960;100:293–302.

185. Dreyfuss UY, Boome RS, Kranold DH. Synovial sarcoma of the hand. A literature study. *J Hand Surg Br* 1986;11:471–472.

186. Pahlos JM, Valdes JC, Garilan F. Bilateral lunate interosseous ganglia. *Skeletal Radiol* 1998;27:708–720.

187. Peh WCG, Ip WY, Wong LLS. Diagnosis of dorsal interosseous pseudotumors by magnetic resonance imaging. *Australas Radiol* 1999;43:394–396.

188. Saitoh S, Hatori M, Ehara S. Ewings sarcoma of the middle finger in an infant. *Orthopedics* 2000;23:379–380.

189. Schajowics F, Aiello CL, Slullitel I. Cystic and pseudocystic lesions of the terminal phalanx with specific references to epidermoid cysts. *Clin Orthop* 1970;68:84–92.

190. Aoki J, Tanakawa H, Ishii K, et al. MR findings indicative of hemosiderin in giant cell tumors of bone: frequency, cause and diagnostic significance. *AJR Am J Roentgenol* 1996;166:145–148.

191. Assorin J, Richardi G, Railhoc JJ, et al. Osteoid osteoma: MR imaging versus CT. *Radiology* 1994;191:217–233.

192. Murphey MD, Flemming DJ, Boyea SR, et al. Enchondroma versus chondrosarcoma in the appendicular skeleton: differentiating features. *Radiographics* 1998;18:1213–1217.

193. Unni KK. *Dahlin's bone tumors. General aspects and data on 11,087 cases*, 5th ed. Philadelphia, PA: Lippincott-Raven, 1996.

194. Yamamoto T, Mizuno K. Chondromyxoid fibroma of the finger. *Kobe J Med Sci* 2000;46:29–32.

195. Cawte TG, Steiner GC, Beltran J, et al. Chondrosarcoma of the short tubular bones of the hands and feet. *Skeletal Radiol* 1998;27:625–632.

196. Beltran J, Simon DC, Katz W, et al. Increased MR signal intensity in skeletal muscle adjacent to malignant tumors: pathologic correlation and clinical relevance. *Radiology* 1987;162:251–255.

197. Drape JL, Idy-Peretti I, Goettmann S, et al. MR imaging of digital mucoid cysts. *Radiology* 1996;200:531–536.

198. Ha D-H, Jung W-H, Yoon C-S. Cutaneous hamartoma of the hand. MR image findings. *Yonsei Med J* 2000;41:147–149.

199. Sundaram M, McGuire MH, Herbold DR, et al. High signal intensity soft tissue masses on T1-weighted pulsing sequences. *Skeletal Radiol* 1987;16:30–36.

200. Sundaram M, McGuire MH, Schajowic ZF. Soft tissue masses: histologic bases for decreased signal (short T2) on T2-weighted images. *AJR Am J Roentgenol* 1987;148:1247–1250.

201. Campanacii M. *Bone and soft tissue tumors.* New York: Springer-Verlag, 1999.

202. Weiss SW, Goldblum JR. *Enzinger and Weiss' soft tissue tumors,* 4th ed. St. Louis: Mosby, 2001.

203. Dooms GC, Hricak H, Sollitto RA, et al. Lipomatous tumors and tumors with fatty component: MR imaging potential and comparison of MR and CT results. *Radiology* 1985;157:479–483.

204. Poznanski AK. *The hand in radiologic diagnosis.* Philadelphia, PA: WB Saunders, 1984.

205. Drape J-L, Idy-Peretti I, Goetturmann S, et al. Standard and high resolution magnetic resonance imagine of glomus tumors of the toes and fingers. *J Am Acad Dermatol* 1996;34:550–555.

206. Blain O, Binda R, Middleton W, et al. The occult dorsal carpal ganglion: usefulness of magnetic resonance imaging. *Am J Orthop* 1998;27:107–110.

207. El-Noueam KI, Schweitzer ME, Blasbalg R, et al. Is a subset of wrist ganglia the sequelae of internal derangements of the wrist joint? MR imaging findings. *Radiology* 1999;212:537–540.

208. Ushijima M, Hashimoto H, Tsuneyoshi M, et al. Giant cell tumor of the tendon sheath (nodular tenosynovitis). A study of 207 cases to compare the large joint group with the common digital group. *Cancer* 1986;57:875–884.

209. Fox MG, Kransdorf MJ, Bancroft LW, et al. MR imaging of fibroma of the tendon sheath. *AJR Am J Roentgenol* 2003;180: 1449–1453.

210. Theumann NH, Bittoun J, Goettmann D, et al. Hemangiomas of the finger: MR imaging evaluation. *Radiology* 2001;218:841–847.

211. Goodman HJB, Richards AM, Klassen MF. Use of magnetic resonance imaging on a large lipoma of the hand. A case report. *Aust N Z J Surg* 1997;67:489–491.

212. Amadio PC, Reiman HM, Dobyns JH. Lipofibromatous hamartoma of nerve. *J Hand Surg Am* 1998;13A:67–75.

213. Meyer B-U, Rorieht S, Schmitt R. Bilateral fibrolipomatous hamartoma of the median nerve with macrocheiria and late onset nerve entrapment syndrome. *Muscle Nerve* 1998;21: 656–658.

214. Wang Y-C, Jeng C-M, Marcantonio DR, et al. Macrodystrophia lipomatosa: MR imaging in three patients. *Clin Imaging* 1997;21: 323–327.

215. Shih TT-F, Sim J-S, Hou K-M, et al. Magnetic resonance imaging of glomus tumor in the hand. *Int Orthop* 1996;20:342–345.

216. Nectcher D, Mosharrofa A, Lee M, et al. Transverse carpal ligament: the effect of flexor tendon excursion, morphologic changes of the carpal canal and on pinch and grip strength after open carpal tunnel release. *Plastic Reconstr Surg* 1997;100: 636–642.

217. Boutin RD, Joachim B, Sartoris DJ, et al. Update on orthopedic infections. *Orthop Clin North Am* 1998;29:41–66.

218. Datz FL, Thorne DA. Effect of chronicity of infection on the sensitivity of the In-111 labeled leukocyte scan. *AJR Am J Roentgenol* 1986;147:809–812.

219. Erdman WA, Towburro F, Joyson HT, et al. Osteomyelitis: characteristics and pitfalls of MR imaging. *Radiology* 1991;180:533–539.

220. Graif M, Schweitzer ME, Deely D, et al. The septic versus nonseptic inflamed joint. *Skeletal Radiol* 1999;28:616–620.

221. Hopkins KL, Li KCP, Bergman G. Gadolinium DTPA-enhanced magnetic resonance imaging of musculoskeletal infectious processes. *Skeletal Radiol* 1995;24:325–330.

222. Jaramillo D, Treves ST, Kasser JR, et al. Osteomyelitis and septic arthritis in children: appropriate use of imaging to guide treatment. *AJR Am J Roentgenol* 1995;265:399–403.

223. Unger E, Moldofsky P, Gatenby R, et al. Diagnosis of osteomyelitis by MR imaging. *AJR Am J Roentgenol* 1988; 150:605–610.

224. DuBuf-Vereijhem PWG, Vander Ven AJAM, Meis JFMG, et al. Swelling of the hand and forearm by mycobacterium bovis. *Neth J Med* 1999;54:70–72.

225. Paajanen H, Grodd W, Revel D, et al. Gadolinium-DTPA enhanced MR imaging of intramuscular abscesses. *Magn Reson Imaging* 1987;5:109–115.

226. Amrami KK, Sundarum M, Shin AY, et al. Mycobacterium marinum infections of the distal upper extremities: clinical course and imaging findings in two cases with delayed diagnosis. *Skeletal Radiol* 2003;32:546–549.

227. Chan MK, Chowchuen P, Workman T, et al. Silicone synovitis: MR imaging in five patients. *Skeletal Radiol* 1998;27:13–17.

228. Lee EY, Rubin DA, Brown DM. Recurrent mycobacterium marinum tenosynovitis of the wrist mimicking extraarticular synovial chondromatosis on MR images. *Skeletal Radiol* 2004;33: 405–408.

229. Theodorou DJ, Theodorou SJ, Kakitubata Y, et al. Imaging characteristics and epidemiologic features of atypical mycobacterial infections involving the musculoskeletal system. *AJR Am J Roentgenol* 2001;176:341–349.

230. Vogler JB III, Murphy WA. Bone marrow imaging. *Radiology* 1988;168:679–693.

231. Sueyoshi E, Uetani M, Hayashi K, et al. Tuberculous tenosynovitis of the wrist: MRI findings in three patients. *Skeletal Radiol* 1996;25:569–572.

232. Albornoz MA, Mezgarzedeh M, Neuman CH, et al. Granulomatous tenosynovitis: a rare manifestation of tuberculosis. *Clin Rheumatol* 1998;17:166–169.

233. Hoffman KL, Bergman AG, Hoffman DK, et al. Tuberculous tenosynovitis of the flexor tendons of the wrist: MR imaging with pathologic correlation. *Skeletal Radiol* 1996;25:186–188.

234. Beltran J, Noto AM, McGhee RB, et al. Infections of the musculoskeletal system: high-field-strength MR imaging. *Radiology* 1987;164:449–454.

235. Bachir T, Souhil Z, Peterfly CG, et al. Rheumatoid arthritis of the hand and wrist: comparison of three imaging techniques. *AJR Am J Roentgenol* 2004;182:937–943.

236. Brower AC. *Arthritis in black and white,* 2nd ed. Philadelphia, PA: WB Saunders, 1997.

237. Chau CHF, Griffith JF, Chan PT, et al. Rice body formation in atypical mycobacterial tenosynovitis and bursitis: findings on sonography and MR imaging. *AJR Am J Roentgenol* 2003;180: 1455–1459.

238. Beltran J, Noto AM, Herman LJ, et al. Joint effusions: MR imaging. *Radiology* 1986;158:133–137.

239. Beltran J, Caudill JL, Herman LA, et al. Rheumatoid arthritis: MR imaging manifestations. *Radiology* 1987;165:153–157.

240. Gasson J, Gandy SJ, Hutton CW, et al. Magnetic resonance imaging of rheumatoid arthritis in the metacarpophalangeal joints. *Skeletal Radiol* 2000;29:324–334.

241. Senac MO, Beutsch D, Bernstein BH, et al. MR imaging in juvenile rheumatoid arthritis. *AJR Am J Roentgenol* 1988;150:873–878.

242. Wongworawat MD, Holton P, Leach TJ, et al. A prolonged case of mycobacterium marinum flexor tenosynovitis: radiographic and histologic correlation and review of the literature. *Skeletal Radiol* 2003;32:542–545.

243. Olivieri I, Barozzi L, Favaro L, et al. Dactyliltis in patients with seronegative spondyloarthropathy: assessment by ultrasound and magnetic resonance imaging. *Arthritis Rheum* 1996;39: 1524–1528.

244. Nakahara N, Uetani M, Hayaski K, et al. Gadolinium-enhanced MR imaging of the wrist in rheumatoid arthritis: value of fat suppression pulse sequences. *Skeletal Radiol* 1996;25:639–647.

245. Lee J, Lee SK, Suh JS, et al. Magnetic resonance imaging of the wrist defining remission in rheumatoid arthritis. *J Rheumatol* 1997;24:1303–1308.

246. Goupille P, Roulot B, Akoka S, et al. Magnetic resonance imaging: a valuable method for detection of synovial inflammation in rheumatoid arthritis. *J Rheumatol* 2001;28:35–40.

247. Osterguaard M, Hansen M, Stoltenberg M, et al. Magnetic resonance imaging determined synovial membrane volume as a marker of disease activity and predictor of progressive joint destruction in wrists of patients with rheumatoid arthritis. *Arthritis Rheum* 1999;42:918–929.

248. Yulish BS, Lieberman JM, Newman AJ, et al. Juvenile rheumatoid arthritis: assessment with MR imaging. *Radiology* 1987;165: 149–152.

249. McQueen FM, Stewart N, Crabbe J, et al. Magnetic resonance imaging of the wrist in early rheumatoid arthritis reveals a high prevalence of erosions four months after symptom onset. *Ann Rheum Dis* 1998;57:350–356.

250. Shin AY, Weinstein LP, Bishop AT. Kienbock's disease and gout. *J Hand Surg Br* 1999;24B:363–365.

251. Poop JD, Bidgood WD, Edwards L. Magnetic resonance imaging of tophaceous gout in the hand and wrist. *Semin Arthritis Rheum* 1996;25:282–289.

252. Mandelbaum BR, Grant TT, Hartzman S, et al. The use of MRI to assist in diagnosis of pigmented villonodular synovitis of the knee joint. *Clin Orthop* 1988;231:135–139.

253. Spritzer CE, Dalinka MK, Kressel HY. Magnetic resonance imaging of pigmented villonodular synovitis: a report of two cases. *Skeletal Radiol* 1987;16:316–319.

254. Carpintero P, Serrano J, Garcia-Frasquet A. Pigmented villonodular synovitis of the wrist invading bone. A report of two cases. *Acta Orthop Scand* 2000;71:424–426.

255. Llauger J, Palmer J, Roson N, et al. Pigmented villonodular synovitis and giant cell tumors of the tendon sheath: radiologic and pathologic features. *AJR Am J Roentgenol* 1999;172:1087–1091.

256. Atkinson RE, Smith RJ. Silicone synovitis following implant arthroplasty. *Hand Clin* 1986;2:291–299.

257. Abascal F, Cerezal L, del Pinal F, et al. Unilateral osteonecrosis in a patient with bilateral os centrale carpi: imaging findings. *Skeletal Radiol* 2001;30:643–647.

258. Amadio PC. Scaphoid fractures. *Orthop Clin North Am* 1992; 23:7–17.

259. Amadio PC, Hanssen AD, Berquist TH. The genesis of Kienbock's disease: Early diagnosis by magnetic resonance imaging. *J Hand Surg Am* 1987;12A:1044–1049.

260. Trumble TE, Irving J. Histologic and magnetic resonance imaging correlation in Kienbock's disease. *J Hand Surg Am* 1990; 15A:879–884.

261. Reinus WR, Conway WF, Totty WG, et al. Carpal avascular necrosis: MR imaging. *Radiology* 1986;160:689–693.

262. Barnes NA, Howes AJ, Jeffers H, et al. Avascular necrosis of the third metacarpal head. *Eur J Radiol* 2000;3:115–117.

263. Wright TC, Dell PC. Avascular necrosis and vascular anatomy of the metacarpal. *J Hand Surg Am* 1991;61A:540–544.

264. Sowa DT, Holder LE, Patt PG. Application of magnetic resonance imaging to ischemic necrosis of the lunate. *J Hand Surg Am* 1989;14A:1008–1016.

265. Greening J, Smart S, Leary R, et al. Reduced movement of median nerve in the capral tunnel during wrist flexion in patients with non-specific arm pain. *Lancet* 1999;354:217–218.

266. Ogose A, Hotta T, Morita T, et al. Tumors of the peripheral nerves: correlation of symptoms, clinical signs, imaging features and histologic diagnosis. *Skeletal Radiol* 1999;28:123–128.

267. Radack DM, Schweitzer ME, Taras J. Carpal tunnel syndrome: are the MR findings a result of population selection bias? *AJR Am J Roentgenol* 1997;169:1649–1653.

268. Rempel D, Dahlin L, Lundborg G. Pathophysiology of nerve compression syndromes: response of peripheral nerves to loading. *J Bone Joint Surg Am* 1999;81A:1600–1610.

269. Zagnoli F, Andre V, LeDraff P, et al. Idiopathic carpal tunnel syndrome: clinical, elecrodiagnostic and magnetic resonance imaging correlation. *Rev Rhum* 1999;66:192–200; Zeiss J, Guilliam-Hardet L. MR demonstration of anomalous muscles on the volar aspect of the wrist and forearm. *Clin Imaging* 1996; 20:219–221.

270. Buchberger W, Judmaier W, Birbamer GC, et al. Carpal tunnel syndrome: diagnosis with high-resolution sonography. *AJR Am J Roentgenol* 1992;159:793–798.

271. Duncan I, Sullivan P, Lomas F. Sonography in the diagnosis of carpal tunnel syndrome. *AJR Am J Roentgenol* 1999;173: 681–684.

272. Mesgarzadeh M, Schneck CD, Bonakdapour A. Carpal tunnel: MR imaging. Part I: normal anatomy. *Radiology* 1989;171: 743–748.

273. Middleton WD, Keeland JB, Kellman GM, et al. MR imaging of the carpal tunnel: normal anatomy and preliminary findings in the carpal tunnel syndrome. *AJR Am J Roentgenol* 1987;148: 307–316.

274. Lanz U. Anatomic variations in the median nerve in the carpal tunnel. *J Hand Surg Am* 1977;2A:44–53.

275. Phalen GS. Carpal tunnel syndrome: clinical evaluation in 598 hands. *Clin Orthop* 1972;83:29–40.

276. Mauer J, Bleochkowski A, Tempka A, et al. High resolution MR imaging of the carpal tunnel and wrist. *Acta Radiol* 2000; 41:78–83.

277. Spinner RJ, Lins RE, Spinner M. Compression of the medial half of the deep branch of the ulnar nerve by an anomalous origin of the flexor digiti minimi. *J Bone Joint Surg Am* 1996;78A: 427–430.

278. Sugimoto H, Miyayi N, Ohsawa T. Carpal tunnel syndrome: evaluation of median nerve circulation with dynamic contrast-enhanced MR imaging. *Radiology* 1994;190:459–466.

279. Cobb TK, Dalley BK, Posteraro RH, et al. Establishment of carpal contents/carpal canal ratio by means of magnetic resonance imaging. *J Hand Surg Am* 1993;17A:843–849.

280. Monagle K, Dai G, Chu A, et al. Quantitative MR imaging of carpal tunnel syndrome. *AJR Am J Roentgenol* 1999;172: 1581–1586.

281. Bigattini D, Daenen B, Dondelinger RF. Osseous sarcoidosis. *J Belge Radiol-Belg Tijdschr/voor Radiol* 1999;82:108.

282. Shum C, Parisien M, Strauch R, et al. The role of flexor tenosynovectomy in operative treatment of carpal tunnel syndrome. *J Bone Joint Surg Am* 2002;84A:221–225.

283. Plancher KD, Peterson RK, Sterchen JB. Compression neuropathies and tendinopathies in the elbow and wrist. *Clin Sports Med* 1996;15:331–371.

284. Barberie JE, Connell DG, Munk PL, et al. Ulnar nerve injuries of the hand producing intrinsic muscle denervation on magnetic resonance imaging. *Australas Radiol* 1999;43:355–357.

285. Rask MR. Anterior interosseous nerve entrapment (Liloh-Nevin Syndrome). *Clin Orthop* 1979;142:176–181.

286. Grainger AJ, Campbell RSD, Stothard J. Anterior interosseous nerve syndrome: appearance at MR imaging in three cases. *Radiology* 1998;208:381–384.

287. Anderson SE, Steinbach LS, DeMonaco D, et al. "Baby wrist": MRI of an overuse syndrome in mothers. *AJR Am J Roentgenol* 2004;182:719–724.

288. Fujita A, Sugimoto H, Kikkawa I, et al. Phalangeal microgeotic syndrome: findings on MR imaging. *AJR Am J Roentgenol* 1999;173:711–712.

289. Kumar PR, Jenkins JPR, Hodgson SP. Bilateral chronic exertional compartment syndrome of the dorsal part of the forearm: the role of magnetic resonance imaging in diagnosis. *J Bone Joint Surg Am* 2003;85A:1557–1559.

290. Yacol ME, Bergman AG, Ladd AL, et al. Dupuytren's contracture: MR image findings and correlation between signal intensity and cellularity of lesions. *AJR Am J Roentgenol* 1993;160:813–817.

Musculoskeletal Neoplasms

Mark J. Kransdorf   Thomas H. Berquist

The imaging evaluation of musculoskeletal tumors has undergone dramatic evolution with the advent of computer-assisted imaging, specifically computed tomography (CT) and magnetic resonance imaging (MRI). Despite these sophisticated imaging modalities, the objectives of initial radiologic evaluation remain unchanged: detecting the suspected lesion; establishing a diagnosis or, more frequently, formulating an appropriate differential diagnosis; and radiologic staging of a lesion (1). This chapter reviews techniques required for MRI in the evaluation of soft tissue and bone tumors, including coil selection, imaging planes, and pulse sequence selection. Particular emphasis is on those soft tissue and bone diagnoses that may be confidently made or suggested by MRI and lesions that are frequently encountered as incidental findings on examinations obtained for unrelated reasons. The use of MRI in differentiating benign from malignant soft tissue lesions, follow-up evaluation for differentiation of recurrent tumors from postoperative or radiation change, and response to therapy are also covered. Imaging evaluation for diagnosis and staging should be done before biopsy.

TECHNIQUES

MRI has emerged as the preferred modality for evaluating musculoskeletal lesions and should be obtained after radiographic evaluation. MRI provides superior soft tissue contrast, allows multiplanar image acquisition, obviates the need for iodinated contrast agents or for ionizing radiation, and is devoid of streak artifact commonly encountered with CT (2–5). Critical assessment by multiple investigators (3,5–11) has demonstrated the superiority of MRI over CT in delineating the extent of a musculoskeletal lesion and in defining its relationship to adjacent neurovascular structures. Recently, however, the superiority of MRI in the staging of musculoskeletal tumors has come into question. In a multiinstitutional study of 316 patients with primary bone and soft tissue malignancies, the Radiology Diagnostic Oncology Group found no statistically significant difference between CT and MRI in determining tumor involvement of muscle, bone, joint, or neurovascular structures (12). Despite this caveat, most radiologists are comfortable with the use of MRI in the evaluation of musculoskeletal tumors, and we believe it is the modality of choice and, when used in conjunction with a systematic approach, can correctly diagnose most masses.

The basic principles of MRI (see Chapter 1) and general techniques (see Chapter 3) have been previously discussed. Certain technical factors, however, require special attention and need to be emphasized: patient positioning, coil selection, imaging planes, pulse sequence selection, and imaging limitations.

Positioning and Coil Selection

Positioning of patients and the choice of proper coils for studies of musculoskeletal neoplasms are essential to minimize motion artifacts and obtain optimal signal-to-noise ratios. Evaluation of the trunk and thighs is most efficacious using the torso coil with the patient supine. If a gluteal soft tissue lesion is suspected, the prone position may be helpful to avoid distortion of the posterior soft tissues. The torso coil also allows comparison of both lower extremities and can provide more complete evaluation of the entire osseous or soft tissue region of interest (i.e., femur, tibia, etc.) (see Fig. 12-1). In certain skeletal neoplasms, imaging the entire bone or region of interest is important to be certain that skip lesions are not overlooked (see Fig. 12-2) (13–15).

The peripheral lower extremities distal to the knee and the upper extremities are usually evaluated using flat surface coils or circumferential volume coils. These coils are important in achieving superior image quality and are selected on the basis of the body part and patient position needed for the examination. For example, a lesion in the shoulder might be easily evaluated using the 5-inch circular coil. A lesion in the humerus should be studied using a larger phased array coil to include a larger area of the upper extremity (see Fig. 12-3). The circumferential volume extremity coil provides a more uniform signal, but it must be positioned in the center of the gantry with most imagers. Positioning is not difficult for evaluating the knee, calf, or foot and ankle, but evaluation of the forearm and wrist may require that the patient place his or her arm above the head (see Chapter 11). The latter position is uncomfortable, leading to motion artifacts that reduce image quality (14,15).

New coils are now becoming available that allow superior image quality and more flexibility in the amount of area covered. These array coils are commonly used for the spine and are very useful for evaluating large segments of the spine in patients with suspected lymphoma, myeloma, or metastatic disease (13–16).

Imaging Planes and Pulse Sequence

In a given clinical setting, numerous pulse sequences could be used to evaluate the musculoskeletal system. These include the commonly used spin-echo (SE) sequences (short echo time [TE], repetition time [TR], and long TE, TR), short TI inversion recovery (STIR) sequences, gradient-echo (GRE) sequences, and fast spin-echo techniques (13–18). For most patients with suspected bone or soft tissue neoplasms, spin-echo sequences are well suited for lesion detection and characterization (13–16,19). With these sequences, normal tissues have predictable signal intensity. Fat and bone marrow have high signal intensity on T1-weighted and intermediate signal on T2-weighted spin-echo MR images. Muscle has intermediate signal intensity, whereas cortical bone, ligaments, tendon, calcium, air, and fibrocartilage appear dark or black. Flowing blood usually gives no signal, but this finding is inconsistent and varies with the flow rate and pulse sequences used. Nerves are usually of slightly lower intensity than muscles (13).

Lesions should be imaged in at least two orthogonal planes, using conventional T1- and T2-weighted spin-echo MR pulse sequences in at least one of these. Standard spin-echo imaging is most useful in establishing a specific diagnosis, when possible, and is the most reproducible technique, and the one most often referenced in the tumor imaging literature. It is the imaging technique with which we are most familiar for tumor evaluation, and it has established itself as the standard by which other imaging techniques must be judged (20). The main disadvantage of spin-echo imaging remains the relatively long acquisition times, especially for double-echo T2-weighted sequences (20). Radiologists are most familiar with conventional axial anatomy, and axial T1- and T2-weighted spin-echo images should be obtained in

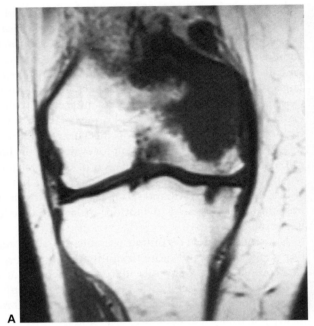

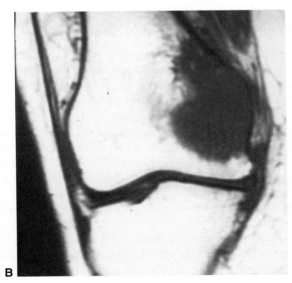

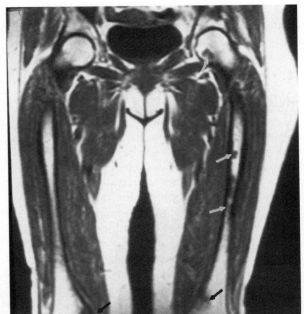

Figure 12-1 A 65-year-old woman with suspected lymphoma and knee pain. Coronal spin-echo (SE) 427/11 images **(A,B)** show low-intensity regions in the medial right knee. Because of the history, both femurs were also examined for comparison and to exclude other lesions. Coronal SE 500/11 **(C)** image demonstrates multiple areas of abnormal signal intensity (*arrows*) due to lymphoma.

almost all cases. The choice of additional imaging plane or planes will vary with the involved body part, the lesion location, and its relationship to crucial structures. In general, the additional plane is sagittal with anterior or posterior masses and coronal with medial or lateral lesions. Oblique planes may also be a useful adjunct to reduce the problems from partial volume effects (see Fig. 12-4). In these additional planes, a combination of conventional T1- and T2-weighted spin-echo (SE) images, turbo (fast) spin-echo images, gradient images, and STIR imaging is useful, as the cases require.

Field of view (FOV) is dictated by the size and location of the lesion. In general, a small field of view is preferred; however, the field of view must be large enough to evaluate the lesion and allow appropriate staging. When an extremity is being evaluated, it is not usually necessary to obtain

the contralateral extremity for comparison, unless no lesion is detected on initial sequences. It is useful to place a marker over the area of clinical concern to ensure it is appropriately imaged. This marker becomes important in evaluation of lesions such as a subcutaneous lipoma or lipomatosis, in which the lesion may not be appreciated as distinct from the adjacent adipose tissue (see Fig. 12-5). When small superficial lesions are being evaluated, care should be taken to ensure the marker or patient position does not compress the mass.

Fast scanning techniques allow for shorter imaging times, decreased motion artifact, and increased patient tolerance and patient throughput (20,21). They may add additional information and may be helpful in specific instances, although fast scanning techniques have not

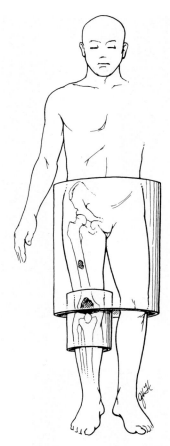

Figure 12-2 A primary sarcoma in the knee with a midfemoral skip lesion. The knee coil would be optimal for imaging the knee, but the skip lesion would not be identified unless the entire femur was examined.

replaced standard spin-echo imaging. Gradient-echo imaging may be a useful supplement in demonstrating hemosiderin because of its greater magnetic susceptibility, and in general, susceptibility artifacts related to metallic material, hemorrhage, and air are accentuated on gradient-echo images (see Fig. 12-6) (22). Gradient-echo images may also be better in some instances to demonstrate the lesion–fat interface and to depict small surrounding vessels (23). Short TI inversion recovery sequences are very useful in evaluating subtle marrow abnormalities and are frequently added in addition to the conventional spin-echo sequences. This technique (inversion recovery time 160, TE 30, TR 1,500) suppresses fat signal while providing an additive effect on T1 and T2 signal enhancement. The superior contrast achieved with this sequence can allow subtle lesions to be more easily identified (17,18). Some authors prefer short TE/TR spin-echo (500/20) and STIR sequences to typical T1- and T2-weighted spin-echo sequences (24). Short TI inversion recovery sequences can be performed more quickly (TR 1,500 compared with TR 2,000 for long TE/TR spin-echo sequence) than T2-weighted spin-echo sequences (13,17). Although STIR imaging increases lesion

conspicuity (18,24), it typically has lower signal-to-noise ratios than does spin-echo imaging and is also more susceptible to degradation by motion (18,20). Short TI inversion recovery imaging can be an adjunct in selective cases but should not replace conventional spin-echo sequences. Lesions are generally well seen on standard imaging, and in our opinion, STIR imaging tends to reduce the variations in signal intensities identified on conventional spin-echo MRI that are most helpful in tissue characterization.

Use of gadolinium as a contrast medium has been suggested to improve characterization of musculoskeletal neoplasms and for evaluating recurrence after surgery, radiation or chemotherapy (25–27). Some authors prefer T1-weighted sequences with and without gadolinium to the more conventional approach of using T1- and T2-weighted images (13). This would obviously reduce the examination time. Gadolinium diethylenetriamine pentaacetic acid (Gd-DTPA) produces increased signal intensity on T1-weighted spin-echo images because of the reduction in T1 relaxation time. Therefore, zones in neoplasms that show a marked increase in signal intensity correlate with highly vascular regions, whereas zones that show low intensity or no intensity are thought to be due to necrosis (13,28,29). These data suggest that gadolinium may be valuable in identifying the areas of viable tumor within a mass, which is useful in determining whether residual tumor is still present. In addition, this information can be useful for selecting biopsy sites (29). One should try to avoid areas of necrosis and biopsy to concentrate only on those areas more likely to contain viable tumors (13,25,26,29).

Early studies with gadolinium have suggested several techniques (static or dynamic using bolus injection and fast scan techniques) to evaluate enhancement rates, enhancement patterns, tumor volume, and other parameters. Results have been inconsistent and confusing, especially to radiologists who have learned morphologic tumor patterns that occur with specific lesions using conventional sequences (see Fig. 12-7) (13,28,29). Benedikt et al. (30) studied 30 patients with soft tissue masses (22 benign and 8 malignant). Eighty-seven percent of lesions enhanced after gadolinium. This occurred in 82% of benign and 100% of malignant lesions. The pattern of enhancement (homogeneous vs. inhomogeneous) was not useful for differentiating benign and malignant lesion (28,31). Dynamic studies using fast scan techniques were initially reported by Erlemann et al. (25,26). Others have also studied these techniques (28,29), but with inconsistent results. In our practice, we reserve the use of gadolinium for selected cases (see below) (see Fig. 12-8).

Spectroscopy or combined imaging and spectroscopic techniques have also been explored to improve lesion characterization and evaluate response to therapy (32,33). Spectroscopic techniques are not commonly used in most clinical settings. These techniques are summarized in Chapter 16.

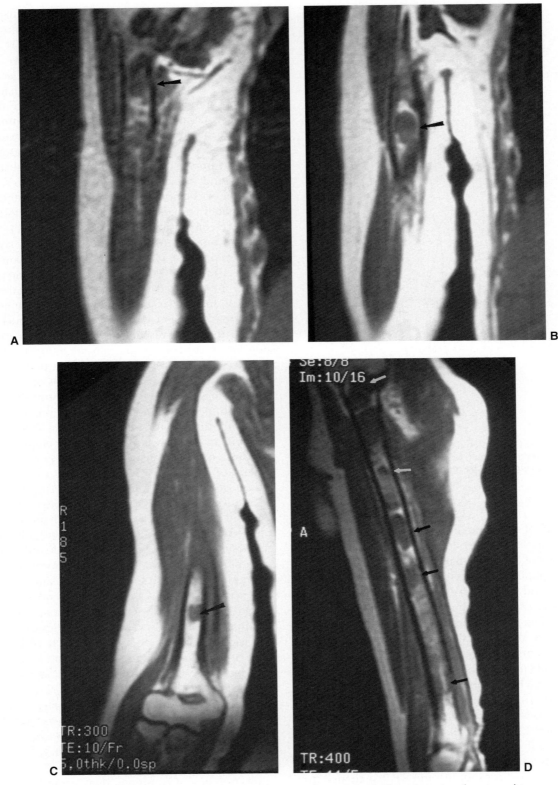

Figure 12-3 Middle-aged man with lymphoma and arm pain. A phased array coil was used to evaluate the right humerus. Coronal SE 427/11 images **(A–C)** do not include the entire structure on a single image plane. Diffuse involvement (*arrows*) is apparent when a sagittal image **(D)**, which shows the entire length of the humerus, is selected.

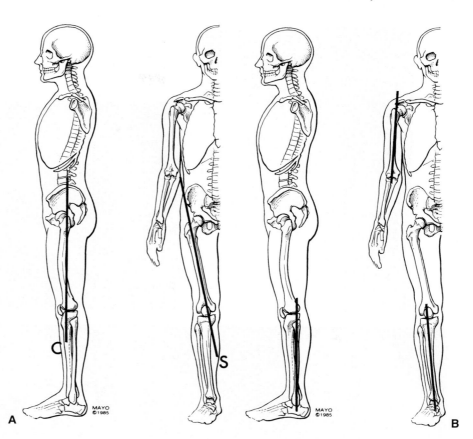

Figure 12-4 Skeletal illustrations demonstrating oblique planes required to accurately access the long bones. **A:** The femur is most easily evaluated in the oblique sagittal plane (*S*) due to the normal anterior bowing, which creates partial volume problems in the coronal plane (*C*). **B:** The oblique sagittal plane is also most useful for the humerus. Either the sagittal or coronal plane can be used for the tibia and fibula.

Limitations of Magnetic Resonance Imaging

An important limitation of MRI is its relative inability to detect soft tissue calcification (3,4,10,34,35); consequently, diagnoses that may be readily apparent on radiographs frequently remain nonspecific on MRI. As an additional caveat, Totty et al. (10) noted that MRI failed to demonstrate soft tissue gas in 1 of 32 patients being evaluated for a soft tissue mass. CT may be useful in specific instances to identify the presence and pattern of subtle

soft tissue mineralization and in those cases in which lesions are not adequately evaluated by radiographs (36). Although initial investigations maintained that CT is superior to MRI in detecting destruction of cortical bone (3,5,11), more recently it has been suggested that these two modalities are comparable in this regard (2,37).

It has also been our experience that nonmetallic foreign bodies may be difficult to identify on MRI. In such cases, MRI will show the changes associated with the foreign body, although the foreign body itself may have no signal

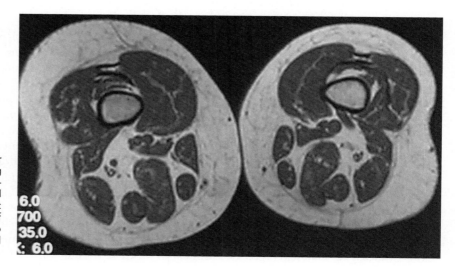

Figure 12-5 Lipomatosis of the right lower extremity in a 54-year-old woman presenting with "fullness" around the knee. Axial T1-weighted SE (700/16) MR image of both distal thighs shows increased adipose tissue on right as compared with contralateral side. Images of both distal thighs were obtained after no cause for clinical findings were found on axial images of right knee.

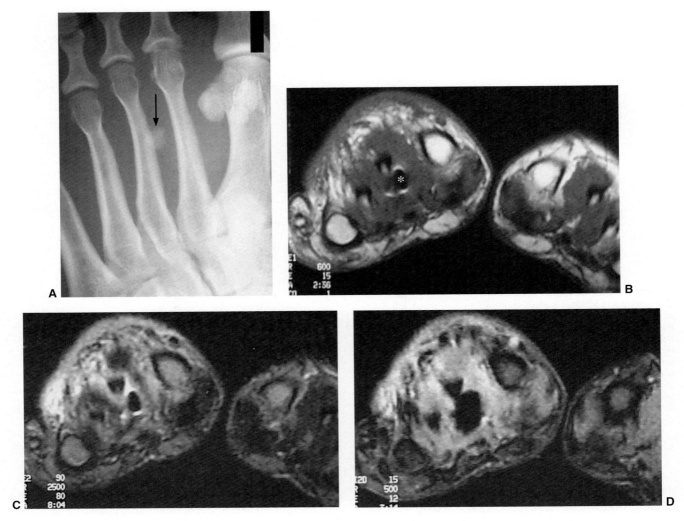

Figure 12-6 Foreign body and associated abscess in a 27-year-old woman. **A:** Oblique radiograph of foot shows irregular opacity (*arrow*) initially interpreted as calcification. **B:** Coronal T1-weighted (600/15, TR/TE) SE MR image shows prominent signal void (*asterisk*), with "parenthetical" artifact, compatible with foreign body. **C:** Corresponding conventional T2-weighted (2,500/80, TR/TE) SE MR image shows foreign body with associated inflammatory change. **D:** Gradient-echo (15/12/15 degrees, TR/TE/flip angle) image shows "blooming" due to greater magnetic susceptibility. (From Kransdorf MJ, Murphey MD. Radiologic evaluation of soft tissue masses: a current perspective. *AJR Am J Roentgenol* 2000;175:575–587.)

and may be difficult to identify. We have found ultrasound a useful adjunct in such cases (see Fig. 12-9) (38).

It must be emphasized that it is essential to interpret MR images in conjunction with appropriate corresponding radiographs (and other imaging studies, if available). Unbending adherence to this principle will minimize interpretive errors.

STAGING

Simply stated, the purpose of a staging system is to provide a standard manner in which to communicate readily the state of a malignancy, defining the local and distant tumor extent. Local staging is best accomplished using MRI, which

can accurately depict the anatomic spaces (compartments) involved by tumor (39). MRI provides valuable information regarding the extent of primary benign and malignant lesions and skeletal metastases. The staging process should include tabulation of clinical data (patient age, location of suspected lesion, type of symptoms) and, importantly, the review of routine radiographs and other imaging techniques. The main role of MRI in staging is to provide information on the extent of a musculoskeletal neoplasm using established standards.

It is essential that the staging process for musculoskeletal neoplasms is understood when evaluating MR images. Staging of skeletal neoplasms has been extensively reviewed by Enneking (40–42). Neoplasms are staged to evaluate risk of local recurrence and distant metastasis,

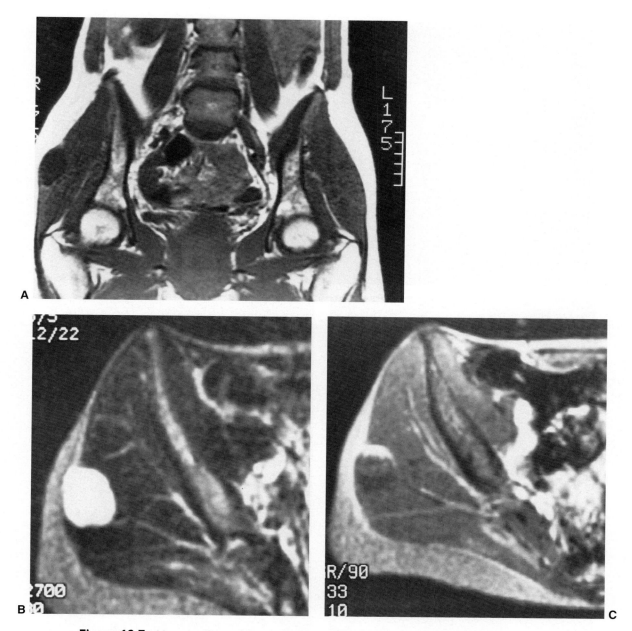

Figure 12-7 Myxoma. Coronal SE 500/20 **(A)** and axial SE 2,700/80 **(B)** images demonstrate a well-defined lesion with low intensity on T1-weighted **A** and high uniform signal intensity on T2-weighted **B** images. These features are characteristic of myxoma. After gadolinium injection **(C)**, the enhancement pattern is inhomogeneous and suggests a more aggressive lesion due to the irregular enhancement pattern.

select the optimal treatment method, and provide guidelines for adjunctive treatment planning (28,41,42). The staging system is based on histologic grading (G), site of tumor (T), and the presence of local or distant metastases (M) (Table 12-1). Low-grade histologic lesions are classified as G1 and high-grade lesions as G2. Tumors that are intracompartmental are considered T1. A tumor is classified as intracompartmental if it is bounded by natural barriers to extension such as bone, fascia, synovium, periosteum, and cartilage (see Figs. 12-10 and 12-11). Once extension

(tumor beyond compartment of origin) has occurred, the lesion is extracompartmental T2. On the basis of these two categories and the presence or absence of metastases, the Enneking classification divides malignant tumors into three different stages. Stage I lesions are low grade (G1) without metastases. These are categorized as A or B based on whether or not the lesion is intra- (T1) or extracompartmental (T2) (Table 12-2). Stage II lesions are high grade without metastases and again are classified as A or B depending on whether they are intra- or extracompartmental

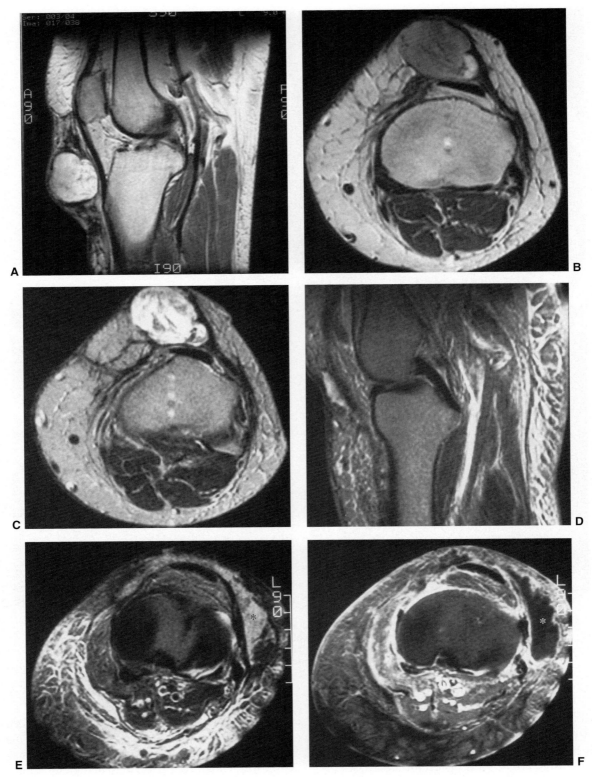

Figure 12-8 Sagittal SE 2,000/80 **(A)** and axial SE 2,000/80 **(B)** and SE 2,000/80 **(C)** images demonstrate an inhomogeneous lesion in the anterior knee. Surgically resected malignant fibrous histocytoma. Sagittal **(D)** and axial **(E)** SE 2,000/80 images 1 year later show an area of increased signal intensity (*asterisk*) anterolaterally. There is a large amount of edema due to radiation therapy. Postgadolinium image **(F)** shows peripheral enhancement with low intensity in the region of interest (*asterisk*) indicating a fluid collection and not a solid mass.

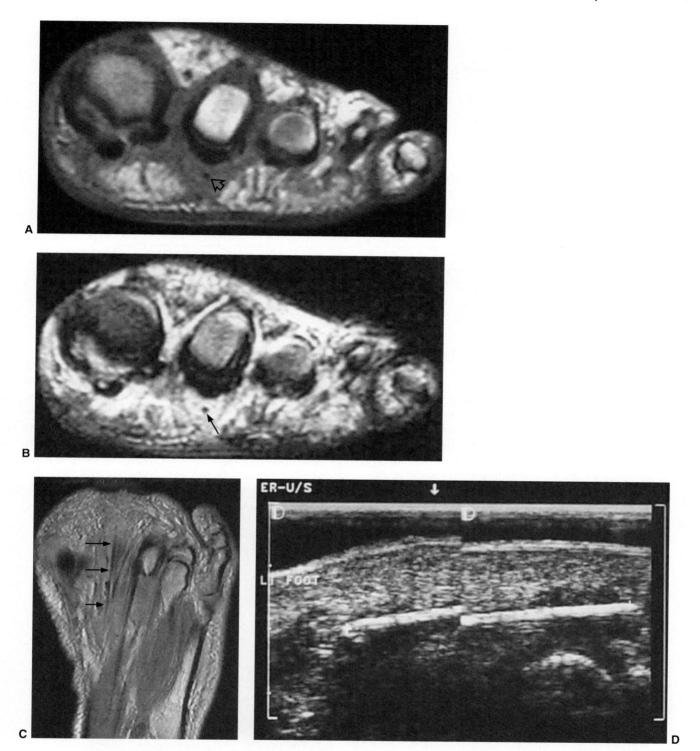

Figure 12-9 Toothpick foreign body in the foot of a 49-year-old woman. Coronal T1-weighted (700/20) SE **(A)** and T2-weighted (2,000/90) **(B)** SE MR images show poorly defined abnormal signal intensity with a small mass below the second toe. The small signal void within the mass is the tooth-pick foreign body (*arrow*). **C:** Axial proton (2,000/30) SE MR image shows the foreign body as a lin-ear signal void (*arrows*). **D:** Follow-up ultrasound shows the toothpick to better advantage.

TABLE 12-1

ENNEKING SYSTEM: STAGING OF MUSCULOSKELETAL NEOPLASMS

Stage	Grade	Site	Metastasis	MR Features
1A	G1	T1	No	Abnormal signal intensity confined to bone or soft tissue compartment
1B	G1	T2	No	Abnormal signal intensity extends beyond the compartment
IIA	G2	T1	No	Abnormal signal intensity with cortex or capsular involvement
IIB	G2	T2	No	Abnormal signal intensity extending beyond bone or compartment
IIIA	G1–G2	T1	Yes	As above with distant metastasis
IIIB	G1–G2	T2	Yes	As above with distant metastasis

G1, low grade; G2, high grade; T1, intracompartmental; T2, extracompartmental.
(Adapted from Berquist TH. Magnetic resonance imaging of musculoskeletal neoplasms. *Clin Orthop Relat Res* 1989;244:101–118; Berquist TH. *MRI of the musculoskeletal system*, 3rd ed. Philadelphia, PA: Lippincott-Raven 1996:735–840; Enneking WF. Staging of musculoskeletal neoplasms. *Skeletal Radiol* 2115;13:196–207; and Enneking WF, Spanier SS, Goodman MA. A system for surgical staging of musculoskeletal sarcoma. *Clin Orthop Relat Res* 1980;153:106–120.)

(see Fig. 12-12). Stage III lesions have either regional or distant metastases (Table 12-2).

Enneking (41) also devised a staging system for benign lesions based on the aggressiveness of the lesion. However, MR features of all lesions have not been thoroughly worked out at this time. Therefore, the staging system used for malignant lesions (Table 12-1) is currently most applicable.

Spanier et al. (44) evaluated the prognosis of stage IIB (high grade with cortical penetration) osteosarcomas. This study demonstrated a poor prognosis for lesions that penetrated the periosteum and involved two or more adjacent soft tissue structures (E6) (44). Tumors in groups E1 to E5 ranged from high grade with no periosteal involvement (E1) to those that involved the periosteum but only one adjacent structure (E5). The probability of disease-free survival was 49% at 5 years for the entire group of patients. Patients with E6 disease had a 17.6% 5-year survival and those who were not E6 a 79.8% 5-year survival (44). This

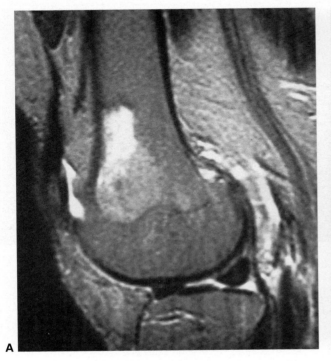

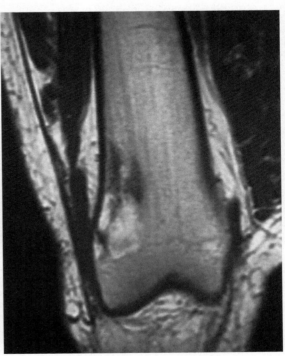

Figure 12-10 Sagittal **(A)** and coronal **(B)** SE 2,000/80 images of the distal femur in a patient with an intraosseous (T1) xanthoma.

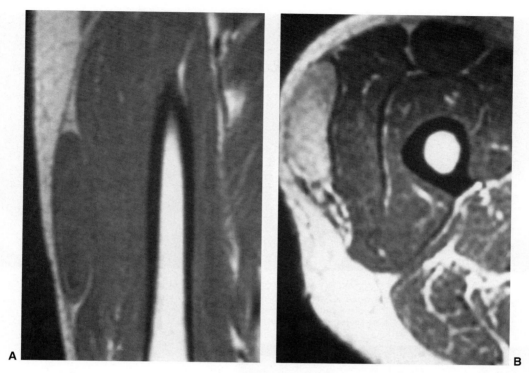

Figure 12-11 Coronal SE 500/20 **(A)** and axial SE 2,000/20 **(B)** image of an encapsulated myxoid sarcoma confined to the anterior compartment (T1).

study points out the importance of MRI in staging osseous and extraosseous tumor involvement (13,14,44).

SOFT TISSUE NEOPLASMS

Patients with a soft tissue tumor or tumorlike mass usually present with nonspecific clinical findings, such as soft tissue swelling or a discrete palpable mass, sometimes with accompanying tenderness or pain (1,45). When clinical findings are equivocal, however, imaging evaluation can confirm the presence of a soft tissue lesion or reassuringly identify a suspected "bump" or "mass" as normal tissue (see Fig. 12-13) or clearly distinguish it as nonneoplastic (see Fig. 12-14).

Initial Evaluation

Despite dramatic technologic advances in computer-assisted imaging, the radiologic evaluation of a suspected soft tissue mass must begin with the radiograph. Radiographs may be diagnostic of a palpable lesion caused by an underlying skeletal deformity (such as exuberant callus related to prior trauma) or bony exostosis that may masquerade as a soft tissue mass. Radiographs may also reveal the presence and nature of soft tissue calcifications, which can be suggestive and at times very characteristic of a specific diagnosis. For example, they may reveal the phleboliths within a hemangioma, the juxtaarticular osteocartilaginous masses of synovial osteochondromatosis, the peripherally more mature ossification of myositis ossificans, or the characteristic bone changes of other processes with associated soft tissue involvement (see Fig. 12-15).

In addition, plain radiographs are the best initial method of assessing coexistent bony involvement, such as osseous remodeling, periosteal reaction, or overt osseous destruction (45). Unlike its intraosseous counterpart,

TABLE 12-2	
STAGING SYSTEM FOR METASTASES	

Tumor sites

Intracompartmental (T1)	Extracompartmental (T2)
Intraosseous	Extraosseous extension
Intraarticular	Extraarticular extension
Intrafascial compartments	Extrafascial extension
Posterior calf	
Anterolateral leg	
Anterior thigh	
Posterior thigh, etc.	

Tumor grade

Low grade (G1)	High grade (G2)
Parosteal osteosarcoma	Classic osteosarcoma
Secondary chondrosarcoma	Paget sarcoma
Giant cell tumor	Malignant fibrous
Myxoid liposarcoma	Histiocytoma
Chondroma	Angiosarcoma
Adamantinoma	Neurofibrosarcoma

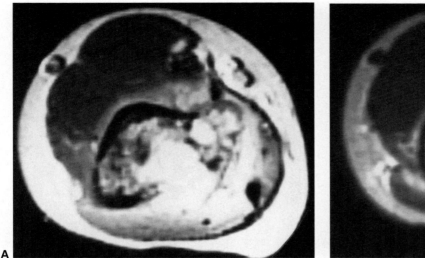
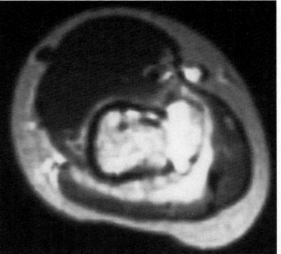

Figure 12-12   Axial SE 2,000/20 **(A)** and SE 2,000/80 **(B)** images of an aggressive osteosarcoma (E2) extending through the bone (T2) and involving more than two structures beyond the periosteum (stage IIB E6) (43). This distal humeral osteosarcoma has a poorer progress due to the extracompartmental extent. There were no distant metastases.

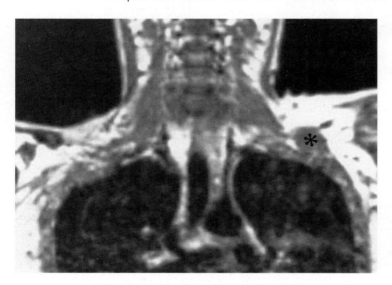

Figure 12-13   Surgically confirmed hypertrophied scalenus anterior muscle in a 35-year-old woman presenting with a palpable left supraclavicular mass. Coronal T1-weighted (700/20) SE MR image shows the lesion (*asterisk*) to image identical to skeletal muscle. Similar findings were seen on all pulse sequences.

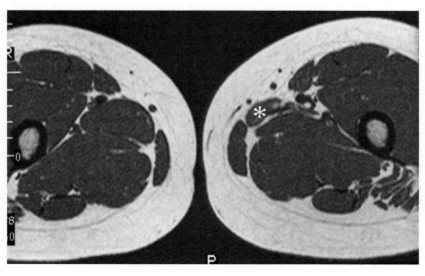

Figure 12-14   Atrophied adductor muscle in a 24-year-old woman presenting with soft tissue asymmetry, suggesting a soft tissue mass. Axial T1-weighted (600/16) SE MR image shows the marked atrophy to the left adductor longus muscle (*asterisk*). Atrophy was secondary to a previous muscle injury.

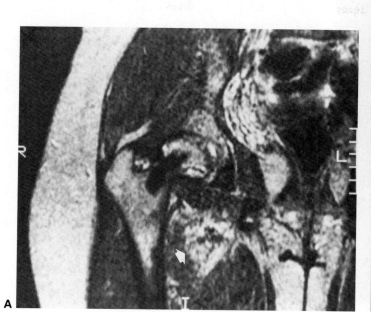 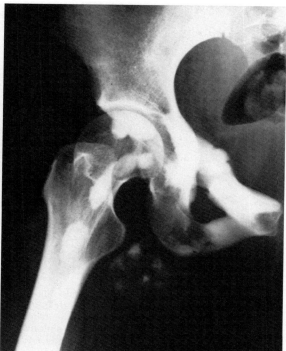

Figure 12-15 Melorheostosis in a 26-year-old woman presenting with hip pain and a soft tissue mass in the right groin. **A:** Coronal T2-weighted (2,000/80) SE MR image of the hip shows a heterogeneous nonspecific soft tissue mass (*arrow*). The lesion showed a signal intensity similar to skeletal muscle on corresponding T1-weighted image (not shown). An associated interosseous abnormality is noted in the proximal femur. **B:** Corresponding radiograph readily confirms the diagnosis of melorheostosis with soft tissue involvement.

however, the biologic activity of a soft tissue mass cannot be reliably assessed by its growth rate. A slow-growing soft tissue mass that may remodel adjacent bone (causing a scalloped area with well-defined sclerotic margins) may still be highly malignant on histologic examination (46).

A soft tissue mass may also be the initial presentation of a primary bone tumor or inflammatory process. In such cases, the radiograph may also be useful. The diagnosis of a malignant bone tumor, such as Ewing sarcoma or primary lymphoma of bone, should be considered when there is a large circumferential soft tissue mass in association with an underlying destructive bone lesion. A subtle radiologic feature that may be used to separate inflammatory and neoplastic processes is that inflammatory processes typically obliterate fascial planes rather than displace them.

Initial radiographs should be obtained with a low kilovoltage technique (i.e., less than 50 kV peak), thereby enhancing radiographic density differences between soft tissues such as fat and muscle (45).

Specific Diagnoses

Despite the superiority of MRI in identifying, delineating, and staging soft tissue tumors, it remains limited in its ability to precisely characterize soft tissue masses, with most lesions demonstrating prolonged T1 and T2 relaxation times

(47,48). There are instances, however, in which a specific diagnosis may be made or strongly suspected: lipoma; liposarcoma; benign vascular lesions such as hemangioma, arteriovenous malformation, and pseudoaneurysm; hemosiderin-laden lesions such as pigmented villonodular synovitis (PVNS); fibromatosis; subacute hematomas; and certain tumorlike lesions (19,49). Clearly, the percentage of cases in which MRI may correctly suggest the diagnosis will vary with the referral population (19). In general, a correct histologic diagnosis can be reached on the basis of imaging studies in approximately one fourth to one third of cases (19,35, 50,51). Significantly higher levels of accuracy may be achieved with common benign lesions and by using a systematic approach to evaluation.

Lipomatous Tumors

Lipoma

Soft tissue tumors are derived predominantly from primitive mesenchyme. Probably the most common mesenchymal tumor is lipoma, a benign tumor composed of mature adipose tissue. Patients with a soft tissue lipoma typically present in middle age (fifth and sixth decades). After an initial period of discernible growth, a lipoma usually stabilizes in size (52). A soft tissue lipoma is categorized by anatomic location as either superficial (cutaneous) or deep. The

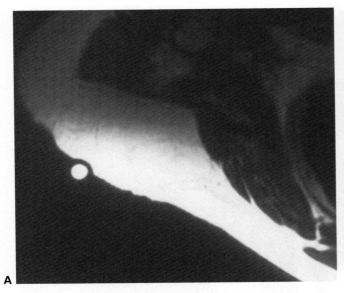

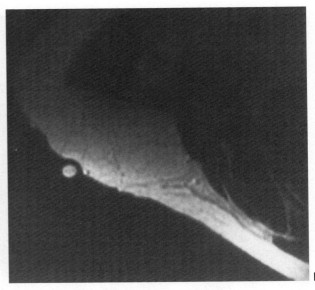

Figure 12-16 Superficial lipoma in the subcutaneous tissue of the shoulder of a 65-year-old woman. **A:** Axial T1-weighted (700/20) SE MR image of the right shoulder shows a poorly defined mass, imaging identical to subcutaneous fat. Such lesions may be inapparent on MRI unless a marker is placed over the palpable abnormality. **B:** Corresponding T2-weighted (2,000/80) SE MR also shows the lesion to image identical to subcutaneous fat.

superficial lipoma occurs more commonly and is more sharply circumscribed and smaller in size than its deep-seated counterpart. A superficial (subcutaneous) lipoma may be inapparent, blending in with the adjacent subcutaneous fat on MRI. Unless a marker is placed over the mass before imaging, it may appear only as a thickening of the subcutaneous fat (see Fig. 12-16). The deep-seated lipoma occurs most commonly in the retroperitoneum, chest wall, and deep soft tissue of the hands and feet. Retroperitoneal lipomas are relatively rare. Most large lipomatous retroperitoneal tumors are liposarcomas. The pathogenesis of a lipoma is unknown, although it is thought to represent a true mesenchymal neoplasm. It is usually a solitary lesion, although a small percentage of patients (5% to 7%) demonstrate multiple tumors, which can vary in number from a few to several hundred (53). A rare entity of familial multiple lipomas has also been reported (53–55). Interestingly, the fat within the lipoma is unavailable for systemic metabolism and, paradoxically, may actually increase in size during starvation (56).

Depending on the size and location of the lesion, the plain radiograph may be either unremarkable or demonstrate a mass of fat density. The lipoma is well characterized on MRI, with the lesion having an appearance identical to that of subcutaneous fat on all pulse sequences, without discernible enhancement after the administration of intravenous gadolinium (see Figs. 12-16 to 12-18) (4,25,57–63).

Lipomas occasionally contain other mesenchymal elements. The most common of these is fibrous connective

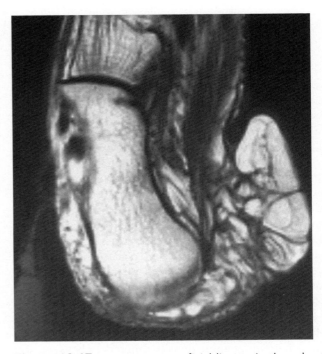

Figure 12-17 Recurrent superficial lipoma in the subcutaneous tissue of the heel in a 69-year-old woman. T1-weighted (600/15) SE MR image shows the mass to have a lobulated contour with a signal intensity identical to subcutaneous fat. The lesion has multiple linear septations of decreased signal intensity coursing through its substance. These showed a similar decreased signal intensity on T2-weighted images (not shown). They corresponded to fibrous tissue on histologic examination. Lesions such as these are often referred to as fibrolipoma.

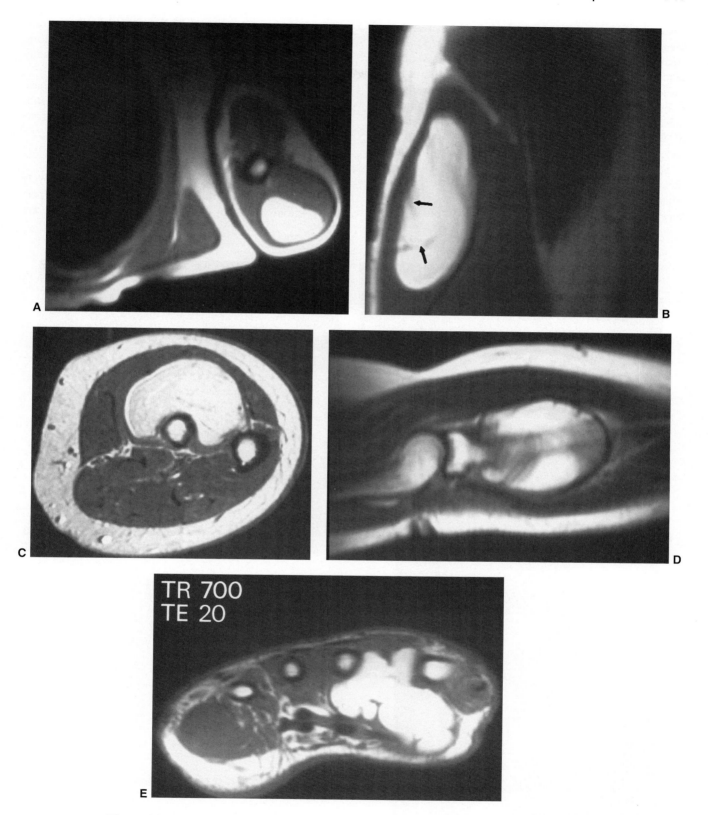

Figure 12-18 Benign lipomas, multiple patients. Axial SE 500/20 **(A)** and sagittal SE 2,000/60 **(B)** images of a benign lipoma in the proximal arm with well-defined fibrous septation (*arrows*). **C,D:** Axial SE 2,000/20 and sagittal SE 500/20 images of a benign lipoma in the supinator muscle. **E:** Axial T1 (700/20) SE MR image of a lobulated lipoma in the hand.

tissue, which may be in the configuration of septa and therefore appear as linear densities on CT (62,63) or linear areas of decreased signal on MRI, regardless of pulse sequence (see Fig. 12-17) (62,63). When significant fibrous tissue is present, these lesions may be termed fibrolipoma. It is important to remember that when a fatty lesion does not meet the imaging requirements for a lipoma, liposarcoma is typically the diagnosis of exclusion; however, lipoma variants are encountered more commonly than liposarcoma (64).

Soft tissue lipoma may be associated with changes in the skeleton. Cortical thickening may be seen in association with adjacent parosteal lipoma, and congenital osseous anomalies have been described adjacent to deep lipomas (65,66).

Chondroid or osseous metaplasia is occasionally encountered within a lipoma, particularly if the lipoma is long standing. The term "benign mesenchymoma" is occasionally used to describe this type of lesion (see Fig. 12-19).

A few cases of malignant transformation of lipoma have been reported, but these may represent cases where the subtle histologic features of malignancy were initially overlooked (46,67).

Intramuscular and Intermuscular Lipomas

Intramuscular and intermuscular lipomas are relatively common benign lipomatous tumors that arise, respectively, either within or between skeletal muscle. They are

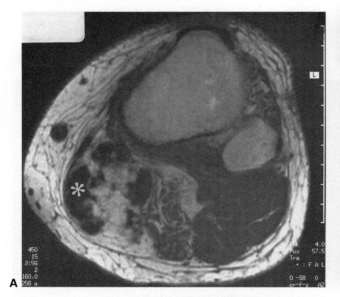
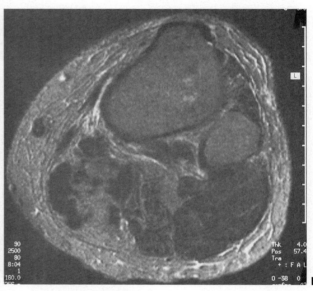
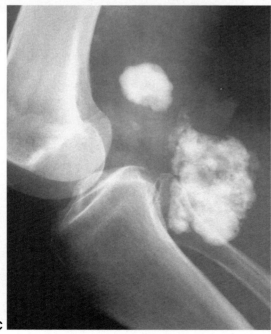

Figure 12-19 Benign mesenchymoma in the popliteal fossa of a 79-year-old man. **A:** Axial T1-weighted (450/15) SE MR image shows a fatty mass with a central region of markedly decreased signal intensity (*asterisk*). **B:** Corresponding T2-weighted (2,500/80) image shows similar findings. **C:** Radiograph shows densely mineralized mass.

members of a subgroup of lesions referred to as "lipomatous tumors" in which the fatty mass is intimately associated with specific nonadipose tissue. The remaining members of this subgroup of lesions are uncommon and include lipoma of the tendon sheath and joint, and lipomatosis of nerve (67,68). Although it arises within the muscle, intramuscular lipoma may actually involve both muscular and intermuscular tissue; however, involvement isolated to the intermuscular region (intermuscular lipoma) is less common. Intramuscular lipoma occurs in patients of all ages but predominantly in adults, with most presenting in patients between 30 and 60 years of age (46). There is a slight male predominance. Patients typically present with a mass in the large muscles of the extremities, especially the thigh, shoulder, and upper arm. The fat within the intramuscular lipoma may infiltrate between skeletal muscle fibers, giving the intramuscular lipoma a striated appearance on gross inspection.

Radiographs may reveal an intramuscular mass of fat density. An intramuscular lipoma may be identified on MRI as a predominantly fatty mass (with signal intensity equal to that of the subcutaneous fat), infiltrating the adjacent skeletal muscle. The mass is usually well defined and sharply circumscribed, with imaging characteristics similar to that of an "ordinary lipoma." This lesion has also been referred to as "infiltrating lipoma." Despite being well defined radiologically, margins are frequently infiltrating at microscopy, with adipose tissue intermingled with skeletal muscle fibers that are variably atrophic (see Figs. 12-20 and 12-21). Matsumoto et al. (69) reported the MR appearance

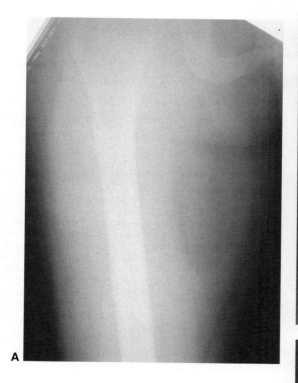

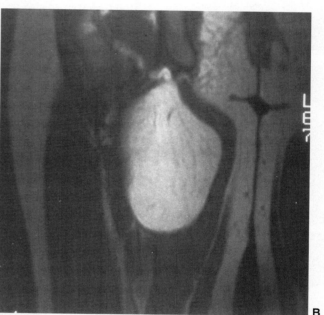

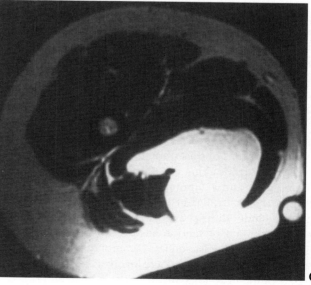

Figure 12-20 Intramuscular lipoma in the thigh of a 29-year-old woman. **A:** Anteroposterior radiograph shows a fat density mass in the medial aspect of the proximal right thigh. **B:** Corresponding coronal T1-weighted (650/20) SE MR image shows the signal intensity of the mass to be identical to that of the subcutaneous fat. **C:** Axial T1-weighted (500/20) localizes the mass to the adductor compartment.

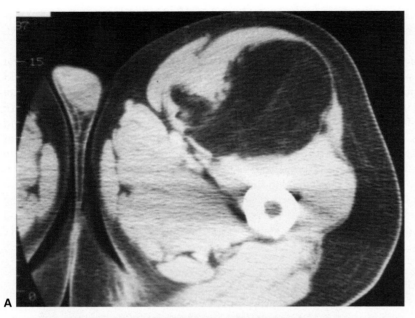

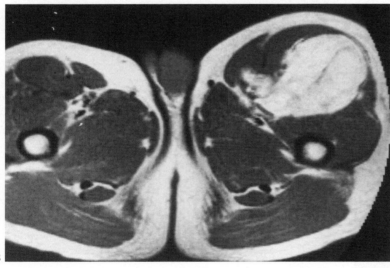

Figure 12-21 Intramuscular lipoma in the thigh of a 50-year-old man. **A:** Axial CT shows a fatty mass in the anterior aspect of the left thigh. There are some small areas of increased attenuation within the lesion. **B:** Corresponding axial T1-weighted (800/20) SE MR image nicely shows the fatty nature of the mass. The area of increased attenuation on CT on the medial aspect of the mass images identical to skeletal muscle and is compatible with muscle infiltrating the margin of the lesion. Similar findings were seen on T2-weighted images (not shown).

of intramuscular lipoma in 17 cases and found the lesion to be homogeneously pure fatty tissue in 12 (71%), with the remainder being fat with intermingled muscle fibers, the latter showing a signal intensity identical to that of skeletal muscle on T1 and T2-weighted pulse sequences. An infiltrative margin was seen in seven cases (41%).

Lipoma of Tendon Sheath and Joint

There are two variants of these rare tumors: a discrete solid fatty mass that extends along the affected tendon or within the affected joint and a "lipomalike" lesion composed of hypertrophic synovial villi distended with fat. Synonyms for the latter include diffuse synovial lipoma or lipoma arborescens. Lipoma of tendon sheath most commonly arises in the hand and wrist and less commonly in the ankle and foot. Lipoma arborescens usually involves the knee (70). About 20% of the time, knee involvement is bilateral (71).

Although it may arise *de novo*, it is frequently associated with degenerative joint disease, chronic rheumatoid arthritis, or prior trauma involving the affected joint (70). It may be a reactive process related to chronic synovitis. Lipoma arborescens of the subacromial–subdeltoid bursa has been reported in association with rotator cuff tear (72). Although all these lesions are rare, the lipoma arborescens form of synovial lipoma is encountered more frequently than the discrete form of synovial lipoma.

Radiologically, a lipoma of tendon sheath or discrete synovial lipoma is a focal lipomatous mass, similar to a superficial or deep lipoma. Patients afflicted with the lipoma arborescens form of synovial lipoma present with soft tissue swelling around the knee, which may or may not be radiolucent on plain radiographs (70). MRI examples of lipoma arborescens are rare, but limited experience has shown a fatty proliferation of the synovium with an associated joint

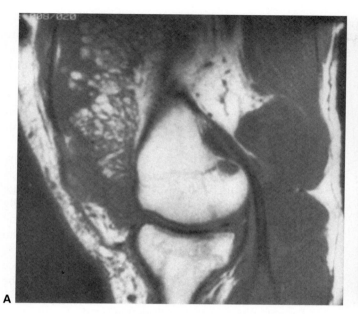
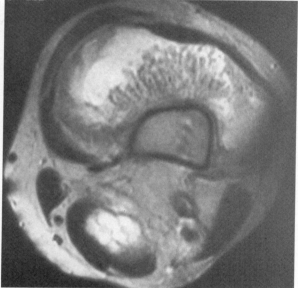

Figure 12-22   Lipoma arborescens in a 58-year-old man. Sagittal T1-weighted (427/20) **(A)** and axial T2-weighted (2,000/80) **(B)** SE MR images show a large joint effusion with fat in a frondlike pattern, representing the synovial villi, distended with adipocytes.

effusion (see Fig. 12-22). Osseous erosions at the articular margins have been reported in up to 38% of cases, associated synovial cysts are seen in 25%, and degenerative change in 13% (71).

Neural Fibrolipoma

Fibrofatty enlargement of the median nerve was initially described in English literature in 1953, with the presentation of two cases to the American Society for Surgery of the Hand (73). This lesion has been reported under a variety of names, which include neural fibrolipoma, fibrolipomatous hamartoma of nerve, perineural lipoma, fatty infiltration of the nerve, and intraneural lipoma (73,74). Currently, the term "neural fibrolipoma" is generally preferred because it better describes the underlying pathology (73). The cause of this disorder remains unclear; it may be related to hypertrophy of mature fat and fibroblasts in the epineurium (74).

Patients with neural fibrolipoma typically present during early adulthood with a soft slowly enlarging mass occurring in the volar aspect of the hand, wrist, or forearm (74). The lower extremity is involved much less frequently (4% to 22% of cases) (75,76). The lesion is typically present at birth or presents within the first 2 years of life (75,76). There is no familial predisposition (74). Approximately 80% of upper extremity lesions originate in the distribution of the median nerve (75,76). Accompanying symptoms include pain, tenderness, decreased sensation, and paresthesia. Carpal tunnel syndrome may be a late symptom (77). Patients may demonstrate macrodactyly (76,78), referred to as macrodystrophia lipomatosa, usually involving the second and third digits of the hand or foot. Macrodactyly was noted in 7 of 26

(27%) cases reported by Silverman and Enzinger (74) and 12 of 18 (67%) lesions reported by Amadio et al. (75). Multiple digits may be involved. Surgical excision is not without risk, and motor and sensory deficits have been reported after resection (77,79).

Grossly, the lesion is described as a fusiform, sausagelike enlargement of the nerve by fibrofatty tissue (74), appearing as a tan yellow mass within the nerve sheath (79). Microscopy demonstrates infiltration of the epineurium and perineurium by fibrofatty tissue (74). Cases in which there is macrodactyly are histologically indistinguishable from those in which there is no macrodactyly (74).

Radiographs of patients with macrodystrophia lipomatosa demonstrate both bone and soft tissue abnormalities. The phalanges are long, broad, and often splayed at their distal ends. The osseous overgrowth may be marked and disproportionately large with extensive secondary degenerative change (see Fig. 12-23) (80). The MR appearance of the nerve is characteristic, reflecting the morphology of the lesion. MRI will demonstrate small longitudinally oriented cylindrical areas, approximately 3 mm in diameter. These cylindrical areas demonstrate a decreased signal intensity on a background of increased signal intensity, thought to represent the nerve fascicles with epineural and perineural fibrosis on a background of fatty tissue (see Fig. 12-24) (79). The amount of fat present varies; however, it tends to be more prominent between the nerve fibers rather than surrounding them peripherally (81).

Amadio et al. (75) reviewed the Mayo Clinic institutional experience with macrodactyly from 1950 to 1985. Neural fibrolipoma was the most common condition associated with macrodactyly of the upper extremity, seen in 10

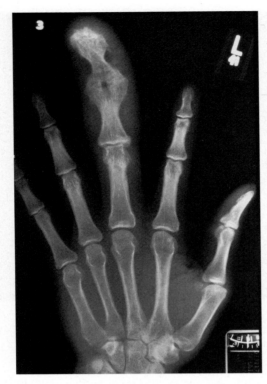

Figure 12-23 Macrodystrophia lipomatosa in the middle finger of a 26-year-old man. The hand demonstrates abnormalities of both bone and soft tissue. The phalanges are long, broad, and splayed at their distal ends. The osseous overgrowth is marked and disproportionately large with extensive secondary degenerative change.

of 22 cases. Other lesions included five vascular cases, five idiopathic cases, and two cases of neurofibromatosis. In contradistinction, it was noted that neural fibrolipoma was the least common cause associated with macrodactyly of the lower extremity, being identified in 1 of 43 cases. In the remaining cases, the cause was vascular in ten, neurofibromatosis in one, and idiopathic in the remaining cases (82). In this study, idiopathic cases were defined as those patients with no stigmata of neurofibromatosis or congenital malformation. The authors also noted nine cases of hemihypertrophy. The differential diagnosis of localized gigantism would also include Proteus syndrome (83).

Parosteal Lipoma

Parosteal lipoma is an unusual lesion that represents about 0.3% of all lipomas (60,66). The lesion was originally described as a "periosteal lipoma" by Seering (84) in 1966, with the term "parosteal lipoma" subsequently suggested by Power (85) to indicate that the lesion does not arise within the periosteum. The term "parosteal lipoma" is generally accepted over periosteal lipoma because the former indicates the juxtaposition of the lesion to the surface of the bone without identifying the tissue of origin (60). Patients are usually adults with an

average age of approximately 50 years (range, 4 to 64 years). There is a male predilection (60,86). Lesions are most common in the thigh, forearm, calf, and arm adjacent to the diaphysis or metadiaphysis of bone (60,86). Virtually all lesions are singular, with the exception of a case reported by Goldman et al. (60) in which there was a coincident intramuscular lipoma. Patients typically present with a painless soft tissue mass. Muscle atrophy is not uncommon (86).

Lesions are encapsulated and adherent to the underlying periosteum (86). Histologically, a parosteal lipoma is identical to a superficial or deep lipoma (60). Cartilage and bone metaplasia may be present. Cartilage is typically hyaline, but small foci of fibrocartilage may be seen at the periphery of large osseous excrescences (86). The septa seen within the lesion contain fibrovascular tissue (86). At the point of attachment there may be a bony excrescence or cortical thickening. The cortical thickening is likely to be secondary to tugging on the periosteum.

Radiographs reveal a well-defined radiolucent mass (60,86). Variable fibrovascular septa may be present within the mass (86). The adjacent bone may demonstrate solid periosteal reaction, cortical thickening, saucerization, or osseous excrescences (60,86). Osseous changes are seen in 67% to 100% of cases (60,86,87), although these may be subtle. The periosteal reaction in two cases reported by Murphey et al. (86) was minimal, being identified only on magnification radiography. The osseous excrescences do not demonstrate the cortical and medullary continuity or hyaline cartilaginous cap seen with a true osteochondroma (60).

MRI demonstrates the fatty nature of the mass with a signal intensity identical to that of subcutaneous fat on all pulse sequences. Fibrovascular tissue septa may demonstrate an increased signal intensity on long TR images, as may hyaline cartilage, which may also be found within lesions (86). In addition, MRI can identify muscle atrophy as increased striations of fat within muscle (see Fig. 12-25).

Lipomatosis

Diffuse lipomatosis is an entity characterized by diffuse overgrowth of mature adipose tissue infiltrating through the soft tissues of an affected extremity or body trunk. Microscopically, this lesion is indistinguishable from lipoma or intramuscular lipoma (see Fig. 12-26).

Patients affected with lipomatosis usually present during the early years of life, often by age 2, although there have been scattered reports of presentation in adulthood (46,88). Coode et al. (88) noted that the designation of diffuse congenital lipomatosis has been suggested on the assumption that adult cases represent delayed presentation. Diffuse lipomatosis typically affects the limbs, although involvement of the trunk and chest wall may be seen (88). Lipomatosis may be associated with coexistent osseous hypertrophy, but unlike macrodystrophia lipomatosa, the nerve is unaffected and the disease is not confined to an extremity. Reported as rare (46), we believe that

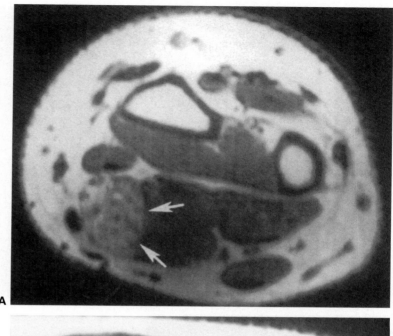

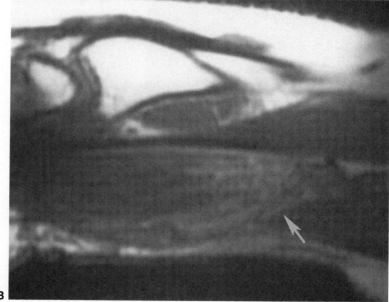

Figure 12-24 Neural fibrolipoma of the median nerve of a 36-year-old woman. Axial **(A)** and sagittal **(B)** T1-weighted SE MR images demonstrate small longitudinally oriented cylindrical areas of decreased signal intensity (*arrows*) on a background of increased signal intensity, representing the nerve fascicles with epineural and perineural fibrosis on a background of fatty tissue.

mild cases of lipomatosis are not uncommon and may be easily overlooked (Fig. 12-5).

Lipomatosis may be distinguished from the rare symmetric lipomatosis, which is also known as Madelung disease or benign symmetric lipomatosis. Symmetric lipomatosis is seen almost exclusively in middle-aged men, often, though not always, with a history of alcoholism or liver disease (89). In such cases, the masses may appear suddenly and grow rapidly, infiltrating the neck and extending into the axilla or extending into the back (89). The growth rate is irregular, and the lesion may cease to grow spontaneously or become intermittently quiescent (89). Involvement may occur in the groin as well (see Fig. 12-27) (89).

Liposarcoma

Liposarcoma is the second most common soft tissue sarcoma encountered in adults, accounting for 16% to 18% of all malignant soft tissue tumors (46). Liposarcomas are classified into four histologic subtypes: well differentiated, myxoid, pleomorphic, and dedifferentiated (46). The well-differentiated variant is considered to be a low-grade malignancy, whereas the pleomorphic and dedifferentiated types are considered to be high grade, with a high rate of local recurrence and metastasis. While the round cell liposarcoma was previously identified as distinct subtypes by the World Health Organization Classification of Soft Tissue Tumors,

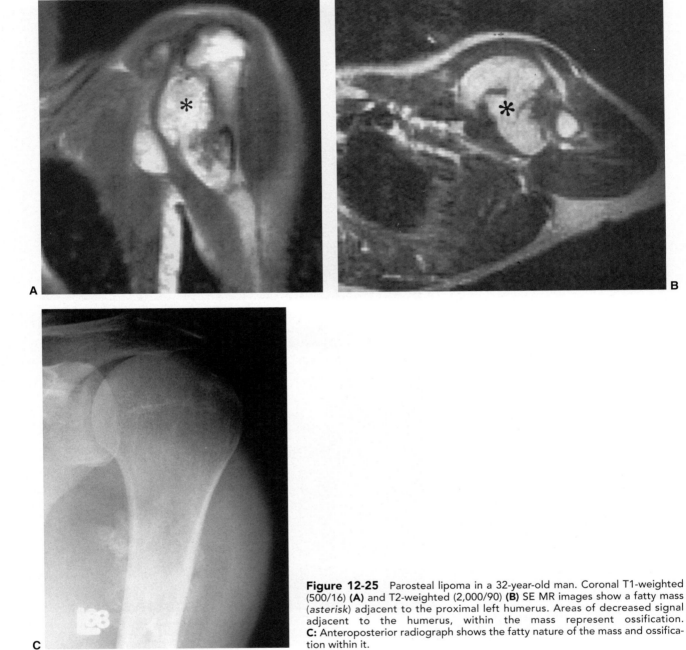

Figure 12-25 Parosteal lipoma in a 32-year-old man. Coronal T1-weighted (500/16) **(A)** and T2-weighted (2,000/90) **(B)** SE MR images show a fatty mass (*asterisk*) adjacent to the proximal left humerus. Areas of decreased signal adjacent to the humerus, within the mass represent ossification. **C:** Anteroposterior radiograph shows the fatty nature of the mass and ossification within it.

the myxoid and round-cell liposarcoma are now combined under the designation of myxoid liposarcoma (68). These lesions were known to form a histological continuum, and represented the ends of a common spectrum (52). Now under a single diagnosis, the pure myxoid lesion is considered an intermediate grade tumor at the low-grade end of this spectrum, while the hypercellular (round cell) morphology represents the histologically similar, high-grade counterpart. The presence of the hypercellular (round cell) component is associated with a more aggressive clinical course and a significantly worse prognosis

(90). Well-differentiated liposarcomas are most common, accounting for about 54% of all classified liposarcomas. Myxoid liposarcoma is next most common, accounting for 28%, followed by dedifferentiated (10%), and pleomorphic liposarcoma (91). Liposarcomas tend to occur in both the retroperitoneum and extremities, with extremity lesions presenting about 10 years earlier than those in the retroperitoneum. Dedifferentiated liposarcomas are most common in the retroperitoneum, whereas the other subtypes are more common in the extremities (91).

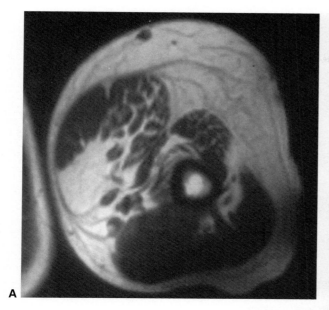

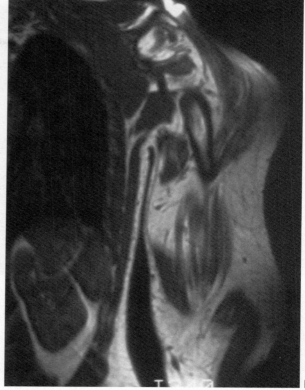

Figure 12-26 Upper extremity lipomatosis in a 23-year-old man. Axial **(A)** and coronal T1-weighted (427/20) **(B)** SE MR images of the left upper extremity show diffuse overgrowth of adipose tissue.

On MRI, a well-differentiated (lipomalike) liposarcoma will image as a predominantly fatty mass with irregularly thickened linear or nodular septa, which demonstrates a nonspecific decreased signal on T1-weighted and increased signal on T2-weighted spin-echo images (see Figs. 12-28 to 12-30) (92,93). Although a lipoma that is completely homogeneous and images identical to fat may be easily distinguished from a well-differentiated liposarcoma, lipoma variants occur with an imaging appearance that will overlap that of a well-differentiated liposarcoma. The distinction of lipoma and well-differentiated liposarcoma is simple when the former is homogeneous with an imaging

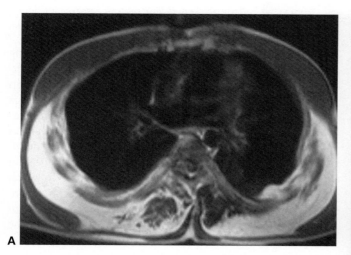

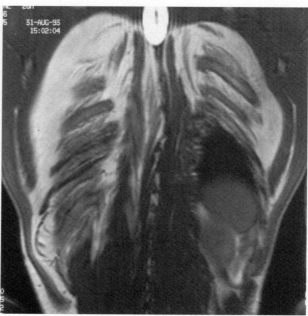

Figure 12-27 Symmetric lipomatosis in a 28-year-old man. Axial T1-weighted (775/20) **(A)** and coronal T1-weighted (700/15) **(B)** SE MR images show extensive, but symmetric, involvement of the chest wall.

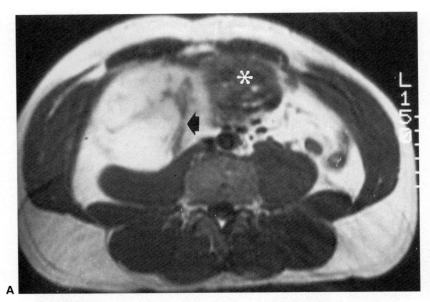

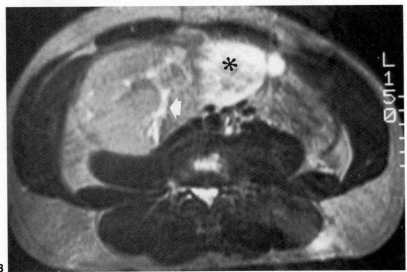

Figure 12-28 Retroperitoneal well-differenti-ated liposarcoma in a 50-year-old man. Axial T1-weighted (600/20) **(A)** and T2-weighted (2,500/80) **(B)** SE MR images show a predominantly fatty retroperitoneal mass. The mass does not meet the criteria for a lipoma, containing nonspecific irregu-larly thickened linear septa (*arrow*). Incidental note is made of a pelvic kidney (*asterisk*).

appearance identical to that of the subcutaneous adipose tissue. When nonadipose elements are present, however, this distinction may be quite problematic. Recent literature has documented a wider spectrum for the imaging features of lipoma than had been previously appreciated, with a small but significant number of lipomas demonstrating prominent nonadipose areas and an imaging and appear-ance that may mimic that traditionally ascribed to well-differentiated liposarcoma (91). In these cases, the non-adipose areas represent fat necrosis and associated calci-fication, fibrosis, inflammation, and myxoid change. As a generalization, lesion size may also be useful, in that well-differentiated liposarcoma tends to be significantly larger than lipoma. In a recent review of 60 well-differentiated fatty tumors, the average largest dimension of malignant lesions was nearly twice that of benign lipomas (24 cm vs. 13 cm) (91). Enhancement pattern may also be useful, with well-differentiated tumors showing contrast enhancement (94).

The dedifferentiated liposarcoma is a rare, interesting variant of the well-differentiated liposarcoma. A "dediffer-entiated" sarcoma is best defined as a bimorphic neoplasm in which a borderline or low-grade malignant neoplasm is juxtaposed with a high-grade histologically different sar-coma (95,96). Although the concept of dedifferentiation was initially described in chondrosarcoma, the term "dedif-ferentiated liposarcoma" was introduced by Evans (95) in 1979 to describe a histologically distinctive lesion in which a well-differentiated liposarcoma is juxtaposed with a high-grade sarcoma, such as a malignant fibrous histiocytoma or fibrosarcoma. Dedifferentiated liposarcoma is probably the most common of all the dedifferentiated sarcomas, with up to half of the deeply situated liposarcomas demonstrating this phenomenon (96). Dedifferentiated liposarcoma occurring outside of the mediastinum, retroperitoneum, or inguinal regions (the inguinal regions can be considered to be an extension of the retroperitoneum) is, however, quite

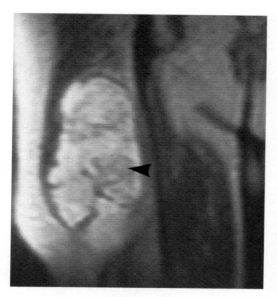

Figure 12-29 Low-grade liposarcoma seen on coronal SE 500/20 image. The tumor is primarily fatty with areas of low signal intensity (*arrowhead*) scattered throughout the lesion.

rare. Although the different types of liposarcoma cannot be reliably distinguished with imaging studies, a well-defined nonlipomatous mass juxtaposed with a predominantly fatty tumor is suggestive of a dedifferentiated liposarcoma (see Figs. 12-31 and 12-32) (97).

Currently, an atypical well-differentiated lipomatous tumor of the extremity is often termed either an atypical lipoma or a well-differentiated liposarcoma. Atypical lipomas and well-differentiated liposarcomas are essentially histologically indistinguishable, and the term "atypical lipoma" has been advocated by some to spare the patient a malignant diagnosis and prevent unnecessary radical surgery for well-differentiated lipomatous tumors of the extremity. However, other investigators prefer the term "well-differentiated liposarcoma" for deep fatty tumors of the extremities because of the propensity of these tumors to recur and because of the remote possibility of dedifferentiation, either *de novo* or in recurrences. One could theoretically categorize both atypical lipoma and well-differentiated liposarcoma as atypical lipomatous tumors, because both have a propensity to recur locally but no tendency to metastasize (95). Lesions with similar histology in the retroperitoneum have retained the designation of well-differentiated liposarcoma because of their association with multiple local recurrences (presumably because they are frequently incompletely resected) and because such lesions may eventually be fatal (98–101).

Accordingly, the new World Health Organization Classification of Tumors notes atypical lipomatous tumor and well-differentiated liposarcoma are identical morphologically and karyotypically, and recommends that the term "well-differentiated liposarcoma" be retained for

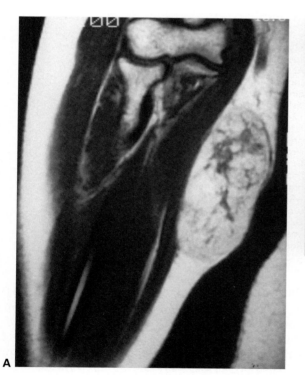

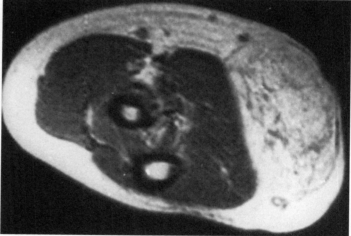

Figure 12-30 Well-differentiated liposarcoma of the upper extremity in a 34-year-old woman. **A:** Coronal T1-weighted (600/20) SE MR image of the forearm shows a fatty subcutaneous mass. The mass is predominantly fatty but shows linear and globular areas of nonfatty tissue within it. **B:** Axial T2-weighted (2,000/80) image shows linear areas of nonfatty tissue, although these are not as conspicuous as that seen in **A**. This is the type of lesion sometimes referred to as an atypical lipoma.

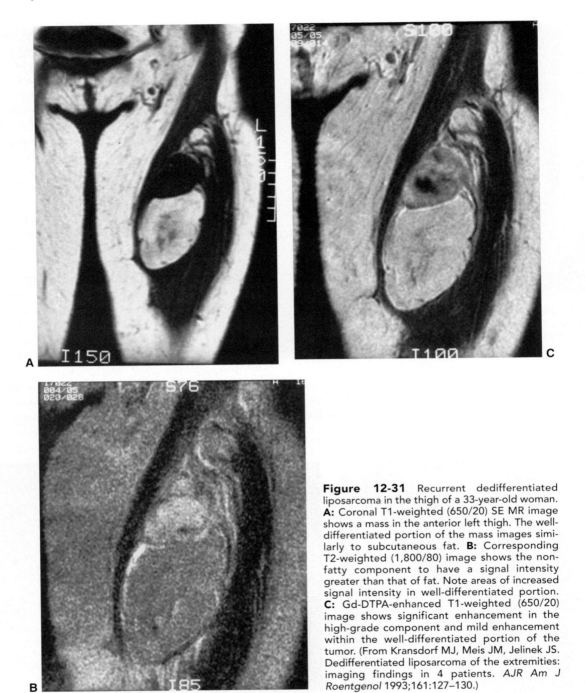

Figure 12-31 Recurrent dedifferentiated liposarcoma in the thigh of a 33-year-old woman. **A:** Coronal T1-weighted (650/20) SE MR image shows a mass in the anterior left thigh. The well-differentiated portion of the mass images similarly to subcutaneous fat. **B:** Corresponding T2-weighted (1,800/80) image shows the non-fatty component to have a signal intensity greater than that of fat. Note areas of increased signal intensity in well-differentiated portion. **C:** Gd-DTPA-enhanced T1-weighted (650/20) image shows significant enhancement in the high-grade component and mild enhancement within the well-differentiated portion of the tumor. (From Kransdorf MJ, Meis JM, Jelinek JS. Dedifferentiated liposarcoma of the extremities: imaging findings in 4 patients. *AJR Am J Roentgenol* 1993;161:127–130.)

lesions located at sites at which a wide surgical margin cannot be obtained (68). Such sites include the retroperitoneum and mediastinum (68). Although there is no agreement on the terminology for lesions in the deep somatic soft tissues, we would agree with Weiss and Goldblum and use the term "atypical lipoma" only for subcutaneous extremity lesions, reserving the term "well-differentiated liposarcoma" for lesions with similar histologies in all remaining sites (46,52).

The myxoid, pleomorphic, and round-cell liposarcomas often do not contain substantial amounts of fat, and only approximately 50% to 80% will demonstrate fat radiologically (see Figs. 12-32 to 12-34) (9,102,103). When fat is present, it is usually in a lacy, amorphous, clumplike, or linear pattern (see Fig. 12-35) (48,103–105). The pleomorphic and round-cell types are more heterogeneous. Myxoid liposarcoma is typically more homogeneous and may appear deceptively benign on MRI, and an appearance

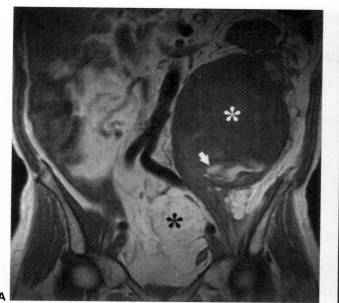

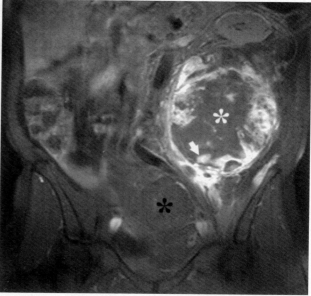

Figure 12-32   Dedifferentiated liposarcoma in the retroperitoneum of a 74-year-old man. Coronal T1-weighted (549/12) **(A)** and postcontrast fat-suppressed coronal T1-weighted (757/12) **(B)** SE MR images show a large mass (*white asterisk*) with a juxtaposed poorly defined predominantly fatty component (*black asterisk*). Note central nonenhancing area in **B** (*asterisk*). Area of high signal intensity inferiorly (*arrow*) represents subacute blood, in keeping with previous hemorrhage and necrosis. Also note superior displacement of kidney.

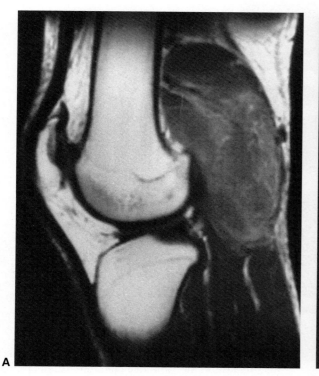

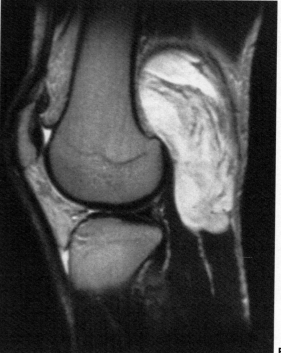

Figure 12-33   Myxoid liposarcoma in the popliteal fossa of a 22-year-old man. Sagittal T1-weighted (650/20) **(A)** and T2-weighted (1,800/80) **(B)** SE MR images show linear and amorphous fatty areas within an otherwise nonspecific mass.

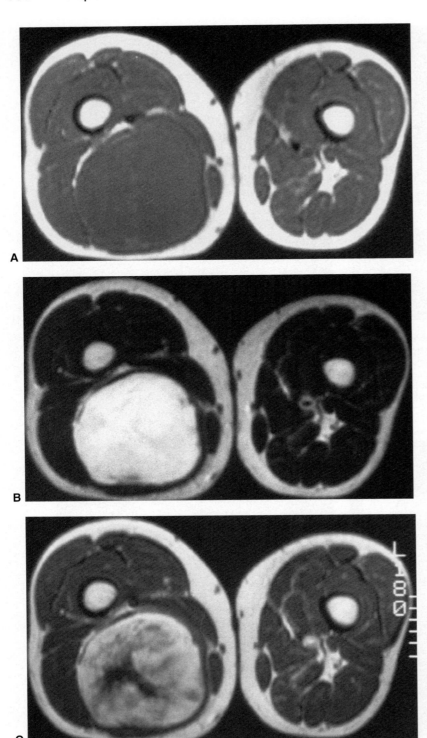

Figure 12-34 Myxoid liposarcoma in the posterior thigh of a 49-year-old man. Axial T1-weighted (600/15) **(A)** and T2-weighted (3,000/102) **(B)** SE MR images show a nonspecific mass in the posterior right thigh. **C:** Corresponding T1-weighted image after Gd-DTPA administration shows marked enhancement.

similar to that of a cyst has been reported in as many as 20% of cases (see Fig. 12-36) (35,57,102,106).

Lipoblastoma

The "ordinary" lipoma is overwhelmingly the most frequently encountered fatty soft tissue tumor; however, there are numerous lipoma variants. Although these variants are

well described in the pathology literature, they have received scant attention in the radiology literature. These lipoma variants differ from the classic soft tissue lipoma with regard to both clinical presentation and microscopic appearance. Lipoblastoma is a relatively immature cellular lipoma that occurs almost exclusively in infancy and early childhood, usually in children under 3 years of age; however, rare cases

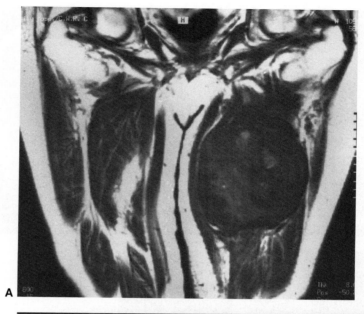

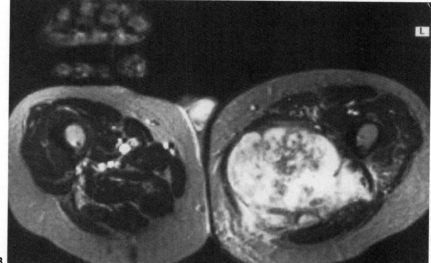

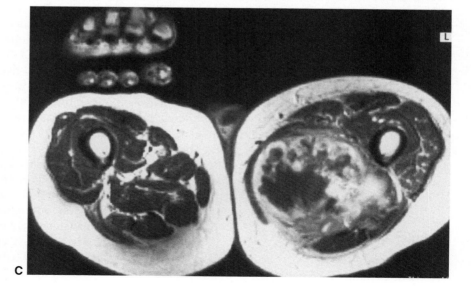

Figure 12-35 Pleomorphic liposarcoma in the posterior thigh of an 85-year-old man. **A:** Coronal T1-weighted (600/15) SE MR image shows a large inhomogeneous mass with central areas of increased signal intensity. **B:** Axial T2-weighted (2,500/90) SE MR image is very inhomogeneous, but otherwise nonspecific. **C:** Corresponding axial T1-weighted image after Gd-DTPA administration shows marked irregular peripheral enhancement.

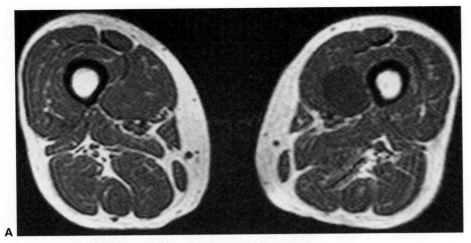

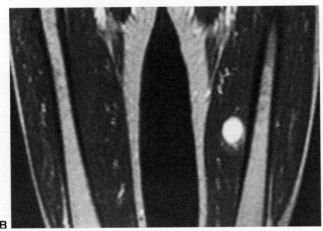

Figure 12-36   Myxoid liposarcoma in the thigh of a 56-year-old woman. Axial T1-weighted (650/20) **(A)** and T2-weighted (2000/80) **(B)** SE MR images show a round well-defined lesion in the medial aspect of the left thigh. The lesion has imaging characteristics identical to a cyst.

have been reported in adults (107–110). Most lipoblastomas are situated in the superficial soft tissue or subcutis of the extremities, although they have also been reported in the neck, trunk, perineum, and retroperitoneum (109). Males are affected two or three times more frequently than are females (108,109). Two thirds of these masses are circumferentially well circumscribed, comprising the classic lipoblastoma. The remaining cases are diffuse, infiltrating both the musculature and the subcutis, and are referred to as diffuse lipoblastomatosis (111).

Radiologically, lipoblastoma and liposarcoma may be indistinguishable (see Figs. 12-28, 12-29, and 12-37). Although the radiologic differential diagnosis is that of liposarcoma, this entity is exceedingly rare in children. In a review of more than 2,500 cases of liposarcoma at the Armed Forces Institute of Pathology, only two (0.08%) occurred in children younger than 10 years of age. Fifteen additional cases were identified in children between the ages of 11 and 15 years (112).

Vascular Lesions

Hemangioma

Soft tissue hemangiomas represent a broad spectrum of benign neoplasms that histologically closely resemble

normal blood vessels. Hemangiomas often contain considerable amounts of nonvascular tissue, the most common of which is adipose tissue. Other nonvascular elements encountered in hemangiomas include smooth muscle, fibrous tissue, thrombi, and bone. Lesions may intermittently change size and may be painful (113). The overlying skin may have a bluish discoloration (113). Hemangiomas may be superficial or deep, with deep-seated lesion more frequently a diagnostic dilemma. This discussion is limited to intramuscular hemangioma in that it is the lesion most likely to be confused clinically with a soft tissue mass. Most occur in young adults, with 80% to 90% presenting by 30 years of age (114). The long duration of symptoms and relatively young age at presentation suggests that many of these lesions are congenital. Both males and females are affected equally (46,114,115). Hemangiomas are usually classified as either cavernous (large-caliber vessels) or capillary (small-caliber vessels), depending on the size of the blood vessels comprising most of the lesion. However, admixtures or mixed capillary and cavernous hemangiomas are not uncommon (114). Nonvascular elements are most commonly encountered in cavernous hemangiomas (116).

Radiographs of patients with soft tissue hemangioma are frequently nonspecific but may reveal phleboliths

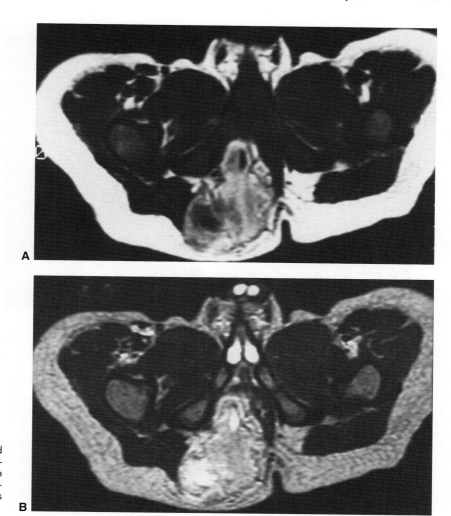

Figure 12-37 Lipoblastoma in a 1-year-old boy. Axial T1-weighted (500/20) **(A)** and T2-weighted (2,000/70) **(B)** SE MR images show a large predominantly fatty mass with a significant nonfatty component. In an adult, this appearance would suggest a liposarcoma.

within a soft tissue mass. Osseous changes may be seen in as many as one third of cases, consisting of periosteal or cortical thickeneng (117). Phleboliths are most common in cavernous hemangiomas and are seen in 30% to 50% of cases. The MRI appearance of an intramuscular hemangioma is frequently characteristic. On T1-weighted images, the intramuscular hemangioma is typically poorly marginated and isointense to skeletal muscle (115). Within the lesion are areas of increased signal (4,118) approximating that of subcutaneous fat (116). These areas vary in appearance from fine, delicate, or lacelike strands to thick coarse bands. On T2-weighted images, the intramuscular hemangioma is typically well marginated and markedly hyperintense as compared with subcutaneous fat (116,119). Segments of the lesion are isointense to either fat and/or muscle. Phleboliths (within the hemangioma) may be detected as small rounded areas of signal void on MRI, but these are more readily apparent on radiographs or CT (see Figs. 12-38 to 12-40) (116). Marrow signal abnormalities may be seen adjacent to large hemangiomas. Although their nature is not known, they are hypothesized to represent either marrow edema or hematopoetic conversion with localized hyperemia (117).

Naturally, the MR appearance reflects the underlying morphology. Areas of hyperintensity on T1-weighted images reflect fatty tissue interspersed between the vessels. The hyperintense signal on T2-weighted spin-echo images reflects the slowly flowing relatively stagnant blood within the hemangioma (116,119). A cavernous hemangioma may be larger than a capillary hemangioma and contains greater amounts of nonvascular tissue, especially adipose tissue. In fact, a cavernous hemangioma can contain such large amounts of adipose tissue that portions may be indistinguishable from a lipoma (114).

Angiolipoma

Angiolipoma is a lesion characterized histologically by adipose tissue, small vessels, and capillaries. Angiolipoma is a cutaneous lesion that typically occurs on the trunk and extremities of young adults, with the forearm being the most common location. As a cutaneous lesion, it is typically not subject to radiologic examination, and the diagnosis is usually established clinically. A rare variant, the infiltrating angiolipoma, has been described as a nonencapsulated infiltrating lesion composed of mature adipose tissue and benign vascular elements (120). This lesion has

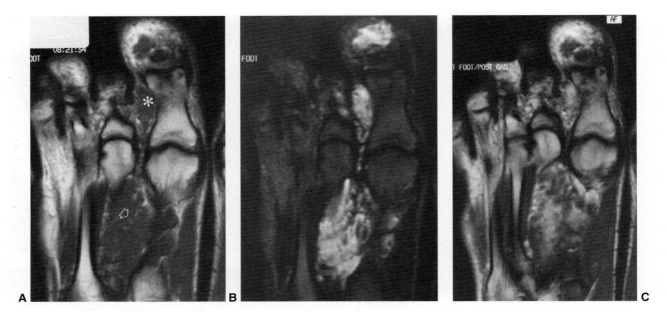

Figure 12-38 Intramuscular hemangioma in the foot of a 40-year-old woman. **A:** Axial T1-weighted (600/15) SE MR image shows areas of increased signal within the lesion (*arrow*), approximating that of subcutaneous fat. The tumor has a very infiltrative pattern of growth, typical of angiomatous lesions, extending to the distal aspects of first and second toes (*asterisk*). **B:** T2-weighted (1,800/80) SE MR image shows the lesion to have a lobular configuration with areas markedly hyperintense to subcutaneous fat. Septations within the lesion are isointense to either fat and/or muscle. Note infiltrative growth pattern, extending between the toes, to the dorsum of the foot. **C:** Corresponding postcontrast T1-weighted image shows marked enhancement.

been separated from the cutaneous (encapsulated) form because of its tendency to recur locally (121–124). Calcium salts, heterotopic bone, and phleboliths may be found within the infiltrating nonencapsulated angiolipoma (64,125). These lesions fall within the spectrum of benign vascular lesions and are probably best classified as an intramuscular hemangioma (see Fig. 12-41) (126).

Arteriovenous Hemangioma (Vascular Malformation)

Although many authors separate benign vascular lesions into hemangiomas and vascular malformations, we do not. The two are not necessarily mutually exclusive, and attempting to separate them assumes that these lesions are always histologically and clinically distinguishable, which they frequently are not. Consequently, we prefer to classify all these benign

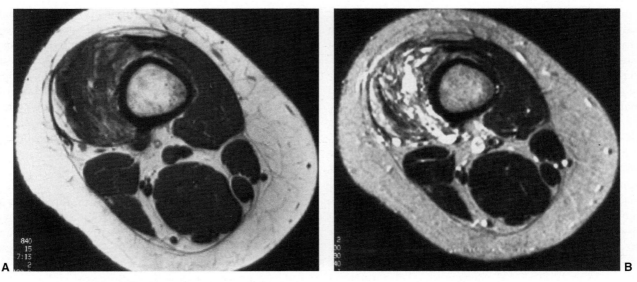

Figure 12-39 Intramuscular hemangioma in the thigh of a 23-year-old woman. **A:** Axial T1-weighted (840/15) SE MR image shows areas of increased signal, in a lacelike pattern, coursing through the lesion. **B:** Corresponding axial T2-weighted (3,000/90) SE MR image shows the lesion to have a lobular configuration with areas markedly hyperintense to subcutaneous fat, and others isointense to fat and skeletal muscle.

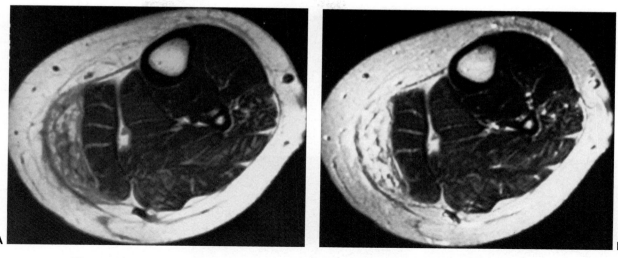

Figure 12-40 Hemangioma in the calf of a 12-year-old boy. Corresponding axial T1-weighted (500/20) **(A)** and T2-weighted (2,500/80) **(B)** MR SE images of the calf show an extensive fatty component to the lesion infiltrating the gastrocnemius muscle.

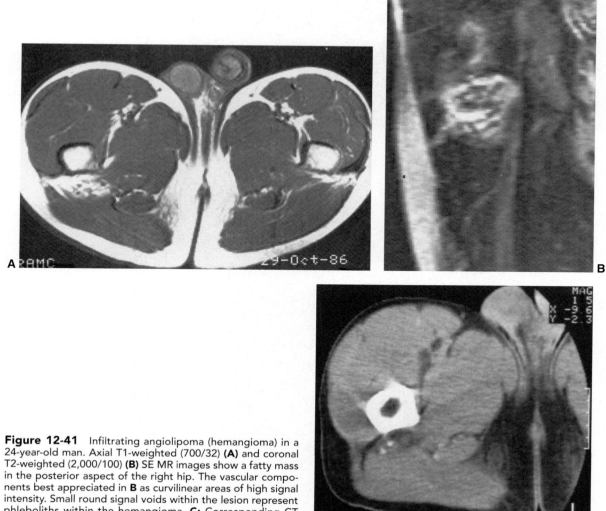

Figure 12-41 Infiltrating angiolipoma (hemangioma) in a 24-year-old man. Axial T1-weighted (700/32) **(A)** and coronal T2-weighted (2,000/100) **(B)** SE MR images show a fatty mass in the posterior aspect of the right hip. The vascular components best appreciated in **B** as curvilinear areas of high signal intensity. Small round signal voids within the lesion represent phleboliths within the hemangioma. **C:** Corresponding CT scan shows the phleboliths to better advantage.

vascular soft tissue lesions as hemangiomas, reserving the term "arteriovenous hemangioma" for those lesions demonstrating unequivocal arterial and venous components. Clearly, those lesions in which there is a significant arterial and/or venous component will behave differently (120). MRI will reflect the rapidly flowing blood within the arterial component as multiple serpiginous flow voids, interdigitating within the interstices of the mass (see Figs. 12-42 and 12-43).

Lymphangioma

A lymphangioma is a lesion made up of tissue resembling normal lymphatic channels, composed of endothelial cells and supporting connective tissue (127). Other mesenchymal elements, typically fat, fibrous tissue, and smooth muscle, are also frequently present (127,128). The etiology of lymphangioma is unknown. It may represent a developmental anomaly of the lymphatic vessels (128) or may be

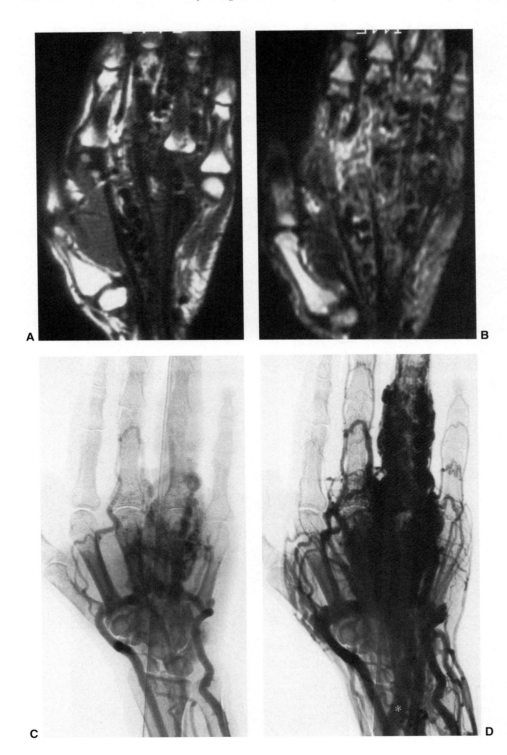

Figure 12-42 Arteriovenous hemangioma (arteriovenous malformation) in the hand of a 21-year-old woman. Coronal T1-weighted (500/20) **(A)** and T2-weighted (1,800/80) **(B)** SE MR images of the hand show multiple serpiginous flow voids, representing rapidly flowing blood within the large caliber vessels of the lesion. Early **(C)** and late **(D)** arterial films show marked vascularity of the lesion. Note early draining veins (*asterisk*).

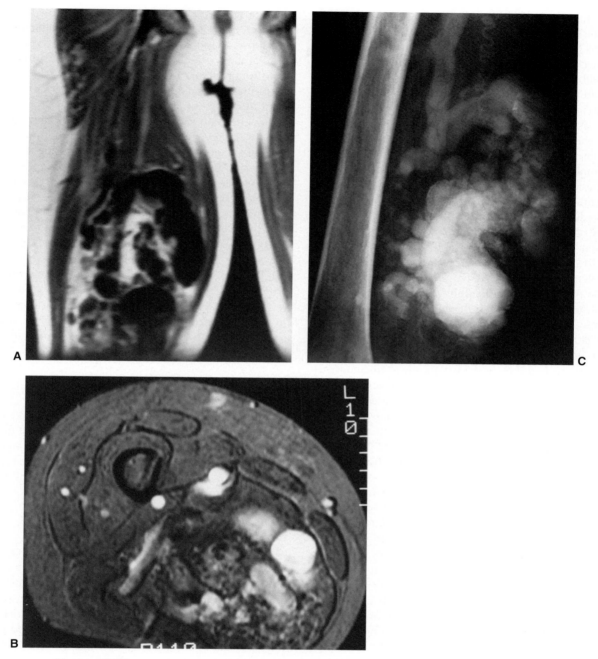

Figure 12-43 Arteriovenous hemangioma (arteriovenous malformation) in the thigh of a 35-year-old man. **A:** Coronal T1-weighted (600/20) SE MR image of the thigh shows prominent flow voids representing rapidly flowing blood in the lesion. **B:** Axial gradient image (33/14/30) shows the lesion to have an infiltrative growth pattern. **C:** Arteriogram shows the marked vascularity of the lesion, with markedly enlarged, tortuous, draining veins.

the sequela of congenital obstruction of lymphatic drainage (129,130). Its progressive nature, however, has suggested that it may be a benign mesenchymal neoplasm (127).

Lymphangiomas are subclassified by the size of the lymphatic vessels that comprise the lesion into simple (capillary) lymphangiomas, cavernous lymphangiomas, and cystic lymphangiomas (cystic hygromas) (127,131,132). The sizes of the vessels within these lesions range from thin-walled capillary-sized vessels, to dilated lymphatic channels, to cysts from a few millimeters to several centimeters in diameter (131). Additionally, one may see vasculolymphatic malformations (133). Lymphangiomas are often an admixture of all histologic subtypes and should be considered as a pathologic spectrum (113,131,133).

The cystic lymphangioma (cystic hygroma) is the most common type of lymphangioma and is characterized by large uniloculated or multiloculated cystic spaces, lined by lymphatic endothelium (127,133). It contains serous or chylous fluid (128). Cystic lymphangiomas are most common in the neck (typically in the posterior cervical space) and axilla, with these locations accounting for 75% and 20% of lesions, respectively (134,135). The prevalence of these locations has been suggested to be the result of sequestered lymphatic anlage, which lack adequate drainage. Other rare locations include the mediastinum, retroperitoneum, bone, omentum, and mesentery (135). Up to 10% of cervical cystic lymphangiomas will extend into the mediastinum (136). Cystic lesions (cystic hygromas) are typically found in regions in which the loose fatty connective tissue allows relatively unlimited growth (131,133). The overwhelming majority of lesions present in children, with more than half present at birth and 90% discovered by the age of 2 years (127,128,136–138). Fewer than 10% are found in adults (133). Retroperitoneal cystic lymphangiomas are usually found in older children and adults. Acute symptoms result from infection, rupture, hemorrhage, or pressure on adjacent structures (128). Cystic lymphangiomas are usually isolated lesions, although posterior neck cystic lymphangiomas may be associated with Turner syndrome (139).

A cavernous lymphangioma is typically a subcutaneous lesion composed of dilated lymphatic spaces, intermediate in size between those of the cystic hygroma and simple lymphangioma (127,133). Cavernous lymphangiomas are more common in areas in which there is a more limited potential for expansion, such as in the floor of the mouth, lips, tongue, cheek, salivary glands, and intramuscular septa (127,131,133).

A simple or capillary lymphangioma is a rare tumor composed of small capillary-sized vessels, lined by a flat or cuboidal epithelium (127,130). It is usually small, well circumscribed, and localized to the dermis and epidermis (127,133). These lesions may be seen in patients of any age, and approximately one fourth are found in patients older than 45 years of age (133). Because of its superficial location and small size, capillary lymphangioma is rarely imaged.

Patients with lymphangioma most commonly present with a discrete soft tissue mass (127,131), although they are otherwise asymptomatic (130). In children, large cervicomediastinal lymphangiomas are commonly associated with respiratory distress (131). Deviation of the trachea and compression of the esophagus may be seen in adults (136). Rarely, infiltrating lesions may give rise to elephantiasis (125). Lymphangiomas have no malignant potential. Surgery remains the treatment of choice, although recurrence is not rare and has been reported to be as high as 15% (131,133,138). Frequently, complete excision may not be possible because of infiltration of adjacent essential structures (see Fig. 12-44) (131). The most common postoperative complication is edema and may be seen in up to 50% of cases (131).

Radiographs may reveal a soft tissue mass. Calcification is rarely seen (140). The lesion may be associated with secondary bone changes and consequently may cause increased tracer accumulation on bone scintigraphy (141). MRI shows a cystic lymphangioma as a unilocular or multilocular mass of water density. Siegel et al. (130) reported the MRI appearance of 17 lymphangiomas in 15 patients, describing a typical appearance: heterogeneous with a low signal intensity, similar to that of muscle, on T1-weighted images and high signal intensity, greater than that of fat, on T2-weighted images, reflecting the preponderance of fluid-filled cystic spaces. Focal inhomogeneities within the lesions are present in nearly all cases and appear as low-intensity linear structures of variable thickness, representing fibrous septa within the lesion (see Fig. 12-45). Four of these lymphangiomas demonstrated a signal intensity similar to that of fat on T1-weighted images. In two of these cases, the lesions were composed of small lymphatic vessels, separated by thick fibrous–fatty septa. One other lesion was composed of both small and large cysts, one filled with fat and the other filled with clotted blood and necrotic debris. Rim and septal enhancement may be seen on MRI after gadolinium administration (78). It is our experience that the fibrous septa within lymphangiomas are seen to better advantage on sonography.

Synovial Lesions

Benign proliferative lesions of the joint, bursa, and tendon sheath are common in clinical practice. The most frequent of these is the localized giant cell tumor of tendon sheath (nodular tenosynovitis), representing the localized form of a spectrum of benign synovial proliferations, which when diffuse and intraarticular is termed PVNS (142).

Giant Cell Tumor of Tendon Sheath

Giant cell tumor of tendon sheath occurs in either a localized or a diffuse form (46). The localized form is often termed nodular tenosynovitis, and, as its name would imply, this lesion clinically presents as a nodular or polypoid mass, most commonly in the hand and wrist. In its diffuse form, the lesion is less well defined and grossly characterized by shaggy beardlike projections (representing hypertrophic synovial villi). Clearly, the distinction between the localized and diffuse form is on occasion blurred and a function of its gross and microscopic appearance. The term "PVNS" is usually reserved for those cases in which there is diffuse involvement of a large joint. The diffuse form of giant cell tumor of tendon sheath usually occurs adjacent to large weight-bearing joints and in most cases, although not all, represents extraarticular extension of PVNS. Ushijima et al. (143), in reporting a 20-year experience with 220 cases, found nodular tenosynovitis to be more than seven times more common than PVNS.

Localized nodular tenosynovitis is one of the most common masses of the hand (135,144), second in frequency only to a ganglion. Patients are typically adults with a peak

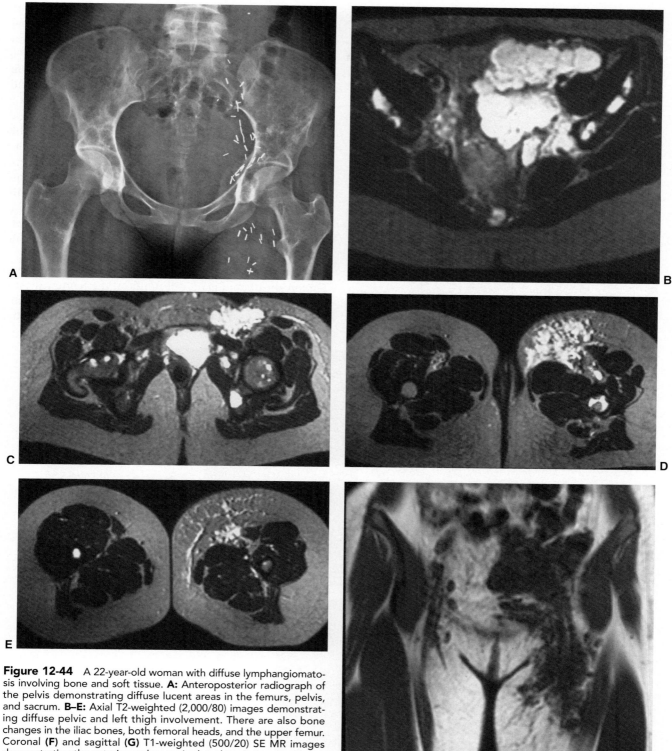

Figure 12-44 A 22-year-old woman with diffuse lymphangiomatosis involving bone and soft tissue. **A:** Anteroposterior radiograph of the pelvis demonstrating diffuse lucent areas in the femurs, pelvis, and sacrum. **B–E:** Axial T2-weighted (2,000/80) images demonstrating diffuse pelvic and left thigh involvement. There are also bone changes in the iliac bones, both femoral heads, and the upper femur. Coronal **(F)** and sagittal **(G)** T1-weighted (500/20) SE MR images demonstrating the anterior and posterior lymphangiomas.

incidence in the third and fourth decade (143,145,146), and there is a slight female predominance (1.5–2.1:1). The lesion affects the volar aspect of the digits, more commonly than the dorsal surface, although lesions may be lateral or circumferential (143,146). Involvement is most usually seen in the first three fingers and first two toes (143,146).

Most patients present with soft tissue swelling (143, 145) or a slowly enlarging painless soft tissue mass, which is freely mobile under the skin but attached to deeper

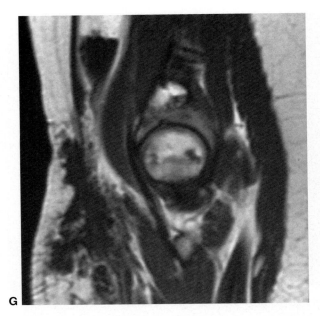

G

Figure 12-44 *(continued)*

structures (135,147). Pain is not uncommon and may be aggravated by activity (145). Multiple lesions are unusual but have been reported (143). Local recurrence is not uncommon and may be seen in approximately 9% to 20% of cases (143,146). A malignant giant cell tumor of tendon sheath with metastases was reported by Carstens and Howell (148); however, such lesions are quite rare.

Radiographs most usually demonstrate a soft tissue mass (145,146). Pressure erosions will be seen on the underlying bone in about 15% of cases (143). Because the diagnosis is usually suggested clinically, CT and MRI are rarely used, and experience with this lesion is quite limited. MRI typically demonstrates a nonspecific well-defined mass adjacent to a tendon, isointense with muscle on T1-weighted, and more inhomogeneous and hyperintense on muscle (but less than fat) on T2-weighted MR spin-echo images (see Fig. 12-46) (104,149,150).

Some investigators have suggested that fibroma of the tendon sheath and giant cell tumor of the tendon sheath make up a spectrum of histiocytic–fibroblastic–myofibroblastic lesions (151,152). Maluf et al. (151) noted that the

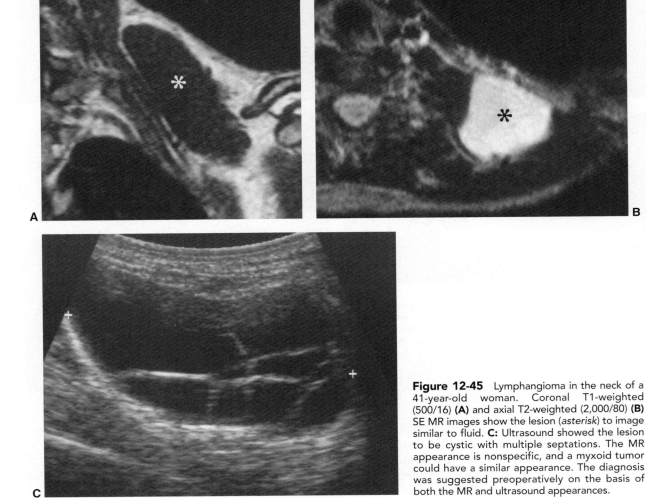

A

B

C

Figure 12-45 Lymphangioma in the neck of a 41-year-old woman. Coronal T1-weighted (500/16) **(A)** and axial T2-weighted (2,000/80) **(B)** SE MR images show the lesion (*asterisk*) to image similar to fluid. **C:** Ultrasound showed the lesion to be cystic with multiple septations. The MR appearance is nonspecific, and a myxoid tumor could have a similar appearance. The diagnosis was suggested preoperatively on the basis of both the MR and ultrasound appearances.

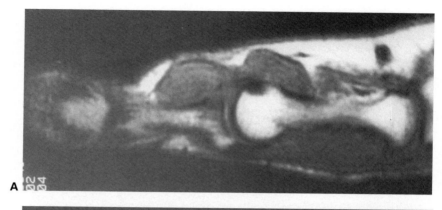

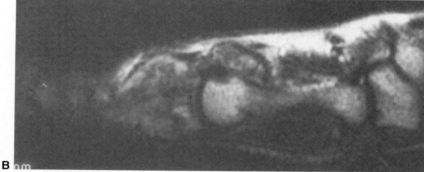

Figure 12-46 Giant cell tumor of tendon sheath in the thumb of a 26-year-old woman. Sagittal T1- **(A)** and T2- **(B)** weighted SE MR images show a nodular mass of relatively decreased signal intensity adjacent to the flexor tendon of the thumb.

lesions have an overlapping clinical presentation, with similar patient age and gender as well as lesion location and distribution. In addition, these lesions share similar growth patterns, showing a lobulated architecture. Although the microscopic appearance varies, both lesions contain spindle cells and multinucleated giant cells and share similar immunohistochemical attributes. Hence, the fibroma and giant cell tumor of tendon sheath may represent end points of a spectrum of cellular proliferation (152). It has been our experience that these lesions will show a similar appearance at MRI (see Fig. 12-47).

Pigmented Villonodular Synovitis

Approximately 80% of PVNS cases affect the knee (153). Other large joints affected in order of decreasing frequency include the hip, ankle, shoulder, and elbow (153,154). Patients usually complain of intermittent pain and swelling with decreased motion. The time interval from onset of symptoms to clinical presentation varies from months to years (153,155). Patients are usually adults and young adults presenting in the third or fourth decade (149), although it has been reported in children as young as 4.5 years (156). Childhood PVNS has been reported in conjunction with synovial hemangioma, and recurrent hemorrhage within the hemangioma has been suggested as a cause (144). Involvement of more than one joint is distinctly unusual (157), although recently Cotton et al. (158) reported 58 patients, 2 (3%) of whom probably had bilateral hip involvement. Malignant transformation is

exceedingly rare. A case of malignant PVNS was reported by Kalil and Unni (159), in which the metastases were identified 64 years after initial presentation.

There is typically an associated joint effusion with serosanguineous or xanthochromic fluid (153,155). Surgery remains the preferred treatment. Recurrence rates are typically quite high, approaching 50% (160). Joint fusion may be required in cases with advanced disease (7). Total joint replacement will relieve pain and restore function in selected patients (153).

Lesions are usually much larger and more irregular in shape than those seen in nodular tenosynovitis. Grossly, the lesion has been likened to a "shaggy red beard" to emphasize the villous or frondlike synovial projections. The reddish or rust color is the result of iron pigment (hemosiderin) within the lesion (76,155).

Radiographs may be normal or show a noncalcified soft tissue mass. Well-defined bone erosions on both sides of a joint and joint effusion may also be seen (153,161). Erosive bone lesions are seen in about 50% of all cases (93), being most common in joints with tight capsules such as the hip (93%) and shoulder (75%) and least common in the knee (26%) (153). These erosive changes are usually geographic lytic lesions with well-defined thinly sclerotic margins. They are most characteristic when they are multiple and are seen on both sides of the joint. The joint space is usually preserved, as is bone density (153). Uncommonly, radiographs will demonstrate an osteoarthritis appearance, with typical osteophytes, sclerosis, cysts, and joint narrowing, or an

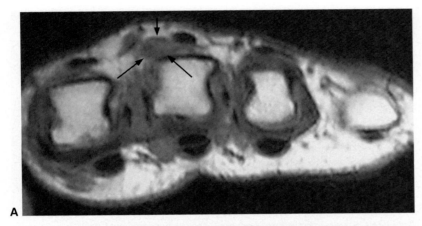

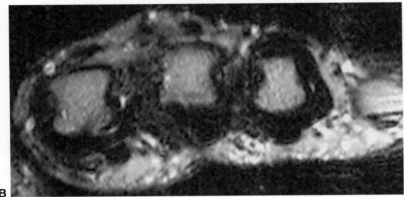

Figure 12-47 Fibroma of tendon sheath of the middle finger in a 38-year-old man. **A:** Axial T1-weighted (700/20) SE MR image of the hand shows a small mass (*arrows*) adjacent to the extensor tendon of the middle finger. **B:** The lesion shows an intermediate signal intensity on corresponding T2-weighted (2,000/90) SE MR image and is not readily identified from the adjacent subcutaneous fat.

arthritis-like appearance, with concentric joint space loss, osteoporosis, and erosions (158). Radiologic calcification within the mass has been reported (162) but is extremely unusual and should suggest an alternative diagnosis. Calcification has also been reported in diffuse giant cell tumor of tendon sheath (163).

The MRI appearance of PVNS is often characteristic. It presents as a heterogeneous synovial process that usually extends away from the joint space (161). The lesions contain areas of intermediate signal intensity and/or hypointensity when compared with skeletal muscle on T1-weighted spin-echo MR images. A similar pattern may be seen on T2-weighted images (161,164). The decreased signal intensity is usually more pronounced on long TR/TE images, due to the preferential shortening of T2 relaxation times of hemosiderin (see Fig. 12-48) (155). This is more pronounced at high field strengths (155,164,165). The lytic bone lesions seen on radiographs and joint effusions are typically well seen on MRI (161). The diffuse giant cell tumor of tendon sheath has a skeletal distribution similar to that of PVNS and is often considered an extraarticular extension of PVNS. Its MRI signal intensity characteristics are similar to PVNS (see Fig. 12-49).

Popliteal (Synovial) Cysts

Popliteal cysts, also known as synovial cysts, probably result from a slit-shaped communication of the knee joint with the normally occurring gastrocnemiosemimembranous bursa (166). This communication is more common in older individuals because of degeneration and reduced elasticity of the joint capsule (166,167). In a study of adult cadaver knees, a communication between the semimembranous and gastrocnemius bursa was found in more than half the cases (168). The incidence of popliteal cyst increases with age (167,169), being demonstrated arthrographically in 16% of patients in the second decade, 36% in the third decade, and 54% beyond the fifth decade (167). The term "Baker cyst" is usually reserved for those cases in which this gastrocnemiosemimembranous bursa is distended by fluid (166). Baker described eight cases of swelling in the popliteal region in 1877 and 1885, hypothesizing that it was the result of synovial membrane herniation and cyst formation due to osteoarthritis (166). While involvement of the gastrocnemiosemimembranous bursa is necessary for diagnosis, popliteal cysts may dissect between muscle planes, and may rarely dissect into the vastus medialis or gastrocnemius muscle (170).

In a recent study of the MRI examinations of 1,113 patients referred for evaluation of internal derangement, the incidence of popliteal cysts was 5% (169). The prevalence of cysts demonstrated by arthrography ranges between 7% and 42% (129,167,169,171,172). This higher incidence is likely due to the distension of the normally collapsed bursa during arthrography (169).

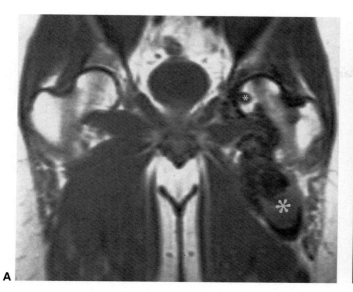
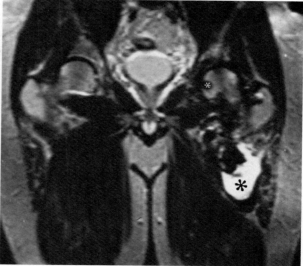

Figure 12-48   Pigmented villonodular synovitis of the left hip in a 42-year-old-man. Coronal T1-weighted (720/34) **(A)** and T2-weighted (2,197/90) **(B)** SE MR image shows a large mass of markedly decreased signal intensity, with a large associated joint effusion (*asterisk*). Note associated erosions on both sides of the hip joint (*small asterisk*).

The relationship between popliteal cysts and meniscal injury, usually to the posterior horn of the medial meniscus, has been previously emphasized. Approximately 80% to 90% of popliteal cysts are associated with a meniscal tear (167,169,173), usually medial, although 10% to 15% are lateral by arthrography and 38% are lateral by MRI (169). There is also an association with previous meniscectomy, articular cartilage damage (chondromalacia patella and degenerative arthritis), collateral and cruciate ligament injury, loose bodies, rheumatoid arthritis, and other arthritides (167,169,174–176). Wolfe and Colloff (167) suggested that it is the production of an effusion producing intraarticular lesion rather than the specific injury that is important in the production of popliteal cysts.

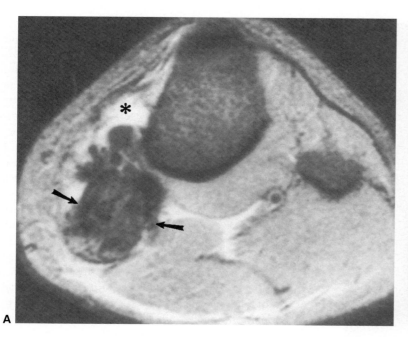
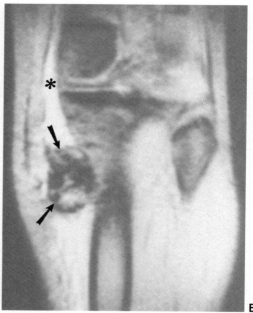

Figure 12-49   Diffuse giant cell tumor of tendon sheath in a 16-year-old girl. **A:** Axial gradient-echo image (342/10/15) shows a lobular nodular mass (*arrows*), adjacent to the posterior medial tibia. High signal intensity extending from the mass represents associated edema (*asterisk*), a nonspecific finding. **B:** Corresponding coronal (467/10/15) image shows similar findings.

Giant synovial cysts have also been reported in association with rheumatoid arthritis and, less often, trauma, involving the large joints (knee, shoulder, and elbow) (177). They have also been reported in pseudarthroses, thought to be due to synovial proliferation with secondary formation of a fluid-filled synovial-lined cavity (178), most likely occurring after trauma.

Patients with popliteal cysts may be asymptomatic or may present with pain or signs and symptoms suggesting internal derangement of the knee and only uncommonly will present for the evaluation of a cyst or mass (129,167,172). Bierbaum (129) noted a popliteal cyst was clinically evident in only 2 of 33 patients identified as having them on arthrography. Popliteal cysts may also be confused with proliferation of adipose tissue, tortuosity, aneurysmal dilatation of the popliteal artery, a thrombosed vessel, or tumor (66,179). Cysts may dissect into the calf or rupture and simulate thrombophlebitis clinically (179–181). Rarely, a dissecting popliteal cyst and thrombophlebitis may coexist (182,183). Mink and Deutsch (183) suggested the term "pseudopseudothrombophlebitis syndrome" to describe a deep vein thrombosis occurring secondary to a ruptured popliteal cyst. Less than half of the lesions noted on arthrography are detectable on clinical examination (64,184).

MRI demonstrates a mass with a low signal on T1-weighted and a high signal on T2-weighted spin-echo MR images (see Figs. 12-50 through 12-52) (163,185). The protein-containing synovial fluid within the cyst may result in an increased signal intensity on T1-weighted images (186). Sundaram et al. (163) also reported a case in which the lesion appeared as intense as fat on T1-weighted images. Blood products within the cyst, from subclinical hemorrhage, have been hypothesized to be responsible for increased signal on T1-weighted images (178).

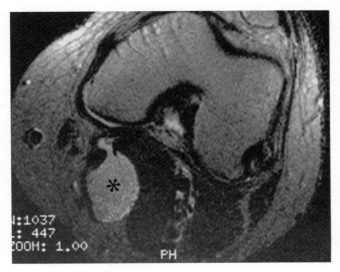

Figure 12-50 Popliteal cyst in a 20-year-old man. Axial T2-weighted (2,213/80) SE MR image shows fluid extending into the gastrocnemiosemimembranous bursa (*asterisk*).

Fibrous Tumors

Fibromatoses

Fibromatosis refers to a family of soft tissue lesions characterized by proliferation of benign fibrous tissue, which is composed of uniform, elongated, fusiform, or spindle-shaped cells surrounded and separated by abundant collagen (46). Their biologic behavior is intermediate between that of benign fibrous lesions (such as fibroma or fasciitis) and that of fibrosarcoma, although they never metastasize (187,188). Synonymous terms include nonmetastasizing fibrosarcoma and aggressive fibromatosis, but these may be misleading because the clinical course of any individual tumor is unpredictable (46).

The fibromatoses are classified on the basis of their anatomic location as either superficial or deep. The superficial group includes palmar fibromatosis (Dupuytren contracture), plantar fibromatosis (Ledderhose disease), penile fibromatosis (Peyronie disease), and knuckle pads. The deep, or musculoaponeurotic, fibromatoses include extraabdominal fibromatosis (aggressive fibromatosis), abdominal fibromatosis, and intraabdominal fibromatosis (189–192). They were initially described in 1962 in the abdominal wall. The descriptive term desmoid tumor was coined in 1968 to emphasize the "bandlike or tendonlike" character of the lesions (46).

Superficial Fibromatosis

The superficial fibromatoses are, in general, small lesions that usually arise from fascia or aponeuroses. They are typically slow growing, in sharp contrast to the deep fibromatoses, which usually grow rapidly and are larger and more aggressive in their biologic behavior.

Dupuytren contracture primarily involves the palmar aponeurosis of the hand and its extensors (193). Patients typically present with a subcutaneous nodule in the palm of the hand, at the level of the distal palmar crease. The fourth ray is the most commonly affected, followed by the fifth, third, and second rays (193). Surgery remains the primary mode of therapy with release of the flexion contracture, although early surgery is generally avoided because of an increased tendency for lesions in the early proliferative stage to recur (193). Recurrence is common, affecting 30% to 40% of patients.

The superficial fibromatoses are usually diagnosed clinically and are only rarely the subject of radiologic examination. Yacoe et al. (193) reported the MR findings in 22 lesions of Dupuytren contracture in ten patients. They noted the lesions to be cords, arising proximally from the palmar aponeurosis and extending distally and superficially, parallel to the flexor tendons. The lesions varied in length from 10 to 55 mm and most often terminated in fine strands extending into the subcutaneous tissue at the level of the distal metacarpals. Less commonly, the lesion terminated as a nodule or other branching configuration. Associated nodules were seen in approximately 64% of cases (see Fig. 12-53).

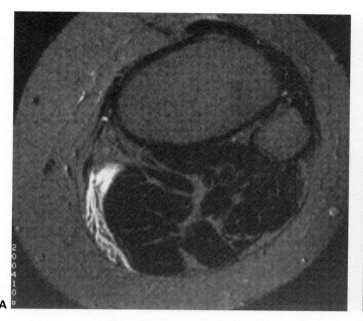
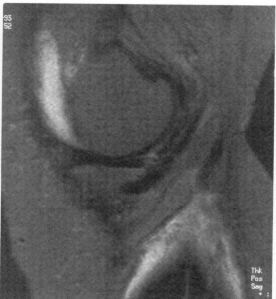

Figure 12-51 Dissecting popliteal cyst in a 46-year-old woman. **A:** Axial T2-weighted (2,500/90) SE MR image shows fluid dissecting down the medial aspect of the medial gastrocnemius muscle. **B:** Sagittal T2-weighted (2,500/90) image shows a joint effusion and fluid dissecting along the medial aspect of the medial gastrocnemius muscle.

Yacoe et al. (193) correlated the cellularity of lesions with their MR appearance. They noted all lesions had low signal intensity on T2-weighted spin-echo MR images: 18 (82%) of 22 cords had uniform decreased signal intensity and 4 (18%) had a low to intermediate signal on T1-weighted images.

These lesions were hypocellular and mostly dense collagen. Eleven nodules, which demonstrated intermediate signal intensity on both T1- and T2-weighted spin-echo MR images, were all either cellular or demonstrated a mixed histologic picture with hypocellular and cellular regions.

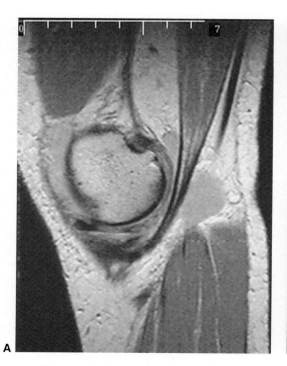
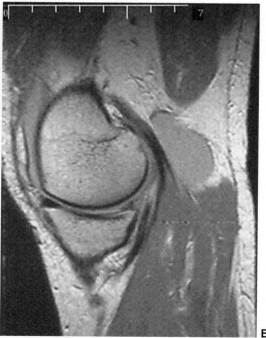

Figure 12-52 Popliteal cyst in a 60-year-old woman with a meniscal tear. **A,B:** Sagittal proton-weighted (2,376/20) SE MR images show a large popliteal cyst posterior to the medial gastrocnemius muscle, with associated meniscal tear. The tear extended into the middle third of the meniscus.

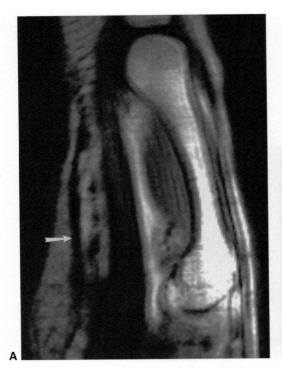
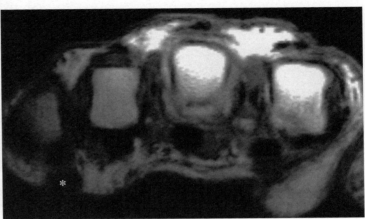

Figure 12-53 Palmar fibromatosis in a 62-year-old man. **A:** Sagittal T1-weighted (633/20) SE MR image of the fifth metacarpal shows a low-signal intensity cord (*arrow*) in the superficial palmar soft tissues. **B:** Axial T1-weighted (633/20) shows a subcutaneous nodule (*asterisk*), which was the termination of the subcutaneous cord.

The MRI appearance of plantar fibromatosis is also relatively characteristic. Lesions are centered in the plantar aponeurosis, typically with infiltrative superficial margin. Extension deep to the aponeurosis is seen in approximately 15%. Lesions are typically heterogeneous with a signal intensity similar to that of skeletal muscle on T1-weighted spin-echo MRI and similar to or slightly hyperintense to that of skeletal muscle on T2-weighted spin-echo images. Short TI inversion recovery images will typically show increased signal intensity. Enhancement is variable, with approximately 60% showing marked enhancement (see Figs. 12-54 and 12-55) (194). There is a wide spectrum, and small lesions may appear as a nodular thickening of plantar aponeurosis, demonstrating decreased signal intensity on all pulse sequences (195).

Deep Fibromatosis

The deep musculoaponeurotic fibromatosis typically present in young adults between puberty and 40 years of age, with a peak incidence between 25 and 35 years. Cases have been reported in infants and children, although these are less common (192). Reports in the literature indicate that men and women are almost equally affected or there is a slight female predominance (189). The fibromatoses may occur anywhere, although more than two thirds of cases occur in the lower extremity (189). Most of the remainder occur in the upper extremity, with about half of these in the shoulder region (189).

These tumors are usually solitary; however, synchronous multicentric lesions have been reported with a prevalence of 10% to 15% in two large series of 205 and 110 patients, respectively (189,196). Synchronous lesions are confined to the same extremity in 75% to 100% of cases (189,196), and a second soft tissue mass in the extremity of a patient with a previously confirmed desmoid tumor should be regarded as a second desmoid tumor until proven otherwise (147).

Local recurrence is common, occurring in as many as 77% of patients, usually within 18 months of the original surgery, although recurrence may not present for several years after the initial surgery (196,197). Fatalities secondary to direct invasion of the chest wall or neck and infiltration of vital organs have been reported (147,196–200).

Prognosis is related to the age of the patient, with younger individuals (those under 20 to 30 years of age) having a longer duration of tumor activity and a higher recurrence rate (196,201). Similarly, younger patients with recurrence require more aggressive treatment to effect a cure (196). Wide local excision is the treatment of choice, although adjuvant radiation has been used. In extremity lesions, amputation may be required for local control.

Fibromatosis of the abdominal wall (abdominal desmoid) is distinguished from other musculoaponeurotic fibromatoses because of its distinct predilection to develop in women of childbearing age (202). Typically,

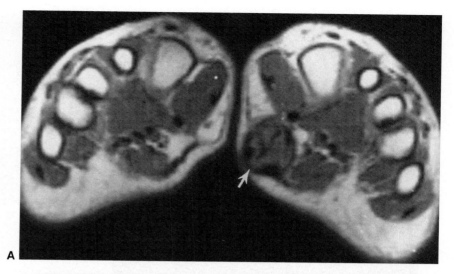

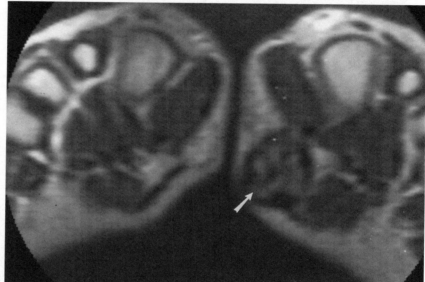

Figure 12-54 Plantar fibromatosis in a 26-year-old woman. Coronal T1-weighted (550/26) **(A)** and T2-weighted (1,800/80) **(B)** SE MR images show a mass arising from the plantar fascia (*arrows*). The mass has a signal intensity equal to or less than that of skeletal muscle.

the lesion develops after, or less often during, pregnancy. Approximately 87% of cases occur in women and 95% in those with at least one child.

Intraabdominal fibromatosis (intraabdominal desmoid) refers to those lesions occurring in the pelvis, mesentery, and retroperitoneum. Of these, the latter two are associated with Gardner syndrome in approximately 15% of patients (203–205). In a study of 15 patients with Gardner syndrome, Healy et al. (206) found 35 lesions, 13 in the abdominal wall and 22 intraabdominal. As a group, these lesions are usually not within the realm of the musculoskeletal radiologist.

Radiographs are usually nonspecific or may reveal a mass. Approximately 6% to 16% of patients will have evidence of bone involvement, which is usually a pressure erosion or a scalloping without invasion or destruction, or a stimulation of the periosteum producing a "frondlike" periosteal reaction (8,14,114,196,207). Bone involvement is more common in patients with multiple recurrences (196).

Disler et al. (189) reported a skeletal dysplasia in 3 of 16 (18.8%) patients with multicentric fibromatosis. In two of these cases, the dysplastic changes were seen in all long bones and consisted predominantly of undertubularization similar to that in Pyle disease or the Erlenmeyer flask deformity of Gaucher disease. In the remaining case, these changes were seen only in the involved limb. Unlike Pyle disease, the skull was normal in all three patients, and in none of the cases was a marrow abnormality detected. Familial cases of fibromatosis have also been reported (147).

On MRI, the deep musculoaponeurotic fibromatoses were initially described as demonstrating decreased signal intensity on all pulse sequences, reflecting the fibrous nature of the tumor (188,208,209). Sundaram et al. (210) described three cases of "aggressive fibromatosis," two demonstrating a decreased signal on T2-weighted pulse sequences and one showing a paradoxical increased signal. Two these tumors were hypocellular and had abundant

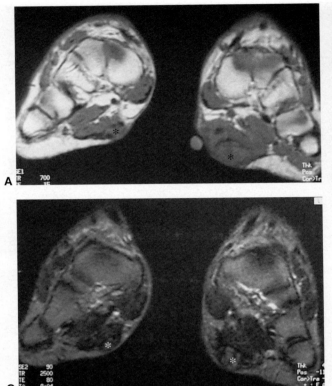

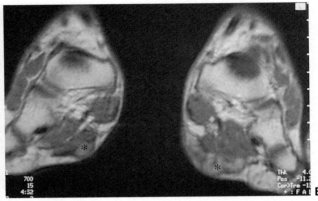

Figure 12-55 Bilateral plantar fibromatosis in a 39-year-old man. Coronal pre- **(A)** and postcontrast **(B)** T1-weighted (700/15) SE MR images show masses (*asterisks*) arising from the plantar fascia bilaterally. The lesions enhance markedly. **C:** Corresponding T2-weighted (2,500/90) SE MR image shows the lesions to be heterogeneous with predominantly intermediate signal intensity.

collagen. The lesion that showed high signal on T2-weighted MR images had marked cellularity and abundant collagen. Sundaram et al. concluded that the combination of marked hypocellularity and abundant collagen produces decreased signal on T2-weighted pulse sequences and that the decreased cellularity is of prime importance. Recently, signal intensity on T2-weighted imaging has been shown to have a prognostic value, with lesions showing increased signal associated with marked interval growth on follow-up evaluation (206).

Subsequent reports have shown great variability of the MRI characteristics of these lesions (9,188,211–214). More typically, the lesion has an inhomogeneous signal intensity approximating that of fat on T2-weighted and that of skeletal muscle on T1-weighted spin-echo images. Considerable variation may be noted. The heterogeneous signal likely reflects varying proportions and distribution of collagen, spindle cells, and mucopolysaccharide within the tumor. Corresponding areas of decreased signal intensity have been noted on all pulse sequences, likely reflecting areas of dense collagen within the lesions (see Fig. 12-56). Fibromatosis will demonstrate moderate to marked enhancement after the administration of intravenous contrast, with enhancement corresponding to the cellular portions of the lesion (see Fig. 12-57) (213). Tumor margins vary greatly, though they are usually well defined at initial presentation (214,215). Bone involvement is less common but has been reported in up to 37% of cases (212). It must be emphasized

that decreased signal intensity on all pulse sequences only reflects the gross morphology of a lesion. Decreased signal may be seen in lesions that are densely mineralized, hemosiderin laden (such as PVNS), or relatively acellular with large amounts of collagen (fibromatosis) (48,210). It is not characteristic for a specific histology and has also been reported in malignant fibrous histiocytoma and other malignancies (48).

Elastofibroma

Elastofibroma is a slowly growing fibroelastic pseudotumor thought to result from mechanical friction between the scapula and chest wall; hence, it is to be considered reactive rather than neoplastic (54,216). Originally described at the Twelfth Congress of Scandinavian Pathologists by Järvi and Saxén in 1959 and subsequently reported in 1961 (54,216), elastofibroma has received little attention in the radiologic literature and is considered to be a rare lesion. However, it is not uncommon and was found in 24% of women and 11% of men in one autopsy series of patients over 55 years old (217). In this autopsy study, lesions were 3 cm or smaller in size, suggesting that most elastofibromas are clinically occult, accounting for the perception that they are rare. In a study of 258 patients undergoing CT examination for reasons unrelated to posteriorlateral chest wall pain, Brandser et al. (218) found five lesions in four patients, for a prevalence of 2%.

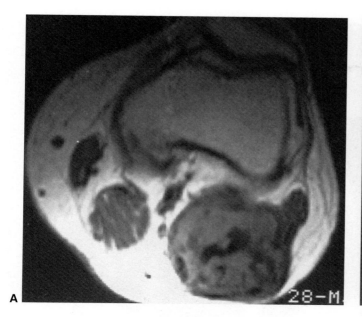
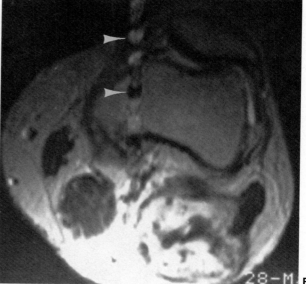

Figure 12-56   Deep (aggressive) fibromatosis in the popliteal fossa of a 22-year-old man. Axial T1-weighted (700/34) **(A)** and T2-weighted (2,000/80) **(B)** SE MR images show a relatively well-defined mass in the popliteal fossa. The mass has a signal intensity slightly higher than that of skeletal muscle on T1-weighted images and approximately equal to that of fat on T2-weighted images. There are central areas of markedly decreased signal intensity centrally on both pulse sequences. Note the flow artifact (*arrowheads*) and signal drop-off due to a flat posterior coil.

Lesions typically occur on the back and are thought to be due to repeated mechanical friction between the chest wall and the tip of the scapula. Patients often have an occupational history of manual labor, such as farming; however, this may be a coincidence (54,205,216,219). Other types of trauma, mechanical stress, chronic irritation, and nutritional derangement have also been suggested as etiologic factors (217,220), but these factors alone may not explain the development of elastofibroma. As many as one third of patients may have a genetic predisposition (221). Barr (222) postulated that "the lesion results from elastic degeneration of collagen following trauma and friction in individuals who possibly have some inherited enzymatic defect related to connective tissue metabolism." However, recent *in situ* hybridization and immunoelectron microscopic studies indicate that active synthesis of elastin occurring within elastofibromas and elastic fibrillogenesis is abnormal rather than a degenerative phenomenon (223).

The location between the chest wall and inferior scapular tip is most characteristic of elastofibroma; it was the site of the lesion in 99% of reported cases (221). Bilateral lesions are common and are seen in 10% to 66% of patients (54,217,219,221,222,224). In a recent study of 21 lesions in 12 patients by Naylor et al. (225), bilateral lesions were found in 100% of nine patients in whom both sides of the chest were imaged. Synchronous infraolecranon lesions are also common. Nagamine et al. (221) found this area to be involved in approximately 16% of patients. They also noted isolated synchronous lesions in the thoracic wall and in the area of the ischial tuberosity. One

patient had lesions in seven different anatomic locations. Isolated rare lesions have been reported in the hand, foot, regions overlying the greater trochanter and ischial tuberosity, deltoid region, temporal bulbar conjunctiva, and cervical epidural space (220,222,226–230).

Most patients are older adults. The mean age is approximately 70 years (221), although elastofibroma has been reported in children as young as 6 years (219). More than half the patients are asymptomatic (219,221). The most common symptom is stiffness, which is seen in approximately one fourth of patients (221). Pain is relatively uncommon and is the presenting symptom in another 10% (221). Large lesions may ulcerate (231). The disorder has a female predominance, usually estimated to be 2:1 (217,220); however, it may range from 1:1 to as high as 13:1 (221,232).

On spin-echo MR images, the typical subscapular lesion is a lenticular well-defined mass with an intermediate signal intensity, approximately equal to that of skeletal muscle, interlaced with areas of signal intensity similar to that of fat on both T1- and T2-weighted images (232,233). Gadolinium-enhanced MR images show areas with and without enhancement (232). Although the origin of the fat within the lesion is unclear, it is thought to be entrapped mature adipose tissue (see Fig. 12-58) (232).

The imaging features of elastofibroma are different from most other soft tissue tumors, reflecting entrapped fat within a predominantly fibrous mass. Although not pathognomonic, recognition of these characteristic imaging features in a subscapular lesion in an older patient

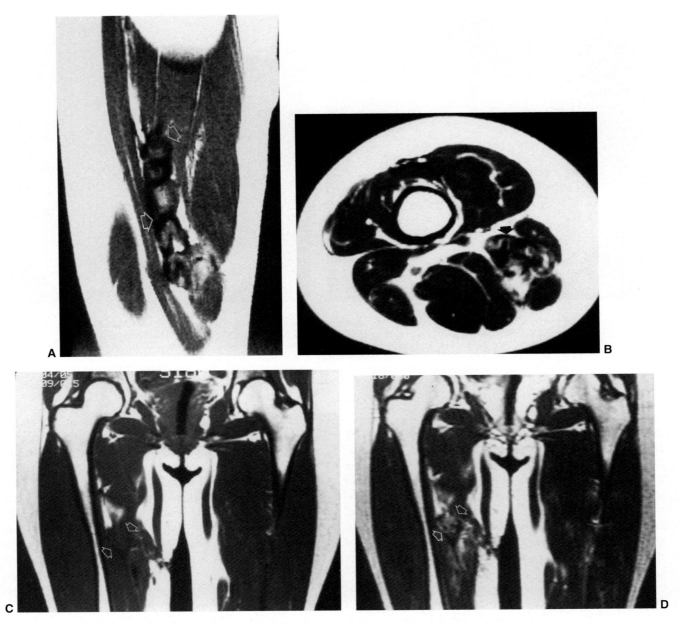

Figure 12-57 Fibromatosis of the thigh in an 18-year-old woman, with recurrence 1 year after initial surgery. Sagittal T1-weighted (500/40) **(A)** and axial T2-weighted (2,000/60) **(B)** SE MR images show the mass (*arrows*) to have a lobular contour, with decreased signal intensity. Coronal T1-weighted (617/20) **(C)** and T2-weighted (1,800/80) **(D)** images, approximately 1 year after resection, show a recurrent mass (*arrows*). The mass is not conspicuous, due the areas of markedly decreased signal intensity. **E:** Coronal T1-weighted (617/20) image following contrast administration shows inhomogeneous enhancement. **F:** Corresponding digital subtraction arteriogram shows the lesion to be moderately vascular.

facilitates making a successful presumptive diagnosis of elastofibroma.

Peripheral Nerve Sheath Tumors

Peripheral nerve sheath tumors are typically divided into two major benign groups, neurofibroma and schwannoma, and malignant peripheral nerve sheath tumor.

Synonyms for the latter include malignant schwannoma, neurogenic sarcoma, malignant neurilemoma, and neurofibrosarcoma (234). Both the neurofibroma and schwannoma contain cells that are closely related to the normal Schwann cell, from which some would speculate they arise (234). The malignant schwannoma is the primary malignancy of peripheral nerve. Its origin is not established, and although a small number arise from preexisting neurofibroma in

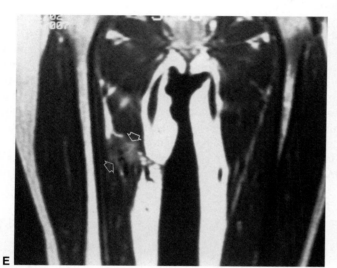

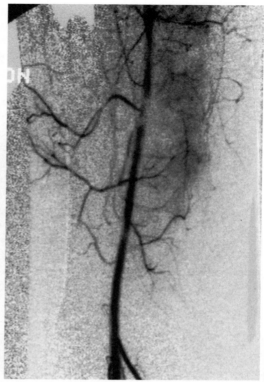

E

F

Figure 12-57 *(continued)*

patients with neurofibromatosis, most likely arise from Schwann cells, perineural cells, and fibroblasts (46). Neurofibroma and schwannoma have a similar prevalence and together comprise about 10% of all biopsied soft tissue tumors (235). Additionally, the traumatic neuroma and Morton neuroma are discussed. These last lesions are not true soft tissue tumors but rather represent pseudotumorous lesions of nerve.

Neurofibroma

Patients with neurofibroma are usually between 20 and 40 years of age and present with a slowly growing mass. Neurofibroma most commonly arises in association with the cutaneous nerves. Symptoms are usually related to the size of the lesion and are similar to those associated with schwannoma (180). Less commonly, neurofibroma arises in association with a major nerve. It is estimated that

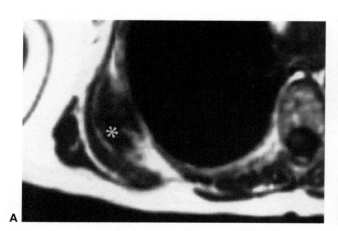

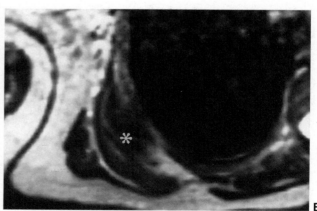

A

B

Figure 12-58 Elastofibroma in the infrascapular region of a 63-year-old woman. Axial T1-weighted (550/22) **(A)** and T2-weighted (2,000/90) **(B)** SE MR images show the lesion (*asterisk*) to be relatively well defined, with a crescentic shape. The mass has a signal intensity similar to skeletal muscle. Within the lesion are curvilinear regions with signal intensity similar to fat, representing fat within the lesion.

approximately 90% of neurofibromas are of the solitary type (236). Sudden onset of pain or enlargement of a neurofibroma in a patient with neurofibromatosis is very suspicious for malignant transformation (234,237).

Microscopically, neurofibroma typically contains interlacing bundles of elongated cells with wavy dark-staining nuclei (46). There are many variations in histologic appearance; however, neurofibroma is not encapsulated and does not display the two characteristic morphologic regions seen with schwannoma. Suh et al. (21), in a review of the MR images of 16 peripheral nerve sheath tumors, found a characteristic target appearance on T2-weighted images in 7 of 10 neurofibromas, with a central zone of low signal intensity and a peripheral zone of higher signal intensity. Sakai et al. (238), in reviewing the MRI appearance of three neurofibromas of the chest, found similar results with a peripheral zone of high signal intensity on T2-weighted images, greater than that of subcutaneous fat, with a central area of lower signal intensity with regional curvilinear or nodular low intensities at the boundary between the two zones. The central area enhances after contrast administration (see Fig. 12-59). Histologically, this corresponded to a peripheral region with loosely arranged myxoid stroma and a solid central, tightly packed, cellular portion with fibrous tissue and xanthomatous areas. Atrophy along the long axis of the muscle is less common than with schwannoma, being seen in only one of seven neurofibromas reported by Stull et al. (234).

A target pattern, which was initially described in neurofibroma, may also be seen in schwannoma. This pattern was seen in 6 of 13 (46%) schwannomas reported by Varma et al. (239). Overall, they noted this sign in 12 of 23 (52%) benign nerve sheath tumors and did not identify it in nine malignant peripheral nerve sheath tumors, suggesting it is helpful in identifying benign nerve sheath tumors when analyzed in conjunction with the anatomic location of a lesion.

It has been our anecdotal experience that plexiform neurofibromas, which may be considered virtually

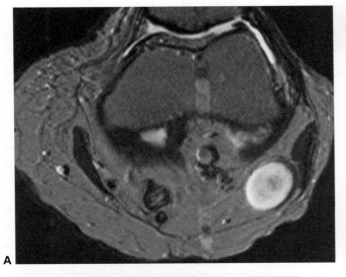

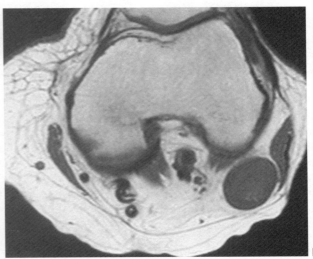

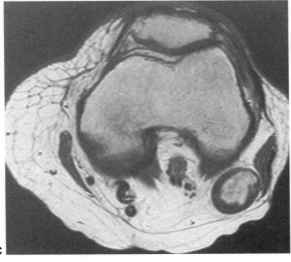

Figure 12-59 Neurofibroma of the peroneal nerve in a 77-year-old woman. **A:** T2-weighted (2,213/80) SE MR image demonstrates the characteristic target appearance, with a central zone of low signal intensity and a peripheral zone of higher signal intensity. **B:** Corresponding T1-weighted (450/16) SE MR image is nonspecific, imaging similar to that of skeletal muscle. **C:** Corresponding axial T1-weighted image after the administration of contrast shows intense central enhancement.

pathognomonic for neurofibromatosis, may occasionally mimic an intramuscular hemangioma. Grossly, the lesion has an irregular convoluted appearance (234). The MRI appearance likely reflects this, with entrapped fat simulating the lacelike pattern of fat interdigitating between the vascular elements of a hemangioma.

Schwannoma

Patients with schwannoma, also known as neurilemoma, typically present between 20 and 50 years of age with a slowly growing mass. Lesions are most common in the soft tissue of the head and neck, flexor surfaces of the extremities, trunk, mediastinum, and retroperitoneum (240). They characteristically involve the posterior spinal nerve roots, producing sensory symptoms (180). Paresthesia, pain, and other symptoms usually occur when the lesion becomes large enough to compress the adjacent nerve. Pain may radiate along the course of the nerve. Small lesions are usually asymptomatic (180). Lesions are almost always solitary, except when associated with neurofibromatosis (46).

Lesions are sharply circumscribed round to oval masses that are usually less than 5 cm in diameter, although mediastinum and retroperitoneal tumors tend to be larger (240). When large, they may show secondary degenerative hemorrhage and cyst formation (240). Schwannomas are well-encapsulated lesions, surrounded by a true capsule of epineurium. They displace nerve fibers and can be dissected and removed from the adjacent nerve without resultant neurologic damage (21,240). This is in contradistinction to neurofibromas, in which the adjacent nerve infiltrates the underlying nerve and cannot be dissected free (240,241).

The schwannoma is characterized histologically as an encapsulated lesion composed of a highly ordered cellular component (Antoni A area) and a loose myxoid component (Antoni B area) (46). Antoni A areas are typically composed of interlacing fascicles of spindle cells with indistinct cytoplasmic borders and twisted nuclei (46). Antoni B areas are hypocellular regions composed of a loose matrix.

On MRI, schwannoma demonstrates a low to intermediate signal intensity on T1-weighted images and a markedly hyperintense signal intensity on T2-weighted images (238,240,241). Suh et al. (21) noted that lesions were inhomogeneous on T2-weighted images, corresponding to a random histologic distribution of dense and scanty cellular area within the tumor (so-called Antoni A and Antoni B areas). Sakai et al. (238) noted inhomogeneity in two of four schwannomas, with areas of very high signal intensity on T2-weighted images corresponding to areas of cystic degeneration within the lesion. Gadolinium enhancement identifies hemorrhagic or necrotic areas within the tumor (see Fig. 12-60) (240). Cerofolini et al. (241) reviewed the MR images of 17 peripheral nerve sheath tumors and found that in 90% of schwannomas, the nerve could be identified along one side of the mass. In neurofibromas, the nerve was either obliterated or no longer visible. Atrophy may be seen along the long axis of the muscle adjacent to the lesion in approximately 25% of cases (234).

Malignant Peripheral Nerve Sheath Tumor

Malignant peripheral nerve sheath tumor accounts for 6% to 10% of all soft tissue sarcomas. Approximately half arise in patients with neurofibromatosis (208,241). Of those patients with neurofibromatosis, 3% to 29% (average approximately 5%) will develop solitary or multiple malignant peripheral nerve sheath tumors, usually after a latent period of 10 to 20 years (234,237,242,243). Patients with neurofibromatosis present at a younger age and have larger higher grade lesions than do those patients in whom lesions occur sporadically (234). The prognosis remains guarded, with a 5-year survival rate between 15% and 30% (237). The prognosis is worse for patients with lesions greater than 5 cm and for those patients with neurofibromatosis (242). Malignant and benign nerve sheath neoplasms cannot be reliably distinguished by MRI, although marked inhomogeneities, infiltrating margins, and irregular bone destruction are more common in malignant neural neoplasms (see Fig. 12-61) (237,239).

Morton Neuroma

Morton neuroma is a pseudotumor of nerve and is a term used to describe perineural fibrosis of the plantar digital nerve (244). The lesion was originally described by Morton (245) in 1876, as a "peculiar and painful affection of the foot . . . localized in the fourth metatarsophalangeal articulation." The lesion is believed to be traumatic and is often attributed to compression of the interdigital nerve against the intermetatarsal ligament, in some cases exacerbated by an enlarged intermetatarsal bursa (244,246). Patients typically present with pain and/or numbness of the forefoot, usually exacerbated by walking and relieved by rest (244,246). The plantar digital nerve is usually affected at the level of the metatarsal head, and there is frequently associated inflammatory response about the lesion. The nerve between the third and fourth metatarsals is most often involved, followed by that between the second and third (245,247–251). Involvement between the first and second metatarsal heads is uncommon, and involvement between the fourth and fifth is rare (249,251).

A palpable mass is usually not identified, although associated synovial cysts may be clinically evident. There is a marked female predilection (as high as 18:1) that has led to the suggestion that the cause is related to irritation from the wearing of high-heeled shoes. The foot position in high-heeled shoes is thought to compress the nerve against the intermetatarsal ligament. Although this seems correct intuitively, it has not been substantiated in biomechanical study, which has shown that the neurovascular bundle moves parallel to the surrounding structures, and other causes, to include ischemia, have been suggested (251).

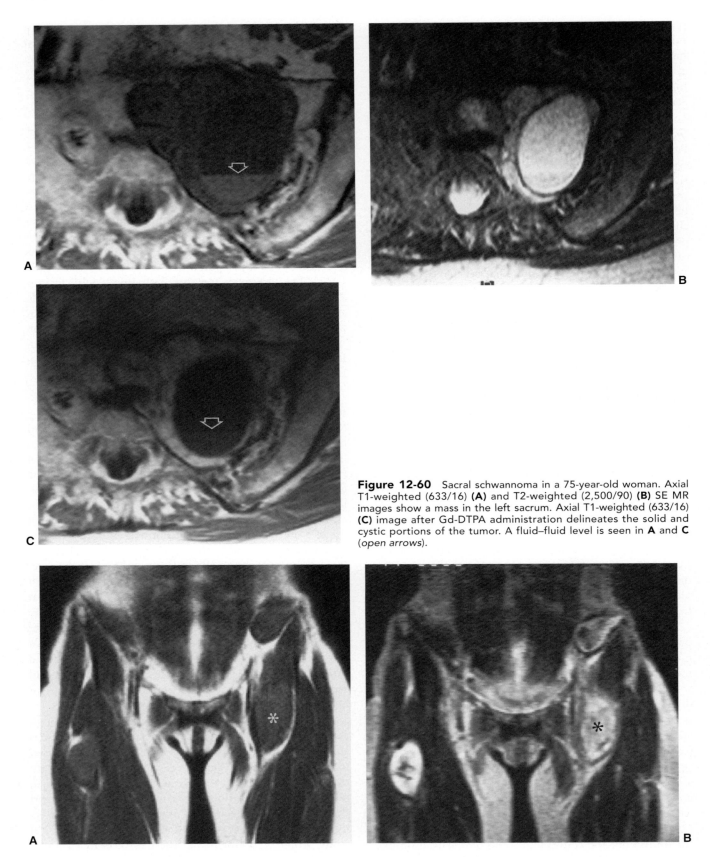

Figure 12-60   Sacral schwannoma in a 75-year-old woman. Axial T1-weighted (633/16) **(A)** and T2-weighted (2,500/90) **(B)** SE MR images show a mass in the left sacrum. Axial T1-weighted (633/16) **(C)** image after Gd-DTPA administration delineates the solid and cystic portions of the tumor. A fluid–fluid level is seen in **A** and **C** (*open arrows*).

Figure 12-61   Neurofibromatosis in a 44-year-old woman. Coronal T1-weighted (700/32) **(A)** and T2-weighted (2,000/80) **(B)** SE MR images show multiple neurofibromas in the lower extremities. The lesion in the left thigh (*asterisk*) was a malignant schwannoma.

Clinically occult lesions may be significantly more common than is generally appreciated, with a prevalence of 30% reported in a review of the MR images of 70 asymptomatic volunteers (251). It is interesting that there is no significant gender predilection in this group, in contradistinction to symptomatic patients. Not surprisingly, clinically occult lesions were also statistically smaller than those on symptomatic patients, with a mean transverse diameter of 4.5 versus 5.6 mm, respectively.

The diagnosis is often made on clinical grounds, and imaging evaluation is often unnecessary (246). Radiologic evaluation is often reserved for atypical cases or when confirmation of diagnosis is required (246). Radiographs are typically normal and are most useful in excluding other causes for pain. MRI is generally the accepted standard for diagnosis and localization, with a reported accuracy of about 90%, a positive predictive value of 100%, and a negative predictive value of 60% (250). Lesions are most evident on T1-weighted images (244,246,250), and additional pulse sequences are best used for purposes of differential diagnosis (250). Zanetti et al. (251) suggested three MR criteria for this diagnosis at MRI. First, the lesion is centered in the region of the neurovascular bundle, within the intermetatarsal space, on the plantar side of the transverse metatarsal ligament. Next, the lesion is well demarcated (excluding partial volume artifact from the adjacent joint capsule). Third, the signal intensity of the lesion should be similar to that of skeletal muscle on T1-weighted images and less than that of fat on T2-weighted images (see Fig. 12-62). It is the fibrous nature of the lesion that likely reflects its decreased signal intensity on MRI.

The conspicuity of the lesion is markedly reduced on T2-weighted MR images, making distinction from surrounding muscle and fat difficult. Fat-suppressed T2 sequences may allow better delineation. Lesions usually, but not invariably, will enhance after intravenous contrast administration (see Fig. 12-63). Terk et al. (246), in a study of six patients with surgically proven Morton neuroma, found fat-suppressed contrast-enhanced MR images best to depict the lesion and were able to identify neuromas with this technique when T1-weighted, T2-weighted, and T2-weighted fat-suppressed MRI sequences failed to detect them in two patients.

MRI is also excellent at detecting fluid in the intermetatarsal bursa, which is characterized by increased signal intensity on T2-weighted images between the metatarsal heads, dorsal to the transverse metatarsal ligament (251). This finding was identified proximal to the neuroma by Erickson et al. (244) in 10 of 15 lesions and in seven intermetatarsal spaces with no adjacent mass. Zanetti et al. (251) found that this may be seen in two thirds of asymptomatic patients, noting that the fluid was in the first through third intermetatarsal spaces and small in transverse diameter, with only 2 of the 81 fluid collections (in 47 of 70 volunteers) larger than 3 mm. Fluid was not identified in the fourth intermetatarsal space in normal volunteers.

Treatment of Morton neuroma is usually initially directed at modifying the patient's footwear. Other modes of therapy include neurolysis, steroid injection, ultrasound therapy, and surgical release of the transverse metatarsal ligament for decompression. Surgical excision of the neuroma and involved nerve segment appears to be the most successful mode of treatment.

Traumatic Neuroma

The traumatic neuroma is not a true neoplasm. It represents a proliferation of nerve tissue, usually related to the proximal end of a severed nerve (252). Typically, this is associated with trauma or surgical amputation. The incidence of traumatic neuroma is markedly reduced, and regeneration is possible if the nerve ends are closely approximated after injury (253). Clinically, traumatic

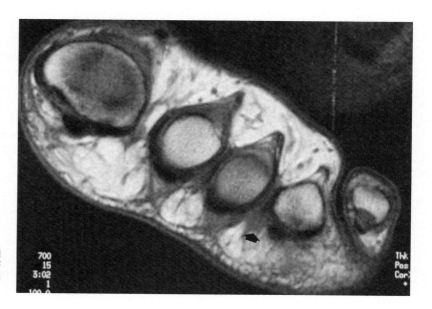

Figure 12-62   Morton neuroma in a 31-year-old man. Coronal T1-weighted (700/15) SE MR image of the left foot shows a 5-mm Morton neuroma (*arrow*) between the third and fourth metatarsal heads.

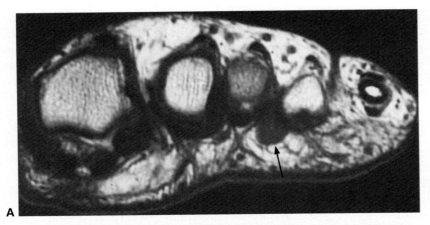

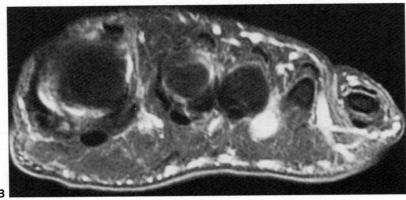

Figure 12-63 Morton neuroma in a 50-year-old man. **A:** Coronal T1-weighted (679/12) SE MR image of the left foot shows a small Morton neuroma (*arrow*) between the third and fourth metatarsal heads. **B:** Corresponding axial fat-suppressed postcontrast image shows marked enhancement.

neuroma may be asymptomatic or painful and presents as a firm nodule. Pathologically, disorganized proliferation of nerve fascicles, including all cellular neurogenic components (axons, Schwann cells, and fibroblasts with significant collagen), is seen. This feature distinguishes traumatic neuroma from neurofibroma (46,253).

Experience with the imaging of traumatic neuroma is limited (254–256). MR images typically show intermediate signal intensity on both T1- and T2-weighted images and with T2-weighting often showing a mild heterogeneous signal (252,256). A high signal intensity on T2-weighted images may occasionally be seen. On closer inspection, long-axis (coronal or sagittal) MR images may demonstrate the entering nerve as a thickened tubular structure (see Fig. 12-64) (252,256).

Synovial Sarcoma

Synovial sarcoma is a well-recognized soft tissue malignancy that typically arises in young adults. First reported in 1893, it is a relatively common primary soft tissue sarcoma, accounting for approximately 10% of all malignant mesenchymal neoplasms. Although the tumor resembles synovium at light microscopy, its origin is likely from undifferentiated mesenchymal tissue. Clinically, presentation spans a wide range in age, although synovial sarcoma is most prevalent between the ages of 15 and 35 years (46). It has been

reported in children and has been noted at birth (257). The patient generally presents with a palpable soft tissue mass, which may be quite slow growing and may clinically simulate a benign process (258). Pain is often present. Additional complaints include sensory and/or motor dysfunction distal to the lesion. The duration of symptoms is quite variable and may be present for days to weeks or as long as 20 years before initial diagnosis (259).

Most (80% to 95%) synovial sarcomas occur in the extremities, with approximately 60% to 70% in the lower limbs (259,260). Fewer than 10% of cases are reported as intraarticular, and in our experience, intraarticular lesions are quite rare. Other rare sites of involvement include the neck, pharynx, larynx, precoccygeal and paravertebral regions, thoracic and abdominal wall, and heart (261–265).

Metastases or local recurrence is seen in approximately 80% of patients (266). Metastases are present at the time of initial diagnosis in about one fourth of patients (266) but have been reported as long as 35 years after initial diagnosis (267). Metastases are predominantly pulmonary, occurring in approximately 59% to 94% of those with metastases (260,266,268). Other common sites include lymph nodes (4% to 18%) and bone (8% to 11%) (260,266,268–270). Soft tissue metastases are rare but have been reported (271). Local recurrence is frequent, seen in about 20% to 26% of patients (260,265,268,270),

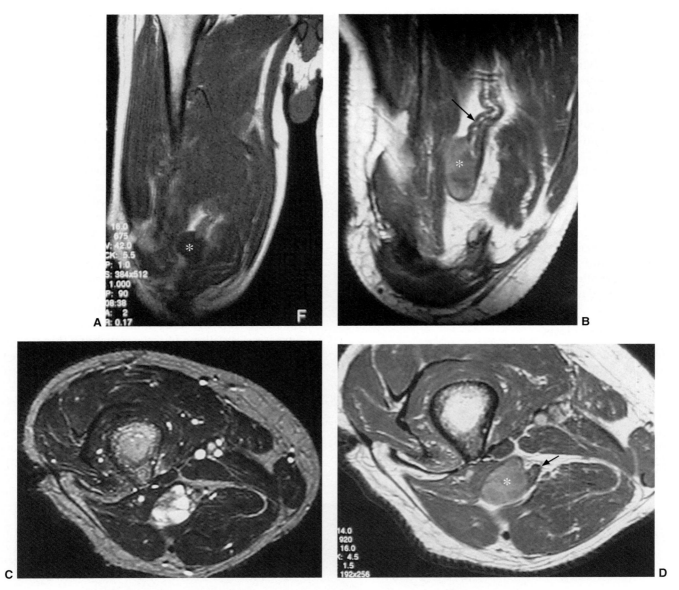

Figure 12-64 Traumatic neuroma in a 41-year-old man, 5 years after above knee amputation. **A:** Coronal T1-weighted (675/16) SE MR image of the thighs shows a small mass (*asterisk*) arising from the distal stump of the right siatic nerve. **B:** Axial T2-weighted (2,700/80) SE MR image shows the lesion to have a mixed signal intensity. Sagittal **(C)** and axial **(D)** contrast enhanced T1-weighted (750/15) SE MR images show the relationship of the enhancing lesion (*asterisk*) to the nerve stump (*arrow*).

occurring in the excision scar or the amputation stump, often within 2 years of initial presentation.

The prognosis remains guarded, although the biologic activity of the tumor is variable. The median survival after diagnosis is 33 months, with the 5-year survival rate approximately 27% to 55% (260,268). Median survival after first recurrence is less than one half that at diagnosis (268). Lesions that demonstrate extensive calcification have a more favorable prognosis (272), as do younger patients, tumors less than 5 cm in diameter, and lesions located in the extremities (260). The size of the tumor is the most important variable in determining prognosis (260).

Routine radiographs may be interpreted as normal in approximately one half of patients (260). When a mass is identified, it is most commonly a well-defined round or lobulated soft tissue mass (273). As many as one third of lesions demonstrate some internal calcification (less commonly ossification), typically in the periphery of the tumor (259,274). Coexistent adjacent bony involvement, manifested by periosteal reaction, bony remodeling (due to pressure from the adjacent tumor), or frank bony invasion, is seen in 11% to 20% of cases (259,260,273).

On MRI, the lesion is usually a nonspecific inhomogeneous mass, with signal intensity approximately equal to that of skeletal muscle on T1-weighted and brighter than that of subcutaneous fat on T2-weighted spin-echo MR images (275–277). The lesion may demonstrate a multi-locular configuration with internal septation (277). Changes compatible with previous hemorrhage, to include fluid–fluid levels, have been reported in 10% to 44% of lesions on MRI (275–279). Fluid–fluid levels are a nonspecific finding and have been reported in other soft tissue lesions, including hemangioma and myositis ossificans (see Fig. 12-65). Portions of the margins are often poorly defined or infiltrating (277), although margins are variable and may be well defined (275). Homogeneous well-defined lesions with signal intensity similar to that of skeletal muscle on both T1- and T2-weighted images have been reported (see Fig. 12-66) (277). The soft tissue calcifications frequently seen on radiographs may not be detected on MRI (276,277), although larger calcifications may be identified as areas of decreased signal intensity on all pulse sequences.

Tumorlike Lesions

Myositis Ossificans

Myositis ossificans is a benign, solitary, self-limiting, ossifying, soft tissue mass typically occurring within skeletal muscle. A history of trauma is often not apparent. The pathogenesis of myositis ossificans is unknown, and the term "myositis" is a misnomer in that no primary inflammation of skeletal muscle is associated with the process (280). Synonyms include pseudomalignant osseous tumor of soft tissue, extraosseous localized nonneoplastic bone and cartilage formation, myositis ossificans circumscripta, pseudomalignant myositis ossificans, and heterotopic ossification (280–283).

The most frequent symptoms are pain, tenderness, and a soft tissue mass; however, the lesion may be an incidental finding. Patients are usually young adults; myositis ossificans is quite rare in children. Approximately 80% of cases arise in the large muscles of the extremities (284). Myositis ossificans is not a premalignant lesion, and there is no convincing evidence that such lesions may undergo malignant transformation. Local excision is generally curative.

Lesions are typically well circumscribed and rimmed by compressed fibrous connective tissue; these are frequently surrounded by or contain atrophic skeletal muscle. Typically, a distinct zoning pattern is present, in which lesional maturation progresses from an immature, central, nonossified cellular focus, to osteoid, to a peripheral rim of mature lamellar bone. Central nodular fasciitis-like areas and chondroosseous nodules may also be seen. As lesions mature, the nodular fasciitis-like areas in the intratrabecular spaces become areas of delicate fibrosis, containing thin-walled ectatic vascular channels that eventually become replaced by both adipose tissue and mature bone in the oldest lesions (285).

Plain radiographs of myositis ossificans show faint calcification within 2 to 6 weeks of onset of symptoms (280). A sharply circumscribed bony mass is usually apparent by 6 to 8 weeks (although it may be seen much earlier), becoming smaller and mature by 5 to 6 months (197,286,287).

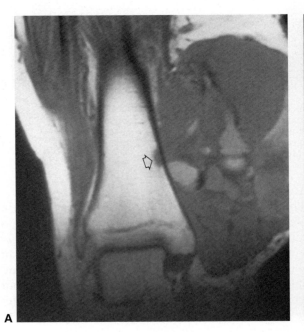
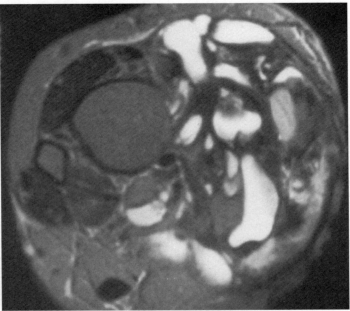

Figure 12-65 Synovial sarcoma in the ankle of a 37-year-old woman. Coronal T1-weighted (600/20) **(A)** and axial T2-weighted (2,000/80) **(B)** SE MR images show a large well-defined mass, with a complex signal intensity compatible with previous hemorrhage. Note subtle area of bone invasion in **A** (*open arrow*).

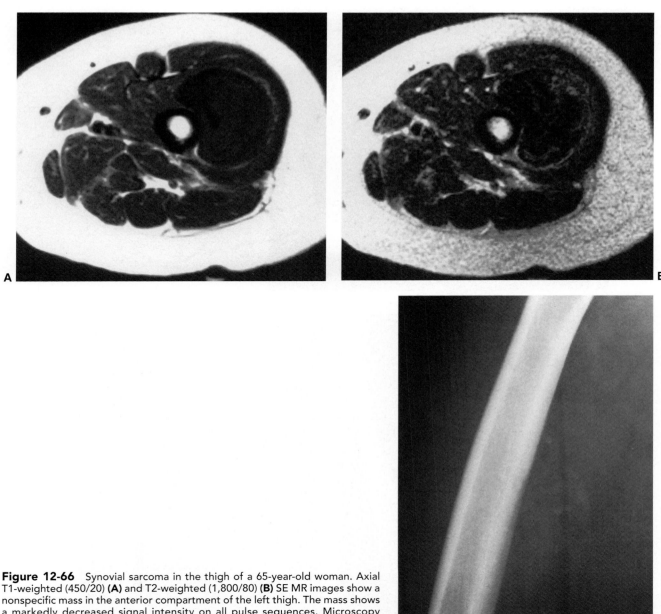

Figure 12-66 Synovial sarcoma in the thigh of a 65-year-old woman. Axial T1-weighted (450/20) **(A)** and T2-weighted (1,800/80) **(B)** SE MR images show a nonspecific mass in the anterior compartment of the left thigh. The mass shows a markedly decreased signal intensity on all pulse sequences. Microscopy revealed monophasic synovial sarcoma, fibrous type, which contained abundant collagen. **C:** Corresponding radiograph shows amorphus calcification within the mass.

Lesions are often deep and may be associated with the periosteum but are usually separated from it by a radiolucent zone (197). The pattern of mineralization with peripheral mature ossification is essential in establishing the radiologic diagnosis and allows differentiation from other mineralized lesions, especially extraskeletal and juxtacortical osteosarcoma.

The MRI appearance of myositis ossificans will change with the lesion's age, reflecting the evolving histology. Early lesions, before radiographically visible mineralization, will demonstrate a signal intensity greater than that of fat on T2-weighted spin-echo MR images. The lesions will be moderately inhomogeneous with diffuse surrounding soft tissue edema (285,288,289). On corresponding T1-weighted images, the lesion is usually isointense to skeletal muscle. Margins are poorly defined and may be recognized only secondarily by mass effect and displacement of fascial planes (285,288). Curvilinear areas of decreased signal intensity may be seen surrounding lesions, corresponding to peripheral mineralization. Intermediate or older lesions are similar but will typically demonstrate a rim of curvilinear decreased signal intensity corresponding to the lesions' peripheral ossification. Irregular areas of decreased signal intensity may

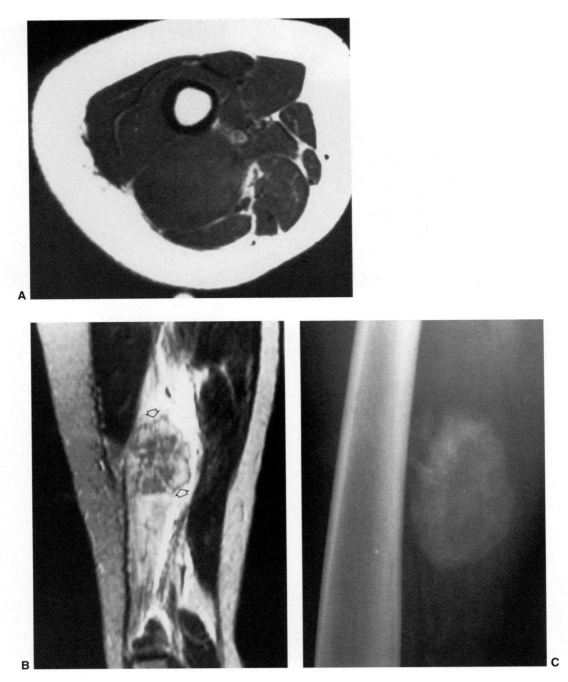

Figure 12-67 Myositis ossificans in a 24-year-old woman. **A:** Axial T1-weighted (427/20) SE MR image shows the lesion to be isointense to skeletal muscle. **B:** Coronal T2-weighted (2,213/80) image shows the lesion (*open arrows*), with extensive surrounding edema. **C:** Corresponding radiograph shows the mass to be densely mineralized.

be seen coursing through lesions as well, again corresponding to areas of mineralization (see Fig. 12-67).

Infrequently, fluid–fluid levels may be detected and are consistent with previous hemorrhage (289,290). This is not an uncommon histologic finding in the inner, most immature portion of the lesion (see Fig. 12-68). MRI signal changes compatible with edema in the adjacent bone marrow (poorly defined areas of increased signal intensity on T2-weighted and decreased signal on T1-weighted spin-echo MR images) have also been infrequently noted (281).

Mature (late) lesions are well-defined inhomogeneous masses with a signal intensity approximating that of fat on both T2- and T1-weighted images without associated edema. On all pulse sequences, a rim of decreased signal intensity surrounds the lesion, and similar areas of decreased signal intensity may be seen within the lesion.

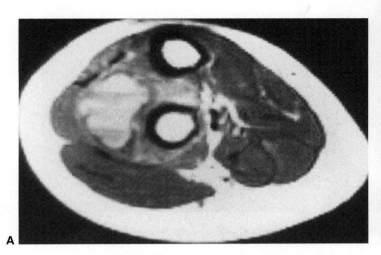

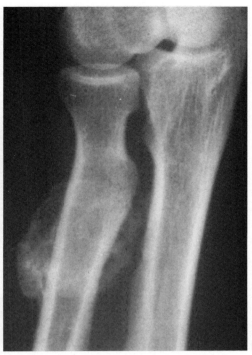

A   B

Figure 12-68 Myositis ossificans in a 31-year-old woman. **A:** Axial proton density (2,000/40) SE MR image shows multiple fluid–fluid levels. Area of increased signal intensity surrounding the lesion is likely from previous hemorrhage. **B:** Corresponding radiograph shows the mass to be densely mineralized, with a more mature peripheral shell. (From Kransdorf MJ, Meis JM, Jelinek JS. Myositis ossificans: MR appearance with radiologic-pathologic correlation. *AJR Am J Roentgenol* 1991;157:1243–1248.)

Mature lesions may also demonstrate relatively decreased signal on all spin-echo MR pulse sequences, secondary to dense ossification and fibrosis (see Fig. 12-69) (288).

The inhomogeneous areas of intermediate signal seen within late myositis ossificans on T2-weighted images reflect areas of mature fat between bone trabeculae of the lesion. These same areas have a high signal intensity on T1-weighted images. The areas of decreased signal intensity on both pulse sequences represent the bone trabeculae of the lesion. Areas of hemosiderin deposition from previous hemorrhage and fibrosis may also contribute to areas of decreased signal intensity on both pulse sequences.

Active lesions demonstrate enhancement after intravenous gadolinium dimeglumine (285). Although understanding of enhancement is incomplete, the vascularity seen arteriographically is likely responsible, at least in part, for the contrast enhancement seen on MRI (291). Surrounding enhancement reflects associated edema (25,291).

Hematoma

The MR appearance of hematomas is variable and will be a function of the age of the lesion and the stage and amounts of the various hemoglobin breakdown products: oxyhemoglobin, deoxyhemoglobin, methemoglobin, and hemosiderin (292). Extracranial hematomas are usually classified by age as acute, subacute, or chronic, although these terms are not rigorously defined. In general usage, acute hematoma is used for a lesion hours to days old. A subacute hematoma is one that is 1 week to about 3 months old, and a chronic hematoma is one older than 3 months. The susceptibility phenomenon is proportional to the square of the magnetic field, and imaging features of degradation products are best demonstrated on high field strength magnets.

On spin-echo MRI, an acute hematoma shows a signal intensity relatively similar to that of skeletal muscle on T1-weighted images, varying from slightly hyperintense to hypointense. A decreased signal intensity, less than that of skeletal muscle, is seen on T2-weighted images corresponding to intracellular deoxyhemoglobin or methemoglobin (292,293). Acute hematomas have considerable variability; a heterogeneous appearance may be seen, and adjacent edema may be a prominent feature (see Fig. 12-70).

Most subacute hematomas (weeks to months old) will demonstrate increased signal on both T1- and T2-weighted spin-echo MR images (293,294), due to the presence of extracellular methemoglobin (see Fig. 12-71). Typically, with time, as the lesion becomes chronic, a rim of decreased signal intensity will be seen with time, due to the accumulation of hemosiderin laden macrophages (293). This will demonstrate marked hypointensity and may eventually encompass the entire lesion (see Fig. 12-72).

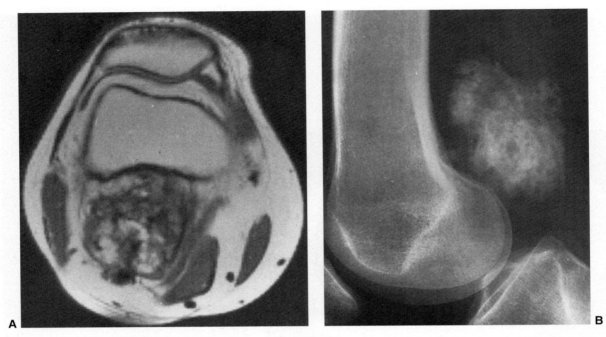

Figure 12-69 Mature myositis ossificans in the popliteal fossa of a 35-year-old man. **A:** Axial T1-weighted (500/30) SE MR image shows a well-defined inhomogeneous mass in the popliteal fossa, with areas imaging identical to subcutaneous fat. **B:** Corresponding radiograph shows the mass to be densely mineralized.

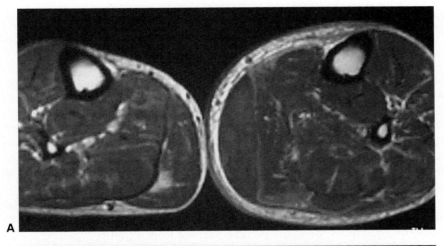

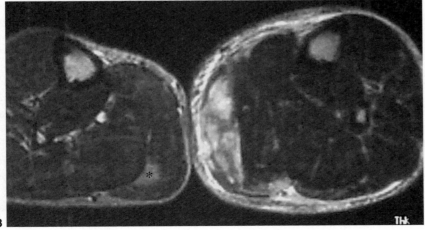

Figure 12-70 Acute hematoma (3 days old) in the calf of a 59-year-old man. Axial T1-weighted (800/15) **(A)** and T2-weighted (2,500/90) **(B)** SE MR image shows a heterogeneous mass on the medial gastrocnemius muscle with associated edema. Incidental note is made of a small intramuscular lipoma in the right medial gastrocnemius (*asterisk*).

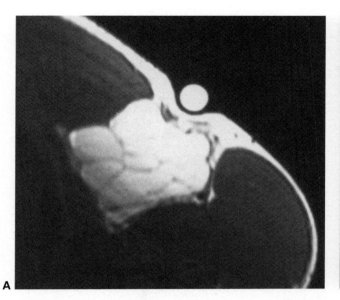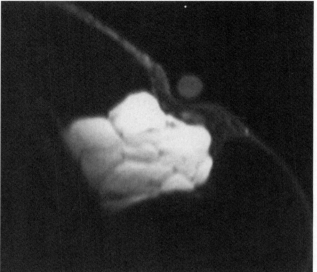

A   **B**

Figure 12-71   Hematoma in the axilla of a 17-year-old boy. **A:** Axial T1-weighted (600/20) SE MR image shows a well-defined lobulated mass, with signal intensity similar to subcutaneous fat. **B:** Corresponding T2-weighted (2,000/80) image shows a similar configuration, with signal intensity greater than fat, compatible with subacute blood.

Hematomas can persist long after initial injury and may slowly enlarge. This situation, termed chronic expanding hematoma, may suggest a malignancy due to a history of a growing soft tissue mass (295). It is postulated that the lesion is the result of the irritant effects of blood and its breakdown products, causing repeated exudation or bleeding from capillaries in granulation tissue (295,296). These lesions typically show a central area of intermixed high and low signal intensity on T2-weighted images, corresponding to hemosiderin deposition, loose connective tissue, granulation tissue, necrotic debris-filled cavities, fibrin, and blood clot (295). This is surrounded by a rim of decreased signal intensity, corresponding to a pseudocapsule of hyaline fibrous tissue. There may be areas of high signal on T1-weighted images or on both T1- and T2-weighted images, as a result of associated acute or subacute hemorrhage. The adjacent osseous structure will typically show erosive change with reactive change and nodular and non-specific calcifications.

Care must be taken to differentiate malignant soft tissue tumor with hemorrhage from hematoma. The presence of a tumor nodule or rim of tumor may be helpful in distinguishing a simple hematoma from a hemorrhagic neoplasm (3).

Pseudoaneurysm

Pseudoaneurysm may also occasionally present as a soft tissue mass. Pseudoaneurysm typically shows a complex pattern with signal voids in regions of flowing blood, marked hyperintense signal on T1- and T2-weighted images in areas of subacute blood, and marked decreased signal intensity in areas of hemosiderin deposition due to chronic bleeding (293,297). Large arteriovenous malformations demonstrate

signal void on spin-echo sequences due to the presence of flowing blood. On gradient-echo images, flowing blood gives a uniform hyperintense signal. The multiplicity of large vessels is usually demonstrated, although visualization of the smaller millimeter vessels is not clearly identified (298). MR arteriography may prove to be a valuable adjunct for evaluation of vascular malformations and peripheral vessels (see Fig. 12-73) (299,300).

Ganglion

Ganglions are tumorlike lesions of unknown origin that arise in the juxtaarticular soft tissue. They have been recognized since antiquity and were described by Hippocrates as a "knot of tissue containing mucoid flesh" (301,302). Synovial herniation and tissue degeneration, as well as repeated trauma, have been suggested as the cause (46). The lesion is most frequently found around the wrist and distal interphalangeal joints of the hand (303) and foot (304). Lesions may also develop adjacent to any joint or tendon sheath (305,306). The pathogenesis is unknown, although they are presumably caused by a coalescence of small cysts formed by the myxomatous degeneration of periarticular connective tissue (307). We prefer the term "ganglion" to "ganglion cyst," in that lesions are uncommonly completely cystic. Typically presenting in young adults (25 to 45 years of age), there is a slight female predominance (46,308). Lesions are often asymptomatic. About half the cases are associated with tenderness, mild pain, or functional impairment (308,309). Lesions may grow, diminish in size, or resolve spontaneously (301). Lesions may compress adjacent structures and may be the cause of nerve palsy (310). Ganglia were reported in 21 of

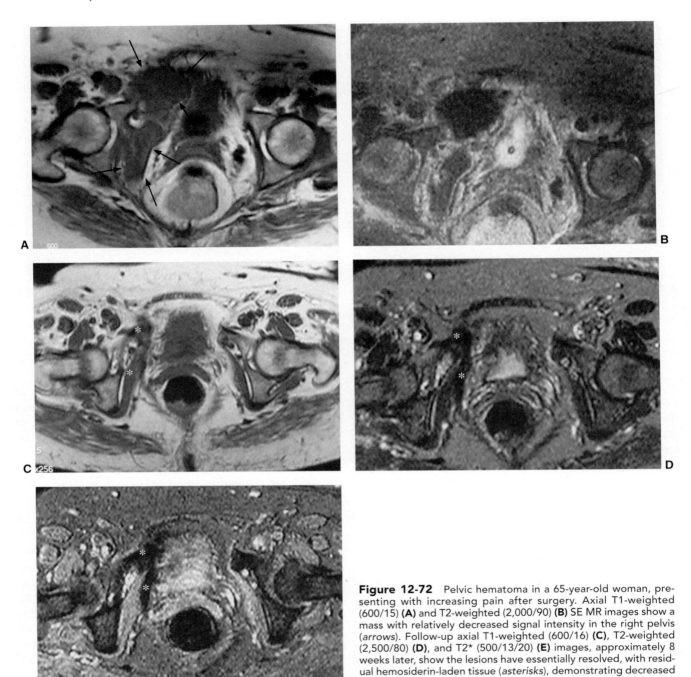

Figure 12-72 Pelvic hematoma in a 65-year-old woman, presenting with increasing pain after surgery. Axial T1-weighted (600/15) **(A)** and T2-weighted (2,000/90) **(B)** SE MR images show a mass with relatively decreased signal intensity in the right pelvis (*arrows*). Follow-up axial T1-weighted (600/16) **(C)**, T2-weighted (2,500/80) **(D)**, and T2* (500/13/20) **(E)** images, approximately 8 weeks later, show the lesions have essentially resolved, with residual hemosiderin-laden tissue (*asterisks*), demonstrating decreased signal with T2-weighting and markedly decreased signal on T2* imaging.

27 patients presenting with entrapment of the suprascapular nerve (132).

Most lesions are small, measuring 1.5 to 2.5 cm, without communication to the joint space (46). Microscopically, one sees thick-walled cystic spaces in association with myxoid areas, which may be outside the cystic spaces (46). There is no discernible internal lining cell type (311). The lesion is surrounded by dense connective tissue and is filled with viscous gelatinous fluid that is rich in hyaluronic acid

and other mucopolysaccharides (312). Lesions may be unilocular or multilocular (301).

Radiographs may be normal or may reveal a soft tissue mass. The adjacent bone may demonstrate evidence of bone resorption or periosteal new bone. Lesions are typically rounded to lobular in shape and located adjacent to joint capsules or tendon sheaths (99). They typically image similar to fluid on MRI with a low signal intensity on T1-weighted images and high signal intensity on T2-weighted

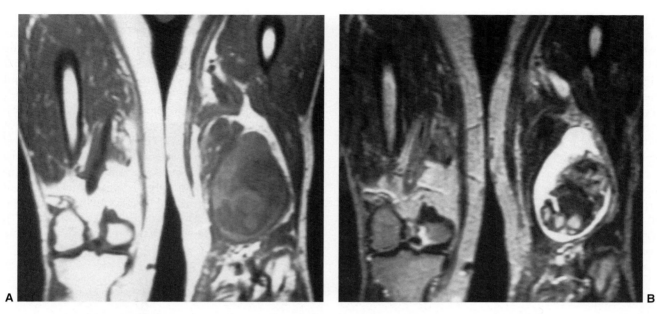

Figure 12-73 Pseudoaneurysm in the popliteal fossa of a 65-year-old man. Coronal T1-weighted (650/20) **(A)** and T2-weighted (2,000/80) **(B)** SE MR image show well-defined mass with a complex pattern of signal intensities, compatible with subacute and chronic hemorrhage.

images (132,209,310–312), or they may be isointense or slightly hyperintense to muscle on T1-weighted spin-echo images (see Fig. 12-74) (301). Feldman et al. (301) noted sharply defined delicate internal septa, creating a characteristic corrugated or compartmentalized appearance in 13 of

17 cases. They also noted small fluid-filled pseudopodia in 11 of 17 cases. MRI clearly localizes the lesion and identifies its relationship to adjacent structures, including vessels, tendons, and nerves (209). The relationship to adjacent joints, capsules, and tendons is best demonstrated

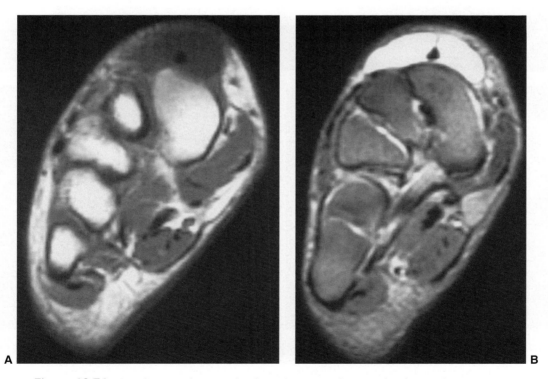

Figure 12-74 Ganglion. Axial T1-weighted (500/20) **(A)** and T2-weighted (2,000/80) **(B)** SE MR images of the foot demonstrating a well-defined ganglion with high signal intensity on T2-weighted **B** and low signal intensity on T1-weighted **A** images.

on long TR/TE or other fluid-sensitive sequences (301). Ganglions may be associated with major vessels in 10% to 20% of cases, making aspiration difficult (209,313).

Caution is required in making the diagnosis of a cyst solely on the basis of MRI signal characteristics, and a small homogeneous malignancy may masquerade as a "cyst." The differentiation between a cyst and a homogeneously solid mass is better made on sonography. On MRI examination, ganglion may show variable enhancement (see Fig. 12-75).

Periosteal Ganglion

Periosteal ganglion is a rare lesion. Abdelwahab et al. (307) reported 4 cases and found 11 previous cases in their review of the English literature. Periosteal ganglion is more common in men, accounting for 12 of the previously reported 15 cases (307). Most (67%) are found in the region of the pes anserinus (307). The remaining lesions mainly affect the ends of long tubular bones, to include the distal shafts of the ulna, radius and femur, and medial malleolus. Patients usually present with swelling and mild tenderness (307).

Radiographs may show scalloping due to extrinsic pressure remodeling (307). These erosions are the hallmark of diagnosis on radiographs. Thick spicules of reactive periosteal new bone may extend from the scalloped area (307). MRI shows a homogeneous, well-defined, juxtacortical mass with signal intensity approximately equal to that of skeletal muscle on T1-weighted images and brighter than fat on T2-weighted spin-echo images (see Fig. 12-76) (307). Peripheral enhancement can be seen after gadopentetate administration.

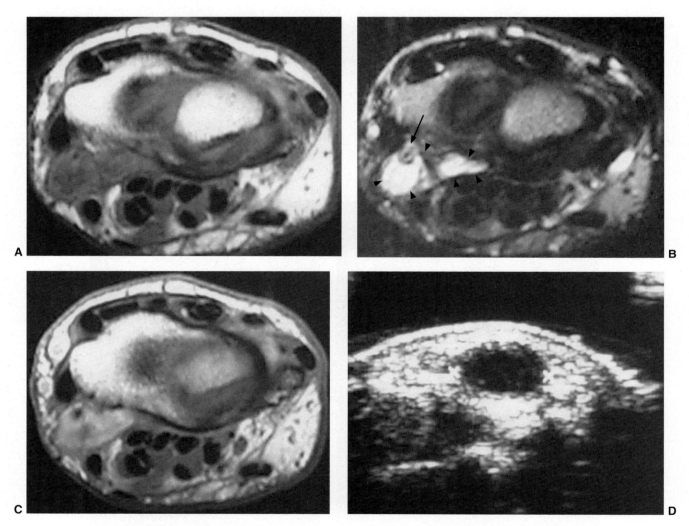

Figure 12-75 Ganglion of the wrist in a 49-year-old woman. Axial T1-weighted (600/20) **(A)** and T2-weighted (2,000/90) **(B)** SE MR images show a lobulated small mass (*arrowheads*) adjacent to the volar aspect of the radiocarpal joint. Note the position of the radial artery (*arrow*). The mass is relatively well defined with heterogeneous signal intensity. **C:** Corresponding axial T1-weighted (600/20) SE MR image after contrast administration shows significant contrast enhancement peripherally. **D:** Ultrasound shows a more cystlike appearance.

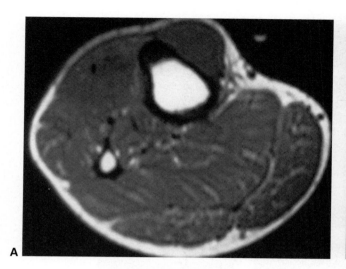
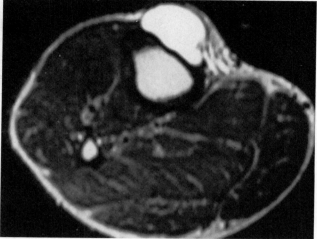

Figure 12-76 Periosteal ganglion in a 45-year-old man. Axial T1-weighted (600/20) **(A)** and T2-weighted (1,800/80) **(B)** SE MR images show a well-defined mass in the region of the pes anserinus. The lesion images similar to fluid. There is mild remodeling of the medial tibial cortex.

Intramuscular Myxoma

Intramuscular myxoma is a distinctive benign mesenchymal lesion that probably arises from altered fibroblasts that produce excessive amounts of mucopolysaccharide, which in turn inhibit the polymerization of normal collagen (314). It is most common in adults in the fifth to seventh decades. This lesion is uncommon in young adults and rare in children (1). Patients typically present with a palpable soft tissue mass, and fewer than one fourth of patients complain of pain or tenderness (314). Growth rate is variable, and lesions may be stable with no apparent growth over long periods of time (46). Lesions are most common in the thigh; other common locations include the shoulder, buttocks, and upper arm (139).

Intramuscular myxoma is usually a solitary lesion, although rare multiple lesions have been reported in association with fibrous dysplasia of bone, usually the polyostotic form (315–317). This is also known as Mazabraud syndrome. As of 1993, only 19 cases of this interesting association were reported (318).

On MR imaging, intramuscular myxoma typically appears as a homogeneous, well-defined, soft tissue mass with signal intensity less than that of skeletal muscle on T1-weighted images and greater than that of fat on T2-weighted images (see Figs. 12-77 and 12-78) (139). This appearance may simulate fluid; therefore, ultrasound may be especially helpful in differentiating the lesion from a true cyst. Intramuscular myxomas frequently have partly ill-defined borders, and a peritumoral fat rind. Additionally, increased signal intensity in the adjacent muscle on fluid sensitive sequences also often present.

The rind of adipose tissue is likely reactive fat, secondary to muscle atrophy associated with the slowly growing mass. This may be so extensive as to simulate fat within the lesion. Intramuscular myxomas have no capsule, and the increased signal intensity on fluid sensitive sequences is the result of myxomatous material infiltrating the adjacent atrophic and edematous striated muscle (319).

Following gadolinium administration, a combined peripheral and central enhancement is seen. The most reliable radiologic features in differentiating an intramuscular myxoma from a myxoid liposarcoma is the identification of the perilesional rind of adipose tissue on T1-weighted images and increased signal intensity in the adjacent muscle on T2-weighted or fluid sensitive sequences (see Fig. 12-79) (319,320). On occasion, an intramuscular myxoma may not be radiologically differentiated from a myxoid liposarcoma.

Juxtaarticular Myxoma

The juxtaarticular myxoma, also known as a periarticular myxoma, is a controversial lesion that is probably a variant of myxoma that usually occurs around large joints, particularly the knee (90%) (321). These lesions have histologic features of a myxoma but are frequently associated with cystic change resembling ganglions (321). The origin of the cystic change is uncertain but is suspected to be the result of motion, friction, or torsion affecting certain joints and juxtaarticular structures (321). The lesion may be related to previous trauma, explaining its predilection for the knee and frequent association with degenerative joint disease (321). There is scant literature on the MRI appearance of juxtaarticular myxoma; however, our experience is that a juxtaarticular myxoma cannot be adequately differentiated from a ganglion (see Fig. 12-80).

Multiple Lesions

Soft tissue tumors are typically solitary, and the identification of multiple lesions significantly limits the differential

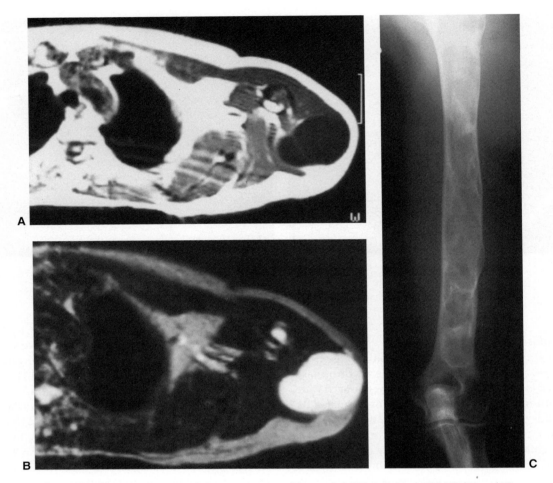

Figure 12-77 Mazabraud syndrome in a 55-year-old man. Axial T1-weighted (600/17) **(A)** and T2-weighted (2670/90) **(B)** SE MR images show a well-defined homogeneous mass in the left shoulder. The signal intensity of the mass suggests it is fluid filled; however, sonogram (not shown) was inconsistent with simple fluid. **C:** Radiograph of the left humerus shows changes compatible with fibrous dysplasia.

diagnosis. Multiple lipomas are seen in 5% to 7% of patients (53). The diagnosis in these cases can be made confidently on the basis of MR signal intensity. Aggressive fibromatosis is multifocal in 10% to 15% of patients, and a second soft tissue mass in a patient with previously confirmed desmoid tumor should be regarded as a second desmoid tumor until proven otherwise (189,196,231). Patients with neurofibromatosis may also have multiple lesions. Although the diagnosis may be known or suggested on clinical grounds, the diagnosis can be suggested on imaging studies by the identification of multiple lesions in major nerve distribution.

Angiomatous lesions are quite common and are multiple in up to 20% of patients (46). In such cases, superficial and deep lesions may coexist. Multiple lesions may also be seen with metastatic disease. The soft tissue is relatively resistant to metastasis, and although it comprises about 40% of total body weight, soft tissue metastases are quite rare. The skin and subcutaneous tissue is also a frequent site of extraosseous involvement in patients with multiple myeloma, with involvement typically as multiple subcutaneous nodules (322). Extraosseous manifestations are found in less than 5% of patients with multiple myeloma and are associated with a more aggressive clinical course (322). Metastatic melanoma may display a similar pattern of multiple nodular subcutaneous metastases (43). These are seen in more than 30% of patients with melanoma metastatic disease (usually in patients with Clark level IV or V disease) and may be the only radiologic manifestation of metastases (43). Finally, multiple myxomas may be seen in association with fibrous dysplasia of bone (Mazabraud syndrome) (317). The myxomas are usually intramuscular, and the association is most typically with polyostotic disease (Fig. 12-77) (317,323).

Benign versus Malignant

Although there is general agreement on the diagnostic value of MRI in many cases, the issue of whether MRI can reliably predict benign from malignant is much less clear (324).

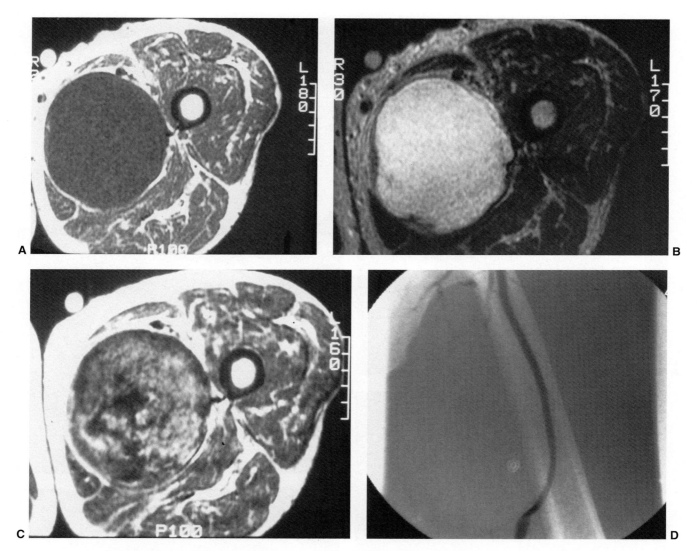

Figure 12-78 Intramuscular myxoma in the thigh of a 69-year-old man. Axial T1-weighted (427/20) **(A)** and T2-weighted (1,800/80) **(B)** SE MR images show a well-defined homogeneous mass with signal intensity similar to fluid. **C:** Corresponding axial T1-weighted (427/20) image after Gd-DTPA administration shows marked inhomogeneous enhancement. **D:** Arteriogram shows the mass to be avascular.

One study has suggested that MRI can differentiate benign from malignant masses in greater than 90% of cases based on the morphology of the lesion (19). Criteria used for a benign lesion included smooth well-defined margin, small size, and homogeneous signal intensity, especially on T2-weighted images. Other studies, however, note that malignant lesions may appear as smoothly marginated homogeneous masses, and MRI cannot reliably distinguish benign from malignant processes (see Figs. 12-81 and 12-82) (4,9,10,22,35,325). This discrepancy may well reflect differences within the populations studied.

When the MR images of a lesion are not sufficiently characteristic to suggest a specific diagnosis, a conservative approach is warranted. Malignancies, by virtue of their very nature and potential for autonomous growth, are generally larger and more likely to outgrow their vascular supply with subsequent infarction and necrosis and heterogeneous signal intensity on T2-weighted spin-echo MR images. Consequently, the larger a mass is, the greater its heterogeneity, the greater is the concern for malignancy (Fig. 12-65). Only 5% of benign soft tissue tumors measure 5 cm or more (326,327). In addition, most malignancies are deep lesions, whereas only about 1% of all benign soft tissue tumors are deep (326,327). Although these figures are based on surgical and not imaging series, these trends are likely still valid for radiologists.

When sarcomas are superficial, they generally have a less aggressive biologic behavior than do deep lesions. As a rule, most malignancies grow as deep space-occupying lesions, enlarging in a centripetal fashion (328), pushing

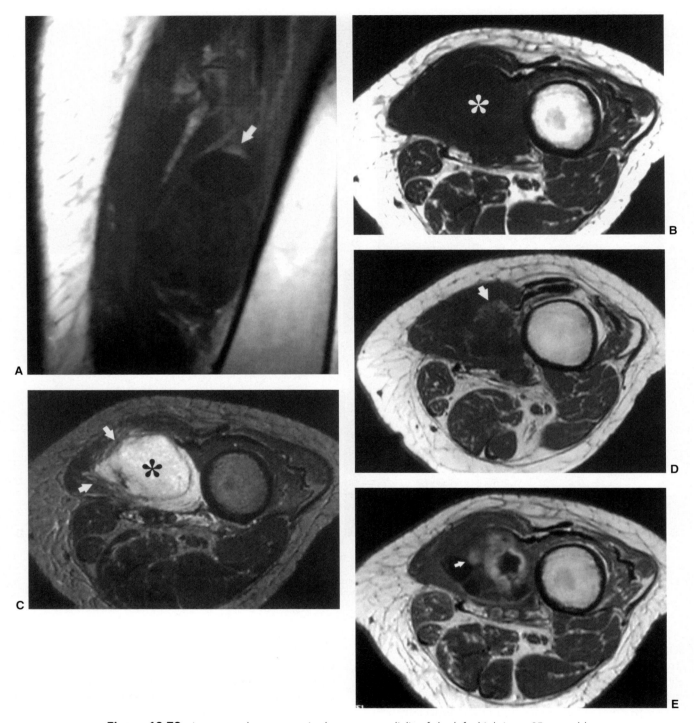

Figure 12-79 Intramuscular myxoma in the vastus medialis of the left thigh in an 85-year-old woman. **A:** Coronal T1-weighted (500/15) SE MR image shows a subtle rind of adipose tissue (*arrow*) at the periphery of the ovoid, heterogeneous lesion. Corresponding axial T1-weighted (600/15) **(B)** and conventional T2-weighted (2140/80) **(C)** SE MR images at the midportion of the lesion (*asterisk*) depicts the lesion's heterogeneous hypointense and intermediate signal intensity. Note the partially ill-defined border of the lesion in **C** (*arrows*), which blends imperceptibly with the adjacent hyperintense muscle. **D:** The rind of adipose tissue (*arrow*) at the inferior aspect of the lesion is easily appreciated on a more inferior axial T1-weighted image. However, in the axial plane, its contour may suggest intermuscular fat, rather than the interface between the lesion and surrounding muscle. **E:** Axial enhanced T1-weighted (600/15) image near the midportion of the lesion shows prominent heterogeneous central and peripheral enhancement (*arrow*).

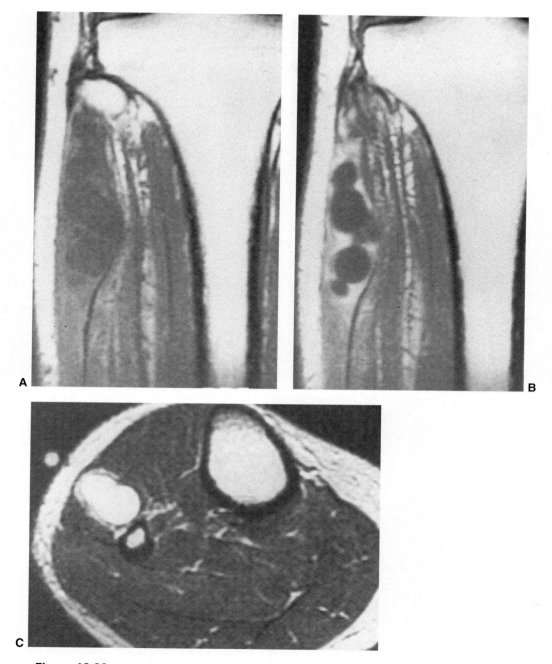

Figure 12-80   Juxtaarticular myxoma in a 49-year-old woman. **A:** Coronal T1-weighted (550/20) SE MR image shows the lesion adjacent to the proximal right fibular. The signal intensity of the lesion is similar to skeletal muscle, making the margins difficult to delineate. **B:** Axial T2-weighted (2,000/80) SE MR image shows a signal intensity greater than fat. **C:** Coronal T1-weighted (550/20) SE MR image after contrast administration shows enhancement at the periphery of the lesion.

rather than infiltrating adjacent structures (although clearly there are exceptions to this general rule). As they enlarge, a pseudocapsule of fibrous connective tissue is formed around them by compression and layering of normal tissue, associated inflammatory reaction, and vascularization (328). Generally, they respect fascial borders and remain within anatomic compartments until late in their course (328). It is this pattern of growth that gives most

sarcomas relatively well-defined margins, in distinction to the general concepts of margins used in the evaluation on osseous tumors.

Although our experience with metastatic carcinoma in soft tissue is limited, we have generally found these lesions to be very infiltrative, with lesions violating fascial planes and anatomic compartments. This pattern of growth is quite different from that seen in most primary soft tissue tumors.

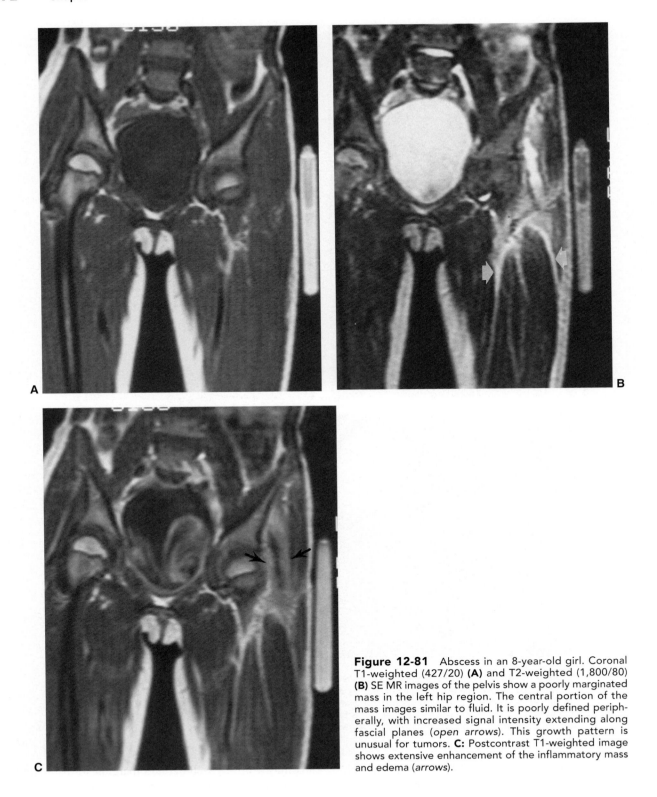

Figure 12-81 Abscess in an 8-year-old girl. Coronal T1-weighted (427/20) **(A)** and T2-weighted (1,800/80) **(B)** SE MR images of the pelvis show a poorly marginated mass in the left hip region. The central portion of the mass images similar to fluid. It is poorly defined peripherally, with increased signal intensity extending along fascial planes (*open arrows*). This growth pattern is unusual for tumors. **C:** Postcontrast T1-weighted image shows extensive enhancement of the inflammatory mass and edema (*arrows*).

Increased signal intensity in the skeletal muscle surrounding a musculoskeletal mass on T2-weighted spin-echo MR images or other fluid-sensitive sequences (i.e., STIR) has also been suggested as a reliable indicator of malignancy (222,329). These results are based on studies in which both bone and soft tissue lesions were evaluated. Although this increased signal intensity may be seen with malignancy, in our experience this finding is quite nonspecific. In fact, prominent high signal intensity surrounding a soft tissue mass more commonly suggests inflammatory

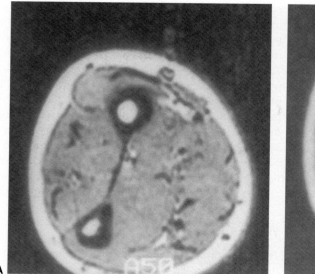
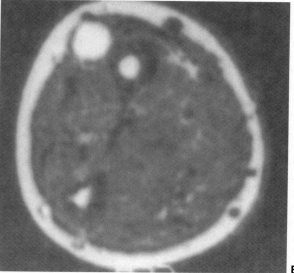

Figure 12-82 Synovial sarcoma in the forearm of a 9-year-old boy. Axial T1-weighted (600/16) **(A)** and T2-weighted (2,000/80) **(B)** SE MR images show an innocent-appearing, small, well-defined, homogeneous mass. The signal intensity is nonspecific.

processes, abscesses, myositis ossificans, local trauma, hemorrhage, biopsy, or radiation therapy rather than a primary soft tissue neoplasm (Figs. 12-67 and 12-81).

Gadolinium imaging has also been proposed as useful in differentiating benign and malignant soft tissue lesions, with malignant lesions showing a greater enhancement and a greater rate of enhancement (25,26,28,31,291, 330–332). Enhancement reflects tissue vascularity and tissue perfusion, and in general, the rate of enhancement of malignant lesions is greater than that seen in benign lesions. However, the overlap between benign and malignant is so great that this is of little practical value in any specific case (28). When a lesion has a nonspecific MR appearance, one is ill advised to suggest a lesion is benign or malignant based solely on its MRI characteristics and rate or degree of enhancement.

DeSchepper et al. (24) performed a multivariate statistical analysis of 10 imaging parameters, individually and in combination. They found that malignancy was predicted with the highest sensitivity when lesions had a high signal intensity on T2-weighted images, was larger than 33 mm in diameter, and had a heterogeneous signal intensity on T1-weighted images. Signs that had the greatest specificity for malignancy included tumor necrosis, bone or neurovascular involvement, and mean diameter of more than 66 mm.

In the final analysis, unfortunately, there are no absolutes. Perhaps Sundaram et al. (4) best summarized the impact of MRI on the evaluation of soft tissue tumors or tumorlike processes when they wrote that despite MRI's superiority over other imaging modalities in anatomic staging of soft tissue tumors, it, like CT, is of limited value in characterizing soft tissue sarcomas.

Gadolinium-enhanced Magnetic Resonance Imaging

Although there is general agreement on the value of MRI in the detection, diagnosis, and staging of soft tissue tumors and tumorlike lesions, the use of intravenous contrast in their evaluation remains controversial. In general, MR contrast agents enhance the signal intensity on T1-weighted spin-echo MR images of many tumors, in some cases enhancing the demarcation between tumor and muscle and tumor and edema and providing information on tumor vascularity (330,332). In actuality, differentiation between tumor and muscle is usually quite well delineated without enhanced imaging on T2-weighted images, and the accurate distinction between tumor and edema is probably of little practical value. Edema, which is infrequent without superimposed trauma or hemorrhage, is considered to be part of the reactive zone around the neoplasm and as such is removed *en bloc* with the tumor (204).

Information on tumor enhancement is not without a price. The use of intravenous contrast substantially increases the length and cost of the examination. Although contrast-enhanced MRI may provide some additional information, it has not been shown to increase lesion conspicuity or to replace conventional T2-weighted imaging (30). Moreover, although the incidence of untoward reaction as a result of contrast administration is small, it is real. Severe reactions have been reported with both gadopentitate dimeglumine (Magnevist, Berlex Laboratories, Wayne, NJ) and gadoteridol (ProHance, Squibb Diagnostics, Princeton, NJ) that include hypotension, laryngospasm, bronchospasm, anaphylactoid reaction, and anaphylactic shock (331,333–336) and a full spectrum of less serious reactions. Recently, Jordan and

Mintz (337) reported a fatal reaction to gadopentetate dimeglumine presumed to be due to anaphylactic reaction with associated bronchospasm. Consequently, gadolinium-enhanced imaging should be reserved for those cases in which the results influence patient management.

One specific circumstance in which gadolinium-enhanced imaging is useful is in the evaluation of hematomas. In such cases, contrast-enhanced imaging may reveal a small tumor nodule that may have been inapparent within the hemorrhage on conventional MRI (338,339). Caution is required, however, in that the fibrovascular tissue in organizing hematomas may show enhancement (101). Gadolinium-enhanced imaging has also been used to differentiate solid from cystic (or necrotic) lesions or to identify cystic or necrotic areas within solid tumors, with these necrotic or cystic areas showing no enhancement (330). This distinction may be difficult or impossible to make on conventional T2-weighted images, when both tumor and fluid show high signal intensity, well-defined margins, and homogeneous signal intensity, and is especially important to guide biopsy (Fig. 12-60). Care is needed, however, in that myxoid lesions such as intramuscular myxoma or myxoid liposarcoma and hyaline cartilage lesions such as synovial chondromatosis may demonstrate little or mild enhancement and may mimic cysts or lesions with cystic components. In general, ultrasound is fast and inexpensive and is an ideal method for differentiating solid and cystic lesions, when the lesion is in an anatomic location accessible to sonographic evaluation. Other potential advantages include assessment of enhancement pattern suggesting overall tumor vascularity (see Fig. 12-83). It must be emphasized, however, that not all lesions that enhance are hypervascular (Fig. 12-78). It is unlikely that enhanced MRI will replace routine spin-echo T1- and T2-weighted images.

Posttreatment Evaluation

Radiologic differentiation of postoperative and postradiation change from that of residual or recurrent tumor can be exceedingly difficult, if not impossible, in the immediate postoperative period (340,341). At least half of patients with soft tissue sarcomas will have local recurrence (27,108,268). Consequently, routine follow-up is essential. MRI and ultrasonography have both been shown to be useful in detecting local recurrence (9). On MRI, the configuration and signal intensity of the lesion within the surgical bed are of prime importance in identifying local recurrence (9,27). Choi et al. suggested that recurrent tumor is characterized by the presence of a discrete nodule with prolonged T1 and T2 relaxation times, with or without deformity of adjacent tissue, whereas fluid collections without nodule or areas of low or intermediate signal intensity suggest postsurgical change (see Fig. 12-84).

Vanel et al. (27) reviewed the finding on follow-up MRI examination in 182 patients, 164 with malignant soft tissue tumors and 18 with fibromatosis. They noted that 24 (96%)

of 25 patients without high signal intensity on T2-weighted images had no recurrence, and only 2 (3%) of 79 patients with high signal intensity on T2-weighted images, without a mass, had recurrence. A mass with high signal intensity on T2-weighted images was found in the remaining patients and was due most commonly to recurrent tumor, less likely to postoperative hygroma, or rarely to radiation-induced pseudotumor. Dynamic gadolinium imaging was useful in differentiating the last group with no enhancement seen in hygromas, postradiation change enhancing at 4 to 7 minutes, and recurrence enhancing at 1 to 3 minutes. We would recommend baseline MRI examination at 3 months after surgery. This will allow time for healing at the surgical site.

When to Biopsy

The question as to whether all clinically apparent lesions need to be biopsied is not easily answered, nor is there uniform agreement. As a general rule, we do not recommend biopsy for an unequivocal superficial lipoma. Our referring orthopedic surgeons have followed selected patients with a presumed hemangioma, intramuscular lipoma, lipomatosis, myositis ossificans, and ganglion in the appropriate clinical setting. Similarly, we would be willing to follow a presumed lipoblastoma, lipoblastomatosis, or elastofibroma. When imaging characteristics are nonspecific, however, a malignancy must be considered.

BONE NEOPLASMS

Patients with osseous tumors or tumorlike processes frequently present with symptoms that are nonspecific, such as pain or tenderness, perhaps with an associated soft tissue mass. However, asymptomatic skeletal lesions are often identified on imaging studies obtained for unrelated reasons (1). MRI can provide valuable information for the evaluation of primary benign and malignant tumors and metastatic lesions (13).

Initial Evaluation

The conventional radiograph remains the initial imaging examination in evaluating bone lesions and is almost invariably the most diagnostic. The radiograph accurately predicts the biologic activity of a lesion, which is reflected in the appearance of the lesion's margin and the type and extent of accompanying periosteal reaction. In addition, the pattern of associated matrix mineralization may be a key to the underlying histology (e.g., cartilage, bone, fibroosseous) (342–345). Although other imaging modalities (MRI and CT) are superior to radiographs in staging a bone lesion, the conventional radiograph remains the best modality for establishing a diagnosis, for formulating a differential, and for accurately assessing the biologic activity (separating benign from malignant lesions).

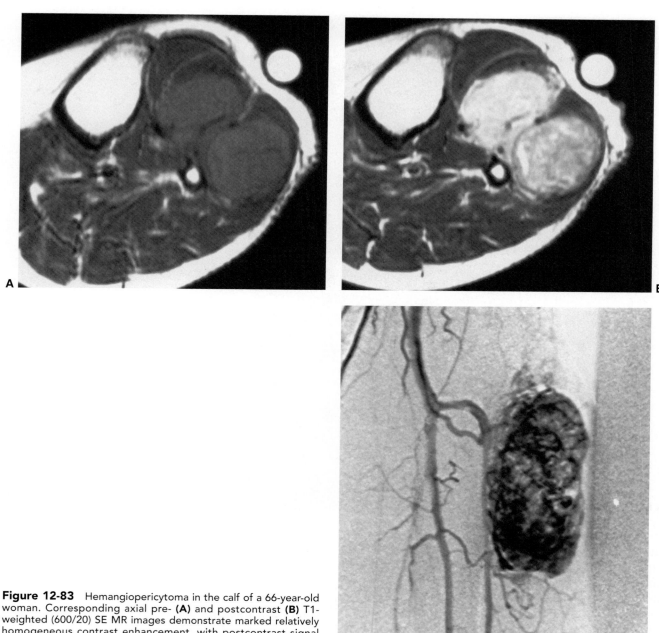

Figure 12-83 Hemangiopericytoma in the calf of a 66-year-old woman. Corresponding axial pre- **(A)** and postcontrast **(B)** T1-weighted (600/20) SE MR images demonstrate marked relatively homogeneous contrast enhancement, with postcontrast signal intensity approaching that of subcutaneous fat. **C:** Late arterial image from a digital subtraction arteriogram shows the lesion to be markedly vascular.

In many cases, as in patients with fibroxanthoma (nonossifying fibroma), fibrous dysplasia, osteochondroma, or enchondroma, radiographs may be virtually pathognomonic, and no further diagnostic imaging is required. In other cases, despite not having an unequivocal diagnosis, a benign-appearing lesion with previous radiographs documenting long-term stability may require only continued radiographic follow-up. MRI is usually reserved for those lesions requiring staging before surgery (aggressive benign, indeterminate, and malignant lesions) or in specific problem-solving situations (a symptomatic patient

with normal or only questionably abnormal radiographs) (48). In this latter situation, it must be emphasized that radiographs are relatively insensitive in detecting bone lysis. Cancellous bone, which is lost more rapidly than cortical bone because of its greater surface area, must be decreased by 30% to 50% before lysis is apparent on radiographs (342). In such situations, MRI may confirm the presence of a space-occupying lesion or underlying marrow abnormality.

MRI is the favored cross-sectional imaging modality for thoroughly assessing bone tumors and should be obtained

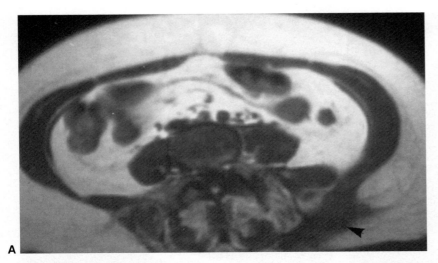

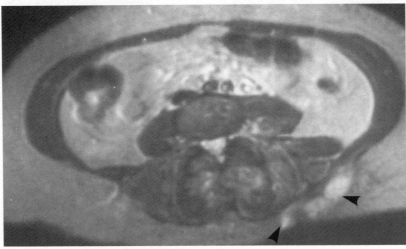

Figure 12-84   Recurrent tumor after surgery. Axial T1-weighted (500/20) **(A)** and T2-weighted (2,000/60) **(B)** SE MR images demonstrate a lobular area of increased signal intensity on T2-weighted **B** compared with T1-weighted **A** (*arrowheads*) due to recurrent tumor.

after plain film examination. MRI is generally accepted as superior to CT in staging tumors (3,13,82,346–349). In a multi-institutional study of 341 patients with primary bone and soft tissue malignancies, however, the Radiology Diagnostic Oncology Group found no statistically significant difference between CT and MRI in determining tumor involvement of muscle, bone, joint, or neurovascular structures (12). Despite this, we prefer MRI because of the improved lesion conspicuity and multiplanar capabilities. We have found CT especially useful in cases in which lesions are not well evaluated on radiographs. This is generally for lesions in which the bony anatomy is complex, such as the pelvis or shoulder girdle. In these instances, CT allows better evaluation of lesion margin, periosteal reaction, and matrix and often supplements MRI.

Specific Diagnoses

Despite the great value of MRI in the staging of bone lesions, it is of little value in diagnosis. There are specific diagnoses, however, that have a relatively characteristic MRI appearance: osteochondroma, enchondroma, chondroblastoma,

central chondrosarcoma, fibroxanthoma (nonossifying fibroma), intraosseous lipoma, bone infarct, and lesions with aneurysmal bone cyst (ABC)-like changes.

Cartilage Lesions

Chondroblastoma

Chondroblastoma is an uncommon primary cartilage tumor of bone. Originally thought to be a variant of giant cell tumor, the designation of chondroblastoma was introduced by Jaffe and Lichtenstein (350) in 1942 to emphasize its distinction from giant cell tumor. Chondroblastoma is usually found in adolescents and young adults, with approximately 70% of lesions occurring in the second decade and 90% occurring in patients between 5 and 25 years of age. Men are more commonly affected than women by a ratio of approximately 2 to 3:1 (351).

Chondroblastoma usually arises in the ends of long bones, typically within the epiphysis or epiphysis and metaphysis. About half of all chondroblastomas are confined to the epiphysis, with the vast majority of the remainder extending from the epiphysis into the metaphysis.

Isolated metaphyseal involvement is rare. Nearly half of all chondroblastomas occur around the knee (351).

Radiographs reveal a round to oval geographic lytic lesion with well-defined margins. A sclerotic rim is usually, though not invariably, present. A small percentage of cases show an ill-defined margin. Mineralized matrix is seen in 50% to 60% of cases (352). Periosteal reaction is seen on radiographs in approximately 50% of cases (353).

On MRI, the lesion demonstrates a distinct lobular pattern on T2-weighted images with signal intensity less than or equal to that of fat in most cases (352). Small foci of hemorrhage or hyaline cartilage within the lesion may show as scattered foci of increased signal intensity. The signal intensity of the lesion on T1-weighted spin-echo MR images is similar to that of muscle, although it is more homogeneous than that demonstrated on T2-weighted images (352). Associated marrow edema was seen in 17 (77%) of 22 cases reported by Weatherall et al. (352). These authors also noted adjacent soft tissue reaction, extending at least 1 cm beyond the margin of the periosteum in 16 (73%) cases. Periosteal reaction (which was identified on MRI as thickening and/or increased signal intensity) was seen in 18 (82%) of 22 cases. On radiographs or CT, periosteal reaction was found in 11 (50%) of 22 cases (see Fig. 12-85).

The cause of the marrow and soft tissue signal abnormalities associated with chondroblastoma remains obscure. Brower et al. (353) suggested they were the result of the propensity of the lesion to cause hyperemia and incite a local tissue reaction.

Enchondroma

Enchondroma is a tumor composed of lobules of hyaline cartilage thought to arise from the growth plate (354). The lesion is usually centrally located in the metaphysis of tubular bone, although great variability may be seen. Enchondroma is quite common and is the most common lesion of the hand. Approximately half of all enchondromas occur in the hands. On the basis of surgical series, osteochondroma is approximately three times as common as enchondroma (355). This statistic must be viewed with caution in that many enchondromas are incidental findings on imaging obtained for nonrelated reasons and histologic confirmation is not obtained.

Radiographs reveal a central geographic lytic lesion, with margins varying from sclerotic to ill defined. A lobulated contour is frequently present as is mineralized matrix. The overlying cortex often shows endosteal scalloping or expansile remodeling, especially in the small bones of the hand. Lesions may infiltrate the medullary canal without scalloping the adjacent cortex and, if not mineralized, may be invisible on radiographs.

Cohen et al. (356) observed a distinctive MRI appearance in chondroid lesions containing a matrix of hyaline cartilage. The unique pattern consisted of homogeneous high signal in a discernible lobular configuration on T2-weighted spin-echo MR images. This MRI appearance

reflects the underlying high ratio of water content to mucopolysaccharide component within the hyaline cartilage (356). On T1-weighted MR images, the lesion typically shows a lobulated intramedullary lesion with a signal intensity approximately equal to that of skeletal muscle. Occasionally, high signal bands may be seen on T1-weighted images, likely due to medullary fat within the lesion (see Fig. 12-86) (357). The signal intensity of the lesion tends to be somewhat less on fast or turbo T2-weighted images than on conventional T2-weighted images (see Fig. 12-87).

The distinction between enchondroma and intramedullary chondrosarcoma of the appendicular skeleton can be quite difficult. MRI may be useful in this regard. In a review of 187 cartilage lesions, 92 enchondromas and 95 chondrosarcomas, Murphey et al. (358) was able to differentiate these lesions successfully in more than 90% of cases. This was done on a basis of clinical and imaging features, including pain related to the lesion, deep endosteal scalloping (greater than two thirds of cortical thickness), cortical destruction and soft tissue mass, periosteal reaction (at radiography), and marked radionuclide uptake (greater than the iliac crest) at scintigraphy (see Fig. 12-88). The presence and pattern of gadolinium enhancement was not statistically significant in differentiating between these lesions.

Periosteal Chondroma

Periosteal chondroma is a relatively rare cartilage tumor arising from the periosteum (359,360). Periosteal chondromas represent about 1% of all cartilage tumors (359–361). The lesion is usually seen in patients less than 30 years old. Lesions are most frequently located in the small bones of the hands and feet, or less commonly in the long bones, most often the proximal humerus and proximal tibia.

Radiographs will demonstrate a juxtacortical lesion that will scallop the adjacent cortex (359). A thin rind or periosteal bone may be seen around the lesion, without intramedullary involvement (359). Radiographs will show matrix calcification in about 50% of patients (360). On CT scanning, the lesion may show calcification and decreased attenuation reflecting calcification within the hyaline cartilage tumor. MR imaging will show a low to intermediate signal intensity on T1-weighted images and high signal intensity on T2-weighted and fluid sensitive pulse sequences (359) (see Fig. 12-89). Areas of calcification and matrix mineralization will show decreased signal intensity on all pulse sequences. Contrast enhancement is variable, but will generally reflect the peripheral and septal pattern seen in other cartilage lesions.

The radiologic distinction between periosteal chondroma and periosteal chondrosarcoma is often quite difficult (362). Periosteal chondrosarcoma is typically a low grade malignancy, and in general, the imaging appearances of periosteal chondroma and periosteal chondrosarcoma overlap significantly (360,363). The most reliable

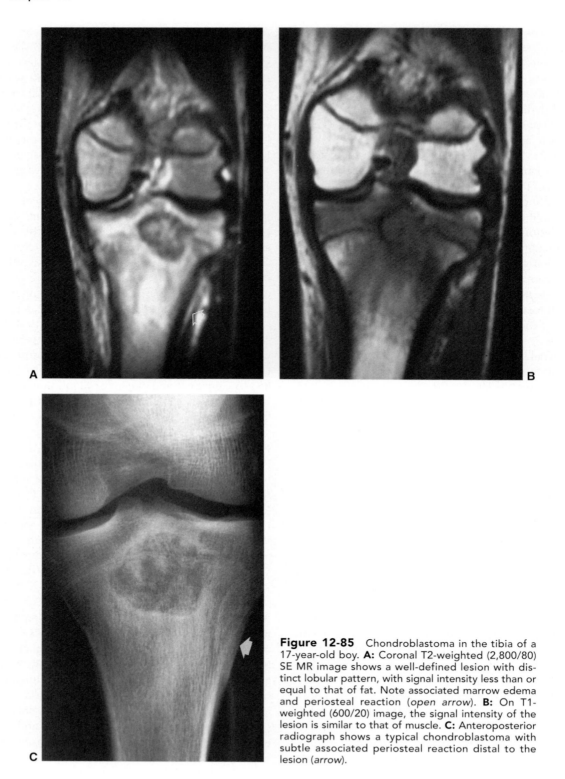

Figure 12-85 Chondroblastoma in the tibia of a 17-year-old boy. **A:** Coronal T2-weighted (2,800/80) SE MR image shows a well-defined lesion with distinct lobular pattern, with signal intensity less than or equal to that of fat. Note associated marrow edema and periosteal reaction (*open arrow*). **B:** On T1-weighted (600/20) image, the signal intensity of the lesion is similar to that of muscle. **C:** Anteroposterior radiograph shows a typical chondroblastoma with subtle associated periosteal reaction distal to the lesion (*arrow*).

indicator in distinguishing between periosteal chondroma and periosteal chondrosarcoma is the size of the lesion, with a size of greater than 3 cm suggesting malignancy.

Osteochondroma

Osteochondroma is the most common benign skeletal neoplasm, comprising 32% of benign lesions in the Mayo

Clinic series (355). The lesion is thought to arise from the periphery of the physis, where an abnormal focus of metaplastic cartilage forms as a consequence of trauma or congenital perichondral deficiency (364). Rarely, an osteochondroma may be the sequela of trauma or radiation (365). Osteochondromas are usually classified as pedunculated or sessile (broad based) on the basis of their

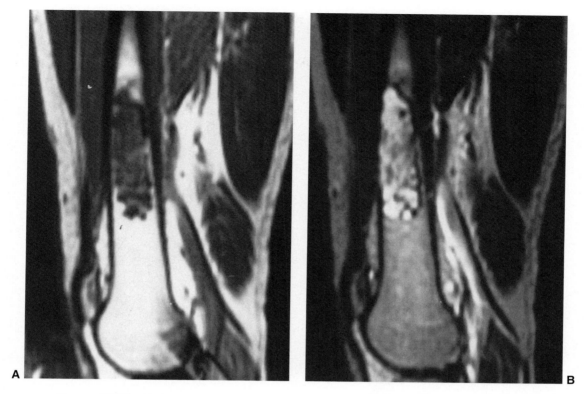

Figure 12-86 Enchondroma in the distal femur of a 28-year-old man. Sagittal T1-weighted (600/20) **(A)** and T2-weighted (2,000/80) **(B)** SE MR images show a lobulated intramedullary lesion with a signal intensity approximately equal to that of skeletal muscle on T1- and brighter than that of fat on T2-weighted images.

morphology. By definition, the lesion arises from the surface bone; the cortex of the host bone is contiguous with the stalk of the lesion, as is the medullary canal. The surface of the lesion consists of *hyaline cartilage of variable thickness.*

Many osteochondromas are asymptomatic and are incidental findings, whereas others present as an asymptomatic mass. Symptoms, when present, are often secondary to the size and location of the lesion or secondary fracture. Rarely, lesions may develop an overlying bursa (366). Malignant transformation is rare.

Radiographs reveal a lesion originating from the surface of a long bone, although any bone preformed in cartilage may be affected. The stalk of a pedunculated lesion is usually directed away from the end of the bone toward the diaphysis. The cap of the osteochondroma is quite variable in appearance, ranging from those that are thick and convoluted with characteristic mineralization, described as spicules, floccules, or arcs and rings, to those that are imperceptibly thin.

MRI is rarely indicated for the evaluation of an osteochondroma. It can be useful, however, in the evaluation of a symptomatic lesion or a lesion suspected of undergoing malignant transformation. The hyaline cartilage of the cap shows a signal intensity approximately equal to that of skeletal muscle on T1-weighted images and greater than that of fat on T2-weighted images. The overlying perichondrium images as a thin peripheral zone of decreased signal intensity on T2-weighted images (367). MRI also allows

precise measurement of the thickness of the cartilage cap of an osteochondroma. This has important clinical implications, because it assists in predicting which osteochondromas are most predisposed to undergoing malignant transformation to "secondary" chondrosarcoma. It is generally agreed that the risk of malignant transformation of an osteochondroma is directly related to the thickness of the cartilage cap, especially when the latter exceeds 2 or 3 cm (see Fig. 12-90) (367,368). Recently, ultrasound has been found to be as accurate as MRI in assessing the thickness of the cartilaginous cap (369).

On MR images obtained after gadolinium administration, cartilaginous tumors may demonstrate curvilinear enhancement representing enhancement of fibrovascular tissue between lobules of paucicellular hyaline cartilage lobules (357,370). Geirnaerdt et al. (370) noted this pattern of enhancement in 24 of 27 low-grade chondrosarcomas and suggested it is a useful imaging finding that may assist in separating low-grade chondrosarcoma (grade I and grade II) from high-grade chondrosarcoma (grade III). The validity of this observation is debated and is still to be proven by others (371), although this pattern of enhancement may be useful in suggesting a cartilage tumor. More recently, Geirnaerdt et al. (87) noted that the rate of enhancement as defined with time–signal intensity curves may be a significant discriminator with early enhancement as seen in chondrosarcoma but not in enchondroma.

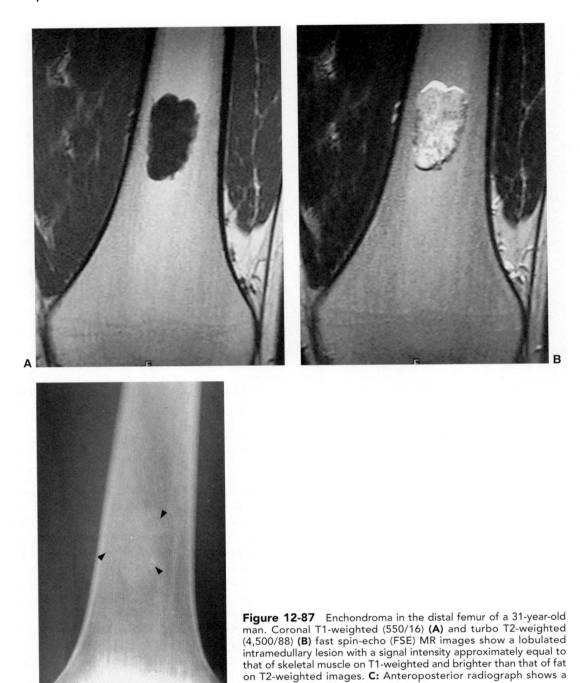

Figure 12-87 Enchondroma in the distal femur of a 31-year-old man. Coronal T1-weighted (550/16) **(A)** and turbo T2-weighted (4,500/88) **(B)** fast spin-echo (FSE) MR images show a lobulated intramedullary lesion with a signal intensity approximately equal to that of skeletal muscle on T1-weighted and brighter than that of fat on T2-weighted images. **C:** Anteroposterior radiograph shows a subtle mineralized lesion (*arrowheads*).

Conventional Chondrosarcoma

Conventional intramedullary chondrosarcoma is the most common type of primary chondrosarcoma. It has also been referred to as central chondrosarcoma (358,372). While there are numerous other subtypes of chondrosarcoma, the conventional intramedullary chondrosarcoma is the most readily diagnosed. Patients with conventional chondrosarcoma most commonly present in the fourth to fifth decades of life, and there is a male predilection. Chondrosarcoma is the third most common primary

malignant tumor of bone, exceeded in frequency only by multiple myeloma and osteosarcoma. Chondrosarcoma accounts for 3.5% of all biopsied primary bone tumors and 20% to 27% of primary malignant osseous neoplasms (347,358,372,373). Clinical symptoms are nonspecific with pain, the most frequent occurring in at least 95% of patients (358,372). The pain is often insidious, progressive, worse at night and has been present for months to years prior to the time of presentation. Pathologic fractures are also common at initial presentation in 3% to

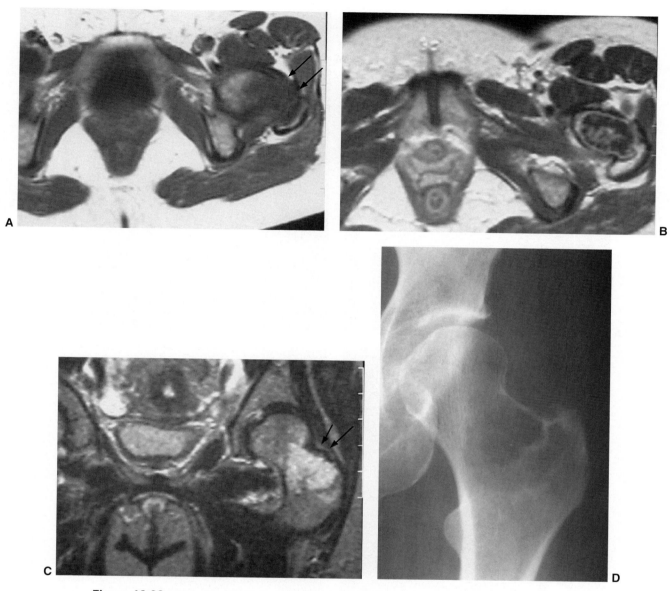

Figure 12-88 Chondrosarcoma in the proximal femur of a 50-year-old woman. Axial pre- **(A)** and post- **(B)** contrast axial T1-weighted (525/25) SE MR images show a lobulated intramedullary carti- lage lesion with peripheral and septal enhancement. The lesion shows deep cortical scalloping with associated soft tissue extension. **C:** Coronal T2-weighted (1,800/90) SE MR shows subtle soft tissue extension (*arrows*). **D:** The lesion radiograph shows a lobulated lytic lesion with variable margins, without periosteal reaction or matrix.

17% of patients with conventional chondrosarcoma (347,358,372–374).

Central chondrosarcoma is most common in the femur, accounting for approximately 20% to 35% of cases, fol- lowed in frequency by the tibia (5%) (358,372). Long tubular bone lesions most commonly involve the metaph- ysis (49% of cases), followed by the diaphysis (36% of cases) (372). Chondrosarcomas involving the humerus and fibula are almost invariably proximal.

Radiographs will typically reveal a mixed lytic and scle- rotic appearance, with areas of sclerosis representing chondroid matrix mineralization. Mineralized matrix is

seen in about two-thirds of lesions, and is characterized by a "ring and arc" pattern of calcification (347,358, 372–374). Higher-grade chondrosarcomas often contain relatively less extensive areas of matrix mineralization. Murphey et al. note that the depth of endosteal scalloping is the best distinguishing feature between long bone enchondroma and chondrosarcoma (358). Endosteal scalloping greater than two thirds the normal thickness of the long bone cortex is strong evidence of chondrosar- coma. Extensive, longitudinal, endosteal scalloping in long bone lesions (along greater than two thirds of lesion length) is also more suggestive of conventional

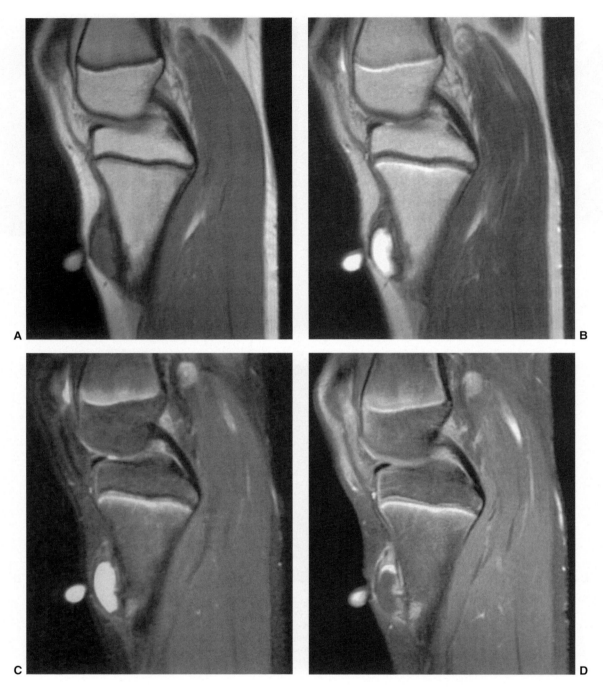

Figure 12-89   Periosteal chondroma in the proximal tibia of an 11-year-old girl. Sagittal T1-weighted (565/20) **(A)** and turbo–T2-weighted (3760/96) **(B)** FSE MR images show mass arising within the cortex. **C:** Sagittal STIR (4247/30/160) MR image shows the lesion to be markedly hyper-intense. **D:** Sagittal fat-supressed contrast-enhanced T1-weighted (448/20) SE MR image shows peripheral enhancement. **E:** Radiograph shows a juxtacortical mass (*arrows*), although the margins of the lesion are not well seen. **F:** Reformatted oblique coronal CT shows the relationship of the lesion to the cortex. Note attenuation of lesion is less than that of the adjacent soft tissue. **G:** Three-dimensional reformatted CT shows the cortical scalloping to better advantage.

chondrosarcoma than enchondroma, although not as distinctive a feature as the depth of scalloping.

MR imaging provides the best method for depiction of the extent of marrow involvement by conventional intramedullary chondrosarcoma (254,325,358,372,375).

MR imaging shows marrow replacement on T1-weighting with low to intermediate signal intensity. Entrapped areas of preexisting yellow marrow may be seen as small speckled punctate regions of high signal intensity on T1-weighted MR imaging in long bone intramedullary

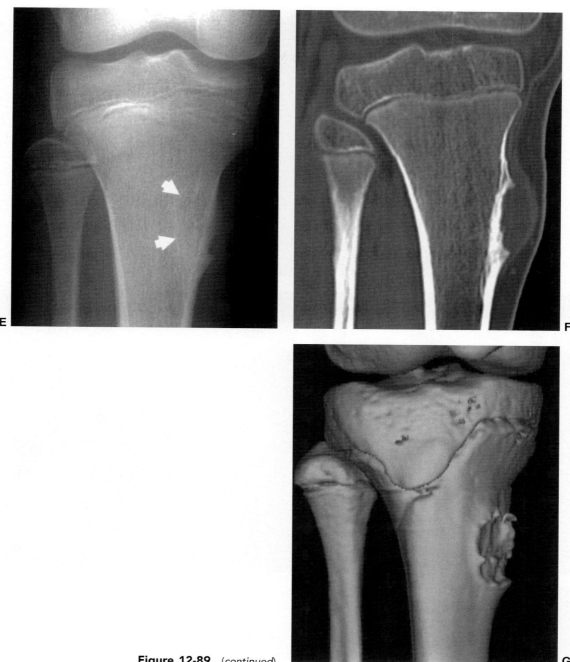

E

F

G

Figure 12-89 *(continued)*

chondrosarcomas (35% of lesions) but are much less common than in enchondromas (65%) (358). The non-mineralized components of chondrosarcoma reveal high signal intensity on T2-weighted MR images, reflection of the high water content of hyaline cartilage (372) (see Fig. 12-91). Areas of matrix mineralization are common and show low signal intensity on all MR pulse sequences, often creating a markedly heterogeneous appearance on T2-weighted MR images (372). The contrast enhancement pattern of conventional intramedullary chondrosarcoma is typically mild in degree and peripheral and septal in pattern

(11A). When there is extensive soft tissue extension, the high signal intensity from the hyaline cartilage, and peripheral and septal enhancement pattern may suggest a complex cytic or myxoid lesion (see Fig. 12-92).

Fibrous Lesions

Fibroxanthoma (Nonossifying Fibroma)

Fibroxanthoma, nonossifying fibroma, and fibrous cortical defect are terms used to describe histologically similar lesions that occur in the metaphysis of long bones. Such

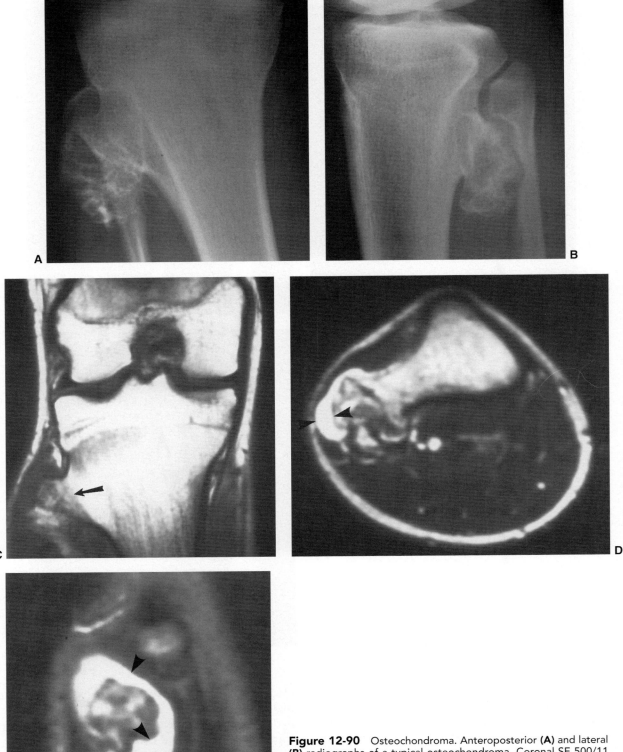

Figure 12-90 Osteochondroma. Anteroposterior **(A)** and lateral **(B)** radiographs of a typical osteochondroma. Coronal SE 500/11 image **(C)** shows the marrow extending into the lesion (*arrow*). Axial **(D)** and sagittal **(E)** SE 2,000/80 images show the thin high signal intensity cartilaginous cap (*arrowheads*).

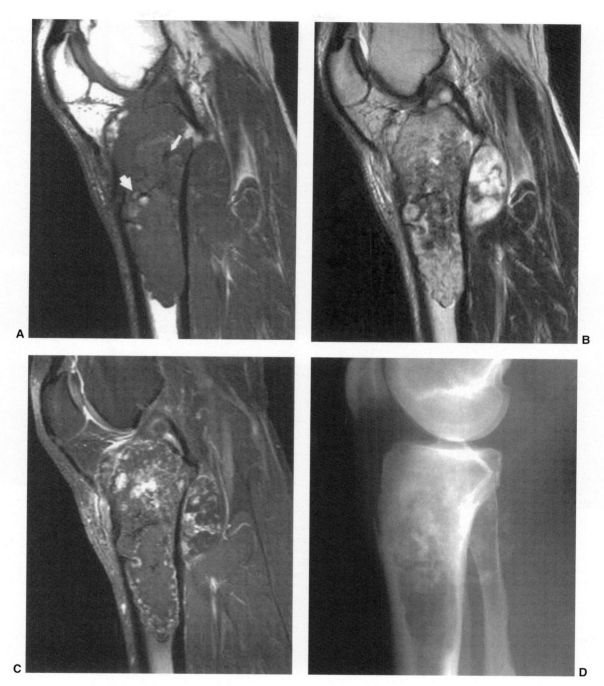

Figure 12-91 Central chondrosarcoma in the proximal tibia of a 56-year-old man. Sagittal T1-weighted (600/13) **(A)** and turbo-T2-weighted (4470/82) **(B)** FSE MR images show a large heterogeneous mass. Note entrapped areas of fatty marrow (**A**, *arrows*), endosteal scalloping of poseterior cortex and posterior soft tissue mass. Central areas of decreased signal intensity correspond to areas of matrix mineralization. **C:** Sagittal fat-supressed enhanced T1-weighted (637/13) MR image shows prominent septal and peripheral enhancement. **D:** Radiograph reveals a mixed lytic and sclerotic lesion with areas of sclerosis representing mineralized chondroid matrix. Note posterior extension.

lesions are quite common, and Caffey (376) noted one or more such lesions in 36% of children studied serially. The clinical variability of the lesion has led to this confusing array of terms. Small, metaphyseal, eccentric lesions that are limited to the cortex are usually termed fibrous cortical defects and likely represent most cases described by Caffey.

Persistent lesions that show interval growth and extend into the medullary cavity are usually referred to as nonossifying fibroma (377,378). The term "fibroxanthoma" is preferred by the authors in that it better reflects the underlying pathology, which is composed of spindle-shaped fibroblasts, scattered giant cells, and foam (xanthoma) cells.

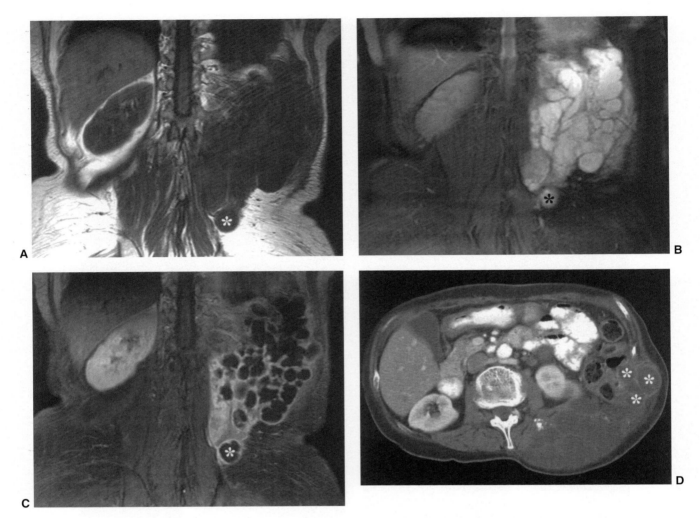

Figure 12-92   Recurrent central chondrosarcoma in posterior left 10th rib in a 70-year-old woman. Coronal T1-weighted (622/13) **(A)** and breath hold fluid-sensative gradient echo (4.3/2.2) **(B)** MR images of the posterior chest wall show a large lobulated mass. The lobules of hyaline cartilage (asterisk) have fluid-like signal characteristics. **C:** Coronal fat-supressed enhanced T1-weighted (660/13) MR image shows areas of prominent enhancement. Nonenhancing areas of hyaline cartilage may mimic a multicystic lesion. **D:** Axial enhanced CT scan of the left flank shows the extensive mass. Note decreased attenuation of the hyaline cartilage loblues (*asterisks*).

Additionally, as these lesions may ossify and become sclerotic, it obviates the need to use the descriptive term ossifying nonossifying fibroma to describe healing lesions.

The radiographic appearance of fibroxanthoma is virtually pathognomonic, demonstrating an eccentric, scalloped, geographic lytic lesion with a sclerotic margin in the metadiaphysis or metaphysis of long bones. Fibroxanthomas are not uncommon incidental findings on MRI. Their MRI appearance parallels their radiographic appearance, typically demonstrating a well-defined, eccentric, scalloped, metadiaphyseal, or metaphyseal lesion. The appearance of the lesion is variable but most frequently demonstrates decreased signal intensity on T1- and T2-weighted spin-echo images, reflecting hemosiderin and fibrous tissue within the tumor (377,379). Collagen and bone formation within the tumor also contribute to the finding of decreased signal intensity

(see Fig. 12-93). The lesion may less frequently show areas with a signal intensity similar to that of fat on all pulse sequences or areas similar to a cyst. Secondary ABC formation may be seen with fluid–fluid levels. After the administration of contrast, intense enhancement is seen in almost 80% of cases, with marginal septal enhancement seen in the remaining (379).

Fibrous Dysplasia

Fibrous dysplasia is not an uncommon skeletal dysplasia, typically encountered in adolescents and young adults. Rather than being a true neoplasm, fibrous dysplasia is a developmental anomaly in which the normal medullary space is replaced by fibroosseous tissue (380). The process may affect a single bone (monostotic fibrous dysplasia) or many bones (polyostotic fibrous dysplasia). Monostotic

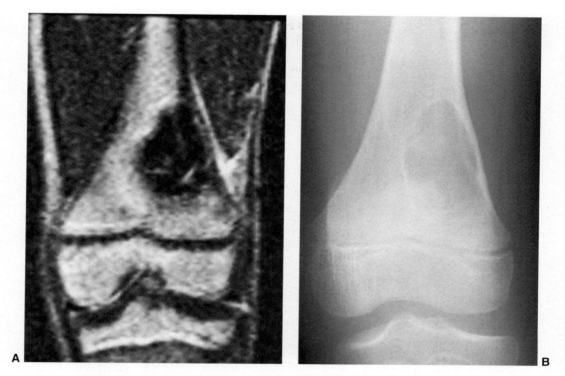

Figure 12-93 Nonossifying fibroma (fibroxanthoma) in the distal femur of a 10-year-old boy. **A:** Coronal T2-weighted (2,213/90) SE MR image of the distal femur shows an eccentric metadiaphyseal lesion with markedly decreased signal intensity. **B:** Corresponding radiograph shows characteristic appearance.

fibrous dysplasia is approximately six times as common as polyostotic disease. The latter is associated with patches of cutaneous pigmentation (cafe-au-lait spots), situated predominantly on the trunk in one third to one half of patients (378,380).

Although patients with fibrous dysplasia may present at any age, typically they are young, in the first and second decades of life. Seventy-five percent of patients present before the age of 30 years (338,380). Patients with polyostotic disease usually present early in life, with a mean age of 8 years. Two thirds of these patients have symptoms by that age (49,98).

Radiographs demonstrate an intramedullary lesion, replacing normal marrow with fibroosseous tissue. The amount of woven bone in the fibroosseous tissue and the extent to which it is mineralized ultimately determine the radiographic density of the lesion. The bone may show an expanded remodeled contour, with thinning of the overlying cortex. There may be a surrounding rind of sclerosis. The lesion is usually well defined and may show a trabeculated appearance due to reinforced subperiosteal ridges of bone.

Initial reports on the MRI appearance of fibrous dysplasia described it as having decreased signal intensity on all MR images obtained with spin-echo pulse sequences (381). More recently, however, fibrous dysplasia has been reported as having a signal intensity similar to that of skeletal muscle on T1-weighted images and variable signal

intensity on T2-weighted images (382,383). This variable appearance on T2-weighted images ranges from a signal intensity greater than that of fat in approximately two thirds of cases to similar to that of fat or skeletal muscle in the remaining one third (382,383). Lesions tend to be relatively homogeneous unless complicated by fracture or secondary ABC (see Fig. 12-94). After contrast administration, approximately 75% of lesions will enhance centrally, with the 25% showing peripheral rim enhancement (382).

Osteoid Osteoma

Osteoid osteoma is a relatively common benign skeletal lesion that accounts for approximately 12% of benign skeletal "neoplasms" (134,233,355). The term "osteoid osteoma" was introduced into the medical literature in 1935 by Jaffe (384) when he described five benign osteoblastic tumors composed of osteoid and atypical bone. In all these cases, surgery was performed on the "assumption that the condition was inflammatory—osteomyelitis or an abscess of the bone—but pus was not found in any instances." Although similar cases were published by Hitzrot and Bergstrand in 1930 and Milch in 1934 (385), these authors were unable to identify the true nature of the lesion, and it was Jaffe who clearly established osteoid osteoma as a distinct clinical and pathologic entity (84,257,386,387). Since then, more than 1,000 cases have

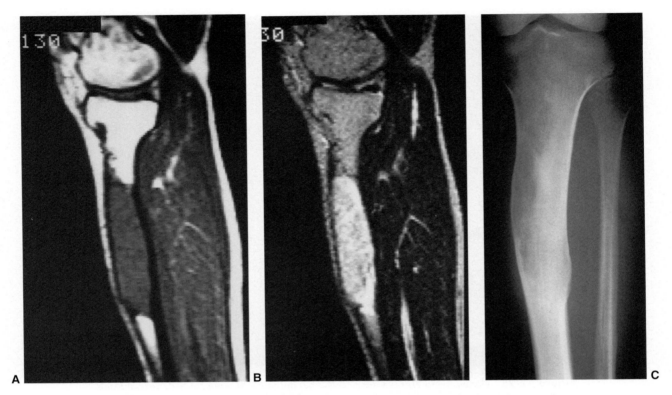

Figure 12-94 Fibrous dysplasia in a 30-year-old man. Sagittal T1-weighted (500/21) **(A)** and T2-weighted (2,000/100) **(B)** SE MR images show a well-defined intramedullary lesion with nonspecific signal intensity. **C:** Corresponding radiograph confirms the diagnosis of fibrous dysplasia.

been reported in the literature, establishing it as a common benign lesion (388).

Osteoid osteoma may occur in virtually any bone, although clearly there is a predilection for the lower extremity with more than 50% of lesions occurring in the femur and tibia (262,355,389). Most lesions arise in the cortex of long bones, where the lesion is usually diaphyseal or metadiaphyseal (389,390). Of the remaining lesions, approximately 30% are equally distributed between the spine, hand, and foot (389,391). When osteoid osteoma occurs in the spine, the most commonly affected area is the lumbar spine, typically involving the neural arch (386,392,393). Lesions limited to the vertebral body are unusual (392). Intraarticular lesions are most commonly encountered in the hip (393,394).

Patients with osteoid osteoma are usually young, with about half presenting between the ages of 10 and 20 years. There is an unmistakable male prevalence. Almost invariably, the presenting complaint is pain, varying in duration from weeks to years. Pain is frequently worse at night (392, 393,395,396) and may awaken the patient from sleep (395). Response to aspirin is clearly not universal (303,394). However, approximately 75% of patients report relief of symptoms after treatment with salicylates (303,355).

In 1966 Edeiken et al. (399) categorized three types of osteoid osteoma, each with differing amounts of associated osteosclerosis, based on radiographic localization of the nidus:

1. Cortical osteoid osteoma, the most common type, typically demonstrates fusiform, sclerotic, cortical thickening in the shaft of a long bone, especially the tibia and femur. A characteristic radiolucency, representing the lesion, is usually located within the center of the osteosclerosis. The latter is reactive and can regress after surgical removal of the osteoid osteoma (355). The lesion, which may be radiolucent or may contain a variable amount of mineralization (sometimes being quite radiopaque), is often referred to as the "nidus" (Fig. 12-94).

2. Cancellous (also referred to as medullary) osteoid osteoma, intermediate in frequency of occurrence, has a site predilection for the femoral neck, small bones of the hand and foot, and the vertebral posterior elements. When present, osteosclerosis is usually mild to moderate and may be distant from the nidus. Unlike its classic cortical counterpart, the nidus of a cancellous osteoid osteoma is not necessarily situated in the center of the accompanying sclerosis. This feature has surgical ramifications, because removal of the nidus is necessary for cure. Initial radiographs may be normal or only retrospectively positive (397). The joint may be widened secondary to synovitis and joint effusion (see Figs. 12-95 and 12-96) (355,389,393,395,398).

3. Subperiosteal osteoid osteoma, the rarest type, arises as a soft tissue mass immediately adjacent to the affected bone. Subperiosteal osteoid osteoma is

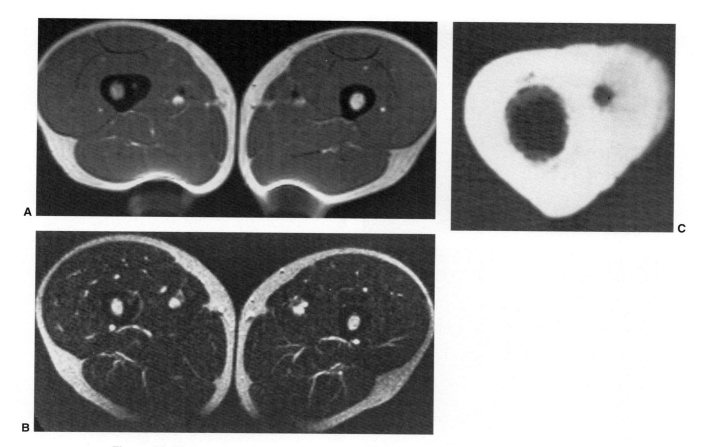

Figure 12-95 Cortical osteoid osteoma in a 19-year-old man with night pain, relieved by aspirin. Axial T1-weighted (700/20) **(A)** and T2-weighted (2,000/80) **(B)** SE MR images of the shaft of the femur show the "nidus" on the right. There is subtle marrow edema and increased signal in the surrounding soft tissue on **B**. **C:** CT remains the best modality to accurately localize the lesion.

typically located along the medial aspect of the femoral neck and in the hands and feet (399). It may be most common in the neck of the talus (400). The subjacent bone may have pressure atrophy or irregular bone resorption (399). Subperiosteal osteoid osteomas produce almost no reactive sclerosis (393). Cancellous and subperiosteal osteoid osteomas typically arise in an intraarticular or juxtaarticular location. As broadly defined by Kattapuram et al. (394), osteoid osteomas occurring at the ends of long bone, in or around the joint, or in the bone surrounded by or very close to the capsule and synovium (although not within the synovial cavity itself such as a loose body) are considered intraarticular osteoid osteomas.

CT remains the diagnostic modality of choice (262,401). On CT, the nidus of a cortical or cancellous osteoid osteoma is a well-defined round or oval lesion of decreased attenuation, with a variable amount of surrounding sclerosis, ranging from mild sclerosis to extensive periosteal new bone. CT has also proven valuable in the surgical localization of osteoid osteoma.

Glass et al. (59) reported the MRI appearance of an intraarticular cancellous osteoid osteoma in the femoral neck. The nidus demonstrated decreased signal intensity on both T1- and T2-weighted images and was surrounded by an area of increased signal intensity on T2-weighted images, likely representing a surrounding intramedullary inflammatory response. There was an associated synovitis and widened joint space (89). Diffuse marrow abnormality was also reported by Yeager et al. (402) in describing an intraarticular osteoid osteoma of the talus. Woods et al. (403) correlated the MRI findings in the associated reactive soft tissue mass with the pathologic findings in three cases of osteoid osteoma and found it to contain inflammatory change on a prominent background of myxomatous change. The marrow space demonstrated "serous atrophy of marrow fat," characterized by depletion of normal marrow elements and replacement with proteinaceous material. The pattern of marrow edema has been verified by others, and Ehara et al. (404) noted that the amount of edema was significantly greater in younger patients (those less than 15 years of age). They also noted no relationship between the amount of edema and the length of symptoms and location of the lesion (see Fig. 12-97).

Houang et al. (405) described the MRI findings in a case of an osteoid osteoma, arising in the uncinate process of C-4. The lesion, which was detected by CT and scintigraphy,

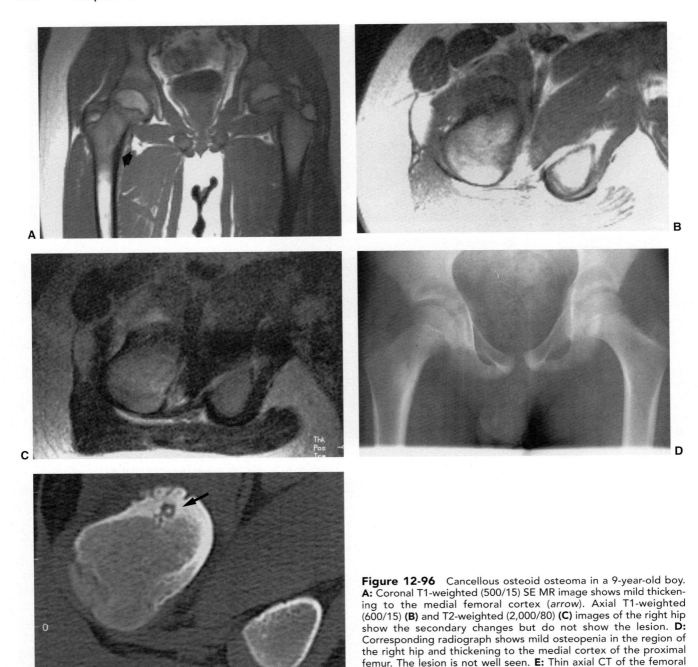

Figure 12-96 Cancellous osteoid osteoma in a 9-year-old boy. **A:** Coronal T1-weighted (500/15) SE MR image shows mild thickening to the medial femoral cortex (*arrow*). Axial T1-weighted (600/15) **(B)** and T2-weighted (2,000/80) **(C)** images of the right hip show the secondary changes but do not show the lesion. **D:** Corresponding radiograph shows mild osteopenia in the region of the right hip and thickening to the medial cortex of the proximal femur. The lesion is not well seen. **E:** Thin axial CT of the femoral neck shows the lesion (*arrow*) to best advantage.

demonstrated abnormal signal in both C-3 and C-4, with decreased signal on T1-weighted and increased signal on T2-weighted spin-echo MR images, a pattern suggesting marrow edema and local inflammation. The nidus demonstrated a low signal intensity on both T1- and T2-weighted images, possibly due to calcification. It is of interest that a similar pattern of marrow abnormality was reported by Crim et al. (406) in describing an osteoblastoma of the T-3 pedicle. In this case, these changes were seen in the adjacent vertebra, ribs, and paraspinal soft tissues, which also showed diffuse enhancement after intravenous gadopentetate

dimeglumine. Histologic correlation from areas of abnormal signal intensity in the bone marrow and soft tissues demonstrated edema and inflammatory infiltrate.

Osteoid osteomas may be difficult to detect on conventional MR imaging and diagnosis may be missed in as many as 35% of cases (407). While CT is still considered the modality of choice for the identification of osteoid osteoma, enhanced MR imaging may also useful. Liu at al (408) showed that lesions imaged with dynamic gadolinium enhanced MR imaging had a conspicuity equal to that or better than that obtained with thin-section CT.

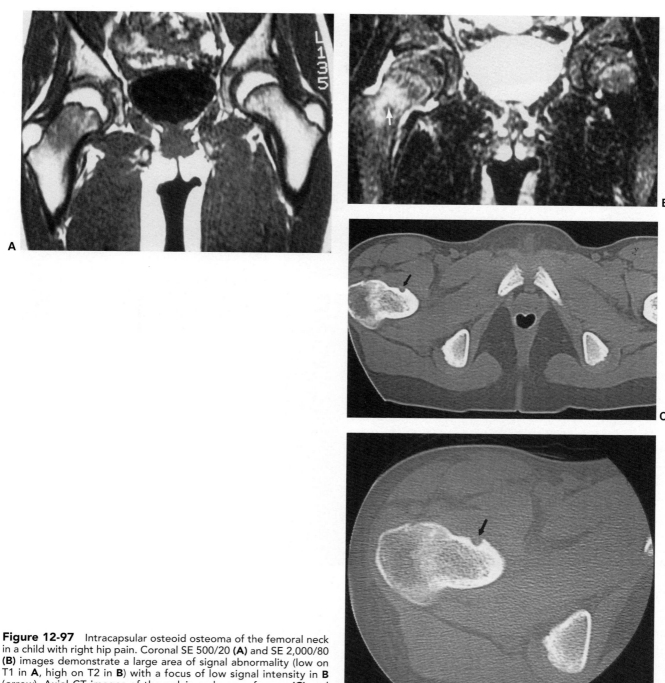

Figure 12-97 Intracapsular osteoid osteoma of the femoral neck in a child with right hip pain. Coronal SE 500/20 **(A)** and SE 2,000/80 **(B)** images demonstrate a large area of signal abnormality (low on T1 in **A**, high on T2 in **B**) with a focus of low signal intensity in **B** (*arrow*). Axial CT images of the pelvis and upper femurs **(C)** and localized image **(D)** of the right femoral neck demonstrate a small cortical focus of low attenuation and a subtle nidus (*arrow*).

Intraosseous Lipoma

Although lipoma is the most common soft tissue lesion by a large margin, intraosseous lipoma is perceived as rare. Ramos et al. (409) noted only approximately 60 cases in their review of the literature in 1985. We suspect these lesions are not uncommon and are occasional incidental findings on examinations obtained for other reasons. Intraosseous lipoma occurs most commonly in the metaphysis

of long bones, especially the fibula, femur, tibia, and in the calcaneus. About two thirds of patients are reported to have symptoms, typically pain and swelling, referable to the lesion (141,389).

The lesion is composed of mature adipocytes. Associated foci of fat necrosis, cystic degeneration, and ischemic ossification may suggest the microscopic diagnosis of bone infarct to the pathologist reviewing material without radiographs (389).

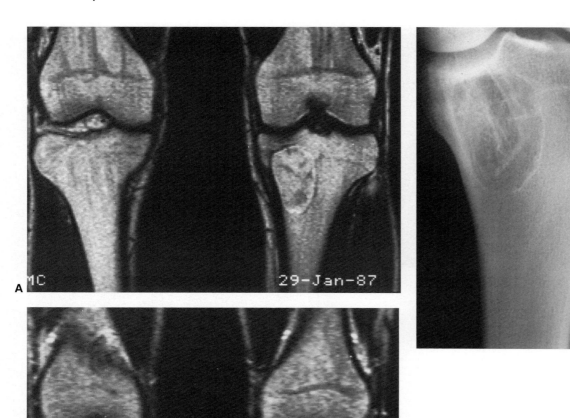

Figure 12-98 Intraosseous lipoma in a 22-year-old man. Coronal T1-weighted (600/32) **(A)** and T2-weighted (2,000/100) **(B)** SE MR images show a well-defined lesion in the proximal left tibia with signal intensity identical to that of marrow fat. **C:** Corresponding radiograph shows a geographic lytic lesion with well-defined sclerotic margins. A small amount of ossification seen in the proximal portion of the lesion.

Radiographs reveal a well-defined lytic lesion with a thin sclerotic margin. A lobulated contour with ridges is often present (389). Foci of ischemic bone may be seen within the lesion, as well as intralesional cysts. In the calcaneus, an intraosseous lipoma is characteristically localized to the anterior portion of the bone. MR images reflect the underlying morphology, with the lesion imaging identical to marrow fat on all pulse sequences (see Fig. 12-98). Areas of ossification or cyst formation within the lesion are also readily detected on MRI (see Fig. 12-99).

Giant Cell Tumor

Giant cell tumor of bone is a relatively common, locally aggressive, benign tumor representing about 5% of primary bone neoplasms undergoing biopsy (410). The lesion is most frequently encountered in patients between ages 20 and 40 years. Although initially described in 1818, it was not until 1940 that it was separated from other giant cell containing lesions and identified as a distinct clinico-pathologic entity (410). The lesion is composed of mononuclear stromal cells and mutinucliated giant cells.

Radiographs will show a geographic lytic lesion, typically with well-defined nonsclerotic margins. Approximately 15% of cases will demonstrate an ill-defined margin. Sclerosis has been reported but is rare. The lesion is localized to the end of the bone, originating in the metaphysis and growing to the subchondral region. Matrix is not seen, and associated periosteal reaction is uncommon. Cortical breakthrough is not uncommon and may be seen in 33% to 50% of cases (151,411).

The diagnosis of giant cell tumor is usually well made on radiographs, and MRI is usually obtained to evaluate the extent of the lesion, the presence or absence of an

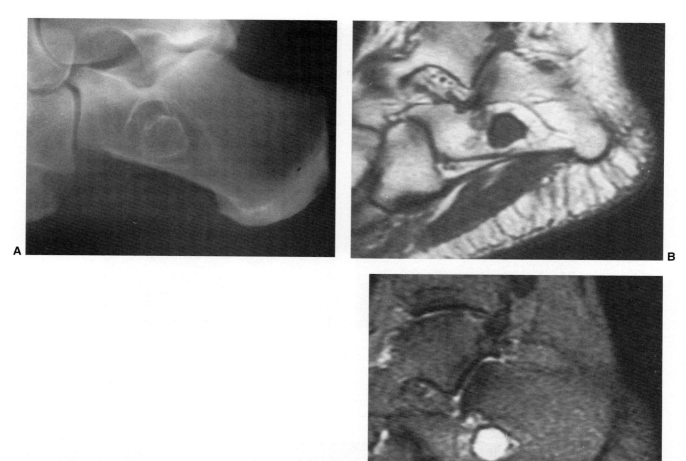

Figure 12-99   Intraosseous lipoma in a 46-year-old woman. **A:** Lateral radiograph shows a well-defined lytic lesion in the anterior aspect of the calcaneous. There is a central rounded density with calcification at its periphery. **B:** Sagittal T1-weighted (650/20) SE MR image through the lesion shows the peripheral signal intensity of the lesion to be identical to that of the subcutaneous fat. **C:** Corresponding T2-weighted (1,800/80) image also shows the peripheral signal intensity of the lesion to be identical to fat. The central rounded density seen of radiographs represents a central cyst, with prolonged T1 and T2 relaxation times.

associated soft tissue mass, and the relationship to critical adjacent structures. The MR signal characteristics are not specific (see Fig. 12-100 and Fig. 12-101) but will typically demonstrate a signal intensity similar to that of skeletal muscle on T1-weighted spin-echo MR images and heterogeneously high signal intensity on T2-weighted images, with areas of hypointense, isointense, and hyperintense to marrow fat (412,413). The areas of decreased signal intensity are due to hemosiderin deposition and are found in approximately 63% of cases (412).

Tumorlike Lesions

Infarct

The term "bone infarct" refers to the pathologic state resulting from the ischemic death of the cellular constituents of bone and marrow (414). By convention, the terms "osteonecrosis," "avascular necrosis," and "aseptic necrosis" are generally reserved for areas of epiphyseal or subarticular involvement, whereas the term "bone infarct" is usually used for metaphyseal or diaphyseal involvement (414). An infarct consists of central cores of dead marrow and bone surrounded by ischemic injured marrow and bone and active hyperemia, in addition to viable marrow and bone. Repair starts at the junction between the ischemic bone and the viable bone and is the cause of the radiodense serpiginous margin seen surrounding an infarct.

Long-standing infarct is often well seen on radiographs, typically showing a well-defined metaphyseal lesion with serpiginous margins. MRI shows a decreased signal on both T1- and T2-weighted images, presumably due to fibrosis within the lesion (415). Alternatively, one may see areas of high signal intensity on T2-weighted images, likely representing cyst formation within old infarcts.

Munk et al. (416) described the findings in eight patients with early infarcts. They noted that radiographs

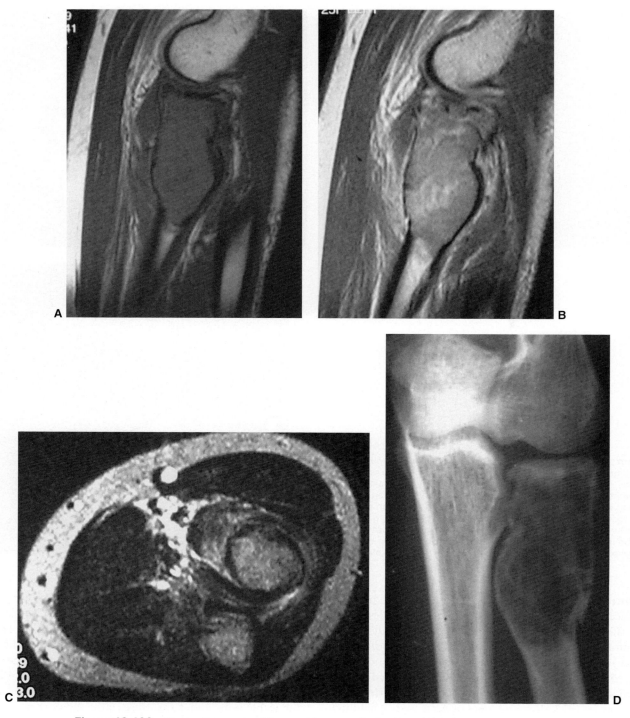

Figure 12-100   Giant cell tumor in a 25-year-old woman. Sagittal pre- **(A)** and postcontrast **(B)** T1-weighted (600/20) SE MR images show an enhancing lesion of the proximal radius, extending to the end of the bone. There is mild expansive remodeling and soft tissue extension. **C:** Axial T2-weighted (2,365/90) SE MR image shows a heterogeneous intermediate signal intensity, making it difficult to appreciate the soft tissue extension. **D:** Radiograph shows a geographic lytic lesion in the proximal radius with pathologic fracture. The lesion extends to the end of the bone and shows mild expansile remodeling, without matrix.

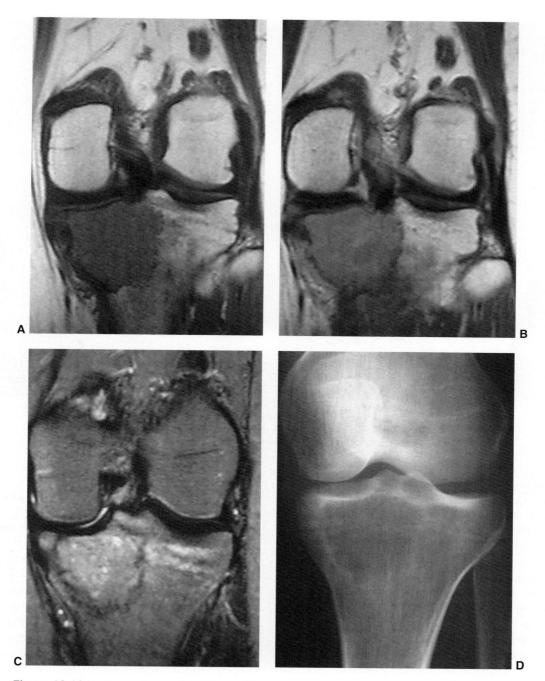

Figure 12-101   Giant cell tumor in a 27-year-old woman. Sagittal pre- **(A)** and postcontrast **(B)** T1-weighted (550/16) SE MR images show an enhancing lesion of the proximal tibia, extending to the end of the bone. Note some abnormal signal in the marrow surrounding the lesion. **C:** Corresponding coronal T2-weighted (2,500/80) SE MR image shows an intermediate signal intensity. **D:** Radiograph shows a geographic lytic lesion in the proximal tibia extending from the metaphysis to the end of the bone.

show mottled radiolucencies in the metadiaphysis with no or only slight sclerosis. MRI in four patients showed a signal intensity of the lesion similar to that of marrow fat, showing intermediate to high signal on all pulse sequences with a thin low-signal serpentine rim on both T1- and T2-weighted spin-echo images (see Fig. 12-102).

Aneurysmal Bone Cyst

The concept of ABC stems from two cases reported by Jaffe and Lichtenstein (417) in their article on unicameral bone cysts in 1942. In that report they noted two "peculiar blood-containing cysts of large size," which they described as aneurysmal cysts. Subsequently, Jaffe chose ABC as the

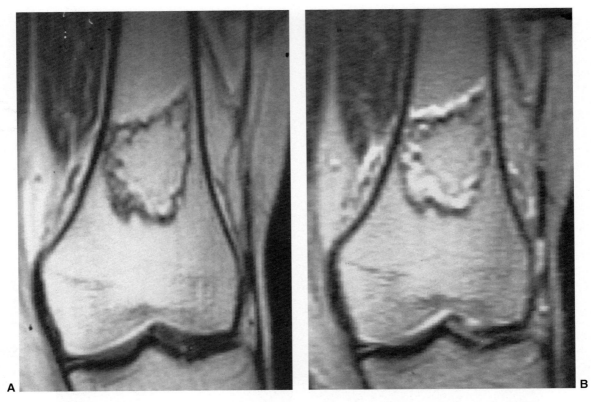

Figure 12-102 Early infarct in the distal femur of a 30-year-old man. Coronal T1-weighted (500/32) **(A)** and T2-weighted (2,000/100) **(B)** SE MR images show the signal intensity of the lesion to be similar to that of marrow fat, with a thin serpentine rim on both T1- and T2-weighted spin-echo images.

descriptive term for this lesion, with aneurysmal emphasizing the "blown out" distended contour of the affected bone and bone cyst underscoring the fact that upon entering the lesion through a thin shell of bone, the lesion appears largely as a blood-filled cavity (286).

As originally described by Jaffe and Lichtenstein (286,417–420), the ABC was sufficiently characteristic to identify it as a distinctive roentgenographic-pathologic entity. However, its nature has remained unclear. In both his original and an ensuing paper on the subject, Jaffe postulated that the ABC may, in fact, be a secondary phenomenon due to a hemorrhagic "blow out" in a preexisting lesion that may have been destroyed in the process (286). The concept of the ABC as a secondary phenomenon occurring in a preexisting lesion has been validated by multiple investigators; in approximately one third (29% to 35%) of cases, the preexisting lesion can be identified (421–424). The most common of these is the giant cell tumor, which accounts for 19% to 39% of those cases in which the preceding lesion is found (421–424). Other common precursor lesions include chondroblastoma, osteoblastoma, fibroxanthoma (nonossifying fibroma), and chondromyxoid fibroma. Less common lesions include solitary bone cyst, fibrous dysplasia, fibrous histiocytoma, eosinophilic granuloma, radiation osteitis, osteosarcoma, trauma (including fracture), fibrosarcoma, and even metastatic carcinoma (390,421–426).

Grossly, the ABC has been likened to a "blood-filled sponge" (419), being composed of blood-filled anastomosing cavernosus spaces, separated by a cystlike wall composed of fibroblasts, myofibroblasts, osteoclast-like giant cells, osteoid, and woven bone (28,425). In approximately one third of cases, a characteristic reticulated, lacy, chondroidlike material is seen (390). Mirra (390) notes this "is strongly suggestive, if not pathognomonic, of repair in an ABC." This supports the concept that ABC may be primarily a reparative process, probably the result of trauma or tumor-induced anomalous vascular process.

Appropriate treatment of an ABC requires the realization that it is the result of a specific pathophysiology, and identification of the preexisting lesion, if possible, is essential. This is especially true for intramedullary lesions. If no coexistent lesion is identified, lesions are usually treated with curettage and bone grafting, with more aggressive treatment reserved for recurrent lesions (390). If a more aggressive lesion is present, treatment must be directed toward the more aggressive component (342). Clearly, an osteosarcoma with superimposed secondary ABC change must be treated as an osteosarcoma, and giant cell tumor with secondary ABC features would be expected to have a greater potential for local recurrence (390).

Most (approximately 80%) patients presenting with ABC-like findings are under 20 years of age, but the lesion is rare in children under 5 years (124,282,390,421–423, 425,427–429). More than half of all such lesions occur in long bones, and approximately 12% to 30% of cases occur in the spine (171,282,371,390). The pelvis accounts for about half of all flat bone lesions (428,430). Most patients present with pain and/or swelling, with symptoms usually present for less than 6 months (428). Vergel De Dios et al. (428) reported multiple bone involvement in 20 (8.4%) of 238 patients with primary ABC, 95% of which involved contiguous spine lesions.

The imaging appearance of ABC reflects the underlying pathophysiologic change. Bonakdarpour et al. (140) noted that in 26 cases of ABC in which a preexisting lesion could be identified, 21 (81%) had the radiologic appearance typical of the primary lesion. In the remaining cases, radiographs show an eccentric lytic lesion with an expanded remodeled blown out or "ballooned" bony contour of the host bone, frequently with a delicate trabeculated appearance (1,93,282,344,431). Radiographs may rarely show flocculent densities within the lesion, which may mimic chondroid matrix (115,430). These densities represent mineralized chondroid within the wall of the cyst, and although this is present histologically in approximately one third of cases, it is seen on radiographs and CT only when abundant (115). Gold and Mirra (115) noted it in 2 (13%) of 15 ABCs, and Vergel De Dios et al. (428) noted faint mineralization in 22 (16%) of 138 cases.

MRI typically shows a well-defined lesion, often with lobulated contour (432,433). Internal septations with multiple fluid–fluid levels may be seen, although adjacent loculations may have markedly different imaging characteristics (432,433). The lesion, as well as internal septations, may demonstrate a thin well-defined rim of decreased signal intensity, thought to be due to fibrous tissue (433). In those regions in which fluid–fluid levels are identified, increased signal on T1-weighted images has been reported in the dependent and nondependent fluid, presumably due to methemoglobin within the fluid (290,431,434). Fluid–fluid levels are less commonly seen on T1-weighted images. Following contrast administration, enhancement will be seen in the fibrous tissue between the internal septations (see Fig. 12-103). One must remember fluid–fluid levels are a nonspecific finding and, when present, only reflect the underlying pathophysiology. They are more readily seen on MRI than on CT (see Fig. 12-104) (290).

The distinction of primary and secondary ABC is critical. In a recent review of 738 consecutive patients with focal bone lesions, O'Donnell and Saifudden (435) identified ABC change in 11.2% of cases, 60% of which were benign (435). Although secondary ABCs are most frequently associated with benign lesions, the telangectatic osteosarcoma may mimic a primary ABC, and the telangiectatic osteosarcoma is the malignant lesion most often confused with an ABC (436). Telangiectatic osteosarcoma must, by definition, be composed of at least 90% hemorrhagic, cystic or necrotic tissue (437). The most

important radiologic feature in distinguishing these two lesions is the identification of a solid enhancing tumor in association with the hemorrhagic tissue as a component of the osteosarcoma (see Fig. 12-105) (436,437).

Solid Aneurysmal Bone Cyst

The term "solid" ABC was coined by Sanerkin et al. (438) in 1983 to describe a lesion that contained the characteristic reticulated, lacy, chondroidlike material seen in ABC but without the cystlike cavities of a typical ABC. In a recent review of 238 patients with primary ABC in the Mayo Clinic files (36), about 5% were the solid variant. This corresponds well with the results of the files of the Rizzoli Institute, in which 15 (7.5%) of 213 cases were the solid variant of ABC (439). The similarity of giant cell reparative granuloma of the jaw to the solid portions of ABC was noted by Dahlin and McLeod (93). More recently, the solid ABC has been equated to the giant cell reparative granuloma in long bone (440,441) and the giant cell reparative granuloma of the small bones of the hands and feet (428). All likely represent responses to intraosseous hemorrhage. There are no differences in clinical or radiologic presentation in patients with classic ABC or the solid variant (428,439).

In a recent report describing the radiologic features of solid variant of aneurysmal bone cyst, Ilaslan et al. noted that one-third of cases were nonaneurysmal (440). They also reported cystic components in one-quarter of their cases with fluid–fluid levels, as well as pronounced perilesional edema-like signal in half of patients.

Bone Cyst

Simple or unicameral bone cysts are fluid-containing lesions that are typically seen in children and young adults. The cause of these lesions remains unknown, although venous outflow obstruction has been postulated to be the cause. Lesions are usually located in the metaphysis, although they are more diaphyseal in older children. The proximal humerus is most commonly affected, followed by the proximal femur and tibia (355,442). Approximately 90% of lesions occur in the humerus and femur (442). Patients usually present in the first two decades of life, with a male predominance as high as 3:1 (442). Approximately two thirds of patients present with pathologic fracture, suggesting most lesions are asymptomatic, and the lesion may represent as many as 5% of all primary bone lesions (442,443).

The bone cyst is lined by a thin layer of fibrous tissue containing scattered benign giant cells (355). Thicker areas may contain vascular connective tissue, osteoid, or bone spicules (442). Occasionally, lesions may contain calcified material resembling a cementoma (355,442). Grossly, a simple cyst will be fluid filled, with the fluid clear or yellowish in color and of low viscosity. Occasionally, fibrous septa may course through the lesion, making the cyst multicameral (355).

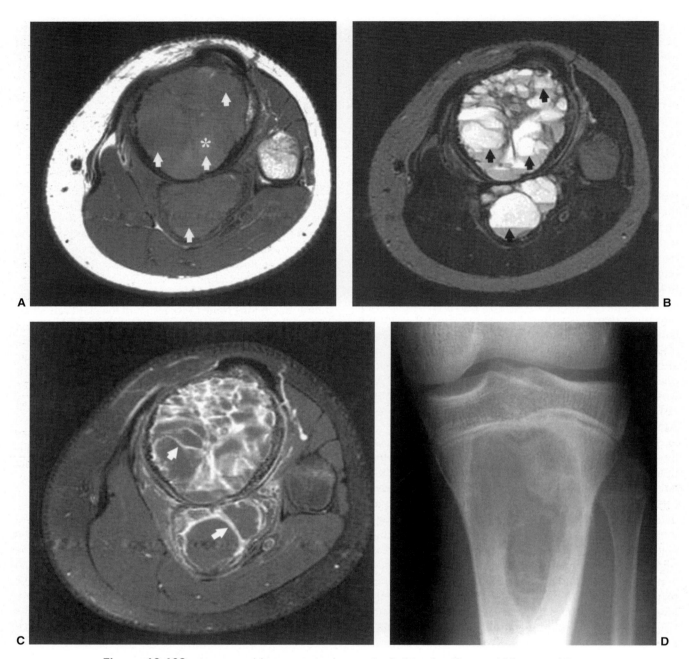

Figure 12-103 Aneurysmal bone cyst in the proximal tibia of a 15-year-old boy. Axial T1-weighted (600/14) **(A)** and T2-weighted (2463/80) **(B)** SE MR images of the proximal tibia show multiple fluid fluid levels (*arrows*). Mildly increased signal intensity is seen in **A** in a few of the hemorrhagic areas (*asterisk*). **C:** Corresponding contrast enhanced fat supressed axial T1-weighted (550/14) SE MR image shows enhancement of the fibrovascular tissue within the septae between the hemorrhagic areas (*arrows*). No mass-like areas of enhancement are noted. **D:** Radiograph shows a geographic lytic lesion in the proximal tibia without identifiable matrix.

Radiographs will show a geographic lytic lesion of bone with variaable margins. Lesions are usually centrally located within the meduallary cavity, thinning the overlying cortex. The long axis of the lesion usually parallels the long axis of the bone shaft. The diaphyseal end of the lesion will show a less well-defined margin than the metaphyseal extent, reflecting the paucity of trabecular bone in the shaft. Peristeal reaction is present only in association with pathologic fracture. Cysts with fracture will demonstrate a "fallen fragment" sign. The fallen fragment sign comprises a small bone fragment that lies in the dependent portion of lesion. This is believed to be virtually pathognomonic and is present in approximately 20% of cysts (443,444).

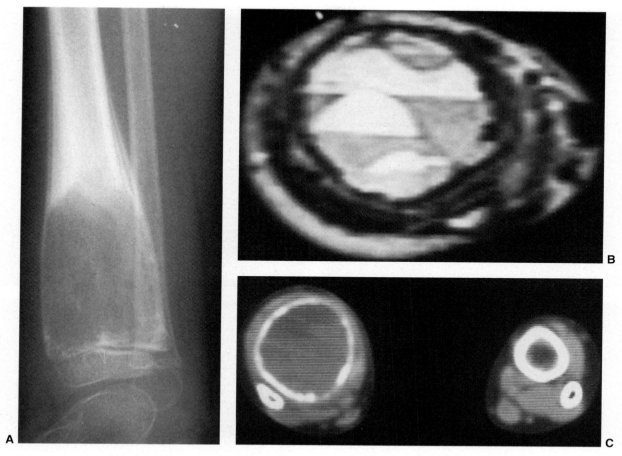

Figure 12-104 Cystic giant cell tumor in the distal tibia of a 4-year-old boy. **A:** Lateral radiograph shows a geographic lytic lesion with an expanded remodeled contour in the metaphysis with an associated laminated periosteal reaction. **B:** Axial T2-weighted (2,000/100) SE MR image shows multiple fluid–fluid level. The diagnosis of giant cell tumor was made on the solid portions of the lesion. **C:** Corresponding axial CT shows the fluid–fluid levels; however, they are more readily appreciated on MRI.

Flat bone lesions are considerably less common and are typically seen in older patients. In the flat bones, cysts are most common in the anterior calcaneous and ilium. In the calcaneus, lesions in the anterior aspect must be differentiated from an intraosseous lipoma and the calcaneus pseudocyst (pseudolesion due to paucity of trabecula in this area).

MRI will show a lesion with a signal intensity similar to that of fluid, with high signal intensity on fluid-sensitive images. Lesions with recent fracture may show a fluid–fluid level or fallen fragment sign. The fibrovascular tissue in the lining of the lesion may show distinct enhancement after contrast administration (see Fig. 12-106).

Malignant Tumors

Most malignant bone tumors have a nonspecific MRI appearance, with lesions typically demonstrating an inhomogeneous prolonged T1 and T2 relaxation time (see Fig. 12-107). The degree of inhomogeneity and the signal intensity often reflect the lesions' matrix, necrosis, hemorrhage, and associated edema (see Fig. 12-108). The primary role of MRI in evaluating malignant tumors is staging the lesion, that is, establishing the extent of marrow involvement (to include identification of skip metastases), soft tissue extension, and neurovascular compromise (see Fig. 12-109) (14,36,37,349). Marrow extent is best established with large field of view T1-weighted images of the entire affected bone, ensuring detection of skip metastases when present. Soft tissue extent is typically best seen on T2-weighted images, and these usually show periosteal and cortical changes better.

Metastases

Radionuclide bone scan and corresponding radiographs are most commonly used for the detection of skeletal metastatic disease. Scintigraphy may be falsely negative in patients with multiple myeloma and may be difficult to accurately interpret in patients with degenerative changes, Paget disease, or previous trauma.

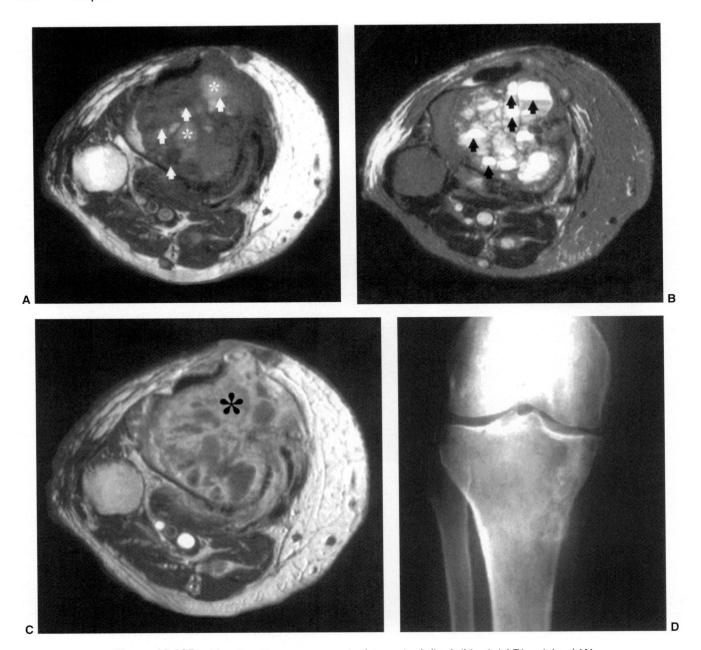

Figure 12-105 Telangiectatic osteosarcoma in the proximal distal tibia. Axial T1-weighted **(A)** and T2-weighted **(B)** SE MR images of the proximal tibia show multiple fluid–fluid levels (*arrows*). **C:** Corresponding contrast-enhanced axial T1-weighted SE MR image shows extensive enhancement within the solid portions of the tumor (*asterisk*), in stark contrast to the appearance of an aneurysmal bone cyst. **D:** Radiograph shows a geographic lytic lesion in the proximal tibia, also simulating the features of an aneursymal bone cyst.

Recently, MRI has proven to be equal to or superior to conventional methods for the detection of subtle metastases, especially in leukemia, lymphoma, small cell carcinoma, and multiple myeloma (see Fig. 12-110) (13,14,445). Daffner et al. (446) evaluated 30 multiple myeloma patients with MRI and found marrow abnormalities, which were confirmed as positive by needle aspiration in all cases. Scintigraphy of this same group showed only six to have positive bone scans. In addition to replacing

normal marrow with tumor nodules, multiple myeloma may diffusely infiltrate with normal marrow elements (447). In such cases, no focal abnormalities may be seen, and it may be impossible to identify patients with myeloma from the variations in fatty marrow distribution seen in normal patients (447).

MRI is especially useful in the evaluation of patients presenting with no history of trauma and new compression fractures of the spine. By analyzing both the signal

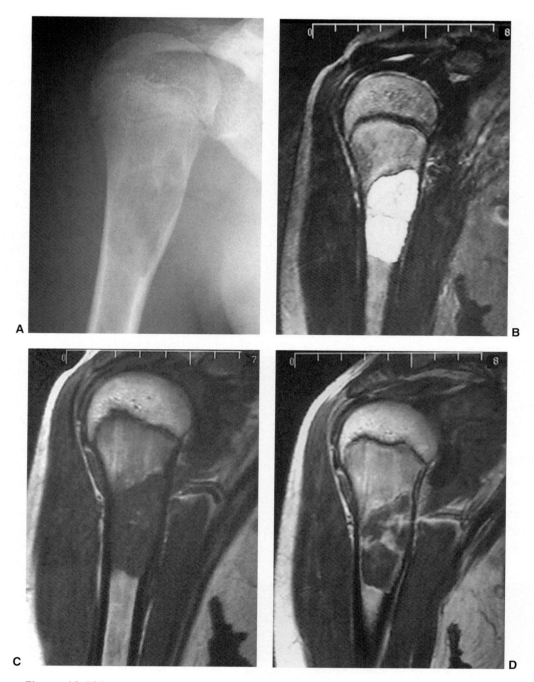

Figure 12-106 Bone cyst in a 12-year-old girl. **A:** Lateral radiograph shows a geographic lytic lesion with a mild expanded remodeled contour in the metaphysis. **B:** Coronal T2-weighted (2,000/90) SE MR image shows a fluid signal intensity lesion with a few subtle internal septa. Corresponding pre- **(C)** and postcontrast **(D)** T1-weighted (550/20) SE MR images show a fluid signal intensity with peripheral and septal enhancement.

intensity of the marrow in the abnormal vertebra and its morphology, MRI has been shown to be approximately 95% accurate in differentiating benign and malignant compression fractures (448).

In general, benign osteoporotic fractures are characterized by preservation of normal bone marrow on both T1- and T2-weighted spin-echo MR images. Malignant

lesions, in contradistinction, typically show complete replacement of normal marrow, often with an associated soft tissue mass and extension into the posterior elements. MRI may identify other lesions in noncompressed vertebrae, further supporting a diagnosis of metastatic disease. Vertebrae in which the marrow is incompletely replaced are more difficult to access; however, when interpreted

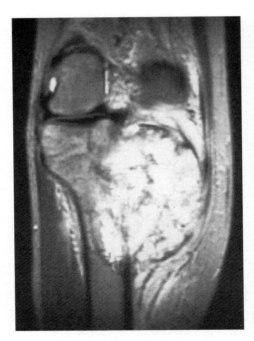

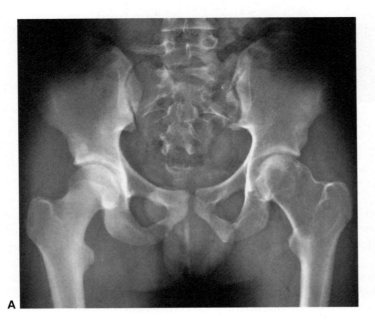

Figure 12-107 Osteosarcoma. T2-weighted (2,000/60) SE MR image of the tibia demonstrating an inhomogeneous high signal intensity lesion extending into the soft tissues.

with secondary findings, they may allow a satisfactory diagnosis (448,449) (see Fig. 12-111).

Multiple Myeloma

Multiple myeloma, also known as plasma cell myeloma, is a malignant disease of plasma cells that usually originates in the bone marrow but may involve other tissue as well. The first recorded patient with this disease was found in 1845 to have pain, and it was noted that his urine contained unusual "animal" matter that became soluble as the urine was heated (450). The term "multiple myeloma" was subsequently coined in 1873 by Rustizky (450).

Multiple myeloma is usually associated with the presence of a monoclonal immunoglobulin in the blood, urine, or both, and with the presence of lytic bone lesions (451). It is a common disease, representing approximately 1% of all malignancies and 10% to 15% of all malignancies of the hematologic system. In the Mayo series, it represented 43% of all malignant bone tumors. The average age of involved patients is 60 to 70 years, and it is unusual below the age of 40 years. It is more common in blacks and somewhat more common in men (single lesions are strikingly more common in men) (450).

The predominant radiographic pattern is one of osteolysis, although sclerotic lesions are seen in 0.5% to 3.0% of patients. Multiple sites of involvement are characteristic; however, solitary lesions (plasmacytomas) may exist for a prolonged period of time. The axial skeleton is involved most commonly, typically including (in descending order) vertebral column, ribs, skull, pelvis, and femur. Plasmacytoma will show a similar distribution with more than 50% of lesions in the vertebrae. Mandibular lesions are seen in about one third of patients (450). Diffuse osteopenia may also be seen, which may simulate osteoporosis.

The lesions of myeloma typically show discrete margins, which appear uniform in size. The more chronic the clinical course, the more discrete and punched out the areas of lysis. Especially characteristic of multiple myeloma is a subcortical or elliptical radiolucency, most often in the long bones. The subcortical defects cause erosion of the inner margins of the cortex and, when extensive, create a scalloped and wavy contour throughout the endosteal bone (450).

This disease is characterized pathologically by infiltration or replacement of the cellular constituents of normal

Figure 12-108 A 16-year-old boy with a clear cell chondrosarcoma. Anteroposterior radiograph **(A)** demonstrates a geographic lytic lesion in the left femoral neck with a variable margin and an expanded remodeled contour. Technetium bone scan **(B)** shows intense tracer uptake in the femoral head and neck. Coronal SE 323/10 images before **(C)** and after **(D)** contrast an inhomogeneous low signal intensity lesion in the femoral head and outer trochanteric region. Note delicate curvilinear enhancement. **E:** Axial SE 2,000/80 image shows the lesion is inhomogeneous with multiple high signal intensity areas.

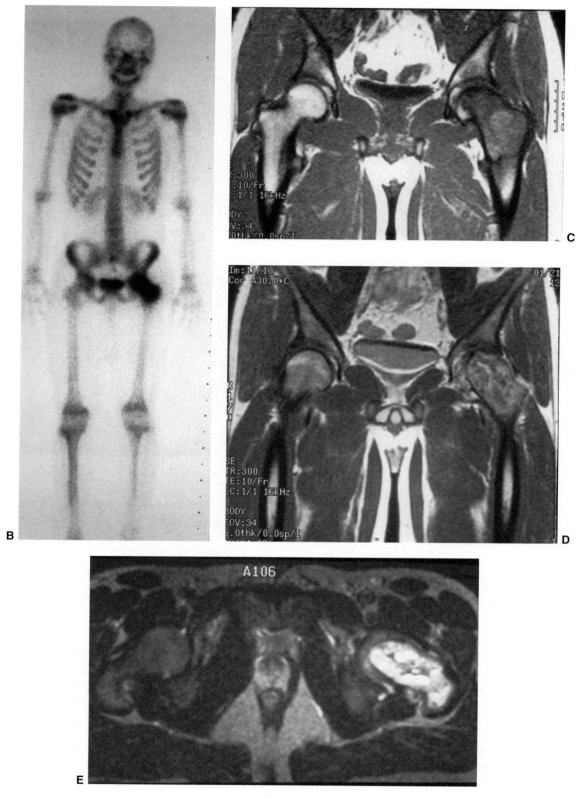

Figure 12-108 (continued)

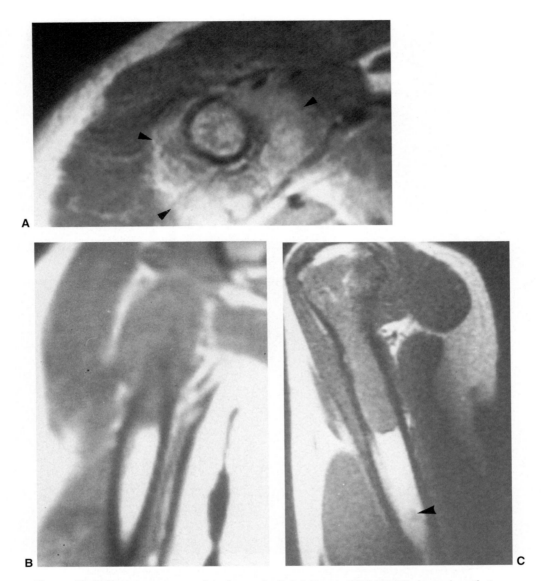

Figure 12-109   Ewing sarcoma of the humerus. **A:** Axial image (SE 2,000/30) shows the soft tissue extension (*arrowheads*) and narrow changes. **B:** Coronal SE 500/20 image does not clearly demonstrate the extent of involvement. **C:** Sagittal SE 500/20 image shows the extent of the lesion and a distal skip lesion (*arrowhead*).

marrow by tumor cells. This replacement may be diffuse and/or focal and predominated in regions of hemopoetic marrow. The MRI features of multiple myeloma reflect this pathophysiology and have been well correlated in the spine (365,450–452). Lecouvet et al. (451) noted three patterns of marrow involvement. Involvement may be characterized by a focal pattern of nodular marrow lesions against a background of normal-appearing marrow (Fig. 12-111). There may be a diffuse pattern of involvement characterized by widespread homogeneous alterations of marrow signal (see Fig. 12-112), or the marrow may appear normal. In a study of 80 patients, Lecouvet et al. (451) noted a normal pattern in 24%, a focal pattern in 44%, and a diffuse pattern in 32%

of patients. In this study, patients with normal marrow pattern responded better to therapy and survived longer than those with abnormal marrow patterns.

It must be emphasized that patients with extensive (stage 3) disease may demonstrate a normal marrow pattern (447). Moreover, in a study of 37 patients with 238 vertebral compression fractures, 67% appeared benign and only 33% appeared malignant, and 14 (38%) patients had only benign-appearing compression fractures at diagnosis, suggesting that most compression fractures in patients with multiple myeloma appear benign at MRI, and their disrtribution is similar to that observed in osteoporotic fractures (451).

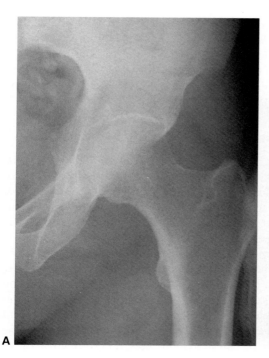

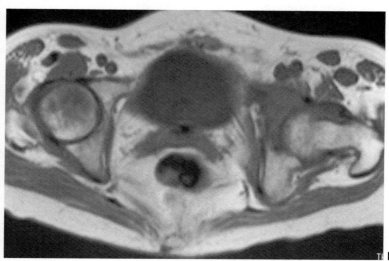

A

B

Figure 12-110 Occult skeletal metastasis in a 67-year-old woman presenting with hip pain. **A:** Radiograph of the left hip is normal. **B:** Axial T1-weighted (600/15) SE MR images shows a destructive lesion in the anterior aspect of the left acetabulum. Biopsy revealed metastatic adenocarcinoma.

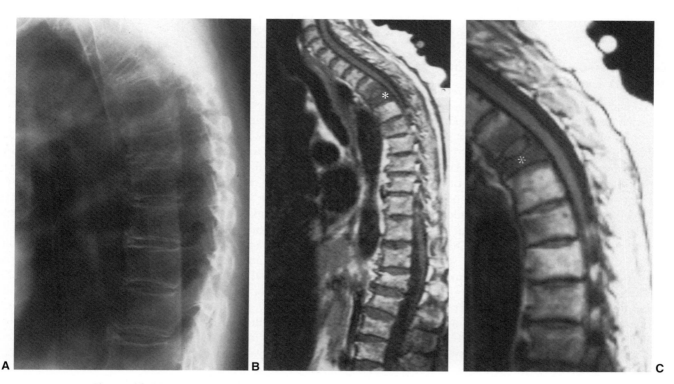

A

B

C

Figure 12-111 Pathologic compression fracture of the T4 vertebral body in a 73-year-old woman being evaluated for metastatic disease after identification of a lung carcinoma. **A:** Lateral thoracic spine radiograph shows marked compression fracture of the T4 vertebral body. No other lesions are seen. **B:** Large field of view T1-weighted (500/15) SE MR image of the spine shows the fracture at T4 (*asterisk*) and as partial replacement of the marrow in the T3 vertebral body and T6 vertebral body. **C:** Corresponding small field of view lateral T1-weighted (500/15) image shows areas of marrow replacement to better advantage. Transpedicular biopsy of the T4 lesion revealed multiple myeloma.

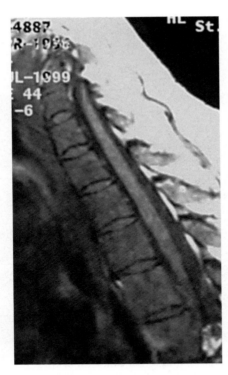

Figure 12-112 Stage III multiple myeloma in a 63-year-old woman. Sagittal T1-weighted (500/14) SE MR image shows complete relatively homogeneous replacement of the normal fatty marrow. Note the signal intensity of the vertebral body is less than that of the intervertebral disc.

Lesions Associated with Marrow and Soft Tissue Changes

Certain benign lesions have associated marrow and soft tissue edema, including chondroblastoma, osteoid osteoma, osteoblastoma, and eosinophilic granuloma (Langerhans cell histiocytosis localized to bone) (406,453). These changes are seen in the absence of a related stress or pathologic fracture and are likely the result of inflammatory and myxomatous changes, which may be seen with these lesions (403,453). Eosinophilic granuloma may also have an associated soft tissue mass, suggesting a more aggressive process, with soft tissue extension. Other lesions to consider with associated marrow and soft tissue changes include osteomyelitis and stress fracture.

The soft tissue and marrow changes may cause the lesion to appear larger on MR images than suspected on radiographs and may decrease the conspicuity of a lesion (453). More importantly, the diffuse inflammatory response may suggest a more aggressive process and simulate a malignancy (406).

Gadolinium-enhanced Magnetic Resonance Imaging

Dynamic MRI studies using gadopentetate dimeglumine have been utilized to distinguish benign and malignant tumors and to assess response to therapy (25,26,291, 330,454). Seeger et al. (339), however, found gadopentetate-enhanced imaging did not assist in defining tumor margins in the preoperative evaluation of 21 patients with osteosarcoma, although it was useful in differentiating intraarticular tumor from effusion in five of these cases.

Response to Therapy

Osteosarcoma and Ewing sarcoma account for most musculoskeletal sarcomas in all patients and almost 90% of those in children and in adolescents (454). Assessment of response to chemotherapy is essential in that initial response is a predictor of outcome and influences subsequent chemotherapy and surgery (454). Recent reports have shown MRI to be useful in this regard (455,456).

Holscher et al. (456) reported that the signal-intensity changes in the extraosseous component of Ewing sarcoma and osteosarcoma on T2-weighted images and changes in tumor volume could be correlated to histopathology and used in evaluating the response to chemotherapy. In the evaluation of osteosarcoma, they noted an increase in tumor volume and increased or unchanged edema were predictive of a poor response. Interestingly, in the same study, a decrease or no change in tumor volume and a decrease in edema were poor predictors of a good response. Lawrence et al. (457) found similar results with no change or an increase in the size of the soft tissue mass and an increase in bone destruction predictive of a poor response. Caution must be exercised to differentiate an increase in soft tissue mass secondary to intralesional hemorrhage from tumor growth. In general, attempts to correlate changes in MRI signal intensity with response to therapy are inconclusive (454).

Recently, gadolinium-enhanced subtraction MRI has been used to evaluate the response to chemotherapy in patients with osteosarcoma. In this technique, subtraction images are created by subtracting precontrast from postgadolinium T1-weighted images (458). Tumor can be separated from inflammation and edema by the rate of enhancement; viable tumor enhancing early, within 1 to 2 minutes; and inflammation and edema enhancing between 4 and 9 minutes after injection (458). Using this fundamental technique on 10 patients with osteosarcoma, De Baere et al. (458) successfully identified four good responders, defining them as patients with nonenhancing masses, with or without enhancing thin lines or nodules less than 3 mm, and five of six nonresponders. Fletcher et al. (459) evaluated 20 pediatric tumor patients, including 12 patients with osteosarcoma and 4 with Ewing's sarcoma, with dynamic time-intensity MRI. They found histologic response correlated well with postchemotherapy enhancement but not very well with changes in tumor size.

The role of MRI in prognosis is less clear. Lawrence et al. (457), in a review of 47 pediatric patients with extremity osteosarcoma, found radiologic imaging of only limited value in predicting prognosis. In this study, images were assessed for the presence of lung metastases, bone expansion, radiologic character of the bone lesion, epiphyseal/articular extension, skip lesions, size of soft tissue mass, and extent of marrow involvement. Of these factors, only the presence of metastases at presentation and a soft tissue mass greater than 20 cm in diameter were predictive of a poor outcome. Others found the clinical course that patients with skip metastases at presentation follow is similar to that of patients presenting with lung metastases (460,461).

REFERENCES

1. Hudson TM. *Radiologic-pathologic correlation of musculoskeletal lesions.* Baltimore, MD: Williams & Wilkins, 1987:1–9, 261–286, 541–604.
2. Dalinka MK, Zlatkin MD, Chao P, et al. The use of the magnetic resonance imaging in the evaluation of bone and soft tissue tumors. *Radiol Clin North Am* 1990;28:461–470.
3. Pettersson H, Gillespy T, Hamlin DJ, et al. Primary musculoskeletal tumors: examination with MR imaging compared with conventional modalities. *Radiology* 1987;164:237–241.
4. Sundaram M, McGuire MH, Herbold DR. Magnetic resonance imaging of soft tissue masses: an evaluation of fifty-three histologically proven tumors. *Magn Reson Imaging* 1988;6:237–248.
5. Tehranzadeh J, Manymneh W, Ghavam C, et al. Comparison of CT and MR imaging in musculoskeletal neoplasms. *J Comput Assist Tomogr* 1989;13:466–472.
6. Chang AE, Matory YL, Dwyer AJ, et al. Magnetic resonance imaging versus computed tomography in the evaluation of soft tissue tumors of the extremities. *Am Surg* 1987;205:240–340.
7. Demas BE, Heelan RT, Lane J, et al. Soft tissue sarcomas of the extremities: comparison of MR and CT in determining the extent of disease. *AJR Am J Roentgenol* 1988;150:615–620.
8. Hudson TM, Hamlin DJ, Enneking MD, et al. Magnetic resonance imaging of bone and soft tissue tumors: early experience in 31 patients compared with computed tomography. *Skeletal Radiol* 1985;13:134–146.
9. Petasnick JP, Turner DA, Charters JR, et al. Soft tissue masses of the locomotor system: comparison of MR imaging with CT. *Radiology* 1986;160:125–133.
10. Totty WG, Murphy WA, Lee JKT. Soft tissue tumors: MR imaging. *Radiology* 1986;160:135–141.
11. Weekes RG, Berquist TH, McLeod RA, et al. Magnetic resonance imaging of soft tissue tumors: comparison with computed tomography. *Magn Reson Imaging* 1985;3:345–352.
12. Panicek DM, Gatsonis C, Rosenthal DI, et al. CT and MR imaging in the local staging of primary malignant musculoskeletal neoplasms: report of the Radiology Diagnostic Oncology Group. *Radiology* 1997;202:237–246.
13. Berquist TH. Magnetic resonance imaging of musculoskeletal neoplasms. *Clin Orthop* 1989;244:101–118.
14. Berquist TH. *MRI of the musculoskeletal system,* 4th ed. Philadelphia, PA: Lippincott Williams & Wilkins, 2001.
15. Berquist TH. Magnetic resonance imaging of primary skeletal neoplasms. *Radiol Clin North Am* 1993;31:411–424.
16. Berquist TH. Magnetic resonance techniques in musculoskeletal diseases. *Rheum Dis Clin North Am* 1991;17:599–616.
17. Dwyer AJ, Frank JA, Sank VJ, et al. Short T1 inversion-recovery pulse sequence: analysis and initial experience in cancer imaging. *Radiology* 1988;168:827–836.
18. Shuman WP, Baron RL, Peters MJ, et al. Comparison of STIR and spin echo MR imaging at 1.5 T in 90 lesions of the chest, liver and pelvis. *AJR Am J Roentgenol* 1989;152:853–859.
19. Berquist TH, Ehman RL, King BF, et al. Value of MR imaging in differentiating benign from malignant soft tissue masses: study of 95 lesions. *AJR Am J Roentgenol* 1990;155:1251–1255.
20. Rubin DA, Kneeland JB. MR imaging of the musculoskeletal system: technical considerations for enhancing image quality and diagnostic yield. *AJR Am J Roentgenol* 1994;163:1155–1163.
21. Suh JS, Abenoza P, Galloway HR, et al. Peripheral (extracranial) nerve tumors: correlation of MR imaging and histologic findings. *Radiology* 1992;183:341–346.
22. Mirowitz SA. Fast scanning and fat-supression MR imaging of musculoskeletal disorders. *AJR Am J Roentgenol* 1993;161:1147–1157.
23. Fujimoto H, Murakami K, Ichikawa T, et al. MRI of soft tissue lesions: opposed-phase T2-weighted gradient echo images. *J Comput Assist Tomogr* 1993;17:418–424.
24. DeSchepper A, Ramon F, Degryse H. Statistical analysis of MRI parameters predicting malignancy in 151 soft tissue masses. *Rofo Fortschr Geb Rontgenstr Neuen Bildgeb Verfahr* 1992;156:587–591.
25. Erlemann R, Reiser MF, Peters PE, et al. Musculoskeletal neoplasms: static and dynamic Gd-DTPA-enhanced MR imaging. *Radiology* 1989;171:767–773.
26. Erlemann R, Vassallo P, Bongartz G, et al. Musculoskeletal neoplasms: fast low-angle shot imaging with and without Gd-DTPA. *Radiology* 1990;176:489–495.
27. Vanel D, Shapeero LG, De Baere T, et al. MR imaging in the follow-up of malignant and aggressive soft tissue tumors: results of 511 examinations. *Radiology* 1994;190:263–268.
28. Mirowitz SA, Totty WG, Lee JKT. Characterization of musculoskeletal masses using dynamic Gd-DTPA enhanced spin echo MRI. *J Comput Assist Tomogr* 1992;16:120–125.
29. Verstraete KL, Dierick A, DeDeene Y, et al. First-pass images of musculoskeletal lesions: a new and useful diagnostic application of dynamic contrast-enhanced MRI. *Magn Reson Imaging* 1994;12:687–702.
30. Beltran J, Simon DC, Katz W, et al. Increased MR signal intensity in skeletal muscle adjacent to malignant tumors: pathologic correlation and clinical relevance. *Radiology* 1987;162:251–255.
31. Benedikt RA, Jelinek JS, Kransdorf MJ, et al. MR imaging of soft tissue masses: role of gadopentetate dimeglumine. *J Magn Reson Imaging* 1994;4:485–490.
32. Sostman HD, Prescott DM, Dewhirst MW, et al. MR imaging and spectroscopy for prognostic evaluation in soft tissue sarcomas. *Radiology* 1994;190:269–275.
33. Zlatkin MB, Lenkinski RE, Shinkwin M, et al. Combined MR imaging and spectroscopy of bone and soft tissue tumors. *J Comput Assist Tomogr* 1990;14:1–10.
34. Cohen MD, Weetman RM, Provisor AJ, et al. Efficacy of magnetic resonance imaging in 149 children with tumors. *Arch Surg* 1986;121:522–529.
35. Kransdorf MJ, Jelinek JS, Moser RP, et al. soft tissue masses: diagnosis using MR imaging. *AJR Am J Roentgenol* 1989;153:541–547.
36. Sundaram M, McLeod RA. Computed tomography or magnetic resonance for evaluation of solitary tumor and tumor-like lesions of bone. *Skeletal Radiol* 1988;17:393–401.
37. Bloem JL, Taminiau AHM, Eulderink F, et al. Radiologic staging of primary bone sarcoma: MR imaging, scintigraphy, angiography, and CT correlated with pathologic examination. *Radiology* 1988;169:805–810.
38. Fornage BD, Rifkin MD. Ultrasound examination of the hand and foot. *Radiol Clin North Am* 1988;26:109–129.
39. Anderson MW, Temple HT, Dussault RG, et al. Compartmental anatomy: relevance to staging and biopsy of musculoskeletal tumors. *AJR Am J Roentgenol* 1999;173:1663–1671.
40. Bertoni F, Present DA, Enneking WF. Staging of bone tumors. In: Unni KK, ed. *Bone tumors.* New York: Churchill Livingstone, 1988:47–83.
41. Enneking WF. Staging of musculoskeletal neoplasms. *Skeletal Radiol* 1985;13:183–194.
42. Enneking WF, Spawer SS, Goodman MA. A system for surgical staging of musculoskeletal sarcoma. *Clin Orthop* 1980;153:106–120.
43. Patten RM, Shuman WP, Teefey S. Subcutaneous metastases from malignant melanoma: prevalence and findings on CT. *AJR Am J Roentgenol* 1989;152:1009–1012.
44. Spanier SS, Shuster JJ, Vander Griend RA. The effect of local tumor extent on prognosis of osteosarcoma. *J Bone Joint Surg Am* 1990;72A:643–653.
45. Madewell JE, Moser RP. Radiologic evaluation of soft tissue tumors. In: Enzinger FM, Weiss SW, eds. *Soft tissue tumors,* 2nd ed. St. Louis, MO: CV Mosby, 1988:43–82.

46. Weiss SW, Goldblum JR. *Enzinger and Weiss's Soft Tissue Tumors*, 4th ed. St. Louis, MO: CV Mosby, 2001.

47. DeSchepper AM, Ramon FA, Degryse HR. Magnetic resonance imaging of soft tissue tumors. *J Belge Radiol* 1992;75:286–296.

48. Sundaram M, McLeod RA. MR imaging of tumor and tumorlike lesions of bone and soft tissue. *AJR Am J Roentgenol* 1990;155:817–824.

49. Harris WD, Dudley R, Barry RJ. The natural history of fibrous dysplasia. *J Bone Joint Surg Am* 1962;44A:207–233.

50. Crim JR, Seeger LL, Yao L, et al. Diagnosis of soft tissue masses with MR imaging: can benign masses be differentiated from malignant ones. *Radiology* 1992;185:581–586.

51. Kransdorf MJ, Murphey MD. Radiologic evaluation of soft tissue masses: a current perspective. *AJR Am J Roentgenol* 2000;175: 575–587.

52. Weiss SW. Lipomatous tumors. In: Weiss SW, Brooks JSJ, eds. *Soft tissue tumors*. Baltimore, MD: Williams & Wilkins, 1996: 207–251.

53. Osment LS. Cutaneous lipomas and lipomatosis. *Surg Gynecol Obstet* 1968;127:129–132.

54. Järvi OH, Saxén AE, Hopsu-Havu VK, et al. Elastofibroma: a degenerative pseudotumor. *Cancer* 1969;23:42–63.

55. Humphrey AA, Kingsley PC. Familial multiple lipomas: a report on a family. *Arch Dermatol* 1938;37:30–34.

56. Lattes R. *Tumors of the soft tissue*. Washington, DC: Armed Forces Institute of Pathology, 1982:53–59. Fascicle 1, second series.

57. Dooms GC, Hricak H, Sollitto RA, et al. Lipomatous tumors and tumors with fatty components: MR imaging potential and comparison of MR and CT results. *Radiology* 1985;157:479–483.

58. Egund N, Ekelund L, Sako M, et al. CT of soft tissue tumors. *AJR Am J Roentgenol* 1981;137:725–729.

59. Glass RBJ, Poznanski AK, Fisher MR, et al. Case report. MR imaging of osteoid osteoma. *J Comput Assist Tomogr* 1986;10: 1065–1067.

60. Goldman AB, DiCarlo EF, Marcove RC. Case report 774. Coincidental lipoma with osseous excrescence and intramuscular lipoma. *Skeletal Radiol* 1993;22:138–145.

61. Ohguri T, Aoki T, Hisaoka M, et al. Differential diagnosis of benign peripheral lipoma from well-differentiated liposarcoma on MR imaging: is comparison of margins and internal characteristics useful? *AJR Am J Roentgenol* 2003;180:1689–1694.

62. Waligore MP, Stephens DH, Soule EH, et al. Lipomatous tumors of the abdominal cavity: CT appearance and pathologic correlation. *AJR Am J Roentgenol* 1981;137:539–545.

63. Weekes RG, McLeod RA, Reiman HM, et al. CT of soft tissue neoplasms. *AJR Am J Roentgenol* 1985;144:355–360.

64. Gonzalez-Crussi F, Enneking WF, Arean VM. Infiltrating angiolipoma. *J Bone Joint Surg Am* 1966;48A:1111–1124.

65. Sauer JM, Ozonoff MD. Congenital bone anomalies associated with lipomas. *Skeletal Radiol* 1985;13:276–279.

66. Fleming RJ, Alpert M, Garcia A. Parosteal lipoma. *AJR Am J Roentgenol* 1962;87:1075–1084.

67. Gaskin CM, Helms CA. Lipomas, lipoma variants, and well-differentiated liposarcomas (atypical lipomas): results of MRI evaluations of 135 consecutive fatty masses. *AJR Am J Roentgenol* 2004;182:733–739.

68. Christopher DM, Unni KK, Mertens F. *WHO classification of tumors. Pathology and genetics: tumors of soft tissue and bone.* Lyon: IARC Press, 2002.

69. Matsumoto K, Hukuda S, Ishizawa M, et al. MRI findings in intramuscular lipomas. *Skeletal Radiol* 1999;28:145–152.

70. Madewell JE, Sweet DE. Tumors and tumor-like lesions in or about joints. In: Resnick D, Niwayama G, eds. *Diagnosis of bone and joint disorders*, 2nd ed. Philadelphia, PA: WB Saunders, 1988:3889–3943.

71. Ryu KN, Jaovisidha S, Schweitzer M, et al. MR imaging of lipoma arborescens of the knee joint. *AJR Am J Roentgenol* 1996;167: 1229–1232.

72. Nisolle JF, Blouard E, Baudrez V, et al. Subacromial-subdeltoid lipoma arborescens associated with a rotator cuff tear. *Skeletal Radiol* 1999;28:283–285.

73. Mason ML. Presentation of cases. Proceedings of the American society for surgery of the hand. *J Bone Joint Surg Am* 1953;35A: 273–275.

74. Silverman TA, Enzinger FM. Fibrolipomatous hamartoma of nerve. A clinicopathologic analysis of 26 cases. *Am J Surg Pathol* 1985;9:7–14.

75. Amadio PC, Reiman HM, Dobyns JH. Lipofibromatous hamartoma of nerve. *J Hand Surg Am* 1988;13A:67–75.

76. Rosenthal DI, Aronow S, Murray WT. Iron content of pigmented villonodular synovitis detected by computed tomography. *Radiology* 1979;133:409–411.

77. Langa V, Posner MA, Steiner GE. Lipofibroma of the median nerve: a report of two cases. *J Hand Surg Br* 1987;12B:221–223.

78. Carpenter CT, Pitcher JD, Davis BJ, et al. Cystic hygroma of the arm: a case report and review of the literature. *Skeletal Radiol* 1996;25:201–204.

79. Cavallaro MC, Taylor JAM, Gorman JD, et al. Imaging findings in a patient with fibrolipomatous hamartoma of the median nerve. *AJR Am J Roentgenol* 1993;161:837–838.

80. Goldman AB. Collagen diseases, epiphyseal dysplasia and related conditions. In: Resnick D, Niwayama G, eds. *Diagnosis of bone and joint disorders*, 2nd ed. Philadelphia, PA: WB Saunders, 1988:3374–3441.

81. Marom EM, Helms CA. Fibrolipomatous hamartoma: pathognomonic on MR imaging. *Skeletal Radiol* 1999;28:260–264.

82. Bohndorf K, Reiser M, Lochner B, et al. Magnetic resonance imaging of primary tumors and tumor-like lesions of bone. *Skeletal Radiol* 1986;15:511–517.

83. Samlaska CP, Levin SW, James WD, et al. Proteus syndrome. *Arch Dermatol* 1989;125:1109–1114.

84. Seering G. Geschicte eines sehr grossen steatoms im hinterhaupte eines 2 und 1/2 jährigen kindes. *Mag Ges Heil* 1836;511–514.

85. Power D. Parosteal lipoma, or congenital fatty tumor, connected with periosteum of femur. *Trans Pathol Soc Lond* 1988;39:270–272.

86. Murphey MD, Johnson DL, Bhatia PS, et al. Parosteal lipoma: MR imaging characteristics. *AJR Am J Roentgenol* 1994; 162:105–110.

87. Geirnaerdt MJA, Hogendoorn PCW, Bloem JL, et al. Cartilage tumors: fast contrast-enhanced MR imaging. *Radiology* 2000;214:539–546.

88. Coode PE, McGuinness FE, Rawas MM, et al. Diffuse lipomatosis involving the thoracic and abdominal wall: CT features. *J Comput Assist Tomogr* 1991;15:341–343.

89. Comings DE, Glenchur H. Benign symmetric lipomatosis [letter]. *JAMA* 1968;203:305.

90. Dei Tos AP. Liposarcoma: new entities and evolving concepts. *Ann Diagn Pathol* 2000;4:252–266.

91. Kransdorf MJ, Bancroft LW, Peterson JJ, et al. Well-differentiated fatty tumors: distinction of lipoma from well-differentiated liposarcoma. *Radiology* 2002;224:99–104.

92. Bush CH, Spanier SS, Gilespy T. Imaging of atypical lipomas of the extremities: a report of three cases. *Skeletal Radiol* 1988;17:472–475.

93. Dahlin DC, McLeod RA. Aneurysmal bone cyst and other non-neoplastic conditions. *Skeletal Radiol* 1982;8:243–250.

94. Yang YJ, Damron TA, Cohen H, et al. Distiction of well-differentiated liposarcoma from lipoma in two patients with multiple well-differentiated fatty masses. *Skeletal Radiol* 2001;30:584–589.

95. Evans HL. Liposarcoma. A study of 55 cases with reassessment of its classification. *Am J Surg Pathol* 1979;3:507–523.

96. Meis JM. "Dedifferentiation" in bone and soft tissue tumors: a histologic indicator of tumor progression. In: Rosen PP, Feckner RE, eds. *Pathology annual*. Norwalk, CA: Appleton and Lange, 1991;37–62.

97. Kransdorf MJ, Meis JM, Jelinek JS. Dedifferentiated liposarcoma of the extremities: imaging findings in 4 patients. *AJR Am J Roentgenol* 1993;161:127–130.

98. Azumi N, Curtis J, Kempson RL, et al. Atypical and malignant neoplasms showing lipomatous differentiation. *Am J Surg Pathol* 1987;11:161–183.

99. Enzinger FM, Winslow DJ. Liposarcoma: a study of 103 cases. *Virchows Arch* 1962;335:367–388.

100. Evans HL, Soule EH, Winkelman RA. Atypical lipoma, atypical intramuscular lipoma, and well differentiated retroperitoneal liposarcoma. *Cancer* 1979;43:574–584.

101. Kindblom L, Angervall L, Fassina AS. Atypical lipoma. *Acta Pathol Microbiol Immunol Scand* 1982;90:27–36.

102. Jelinek JS, Kransdorf MJ, Shmookler BM, et al. Liposarcoma of the extremities: MR and CT findings of the histologic subtypes. *Radiology* 1993;186:455–459.

103. London J, Kim EE, Wallace S, et al. MR imaging of liposarcomas: correlation of MR features and histology. *J Comput Assist Tomogr* 1989;15:832–835.

104. Jelinek JS, Kransdorf MJ, Shmookler BM, et al. MR imaging of giant cell tumor of tendon sheath. *AJR Am J Roentgenol* 1994;162:919–922.

105. Sundaram M, Baran G, Merenda G, et al. Myxoid liposarcoma: magnetic resonance imaging appearances with clinical and histological correlation. *Skeletal Radiol* 1990;19:359–362.

106. Friedman AC, Hartman DS, Sherman J, et al. Computed tomography of abdominal fatty masses. *Radiology* 1981;139:415–429.

107. Carrcassome F, Bonneau H, Peschard JJ, et al. Le lipoblastome. *J Int Coll Surg* 1964;42:311–331.

108. Chung EB, Enzinger FM. Benign lipoblastomatosis: an analysis of 35 cases. *Cancer* 1973;32:482–492.

109. Jimenez JF. Lipoblastoma in infancy and childhood. *J Surg Oncol* 1986;32:238–244.

110. Van Meurs DP. The transformation of an embryonic lipoma to a common lipoma. *Br J Surg* 1947;34:282–284.

111. Black WC, Burke JW, Feldman PS, et al. CT appearance of cervical lipoblastoma. *J Comput Assist Tomogr* 1986;10:696–698.

112. Shmookler BM, Enzinger FM. Liposarcoma occuring in children. *Cancer* 1983;52:567–574.

113. Murphey MD, Fairbairn KJ, Parman LM, et al. Musculoskeletal angiomatous lesions: radiologic-pathologic correlation. *Radiographics* 1995;15:893–917.

114. Allen PB, Enzinger RM. Hemangioma of skeletal muscle: analysis of 89 cases. *Cancer* 1972;29:8–22.

115. Greenspan A, McGahan JP, Vogelsang P, et al. Imaging strategies in the evaluation of soft tissue hemangiomas of the extremities: correlation of finding on plain radiography, angiography, CT, MRI and ultrasonography in twelve histologically proven cases. *Skeletal Radiol* 1992;21:11–18.

116. Buetow PC, Kransdorf MJ, Moser RP, et al. Radiologic appearance of intramuscular hemangioma with emphasis on MR imaging. *AJR Am J Roentgenol* 1990;154:563–567.

117. Ly JQ, Sanders TG, Mulloy JP. Osseous change adjacent to soft-tissue hemengiomas of the extremities: correlation with lesion size and proximity to bone. *AJR Am J Roentgenol* 2003;180:1695–1700.

118. Sundaram M, McGuire MH, Herbold DR, et al. High signal intensity soft tissue masses on T1 weighted pulsing sequences. *Skeletal Radiol* 1987;16:30–36.

119. Cohen EK, Kressel HY, Perosio T, et al. MR imaging of soft tissue hemangiomas: correlation with pathologic findings. *AJR Am J Roentgenol* 1988;150:1079–1081.

120. Kransdorf MJ, Moser RP, Meis JM, et al. Fat containing soft tissue masses of the extremities. *Radiographics* 1991;11:81–106.

121. Chew FS, Hudson TM, Hawkins IF. Radiology of infiltrating angiolipoma. *AJR Am J Roentgenol* 1980;135:781–787.

122. DeOrchis DD, Ozonoff MB. Infiltrating angiolipoma with phlebolith formation. *Skeletal Radiol* 1986;15:464–467.

123. Hanna SL, Magill HL, Brooks MT, et al. Case of the day. Pediatric. Myositis ossificans circumscripta. *Radiographics* 1990;10:945–949.

124. Lin JJ, Lin F. Two entities in angiolipoma: a study of 459 cases of lipoma with review of literature on infiltrating angiolipoma. *Cancer* 1974;34:720–727.

125. Castillo M, Dominguez R. Congenital lymphangiectatic elephantiasis. *Magn Reson Imaging* 1992;10:321–324.

126. Pribyl C, Burke SW, Roberts JM, et al. Infiltrating angiolipoma or intramuscular hemangioma? A report of five cases. *J Pediatr Orthop* 1986;6:172–176.

127. Kittredge RD, Finby N. The many facets of lymphangioma. *AJR Am J Roentgenol* 1965;95:56–66.

128. Munechika H, Honda M, Kushihashi T, et al. Computed tomography of retroperitoneal cystic lymphangiomas. *J Comput Assist Tomogr* 1987;11:111–119.

129. Bierbaum BE. Double contrast knee arthrography. A safe and reliable aid to diagnosis of "internal derangement." *J Trauma* 1968;8:165–176.

130. Siegel MJ, Glazer HS, St. Amour TE, et al. Lymphangiomas in children: MR imaging. *Radiology* 1989;170:467–470.

131. Bill AH, Sumner DS. A unified concept of lymphangioma and cystic hygroma. *Surg Gynecol Obstet* 1965;120:79–86.

132. Godart S. Embryological significance of lymphangioma. *Arch Dis Child* 1966;41:204–206.

133. Zadvinskis DP, Benson MT, Kerr HH, et al. Congenital malformations of the cervicothoracic lymphatic system: embryology and pathogenesis. *Radiographics* 1992;12:1175–1189.

134. Klein MH, Shankman S. Osteoid osteoma: radiologic and pathologic correlation. *Skeletal Radiol* 1992;21:23–31.

135. Radin R, Weiner S, Koenigsberg M, et al. Retroperitoneal cystic lymphangioma. *AJR Am J Roentgenol* 1983;140:733–734.

136. Shin MS, Berland LL, Ho K. Mediastinal cystic hygromas: CT characteristics and pathologic consideration. *J Comput Assist Tomogr* 1985;9:297–301.

137. Buonomo C, Griscom NT. Pediatric case of the day. *Radiographics* 1991;11:1156–1158.

138. Singh S, Baboo ML, Pathak IC. Cystic lymphangioma in children: report of 32 cases including lesions at rare sites. *Surgery* 1971;69:947–951.

139. Peterson KK, Renfrew DL, Feddersen RM, et al. Magnetic resonance imaging of myxoid containing tumors. *Skeletal Radiol* 1991;20:245–250.

140. Bogumill GP, Sullivan DJ, Baker GI. Tumors of the hand. *Clin Orthop Relat Res* 1975;108:214–222.

141. Pilla TJ, Wolverson MK, Sundaram M, et al. CT evaluation of cystic lymphangiomas of the mediastinum. *Radiology* 1982;144:841–842.

142. Jaffe HL, Lichtenstein L, Sutro CJ. Pigmented villonodular synovitis, bursitis and tenosynovitis. *Arch Pathol Lab Med* 1941;31:731–765.

143. Ushijima M, Hashimoto H, Tsuneyoshi M, et al. Giant cell tumor of the tendon sheath (nodular tenosynovitis). A study of 220 cases to compare the large joint group with the common digit group. *Cancer* 1986;57:875–884.

144. Bobechko WP, Kostuik JP. Childhood villonodular synovitis. *Can J Surg* 1968;11:480–486.

145. Oyemade GAA, Abioye AA. A clinicopathologic review of benign giant cell tumors of tendon sheaths in Ibadan, Nigeria. *Am J Surg* 1977;134:392–395.

146. Savage RC, Mustafa ED. Giant cell tumor of tendon sheath (localized nodular tenosynovitis). *Ann Plast Surg* 1984;13:205–210.

147. Sundaram M, Duffrin H, McGuire MH, et al. Synchronous multicentric desmoid tumors (aggressive fibromatosis) of the extremities. *Skeletal Radiol* 1988;17:16–19.

148. Carstens HP, Howell RS. Case report. Malignant giant cell tumor of tendon sheath. *Virchows Arch* 1979;382:237–243.

149. Balsara ZN, Stainken BF, Martinez AJ. Case report. MR imaging of localized giant cell tumor of the tendon sheath involving the knee. *J Comput Assist Tomogr* 1989;13:159–162.

150. Karasick D, Karasick S. Giant cell tumor of tendon sheath: spectrum of radiographic findings. *Skeletal Radiol* 1992;12:219–224.

151. Maluf HM, DeYoung BR, Swanson PE, et al. Fibroma and giant cell tumor of tendon sheath: a comparative histological and immunohistological study. *Mod Pathol* 1995;8:155–159.

152. Satti MB. Tendon sheath tumors: a pathological study of the relationships between giant cell tumor and fibroma of tendon sheath. *Histopathology* 1992;20:213–220.

153. Dorwart RH, Genant HK, Johnston WH, et al. Pigmented villonodular synovitis of synovial joints: clinical, pathologic and radiologic features. *AJR Am J Roentgenol* 1984;143:877–885.

154. Dorwart RH, Genant HK, Johnston WH, et al. Pigmented villonodular synovitis of the shoulder: radiologic-pathologic assessment. *AJR Am J Roentgenol* 1984;143:886–888.

155. Spritzer CE, Dalinka MK, Kressel HY. Magnetic resonance imaging of pigmented villonodular synovitis: a report of two cases. *Skeletal Radiol* 1987;16:316–319.

156. Sundaram M, Chalk D, Merenda J, et al. Case report 563. Pigmented villonodular synovitis (PVNS) of knee. *Skeletal Radiol* 1989;18:463–465.

157. Wagner ML, Spjut HJ, Dutton RV, et al. Polyarticular pigmented villonodular synovitis. *AJR Am J Roentgenol* 1981;136:821–823.

158. Cotten A, Flipo RM, Chastanet P, et al. Pigmented villonodular synovitis of the hip: review of radiographic features in 58 patients. *Skeletal Radiol* 1995;24:1–6.

159. Kalil RK, Unni KK. Malignancy in pigmented villonodular synovitis. *Skeletal Radiol* 1998;27:392–395.

160. Byers PD, Cotton RE, Deacon OW, et al. The diagnosis and treatment of pigmented villonodular synovitis. *J Bone Joint Surg Br* 1968;50B:290–305.

161. Jelinek JS, Kransdorf MJ, Utz JA, et al. Imaging of pigmented villonodular synovitis with emphasis on MR imaging. *AJR Am J Roentgenol* 1989;152:337–342.

162. Lindenbaum BL, Hunt T. An unusual presentation of pigmented villonodular synovitis. *Clin Orthop* 1977;122:263–267.

163. Sundaram M, McGuire MH, Fletcher J, et al. Magnetic resonance imaging of lesions of synovial origin. *Skeletal Radiol* 1866;15:110–116.

164. Kottal RA, Vogler JB, Matamoros A, et al. Pigmented villonodular synovitis: a report of MR imaging in two cases. *Radiology* 1987;163:551–553.

165. Stark DD, Mosley ME, Brown BR, et al. Magnetic resonance imaging and spectroscopy of hepatic iron overload. *Radiology* 1985;154:137–142.

166. Lindgren PG, Willén R. Gastrocnemio-semimembranosus bursa and its relation to the knee joint. Anatomy and histology. *Acta Radiol* 1977;18:497–512.

167. Wolfe RD, Colloff B. Popliteal cysts. An arthrographic study and review of the literature. *J Bone Joint Surg Am* 1972;54A:1057–1063.

168. Wilson PD, Eyre-Brook AL, Francis JD. A clinical and anatomic study of the semimembranosis bursa in relation to popliteal cyst. *J Bone Joint Surg* 1938;20:963–984.

169. Fielding JR, Franklin PD, Kustan J. Popliteal cysts: a reassessment using magnetic resonance imaging. *Skeletal Radiol* 1991;20:433–435.

170. Fang CSJ, McCarthy CL, McNally EG. Intramuscular dissection of Baker's cysts: report of three cases. *Skeletal Radiol* 2004;33:367–371.

171. Butt WP, McIntyre JL. Double-contrast arthrography of the knee. *Radiology* 1969;92:487–499.

172. Nicholas JA, Freiberger RH, Killoran PJ. Double-contrast arthrography of the knee. *J Bone Joint Surg Am* 1970;52A:203–220.

173. Miller TT, Staron RB, Koenigsberg T, et al. MR imaging of Baker cysts: association with internal derangement, effusion, and degenerative arthropathy. *Radiology* 1996;201:247–250.

174. Hermann G, Yeh HC, Lehr-Janus C, et al. Diagnosis of popliteal cyst: double-contrast arthrography and sonography. *AJR Am J Roentgenol* 1981;137:369–372.

175. Richardson ML, Selby B, Montana MA, et al. Ultrasonography of the knee. *Radiol Clin North Am* 1988;26:63–75.

176. Good AE. Rheumatoid arthritis, Baker's cyst and "thrombophlebitis." *Arthritis Rheum* 1964;7:56–64.

177. Fedullo LM, Bonakdarpour A, Moyer RA, et al. Giant synovial cysts. *Skeletal Radiol* 1984;12:90–96.

178. Morris CS, Beltran JL. Giant synovial cyst associated with a pseudarthrosis of a rib: MR appearance. *AJR Am J Roentgenol* 1990;155:337–338.

179. Hudson TM, Bertoni F, Enneking WF. Scintigraphy of aggressive fibromatosis. *Skeletal Radiol* 1985;13:26–32.

180. Harkin JC, Reed RJ. *Atlas of tumor pathology. Second series, fascicle 3. Tumors of the peripheral nervous system.* Washington, DC: Armed Forces Institute of Pathology, 1968:29–59.

181. McDonald DG, Leopold GR. Ultrasound B-scanning in the differentiation of Baker's cyst and thromophlebitis. *Br J Radiol* 1972;45:729–732.

182. Lazarus ML, Ray CE, Maniquis CG. MRI findings on concurrent acute DVT and dissecting popliteal cyst. *Magn Reson Imaging* 1994;12:155–158.

183. Mink JH, Deutsch AL. *MRI of the musculoskeletal system. A teaching file.* New York: Raven Press, 1990:352–353.

184. Moore CP, Sarti DA, Louie JS. Ultrasonic demonstration of popliteal cysts in rheumatoid arthritis. *Arthritis Rheum* 1975;18:577–580.

185. Langer JE, Meyer SJF, Dalinka MK. Imaging of the knee. *Radiol Clin North Am* 1990;28:975–990.

186. Hartzman S, Reicher MA, Bassett LW, et al. MR imaging of the knee. Part II. Chronic disorders. *Radiology* 1987;162:553–557.

187. Francis IR, Dorovini-Zis K, Glazer GM, et al. The fibromatoses: CT-pathologic correlation. *AJR Am J Roentgenol* 1986;147:1063–1066.

188. Hudson TM, Vandergriend RA, Springfield DS, et al. Aggressive fibromatosis: evaluation by computed tomography and angiography. *Radiology* 1984;150:495–501.

189. Disler DG, Alexander AA, Mankin HJ, et al. Multicentric fibromatosis with metaphyseal dysplasia. *Radiology* 1993;187:489–492.

190. Macfarlane J. *Clinical reports of the surgical practice of the Glasgow royal infirmary.* Glasgow: Robertson, 1832:63–66.

191. Mueller J. *Uber den feineren Bau der Krankhaften Geschwukste.* Berlin: Breicht, 1836:107–113.

192. Taylor LJ. Musculoaponeurotic fibromatosis. A report of 28 cases and review of the literature. *Clin Orthop* 1987;224:294–302.

193. Yacoe ME, Bergman AG, Ladd AL, et al. Dupuytren's contracture: MR imaging findings and correlation between MR signal intensity and cellularity of lesions. *AJR Am J Roentgenol* 1993;160:813–817.

194. Morrison WB, Schweitzer ME, Wapner KL, et al. Plantar fibromatosis: a benign aggressive neoplasm with a characteristic appearance on MR images. *Radiology* 1994;193:841–845.

195. Wetzel LH, Levine E. Soft tissue tumors of the foot: value of MR imaging for specific diagnosis. *AJR Am J Roentgenol* 1990;155:1025–1030.

196. Rock MG, Pritchard DJ, Reiman HM, et al. Extra-abdominal desmoid tumors. *J Bone Joint Surg Am* 1984;66A:1369–1374.

197. Griffiths HJ, Robinson K, Bonfiglio TA. Aggressive fibromatosis. *Skeletal Radiol* 1983;9:179–182.

198. Ashby MA, Harmer CL, McKinna JA, et al. Case report. Infiltrative fibromatosis: a rare cause of fatal hemorrhage. *Clin Radiol* 1986;37:193–194.

199. Musgrove JE, McDonald JR. Extra-abdominal desmoid tumors. Their differential diagnosis and treatment. *Arch Pathol* 1948;45:513–540.

200. Wara WM, Phillips TL, Hill DR, et al. Desmoid tumors, treatment and prognosis. *Radiology* 1977;124:225–226.

201. Enzinger FM, Shiraki M. Musculo-aponeurotic fibromatosis of the shoulder girdle (extra-abdominal desmoid). *Cancer* 1967;20:1131–1140.

202. Shiu MH, Flancbaum L, Hajdu SI, et al. Malignant soft tissue tumors of the anterior abdominal wall. *Arch Surg* 1980;115:152–155.

203. Burke AP, Sobin LH, Shekitka KM. Mesenteric fibromatosis. *Arch Pathol* 1990;114:832–835.

204. McAdam WAF, Goligher JC. The occurrence of desmoid tumors in patients with familial polyposis coli. *Br J Surg* 1970;57:618–631.

205. Nichols RW. Desmoid tumors: a report of 31 cases. *Arch Surg* 1923;7:227.

206. Healy JC, Reznek RH, Clark SK, et al. MR appearances of desmoid tumors in familial adenomatous polyposis. *AJR Am J Roentgenol* 1997;169:465–472.

207. Abramowitz D, Zornoza J, Ayala AG, et al. Soft tissue desmoid tumors: radiographic bone changes. *Radiology* 1983;146:11–13.

208. Aisen AM, Martel W, Braunstein EM, et al. MRI and CT evaluation of primary bone and soft tissue tumors. *AJR Am J Roentgenol* 1986;146:749–756.

209. Weiss KL, Beltran J, Lubbers LM. High-field MR surface-coil imaging of the hand and wrist. Part II. Pathologic correlation and clinical revelance. *Radiology* 1986;160:147–152.

210. Sundaram M, McGuire MH, Schajowicz F. Soft tissue masses: histologic basis for decreased signal (short T2) on T2-weighted MR images. *AJR Am J Roentgenol* 1877;148:1247–1250.

211. Feld R, Burk L, McCue P, et al. MRI of aggressive fibromatosis: frequent appearance of high signal intensity on T2-weighted images. *Magn Reson Imaging* 1990;8:583–588.

212. Hartman TE, Berquist TH, Fetsch JF. MR imaging of extraabdominal desmoids: differentiation from other neoplasms. *AJR Am J Roentgenol* 1992;158:581–585.

213. Hawnaur JM, Jenkins JPR, Isherwood I. Magnetic resonance imaging of musculoaponeurotic fibromatosis. *Skeletal Radiol* 1990;19:509–514.

214. Quinn SF, Erickson SJ, Dee PM, et al. MR imaging in fibromatosis: results in 26 patients with pathologic correlation. *AJR Am J Roentgenol* 1991;156:539–542.

215. Kransdorf MJ, Jelinek JS, Moser RP, et al. MR appearance of fibromatosis: a report of 14 cases and review of the literature. *Skeletal Radiol* 1990;19:495–499.
216. Järvi OH, Saxén AE. Elastofibroma dorsi. *Acta Pathol Microbiol Scand* 1961;144(Suppl. 51):83–84.
217. Järvi OH, Länsimies PH. Subclinical elastofibromas in the scapular region in an autopsy series: additional notes on the aetiology and pathogenesis of elastofibroma pseudoneoplasm. *Acta Pathol Microbiol Scand* 1975;83:87–108.
218. Brandser EA, Goree JC, El-Khoury GY. Elastofibroma dorsi: prevalence in an elderly patient population as revealed by CT. *AJR Am J Roentgenol* 1998;171:977–980.
219. Marin ML, Perzin KH, Markowitz AM. Elastofibroma dorsi: benign chest wall tumor. *J Thorac Cardiovasc Surg* 1989;98:234–238.
220. Mirra JM, Straub LR, Järvi OH. Elastofibroma of the deltoid. *Cancer* 1974;33:234–238.
221. Nagamine N, Nohara Y, Ito E. Elastofibroma in Okinawa: a clinicopathologic study of 180 cases. *Cancer* 1982;50:1794–1805.
222. Barr JR. Elastofibroma. *Am J Clin Pathol* 1996;45:679–683.
223. Kumaratilake JS, Krishnan R, Lomax-Smith J, et al. Elastofibroma: disturbed elastic fibrillogenesis by periosteal-derived cells? An immunoelectron microscopic and in situ hybridization study. *Hum Pathol* 1991;22:1017–1029.
224. Gould ES, Javors BR, Morrison J, et al. Case report. MR appearance of bilateral periscapular elastofibroma. *J Comput Assist Tomogr* 1989;13:701–703.
225. Naylor MF, Nascimento AG, Sherrick AD, et al. Elastofibroma dorsi: radiologic findings in 12 patients. *AJR Am J Roentgenol* 1996;167:683–687.
226. Austin P, Jakobiec FA, Iwamoto T, et al. Elastofibroma oculi. *Arch Ophthalmol* 1983;101:1575–1579.
227. Cross DL, Mills SE, Kulund DN. Elastofibroma arising in the foot. *South Med J* 1984;77:1194–1196.
228. Kapff PD, Hocken DB, Simpson RHW. Elastofibroma of the hand. *J Bone Joint Surg Br* 1987;69B:468–469.
229. Prete PE, Henbest M, Michalski JP, et al. Intraspinal elastofibroma: a case report. *Spine* 1983;8:800–802.
230. Waisman J, Smith DW. Fine structure of an elastofibroma. *Cancer* 1968;22:671–677.
231. Schwarz T, Opplzer G, Duschet P, et al. Ulcerating elastofibroma dorsi. *J Am Acad Dermatol* 1989;21:1142–1144.
232. Kransdorf MJ, Meis JM, Montgomery E. Elastofibroma: MR and CT appearance with radiologic-pathologic correlation. *AJR Am J Roentgenol* 1992;159:575–579.
233. Greenspan A. Benign bone forming lesions: osteoma, osteoid osteoma, osteoblastoma. *Skeletal Radiol* 1993;22:485–500.
234. Stull MA, Moser RP, Kransdorf MJ, et al. Magnetic resonance appearance of peripheral nerve sheath tumors. *Skeletal Radiol* 1990;20:9–14.
235. Kransdorf MJ. Benign soft tissue tumors in a large referral population: distribution of diagnoses by age, sex and location. *AJR Am J Roentgenol* 1995;164:395–402.
236. Geschickter CF. Tumors of the peripheral nerves. *Am J Cancer* 1935;25:377–410.
237. Levine E, Huntrakoon M, Wetzel LH. Malignant nerve-sheath neoplasms in neurofibromatosis: distinction from benign tumors by using imaging techniques. *AJR Am J Roentgenol* 1987;149:1059–1064.
238. Sakai F, Sone S, Kiyono K, et al. Intrathoracic neurogenic tumors: MR-pathologic correlation. *AJR Am J Roentgenol* 1992;159:279–283.
239. Varma DGK, Moulopoulos A, Sara AS, et al. MR imaging of extracranial nerve sheath tumors. *J Comput Assist Tomogr* 1992;16:448–453.
240. Kim SH, Choi BI, Han MC, et al. Retroperitoneal neurilemoma: CT and MR findings. *AJR Am J Roentgenol* 1992;159:1023–1026.
241. Cerofolini E, Landi A, DeSantis G, et al. MR of benign peripheral nerve sheath tumors. *J Comput Assist Tomogr* 1991;15:593–597.
242. Ducatman BS, Scheithauer BW, Piepgras DG, et al. Malignant peripheral nerve sheath tumors: a clinicopathologic study of 120 cases. *Cancer* 1986;57:2006–2021.
243. Murphey MD, Smith SW, Smith SE, et al. Imaging of musculoskeletal neurogenic tumors: radiologic-pathologic correlation. *Radiographics* 1999;19:1253–1280.

244. Erickson SJ, Canale PB, Carrera GF, et al. Interdigital (Morton) neuroma: high-resolution MR imaging with a solenoid coil. *Radiology* 1991;181:833–836.
245. Morton TG. A peculiar and painful affliction of the fourth metatarsophalangeal articulation. *Am J Med Sci* 1876;71:37–45.
246. Terk MR, Kwong PK, Suthar M, et al. Morton neuroma: evaluation with MR imaging performed with contrast enhancement and fat suppression. *Radiology* 1993;189:239–241.
247. Alexander IJ, Johnson KA, Parr JW. Morton's neuroma: a review of recent concepts. *Orthopedics* 1987;10:103–106.
248. Mann RA, Reynolds JC. Interdigital neuroma: a critical analysis. *Foot Ankle* 1983;3:238–243.
249. Redd RA, Peters VJ, Emery SF, et al. Moron neuroma: sonographic evaluation. *Radiology* 1989;171:415–417.
250. Zanetti M, Ledermann T, Zollinger H, et al. Efficacy of MR imaging in patients suspected of having Morton's neuroma. *AJR Am J Roentgenol* 1997;168:529–532.
251. Zanetti M, Strehle JK, Zollinger H, et al. Morton neuroma and fluid in the intermetatarsal bursae on MR images of 70 asymptomatic volunteers. *Radiology* 1997;203:516–520.
252. Donnal JF, Blinder RA, Coblentz CL, et al. MR imaging of stump neuroma. *J Comput Assist Tomogr* 1990;14:656–657.
253. Huber GC, Lewis D. Amputation neuromas: their development and prevention. *Arch Surg* 1920;1:85–113.
254. De Beuckeleer LHL, De Schepper AMA, Ramon F. Magnetic resonance imaging in cartilaginous tumors: retrospective study of 79 patients. *Eur J Radiol* 1995;21:34–40.
255. Singson RD, Feldman F, Slipman C, et al. Post amputation neuromas and other symptomatic stump abnormalities: detection with CT. *Radiology* 1987;162:743–745.
256. Singson RD, Feldman F, Staron R, et al. MRI of postamputation neuromas. *Skeletal Radiol* 1990;19:259–262.
257. Israels SJ, Chan HSL, Daneman A, et al. Synovial sarcoma in childhood. *AJR Am J Roentgenol* 1983;142:803–806.
258. Bogumill GP, Bruna PD, Barrick EF. Malignant lesions masquerading as popliteal cysts. *J Bone Joint Surg Am* 1981;63A:474–477.
259. Cadman NL, Soule EH, Kelley PJ. Synovial sarcoma: an analysis of 144 tumors. *Cancer* 1965;18:613–627.
260. Wright PH, Sim FH, Soule EH, et al. Synovial sarcoma. *J Bone Joint Surg Am* 1982;64A:112–131.
261. Atsakis JG, Nishiyama RH, Sullinger GD. Synovial sarcoma of the neck. *Arch Otolaryngol* 1961;85:327–331.
262. Goldman AB, Schneider R, Pavlov H. Osteoid osteomas of the femoral neck: report of four cases evaluated with isotope bone scanning, CT and MR imaging. *Radiology* 1993;186:227–232.
263. Roth JA, Enzinger FM, Tannenbaum MT. Synovial sarcoma of the neck: a follow up study of 24 cases. *Cancer* 1975;35:1243–1253.
264. Tahir T, Sanjiv G. Synovial sarcoma of the right ventricle. *Am Heart J* 1991;121:933–938.
265. Treu EBWM, de Slegte RGM, Golding RP, et al. CT findings in paravertebral synovial sarcoma. *J Comput Assist Tomogr* 1986;10:460–462.
266. Ryan JR, Baker LH, Benjamin RS. The natural history of metastatic synovial sarcoma. The experience of the southwest oncology group. *Clin Orthop* 1982;164:257–260.
267. Sutro J. Synovial sarcoma of the soft parts in the first toe: recurrence after thirty-five year interval. *Bull Hosp Joint Dis* 1976;37:105–109.
268. Vezeridis MP, Moore R, Karakousis CP. Metastatic patterns in soft tissue sarcomas. *Arch Surg* 1983;118:915–918.
269. Mazeron JJ, Suit HD. Lymph nodes as sites of metastases from sarcomas of soft tissue. *Cancer* 1987;60:1800–1808.
270. Pack GT, Ariel IM. Treatment of cancer and allied diseases. In: Pack GT, Ariel IM, eds. *Tumors of the soft somatic tissues and bone*, Vol. 8. New York: Harper & Row, 1965:8–39.
271. Meyer CA, Kransdorf MJ, Jelinek JS, et al. Case report 716. Soft tissue metastasis in synovial sarcoma. *Skeletal Radiol* 1992;21:128–131.
272. Varela-Duram J, Enzinger FM. Calcifying synovial sarcoma. *Cancer* 1982;50:345–352.
273. Horowitz AL, Resnick D, Watson RC. The roentgen features of synovial sarcoma. *Clin Radiol* 1973;24:481–484.
274. Genest P, Kim TH, Katsarkas A, et al. Calcified synovial sarcoma of the oropharynx. *Br J Radiol* 1983;56:580–582.

275. DeCoster TA, Kamps BS, Craven JP. Magnetic resonance imaging of a foot synovial sarcoma. *Orthopedics* 1991;14:169–171.

276. Mahajan H, Lorigan JG, Shirkhoda A. Synovial sarcoma: MR imaging. *Magn Reson Imaging* 1989;7:211–216.

277. Morton MJ, Berquist TH, McLeod RA, et al. MR imaging of synovial sarcoma. *AJR Am J Roentgenol* 1990;156:337–340.

278. Jones BC, Sundaram M, Kransdorf MJ. Synovial sarcoma: imaging findings in 34 patients. *AJR Am J Roentgenol* 1993;161:827–830.

279. Nakanishi H, Araki N, Sawai Y, et al. Cystic synovial sarcomas: imaging features with clinical and histopathologic correlation. *Skeletal Radiol* 2003;32:701–707.

280. Ackerman LV. Extra-osseous localized non-neoplastic bone and cartilage formation (so-called myositis ossificans). *J Bone Joint Surg Am* 1958;40A:279–298.

281. Heinrich SD, Zembo MM, MacEwen GD. Pseudomalignant myositis ossificans. *Orthopedics* 1989;12:599–602.

282. Hudson TM. Fluid levels in aneurysmal bone cysts: a CT feature. *AJR Am J Roentgenol* 1984;141:1001–1004.

283. Ogilvie-Harris DJ, Fornasier VL. Pseudomalignant myositis ossificans: heterotopic new-bone formation without a history of trauma. *J Bone Joint Surg Am* 1980;62A:1274–1283.

284. Nuovo MA, Norman A, Chumas J, et al. Myositis ossificans with atypical clinical, radiographic, or pathologic findings: a review of 23 cases. *Skeletal Radiol* 1992;21:87–101.

285. Kransdorf MJ, Meis JM, Jelinek JS. Myositis ossificans: MR appearance with radiologic-pathologic correlation. *AJR Am J Roentgenol* 1991;157:1243–1248.

286. Jaffe HL. Aneurysmal bone cyst. *Bull Hosp Joint Dis* 1950;11:3–13.

287. Norman A, Dorfman HP. Juxtacortical circumscribed myositis ossificans: evolution and radiographic features. *Radiology* 1979;96:301–306.

288. De Smet AA, Norris MA, Fisher DR. Magnetic resonance imaging of myositis ossificans: analysis of seven cases. *Skeletal Radiol* 1992;21:503–507.

289. Goldman AB. Myositis ossificans circumscripta: a benign lesion with a malignant differential diagnosis. *AJR Am J Roentgenol* 1976;126:32–40.

290. Tsai JC, Dalinka MK, Fallon MD, et al. Fluid–fluid level: a nonspecific finding in tumors of bone and soft tissue. *Radiology* 1990;175:779–782.

291. Pettersson H, Eliasson J, Egund N, et al. Gadolinium-DTPA enhancement of soft tissue tumors in magnetic resonance imaging-preliminary clinical experience in five patients. *Skeletal Radiol* 1988;17:319–323.

292. Bush CH. The magnetic resonance imaging of musculoskeletal hemorrhage. *Skeletal Radiol* 2000;29:1–9.

293. Rubin JI, Gomori JM, Grossman RI, et al. High-field MR imaging of extracranial hematomas. *AJR Am J Roentgenol* 1987;148:813–817.

294. Unger EC, Glazer HS, Lee JKT, et al. MRI of extracranial hematomas: preliminary observations. *AJR Am J Roentgenol* 1986;146:403–407.

295. Aoki J, Nakata H, Watanabe H, et al. The radiological findings in chronic expanding hematoma. *Skeletal Radiol* 1999;28:396–401.

296. Reed JD, Kommareddi S, Lankerani M, et al. Chronic expanding hematomas: a clinicopathologic entity. *JAMA* 1980;244:2441–2442.

297. Dooms GC, Fisher MR, Hricak H, et al. MR imaging of intramuscular hemorrhage. *J Comput Assist Tomogr* 1985;9:908–913.

298. Cohen JM, Weinreb JC, Redman HC. Arteriovenous malformations of the extremities: MR imaging. *Radiology* 1986;158:475–479.

299. Edelmam RR, Mattle HP, Atkinson DJ, et al. MR angiography. *AJR Am J Roentgenol* 1990;154:937–946.

300. Mitchell DG, Carabasi A. Vascular applications of magnetic resonance imaging. *Magn Reson Imaging* 1989;3:400–419.

301. Feldman F, Singson RD, Staron RB. Magnetic resonance imaging of para-articular and ectopic ganglia. *Skeletal Radiol* 1989;18:353–358.

302. Hippocrates. *On joints*. Translated by Withington ET. London: W Heinemann, 1927:200–397.

303. Healey JH, Ghelman B. Osteoid osteoma and osteoblastoma. Current concepts and recent advances. *Clin Orthop* 1986;204:76–85.

304. Kirby EJ, Shereff MJ, Lewis MM. Soft tissue tumors and tumor-like lesions of the foot. *J Bone Joint Surg Am* 1989;71A:621–626.

305. Genovese GR, Joyson MIV, Dixon ASJ. Protective value of synovial cysts in rheumatoid arthritis. *Ann Rheum Dis* 1972;31:179–182.

306. Haller J, Resnick D, Greenway G, et al. Juxtaacetabular ganglionic (or synovial) cysts: CT and MR features. *J Comput Assist Tomogr* 1989;13:976–983.

307. Abdelwahab IF, Kenan S, Hermann G, et al. Periosteal ganglia: CT and MR imaging features. *Radiology* 1993;188:245–248.

308. Conrad EU, Enneking WF. Common soft tissue tumors. *Clin Symp* 1990;42:1–21.

309. Fritz RC, Helms CA, Steinbach LS, et al. Suprascapular nerve entrapment: evaluation with MR imaging. *Radiology* 1992;182:437–444.

310. Ogino T, Minami A, Kato H. Diagnosis of radial nerve palsy caused by ganglion with use of different imaging techniques. *J Hand Surg Am* 1991;16A:230–235.

311. Burk DL, Dalinka MK, Kanal E, et al. Meniscal and ganglion cysts of the knee: MR evaluation. *AJR Am J Roentgenol* 1988;150:331–336.

312. Tom BM, Rao VM, Farole A. Bilateral temporomandibular joint ganglion cysts: CT and MR characteristics. *AJNR Am J Neuroradiol* 1990;11:746–748.

313. Johnson J, Kilgore E, Newmeyer W. Tumorous lesions of the hand. *J Hand Surg Am* 1985;10:284–286.

314. Enzinger FM. Intramuscular myxoma. A review and follow-up study of 34 cases. *Am J Pathol* 1965;43:104–113.

315. Greenfield GB, Arrington JA, Kudryk BT. MRI of soft tissue tumors. *Skeletal Radiol* 1993;22:77–84.

316. Ireland DCR, Soule EH, Ivins JC. Myxoma of somatic soft tissue. A report of 58 patients, 3 with multiple tumors and fibrous dysplasia of bone. *Mayo Clin Proc* 1973;48:401–410.

317. Sundaram M, McDonald DJ, Merenda G. Intramuscular myxoma: a rare but important association with fibrous dysplasia of bone. *AJR Am J Roentgenol* 1989;153:107–108.

318. Gober GA, Nicholas RW. Case report 800. Skeletal fibrous dysplasia associated with intramuscular myxoma (Mazabraud's syndrome). *Skeletal Radiol* 1993;22:452–455.

319. Bancroft LW, Kransdorf MJ, Menke DM, et al. Intramuscular myxoma: characteristic MR imaging features. *AJR Am J Roentgenol* 2002;178:1255–1259.

320. Murphey MD, McRae GA, Fanburg-Smith JC, et al. Imaging of soft-tissue myxoma with emphasis on CT and MR and comparison of radiologic and pathologic findings. *Radiology* 2002;225:215–224.

321. Meis JM, Enzinger FM. Juxta-articular myxoma: a clinical and pathologic study of 65 cases. *Hum Pathol* 1992;23:639–646.

322. Moulopoulos LA, Granfield CAJ, Dimopoulos MA, et al. Extraosseous multiple myeloma: imaging features. *AJR Am J Roentgenol* 1993;161:1083–1087.

323. Wirth WA, Leavitt D, Enzinger FM. Multiple intramuscular myxoms: another extraskeletal manifestation of fibrous dysplasia. *Cancer* 1971;27:321–340.

324. Kransdorf MJ. Malignant soft tissue tumors in a large referral population: distribution of diagnoses by age, sex and location. *AJR Am J Roentgenol* 1995;164:129–134.

325. Aoki J, Watanabe H, Shinozaki T, et al. FDG-PET for preoperative differential diagnosis between benign and malignant soft tissue masses. *Skeletal Radiol* 2003;32:133–138.

326. Myhre-Jensen O. A consecutive 7-year series of 1457 benign soft tissue tumors. *Acta Orthop Scand* 1981;52:587–593.

327. Rydholm A. Management of patients with soft tissue tumors. Strategy developed at a regional oncology center. *Acta Orthop* 1983;54(Suppl. 203):1–77.

328. Peabody TD, Simon MA. Principles of staging of soft tissue sarcomas. *Clin Orthop* 1993;289:19–31.

329. Hanna SL, Fletcher BD, Parham DM, et al. Muscle edema in musculoskeletal tumors: MR imaging characteristics and clinical significance. *J Magn Reson Imaging* 1991;1:441–449.

330. Beltran J, Chandnani V, McGhee RA, et al. Gadopentetate dimeglumine-enhanced MR imaging of the musculoskeletal system. *AJR Am J Roentgenol* 1991;156:457–466.

331. Tardy B, Guy C, Barral G, et al. Anaphylactic shock induced by intravenous gadopentetate dimeglumine. *Lancet* 1992;339:494.

332. Verstraete KL, De Deene Y, Roels H, et al. Benign and malignant musculoskeletal lesions: dynamic contrast-enhanced MR

imaging-parametric "first pass" images depict tissue vascularization and perfusion. *Radiology* 1994;192:835–843.

333. Omohundro JE, Elderbrook MK, Ringer TV. Laryngospasm after administration of gadopentetate dimeglumine. *J Magn Reson Imaging* 1992;2:729–730.

334. Shellock FG, Hahn HP, Mink JH, et al. Adverse reaction to intravenous gadoteridol. *Radiology* 1993;189:151–152.

335. Takebayashi S, Sugiyama M, Nagase M, et al. Severe adverse reaction to IV gadopentetate dimeglumine. *AJR Am J Roentgenol* 1993;160:659.

336. Tisher S, Hoffman JC. Anaphylactoid reaction to IV gadopentetate dimeglumine. *AJNR Am J Neuroradiol* 1990;174:17–23.

337. Jordan RM, Mintz RD. Fatal reaction to gadopentetate dimeglumine. *AJR Am J Roentgenol* 1995;164:743–744.

338. Henry A. Monostotic fibrous dysplasia. *J Bone Joint Surg Br* 1969;51B:300–306.

339. Seeger LL, Widoff BE, Bassett LW, et al. Preoperative evaluation of osteosarcoma: value of gadopentetate dimeglumine-enhanced MR imaging. *AJR Am J Roentgenol* 1991;157:347–351.

340. Fletcher BD. Response of osteosarcoma and Ewing sarcoma to chemotherapy: imaging evaluation. *AJR Am J Roentgenol* 1991;157:825–833.

341. Choi H, Varma DGK, Fornage BD, et al. Soft tissue sarcoma: MR imaging vs sonography for the detection of local recurrence after surgery. *AJR Am J Roentgenol* 1991;157:353–358.

342. Madewell JE, Ragsdale BD, Sweet DE. Analysis of solitary bone lesions. Part I. Internal margins. *Radiol Clin North Am* 1981;19:715–748.

343. Moser RP, Madewell JE. An approach to primary bone tumors. *Radiol Clin North Am* 1987;25:1049–1093.

344. Ragsdale BD, Madewell JE, Sweet DE. Analysis of solitary bone lesions. Part II. Periosteal reactions. *Radiol Clin North Am* 1981;19:749–783.

345. Sweet DE, Madewell JE, Ragsdale BD. Analysis of solitary bone lesions. Part III. Matrix patterns. *Radiol Clin North Am* 1981;19:785–814.

346. Bloem JL, Bluemm RG, Taminiau AHM, et al. Magnetic resonance imaging of primary malignant bone tumors. *Radiographics* 1987;7:425–445.

347. Hudson TH, Moser RP Jr, Gilkey FW, et al. Chondrosarcoma. In: Moser RP Jr, ed. *Cartilaginous tumors of the skeleton*. Philadelphia, PA: Hanley & Belfus, 1990:155–205.

348. Wetzel LH, Levine E, Murphey MD. A comparison of MR imaging and CT in the evaluation of musculoskeletal masses. *Radiographics* 1987;7:851–874.

349. Zimmer WD, Berquist TH, McLeod RA. Bone tumors: magnetic resonance imaging versus computed tomography. *Radiology* 1985;155:709–718.

350. Jaffe HL, Lichtenstein L. Benign chondroblastoma of bone. A reinterpretation of the so-called calcifying of chondromatous giant cell tumor. *Am J Pathol* 1942;18:969–992.

351. Brower AC, Moser RP, Gilkey FW, et al. Chondroblastoma. In: Moser RP, ed. *Cartilaginous tumors of the skeleton*. Philadelphia, PA: Hanley & Belfus, 1990:74–113.

352. Weatherall PT, Maale GE, Mendelsohn DB, et al. Chondro-blastoma: classic and confusing appearance at MR. *Radiology* 1994;190:467–474.

353. Brower AC, Moser RP, Kransdorf MJ. The frequency and diagnostic significance of periostitis in chondroblastoma. *AJR Am J Roentgenol* 1990;154:309–314.

354. Milgram JW. The origins of osteochondromas and enchondromas. A histopathologic study. *Clin Orthop* 1983;174:264–284.

355. Unni KK. *Dahlin's bone tumors. General aspects and data on 11,087 cases*, 5th ed. Philadelphia, PA: Lippincott–Raven, 1996:11–24, 121–130, 355–432.

356. Cohen EK, Kressel HY, Frank TS, et al. Hyaline cartilage-origin bone and soft tissue neoplasms: MR appearance and histologic correlation. *Radiology* 1988;167:477–481.

357. Aoki J, Sone S, Fujioka F, et al. MR of enchondroma and chondrosarcoma: rings and arcs of Gd-DTPA enhancement. *J Comput Assist Tomogr* 1991;15:1011–1016.

358. Murphey MD, Flemming DJ, Boyea SR, et al. Enchondroma versus chondrosarcoma in the appendicular skeleton: differentiating features. *Radiographics* 1998;18:1213–1237.

359. Brien EW, Mirra JM, Luck JV. Benign and malignant cartilage tumors af bone and joint: their anatomic and theoretical basis with an emphasis on radiolgy, pathology and clinical biology. II. Juxtacortical cartilage tumors. *Skeletal Radiol* 1999;28:1–20.

360. Robinson P, White LM, Sundaram M, et al. Periosteal chondroid tumors: radiologic evaluation with pathologic correlation. *AJR Am J Roentgenol* 2001;177:1183–1188.

361. Nojima T, Unni KK, McLeod RA, et al. Periosteal chondroma and periosteal chondrosarcoma. *Am J Surg Pathol* 1985;9:666–677.

362. Vanal D, De Paolis M, Monti C, et al. Radiological features of 24 periosteal chondrosarcomas. *Skeletal Radiol* 2001;30:208–212.

363. Ishida T, Iijima T, Goto T, et al. Concurrent enchondroma and periosteal chondroma of the humerus mimicking chondrosarcoma. *Skeletal Radiol* 1998;27:337–340.

364. D'Ambrosia R, Ferguson AB. The formation of osteochondroma by epiphyseal cartilage transplantation. *Clin Orthop* 1968;61:103–115.

365. Libshitz HI, Cohen MA. Radiation-induced osteochondromas. *Radiology* 1982;142:643–647.

366. Griffiths HJ, Thompson RC, Galloway HR, et al. Bursitis in association with solitary osteochondromas presenting as mass lesions. *Skeletal Radiol* 1991;20:513–516.

367. Lee JK, Yao L, Wirth CR. MR imaging of solitary osteochondromas: report of eight cases. *AJR Am J Roentgenol* 1987;149:557–560.

368. Hudson TM, Springfield DS, Spanier SS, et al. Benign exostoses and exostotic chondrosarcomas: evaluation of cartilage thickness by CT. *Radiology* 1984;151:595–599.

369. Malghem J, Vande Berg B, Noel H, et al. Benign osteochondromas and exostotic chondrosarcomas: evaluation of cartilage cap thickness by ultrasound. *Skeletal Radiol* 1992;21:33–37.

370. Geirnaerdt MJA, Bloem JL, Eulderink F, et al. Cartilaginous tumors: correlation of gadolinium-enhanced MR imaging and histologic findings. *Radiology* 1993;186:813–817.

371. Crim JR, Seeger LL. Diagnosis of low-grade chondrosarcoma. *Radiology* 1993;189:503–504.

372. Murphey MD, Walker EA, Wilson AJ, et al. From the archives of the AFIP: imaging of primary chondrosarcoma: radiologic-pathologic correlation. *Radiographics* 2003;23:1245–1278.

373. Lichtenstein L, Jaffe GL. Chondrosarcoma of the bone. *Am J Pathol* 1943;10:553–589.

374. Brien EW, Mirra JM, Kerr R. Benign and malignant cartilage tumors of bone and joint: their anatomic and theoretical basis with an emphasis on radiology, pathology, and clinical biology. I. The intramedullary cartilage rumors. *Skeletal Radiol* 1997;26:325–353.

375. De Beuckeleer LHL, De Schepper AMA, Ramon F. Magnetic resonance imaging in cartilaginous tumors: is it useful or necessary? *Skeletal Radiol* 1995;25:137–141.

376. Caffey J. On fibrous defects in cortical walls of growing tubular bones. *Adv Pediatr* 1955;7:13–51.

377. Kransdorf MJ, Utz JA, Gilkey FW, et al. MR appearance of fibroxanthoma. *J Comput Assist Tomogr* 1989;12:612–615.

378. Wilner D. *Radiology of bone tumors and allied disorders*. Philadelphia, PA: WB Saunders, 1982:551–611.

379. Jee W, Choe B, Kang H, et al. Nonossifying fibroma: characteristics at MR imaging with pathologic correlation. *Radiology* 1998;209:197–202.

380. Mirra JM, Gold RH. Fibrous dysplasia. In: Mirra JM, Piero P, Gold RH, eds. *Bone tumors*, Philadelphia, PA: Lea & Febiger, 1989:191–226.

381. Harms SE. Musculoskeletal system. In: Stark DD, Bradley EG, eds. *Magnetic resonance imaging*, 3rd ed. St. Louis, MO: CV Mosby, 1999:931–976.

382. Jee W, Choi K, Choe B, et al. Fibrous dysplasia: MR imaging characteristics with radiopathologic correlation. *AJR Am J Roentgenol* 1996;167:1523–1527.

383. Utz JA, Kransdorf MJ, Jelinek JS, et al. MR appearance of fibrous dysplasia. *J Comput Assist Tomogr* 1989;13:845–851.

384. Jaffe HL. Osteoid-osteoma. A benign osteoblastic tumor composed of osteoid and atypical bone. *Arch Surg* 1935;31:709–728.

385. Milch H. Osteoid-tissue-forming tumor simulating annular sequestrum. *J Bone Joint Surg* 1934;16:681–688.

386. Sabanas AO, Bickel WH, Moe JH. Natural history of osteoid osteoma of the spine. Review of the literature and report of three cases. *Am J Surg* 1956;91:880–889.

387. Shmookler BM, Enzinger FM, Brannon RB. Orofacial synovial sarcoma: a clinicopathologic study of 11 new cases and review of the literature. *Cancer* 1982;50:269–276.

388. Reicher MA, Hartzman S, Bassett LW, et al. MR imaging of the knee. Part I. Traumatic disorders. *Radiology* 1987;162:547–551.

389. Resnick D, Kyriakos M, Greenway GD. Tumor and tumor-like lesions of bone: imaging of specific lesions. In: Resnick D, ed. *Diagnosis of bone and joint disorders*, 3rd ed. Philadelphia, PA: WB Saunders, 1995:3628–3938.

390. Mirra JM. *Bone tumors. Clinical, radiologic and pathologic correlations.* Philadelphia, PA: Lea & Febiger, 1989:1233–1334.

391. Jackson RP, Reckling FW, Mantz FA. Osteoid osteoma and osteoblastoma. Similar histologic lesions with different natural histories. *Clin Orthop* 1977;128:303–313.

392. Pettine KA, Klassen RA. Osteoid-osteoma and osteoblastoma of the spine. *J Bone Joint Surg Am* 1986;68A:354–361.

393. Swee RG, McLeod RA, Beabout JW. Osteoid osteoma. Detection, diagnosis and localization. *Radiology* 1979;130:117–123.

394. Kattapuram SV, Kushner DC, Phillips WC, et al. Osteoid osteoma: an unusual cause of articular pain. *Radiology* 1983;147:383–387.

395. Sherman MS. Osteoid osteoma. Review of the literature and report of thirty cases. *J Bone Joint Surg* 1947;29:918–930.

396. Sim FH, Dahlin DC, Beabout JW. Osteoid-osteoma: diagnostic problems. *J Bone Joint Surg Am* 1975;57:154–159.

397. Capusten BM, Azouz EM, Rosman MA. Fibromatosis of bone in children. *Radiology* 1984;152:693–694.

398. Biebuyck FC, Katz LD, McCauley T. Soft tissue edema in osteoid osteoma. *Skeletal Radiol* 1993;22:37–41.

399. Edeiken J, DePalma AF, Hodes PJ. Osteoid osteoma (roentgenographic emphasis). *Clin Orthop* 1966;49:201–206.

400. Capanna R, Van Horn JR, Ayala A, et al. Osteoid osteoma and osteoblastoma of the talus. A report of 40 cases. *Skeletal Radiol* 1986;15:360–364.

401. Assorin J, Richardi G, Railhac JJ, et al. Osteoid osteoma: MR imaging versus CT. *Radiology* 1994;191:217–233.

402. Yeager BA, Schiebler ML, Wertheim SB, et al. Case report. MR imaging of osteoid osteoma of the talus. *J Comput Assist Tomogr* 1987;11:916–917.

403. Woods ER, Martel W, Mandell SH, et al. Reactive soft tissue mass associated with oseoid osteoma: correlation of MR imaging features with pathologic findings. *Radiology* 1993;186:221–225.

404. Ehara S, Rosenthal DI, Aoki J, et al. Peritumoral edema in osteoid osteoma on magnetic resonance imaging. *Skeletal Radiol* 1996;28:265–270.

405. Houang B, Grenier N, Gréselle JF, et al. Osteoid osteoma of the cervical spine. Misleading MR features about a case involving the uncinate process. *Neuroradiology* 1990;31:549–551.

406. Crim JR, Mirra JM, Eckardt JJ, et al. Widespread inflammatory response to osteoblastoma: the flare phenomenon. *Radiology* 1990;177:835–836.

407. Davies M, Cassar-Pullicino VN, Davies AM, et al. The diagnostic accuracy of MR imaging in osteoid osteoma. *Skeletal Radiol* 2002;31:559–569.

408. Liu PT, Chivers FS, Roberts CC, et al. Imaging of osteoid osteoma with dynamic gadolinium-enhanced imaging. *Radiology* 2003;227:691–700.

409. Ramos A, Castello J, Sartoris DJ, et al. Osseous lipoma: CT appearance. *AJR Am J Roentgenol* 1985;157:615–619.

410. Manaster BJ, Doyle AJ. Giant cell tumors of bone. *Radiol Clin North Am* 1993;21:299–323.

411. Levine E, DeSmet AA, Neff JR. Role of radiologic imaging in management planning of giant cell tumor of bone. *Skeletal Radiol* 1984;12:79–89.

412. Aoki J, Tanikawa H, Ishii K, et al. MR findings indicative of hemosiderin in giant-cell tumor of bone: frequency, cause and diagnostic significance. *AJR Am J Roentgenol* 1996;166:145–148.

413. Herman SD, Mesgarzadeh M, Bonakdarpour A, et al. The role of magnetic resonance imaging in giant cell tumor of bone. *Skeletal Radiol* 1987;16:635–643.

414. Sweet DE, Madewell JE. Pathogenesis of osteonecrosis. In: Resnick D, Niwayama G, eds. *Diagnosis of bone and joint disorders*, Philadelphia, PA: WB Saunders, 1988:3188–3237.

415. Rao VM, Fishman M, Mitchell DG, et al. Painful sickle cell crisis: bone marrow patterns observed with MR imaging. *Radiology* 1986;161:211–215.

416. Munk PL, Helms CA, Holt RG. Immature bone infarcts: findings on plain radiographs and MR scans. *AJR Am J Roentgenol* 1989;152:547–549.

417. Jaffe HL, Lichtenstein L. Solitary unicameral bone cyst with emphasis on the roentgen picture, the pathologic appearance, and the pathogenesis. *Arch Surg* 1942;44:1004–1025.

418. Lichtenstein L. Aneurysmal bone cyst. A pathological entity commonly mistaken for giant cell tumor and occasionally for hemangioma and osteogenic sarcoma. *Cancer* 1950;3:279–289.

419. Lichtenstein L. Aneurysmal bone cyst. Further observations. *Cancer* 1953;6:1228–1237.

420. Lichtenstein L. Aneurysmal bone cyst. Observations on fifty cases. *J Bone Joint Surg Am* 1957;39A:873–882.

421. Biesecker JL, Marcove RC, Huvos AG, et al. Aneurysmal bone cyst. A clinicopathologic study of 66 cases. *Cancer* 1970;26:615–625.

422. Bonakdarpour A, Levy WM, Aegerter E. Primary and secondary aneurysmal bone cyst: a radiological study of 75 cases. *Radiology* 1978;126:75–83.

423. Levy WM, Miller AS, Bonakdarpour A, et al. Aneurysmal bone cyst secondary to other lesions. Report of 57 cases. *Am J Clin Pathol* 1975;63:1–8.

424. Martinez V, Sissons HA. Aneurysmal bone cyst. A review of 132 cases including primary lesions and those secondary to other bone pathology. *Cancer* 1988;61:2291–2304.

425. Dagher AP, Magid D, Johnson CA, et al. Aneurysmal bone cyst developing after anterior cruciate ligament tear and repair. *AJR Am J Roentgenol* 1992;158:1289–1291.

426. Mintz MC, Dalinka MK, Schmidt R. Aneurysmal bone cyst arising in fibrous dysplasia during pregnancy. *Radiology* 1987;165:549–550.

427. Ruiter DJ, Van Rijssel TG, Van der Velde EA. Aneurysmal bone cysts. A clinicopathological study of 105 cases. *Cancer* 1977;39:2231–2239.

428. Vergel De Dios AM, Bond JR, Shives TC, et al. Aneurysmal bone cyst. A clinicopathologic study of 252 cases. *Cancer* 1992;69:2921–2931.

429. Capanna R, Springfield DS, Biagini R, et al. Juxtaepiphyseal aneurysmal bone cyst. *Skeletal Radiol* 1985;13:21–25.

430. Gold RH, Mirra JM. Case report 248. Aneurysmal bone cyst (ABC) of left scapula with intramural calcified chondroid. *Skeletal Radiol* 1983;10:57–60.

431. Cory DA, Fritsch SA, Cohen MD, et al. Aneurysmal bone cysts: imaging findings and embolotherapy. *AJR Am J Roentgenol* 1991;153:369–373.

432. Beltran J, Simon DC, Levey ML, et al. Aneurysmal bone cyst: MR imaging at 1.5 T. *Radiology* 1986;158:689–690.

433. Munk PL, Helms CA, Holt RG, et al. MR imaging of aneurysmal bone cysts. *AJR Am J Roentgenol* 1989;153:99–101.

434. Pierre Revel M, Vanel D, Sigal R, et al. Aneurysmal bone cysts of the jaws: CT and MR findings. *J Comput Assist Tomogr* 1992;16:84–86.

435. O'Donnell P, Saifuddin A. The prevalence and diagnositic significance of fluid–fluid levels in focal lesions of bone. *Skeletal Radiol* 2004;33:330–336.

436. Murphey MD, wan Jaovisidha S, Temple HT, et al. Telangiectatic osteosarcoma: radiologic-pathologic camparison. *Radiology* 2003;229:545–553.

437. Murphey MD, Robin MR, McRae GA, et al. The many faces of osteosarcima. *Radiographics* 1997;17:1205–1231.

438. Sanerkin NG, Mott MG, Roylance J. An unusual intraosseous lesion with fibroblastic, osteoblastic, aneurysmal and fibromyxoid elements. "Solid" variant of aneurysmal bone cyst. *Cancer* 1983;51:2278–2288.

439. Bertoni F, Bacchini R, Capanna R, et al. Solid variant of aneurysmal bone cyst. *Cancer* 1993;71:729–734.

440. Ilaslan H, Sundaram M, Unni KK. Solid variant of aneurysmal bone cysts in long tubular bones: giant cell reparative granuloma. *AJR Am J Roentgenol* 2003;180:1681–1687.

441. Oda Y, Tsuneyoshi M, Shinohara N. "Solid" variant of aneurysmal bone cyst (extragnathic giant cell reparative granuloma) in the axial skeleton and long bones: a study of its morphologic spectrum and distinction from allied giant cell tumors. *Cancer* 1992;70:2641–2649.

442. Conway WF, Hayes CW. Miscellaneous lesions of bone. *Radiol Clin North Am* 1993;31:299–323.

443. Killeen KL. The fallen fragment sign. *Radiology* 1998;207:261–262.
444. Struhk A, Edelson C, Pritzker H, et al. Solitary (unicameral) bone cysts: the fallen fragment sign revisited. *Skeletal Radiol* 1989;18:261–265.
445. Jelinek JS, Redmind J, Perry JJ, et al. Small cell cancer: staging with MR imaging. *Radiology* 1990;177:837–842.
446. Daffner RH, Lupetin AP, Dash N, et al. MRI in the detection of malignant infiltration of bone marrow. *AJR Am J Roentgenol* 1986;146:353–358.
447. Libshitz HI, Malthouse SR, Cunningham D, et al. Multiple myeloma: appearance at MR imaging. *Radiology* 1992;182:833–837.
448. Yuh WTC, Zachar CK, Barloon TJ, et al. Vertebral compression fractures: distinction between benign and malignant causes with MR imaging. *Radiology* 1989;172:215–218.
449. Baker LL, Goodman SB, Perkash I, et al. Benign versus pathologic compression fractures of vertebral bodies: assessment with conventional spin echo, chemical-shift, and STIR MR imaging. *Radiology* 1990;174:495–502.
450. Resnick D. Plasma cell dyscrasias and dysgammaglobulinemias. In: Resnick D, ed. *Diagnosis of bone and joint disorders*, 3rd ed. Philadelphia, PA: WB Saunders, 1995:2147–2189.
451. Lecouvet FE, Vande Berg BC, Michaux L, et al. Stage III multiple myeloma: clinical and prognostic value of spinal bone marrow MR imaging. *Radiology* 1998;209:653–660.
452. Moulopoulos LA, Varma DG, Dimopoulos MA, et al. Multiple myeloma: spinal MR imaging in patients with untreated newly diagnosed disease. *Radiology* 1992;185:833–840.
453. Hayes CW, Conway WF, Sundaram M. Misleading aggressive MR imaging appearance of some benign musculoskeletal lesions. *Radiographics* 1992;12:1119–1134.
454. Genant HK, Helms CA. Computed tomography of the appendicular musculoskeletal system. In: Moss AA, Gamsu G, Genant HK, eds. *Computed tomography of the body*. Philadelphia, PA: WB Saunders, 1983:475–534.
455. Holscher HC, Bloem JL, Nooy MA, et al. The value of MR imaging in monitoring the effect of chemotherapy on bone sarcomas. *AJR Am J Roentgenol* 1990;154:763–769.
456. Holscher HC, Bloem JL, Vanel D, et al. Osteosarcoma: chemotherapy-induced changes at MR imaging. *Radiology* 1992;182:839–844.
457. Lawrence JA, Babyn PS, Chan HSL, et al. Extremity osteosarcoma in childhood: prognostic value of radiologic imaging. *Radiology* 1993;189:43–47.
458. De Baere T, Vanel D, Shapeero LG, et al. Osteosarcoma after chemotherapy: evaluation with contrast material-enhanced subtraction imaging. *Radiology* 1992;185:587–592.
459. Fletcher BD, Hanna SL, Fairclough DL, et al. Pediatric musculoskeletal tumors: use of dynamic, contrast-enhanced MR imaging to monitor response to chemotherapy. *Radiology* 1992;184:243–248.
460. Malawer MM, Dunham WK. Skip metastases in osteosarcoma: recent experience. *J Surg Oncol* 1983;22:236–245.
461. Wuisman P, Enneking WF. Prognosis for patients who have osteosarcoma with skip metastasis. *J Bone Joint Surg Am* 1990;72A:60–68.

Musculoskeletal Infection

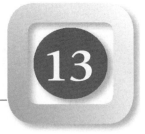

13

Thomas H. Berquist   Daniel F. Broderick

Musculoskeletal infections may present with an acute, rapidly progressing course or in a more insidious fashion. The latter often follow trauma or surgery, such as after placement of orthopedic appliances. Presentation is also highly dependent upon age, virulence of the organism, patient condition, site of involvement, and circulation (1–3). Early treatment, particularly in children with articular infections, is essential to prevent growth defects, joint ankylosis, or other complications (3–6).

Infections may involve osseous, articular, and soft tissues, either isolated or as multisite involvement. Terminology used for different categories of infection is important when considering imaging approaches and treatment (Table 13-1). Osseous infection may involve marrow, cortex, or periosteum. Multiple osseous structures are commonly involved (6–11). Similarly, it is not uncommon for soft tissue, osseous, and articular structures to be simultaneously involved (Table 13-1).

MECHANISMS OF INFECTION

Musculoskeletal tissue may become infected by hematogenous spread, spread from a continuous source, by direct implantation (i.e., skin puncture wound), or following surgery or trauma (6,7,10–12).

Hematogenous spread is common in osteomyelitis and joint space infections. In children, osteomyelitis is almost always hematogenous. The source is commonly the throat, middle ear, or indwelling catheters in infants. Infections typically occur in the metaphysis of long bones or near the physis in flat bones such as the ilium (7,10,12). Involvement of the joint space depends upon capsular attachment in relation to the physis and patient age. In neonates or infants (up to age 2) and adults, the growth plate does not protect the epiphysis. Vascular channels cross the growth plate, allowing metaphyseal and epiphyseal involvement that increases the incidence of associated joint space infection (5,7,10,15). In patients ages 1 or 2 and up to 16 years of age, the growth plate prevents spread to the epiphysis. Therefore, joint space involvement is less common unless the metaphysis is intracapsular (see Fig. 13-1) (7,12,16).

Spread from a contiguous source may result in osseous infection extending into the joint or soft tissues, or vice-versa (16). In soft tissue infection, spread may be

TABLE 13-1

INFECTIONS: TERMINOLOGY AND CATEGORIES

Term/Conditions	Clinical/Image Features
Osteomyelitis	Infections of bone and bone marrow. Bacterial most common
Infective osteitis	Cortical infection. Often associated with marrow or soft tissue infection
Infective periostitis	Periosteal infection. Frequently, cortex and marrow also involved
Soft tissue infection	Involves shin, subcutaneous tissues, muscles, tendons, ligaments, fascia,or bursae
Sequestrum	Segment of necrotic bone separated from viable bone by granulation tissue
Involucrum	Living bone surrounding necrotic bone
Cloaca	Tract through viable bone
Sinus	Tract from infected region to skin
Fistula	Abnormal communication between two internal organs or internal organ and skin
Brodie abscess	Sharply delineated focus of osteomyelitis
Garre sclerosing osteomyelitis	Sclerotic nonpurulent infection with intense periosteal reaction
Chronic recurrent multifocal osteomyelitis (CRMO)	Subacute or chronic osseous infection common in children. May be associated with SAPHO
Synovitis, acne pustulosis, hyperostosis, and osteitis (SAPHO)	Palmoplantar pustulosis, articular and periosteal inflammation. Chronic course involving chest wall, spine, long and flatbones, large and small joints

From references 1,11–14.

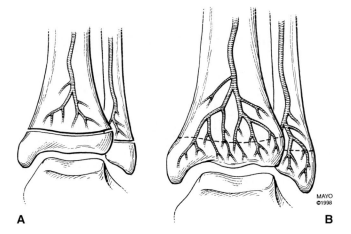

Figure 13-1 Illustrations of vascular patterns at the metaphyseal–epiphyseal junction in a child **(A)** and adult **(B)**. The physis is protected by the growth plate in patients 1 to 16 years of age. (From Berquist TH. *Radiology of the foot and ankle*. Philadelphia, PA: Lippincott Williams & Wilkins, 2000.)

along tendon sheaths or in soft tissue compartments. Spread along the tendon sheaths in the upper extremity may result in involvement of the forearm to hand and wrist (6,17). Osseous involvement in the foot (see Chapter 8) is most commonly due to spread from a contiguous source (18,19). Most patients develop soft tissue infection due to diabetes, skin ulceration, or puncture wounds (20–23). Lederman et al. (21) reported contiguous spread to osseous structures in the forefoot in 16% of 161 feet imaged by magnetic resonance imaging (MRI). Joint space infection occurred in 33%. The first and fifth digits and metatarsals were most commonly involved (21).

Direct implantation is usually related to a puncture wound, bite, or scratch (see Fig. 13-2) (6,7,12). Puncture wounds in the foot occur with stepping on sharp objects, usually when barefoot. Puncture wounds in the hand (i.e., thorns) occur when working with plants or gardening. Direct implantation may also occur when working in contaminated water or soil in the presence of skin abrasions (17,24–26).

Infection may also result from surgical or other minimally invasive procedures such as diagnostic injections (2,6,15,27–29). Symptoms are often insidious, resulting in delayed diagnosis. Imaging evaluation may also be more complicated when anatomy is distorted (trauma) or orthopedic implants are in place.

Organisms

Most musculoskeletal infections are bacterial (Table 13-2). Staphylococcal infections account for 80% to 90% of cases of osteomyelitis (6). In newborns and infants, Group B streptococcal infections are common (4,6,8,30,31). Other organisms, such as pseudomonas, have been associated with puncture wounds to the foot (4,7,8,16). Salmonella infections have been associated with sickle cell disease, hemoglobinopathies, systemic lupus erythematosus, leukemia, and lymphoma (31). *Haemophilus* influenza is most common in children 7 months to 4 years of age and in adults with diabetes or immunodeficiency.

Brucella, cryptococcus, coccidiomycosis, histoplasmosis, and echinococcosis tend to be endemic in certain regions of the United States and the world. However, infections have become less geographic due to immigration and world travel (4,32–35).

Typical (*Mycobacterium tuberculosis*) and atypical (*M. marinum, M. avium, M. fortuitum, M. chelonaes*, etc.) mycobacterial (tuberculosis) infections have become more common over the past decade due to immigration, human immunodeficiency virus (HIV), alcohol and drug abuse, and the aging population (17,23,25,26,36–38). Musculoskeletal tuberculosis is evident in 19% to 20% of infections with extrapulmonary pulmonary involvement (38). Atypical mycobacterial infections involve the musculoskeletal system in 5% to 10% of patients (25,26). Infections may be hematogenous or from dealing with

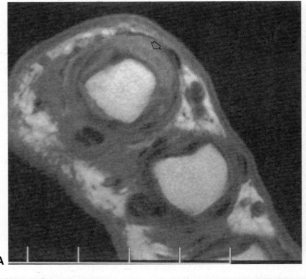

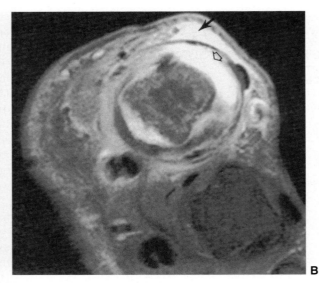

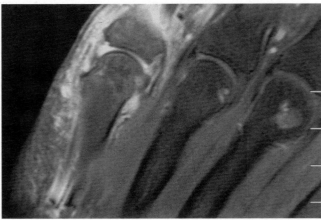

Figure 13-2 Fish hook injury with soft tissue infection extending into the 5th metacarpophalangeal joint. Axial T1- **(A)** and T2- **(B)** weighted images demonstrate soft tissue edema (*arrow,* **B**) and joint distention (*open arrow*). Fat-suppressed contrast-enhanced coronal T1-weighted image **(C)** shows enhancement of the soft tissues and synovial fluid.

animals or contaminated water or soil (26,39) (Table 13-3). In the latter setting, infection is usually related to skin lesions or abrasions (26). Symptoms are nonspecific and insidious resulting in delayed diagnosis (17,25,26).

Multiple imaging approaches may be required for detection and staging of musculoskeletal infections. MRI is a sensitive technique for early detection of musculoskeletal infection. Skeletal infections typically begin in medullary bone. The resulting hyperemia and inflammation cause alterations in signal intensity of medullary bone on MR images. The excellent tissue contrast and multiplanar imaging provided by MRI may allow earlier diagnosis and more accurate assessment of the extent of osseous, articular, and soft tissue infections than other imaging techniques (7,14,40–44). Therefore, acute osteomyelitis may be evident on MR images when radiographs and other modalities are negative (7,45). Multimodality approaches using MRI, conventional isotopes, and positron emission tomography (PET) imaging may be required in certain situations (28,39,46–50).

Discussion of the utility of MRI is facilitated by categorizing patients in the following manner: a) infection in nonviolated tissue; b) infection in violated tissue (previous fracture or surgery, puncture, soft tissue injury); and

c) evaluation of surgical techniques for treatment. The latter category includes patients treated with muscle or omental flaps and vascularized fibular grafts.

INFECTION IN NONVIOLATED TISSUE

Osteomyelitis presents a diagnostic and therapeutic challenge regardless of the age group. Early diagnosis and management are essential to avoid irreversible bone, joint, and soft tissue damage. Hematogenous osteomyelitis, which occurs more commonly in children than adults, may be acute, subacute, or chronic, and most commonly involves the long bones of the lower extremities. In infants (<2 years) and adults, the epiphysis is not protected; vascular channels cross the growth plate allowing infection to involve both the metaphysis and epiphysis with a high incidence of joint space involvement (10,15). In patients from age 1 to 2 years up to 16 years, the growth plate prevents spread of infection to the epiphysis and joint space involvement is less common unless the metaphysis is intracapsular (Fig. 13-1) (12).

Infections typically involve the metaphyseal portion of long bones or areas near the physis in flat bones, such as the

TABLE 13-2

COMMON ORGANISMS IN MUSCULOSKELETAL INFECTIONS

Batcerial Infection

Gram-positive

Staphylococcal
Streptococcal
Meningococcal
Gonococcal

Gram-negative

Coliform bacterial infection
Proteus
Pseudomonas
Klebsiella
Salmonella
Haemophilus
Brucella

Mycobacteria

Tuberculosis
Atypical mycobacterial infection

Fungal and higher bacterial infection

Actinomycosis
Nocardiosis
Cryptococcosis
Coccidioidomycosis
Histoplasmosis
Sporotrichosis

Parasitic infections

Hookworms
Cysticercosis
Echinococcosis

From Resnick D. Osteomyelitis, septic arthritis and soft tissue infections: organisms. In: Resnick D, ed. *Diagnosis of bone and joint disorders.* Philadelphia, PA: WB Saunders, 2002:2510–2624.

TABLE 13-3

ATYPICAL MYCOBACTERIAL INFECTIONS

Mycobacterium	Reservoir/ Transmission	Common Musculoskeletal Involvement
Avium	Soil, water, hogs, cattle, birds	Osseous
Marinum	Water, fish	Soft tissue, hand and wrist
Bausaaii	Water, cattle, hogs	Osseous
Fortuitum	Soil, water, animals, marine life	Osseous
Scrofulaceum	Soil, water, liquid foods	Osseous
Balnei	Water, fish	Soft tissue

From Theodorou DJ, Theodorou SJ, Kakitsubata Y, et al. Imaging characteristics and epidemiologic features of atypical mycobacterial infections involving the musculoskeletal system. *AJR Am J Roentgenol* 2001;176:341–349. Wongworawt MD, Holton P, Learch TJ, et al. A prolonged case of Mycobacterium marinum flexor tenosynovitis: radiographic, and histological correlation, and review of the literature. *Skeletal Radiol* 2003;32:542–545. Amrami KK, Sundaram M, Shin AY, et al. Mycobacterium marinum infections of the distal upper extremities: clinical course and imaging findings in two cases with delayed diagnosis. *Skeletal Radiol* 2003;32:546–549.

the anatomic extent may be inaccurate, especially in the articular regions, and differentiation of soft tissue from bone involvement is not always possible (7). Also, in complex clinical settings such as previous surgery or instrumentation, neurotrophic changes or other conditions that create bone remodeling radionuclide imaging is less specific (16,53). This will be discussed more fully later in this chapter.

In recent years, PET has been effectively used to identify active infection (32,48,50).

Acute Osteomyelitis

MRI is particularly suited to evaluate osteomyelitis due to superior soft tissue contrast and multiple image plane capabilities. Anatomic detail is superior to that provided by isotope studies. Subtle bone and soft tissue changes are more easily appreciated than on radiographs or CT examinations (3,4,51,54). In recent years, new pulse sequences and the use of intravenous contrast have improved the utility of MRI for evaluating infection.

As with other musculoskeletal pathology, examination of patients with suspected infection requires at least T1-weighted and T2-weighted sequences; conventional spin-echo (SE) or fast spin-echo (FSE) sequences can be used (6,7,54). These sequences are needed to provide the necessary contrast between normal and abnormal tissues. T1-weighted sequences (SE or FSE) can be performed quickly and provide high spatial resolution (4,7,34). Infection is demonstrated as an area of decreased signal intensity compared to the high signal intensity of normal marrow (see Fig. 13-4). Changes

ilium. Radiologic changes are nonspecific in the early stages of infection. Localized swelling and distortion of the tissue planes may be the only findings (6,7). This may be followed with osteopenia in the area of marrow involvement or subtle lytic areas in the cortex. More defined bone destruction is usually not appreciated until 35% to 40% of the involved bone is destroyed, and thus is generally not evident for 10 to 14 days (10,12). Periosteal elevation may also be evident. The degree of involvement is often underestimated on routine radiographs. In this situation, computed tomography (CT) may be useful to more clearly define the extent of involvement. CT (see Fig. 13-3) has been especially useful in determining the extent of disease prior to planning operative therapy and for detection of sequestra, cloaca (see Table 13-1), and soft tissue changes (5,6,8,10,34,51).

Radioisotope studies provide a sensitive tool for early detection of osteomyelitis. Technetium-99m, indium-111 labeled leukocytes, and technetium white cells or antigranulocyte antibodies provide sensitive and fairly specific methods for diagnosis of infection (2,5,7,12,27,38,52). However,

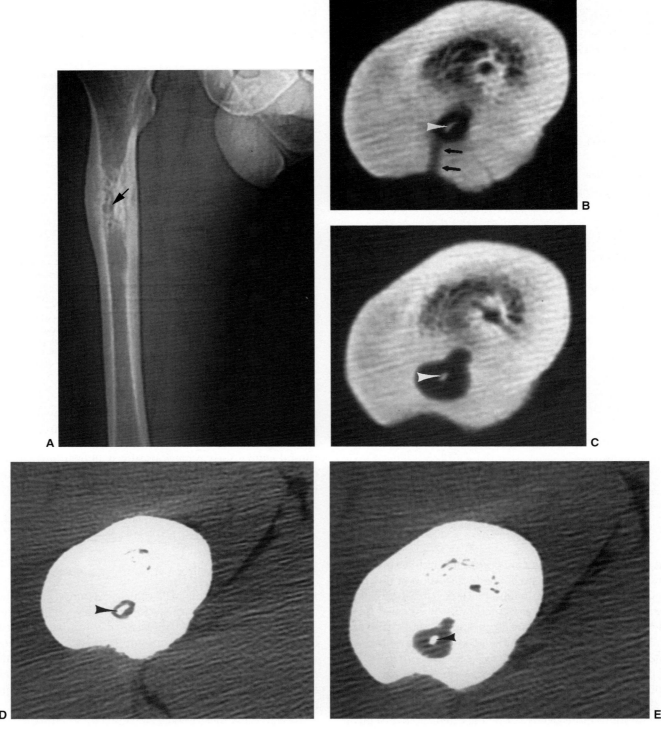

Figure 13-3 Chronic osteomyelitis with sequestrum and cloaca. **A:** CT scout images show medullary sclerosis and cortical thickening in the femur with a central lucency (*arrow*). Axial CT images with bone **(B,C)** and soft tissue **(D,E)** settings show a local abscess with a sequestrum (*arrowheads in C and D*) and cloaca (*arrows*). Beam hardening artifact degrades the image quality of the adjacent soft tissues.

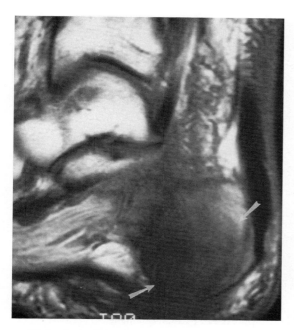

Figure 13-4 Sagittal SE 500/15 image of the calcaneus demonstrating low signal intensity (*arrows*) due to osteomyelitis in a diabetic. Routine radiographs were normal.

in cortical bone, periosteum, and muscle are often less obvious on T1-weighted sequences (Fig. 13-4). T2-weighted sequences (SE or FSE) demonstrate infection as areas of high signal intensity. We use fat suppression with FSE T-2 weighted sequences. Fat signal is reduced so areas of marrow inflammation are increased in signal intensity compared to normal marrow (see Fig. 13-5). In certain situations, more than two sequences may be required to improve tissue characterization. For example, short TI inversion recovery (STIR) sequences (see Fig. 13-6) may provide valuable information about fat, water (cellular elements), or subtle inflammatory changes in bone marrow and soft tissues (6,7,15,34). We routinely add gadolinium-enhanced fat-suppressed T1-weighted images in

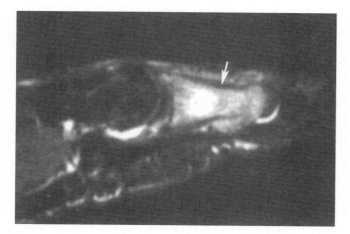

Figure 13-5 Osteomyelitis in the great toe. Fat-suppressed fast spin-echo T2-weighted sequence demonstrates increased signal intensity in the proximal phalanx (*arrow*).

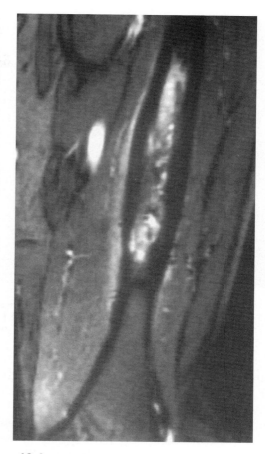

Figure 13-6 Osteomyelitis in the left femur. Coronal STIR sequence shows subtle thickening of the cortex with increased signal intensity in the marrow and adjacent soft tissues.

patients with suspected osteomyelitis (0.1 mmol/kg b.w. intravenously) (see Fig. 13-7).

The anatomic extent of osteomyelitis can be clearly demonstrated by MRI (4,6,7,31). The extent of disease, including detection of skip areas, is easily established using multiple image planes. This information is particularly valuable when planning surgical debridement.

There have also been several studies comparing isotope studies, CT, and MRI in detection of early osteomyelitis. Chandnani et al. (55) compared CT and MRI. MRI demonstrated a 94% sensitivity compared to 66% for CT. Both techniques were equally specific for excluding osteomyelitis. Gallium-67 and indium-111 labeled white blood cells are more specific for infection than technetium scans (28, 56). Beltran et al. (56) compared technetium-99m methylene diphosphonate (MDP), gallium-67, and MRI for evaluating musculoskeletal infection. All techniques were equally effective in detecting osseous infection. However, MRI was more sensitive (100% compared to 69% for isotope scans) in identifying abscesses and distinguishing abscesses from cellulitis (see Fig. 13-8) (54).

The specificity of MRI for diagnosis of osteomyelitis needs to be more clearly defined. Increased signal intensity

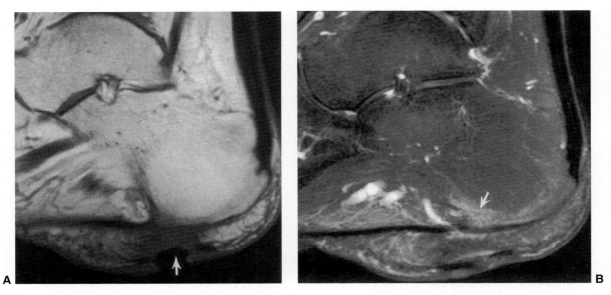

Figure 13-7   Diabetic with calcaneal osteomyelitis. **A:** Sagittal T1-weighted image demonstrates a soft tissue ulcer (*arrow*) and swelling. **B:** Contrast-enhanced fat-suppressed T1-weighted image demonstrates an area of enhancement (*arrow*) due to infection.

in marrow, cortical bone, periosteum, and soft tissue is noted on T2-weighted, STIR, and gradient-echo (T2*) sequences (Figs. 13-4 to 13-7) (5,7,16,53,57).

Morrison et al. (53) evaluated fat-suppressed gadolinium-enhanced imaging in 51 patients with suspected osteomyelitis. These studies were compared with conventional T1- and T2-weighted MR images and technetium-99m MDP bone scintigrams. Focal enhancement with gadolinium was considered indicative of osteomyelitis. In 73% of patients, the diagnosis was complicated by postoperative change, chronic osteomyelitis or neurotrophic arthropathy. Despite this, enhanced fat-suppressed T1-weighted MR images demonstrated a sensitivity of 88% and specificity of 93% compared to a sensitivity of 79% and specificity 53% for non-gadolinium MR images (see Fig. 13-9). Bone scans were 61% sensitive and 33% specific (53). Most agree that sensitivity for detection of infection is improved by contrast-enhanced imaging. However, findings are not specific in differentiating infection from inflammation or neoplasms (47). Lack of bone enhancement effectively excludes infection (47,53,58).

Chronic Osteomyelitis

With acute infections, the clinical features combined with MR features are used to make the diagnosis. With subacute, chronic, or long-standing infections, image features may be more difficult to interpret. MR features combined with radionuclide scans or PET imaging may be required to define active infection. Chronic infection may be related to inadequate treatment, specific organisms, and other clinical features such as immunodeficiency (1,21,22,39,46).

This section will consider low-grade and subtle infections such as tuberculosis, atypical mycobacterial infections, fungal infections, and specific conditions such as chronic relapsing multifocal osteomyelitis (CRMO) and SAPHO (Table 13-1) (6,27,59).

Diagnosis of chronic osteomyelitis is often delayed significantly due to nonspecific symptoms and radiographic features (25,27,38,59).

Mycobacterium Tuberculosis

Extra spinal osteomyelitis accounts for 19% of musculoskeletal tuberculosis. Spinal involvement and tuberculous arthritis respectively remain the most common sites of involvement (60). Tuberculous osteomyelitis involves the metaphysis or epiphysis similar to pyogenic osteomyelitis. Periosteal reaction, bone sclerosis, and sequestra are less common than pyogenic infection (59,60). Changes may resemble a benign bone tumor or, if more aggressive, round cell lesions such as Ewing sarcoma, lymphoma, or leukemia (6,31). CT, radionuclide scans, and MRI frequently add little to the specificity of the pathology (60). Therefore, biopsy and culture are required.

In children, multiple lytic lesions may mimic fungal infection, pyogenic osteomyelitis, or neoplasms. The latter include eosinophilic granuloma, neuroblastoma or lymphoma (38).

Recently, Sharma (59) described MR features of tuberculous osteomyelitis. Two types of lesions were described. Lesions might have predominantly low or intermediate signal intensity on T2-weighted sequences and low signal intensity on T1-weighted sequences. Features are related to central caseating necrosis in tubercular granulomas.

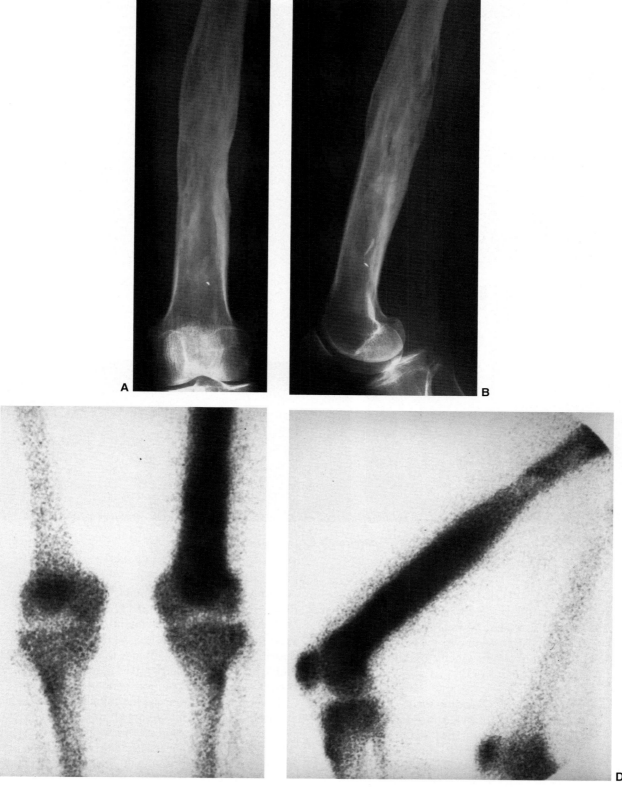

Figure 13-8   Anteroposterior **(A)** and lateral **(B)** radiographs of the femur in a patient with suspected osteomyelitis. Technetium-99m MDP scans **(C,D)** show marked increased uptake in the distal femur. Indium-111 labeled white blood cell images in the anteroposterior. **(E)** and lateral **(F)** projections show scattered areas of uptake in the femur. Soft tissue involvement? Coronal SE 500/15 image **(G)** demonstrates decreased signal intensity in the femur. Note the metal artifact (*arrows*). Axial T2-weighted image **(H)** shows increased signal intensity in the marrow with a localized (*arrow*) juxtacortical abscess.

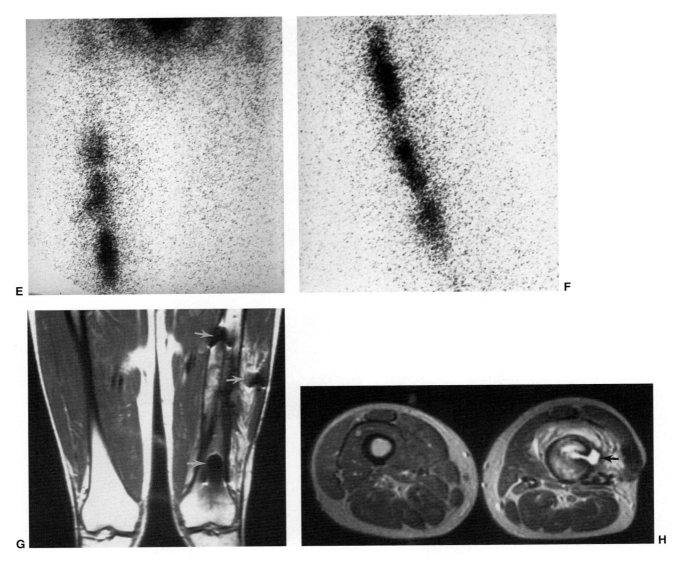

Figure 13-8 (continued)

The second image feature described was low intensity with marginally higher intensity peripherally on T1-weighted images. Surrounding edema was common in this setting (see Fig. 13-10). Extraosseous soft tissue edema and abscess formulation were evident in about 80% of cases (59).

Atypical Mycobacterial Osteomyelitis

Atypical mycobacteria (Table 13-3) are frequently drug resistant and account for up to 30% of all mycobacterial infections (25). The musculoskeletal system is involved in 5% to 10%. Infections may be caused by hematogenous spread or soft tissue contamination from soil, water, fish, birds and other animals (Table 13-3) (17,25). In adults, symptoms are typically mild compared to tuberculosis. However, in children, clinical features are more aggressive (25). Symptoms are nonspecific (local pain,

swelling, low-grade fever, malaise) resulting in delay of diagnosis for up to 10 months (25).

Radiographic features resemble pyogenic infection except that the progression occurs more slowly. Bone destruction takes weeks longer than pyogenic infection. Unlike tuberculosis, sinus tracts, sequestra, abscesses, and periosteal reaction occur more commonly (25).

Image features are nonspecific. MR features may be similar to chronic pyogenic infection with marrow edema, cloacae, periosteal thickening, and soft tissue abscesses. Diagnosis of active infection may be assisted with PET imaging or combined technetium bone scans with technetium 99m antigranulocyte antibodies (32,39,48).

Miscellaneous Organisms

Other organisms (Table 13-2) less commonly involve the musculoskeletal system.

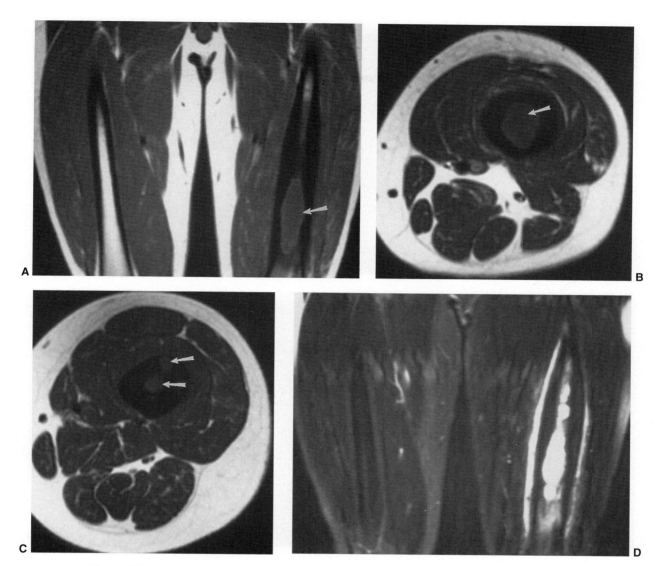

Figure 13-9   Osteomyelitis in the femur. Coronal **(A)** and axial **(B,C)** T1-weighted images demonstrate loss of normal fatty marrow in the femur (*arrows*). Signal intensity is increased on T2-weighted coronal image **(D).** Postcontrast fat-suppressed T1-weighted images. **(E–H)** demonstrate areas of peripheral enhancement in bone due to abscess formation. There is also juxtacortical soft tissue enhancement.

Coccidioidomycosis is endemic in the Southwestern United States and Central and South America (31,35). Most patients present with respiratory or flulike symptoms. With dissemination, osseous involvement may occur with lytic bone lesions and soft tissue inflammation. The axial and appendicular skeleton may be involved (34,61). The diagnosis should be considered in endemic and non-endemic regions. Up to 20% of cases are reported outside endemic regions due to increased travel (62). MR features are nonspecific but useful for staging the extent of osseous and soft tissue involvement.

Echinococcus granulosis, E. multilocularis, and, less frequently, *E. vogeli* and *E. oligarthus,* may also cause osteomyelitis. The liver (65%) and lung (15%) are most commonly involved. However, 1% to 4% of patients also have musculoskeletal

involvement (31,54). The osseous involvement occurs most frequently in the spine (35%) followed by pelvic (21%), femoral (16%), tibial (10%), rib (6%), calvarial (4%), scapular (4%), and humeral and fibular (2%) involvement. Osseous lesions are cystic or multilocular which may resemble bone neoplasms (54).

Chronic Recurrent Multifocal Osteomyelitis (CRMO)

This condition is a chronic osteomyelitis characterized by exacerbations and remissions. Though patients may be affected at any age, the condition is more common at 5 to 10 years of age. Patients typically present with pain, swelling, and tenderness in the areas of skeletal involvement.

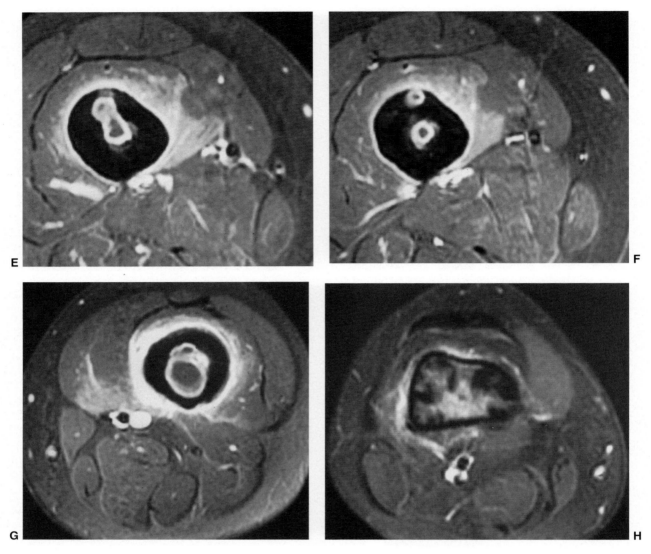

Figure 13-9   (continued)

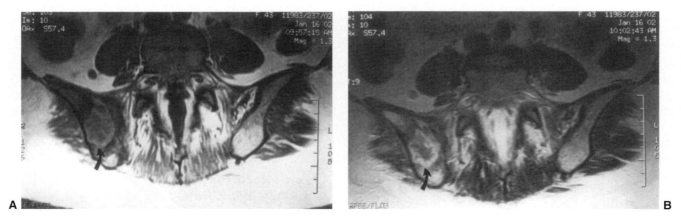

Figure 13-10   Coronal T1-weighted image **(A)** and T2-weighted image **(B)** of the right ilium demonstrate a lesion with a hyperintense rim (*curved arrow*) and hypointense center. The rim appears thicker on the T2-weighted image in **B.** (From Sharma P. MR features of tuberculous osteomyelitis. *Skeletal Radiol* 2003;32:279–285.)

Skin lesions such as acne and pustulosis of the palms and plantar aspects of the feet are not uncommon (63,64). Therefore, CRMO has been considered part of the SAPHO syndrome (6,46,64).

Radiographically, the metaphyses of the femur, tibia, and medial clavicles are most commonly involved. Osteosclerosis with prominent periosteal reaction are characteristic of CRMO. Changes in the clavicle may mimic Paget disease, fibrous dysplasia, or sarcoma. Two additional conditions may be considered with sclerosis of the medial clavicles. The first is hyperostosis, commonly seen in women (osteitis condensans); and the second, sternoclavicular hyperostosis, which is typically seen in patients in their 50s and 60s. Males and females are affected equally (6,46,63–65).

Organisms are difficult to isolate in CRMO. However, when isolated, *Propionibacterium acnes*, corynebacterium, or pneumococci may be cultured. MRI features are not specific. However, based upon radiographic features, it is not surprising that signal intensity is reduced on T1-weighted sequences and variable (low, intermediate, high) on T2-weighted sequences (see Fig. 13-11) (6,46). During quiescent phases, bone sclerosis typically results in low signal intensity on both T1- and T2-weighted sequences (46).

Synovitis, Acme, Pustulosis, Hyperostosis, Osteitis (SAPHO)

Chamot (13) initiated the term SAPHO in 1987 to designate a group of disorders with anterior chest wall osteitis. There is still controversy as to whether SAPHO represents a syndrome or group of disorders. Up to 50 different terms have been used to describe combined cutaneous and osteoarticular disorders (66). Kahn and Chamot (67) emphasized that different skin and osteoarticular disorders fall into the SAPHO syndrome. This rationale was based upon five criteria. First, pustulosis and severe acne share the same histologic features. Second, bone involvement is identical. Third, osteoarticular involvement has a predilection for the anterior chest wall. Fourth, acute arthropathy is observed with skin lesions; and fifth, sacroiliac joint involvement is consistently present (67).

Most would consider SAPHO six groups of disorders that includes CRMO (42,46,64). Skin lesions may not be evident for up to 2 years before osteoarticular findings become evident (46).

Earwalker and Cotton (46) described features of this disorder based upon age. Children, young adults, and older adults have differing presentations.

Anterior chest wall osteitis is evident in 69% to 90% of adults. Nonspecific discitis or vertebral or paravertebral sclerosis is evident in 33% of patients. Unilateral sacroiliitis is present in 13–52%. The long bones are involved in 30% and fat bones (ilium and mandible) in 10% (see Fig. 13-12) (42,46).

Arthropathy involves the spine in 91% and peripheral joints, typically the hips, knees, and ankles, in 36% (42).

In children and some younger adults, patients present with features more in keeping with CRMO. During the early phases, there are lytic changes in the metaphyses of the lower extremities. The tibia, femur, and fibula are most commonly involved. Similar changes are evident in the medial clavicles. The spine and sacroiliac joints may also be involved (42,46,64).

Over time, lesions become sclerotic, with minimal periostitis compared to changes in older adults. Lesions are characteristically sclerotic during phases of remission. Radiographically, the diagnosis is not difficult in children or adults when anterior chest wall and characteristic spine and extremity sites are involved. The diagnosis is more difficult with atypical distribution. Lesions may be confused with Paget disease in adults; eosinophilic granuloma, osteosarcoma, Ewing sarcoma, or typical osteomyelitis in younger patients (42,46).

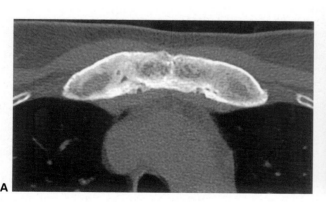
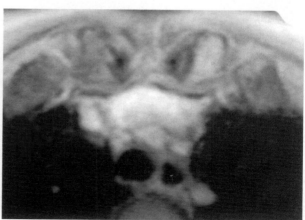

Figure 13-11   Chronic relapsing multifocal osteomyelitis (CRMO). Axial CT **(A)** and T1-weighted MR image **(B)** demonstrate thickening and sclerosis at the costosternal and sternoclavicular junctions.

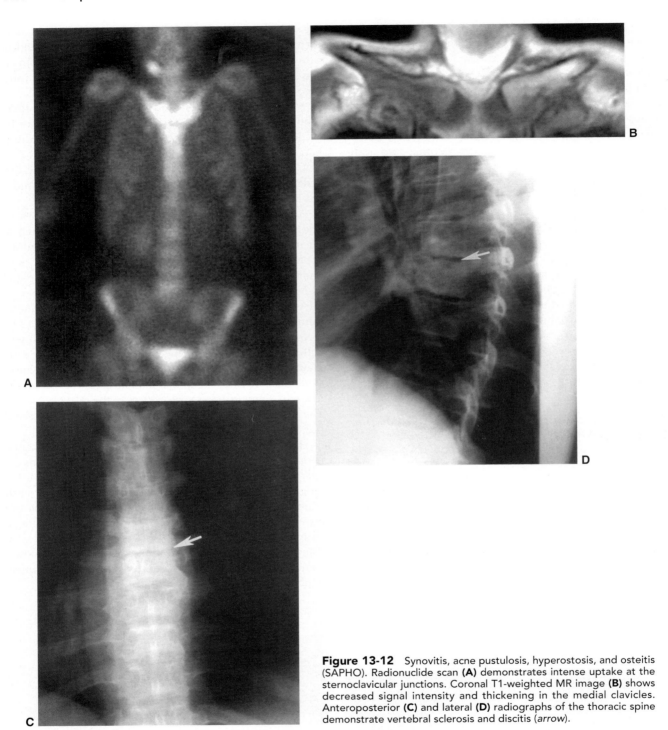

Figure 13-12 Synovitis, acne pustulosis, hyperostosis, and osteitis (SAPHO). Radionuclide scan **(A)** demonstrates intense uptake at the sternoclavicular junctions. Coronal T1-weighted MR image **(B)** shows decreased signal intensity and thickening in the medial clavicles. Anteroposterior **(C)** and lateral **(D)** radiographs of the thoracic spine demonstrate vertebral sclerosis and discitis (*arrow*).

MRI is useful for demonstrating the extent of involvement that is often underestimated on radiographs. Active disease can also be more easily appreciated. During active stages, there is low signal intensity on T1-weighted sequences, with scattered areas of high signal intensity on T2-weighted sequences. There may be associated soft tissue edema without abscess formation. During remission, signal intensity is low on both T1- and T2-weighted sequences. Thus, increased signal intensity on T2-weighted sequences indicates active disease (46,68).

Patients with SAPHO have been treated with anti-inflammatory medications and, in some cases, long-term antibiotics (46).

Infections in the diabetic, specifically the foot (Figs. 13-4, 13-5, and 13-7), present a complex clinical and imaging dilemma (19,21,23,41,69–71). Studies comparing MR

Imaging Approaches for Osteomyelitis

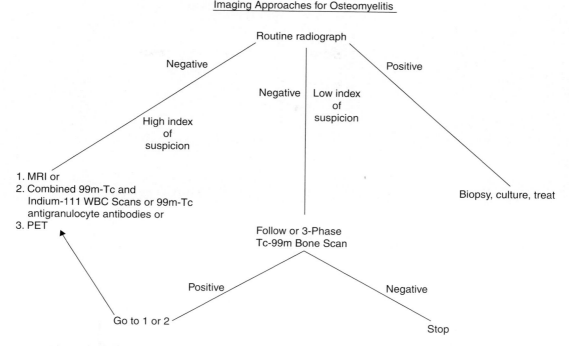

Figure 13-13   Imaging approaches for osteomyelitis. From references 7, 8, 30, 32, 39, and 48.

imaging in diabetic and nondiabetic feet show reduced sensitivity and specificity in diabetic patients. Sensitivity for infection is 89% in nondiabetics compared to diabetics, and specificities are 94% and 80%, respectively. The diabetic foot is discussed more completely in Chapter 8.

Several authors have suggested algorithms for imaging of osteomyelitis in children and adults (7,8,12,30,57). Most include routine radiographs as the initial screening technique followed by radionuclide scans or MRI if radiographs are negative and there is a significant index of suspicion clinically. Figure 13-13 suggests an imaging approach for suspected osteomyelitis.

Joint Space Infection

Joint space infections may present with rapid progressive onset with pyogenic organisms or a more insidious onset when fungal or tubercular organisms are involved. Early diagnosis is essential to prevent loss of joint function (6,72). Infectious arthritis is generally monoarticular and, like osteomyelitis, commonly involves the lower extremities (29,62,73). Nonseptic inflammatory disease, or in children, transient synovitis of the hip, must be included in the differential diagnosis (51,74,75). Differentiation of infection from other inflammatory arthropathies may be difficult. Clinical features and laboratory data are useful. Children with septic arthritis are more likely to have chills, inability to bear weight, an elevated erythrocyte sedimentation rate, and

elevated white count compared to those with transient synovitis of the hip or adults (8,72).

Lee et al. (75) reported mean white counts of 13,850/mm (76) with pyogenic arthritis, compared to 8,660/mm (76) with transient synovitis of the hip. Erythrocyte sedimentation rates had a mean of 75.3 mm/hr with infection compared to 20.6 mm/hr in patients with transient synovitis of the hip.

Image features of joint space infection on radiographs, ultrasound, CT, and MRI have been described (51,74). Early detection is important so therapy can be instituted and joint deformity and bone loss prevented (73,77). Joint space changes and soft tissue swelling may be noted on radiographs, but early bone changes are not appreciated for 1 to 2 weeks with pyogenic infection, and may take months to develop with tuberculous arthritis (12,72,73,75). Isotope scans using technetium-99m MDP are sensitive in detecting early changes, but nonspecific. Gallium-67 and indium-111 WBC or technetium-99m antigranulocyte antibody scans are more specific in this regard (12,28,48).

In recent years, PET has also demonstrated increased sensitivity and specificity for diagnosis of infection (48,49). Ultrasound is useful for detecting effusions, but is not specific for the underlying etiology (75). The role of MRI in joint space infection is more clearly defined today (25,40,66,72, 74,78). Early bone and soft tissue changes and effusions are easily detected (see Fig. 13-14). However, the early erosive changes may not be specific and could be noted with many

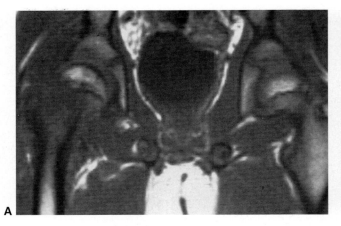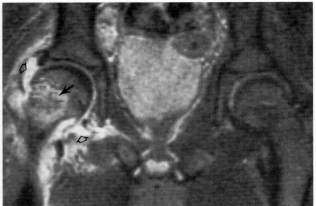

Figure 13-14 Coronal SE 500/15 **(A)** and SE 2,000/80 **(B)** images of the hips in a child with joint space infection and osteomyelitis of the right femoral neck. The joint fluid (*open arrows*) and abnormal marrow signal intensity (*arrow*) are more easily appreciated on the T2-weighted sequence in **B**.

other arthropathies (25). Characterization of the type of fluid present in the joint would be useful. Generally, the T1- and T2- relaxation times of transudates are longer than exudates (11,62,79). Infected fluid and blood in the joint tend to have more intermediate signal intensity and may be inhomogeneous on T2-weighted images. Normal synovial fluid has a uniformly high signal intensity using this sequence (see Figs. 13-14 and 13-15) (80). This information is obviously not sufficient to avoid joint aspiration or synovial biopsy to identify the offending organism (7,25,72).

Multiple studies have been performed to evaluate the MR image findings in pyogenic, tubercular, and non-infectious arthropathies (23,34,40,47,50,72,78). Evaluations studied synovial changes, joint effusions, cartilage loss, and osseous changes.

Graif et al. (47) evaluated image features in infected joints to determine which, if any, might be most useful to confirm infection. Factors included effusion, signal intensity of fluid, synovial thickening, and enhancement after intravenous gadolinium, bone erosions, and marrow edema. The presence of bone erosions and edema were most useful for predicting infection. Synovial thickening or enhancement were also helpful features (47) (Table 13-4).

Similarly, Lee et al. (75) evaluated 23 patients with septic arthritis (9) and transient synovitis of the hip (14). Effusions, marrow, and soft tissue changes were evaluated. Studies were performed using T1-weighted SE, fat-suppressed T2-weighted FSE (2,500–3,500/96–108, ET8), and postcontrast fat-suppressed T1-weighted images (75).

Effusions were graded 0 to 3. Grade 0 was no joint fluid; grade 1, minimal; grade 2, sufficient fluid to surround the femoral neck; and grade 3, joint distention. Grade 3 effusions were evident in 8 of 9 septic joints and 10 of 14 patients with transient synovitis. Therefore, joint distention by effusion was not considered useful. Soft tissue inflammation occurred equally with both conditions.

However, marrow signal intensity abnormalities (↓T1-weighted, ↑T2-weighted, ↑contrast enhancement) were evident in 8 of 9 septic hips and no patients with transient

synovitis of the hip. This would support the utility of marrow changes described by Graif et al. (47) However, it would not be useful in differentiating infection from marrow edema or transient osteoporosis of the hip in adults.

In a more recent study, Karchevsky et al. (81) evaluated synovial changes and effusions in 50 consecutive patients with septic arthritis. Synovial enhancement, perisynovial edema, and effusion had the highest correlation with infection. Reduced marrow signal intensity on T1-weighted sequences had the highest correlation with associated osteomyelitis (81).

Diffusion imaging may be useful for characterizing synovial fluid changes in the future (78). To date, there is not

TABLE 13-4

MR IMAGE FEATURES IN INFECTED AND NONINFECTED JOINTS

Image Features	Infected Joint (%)	No Infection (%)
Joint effusion	79	82
Fluid outpouching from capsule	79	73
Inhomogeneous fluid signal intensity	21	27
Synovial thickening	68	55
Soft tissue edema	63	55
Synovial enhancement after gadolinium	94	88
Bone erosions	79	38
Bone marrow edema	74	38
Marrow enhancement after gadolinium	67	50
Soft tissue enhancement after gadolinium	67	71
Periosteal edema	11	10

From Graif M, Schweitzer MR, Deely D, et al. The septic versus non-septic inflamed joint: MR characteristics. *Skeletal Radiol* 1999;28:616–620.

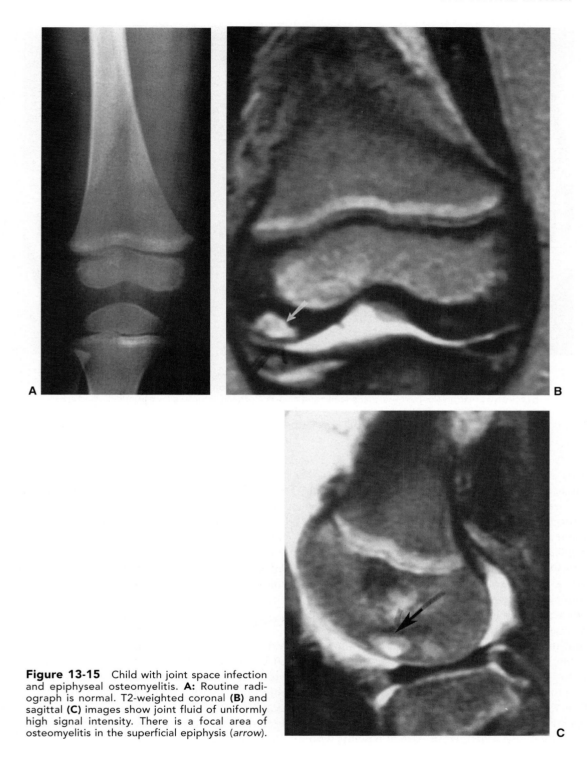

Figure 13-15 Child with joint space infection and epiphyseal osteomyelitis. **A:** Routine radiograph is normal. T2-weighted coronal **(B)** and sagittal **(C)** images show joint fluid of uniformly high signal intensity. There is a focal area of osteomyelitis in the superficial epiphysis (*arrow*).

sufficient data to support this approach for routine clinical imaging.

Differentiating pyogenic from tuberculosis, atypical mycobacterial, and fungal infections is also difficult. Phemister and Hatcher (77) described a radiographic triad for tuberculous arthritis including marginal erosions, osteopenia, and joint space preservation until late in the disease. Tuberculosis also tends to involve the hip, knee, or sacroiliac joint in a monoarticular fashion. Features of tuberculosis and atypical mycobacteria are similar (25). However, in children, atypical mycobacteria are more often implicated in early physeal closure, epiphyseal overgrowth, and leg length discrepancy (25). Differential diagnosis should include rheumatoid arthritis, fungal infection, gout, calcium pyrophosphate dihydrate deposition disease, and idiopathic chondrolysis (25,72).

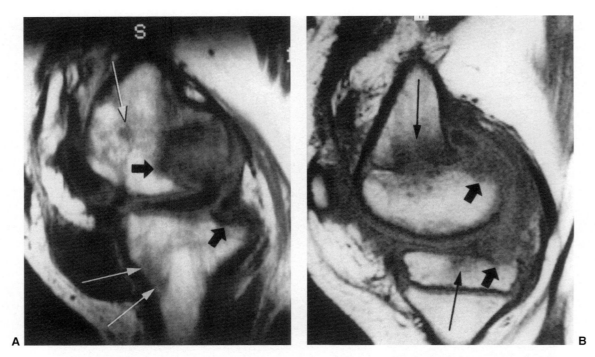

Figure 13-16 Sagittal T1-weighted MR images show bone erosion and marrow signal intensity abnormality. **A:** Tuberculous arthritis shows erosions with well-defined low intensity (*short arrows*) and hypointense marrow (*long arrows*) in the femur and tibia. **B:** Pyogenic arthritis shows poorly defined erosions (*short arrows*) and hypointense marrow (*long arrows*). (From Hong SH, Kim SM, Ahn JM, et al. Tuberculous versus pyogenic arthritis: MR imaging evaluation. *Radiology* 2001;218:848–853.)

Hong et al. (72) compared MR image features of tuberculosis and pyogenic infection. They evaluated joint effusions, cartilage and marrow changes, and soft tissue inflammation and abscesses. Bone erosions (marginal) were evident in 83% of patients with tuberculosis compared to 46% with pyogenic arthritis (see Fig. 13-16). Keep in mind, timing of the examination is critical, as proteolytic enzymes seen with pyogenic infection can cause rapid cartilage destruction on weight-bearing surfaces. Tuberculosis is not associated with proteolytic enzymes, so erosions are marginal due to inflamed synovium, and the joint space can be preserved for months (66,72). Marrow signal intensity abnormalities were more common with pyogenic infection (92%) compared to 59% in tuberculous arthritis. Soft tissue extension occurred in 79% of patients with tuberculosis and 92% with pyogenic arthritis. When abscesses were present, the walls were thin and well-defined in 70% of patients with tuberculosis, but thick and irregular in 83% of pyogenic infections (see Fig. 13-17) (72).

We recommend T1-weighted, fat-suppressed FSE T2-weighted or STIR and contrast-enhanced fat-suppressed T1-weighted images in patients with suspected joint space infection (7,40,58,72,75). The number of image planes will vary with the anatomic region; however, postcontrast image planes should be selected to best compare pathology on precontrast images (7).

Synovial enhancement, marrow changes, cartilage erosion, and soft tissue abscesses appear to be most useful at the time for evaluation of patients with joint space infection (25,47,72,75). However, features are not specific. Therefore, joint aspiration and/or synovial biopsy are still required to establish the diagnosis and isolate the organism (72,75). Figure 13-18 suggests an imaging approach to joint space infection (7,8).

Infectious Spondylitis (Spondylodiscitis)

Various terms have been applied to inflammatory changes in the disc space or vertebra. Disk space narrowing with an elevated sedimentation rate has been termed "discitis, infectious discitis, and intervertebral disk space inflammation" (12,79). Infectious spondylitis is a general term that includes the spectrum of childhood and adult disorders (6,12,82–84).

Infectious spondylitis accounts for 4% to 7% of all cases of osteomyelitis (6,84). The clinical course varies with patient age, location, type of organism, route of infection, and associated diseases or immunocompromise (84,85). Males are affected nearly twice as frequently as females. Infectious spondylitis is most commonly seen in the sixth decade of life (6,84). Patients typically present with fever, malaise, weight loss, and back pain. The pain is typically worse with activity and relieved by rest. Neurologic deficits

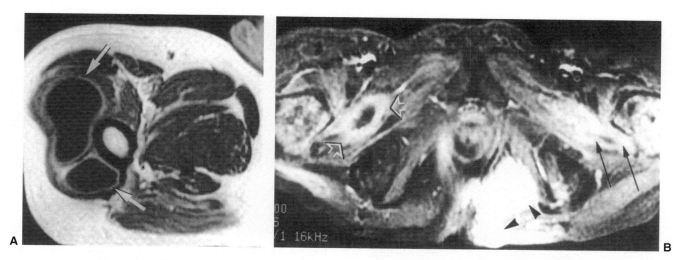

A   B

Figure 13-17   Gadolinium-enhanced T1-weighted images associated with joint space infection in the hip. **A:** Tuberculous abscesses with smooth, thin enhancing walls (*arrows*). **B:** Pyogenic abscess (*open arrows*) with thick, irregular walls. Poorly defined soft tissue enhancement (*arrowheads*) and cellulitis (*long arrows*) are also evident. (From Hong SH, Kim SM, Ahn JM, et al. Tuberculous versus pyogenic arthritis: MR imaging evaluation. *Radiology* 2001;218:848–853.)

may be evident in patients with epidural abscesses or paraspinal involvement (25,37,84). Paravertebral abscesses, such as psoas muscle abscess, may cause leg and hip pain (84).

The intervertebral disc is extremely vascular in neonates and infants up to 2 years of age. This vascularity reduces rapidly, so that by age 13 the disc becomes avascular. Therefore, in infants, the disc may be infected without vertebral involvement. In adults, infection typically involves the vertebral body initially with secondary involvement of the disc and adjacent vertebral body. Infection can spread to involve all components of a vertebra (6,37,84). Ledermann et al. (37) reported involvement of the disc and two adjacent vertebrae in 41 of 46 (89%), an isolated vertebral body and disc in 3 of 46 (6.5%), and isolated vertebral involvement in 1 of 46 (2%). One patient had an abscess (see Fig. 13-19) without disc or vertebral involvement. Excluding tuberculosis and postoperative infections, 52% of infections involved the

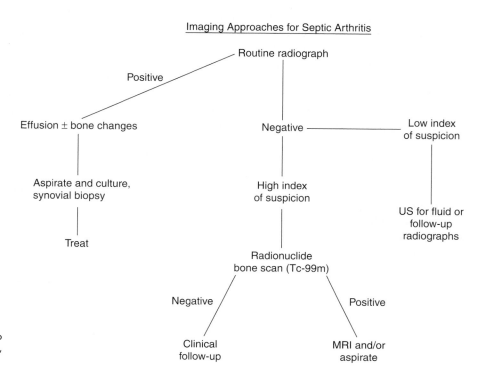

Figure 13-18   Imaging approaches to septic arthritis. From references 7, 8, 25, 40, and 75.

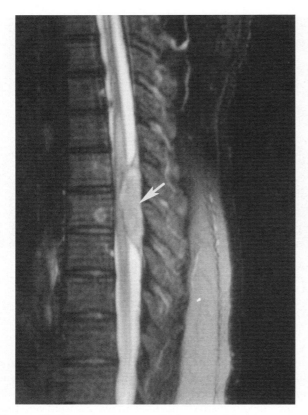

Figure 13-19 Sagittal T2-weighted image of the thoracic spine demonstrating an epidural abscess (*arrow*) with cord compression, but no discitis.

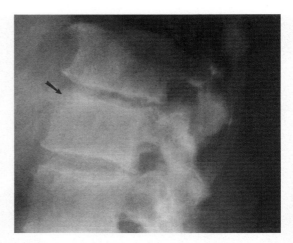

Figure 13-20 Lateral radiograph of the upper lumbar spine demonstrates disc space narrowing and anterior bone loss (*arrow*).

lumbar spine, 22% the thoracic spine, and 26% the cervical spine (37). About 50% of patients with cervical spine involvement demonstrate infection at three or more levels. In the thoracic and lumbar spine, one disc and adjacent vertebrae are most commonly involved (84).

Infectious spondylitis is most often hematogenous, but can occur following procedures (discectomy, CT-guided aspirations or biopsies, and spinal instrumentation) or rarely spread from an adjacent soft tissue source (6,84).

Any organism including bacterial, tuberculosis, atypical mycobacteria, *Brucella*, fungi, and parasites may be isolated from blood culture or biopsy (12,54). However, up to 80% of cases are caused by *Staphylococcus aureus* (6,84). Certain organisms are more commonly involved due to underlying disorders, region, or occupation. For example, pseudomonas infections tend to occur in patients with drug abuse; salmonella species with sickle cell anemia; and *Brucella* in farmers, veterinarians, and meat handlers. Tuberculosis and atypical mycobacteria infections have also become more common in recent years (Table 13-3) (6,25,84).

Early diagnosis and treatment are critical to prevent complications such as vertebral collapse; neurologic compromise, including paralysis; and meningitis or meningoencephalitis (84).

Routine radiographs are typically normal initially. Poorly defined vertebral end plates may be seen at 2 to 3 weeks. Loss of substantial bone typically occurs later and

most often involves the anterior vertebral body (see Fig. 13-20). Serial images will demonstrate progressive disc space narrowing and bony irregularity, which is useful to separate infection from degenerative disease or trauma (12,25,82–84). Radiographic changes can occur over weeks with pyogenic infections or have a more indolent course with tuberculosis, atypical mycobacteria, and fungal infections (31,84). Patients with tuberculosis or atypical mycobacterial infections have a similar presentation, with frequent paraspinal abscesses and soft tissue calcification in addition to changes described above (25,85).

Radionuclide imaging, including PET, may also play a role in early detection. Technetium-99m MDP studies are sensitive but not specific. Fractures, degenerative disease, and tumor may have a similar appearance. Increased specificity may be obtained using indium-111 labeled white blood cells, technetium labeled white blood cells, or technetium labeled antigranulocyte antibody studies (48, 59,85). More recently, PET imaging has become a useful tool for diagnosis of infection. Studies may also differentiate infection from degenerative end plate changes (84).

Computed tomography can play a valuable role for evaluating the vertebral body, disc, and surrounding soft tissues. Soft tissue abscess and subtle calcifications are easily detected. Early end plate changes may be overlooked unless axial images are reformatted into sagittal and/or coronal images (59). Computed tomography is a useful tool for guidance of biopsy and aspiration procedures.

MRI is the technique of choice for detection and staging of spinal infections (9,21,33,59,82). MRI can demonstrate changes earlier than CT or radiographs. Superior tissue contrast allows osseous changes, spinal canal involvement, and paraspinal soft tissue changes to be more easily appreciated (21,33,50,59).

Pulse sequences for evaluating suspected infectious spondylitis do not differ significantly from those used for extraspinal osteomyelitis. T1-, T2- and postcontrast fat-suppressed T1-weighted images are required (see Fig. 13-21). Fast spin-echo sequences can be used instead of conventional

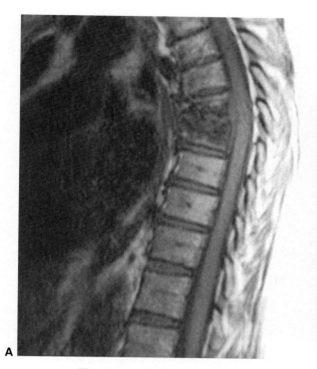
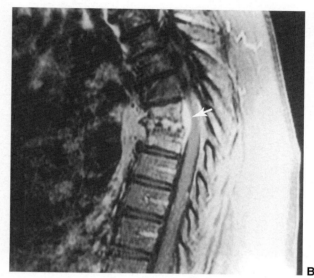

Figure 13-21 Sagittal T1- **(A)** and T2-weighted **(B)** images in a patient with disc space infection, kyphosis, and epidural extension (*arrow*).

SE sequences. Short TI inversion recovery or new FSE STIR (3,000–6,000/20–78, 150–160 TI) sequences are also useful (21,50,59).

Bone marrow edema may be the earliest finding with vertebral osteomyelitis. Edema is low signal intensity on T1-weighted images and high intensity on T2-weighted and STIR sequences (21,50,59). With FSE T2-weighted images, fat suppression should be used. Edema is less specific than end plate destruction. Therefore, loss of the normal low signal intensity end plate on T1-, STIR, or postcontrast fat-suppressed T1-weighted images is the earliest specific feature (59).

Signal intensity in the involved disc is typically low on T1- and high on T2-weighted or STIR sequences. However, in early stages, 9% to 13% of discs may be low intensity on T2-weighted and STIR sequences (see Fig. 13-22). The disc space is also narrowed in most cases (37,84). When a disc abscess is present, the disc height can be increased (37). The normal intranuclear cleft that is evident in 94% of normal discs is not detected in most discs involved with infection (see Fig. 13-23) (84).

Soft tissue inflammation and paraspinal and epidural abscesses are easily demonstrated on MR images. Contrast-enhanced fat-suppressed T1-weighted images are essential and can differentiate granulation tissue or inflammation from abscess formation (58,84).

The differential diagnosis of infectious spondylitis includes degenerative end plate changes, inflammatory spondyloarthropathy, hemodialysis spondylopathy, neuropathic changes, and erosive intervertebral osteochondrosis (37,84). With this in mind, Ledermann et al. (37) recently evaluated the sensitivity of commonly accepted MR features

of infection. Tuberculosis and postoperative infections were excluded (37).

Table 13-5 summarizes MRI features and their sensitivity. The most useful criteria were paraspinal or epidural inflammation (97.7%) (Figs. 13-21 and 13-22), disc enhancement after contrast injection (95.4%), end plate destruction (84.1%), and loss of the nuclear cleft (83.3%) (Fig. 13-23). If two criteria were combined, all combinations except end plate destruction on T1-weighted image and loss of the nuclear cleft (88%) exceeded 95% sensitivity. The combinations of disc enhancement with increased signal intensity on T2-weighted image, disc enhancement with loss of the nuclear cleft, disc enhancement with paraspinal, or epidural inflammation demonstrated 100% sensitivity (37).

TABLE 13-5

MR FEATURES IN INFECTIOUS SPONDYLODISCITIS

Image Finding	Sensitivity
Paraspinal or epidural inflammation	97.7%
Disc enhancement	95.4%
↑ Signal intensity in disc on T2-weighted image	93.2%
End plate destruction	84.1%
Positive nuclear cleft sign	83.3%
Decreased disc space	52.3%
Disc low signal on T1-weighted image	29.5%

From Ledermann HP, Schweitzer ME, Morrison WB, et al. MR imaging findings in spinal infections: rules or myths. *Radiology* 2003;228(2): 506–514.

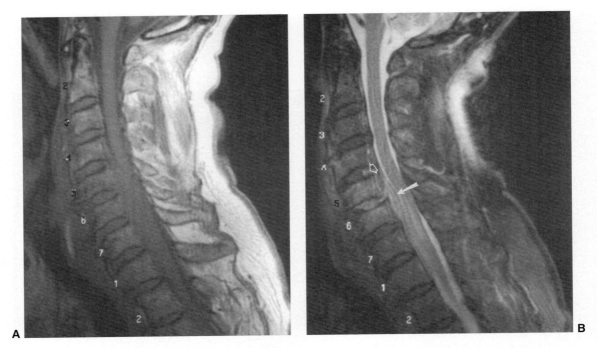

Figure 13-22 Sagittal T1- **(A)** and T2- **(B)** weighted images demonstrate osteomyelitis and disc space infection C4–C6 with epidural abscess (*arrow*). Note the disc height at C4–5 is normal to slightly increased without high signal intensity except posteriorly (*open arrow*).

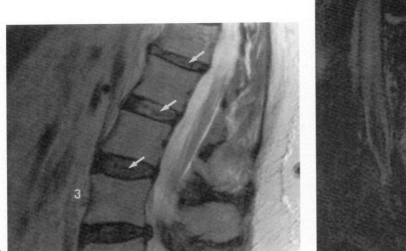

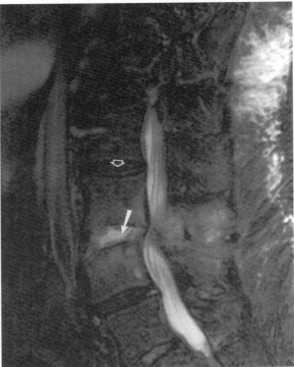

Figure 13-23 **A:** Normal T2-weighted MR image demonstrating the normal nuclear cleft (*arrows*). **B:** Contrast-enhanced fat-suppressed sagittal image demonstrates disc space infection (*arrow*) and a normal nuclear cleft (*open arrow*) in the disc above.

Tuberculosis (*Mycobacterium tuberculosis*) and atypical mycobacterial infections are becoming more common (17,25,72,84,86,87). Therefore, the MR imaging features have been better defined. Tuberculous spondylitis is the most common site of musculoskeletal involvement. The thoracic spine is most frequently involved (84). The course of the disease progresses more slowly, and though some of the same features seen with pyogenic infections (Table 13-5) occur, the changes may be less dramatic. The disc space is maintained for a longer time and end plate destruction is less obvious. Interosseous and paraspinal abscess are common (see Fig. 13-24). These show peripheral enhancement

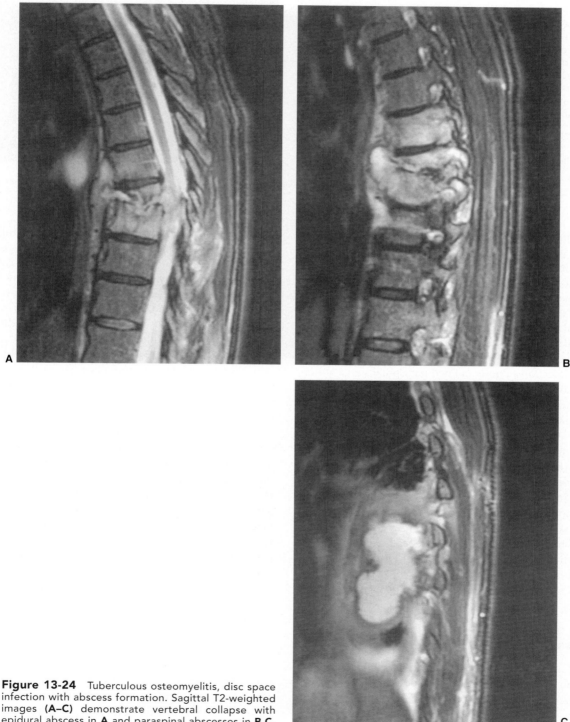

Figure 13-24 Tuberculous osteomyelitis, disc space infection with abscess formation. Sagittal T2-weighted images **(A–C)** demonstrate vertebral collapse with epidural abscess in **A** and paraspinal abscesses in **B,C.**

TABLE 13-6
TUBERCULOSIS VS. PYOGENIC SPONDYLITIS MRI FEATURES

MR Features	Tuberculosis (%)	Pyogenic (%)
Well-defined paraspinal signal abnormalities	95	5
Poorly defined paraspinal signal abnormalities	5	75
Thin-walled abscesses	95	15
Thick-walled abscesses	0	35
Paraspinal or osseous abscesses	95	50
No abscesses	5	50
Subligamentous spread greater than 3 vertebrae	85	40

From Jung NY, Jee WH, Ha KY, et al. Discrimination of tuberculous spondylitis from pyogenic spondylitis on MRI. *AJR Am J Roentgenol* 2004;182:1405–1410.

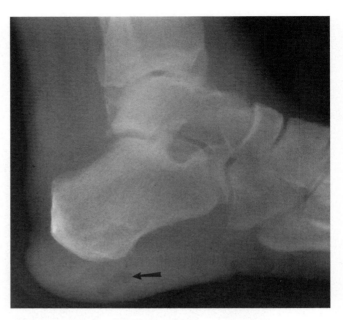

Figure 13-25 Lateral radiograph of the heel shows air in the soft tissues (*arrow*) due to soft tissue infection.

on fat-suppressed postcontrast T1-weighted images. Over time, the anterior end plates are destroyed, resulting in a gibbous deformity (Figs. 13-21 and 13-24) (25,84).

Jung et al. (88) evaluated MRI features of pyogenic and tuberculous spondylitis to determine if image features could differentiate the different infectious processes. Spinal and paraspinal features were studied (Table 13-6). Well-defined paraspinal signal abnormality was evident in 95% of patients with tuberculosis compared with only 23% of patients with pyogenic infections. Poorly defined paraspinal signal abnormality was seen in 75% of pyogenic infections and only 5% of patients with tuberculosis. Thin-walled abscesses (Fig. 13-24C) occurred in 95% of patients with tuberculosis, but only 5% of pyogenic infections. When abscesses were present in pyogenic infection, the walls were thick and irregular in 50%. Multilevel subligamentous involvement is also more common with tuberculosis (85%) compared to pyogenic (40%) infections.

The thoracic spine is also more frequently involved in patients with tuberculosis (40% compared to 10% with pyogenic infection). Using the above features, the sensitivity, specificity, and accuracy for identifying tuberculous spondylitis were 100%, 80%, and 90%, respectively. Sensitivity, specificity, and accuracy for pyogenic infection were 80%, 100%, and 90% (88).

Soft Tissue Infection

Most soft tissue infections are related to direct inoculation by a puncture wound or contamination in a region of skin abrasion (17,24,25,89). Symptoms vary depending upon the organism, host condition, location, and circulation (3). Soft tissue infections may be deep or superficial. Cellulitis is an infection of the skin and subcutaneous tissues. The offending organism is usually *Staphylococcus* or *Streptococcus* (7,51). Deep infections may involve muscle (myositis) or fascia (necrotizing fasciitis). Necrotizing fasciitis is a severe infection that involves the fascial planes (24,75). When superficial fascia is involved, this condition may be difficult to differentiate from cellulitis (51).

Soft tissue abscesses are usually well-defined fluid collections that may be deep or superficial. The walls may be thick compared to a cyst and there is surrounding soft tissue inflammation (7,22,54,80,90). Infection may also involve the tendons, tendon sheaths, or bursae (23–25,43).

Ultrasound, CT, or MRI may be used to evaluate soft tissue infections (7,30,51). Routine radiographs (see Fig. 13-25) may also provide useful information or assist in selecting the next modality to confirm soft tissue or bone infection. Ultrasound is useful for localizing foreign bodies and for detection and aspiration of fluid collections. However, MRI (see Fig. 13-26) provides more information regarding anatomy, extent of the infection, presence of abscesses or necrotic tissue, and involvement of adjacent osteoarticular structures (6,24,45).

MR images should be obtained using T1-weighted, T2-weighted and contrast-enhanced fat-suppressed T1-weighted images; STIR sequences are also useful in certain situations (3,7,22,45,75).

Cellulitis is an acute inflammatory process involving the deeper subcutaneous tissues. Staphylococcal organisms are commonly implicated. Patients may be affected at any age. This infection is particularly common in drug addicts (6,90). Patients with cellulitis demonstrate diffuse low signal

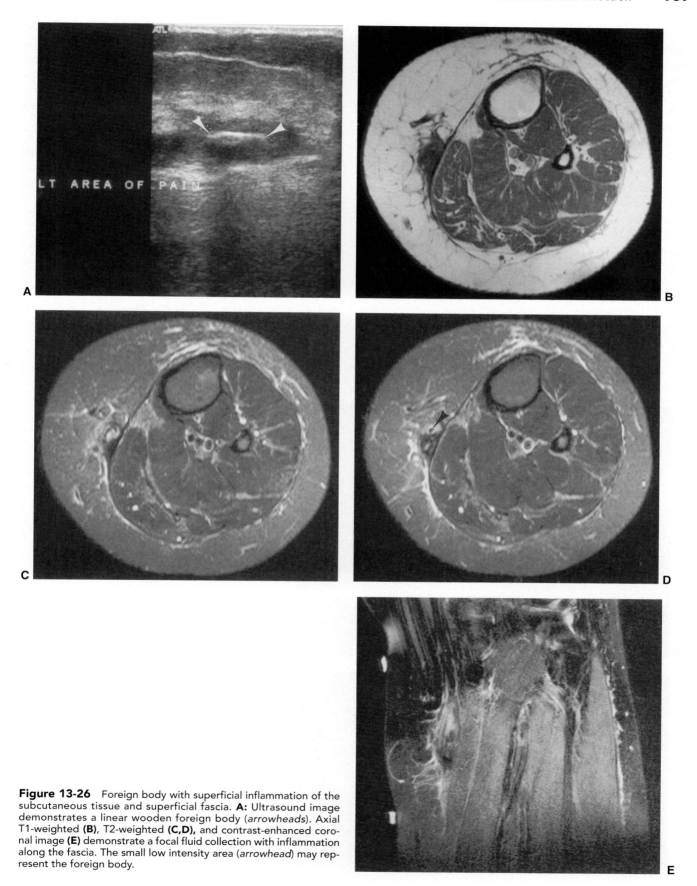

Figure 13-26 Foreign body with superficial inflammation of the subcutaneous tissue and superficial fascia. **A:** Ultrasound image demonstrates a linear wooden foreign body (*arrowheads*). Axial T1-weighted **(B)**, T2-weighted **(C,D)**, and contrast-enhanced coronal image **(E)** demonstrate a focal fluid collection with inflammation along the fascia. The small low intensity area (*arrowhead*) may represent the foreign body.

intensity in the subcutaneous tissues in the involved region. Signal intensity is increased on T2-weighted sequences (see Fig. 13-27). Tissues enhance with contrast, and adjacent superficial fascia may also enhance (3,20,24).

Necrotizing fasciitis is a severe infection involving the subcutaneous tissues and fascia. Group A streptococci alone or in combination with other organisms is commonly implicated. Systemic toxicity is common. Increased creatine phosphokinase is an indicator of progression from cellulites to necrotizing fasciitis (1,31). Necrotizing fasciitis involves the deep fascia (1). Increased signal intensity of the fascia on T2-weighted sequences is not specific (1,90). Thickening of the deep fascia associated with fluid collections and/or small abscesses are more specific features. Fascia enhances on postcontrast fat-suppressed T1-weighted images (see Fig. 13-28) (1).

Additional soft tissue changes may include areas of tissue necrosis, abscesses (see Figs. 13-29 and 13-30), granulomata, mycetomas, and cysts in echinococcal infections (28,32,37,50,74). Abscesses vary in size. However, signal intensity is low on T1-weighted and high on T2-weighted sequences (Fig. 13-29). Signal intensity may vary if there is debris within the abscess (11,62). The wall thickness varies, but enhancement is demonstrated on postcontrast images (Fig. 13-30) (22). In the foot, abscesses are commonly seen in diabetic patients and adjacent ulceration may be noted in up to 97% of cases (22).

Granulomas have mixed signal intensity on T1- and T2-weighted sequences. Histoplasmosis may present with small microabscesses with surrounding granulation tissue that enhances on postcontrast images. Mycetomas have a similar appearance to granulomas and typically are 2 to 5 mm in size (24,32,61).

Infection involving the muscle, tendons, tendon sheath, and bursae may be difficult to differentiate from other inflammatory disorders such as gout, rheumatoid arthritis, or foreign body reactions (17).

Tuberculosis tends to form soft tissue abscesses in the paraspinal region (Fig. 13-24) and also should be considered with greater trochanteric bursa infections or tendon

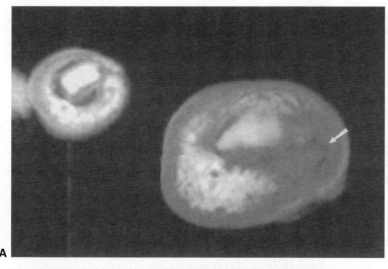

A

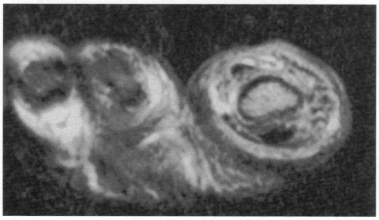

B

Figure 13-27 Soft tissue swelling and cellulitis due to a puncture wound. **A:** T1-weighted image shows swelling with low signal intensity (*arrow*). **B:** T2-weighted image demonstrates swelling with increased signal intensity in the subcutaneous tissues.

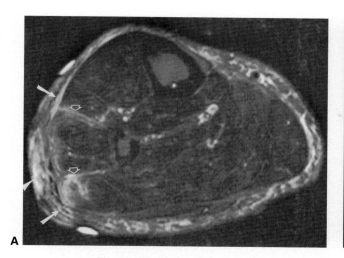

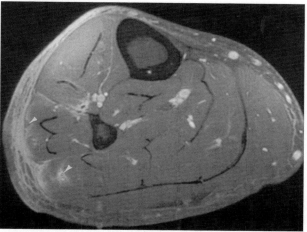

Figure 13-28 Fasciitis. **A:** Axial T2-weighted image demonstrates high signal intensity inflammation along the superficial fascia (*arrows*) with extension (*open arrows*) into the deep fascia. There is a superficial abscess (*arrowhead*). **B:** Contrast-enhanced fat-suppressed T1-weighted image demonstrates enhancement along the fascia with small microabscesses (*arrowheads*).

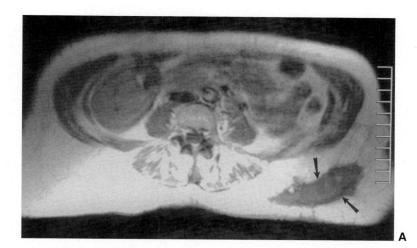

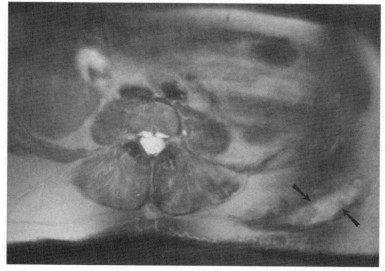

Figure 13-29 Axial T1- **(A)** and T2- **(B)** weighted images of a thick-walled pyogenic abscess (*arrows*).

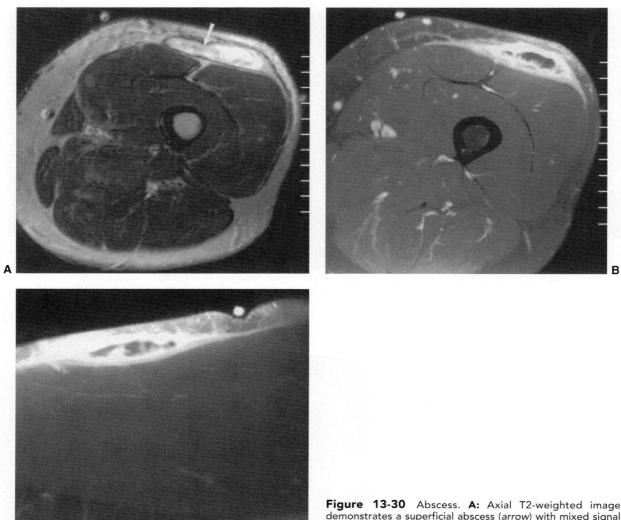

Figure 13-30 Abscess. **A:** Axial T2-weighted image demonstrates a superficial abscess (*arrow*) with mixed signal intensity due to debris. There is peripheral contrast enhancement on axial **(B)** and sagittal **(C)** fat-suppressed T1-weighted images.

sheath inflammation in the hand and wrist (see Fig. 13-31). Tuberculosis in the tendon sheaths of the hand and wrist demonstrates synovial thickening with enhancement. Low intensity densities (rice bodies) may be evident on T2-weighted sequences (Fig. 13-31) (91). Atypical mycobacterial infections have a similar presentation. However, carpal tunnel syndrome is a characteristic feature. Also, tuberculosis may involve any bursa while atypical mycobacterial infections tend to involve the superficial bursae of the elbow and knee (25). Diagnosis is often delayed due to misdiagnosis. Synovial biopsy and culture are necessary to confirm the diagnosis (17,25,26).

INFECTION IN VIOLATED TISSUE

Detection of infection in patients with violated bone and soft tissue presents a difficult diagnostic challenge. This includes patients with previous fracture or surgical intervention, either for fracture reduction or joint replacement (2,92–94). Radiographs and conventional or CT may be difficult to interpret in the early phases of infection due to the changes of fracture healing (Fig. 13-8). Radiographs may not demonstrate subtle changes adjacent to metal fixation devices and joint replacements for weeks. The usually reliable technetium-99m MDP scan can remain positive for more than 10 months following fracture or surgery, but technetium-99m or indium-111 labeled leukocytes and technetium-99m labeled antigranulocyte antibody scans have been more successful in these patients (28,48). Recently, PET studies have been sensitive and specific for demonstrating infection around metal implants (49). The anatomic detail and combination of joint aspiration and anesthetic injection have made subtraction arthrography a very useful technique for patients with joint replacement and suspected infection.

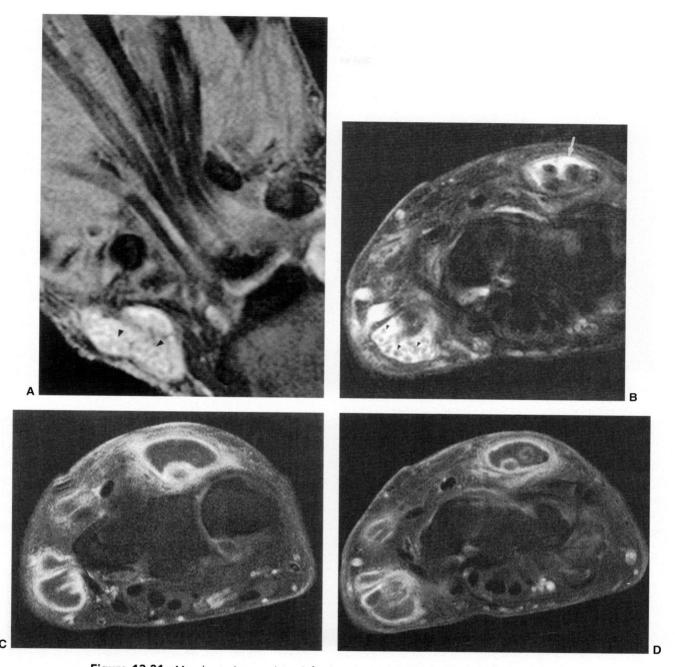

Figure 13-31 Mycobacterium marinum infection. Coronal DESS **(A)** image demonstrates fluid collections with multiple low intensity rice bodies (*arrowheads*). Axial fat-suppressed T2-weighted image **(B)** shows fluid around the extensor tendons (*arrow*) and rice bodies (*arrowheads*). Axial postcontrast fat-suppressed T1-weighted images **(C,D)** demonstrate synovial enhancement and distention of tendon sheaths.

In a review of the MRI studies in over 50 patients with infection in violated bone and soft tissues, we observed abnormalities in all examinations. However, in many cases it was difficult to differentiate areas of osteomyelitis from zones of fracture healing. Fracture healing results in cortical thickening with granulation tissue and fibrocartilage in the region of the fracture. T2-weighted images are most useful because they provide the best contrast between cortical bone and granulation tissue or fibrocartilage. Subtle changes in medullary bone can be seen with STIR sequences or postcontrast fat-suppressed T1-weighted images.

Routine radiographs, tomography, and CT are clearly very useful for identifying sequestra, which appear as areas of decreased signal on MR images (see Fig. 13-32). The artifact created by metal implants (on MR images), though often minimal, may prohibit evaluation of subtle bone

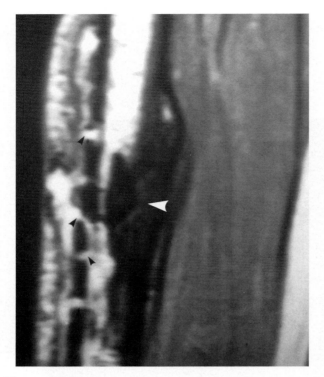

Figure 13-32 Sagittal T2-weighted image demonstrates a large, triangular, low signal intensity sequestrum (*arrowhead*) with fluid extending through old pin tracts (*small arrowheads*) and a superficial abscess.

changes immediately adjacent to the metal. However, we have found that periosteal changes and soft tissue abnormalities can be easily detected even in the region of the hip, where the amount and configuration of the metal tends to cause more artifact (Fig. 13-8) (7,57,80).

Kaim et al. (92) compared MRI with combined techneticum-99m MDP and antigranulocyte antibody scans in patients with chronic posttraumatic osteomyelitis. Assessment on MR images was limited by metal artifact in 17%. Four of 19 false-positive MR studies occurred due to enhancing granulation tissue. There were also four false-positive nuclear studies due to hemopoeitic marrow. MRI demonstrated infection as high signal intensity on T2- and contrast-enhanced T1-weighted fat-suppressed images (Fig. 13-32). Sequestra, sinus tracts, fistulae, and abscesses were also clearly demonstrated (Figs. 13-8 and 13-32). There were no false-negative studies. MRI demonstrated 100% sensitivity, 60% specificity, and 79% accuracy with a positive predictive value of 69% and negative predictive value of 100%. Nuclear scans demonstrated a sensitivity of 77%, specificity of 50%, and accuracy of 61%. The positive predictive value was 58% and negative predictive value 71% for nuclear studies (92). When both studies were combined, the data was improved. Specificity increased to 80% (MRI 60%, nuclear 50%), accuracy to 89% (MRI 79%, nuclear 61%), and the positive predictive value increased to 82% (MRI 69%, nuclear 58%).

In the first year following surgery, marrow edema with contrast enhancement are not useful MR image features compared to similar findings in nonviolated (no prior surgery or trauma) osseous structures (27,92).

A high percentage of adult patients with chronic osteomyelitis require surgical therapy for excision of necrotic or infected tissue. The use of free vascularized muscle, omental, and bone grafts is increasing in the treatment of patients with chronic osteomyelitis (45,69,76, 94–97). Reconstructive procedures may be needed depending on the vascularity of adjacent tissue and the size and type of defect (69). There are several basic goals

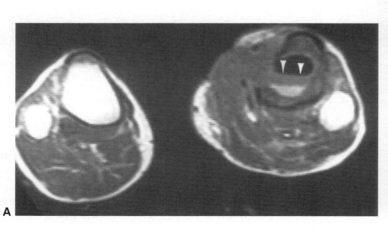
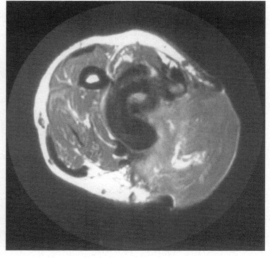

Figure 13-33 Postoperative muscle grafts following surgery for chronic infection. **A:** Axial T1-weighted image after muscle graft demonstrates an air–fluid level (*arrowheads*) indicating residual dead space that will result in recurrent infection. **B:** Axial T1-weighted image of the distal leg demonstrates the muscle graft fills the curetted dead space.

regardless of the tissue or technique used. These include wound coverage, obliteration of dead space (which may permit survival of existing organisms or provide a medium for recurrent infection), and provision of optimal vascular supply to the described area (69,94,96).

Preoperative assessment should include review of the necessary information and planning of the surgical approach; postoperative assessment should determine whether or not the surgical goals have been achieved. Preoperatively, MRI is an ideal technique to assess the extent of bone and soft tissue involvement, as well as detect skip areas. Preoperative images also serve as a valuable baseline to determine later whether the surgical goals have been achieved.

MRI is well suited to evaluate defect coverage or dead space, residual infection, and hematomas or fluid collections, which may serve as media for recurrent infection (see Fig. 13-33). MRI is particularly useful in the evaluation of omental and muscle flaps. Keep in mind that over time, muscle becomes mainly fatty tissue due to disuse. Vascularized fibular grafts can be evaluated, but the small amount of marrow presents certain problems, since there is little fibular marrow to image in the axial plane. This can be improved by using coronal and sagittal views that increase the marrow volume imaged and permit the position, as well as the proximal distal attachments of the grafts, to be more easily evaluated.

Intravenous, Gd-DTPA has been used to confirm viability of vascularized grafts. Varnell et al. (98) demonstrated that viable grafts enhanced, while those with early vascular occlusion did not enhance. Lomasney et al. (99) studied vascularized fibular grafts 1 week after surgery with gadolinium and two-dimensional time of flight (TOF) MR angiography. Gadolinium was useful for evaluating surgical success as enhancement occurred in viable grafts. MR angiographic sequences were not as useful.

Further studies and follow-up of these patients will be needed to determine the effectiveness of MRI in evaluating viability and flow factors in the grafts. Spectroscopy may also play a role in graft evaluation, especially of early ischemic changes (see Chapter 16).

REFERENCES

1. Schmid MR, Kossmann T, Duewells S. Differentiation of necrotizing fasciitis and cellulitis using MR imaging. *AJR Am J Roentgenol* 1998;170(3):615–620.
2. Seabold JE, Nepola JV, Conrad GR, et al. Detection of osteomyelitis at fracture nonunion sites: comparison of two scintigraphic methods. *AJR Am J Roentgenol* 1989;152:1021–1027.
3. Tower JD. The use of intravenous contrast in MRI of extremity infection. *Semin Ultrasound CT MR* 1997;18(4):269–275.
4. Fletcher BD, Scoles PV, Nelson AD. Osteomyelitis in children: detection by magnetic resonance. *Radiology* 1984;150:57–60.
5. Gold RH, Hawkins RA, Katz RD. Bacterial osteomyelitis: findings on plain radiography, CT, MR and scintigraphy. *AJR Am J Roentgenol* 1991;157:365–370.
6. Resnick D. Osteomyelitis, septic arthritis and soft tissue infections: mechanisms and situations. In: Resnick D, ed. *Diagnosis of bone and joint disorders*. Philadelphia, PA: WB Saunders, 2002:2377–2480.
7. Berquist TH. *Radiology of the foot and ankle*, 2nd ed. Philadelphia, PA: Lippincott Williams & Wilkins, 2000.
8. Jaramillo D, Treves ST, Kasser JR, et al. Osteomyelitis and septic arthritis in children: appropriate use of imaging to guide treatment. *AJR Am J Roentgenol* 1995;165:399–403.
9. Rahmouni A, Chosidow O, Mathieu D, et al. MR imaging of acute infectious cellulitis. *Radiology* 1994;192:493–496.
10. Waldvogel FA, Medoff G, Sehwartz MN. Osteomyelitis: a review of clinical features, therapeutic considerations, and unusual aspects. *N Engl J Med* 1970;282:198–206.
11. Wall SD, Fisher MR, Amparo EG, et al. Magnetic resonance imaging in the evaluation of abscesses. *Am J Roentgenol* 1985;144:1217–1221.
12. Bonakdapour A, Gaines VD. The radiology of osteomyelitis. *Orthop Clin North Am* 1983;14:21–37.
13. Chamot A, Benhanaou CL, Morris CS, et al. The syndrome of acne hyperostose osteite (SAPHO). *Rev Rhum* 1987;54:187–196.
14. Erdman WA, Tomburro F, Jayson HT, et al. Osteomyelitis: characteristics and pitfalls of MR imaging. *Radiology* 1991;180:533–539.
15. Quinn SF, Murray W, Clark RA, et al. MR imaging of chronic osteomyelitis. *J Comput Assist Tomogr* 1988;12:113–117.
16. Morrison WB, Schweitzer ME, Wapner KL, et al. Osteomyelitis in feet of diabetics: clinical accuracy, surgical utility and cost-effectiveness of MR imaging. *Radiology* 1995;196:557–564.
17. Amrami KK, Sundaram M, Shin AY, et al. Mycobacterium marinum infections of the distal upper extremities: clinical course and imaging findings in two cases with delayed diagnosis. *Skeletal Radiol* 2003;32:546–549.
18. Ledermann HP, Morrison WB, Schweitzer ME. Is soft tissue inflammation a pedal infection contained by fascial planes? Analysis of compartmental involvement in 115 feet. *AJR Am J Roentgenol* 2002;178(3):605–612.
19. Moore TE, Yuh WTC, Kathol MH, et al. Abnormalities of the foot in patients with diabetes mellitus: findings on MR imaging. *AJR Am J Roentgenol* 1991;157:813–816.
20. Ledermann HP, Schweitzer ME, Morrison WB. Non-enhancing tissue on MR imaging of pedal infection: characterization of necrotic tissue and associate limitations for diagnosis of osteomyelitis and abscess. *AJR Am J Roentgenol* 2002;178(1):215–222.
21. Ledermann HP, Morrison WB, Schweitzer ME. MR image analysis of pedal osteomyelitis: distribution patterns of spread and frequency of associated ulceration and septic arthritis. *Radiology* 2002;223(3):747–755.
22. Ledermann HP, Morrison WB, Schweitzer ME. Pedal abscesses in patients suspected of having pedal osteomyelitis: analysis with MR imaging. *Radiology* 2002;224(3):649–655.
23. Ledermann HP, Morrison WB, Schweitzer ME, et al. Tendon involvement in pedal infection: MR analysis of frequency, distribution and spread of infection. *AJR Am J Roentgenol* 2002;179(4):939–947.
24. Sarris I, Berendt AR, Athanosous N, et al. MRI of mycetoma of the foot: two cases demonstrating the dot-in-circle sign. *Skeletal Radiol* 2003;32(3):179–183.
25. Theodorou DJ, Theodorou SJ, Kakitsubata Y, et al. Imaging characteristics and epidemiologic features of atypical mycobacterial infections involving the musculoskeletal system. *AJR Am J Roentgenol* 2001;176:341–349.
26. Wongworawt MD, Holton P, Learch TJ, et al. A prolonged case of Mycobacterium marinum flexor tenosynovitis: radiographic, and histological correlation, and review of the literature. *Skeletal Radiol* 2003;32:542–545.
27. Kaim A, Ledermann HP, Bongartz G, et al. Chronic post-traumatic osteomyelitis of the lower extremity: comparison of magnetic resonance imaging and combined bone scintigraphy/immune-scintigraphy with radio labeled monoclonal antigranulocyte antibodies. *Skeletal Radiol* 2000;29:378–386.
28. Merkel KD, Brown ML, Dewanjee MK, et al. Comparison of indium-labeled leukocyte imaging with sequential technetium-gallium scanning in diagnosis of low-grade musculoskeletal sepsis: a prospective study. *J Bone Joint Surg Am* 1985;67A:465–476.
29. Orpen NM, Birch NC. Delayed presentation of septic arthritis of a lumbar facet joint after diagnostic facet injection. *J Spinal Disord Tech* 2003;16(3):285–287.
30. Boutin RD, Joachim B, Sartoris DJ, et al. Update of imaging of orthopedic infections. *Orthop Clin North Am* 1998;29:41–66.

31. Resnick D. Osteomyelitis, septic arthritis and soft tissue infections: organisms. In: Resnick D, ed. *Diagnosis of bone and joint disorders*. Philadelphia, PA: WB Saunders, 2002:2510–2624.

32. Guhlmann A, Brecht-Krause D, Suger S, et al. Chronic osteomyelitis detection with FDG PET and correlation with histopathologic findings. *Radiology* 1998;206:749–754.

33. Merkele EM, Schulte M, Vogel J, et al. Musculoskeletal involvement in cystic echinococcosis: report of eight cases and review of the literature. *AJR Am J Roentgenol* 1997;168(6):1531–1534.

34. Nakamura H, Nakamura T, Suzuki M, et al. Disseminated coccidioidomycosis with intra- and para-vertebral abscesses. *J Infect Chemother* 202;8(2):178–181.

35. Garvin GJ, Peterfly CG. Soft tissue coccidiodomycosis on MRI. *J Comput Assist Tomogr* 1995;19(4):612–614.

36. Kim HY, Song K-S, Guo JM, et al. Thoracic sequalae and complications of tuberculosis. *Radiographics* 2001;21:839–860.

37. Ledermann HP, Schweitzer ME, Morrison WB, et al. MR imaging findings in spinal infections: rules or myths. *Radiology* 2003; 228(2):506–514.

38. Morris BS, Varma R, Grag A, et al. Multifocal musculoskeletal tuberculosis in children: appearances on computed tomography. *Skeletal Radiol* 2002;31:1–8.

39. Robiller FC, Stumpe KDM, Kossmann T, et al. Chronic osteomyelitis of the femur: value of PET imaging. *Eur Radiol* 2000;10:855–858.

40. Bellussi A, Busi Rizzi E, Schinina V, et al. STIR sequence in infectious sacroiliitis in three patients. *Clin Imaging* 2002;26(3):212–215.

41. Beltran J, Campanini S, Knight C, et al. The diabetic foot: magnetic resonance imaging evaluation. *Skeletal Radiol* 1990;19:37–41.

42. Hayem G, Bouchard-Chabot A, Benali K, et al. SAPHO Syndrome: long term following study of 120 cases. *Semin Arthritis Rheum* 1999;293:159–171.

43. Jaovisidha S, Chen C, Ryu KN, et al. Tuberculous tenosynovitis and bursitis: Imaging findings in 21 cases. *Radiology* 1996;201:507–513.

44. Longo M, Granata F, Ricciardi K, et al. Contrast enhanced MR imaging with fat suppression in adult-onset septic spondylodiscitis. *Eur Radiol* 2003;13(3):626–637.

45. Fleckenstein JL, Burns DK, Murphy FK, et al. Differential diagnosis of bacterial myositis in AIDS: evaluation with MR imaging. *Radiology* 1991;179:653–658.

46. Earwalker JWS, Cotton A. SAPHO: syndrome or concept? Imaging findings. *Skeletal Radiol* 2003;32:311–327.

47. Graif M, Schweitzer MR, Deely D, et al. The septic versus non-septic inflamed joint: MR characteristics. *Skeletal Radiol* 1999;28:616–620.

48. Guhlmann A, Brecht-Krause D, Suger G, et al. Fluorine-18-FDG PE and technetium-99m antigranulocyte antibody scintigraphy in chronic osteomyelitis. *J Nucl Med* 1998;39:2145–2152.

49. Schiesser M, Stumpe KDM, Trentz O, et al. Detection of metallic implant associated infections with FDG PET in patients with trauma: correlation with microbiological results. *Radiology* 2003;226:391–398.

50. Stumpe KDM, Zanetti M, Weisharpt D, et al. FDG position emission tomography for differentiation of degenerative and infectious end plate abnormalities in the lumbar spine detected on MR imaging. *AJR Am J Roentgenol* 2002;179:1151–1157.

51. Ma LD, Frassica FJ, Bluemke DA, et al. CT and MRI evaluation of musculoskeletal infection. *Crit Rev Diagn Imaging* 1997;36(5):535–568.

52. Jacobson AF, Harley JD, Lipsky BA, et al. Diagnosis of osteomyelitis in the presence of soft tissue infection and radiographic evidence of osseous abnormalities: value of leukocyte scintigraphy. *AJR Am J Roentgenol* 1991;157:807–812.

53. Morrison WB, Schweitzer ME, Bock GW, et al. Diagnosis of osteomyelitis. Utility of fat-suppressed contrast-enhanced MR imaging. *Radiology* 1993;189:251–257.

54. Cohen MD, Klatte EC, Baehner R, et al. Magnetic resonance imaging of bone marrow disease in children. *Radiology* 1984;151:715–718.

55. Chandnani VP, Beltran J, Morris CS, et al. Acute experimental osteomyelitis and abscesses: detection with MR imaging versus CT. *Radiology* 1990;174:223–226.

56. Beltran J, McGhee RB, Shaffer PB, et al. Experimental infections of the musculoskeletal system: evaluation with MR imaging and Tc-99m MDP and Ga-67 scintigraphy. *Radiology* 1988;167:167–172.

57. Beltran J, Nato AM, McGhee RB, et al. Infections of the musculoskeletal system: high-field-strength MR imaging. *Radiology* 1987;164:449–454.

58. Hopkins KL, Li KCP, Bergman G. Gadolinium-DTPA-enhanced magnetic resonance imaging of musculoskeletal infectious processes. *Skeletal Radiol* 1995;24:325–330.

59. Sharma P. MR features of tuberculous osteomyelitis. *Skeletal Radiol* 2003;32:279–285.

60. Ridely N, Shaikh MI, Remedios D, et al. Radiology of skeletal tuberculosis. *Orthopedics* 1998;21:1213–1220.

61. Holley K, Muldoon M, Tasker S. Coccidioides immitis osteomyelitis: a case series review. *Orthopedics* 2002;25(8):827–831.

62. Cohen JM, Weinreb JC, Maravilla KR. Fluid collections in the intraperitoneal and extraperitoneal spaces: comparison of MR and CT. *Radiology* 1985;155:705–708.

63. Demharter J, Bohndorf K, Michl W, et al. Chronic recurrent multifocal osteomyelitis: a radiological and clinical investigation of five cases. *Skeletal Radiol* 1997;26:579–588.

64. Resnick D. Enostosis, hyperostosis and periostitis. In: Resnick D, ed. *Diagnosis of bone and joint disorders*. Philadelphia, PA: WB Saunders, 2002:4844–4919.

65. Gerscovich EO, Greenspan A. Osteomyelitis of the clavicle: clinical radiologic and bacterial findings in 10 patients. *Skeletal Radiol* 1994;23:205–210.

66. Duzgun N, Peksari Y, Sonel B, et al. Localization of extra pulmonary tuberculosis in the synovial membrane, skin, and meninges in a patient with systemic lupus erythematosis and IgG deficiency. *Rheumatol Int* 2002;22(1):41–44.

67. Kahn MF, Chamot A-M. SAPHO syndrome. *Rheum Dis Clin North Am* 1992;18:225–246.

68. Nachtigal A, Cardinal E, Burlase BL, et al. Vertebral involvement with SAPHO: MRI findings. *Skeletal Radiol* 1999;28:163–168.

69. Weiland AJ. Symposium: the use of muscle flaps in the treatment of osteomyelitis in the lower extremity. *Contemp Orthop* 1985;10:127–159.

70. Santoro JP, Cachia VV, Sartoris DJ, et al. Nonspecific inflammation in the foot demonstrated by magnetic resonance imaging. *J Foot Surg* 1988;27:478–483.

71. Yuh WTC, Corson JD, Baraniewski HM, et al. Osteomyelitis of the foot in diabetic patients: evaluation with plain film, 99mTc-MDP bone scintigraphy and MR imaging. *AJR Am J Roentgenol* 1989;152:795–800.

72. Hong SH, Kim SM, Ahn JM, et al. Tuberculous versus pyogenic arthritis: MR imaging evaluation. *Radiology* 2001;218:848–853.

73. Kelly PJ, Martin WJ, Coventry MB. Bacterial arthritis in the adult. *J Bone Joint Surg Am* 1970;52A:1595–1602.

74. Kocher MS, Zurakowski D, Kasser JR. Differentiating between septic arthritis and transient synovitis of the hip in children: an evidence-based clinical prediction algorithm. *J Bone Joint Surg Am* 1999;81A:1662–1670.

75. Lee SW, Suh KJ, Kun YW, et al. Septic arthritis versus transient synovitis at MR imaging: preliminary assessment with signal intensity alterations in bone marrow. *Radiology* 1999;211:459–465.

76. Arnold PG, Irons GB. Lower extremity muscle flaps. *Orthop Clin North Am* 1984;15:441–449.

77. Phemister DB, Hatcher CH. Correlation of pathological and recent roentgenographic findings in diagnosis of tuberculosis arthritis. *AJR Am J Roentgenol* 1933;29:736–738.

78. Eustace S, DiMai M, Adams J, et al. In vitro and in vivo spin-echo diffusion imaging characteristics of synovial fluid: potential non-invasive differentiation of inflammatory and degenerative arthritis. *Skeletal Radiol* 2000;29:320–323.

79. Brown JJ, vanSonnenberg E, Gerber KH, et al. Magnetic resonance relaxation times of percutaneously obtained normal and abnormal body fluids. *Radiology* 1985;154:727–731.

80. Beltran J, Noto AM, Herman LJ, et al. Joint effusions: MR imaging. *Radiology* 1986;158:133–137.

81. Karchevsky M, Schweitzer ME, Morrison WB, et al. MRI findings of septic arthritis and associated osteomyelitis in adults. *AJR Am J Roentgenol* 2004;182:119–122.

82. Modic MT, Feiglin DH, Piraino DW, et al. Vertebral osteomyelitis: assessment using MR. *Radiology* 1985;157:157–166.

83. Modic MT, Pflanze W, Feiglin DHI, et al. Magnetic resonance imaging of musculoskeletal infections. *Radiol Clin North Am* 1986;24:247–258.

84. Stabler A, Reiser MF. Imaging of spinal infection. *Radiol Clin North Am* 2001;39(1):115–135.

85. Mehta JS, Bhojraj SY. Tuberculosis of the thoracic spine. A classification based upon surgical strategies. *J Bone Joint Surg Br* 2001; 83(6):859–863.

86. Akman S, Sirvanci M, Talu U, et al. Magnetic resonance imaging of tuberculous spondylitis. *Orthopedics* 2003;26(1):69–73.

87. Lolge S, Maheshwari M, Shah J, et al. Isolated solitary vertebral body tuberculosis—study of seven cases. *Clin Radiol* 2003;58(7): 545–550.

88. Jung N-Y, Jee W-H, Ha K-Y, et al. Discrimiation of tuberculous spondylitis from pyogenic spondiytis on MRI. *AJR Am J Roentgenol* 2004;182:1405–1410.

89. Weishaupt D, Schweitzer ME, Alain F, et al. MR imaging of inflammatory joint diseases of the foot and ankle. *Skeletal Radiol* 1999;28:663–669.

90. Loh NN, Chen IY, Cheung LP, et al. Deep fascial hyperintensity in soft tissue abnormalities as revealed by T2-weighted MR imaging. *AJR Am J Roentgenol* 1997;168(5):1301–1304.

91. Hoffman KL, Bergman AG, Hoffman DK, et al. Tuberculosis tenosynovitis of the flexor tendons of the wrist: MR imaging with pathologic correlation. *Skeletal Radiol* 1996;25:180–188.

92. Kaim AH, Gross T, von Schulthess GK. Imaging of chronic post-traumatic osteomyelitis. *Eur Radiol* 202;12(5):1193–1202.

93. Sandrasegaran K, Scifuddin MB, Coral A, et al. Magnetic resonance imaging of septic sacroiliitis. *Skeletal Radiol* 1994;23:289–292.

94. Wood MB, Cooney WP III. Vascularized bone segment transfers for management of chronic osteomyelitis. *Orthop Clin North Am* 1984;15:401–472.

95. Irons GB, Fisher J, Schmitt EH. Vascularized muscular and musculo-cutaneous flaps for management of osteomyelitis. *Orthop Clin North Am* 1984;15:473–480.

96. Weiland AJ, Moore JR, David RK. The efficacy of free tissue transfer in treatment of osteomyelitis. *J Bone Joint Surg* 1984;66A:181–193.

97. Fitzgerald RH, Ruttle PE, Arnold PG, et al. Local muscle flaps in the treatment of chronic osteomyelitis. *J Bone Joint Surg Am* 1985;67A:175–185.

98. Varnell RM, Flint DW, Dalley RW, et al. Myocutaneous flap failure: early detection with Gd-DTPA-enhanced MR imaging. *Radiology* 1989;173:755–758.

99. Lomasney LM, Madden JF, Rizk WS, et al. Dynamic contrast-enhanced MR imaging assessment of vascularized free fibular grafts. *J Magn Reson Imaging* 1994;4:441–449.

Diffuse Marrow Diseases

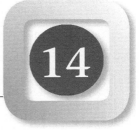

14

James B. Vogler, III   William A. Murphy, Jr.

As one of the larger and more important organs in the human body, bone marrow plays important physiologic roles in both health and disease. In healthy individuals, its function is to provide a continual supply of red cells, platelets, and white cells to meet the body's demands for oxygenation, coagulation, and immunity. As such, bone marrow frequently becomes a target, either directly or indirectly, of many varied disease processes. The way in which marrow responds can, at times, be dramatic.

Until recently, *in vivo* imaging of certain physiologic functions and anatomic features of bone marrow has been limited. Historically, many methods have been utilized and still remain useful, despite shortcomings. Plain film radiography provides an excellent anatomic overview but is limited in detecting even considerable amounts (30% to 50%) of trabecular bone loss that might result from an intramedullary process. More importantly, a radiograph does not detect cellular changes in marrow. Scintigraphy using 99m-technetium phosphate or sulfur colloid tracers affords a physiologic survey of either marrow constituents themselves or the surrounding osseous elements. Physiologic processes such as hematopoietic and phagocytosis can be evaluated (1). Lack of anatomic detail and low specificity, however, are recognized shortcomings. Fluorine-18-fluorodeoxyglucose positron emission tomography (FDG PET) relies on increased glucose metabolism of tumor cells to identify early bone marrow infiltration by malignant neoplasms (2,3). Sensitivities of this modality rival or exceed those of routine MR pulse sequences (2); however, specificity has yet to be established. Computed tomography (CT) provides excellent in-plane spatial resolution (on the order of 0.35 mm) and contrast resolution (on the order of 0.5%) (4). These capabilities allow excellent definition of cortical bone, trabecular bone, and, to a lesser degree, the intramedullary space. The nature of CT is such that extended anatomic regions cannot be evaluated without sacrificing resolution or substantially increasing radiation exposure.

By combining multiplanar images, excellent spatial resolution, superior contrast discrimination and high sensitivity, magnetic resonance imaging (MRI) has greatly improved the ability for *in vivo* assessment of normal and abnormal bone marrow. With this imaging method, the continuous change of normal bone marrow patterns throughout life, the varied responses of marrow cell populations to disease and the introduction of nonmarrow cell populations can be monitored (5).

NORMAL BONE MARROW

Anatomy and Physiology

The basic microstructure of bone marrow consists of an osseous framework housing fat cells and hematopoietic cells both supported by a system of reticulum cells, nerves, and vascular sinusoids (6). The trabecular or cancellous bone is composed of primary and bridging secondary trabeculae. By volume, this osseous tissue occupies 15% of the bone cavity and provides both architectural support and a mineral depot (7). Cellular constituents of marrow occupy the remaining 85%. These constituents include all stages of erythrocytic and leukocytic development, as well as fat cells and reticulum cells (8). Erythrocytic, granulocytic, and megakaryocytic cell lines replenish the body's supply of red cells, white cells, and platelets. The role of fat cells in marrow function is unclear. Speculation suggests that fat cells provide surface and nutritional support and possibly growth factors for hematopoiesis (6,9). Reticulum cells consist of both phagocytic cells (macrophages) that play a role in immunity and undifferentiated nonphagocytic cells (10) whose role is yet to be fully defined. In red marrow, these nonphagocytic reticulum cells occur in greater abundance in perivascular locations and form a reticular meshwork that provides nutritional and mechanical support to the hematopoietic cells (11,12). These reticular cells appear to have the capacity to accumulate lipid and transform into the fat cells of red and yellow marrow. The capability of these cells to become either red or yellow marrow components aids in explaining the capacity of red marrow to expand or retract in response to various physiologic stimuli as will be discussed later (12,13).

The various components of normal marrow (fat cells, hematopoietic cells, reticulum cells, trabeculae, vessels, and nerves) may be simplified into a unifying concept—that of red and yellow marrow. That fraction of bone marrow actively involved in the production of blood cells is termed hematopoietic or "red marrow." The remaining fraction, which is hematopoietically inactive, is termed "yellow marrow." Important anatomic and compositional differences exist between these two types of marrow (8). On average, the chemical composition of red marrow is approximately 40% water, 40% fat, and 20% protein (8). The cellular composition of red marrow is 60% hematopoietic cells and 40% fat cells (8,14). Red marrow has a rich, arborized vascular network. Yellow marrow's chemical composition is approximately 15% water, 80% fat, 5% protein (8). Its cellular composition is 95% fat cells and 5% nonfat cells (8,14). Physiologically, the fat cells in yellow marrow are relatively stable, while those in red marrow appear to be labile (15). Yellow marrow has a sparse vascular network.

At birth, virtually the entire marrow space contains red marrow. During growth and development, conversion of red to yellow marrow occurs throughout the skeleton. This is a normal physiologic process and has a predictable and orderly pattern. This conversion begins in the immediate postnatal period and is first evident in the terminal phalanges of the hands and feet (16). The process then progresses from peripheral (appendicular) toward central (axial), with respect to the skeleton as a whole, and from diaphyseal to metaphyseal in individual long bones (see Fig. 14-1). Within the marrow cavity of long bones, conversion is seen first in the central medullary space from where it progresses toward the diaphyseal and then the metaphyseal subcortical bone. Flat bones and vertebral

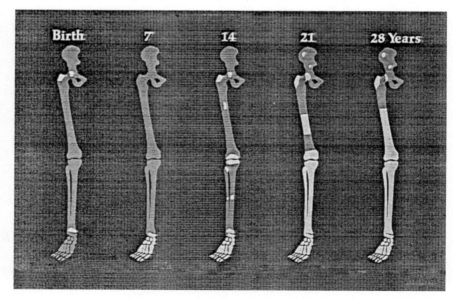

Figure 14-1 Age-related changes in red/yellow marrow distribution based on histologic studies. The natural conversion of red to yellow marrow is illustrated by drawings of the right lower extremity at seven-year increments. At birth, virtually the entire ossified skeleton contains red marrow. Conversion of red to yellow marrow begins shortly after birth and is first evident in the distal appendicular skeleton (hands and feet). Through the ensuing years, the process gradually progresses from distal to proximal with respect to the skeleton as a whole and from diaphyseal to epiphyseal in individual long bones. (Adapted from Hashimoto M. Pathology of bone marrow. *Acta Haematol* 1962;27:193–216 and Chen W, Shih TT, Chen R, et al. Vertebral bone marrow perfusion evaluated with dynamic contrast-enhanced MR imaging: significance of aging and sex. *Radiology* 2001;220:213–218; and Kricun ME. Red-yellow marrow conversion: its effect on the location of some solitary bone lesions. *Skeletal Radiol* 1985;14:10–19.)

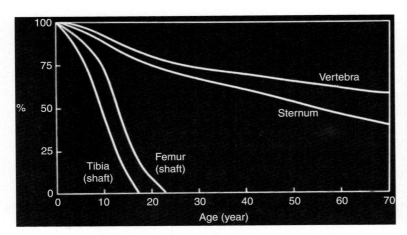

Figure 14-2 Conversion of red to yellow marrow. Changes in the red marrow fraction (percentage cellularity red marrow) at specific anatomic sites are illustrated on this graph. The rate and extent of conversion differs between axial (vertebra and sternum) and appendicular (tibia and femur) sites. The axial skeleton demonstrates a more gradual decline in the red marrow fraction with substantial amounts of red marrow persisting throughout life. The rate of red to yellow marrow conversion in the appendicular skeleton is more rapid with little red marrow persisting in the tibial and femoral shafts beyond 25 years of age. (Adapted from Custer RP. Studies on the structure and function of bone marrow. I. Variability of the hemopoietic pattern and consideration of method for examination. *J Lab Clin Med* 1932;17:951–959.)

bodies show similar patterns with conversion moving from the central medullary space toward the metaphyseal equivalents. Although generally symmetric, the rate and extent of conversion is not uniform but varies according to site in a particular bone as well as among bones (see Fig. 14-2).

Epiphyses and apophyses must be considered independently. These structures lack marrow until they begin to ossify. What remains unclear is how much red marrow appears at these sites and how long it persists. Undoubtedly, any red marrow contained in these structures undergoes rapid, although not necessarily complete, conversion to yellow marrow. The conversion begins in the central marrow cavity and progresses toward the subchondral or peripheral subcortical bone. Thus, as a general rule, epiphyseal and apophyseal ossification centers can be thought of as containing yellow marrow from very early in growth and development. Yellow marrow persists in epiphyses and apophyses throughout life, with the proximal femoral and proximal humeral epiphyses/apophyses being limited exceptions to this rule. Other exceptions may exist; however, to date they remain unidentified.

Usually by 25 years of age, the process of primary red marrow conversion to yellow marrow is complete and a balanced distribution of red and yellow marrow has been achieved (17–20). This balance will vary from person to person as it is influenced by at least age, gender, and health. Similarly, the balance between red and yellow marrow achieved in individual bones varies by location. Red marrow is predominately concentrated in the axial skeleton (skull, vertebrae, ribs, sternum, and pelvis) and the proximal appendicular skeleton (proximal femora and humeri) (see Fig. 14-3). Yellow marrow dominates the remaining portion of the appendicular skeleton and is variably admixed throughout the axial skeleton. Physiologic conversion of red to yellow marrow continues after 25 years of age, albeit at a slower pace, as evidenced by the declining fraction of red marrow at axial sites throughout adult life (Fig. 14-2) (21). This process can also be observed in the proximal femoral and humeral metaphyses (22). In men, most of the red marrow conversion that will

occur at these sites is nearly complete by 35 years of age, while women may display predominantly red marrow at these locations until 55 years of age (23–25).

The boundaries of red and yellow marrow are not absolute and variations in this generally accepted adult pattern do exist. Islands of hematopoietic tissue may be found in areas dominated by fatty marrow and vice versa. Likewise, it is considered normal to find red marrow occupying up to two thirds of the proximal femoral and humeral shafts (8,18,26,27). The red/yellow marrow distribution continues to change slowly with advancing age as the red marrow fraction in individual bones declines (28). Factors modulating this conversion of red to yellow marrow are largely unknown; however, temperature (29), vascularity (20), and low oxygen tension (30) have been implicated.

The process of red to yellow marrow conversion is, at times, halted or reversed as alterations in the body's demand for hematopoiesis provoke a "reconversion" of yellow marrow to red marrow. During this reconversion, yellow marrow is transformed to red marrow throughout the skeleton in the reverse sequence of the primary red to yellow marrow conversion described above. Thus, the process occurs first in the axial skeleton followed by the appendicular skeleton in a proximal to distal sequence (19–21,31) (see Fig. 14-4). Within individual bones, reconversion is first seen at endosteal locations in metaphyses or epiphyses or their equivalents. From there, it progresses toward the central marrow space and toward the diaphyseal subcortical bone, ultimately extending into the central diaphyseal marrow cavity. Temperature (29), low oxygen tension (30), and elevated erythropoietin (32) are again implicated in initiating and modulating this process, although the actual mechanisms and controlling factors remain largely unknown.

MAGNETIC RESONANCE FEATURES

Red and Yellow Marrow

Fat, water, protein, and minerals are the basic constituents of bone marrow that contribute to the formation of its MR

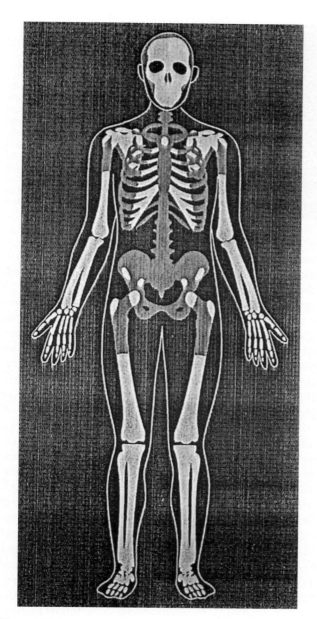

Figure 14-3 Adult pattern of red/yellow marrow based on histologic studies. Usually by 25 years of age, the primary conversion of red to yellow marrow has been accomplished and the adult distribution of red/yellow marrow established. Red marrow is concentrated in the axial and proximal appendicular skeleton while yellow marrow occupies the remainder of the appendicular skeleton. (Adapted from Hashimoto M. Pathology of bone marrow. *Acta Haematol* 1962;27:193–216 and Chen W, Shih TT, Chen R, et al. Vertebral bone marrow perfusion evaluated with dynamic contrast-enhanced MR imaging: significance of aging and sex. *Radiology* 2001;220:213–218 and Kricun ME. Red-yellow marrow conversion: its effect on the location of some solitary bone lesions. *Skeletal Radiol* 1985; 14:10–19.)

image (27). As relative amounts of these constituents change, the signal intensity of marrow is altered accordingly. Fat cells are responsible for the greatest fraction of marrow signal on T1-weighted images. Most protons in fat are contained in hydrophobic CH2 groups and

demonstrate very efficient spin-lattice relaxation, resulting in a particularly short T1 relaxation time and thus high signal intensity on T1-weighted spin-echo images (33,34). Spin–spin relaxation of fat is less efficient, resulting in some prolongation of its T2 relaxation time and thus moderate signal intensity on T2-weighted spin-echo images.

Water in tissue is thought to exist in different forms. Tissues rich in free water (extracellular water) show longer T1 and T2 relaxation times, while those having greater amounts of bound (intracellular) water demonstrate a shortening of T1 and T2 relaxation values (35). The relative contribution of each type of water to overall marrow signal is not clearly defined. Nevertheless, as the amount of marrow water increases, it is logical to expect lower signal intensity on T1-weighted images and higher signal intensity on T2-weighted images.

The contribution of protein to marrow signal intensity is poorly understood. Protein in general has a long T1 relaxation time due to the large size of the molecules (35). Yet, protein in solution will result in a shortening of the T1 relaxation time of that solution. The individual contribution of these competing signal patterns to overall marrow signal intensity remains unclear.

Mineral contributes in a negative fashion to bone marrow signal intensity through two different mechanisms. First, due to a lack of mobile protons, the mineral matrix produces little or no signal; second, inhomogeneous susceptibility where mineral matrix interfaces with water or fat results in local field gradients and signal loss. The mineral matrix of bone marrow is contained in trabecular bone. Since metaphyses and epiphyses contain greater amounts of trabecular bone, signal intensity at these sites is altered accordingly.

Signal characteristics of red and yellow marrow will vary among the different pulse sequences. The vast majority of clinical studies and most of the basic knowledge of MR marrow patterns to date have been based on routine spin-echo pulse sequences with T1- and T2-weighted images. More recently, fast spin-echo techniques have gained popularity in clinical MR imaging and have replaced conventional proton density and T2-weighted sequences in many routine protocols. Because of these considerations, spin-echo pulse sequences (both conventional and fast) will be used to describe typical signal patterns of yellow and red marrow in this chapter (17,27,36,37). These T1 and T2 signal patterns also form the basis for understanding many of the newer pulse sequences discussed later in this chapter.

Yellow marrow, owing to its high fat chemical composition (80%), displays signal intensity comparable to that of subcutaneous fat on T1- and T2-weighted images using both conventional and fast techniques without fat saturation (see Figs. 14-5, 14-6, and 14-7). For comparison purposes, yellow marrow is higher in signal intensity than muscle on both pulse sequences. Having larger fractions of water (40%) and protein (40%) with a smaller fraction of fat (20%), red marrow displays signal intensity lower than

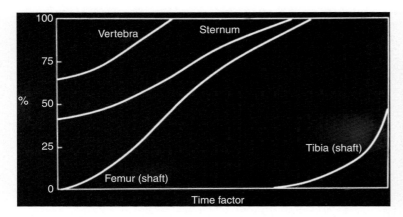

Figure 14-4 Reconversion of yellow to red marrow. Yellow marrow is reconverted to red marrow in response to the body's demand for increased hematopoietic capacity. This reconversion process is first evident in the axial skeleton (vertebra and sternum), where the rate and extent of the process usually exceeds that of the appendicular skeleton (femur and tibia). The extent of axial and appendicular involvement is influenced by the severity and duration of the inciting stimulus. (Adapted from Custer RP. Studies on the structure and function of bone marrow. I. Variability of the hemopoietic pattern and consideration of method for examination. *J Lab Clin Med* 1932;17:951–959.)

that of yellow marrow on T1-weighted images (Figs. 14-5, 14-6, and 14-7). As a reference, red marrow signal intensity is generally slightly greater than normal muscle or nondegenerated intervertebral disks on T1-weighted images (38). The only exception to this rule occurs in infants. At birth, red marrow contains very little fat. As a result, red marrow signal intensity on T1-weighted images will be lower than that of muscle or intervertebral disk until approximately 2 months of age (39). As cellularity of red marrow decreases, its T1 signal intensity rises such that at 1 year of age it is roughly equal to the signal intensity of intervertebral disk. Above 1 year of age, the T1 signal intensity of red marrow should not be lower than that of intervertebral disk, and by 5 years of age, red marrow signal intensity should exceed that of intervertebral disk (39). On proton density and T2-weighted images, the signal intensity of red marrow increases (probably as a result of its water fraction) and approaches that of yellow marrow on both conventional and fast spin pulse sequences (Figs. 14-6 and 14-7). With short TI inversion recovery (STIR) imaging or heavy T2-weighting (repetition time exceeding 3,000 ms and echo time greater than 90 ms), red marrow signal intensity may even exceed that of yellow marrow (see Fig. 14-8). Similarly, adding fat saturation techniques to either conventional or fast spin pulse sequences causes red marrow to appear higher in signal intensity than yellow marrow on proton density and T2-weighted images (even with TRs as low as 1,500 ms and TEs as low as 60 ms) (Fig. 14-7). Red marrow will appear approximately equal to or slightly lower in signal intensity than muscle on proton density images with fat saturation, and will typically appear higher in signal intensity than muscle on T2-weighted images with fat saturation. Thus, on T1-weighted pulse sequences in normal individuals 5 years of age or older, yellow marrow will be higher in signal intensity than red marrow, which in turn is higher in signal intensity than muscle or nondegenerated intervertebral disks. With increasing repetition times and echo delays on conventional sequences without fat saturation, the signal intensity of red marrow approaches that of yellow marrow and both remain higher in signal than muscle, but lower in signal than fluid. The relative signal

intensities of red marrow, yellow marrow, muscle, and fluid remain the same on both conventional and fast spin-echo techniques. On fast spin-echo proton density and T2 sequences without fat saturation, however, the difference in signal intensity between red and yellow marrow can appear greater than that on conventional sequences, since yellow marrow maintains much of its high signal on fast spin-echo proton density and T2 images (Figs. 14-6, 14-7). Adding fat saturation to either conventional or fast spin-echo techniques causes red marrow to become more conspicuous against the black background of fatty marrow.

Having a more extensive blood supply, hematopoietic marrow enhances to a greater degree than fatty marrow following intravenous administration of gadolinium-containing agents, thus reducing the normal contrast between red and yellow marrow on enhanced T1-weighted images (without fat suppression) (40). As a result, the signal intensity changes that occur with normal marrow conversion also become less apparent (40). This differential enhancement is more evident in younger individuals and decreases with age as the cellularity of red marrow declines (41). Advancing age also produces atherosclerotic changes, causing vascular deterioration and further decline in marrow perfusion (42). In adults, visual detection of marrow enhancement on T1-weighted images (without fat saturation) is not possible despite measurable signal intensity changes between unenhanced and enhanced images (43). Since maximum marrow enhancement occurs within the first minute after bolus injection and washes out thereafter, the process cannot be appreciated on standard spin-echo pulse sequences (44). The use of dynamic ultrafast MR sequences overcomes this limitation and allows for identification of marrow enhancement. Adding fat suppression to gadolinium-enhanced T1-weighted pulse sequences also results in the differential enhancement of red and yellow marrow becoming more conspicuous at any age.

The T1-weighted MR appearance of marrow in any particular bone will be determined by the relative fractions of red marrow, yellow marrow, and trabecular bone. At locations where the red marrow fraction is high, overall marrow signal intensity will be lower than at sites where little

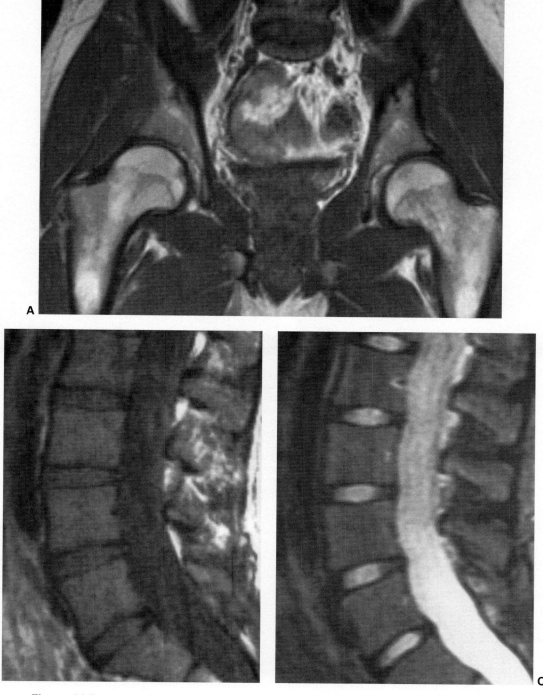

Figure 14-5 Normal red/yellow marrow signal intensities in the axial skeleton (conventional spin echo) of a 24-year-old woman. **A:** On a coronal, Tl-weighted image (SE 600/20) of the pelvis, signal characteristics of red and yellow marrow are apparent. Yellow marrow (seen in the proximal femoral shafts and femoral epiphyses) is roughly isointense to subcutaneous fat. Red marrow (present in the femoral metaphyses, pelvis, and lumbar vertebrae) is lower in signal intensity than yellow marrow but slightly higher in signal intensity than muscle. Note that regions containing higher fractions of red marrow in the axial skeleton (lumbar vertebra) demonstrate lower signal intensity than areas in the appendicular skeleton where the red marrow fraction is less (femurs). Sagittal Tl- (SE 500/20) **(B)** and T2-weighted (SE 2,000/80) **(C)** images of the lumbar spine show red marrow as having slightly higher signal intensity than fluid (cerebrospinal fluid) or intervertebral disks on Tl-weighted images. Due to the young age of the patient, the red marrow fraction is high, making the T1 signal intensity of vertebral marrow close to that of intervertebral disk. Note also that the signal intensity of red marrow is approaching that of subcutaneous fat on the T2-weighted image and is lower than spinal fluid.

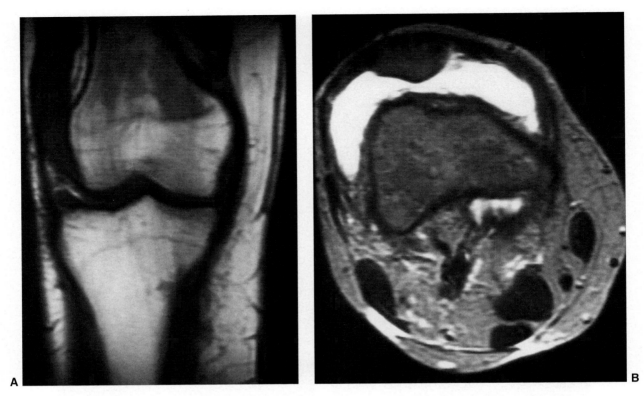

A

B

Figure 14-6 Normal red/yellow marrow signal intensities in the appendicular skeleton (conventional spin echo) of a 28-year-old woman. **A:** T1-weighted (SE 500/20) coronal and **(B)** T2-weighted (SE 2,000/80) axial images of the knee in a 28-year-old woman display signal patterns of normal red and yellow marrow in the appendicular skeleton. On the T1-weighted image **A,** red marrow in the distal femoral metaphysis is lower in signal intensity than yellow marrow seen in the adjacent femoral epiphysis and tibia. Yellow marrow is roughly isointense with subcutaneous fat. Red marrow is higher in signal intensity than muscle (seen in the distal thigh) or fluid (present in the joint). On the T2-weighted axial image **B,** yellow marrow remains roughly isointense with subcutaneous fat. The signal intensity of red marrow approaches that of yellow marrow but typically is slightly hypointense, as in this example. Both red and yellow marrow are higher in signal intensity than muscle but lower in signal intensity than fluid (present in the suprapatellar bursa).

red marrow is found (Fig. 14-5). In the absence of significant differences of other mitigating factors (protein, mineral), it appears that the percentage of fat in the marrow is the controlling factor as to whether voxel signal intensity will reflect red or yellow marrow. As little as 10% histologic fat in a region of red marrow may result in slightly increased signal intensity on T1-weighted images. When the histologic fat fraction reaches 20%, the MR appearance approaches that of fatty marrow (45,46). This phenomenon helps to explain the consistent overestimation of the fat fraction on MR images and differences in the distribution of red and yellow marrow throughout the skeleton observed on histologic (Figs. 14-1 and 14-3) and MR studies (Figs. 14-11, 14-14, and 14-17).

The boundaries between red and yellow marrow change rapidly in the first two decades of life and then more slowly thereafter, but continual change is the general rule. Varying fractions of cellular and fatty marrow can produce a spectrum of signal alterations on MR images. These changes at times result in an inhomogeneous appearance of the marrow, raising concern for the presence of disease.

Several features of normal marrow may be helpful in its identification on T1-weighted images (47). Localized areas of high or low signal intensity probably reflect regions of focal fatty conversion or islands of increased marrow cellularity respectively (48,49). Areas of focal fatty conversion generally have a characteristic appearance and do not present diagnostic dilemmas (see Fig. 14-9). Islands of red marrow can be more problematic. These tend to be geographic or elongated in shape but generally do not have a large, round appearance. They have indistinct margins in younger patients (when marrow conversion is less advanced) and distinct margins in older patients (when marrow conversion is more advanced) (50). The red marrow islands predominate in endosteal locations and tend to be symmetric within individual bones (and in the skeleton as a whole), absent complicating factors such as degenerative change. Histologic studies have demonstrated that conversion to fatty marrow first occurs centrally within a region of red marrow leaving a focus of fat surrounded by a rim of cellular marrow (20,21). The MR equivalent of this histologic process is a central focus of high signal intensity

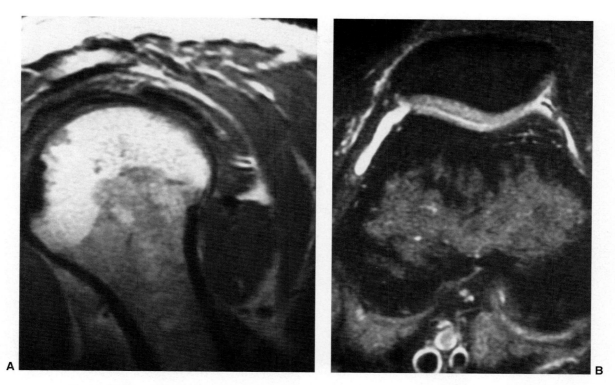

Figure 14-7   Normal red/yellow marrow signal intensities in the appendicular skeleton [fast spin-echo (FSE) images without and with fat saturation] of a 36-year-old woman. **A:** An FSE T2-weighted (2,900/96, 6 echo train) sagittal image of the shoulder in a 36-year-old woman illustrates typical features of red and yellow marrow on this sequence. Fatty marrow (seen in the humeral epiphysis) remains relatively high in signal intensity on FSE T2-weighted images. Red marrow (present in the humeral metaphysis) displays signal intensity lower than fatty marrow but higher than muscle. **B:** Adding fat-saturation, as on this FSE proton density (3,000/28) axial image of the knee in a different patient, results in nulling of the fatty marrow. The signal intensity of red marrow is higher than that of yellow marrow and roughly similar to muscle but lower in signal intensity than fluid (present in the suprapatellar bursa).

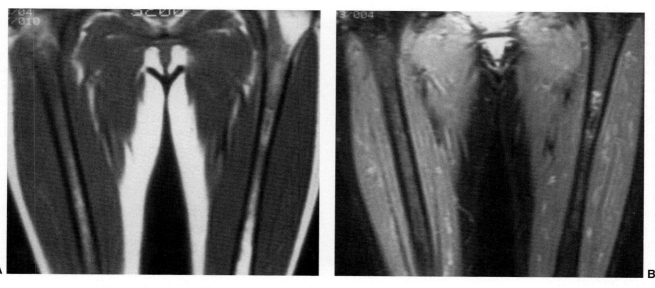

Figure 14-8   Normal marrow in a 30-year-old woman. **A:** On a coronal, Tl-weighted image (SE 500/20) of the thighs, red marrow can be seen occupying the mid- and proximal femoral shafts. Yellow marrow is evident in the distal femoral shafts and left greater trochanter (right greater trochanter not included on this section). **B:** A coronal STIR image at approximately the same level demonstrates the red marrow to have signal intensity exceeding that of the nulled yellow marrow. (The focal area of increased signal intensity in the proximal left femur has been described as a normal variant).

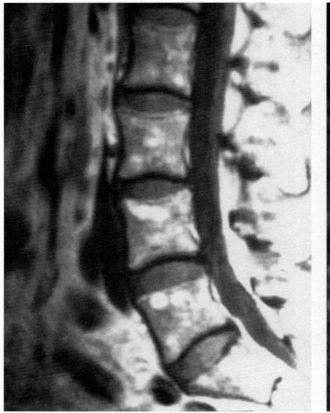
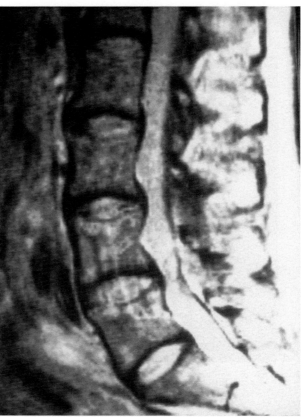

Figure 14-9 Focal fatty conversion of red marrow in the lumbar spine of a 56-year-old man. **A:** A sagittal Tl-weighted image (SE 500/20) of the lumbar spine demonstrates focal areas of increased signal intensity (comparable to subcutaneous fat) subjacent to the superior end plates of L-4 and L-5 and centrally in the L-3 vertebral body. **B:** These areas show some loss of signal intensity on a T2-weighted image (SE 2,000/60) and are representative of focal fatty conversion of vertebral red marrow.

(fat) within an island of low signal intensity (red marrow). This finding has been termed a bull's-eye sign. Although often subtle, when present, this sign becomes a useful indicator of normal marrow (51). Finally, areas of low signal intensity in the marrow space that are presumed to represent normal red marrow should show appropriate signal changes on T2-weighted images and follow gadolinium enhancement as described previously. When the area of signal alteration in question falls within these parameters it can be presumed to represent normal marrow, realizing that, infrequently, some pathologic conditions (i.e., myeloma) can be present when the marrow has a normal MR appearance. Thus, at times, confirmation of MR findings may be necessary with either bone marrow biopsy or follow-up examinations when the clinical situation warrants.

Axial Skeleton

In the skull, MR conversion of red to yellow marrow occurs early, generally before 20 years of age (52), and appears to be more prominent in the frontal and occipital bones. MR evidence of red marrow in the parietal bones persists later in life in some individuals. Many patients, however, will demonstrate only fatty marrow in the entire diploic space on MR imaging as early as the second decade of life.

Marrow signal intensity in vertebral bodies (sites where the red marrow fraction remains relatively high throughout life) is lower than marrow signal intensity in the distal appendicular skeleton, where little red marrow persists in adulthood. In the normal individual, the red/yellow marrow and trabecular bone fractions turn over continuously, but change slowly throughout life. This is reflected by the changing marrow appearance seen on MR images in patients of various ages. The general pattern of change observed on T1-weighted images is one that begins with vertebral marrow displaying diffuse low signal intensity (lower than intervertebral disks) in patients up to 1 year of age (39). From 1 to 5 years of age, the marrow is roughly equal in signal intensity with intervertebral disk. Conversion of red marrow then proceeds focally and diffusely within the vertebral body. Described focal patterns include basivertebral and band patterns (39,52). In the former, a triangular area of fat conversion appears around the exit site of the basivertebral vein, while the latter (possibly a variation of the basivertebral pattern) displays a band of high signal fat conversion centrally in the vertebral body

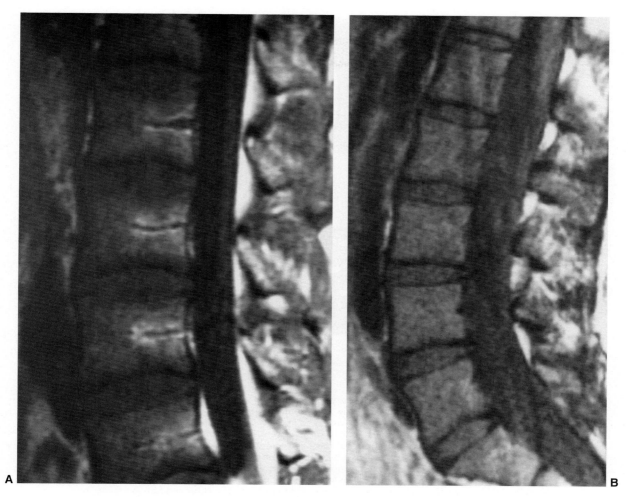

Figure 14-10   Focal and diffuse red to yellow marrow conversion in the lumbar spine. Sagittal T1-weighted images (SE 500/20) of the lumbar spine in a 19-year-old woman **(A)** and a 32-year-old man **(B)** demonstrate different patterns of red to yellow marrow conversion. **A** illustrates focal conversion around the basivertebral plexus while **B** demonstrates diffuse conversion throughout the vertebral marrow. Note that the vertebral marrow in **B** is generally higher in signal intensity than that in figure **A.** This reflects diffuse red to yellow marrow conversion and a lower fraction of red marrow present in the older patient.

(Figs. 14-10A and 14-11A). Disappearance of this basivertebral fat dorsally in the vertebral body has been reported as one of the earliest signs of malignant invasion of marrow (53). These focal patterns of conversion are generally observed in children (older than 5 years) and young adults. Other age-related MR patterns of hematopoietic and fatty marrow in the spine have been described and generally occur in older adults (Figs. 14-10B and 14-11B–D) (52). Fatty marrow can appear near the end plates, presumably due to mechanical stress or degenerative disk disease (Figs. 14-11B and 14-12). This pattern is seen more commonly in the cervical and lumbar regions. Variably sized foci of fatty marrow can also occur diffusely distributed throughout the vertebral body (Fig. 14-11C and D). These patterns occur with greater frequency in patients older than 40 years and may both be present at the same time. There seems to be no orderly progression between the different adult patterns of

focal conversion. Diffuse conversion in the vertebral body is evidenced by a gradual increase in T1 signal intensity (Fig. 14-10B). For example, measured T1 relaxation times of vertebral bodies decline with age (54), probably reflecting a decreasing fractional volume of hematopoietic marrow with concomitant increase in fatty marrow. Supporting this finding is an age-dependent linear increase in fat content of vertebral bodies measured by proton MR spectroscopy (10). The shortening of T1 values is most pronounced in the first four decades of life when normal conversion of red to yellow marrow occurs. Beyond the fourth decade, loss of trabecular bone mass and the resultant reduction of vertebral mineral content (by approximately 40% in men and 55% in women by age 75) (55) contributes to the decline in T1 values. T2 relaxation times show a similar decline with age. Differential loss of trabecular bone with replacement by fat cells, as occurs in osteoporosis, may help explain

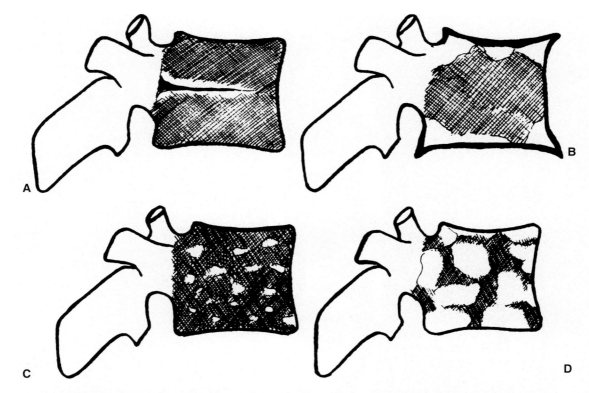

Figure 14-11   Age-related patterns of red/yellow marrow in the spine based on MR studies. **A:** In *pattern 1*, a larger fraction of cellular marrow is present throughout the vertebral body resulting in an overall lowering of signal intensity on T1-weighted images. Conversion of red to yellow marrow is observed around the central venous plexus. This pattern is seen most commonly in younger patients. **B:** *Pattern 2* reflects the effects of mechanical stress on vertebral marrow subjacent to endplates, where conversion of cellular to fatty marrow is observed. **C,D:** *Patterns 3a and b.* Foci of yellow marrow are diffusely distributed throughout the vertebral body. These foci range from being only a few millimeters in size (*pattern 3a*) to larger geographic areas of 0.5 to 1.5 cm (*pattern 3b*). (From Ricci C, Cova M, Kang YS, et al. Normal age-related patterns of cellular and fatty bone marrow distribution in the axial skeleton: MR imaging study. *Radiology* 1990;177:83–88.)

differences in the range of T1 and T2 values for men and women, which is similar under the age of 40 years but slightly higher in women after 50 years of age (54). Declining vertebral bone marrow perfusion due to atherosclerosis also contributes to this phenomenon. The rate of bone marrow perfusion decreases significantly in individuals older than 50 years (42). Despite having higher rates of vertebral bone marrow perfusion before 50 years of age, women show a more marked decrease than men after the fifth decade.

Other factors can influence the MR appearance of vertebral marrow through mechanisms that are, at present, incompletely understood. As the normal age-related conversion of red to yellow marrow occurs in the spine, the process may progress along a more focal (rather than diffuse) pattern in adults (56). This focal conversion to fatty marrow is more evident in the posterior elements, about the central venous channels, and at the periphery of vertebral bodies, particularly adjacent to the end plates (Fig. 14-9). Marrow affected by this process assumes a spotty appearance (particularly on T1-weighted images) as the bright foci of fat contrast with the lower signal-intensity background of red marrow.

The process of focal fat deposition is more prevalent with increasing age and may be present in up to 60% of patients. Among the hypotheses put forward to explain this phenomenon of focal fat distribution is that chronic stress and biomechanical stimuli cause diminished vascularity at involved sites. Insufficient blood flow prompts the conversion of red to yellow marrow.

Certain common diseases cause typical alterations in the MR appearance of vertebral marrow. Adjacent to degenerating intervertebral disks, marrow can assume a bandlike configuration of variable signal intensity (57). Bands of decreased signal intensity on short and long TR/TE images are occasionally observed and probably reflect medullary sclerosis and/or fibrosis adjacent to the end plate. A common juxtaendplate pattern is a band of increased signal intensity (similar to fat) on short TR/TE and long TR/TE images. This focal conversion of hematopoietic to fatty marrow probably results from ischemia associated with degenerative disk disease (Fig. 14-12). Rarely, a juxtaendplate pattern of decreased signal intensity on short TR/TE images and increased signal intensity on long TR/TE

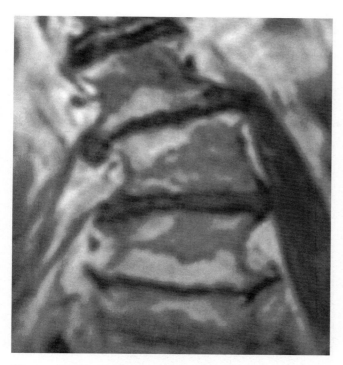

Figure 14-12 Vertebral marrow alterations associated with degenerative disc disease in a 79-year-old woman. On a coronal T1-weighted image (SE 600/20) of the lumbar spine, bands of high signal intensity (comparable to fat) are noted subjacent to the vertebral end plates. These bands indicate areas of focal conversion of red to yellow marrow seen in association with degenerative disc disease. Note the residual areas of red marrow located in the central portions of the vertebral bodies.

images is observed (Fig. 14-13). This pattern probably indicates increased local extracellular marrow water content possibly as a result of focal inflammation or ischemia.

Age-related marrow changes in the pelvis manifest as early conversion of red to yellow marrow in the acetabular regions and anterior ilium and more gradual conversion throughout the remainder of the pelvis (52,58). Fatty marrow appears in the anterior ilium and acetabular areas before 5 years of age, resulting in a heterogeneous MR pattern of the marrow at these sites (Fig. 14-14A). This conversion of red to yellow marrow occurs with such reliability that the absence of such a finding by 5 years of age should prompt further investigation. Marrow signal intensity and heterogeneity on T1-weighted images in the remainder of the pelvis increase with age and correlate with increased fractions of microscopic fat in the marrow (Fig. 14-14B). Areas of confluent red marrow evolve to increasingly well-defined islands in older patients (50). At or around the sixth decade, residual hematopoietic marrow is found predominately in the posterior iliac crests and sacrum (sacral vertebral bodies and sacral ala adjacent to the sacroiliac joints) with very little identifiable cellular marrow remaining in the acetabular regions and symphysis pubis (50,59). The reverse pattern (higher fractions of red marrow being observed in symphyseal and acetabular areas than in the

sacrum and posterior iliac regions) is uncommon in normal individuals and should raise concern for pathologic marrow processes (50). Gender-related differences of red and yellow marrow in the sacrum have been described and generally identify the red marrow fraction as being larger and more cellular in women (59).

Appendicular Skeleton

At sites where red marrow is present, a variety of signal patterns may be observed reflecting relative red/yellow marrow fractions and distribution. A common pattern observed is islands of red marrow scattered throughout a background of fatty marrow (see Fig. 14-15). The islands may have a variety of configurations ranging from small and elongated to large and geographic. Less commonly in the long bones, foci of yellow marrow are evident in a background of red marrow resembling the phenomena of focal fat conversion in the vertebral bodies.

In the appendicular skeleton and in individual long bones, common local MR marrow patterns also exist. The humerus and femur warrant special attention. They represent the long bones that consistently contain the greatest residual concentration of hematopoietic marrow in adults and, in essence, are the sites of transition between the "fatty" appendicular marrow and the "hematopoietic" axial marrow. In these bones, red marrow is commonly found in the proximal two thirds (Fig. 14-15), with the greatest fraction usually in the proximal one third. Less commonly, foci of red marrow may be evident in the distal one third of these bones. This finding, by itself, should not be considered abnormal.

MR patterns reflecting the balance of red and yellow marrow fractions in the shoulder and humerus change throughout life (23,24,60). Normal red to yellow marrow conversion in the humerus occurs early in the distal epiphysis, distal metaphysis, and diaphysis and is often complete by age 6 years (60). Red marrow persists in the proximal humeral metaphysis in a majority of patients until late in life (at least the seventh decade) (24). In a smaller number of normal individuals, it can be found in the proximal humeral epiphysis. This occurs more frequently in younger patients (see Fig. 14-16). Similarly, although red to yellow marrow conversion begins early in the acromion (an epiphyseal equivalent) and continues throughout life, residual red marrow may also be found at this site. In the glenoid, conversion begins later, progresses more slowly, and remains incomplete throughout life.

In the femora, increased signal intensity reflecting the beginning of conversion of hematopoietic to fatty marrow can be seen in the diaphyseal marrow as early as 3 months of age (22,61). As the fat fraction increases, the marrow shows varying degrees of heterogeneity on MR imaging. This feature is always present by 1 year of age. Between 5 and 10 years of age, unequivocal fatty marrow is present in the diaphysis (Fig. 14-17) (46). The absence of diaphyseal

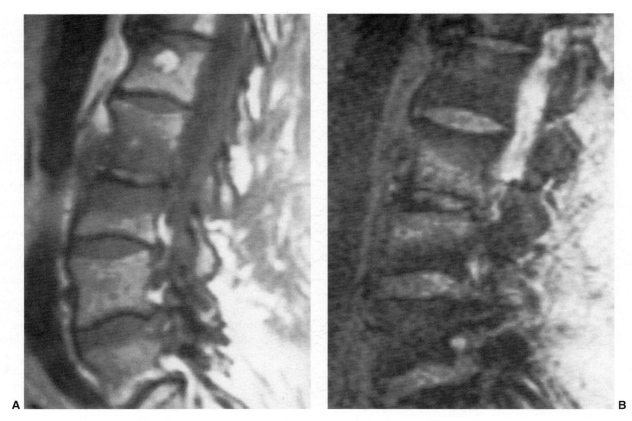

A   B

Figure 14-13   Vertebral marrow alterations associated with degenerative disc disease in a 68-year-old man. Bands of low signal intensity are noted subjacent to the end plates at the L2-3 interspace on a sagittal Tl-weighted image (SE 600/20) **(A).** These bands show increased signal intensity on a T2-weighted image (SE 2000/80) **(B),** presumably reflecting increased local marrow water in response to degenerative disc disease.

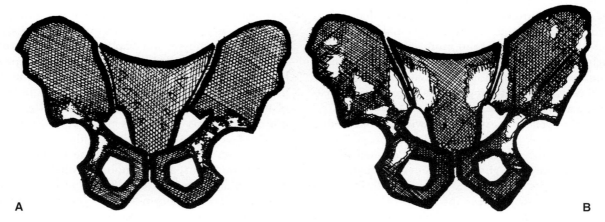

A   B

Figure 14-14   Age-related marrow patterns in the pelvis. **A:** Fatty marrow is observed in the acetabular regions early in life, usually before 5 years of age. **B:** With age, fatty marrow appears in larger fractions at other locations throughout the pelvis, particularly adjacent to the sacroiliac joints. (From Ricci C, Cova M, Kang YS, et al. Normal age-related patterns of cellular and fatty bone marrow distribution in the axial skeleton: MR imaging study. *Radiology* 1990;177:83–88.)

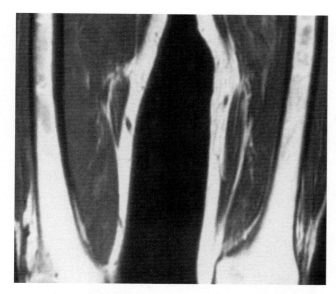

Figure 14-15 Normal marrow distribution in a 48-year-old man. Islands of red marrow (identified as foci of decreased signal intensity in the bright fatty marrow) can be seen to extend to the junction of the middle and distal thirds of the femora. This finding is not unusual and should not by itself be considered abnormal.

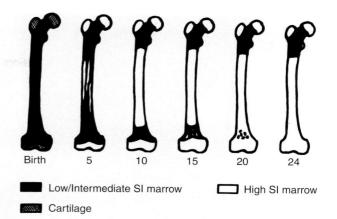

■ Low/Intermediate SI marrow   □ High SI marrow
▨ Cartilage

Figure 14-17 Age-related changes in the MR pattern of red/yellow marrow in the femur. On MR imaging, conversion of cellular to fatty marrow is observed earlier than on histologic studies (Fig. 14-1). The sequence of this conversion, however, appears to be similar between the two methods. Conversion to fatty marrow occurs first in the diaphysis and then progresses to the distal metaphysis followed by the proximal metaphysis. Note that the diaphysis displays a MR pattern of fatty marrow by 10 years of age. (From Moore SG, Dawson KL. Red and yellow marrow in the femur: age-related changes in appearance at MR imaging. *Radiology* 1990;175:219–223.)

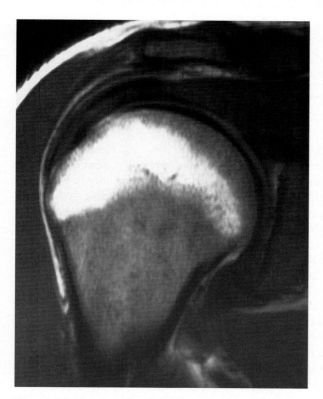

Figure 14-16 Normal red marrow in the proximal humeral epiphysis in a 22-year-old woman. An oblique coronal T1-weighted (SE 600/20) image of the shoulder demonstrates evidence of red marrow in subcortical locations of the proximal humeral epiphysis. This should be considered a normal finding when the red marrow displays expected signal intensities on T1- and T2-weighted images.

fatty marrow at age 10 years or older is distinctly unusual and requires further investigation to exclude underlying marrow disease. In the distal femoral metaphysis, a homogeneous red marrow MR pattern after 25 years of age is atypical and requires explanation if encountered. However, geographic or spotty areas of red marrow can be observed in the distal femoral metaphyses of men and women at almost any age (62). This finding can be encountered in approximately one half of female and one sixth of male patients. Metaphyseal red marrow has a higher prevalence in women between the ages of 40 and 60 years while no age prevalence appears to exist in men (see Fig. 14-18). Other settings in which persistent or reconverted foci of red marrow have been recognized in the distal femoral metaphysis include young patients (under 39 years of age), marathon runners, heavy smokers (more than one pack per day), and obese women (>78 kg) who smoke (see section on reconversion) (62,63).

In the proximal femur, age-related MR patterns of progressive conversion to fatty marrow have been reported (see Fig. 14-19). These patterns can be monitored using a marrow conversion index (52,64). This index is based on a ratio of the measured T1 signal intensity of the greater trochanter to that of the proximal femoral metaphysis (64). Results indicate a linear association of the index with patient age; however, the value of this index in detecting disease is yet to be determined. Red to yellow conversion within the proximal metaphysis occurs first around the greater trochanter and inferomedial to the femoral epiphysis. This is followed by fatty conversion in the region of Ward triangle (generally seen in middle-aged patients).

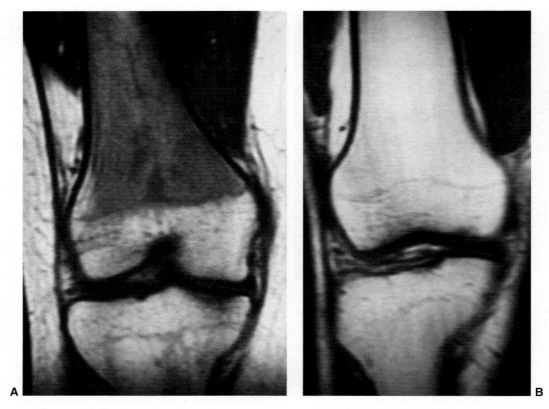

Figure 14-18 The spectrum of normal red/yellow patterns in the distal femoral metaphysis. Coronal T1-weighted (SE 600/20) images of the knee in an 18-year-old woman **(A)** and 65-year-old man **(B)** demonstrate the range of normal marrow signal patterns that can be encountered in the distal femoral metaphysis. These patterns reflect varying fractions of red and yellow marrow that can be present at this location. When the red marrow fraction is high (as generally occurs in younger patients), the MR appearance will resemble **A**. If little or no red marrow is present (as generally seen in older patients), the MR appearance is more likely to resemble **B**.

The conversion process is relentless, leaving only small fractions of red marrow present in the proximal femoral metaphysis of older individuals. Similar to the proximal humeral epiphysis, nonfatty marrow can be identified in the proximal femoral epiphysis in normal individuals (25, 61). Age parameters for this finding are not clearly established, but the prevalence is probably higher in younger individuals. Nevertheless, it can be encountered in middle-aged individuals. This cellular marrow should be subcortical in location with the central epiphyseal marrow cavity appearing predominately fatty (see Fig. 14-20). Gender-related differences showing women as having larger areas of red marrow containing higher proportions of nonfat cells in the proximal femur have been described (25).

Although generally viewed as displaying only yellow marrow signal patterns in the adult, foci of red marrow can be identified in the proximal tibial metaphysis in normal individuals. The settings and prevalence of this finding are similar to those described above for the distal femoral metaphysis; however, the prevalence of tibial hematopoietic marrow is lower in all settings, occurring in only approximately one third of patients with distal femoral red marrow

(62,63). When found in the proximal tibial metaphysis, hematopoietic marrow is also generally present in the distal femoral metaphysis. To find red marrow only in the proximal tibial metaphysis without a similar finding in the distal femur is so unusual that concern would be raised for an underlying marrow disorder. As in the distal femoral epiphysis, red marrow is not normally observed in the proximal tibial epiphysis on MR images.

In the bones of the feet, red marrow has converted to yellow marrow by 2 years of age. Expected MR signal patterns would be of homogeneous fatty marrow on all pulse sequences. Yet heterogeneous signal patterns have been observed in asymptomatic children with no known bone marrow disorders (65). The signal patterns consist of multiple small foci of low signal on T1-weighted images that show increased signal on T2-weighted and especially STIR sequences (see Fig. 14-21). Confluent areas of high signal can also be present on the T2-weighted and STIR sequences. Of the bones in the feet, the calcaneus and talus are most frequently involved. The changes are bilateral and symmetric in extent of involvement and degree of signal alteration. These heterogeneous signal changes are presumed

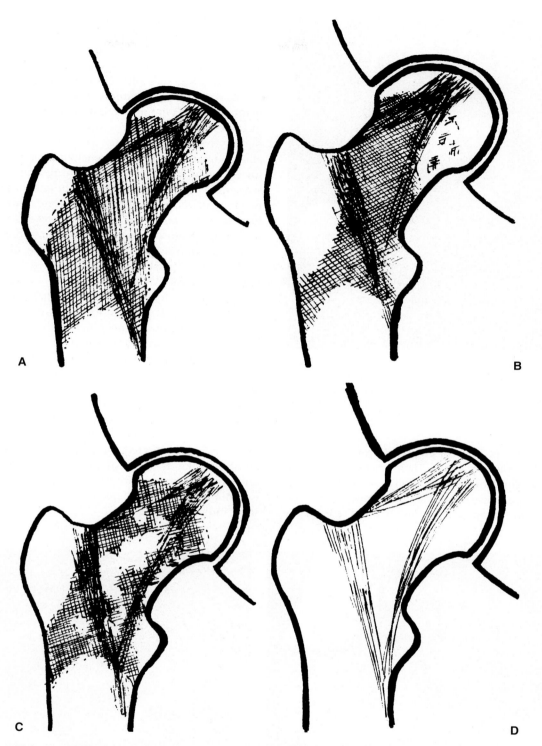

A

B

C

D

Figure 14-19 Age-related patterns of red/yellow marrow in the proximal femur based on MR studies. Conversion of red to yellow marrow occurs first in the inferomedial portion of the femoral neck and around the greater trochanter **(A,B)**. With age, conversion is seen in the region of Ward triangle **(C)**. The process of conversion continues to progress toward a uniform appearance of fatty marrow in some elderly patients **(D)**. (From Ricci C, Cova M, Kang YS, et al. Normal age-related patterns of cellular and fatty bone marrow distribution in the axial skeleton: MR imaging study. *Radiology* 1990;177:83–88.)

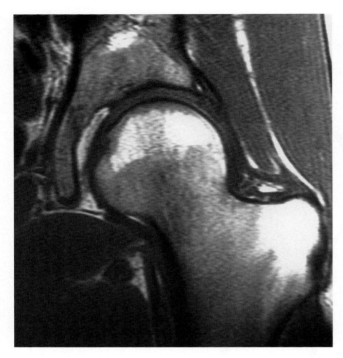

Figure 14-20 Normal red marrow in the proximal femoral epiphysis in a 29-year-old woman. Normal red marrow is identified in the proximal femoral epiphysis. Note that it is subcortical in location and that the central marrow cavity contains fatty marrow. Vertical, linear, low signal intensities in the central cavity of the epiphysis represent compressive trabeculae.

to represent sites of marrow edema despite the lack of identifiable precipitating events. Their exact etiology, however, is unclear. Similar signal alterations have been observed in the feet and ankles of cross-country runners and also attributed to bone marrow edema (66). In the absence of any

systemic illness, the above-described marrow signal alterations in the feet and ankles of children and runners should be considered normal variations. Concern should be raised if the extent of involvement is not symmetric or if signal patterns of involved sites differ from side to side.

Known anatomic features that alter these red/yellow marrow patterns in the extremities include local variations in trabecular bone content and remnants of the growth plate (physeal scar). At sites where trabecular bone is in abundance, the marrow will generally demonstrate slightly lower signal intensity on both long and short TR/TE sequences. This is most commonly encountered in the metaphyseal/epiphyseal regions of long bones. Likewise, load-bearing trabeculae that are thickened and more numerous produce bands of lower signal intensity in the marrow. Compressive and tensile trabeculae coursing through the femoral head and neck are good examples of this. The physeal scar appears as a thin, transverse band of low signal intensity on T1- and T2-weighted images. It is a constant finding at expected locations in the appendicular skeleton. Bone reinforcement lines, if thick enough, would be expected to produce a similar appearance.

The amount and distribution of red marrow is not identical among individuals. At the extremes, some individuals demonstrate virtually no red marrow in the femora or humeri while others display large amounts. Most individuals fall somewhere between. Minor differences in the amount and distribution of red marrow from side to side are expected. However, marked asymmetry in an individual is unusual and warrants explanation. Likewise, the signal intensity of red marrow, although variable among individuals, is roughly symmetric in the same individual.

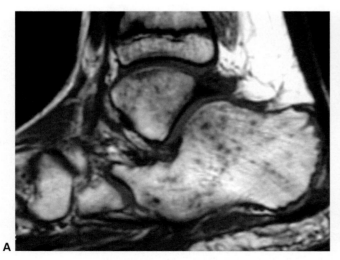
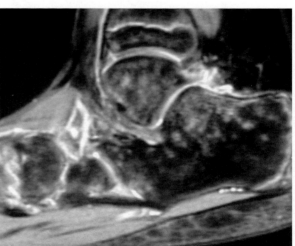

Figure 14-21 Normal variant of marrow signal intensity pattern in a 12-year-old boy. **A:** Multiple small foci of low signal intensity are seen scattered throughout the marrow of the tarsal bones on this sagittal T1-weighted image (SE 500/12). **B:** The foci display high signal intensity on a corresponding proton density image with fat saturation (FSE 2,900/20). This marrow pattern is now recognized as a normal variant in children and runners. The foci are believed to represent marrow edema although their etiology is unclear.

TECHNICAL CONSIDERATIONS

In the MR evaluation of bone marrow and bone marrow disorders, the major technical considerations to be addressed are pulse sequences, slice parameters, imaging planes, contrast agents, and types of coils to be utilized.

The MR appearance of bone marrow varies greatly between pulse sequences. Numerous pulse sequences have been and continue to be developed, each with nuances aimed at improving some aspect of MR imaging. What role, if any, many of these will play in bone marrow evaluation is unclear. Spin-echo pulse sequences (both conventional and fast) with T1- and T2-weighted images have traditionally been the method utilized in MR imaging of marrow and, as such, much of the current knowledge about normal and abnormal bone marrow is based on these sequences.

Evaluating bone marrow with conventional and FSE pulse sequences usually requires both T1- and T2-weighted images. Repetition times utilized in obtaining these images need not be absolute but can vary depending on the anatomic region to be covered. Larger anatomic areas require longer repetition times. As a general guideline, however, the TR for a T1-weighted sequence should be kept below 700 ms and the TR for a T2-weighted sequence should exceed 2,000 ms. Accepted echo delays for T1-weighted images are less variable, generally less than 30 ms and preferably 20 ms. To achieve adequate T2-weighting, TEs of 80 ms or greater are necessary. Thus, utilizing these guidelines, a routine MR evaluation of bone marrow might include T1-weighted images using a TR of 500 ms and TE of 20 ms as well as T2-weighted images obtained with a TR of 2,000 ms and a TE of 80 ms. Studies obtained in this manner take advantage of many inherent marrow properties. On the T1-weighted images, contrast is predominately a function of T1 relaxation time. Due to the short T1 of lipid, the signal from fatty marrow is optimized (see Fig. 14-22). Tissues containing lesser amounts of fat or having longer T1 relaxation times become conspicuous against the background of high-signal fatty marrow. Thus, bone, red marrow, muscle, and most pathologic processes can be readily identified. T1-weighted images also provide excellent anatomic detail.

On conventional spin-echo T2-weighted images, contrast predominately reflects differences in T2 relaxation times (Fig. 14-22). With progressive T2-weighting, the signal intensity of red marrow slowly increases while that of yellow marrow slowly declines making it more difficult to discriminate between the two. Because many pathologic processes have very long T2 relaxation times (greatly exceeding those of red and yellow marrow), they are conspicuous in the marrow. Difficulty arises, however, when an insufficiently T2-weighted pulse sequence is utilized. Narrowing the T2 contrast difference between a pathologic process and normal marrow makes the pathologic process less conspicuous. Adding fat-saturation to T2-weighted images significantly increases lesion detection and should be incorporated into bone marrow MR studies when available.

Fast spin-echo techniques are being used with increased frequency in all areas of MR imaging. The main advantage of these pulse sequences is shorter imaging time. On FSE T2-weighted images, fat (including fatty marrow) remains high in signal intensity, potentially obscuring marrow disease. Incorporating fat saturation with T2-weighted FSE sequences overcomes this potential pitfall. On MR units where fat saturation is not possible, inversion recovery sequences should be considered.

Addition of other pulse sequences to routine spin-echo evaluation of bone marrow provides benefit in certain instances. Chemical shift imaging may improve lesion detection and red/yellow marrow discrimination on spin-echo and gradient-echo(GRE) sequences (67). These forms of imaging are based on the differing precession rates or resonant frequencies of fat and water protons in biologic tissue—about 3.5 ppm or 75 to 150Hz for scanners operating in the range of 0.5 to 1 T (68). Using chemical shift techniques like the one described by Dixon (69), fat and water molecules present in the same voxel will cancel, producing no net signal in the respective pixel. Thus, when tissues containing excess water (most pathologic processes) occur in fatty marrow, a dark interface appears along the perimeter making that tissue more conspicuous. Red marrow, due to its higher water content, is also more conspicuous. Some chemical shift sequences allow for selective fat or water images. Use of these sequences shows initial promise in predicting whether bone marrow signal abnormalities result from neoplastic or nonneoplastic causes (70).

A particular form of the inversion recovery pulse sequence, STIR, can also improve lesion detection. In this specialized pulse sequence, the signal from fat is nulled making it appear dark on the images (Fig. 14-22) (71,72). Tissues having T1 or T2 relaxation values that differ from fat will have greater signal intensity than fat. In fact, due to the nature of inversion recovery sequences, T1 and T2 values are additive making STIR imaging perhaps the most sensitive of all pulse sequences for detecting marrow abnormalities. Limitations of this sequence include lesser anatomic definition than T1-weighted spin-echo images secondary to loss of the fat signal, restrictions in the size of the anatomic region that can be covered, and long scan times. Some of these limitations can be overcome by the use of inversion recovery (IR) FSE pulse sequences. These pulse sequences can be obtained at short scan times (comparable to T1-weighted spin-echo) and allow for greater anatomic coverage. Lesion conspicuity is high but anatomic definition remains limited.

Gradient-echo pulse sequences provide an alternative to STIR and T2-weighted spin-echo sequences yet at much shorter scan times (Fig. 14-22) (73). Numerous GRE sequences exist (GRASS, FLASH, FISP, etc.). All are based on the generation of a GRE rather than the classic 180° refocusing pulse used in spin-echo pulse sequences. The flip angle

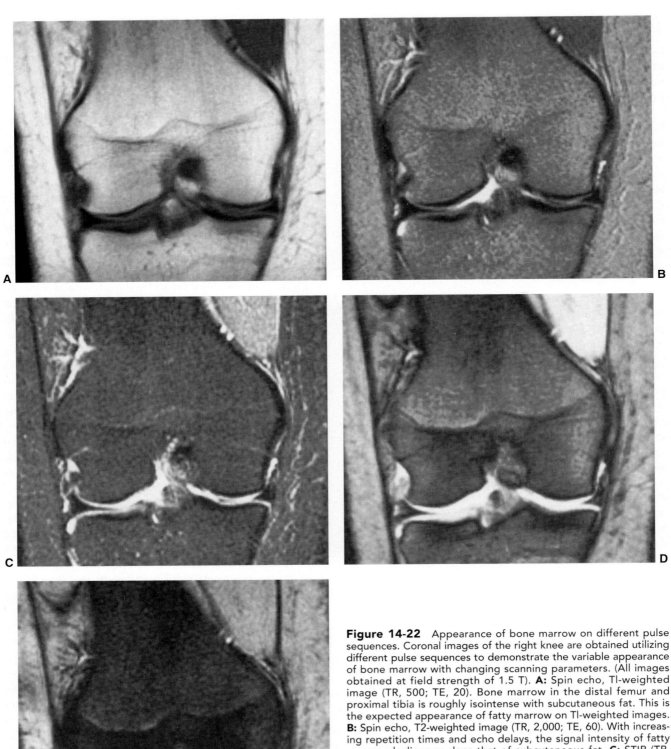

Figure 14-22 Appearance of bone marrow on different pulse sequences. Coronal images of the right knee are obtained utilizing different pulse sequences to demonstrate the variable appearance of bone marrow with changing scanning parameters. (All images obtained at field strength of 1.5 T). **A:** Spin echo, Tl-weighted image (TR, 500; TE, 20). Bone marrow in the distal femur and proximal tibia is roughly isointense with subcutaneous fat. This is the expected appearance of fatty marrow on Tl-weighted images. **B:** Spin echo, T2-weighted image (TR, 2,000; TE, 60). With increasing repetition times and echo delays, the signal intensity of fatty marrow declines as does that of subcutaneous fat. **C:** STIR (TR, 1,500; TE, 30; TI, 140). Since the signal of fat is nulled on STIR images, fatty marrow will appear dark. **D:** Gradient-recalled steady state (GRASS) (TR, 700; TE, 31; flip angle 25°). Gradient-echo (GRE) sequences at low flip angles (theta) tend to accentuate T2 characteristics of tissues and fluids. Note that the fatty marrow is not as bright as on the Tl-weighted image **A** and the synovial fluid displays increased signal intensity. **E:** GRASS (TR, 700; TE, 31; flip angle 25°). Many factors contribute to signal intensity on GRE sequences. Susceptibility effects and field inhomogeneities may in part account for the marked decrease in fatty marrow signal on this image.

(theta) can be kept small in GRE pulse sequences enabling substantial reduction in imaging time. Contrast in these pulse sequences is a function of many different factors including T1, T2, T2*, TR, TE, and theta (33,74). These sequences are very sensitive to field inhomogeneities and chemical shift and susceptibility effects. By varying TR, TE, and theta, the contrast between marrow and most pathologic processes can be increased. Gradient-echo sequences do not suffer the same restrictions in anatomic detail and amount of anatomic coverage as do STIR sequences.

Clinical studies comparing lesion conspicuity on different pulse sequences generally identify STIR or IR–FSE techniques as being superior in this regard (75,76). Adding fat saturation to T2-weighted sequences (conventional, FSE, or GRE) improves lesion detection in these settings. Diffusion-weighted echo-planar imaging appears to offer no advantage over STIR or FSE STIR sequences with regard to sensitivity and specificity of detecting marrow pathology (77).

Techniques aimed at quantifying bone marrow cellularity have been identified, including chemical-shift misregistration, parametric MRI, and H-1 localized spectroscopy (10,78–83). These techniques show good correlation with histomorphometrical data in small numbers of patients and may potentially be beneficial in monitoring some marrow disorders. Quantification of the fat component of bone marrow is now possible and could provide insight into the changing fractions of red and yellow marrow in health and disease (10). Currently, however, these methods have not been validated in large clinical studies and their future role remains unclear.

To date, MR contrast agents (e.g., gadolinium) have not developed a defined utility in evaluation of diffuse marrow disease. These agents hold promise for demonstration of marrow involvement by neoplastic processes in certain settings and may improve the specificity of MR for separation of benign from malignant disorders. Dynamic gadolinium-enhanced MR imaging using fast scan techniques (turbo FLASH, FSE, GRASS, etc.) has shown promise in this regard (84,85). These techniques provide heavy T1 weighting and high temporal resolution. This is of particular importance in evaluating marrow enhancement, which reaches its maximum within the first minute after bolus injection. With this added capability, the potential for separating hematopoietic marrow from pathologic conditions is improved. The decision to use contrast agents is influenced by clinical parameters and findings on initial noncontrast images.

Size of the anatomic region to be evaluated influences many of the MR scanning parameters, including surface coil selection, slice thickness, and interslice gap. Smaller anatomic regions may be better imaged with surface coils whereas larger regions require body coils. Comparison with the contralateral extremity is generally desirable, necessitating use of a body coil. Slice thicknesses on the order of 3 to 5 mm with no interslice gap usually provide the resolution necessary in small anatomic areas. However, 5-mm slices with 5- to 10-mm gaps are often needed to cover larger regions. Signal-to-noise considerations also influence slice thickness and interslice gap in addition to matrix size and number of excitations (NEX). Generally, matrices on the order of 192 × 256 with two excitations provide adequate signal-to-noise for evaluating large anatomic regions.

Clinical settings that account for the majority of MR examinations for diffuse marrow disease include: (i) a problem-solving study to define further the abnormalities encountered on other radiologic procedures or other MR exams; (ii) a screening study of the marrow to detect involvement by processes (e.g., myeloma) not readily imaged with other modalities; (iii) a screening study of the marrow to identify early metastatic disease not detectable by other modalities; (iv) a follow-up study for assessment of response to therapy; and (v) a guidance study to localize potential sites for biopsy.

The sensitivity of MR for detection of marrow abnormalities may indicate a future role for this modality in the initial staging of certain tumors likely to metastasize to bone (breast, prostate, and lung). The MR examination would need to be tailored in each of these situations as it is currently not feasible to image the entirety of an individual's bone marrow. Thus, any screening protocol should be directed at evaluation of skeletal sites where the likelihood of involvement is highest. In adults, this would mean evaluation of the axial skeleton because most diffuse marrow disorders tend to follow the distribution of red marrow. Imaging of marrow in the ribs and skull is limited due to the size and shape of these bones. Time and cost limitations usually prohibit evaluation of all at-risk sites. As a reasonable compromise, one could consider evaluating the pelvis (including proximal femora) and the lumbar spine (including portions of the lower thoracic spine). The study should include T1-weighted images and FSE–IR, STIR, or fat-saturated T2-weighted images. Addition of nondynamic or dynamic gadolinium-enhanced sequences would seem reasonable based on the clinical situation and the appearance of the noncontrast portion of the study.

DIFFUSE MARROW DISORDERS

Bone marrow responds to insult and disease through a select number of mechanisms (27). These pathophysiologic responses can be identified and categorized on MR images. The concept provides a useful means of grouping the various disorders that affect marrow and for understanding associated marrow signal patterns. Five pathophysiological mechanisms are considered. First is reconversion wherein the normal pathophysiologic process of converting red marrow to yellow marrow is reversed such that yellow marrow is "reconverted" to red marrow. Red marrow hyperplasia is a subcategory of this mechanism. The second is myeloid depletion in which all marrow cells other than fat are destroyed or disappear. In the third, ischemia, all marrow elements die and are repaired to a greater or lesser degree. Infiltration, the fourth process, is when pathologic cells invade normal marrow. And finally, the fifth process is marrow edema, wherein excess water appears in the marrow tissue.

An alternative classification system has been proposed (86). In this system T1-weighted images are used to classify marrow disorders into four patterns: marrow depletion, infiltration, replacement and signal void. These four patterns can be observed alone or together in a focal, regional or diffuse skeletal distribution. Marrow disorders are then grouped according to their typical MR signal characteristics and distribution.

In this chapter, marrow disorders will be classified by their pathophysiologic mechanism (reconversion, depletion, ischemia, infiltration, and edema). This conceptualized categorization is imperfect but provides a useful framework for discussion.

Reconversion

When the demand for hematopoiesis exceeds the ability of existing red marrow to meet the required level of cell production, a process is initiated whereby a portion of yellow marrow is reconverted to red marrow. The reconversion sequence is the reverse of normal red to yellow marrow conversion. Reconversion is initiated in the axial skeleton and then progresses toward the distal appendicular skeleton in a proximal to distal pattern. Thus, in a given individual, if reconversion is encountered in the appendicular skeleton, then it should be evident, often to a greater degree, in the axial skeleton. Within individual bones, the process begins in the subcortical marrow of proximal metaphyses or metaphyseal equivalents. It then progresses centrally into the marrow cavity while at the same time moving toward diaphyses and epiphyses or epiphyseal equivalents. Generally, reconversion will become evident in distal metaphyses of long bones before it has been completed in the diaphyses. Pathologically, capillary proliferation and sinusoid formation in the subendosteal portions of the fatty marrow (87) herald the process. A greater blood supply is required to sustain red marrow than yellow marrow.

The process of reconversion is generally symmetric throughout the skeleton, although not necessarily uniform in any particular bone. The extent of reconversion depends on the severity and duration of the stimulus. Mild cases may show only selective hyperplasia of axial marrow and proximal appendicular sites, while in extreme cases, involvement may be evident in distal appendicular regions.

Causes of reconversion and red marrow hyperplasia vary and span a spectrum of diverse disorders from specific disease processes to life style factors. Chronic anemias (sickle cell, thalassemia, etc.), chronic infection, cyanotic heart disease, marrow replacement disorders (metastatic disease, etc.), and myeloproliferative conditions (myeloma, leukemia) are among the processes that may incite this phenomenon. In

hematopoietic conditions, the severity and chronicity of the stimulus (i.e., anemia, infection, hypoxia) will determine the extent of reconversion and/or the degree of persistent red marrow hyperplasia. In patients with sickle cell disorders, the amount of productive marrow volume lost due to osteonecrosis also influences the distribution and degree of reconversion. In a similar fashion, metastases and myeloproliferative disorders cause reconversion of more distal marrow space because hematopoietic capacity in proximal marrow is replaced by pathologic cells. Since neoplastic disorders generally follow the distribution of red marrow (involving the axial skeleton before appendicular sites), identification of hyperplastic red marrow in the extremities of a person with a known neoplastic condition is an ominous sign suggesting extensive replacement of axial marrow by tumor. Extensive appendicular reconversion to red marrow is not common, however, and care must be taken when trying to diagnose reconversion on the basis of MR imaging. To date, there is no reliable means of differentiating reconverted or hyperplastic marrow from other marrow infiltrative disorders. In most cases, bone marrow biopsy is the only reliable method of confirmation.

The MR appearance and diagnostic criteria for determination of reconversion are not firmly established and, as such, the process is probably underdiagnosed. MR images of patients in whom the process of reconversion is operative, display findings indicative of an expanded red marrow fraction (36). The signal intensity of hyperplastic marrow at any particular location is dependent upon the degree of hyperplasia (cellularity). On short TR/TE sequences, involved sites display decreased marrow signal intensity (see Fig. 14-23), while on longer TR/TE and STIR images the signal intensity increases relative to that of fatty marrow. Actual signal intensity observed is influenced by the degree of cellularity, the amount of water residing in the red marrow and the scanning parameters chosen. When extensive red marrow hyperplasia is present, its signal intensity on T1-weighted images can be equal to or slightly lower than that of muscle (see Fig. 14-24). On T2-weighted images, the signal intensity of hyperplastic marrow can exceed the signal intensity of fatty marrow. The process of reconversion involves individual bones to varying degrees, producing a spectrum of MR appearances. In early or mild cases, islands of regenerating red marrow are scattered throughout the marrow space producing a "spotty" or geographic appearance while in severe cases, diffuse and homogeneous involvement of the entire marrow compartment is observed.

In a select number of disorders, the combination of two unique MR signal patterns allows for a short list of differential considerations. MR signal patterns associated with reconversion along with marrow hemosiderosis identify chronic hemolytic anemias (88), a history of multiple blood transfusions (see Fig. 14-25), acquired immunodeficiency syndrome (AIDS) (89,90), Gaucher, (91) or myelofibrosis (92) as the most likely etiologies. Expected MR signal

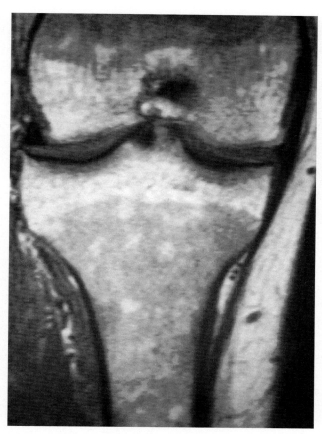

Figure 14-23 Reconversion/persistent red marrow hyperplasia in anemia in a 20-year-old man. A coronal, T1-weighted image (SE 600/17) of the right knee illustrates many features of the reconversion process in a patient with anemia (believed to be alpha thalassemia minor). The fatty marrow that is typically present in the distal femur and proximal tibia of a patient this age has been largely reconverted to (or persists from childhood as) hematopoietic marrow. The large fraction of red marrow present in the distal femur and proximal tibia is evidenced by decreased overall marrow signal intensity at these sites (compared to the normal pattern in Fig. 14-14). Note that there has even been some reconversion of yellow marrow to red marrow in the epiphyses.

changes include red marrow distribution patterns like those described above for reconversion along with diffuse lowering of red marrow signal intensity on T1-weighted images and greater lowering of signal intensity on T2-weighted images (susceptibility changes) resulting from hemosiderin in the marrow cavity.

Some patients without known bone marrow disorders can display evidence of expanded red marrow fractions in the axial and appendicular skeleton (48,63,93). This has been called hematopoietic hyperplasia (63). The term is gaining usage in describing situations where increased red marrow presence is observed in otherwise normal individuals. Sites where this phenomenon has been reported include the spine and knee (see Fig. 14-26), however, it probably occurs at many other locations yet to be specified. This focal red marrow presence is now recognized as physiologic in certain groups of patients. Among these are marathon runners,

heavy smokers (greater than one pack/day), obese women who smoke, and patients under the age of 39 years (63,93). This finding is also associated with menstruation and living at high altitudes. There probably are other unrecognized settings where this phenomenon occurs. Depleted iron reserves and stimulation of red blood cell production caused by anemia, tissue hypoxia, elevated erythropoietin levels, and reticulocyte count are speculated reasons for this finding in most instances. The frequency of observed hematopoietic hyperplasia in endurance athletes is approximately 40% (48,63).

Persistent distal femoral red marrow requires further investigation when the patient's clinical history does not conform to one of the above situations or when the morphologic or signal pattern is atypical for normal hematopoietic marrow. The presence of red marrow in the epiphyseal regions of the knee, even in the setting of hematopoietic hyperplasia, is abnormal and, if substantial, requires further investigation.

The MR signal pattern and distribution of the regenerated red marrow are nonspecific. Differentiation of stimulated red marrow hypertrophy from normal variation in red marrow distribution can be difficult. Of greater concern, however, is the possibility that some neoplastic processes (metastases, myeloma, leukemia, lymphoma) can display T1 and T2 signal characteristics and distribution patterns similar to normal red marrow. This potential problem is theoretically more serious when dealing with hyperplastic or reconverted marrow as the regenerated red marrow and its water fraction can appear very similar to neoplastic infiltration.

Myeloid Depletion

With depletion of the myeloid (hematopoietic) cell fraction within bone marrow, the marrow space previously occupied by these cells becomes filled with fatty marrow. MR images reflect this transition to a high percentage fat cell concentration as the marrow assumes signal characteristics of fat or approaching fat on both T1- and T2-weighted sequences. The magnitude and duration of the inciting process influence the degree to which this occurs. In advanced cases, involved sites assume an appearance of yellow marrow exclusively. Less advanced cases may show variably sized foci of nonfat cells scattered throughout the marrow space. Conditions that result in myeloid depletion include aplastic anemia, radiation therapy, chemotherapy, and exposure to other marrow toxins including drugs (chloramphenicol), toxic substances (organic solvents), and viruses (90,94).

In patients with aplastic anemia, the marrow becomes hypocellular or, in extreme cases, acellular with respect to myeloid cells. In hypocellular cases, residual amounts of red marrow are evident as small areas of decreased signal intensity against a background of bright fatty marrow on T1-weighted sequences (95). In acellular regions, the marrow demonstrates diffuse high T1 signal or low STIR signal

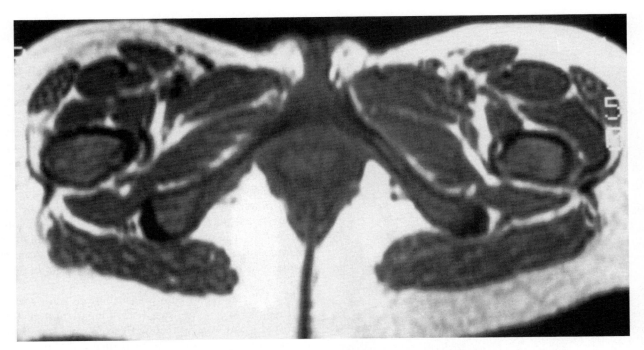

Figure 14-24 Reconversion in anemia in a 29-year-old woman. This patient has chronic anemia due to blood loss from untreated cervical carcinoma. An axial, T1-weighted image (SE 500/20) below the level of the lesser trochanters demonstrates the femoral bone marrow to have decreased signal intensity, comparable to that of muscle. This appearance has resulted from a combination of reconversion of yellow to red marrow and red marrow hyperplasia. The degree of hyperplasia has caused the marked lowering of the marrow signal intensity.

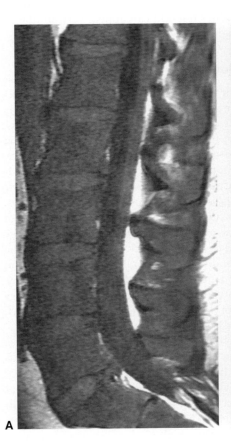

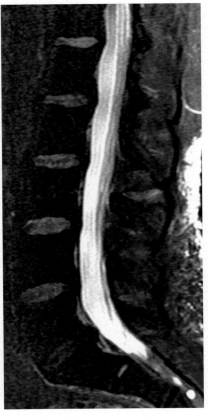

Figure 14-25 Marrow reconversion and hemosiderosis in a 49-year-old man with polycystic kidney disease, chronic anemia, and multiple blood transfusions. **A:** There is diffuse lowering of the marrow signal intensity on this T1-weighted sagittal image (SE 500/18) of the lumbar spine. Notice how the lumbar marrow is lower in signal intensity than the intervertebral discs. The loss of marrow T1 signal intensity is the result of profound reconversion of the marrow due to the patient's chronic anemia. Marrow siderosis contributes to the decreased T1 signal. **B:** The lumbar marrow shows susceptibility to signal changes and becomes even darker on the T2-weighted image (FSE 3,000/105 with fat saturation) due to marrow siderosis stemming from the patient's multiple blood transfusions.

A

B

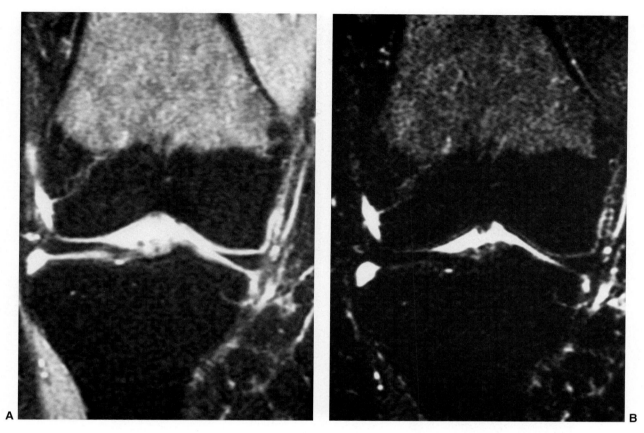

Figure 14-26 Red marrow hyperplasia in a 41-year-old woman. **A:** Coronal proton density (FSE 2,800/28 with fat saturation) and **(B)** coronal T2-weighted (FSE 2,800/98 with fat saturation) images of the knee in a 41-year-old obese woman who smokes more than one pack of cigarettes per day demonstrate evidence of red marrow hyperplasia. Note the presence of diffuse red marrow throughout the distal femoral metaphysis. This hyperplastic red marrow displays the expected signal patterns of normal red marrow on proton density and T2-weighted fat saturation images. As is characteristic of this condition, the epiphyses are not involved.

intensity due to the preponderance of fatty marrow (96–98). With successful treatment, islands of regenerated hematopoietic tissue begin to reappear within the fatty marrow (95) and become evident as foci of decreased signal intensity on T1-weighted images or increased signal intensity on STIR images. With time, these small areas of red marrow can increase in size, coalesce, and become diffuse. In contradistinction to normal hematopoietic marrow, the regenerating red marrow in these individuals shows significant enhancement on spin-echo T1-weighted images following intravenous administration of gadolinium compounds (99). Thus, in this setting, the finding of enhancing red marrow should not be mistaken for more worrisome marrow pathology. Evidence of therapeutic response can be regionally limited at any particular time. Response in the axial skeleton is expected to precede that in the appendicular skeleton. The precise sequence of response throughout the skeleton has been incompletely defined. STIR sequences of the thoracolumbar spine have been shown to be more sensitive than T1-weighted images or bone marrow biopsies for assessing

bone marrow activity as reflected by peripheral blood counts in patients undergoing therapy (100–102).

Radiation therapy exerts toxic effects on red marrow. Early pathologic alterations following these insults include marrow vascular congestion, capillary injury, hemorrhage, and edema (103). Sinusoidal dilatation and hemorrhage in the irradiated marrow can be detected as early as 1 to 3 days after initiation of therapy (104). As these acute changes subside, the hematopoietic tissue and blood vessels gradually disappears leaving predominately poorly vascularized fatty marrow. From weeks to months following this phase, on a dose-dependent basis, small foci of red marrow may begin to regenerate. MR findings reflecting the pathologic alterations and the timing of their appearance are not firmly established. Reports of radiation changes in vertebral marrow as assessed by MR imaging (105–108) describe either no change or slight change within the first week of therapy. Slight marrow change is manifested by decreased signal intensity on T1-weighted images and increased signal intensity on T2-weighted and STIR images presumably due to edema. Generally, at 2 weeks following the initiation of therapy,

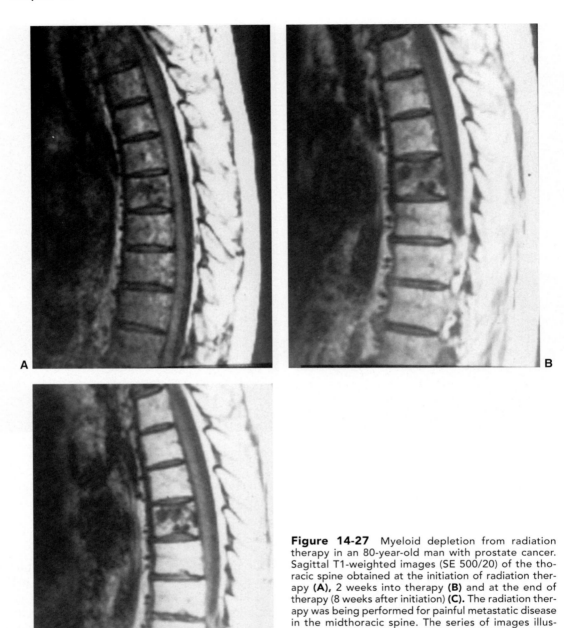

A

B

C

Figure 14-27 Myeloid depletion from radiation therapy in an 80-year-old man with prostate cancer. Sagittal T1-weighted images (SE 500/20) of the thoracic spine obtained at the initiation of radiation therapy **(A),** 2 weeks into therapy **(B)** and at the end of therapy (8 weeks after initiation) **(C).** The radiation therapy was being performed for painful metastatic disease in the midthoracic spine. The series of images illustrates progressive myeloid depletion in the thoracic spine. As the red marrow is depleted in **B** and **C,** the thoracic marrow assumes an appearance of predominately fatty marrow. The persistent foci of low signal intensity in one of the midthoracic vertebrae represent the site of metastatic disease.

vertebral marrow begins to show signs of increased fat content by appearing either mottled or displaying a central fatty component (see Fig. 14-27). Dynamic gadolinium-enhanced sequences show increased marrow enhancement at this time, presumably reflecting the dilatation of vascular sinusoids observed histologically in the acute marrow response to radiation (107). From 3 to 8 weeks after the start of therapy and possibly continuing for months thereafter, MR imaging of patients receiving higher radiation doses tend to show

progressive fat signal intensity throughout the involved vertebral bodies (Fig. 14-27), accompanied by a significant decrease in marrow enhancement as assessed by quantitative dynamic gadolinium-enhanced MR sequences (107). These MR findings probably reflect histologic changes observed in the chronic phase of irradiated marrow including microvascular occlusion and fibrosis resulting in decreased vascularity and depletion of hematopoietic cells with replacement by fatty cells. By comparison, patients receiving lower doses can show a band pattern of fatty marrow centrally and what is presumed to be red marrow at the periphery of the vertebral body. This pattern has been interpreted as regenerating red marrow supported by sinusoids juxtaposed to the vertebral body endplates. Factors affecting the ability of hematopoietic marrow to regenerate following potentially ablative doses include the absorbed dose, the volume of hematopoietic marrow treated, and the patient's age. With doses below 30 Gy, recovery is likely. Between 20 and 40 Gy, recovery may be seen up to 30 months after therapy (106). The extent of this recovery correlates with the length of time since completion of therapy. When doses exceed 50 Gy, the marrow changes appear to be irreversible (109).

Bone marrow outside the field of radiation therapy can also show signal changes on MR imaging (105,107,110). These signal changes presumably reflect the effects of a low scatter dose of radiation on the adjacent marrow. The net result is a small but measurable increase in the marrow fat signal on both quantitative and nonquantitative MR studies causing the involved marrow to display slightly higher T1 signal intensity than unaffected marrow. The involved marrow also shows a significant progressive decrease in contrast enhancement as identified on dynamic gadolinium-enhanced MR imaging (107). This finding suggests an increased sensitivity of marrow microvascular structure over hematopoietic cells to low-dose radiation effects, but this has yet to be verified.

Systemic and/or regional chemotherapy also result in myeloid depletion. As with radiation therapy, the net effect will be a loss of hematopoietic marrow with fatty marrow replacement. The time course and dose relationships of this change have not been established. Also unclear is to what degree, if any, marrow exposed to chemotherapy will undergo changes similar to those encountered in the early phases of radiation therapy (vascular congestion, marrow edema, and infarction).

MR findings at more complete stages of marrow ablation are as expected. Involved marrow manifests the signal pattern of fatty marrow on STIR, T1- and T2-weighted sequences. These changes are typically diffuse throughout the skeleton in the setting of systemic chemotherapy but regionally limited in radiation therapy (see Fig. 14-28) or local chemotherapy (e.g., intraarterial chemotherapy).

The effects of marrow depletion can be blunted or reversed in some settings by the use of recombinant human hematopoietic growth factors such as granulocyte colony-stimulating factor. This substance stimulates proliferation and differentiation of neutrophil precursors. When used during and/or after chemotherapy or radiation therapy, these factors result in signal patterns consistent with reconversion of fatty to hematopoietic marrow in diaphyseal and metaphyseal regions of long bones on a dose dependent basis (80,111). The time frame for this to occur is not established but may begin as soon as 6 to 7 weeks following initiation of therapy.

Bone Marrow Ischemia

Although usually focal in nature, bone marrow ischemia may be present at multiple sites throughout the skeleton in select individuals. Settings that predispose to this occurrence include trauma, collagen vascular diseases (systemic lupus erythematosus), exogenous steroid administration, marrow packing diseases (Gaucher), sickle cell anemia, pancreatitis, radiation therapy, Caisson disease, pregnancy, and idiopathic causes, among others. More recently, patients with leukemia undergoing therapy have been identified as being at increased risk for developing multifocal osteonecrosis (112). Osteonecrosis seen in association with some of the above disorders has a predilection for certain anatomic sites. Favored sites include the shoulder in patients with sickle cell anemia, the hip in settings of exogenous steroids, the talus in patients with systemic lupus erythematosus, and the medial femoral condyle with extension into the posterior intercondylar region in patients with idiopathic osteonecrosis of the knee (113). In the absence of disease-specific findings, the distribution and appearance of osteonecrosis in these diverse disorders may be identical and thus differentiation of the disorders on the basis of MR findings may not be possible. Two basic types of marrow ischemia are to be considered: avascular necrosis (AVN) and bone infarction. Details of the basic pathophysiology of marrow ischemia have been discussed elsewhere in this text and only portions will be reemphasized in this chapter.

Avascular necrosis is most frequently encountered in the subarticular regions of long bones (114). Anatomic sites particularly prone to this process include femoral heads, humeral heads, femoral condyles and tibial plateaus. The appendicular skeleton is more often involved than the axial skeleton probably reflecting the propensity of osteonecrosis to affect fatty marrow in preference to hematopoietic marrow. This propensity presumably reflects the difference between the vascular systems of red and yellow marrow (rich in red marrow and sparse in yellow marrow). This concept has been supported by identification of an increased prevalence of fatty marrow in the proximal femora of patients with nontraumatic AVN as compared to patients without AVN (17); however, the concept is yet to be substantiated on subsequent studies involving large patient populations.

Bone infarction occurs most frequently in the metadiaphyseal regions of long bones. Favored anatomic sites include femora, humeri, and tibiae. While flat bones are by no means immune, occurrence at these sites is less frequently detected. As with AVN, the appendicular skeleton is more often involved than the axial skeleton.

Regardless of the cause or site of involvement, the histopathologic changes in all forms of ischemic marrow are similar, therefore producing similar MR appearances. Though the cause is ischemia, manifestations of the process represent a balance of progressive cell death and host response through repair (115–117).

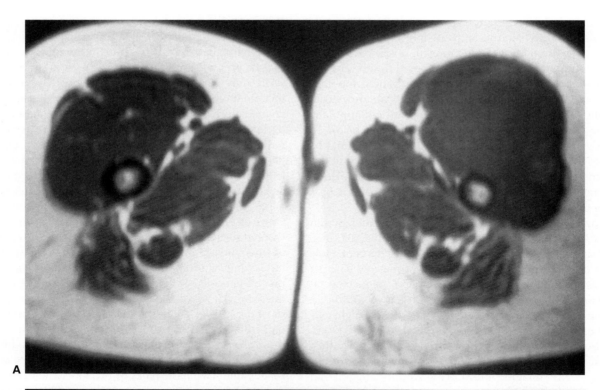

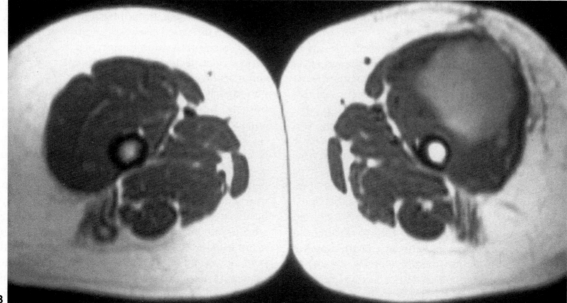

Figure 14-28 Myeloid depletion from radiation therapy in a 28-year-old woman. **A:** An axial, T1-weighted image (SE 500/20) of the proximal thighs in this patient with a malignant fibrous histiocytoma (anterior compartment of the left thigh) demonstrates normal red/yellow marrow signal intensity in both femoral shafts. Note the symmetrical intermediate signal intensity of both medullary spaces. **B:** Following radiation therapy to the left thigh, there has been a significant change in the signal intensity of the left femoral marrow. An axial, T1-weighted image (SE 500/20) obtained at the same level as A demonstrates marked increase in the signal intensity of the left femoral marrow such that it is now isointense with subcutaneous fat. This change reflects loss of red marrow or myeloid depletion due to radiation therapy. Only fatty marrow is evident on the left following the therapy. Note also how the soft tissue tumor has become necrotic.

Controversy exists as to just how early MRI can detect signal alterations in ischemic marrow. Since fat cells provide the high signal intensity of normal marrow, the speculation is that marrow signal changes begin with the death of fat cells (approximately 2 to 5 days following the ischemic event) (118). However, it is possible that the death of fat cells does not immediately alter signal intensity since signal derived from depot lipid can persist for an extended time after fat cell death (119). If that is the case, then signal changes will not develop until later in the process when depot lipid is altered. To date, this issue has not been resolved.

A variety of morphologic and signal patterns are produced in the setting of AVN of the femoral head. Morphologic configurations include oval, ring, geometric, and band patterns (118). Involved marrow can display homogeneous or inhomogeneous signal patterns; however, some component of diminished signal intensity on T1-weighted images is usually present. This reflects partial replacement of fatty marrow by a balance of edema, amorphous cellular debris, granulation tissue, and fibrosis. Infrequently, MR signal alterations identifying hemorrhage may be encountered on T1- weighted images. Variable signal changes are evident on T2-weighted images ranging from low to high signal intensity when compared to normal fatty marrow.

Uncommonly, AVN presents as diffuse signal abnormality in the femoral head with extension into the femoral neck and intertrochanteric region (120). The abnormal areas demonstrate low signal intensity on short TR/TE images and increased signal intensity on long TR/TE images—a pattern associated with bone marrow edema and similar to that encountered in patients with several other conditions (see section on edema).

Also, there probably are cases in which MR imaging yields normal results yet the patient goes on to develop AVN. As with other marrow disorders, biopsy may be necessary to establish a diagnosis when MR imaging is equivocal. Despite recognized limitations, there is general agreement that MR imaging remains the most sensitive imaging method for detecting AVN.

In theory, the different morphologic and signal patterns encountered in osteonecrosis reflect chronologic stages of the ischemic process. Signal patterns that indicate a preponderance of edema and/or hemorrhage in the involved area suggest an earlier stage of AVN while patterns associated with fibrosis and sclerosis imply a more advanced process. In the hip, areas of focal osteonecrosis (without subchondral fracture or collapse) combined with marrow edema extending into the proximal femur correlate with hip pain in an early stage of disease (121). Evidence of periosteal response, seen more commonly in bone infarcts than AVN, also signifies early disease (113). In both AVN and bone infarcts, the presence of marrow edema has a high correlation with pain (36,121). In these settings, the pain is usually transient and improves in conjunction with the marrow edema. The etiology of this marrow edema is unclear. Tissue ischemia is a possible explanation. Involved regions often

do not progress to osteonecrosis (121). Signal intensities identifying fat may reflect either very early or late stages. When a reactive interface forms between viable and necrotic tissue, the MR image may demonstrate a "double-line sign" (a band of low signal intensity on T1-weighted images that is partially hyperintense on T2-weighted images) (see Fig. 14-29). Presumably, the high signal component of this double line represents vascularized fibroblastic repair tissue that contains increased amounts of water. Widening and geographic change of this interface within the boundaries of the involved area could indicate progressive repair or progressive ischemia. Developing areas of signal void reflecting sclerosis imply chronicity. Likewise, subchondral fractures (indicating a more advanced stage of disease) produce signal changes in the subchondral marrow consisting of decreased signal intensity on T1-weighted images and increased linear signal on T2-weighted images (122).

Occasionally, additional marrow abnormalities are present in patients with avascular alterations (such as hyperplastic marrow and hemosiderosis in a patient with sickle cell anemia or diffuse infiltrative disease in patients with Gaucher or leukemia) that point to a specific disorder as the etiology of the ischemic condition. Often, however, no disease-specific markers can be found and the differential diagnosis is formulated on the basis of the patient's clinical setting.

Marrow Infiltration or Replacement

A wide variety of disorders alter marrow by infiltrating or replacing normal components. Included in this group are neoplastic processes, inflammatory conditions, myeloproliferative disorders, lipidoses, and histiocytoses. The effect of these different processes on marrow signal patterns depends largely upon the type of cells or tissues infiltrating the marrow and the degree of cellularity of the process. Other factors affecting the signal patterns include neovascularity, hemorrhage, necrosis, fibrosis, sclerosis, and inflammatory debris with associated water content or edema. Substantial overlap among these disorders exists. Therefore, histologic prediction based on MR findings is unreliable. Bone marrow biopsy is required to make that determination if necessary.

Neoplastic processes, whether primary or metastatic, alter marrow by infiltration. With rare exception, tumor cells have long T1 values and variable T2 values (105,123,124). Measured T1 and T2 relaxation times for a spectrum of infiltrative processes (15,125–127) demonstrate no reliable means to identify specific histologic types or to differentiate benign from malignant tumors. In certain settings (e.g., leukemia), when the diagnosis is established, however, sequential measurement of T1 relaxation values may be helpful for documentation of new disease, remission, and relapse (128,129).

MR signal characteristics of infiltrative lesions vary. With the exception of melanoma and rarely myeloma (10,130), however, all demonstrate a degree of decreased

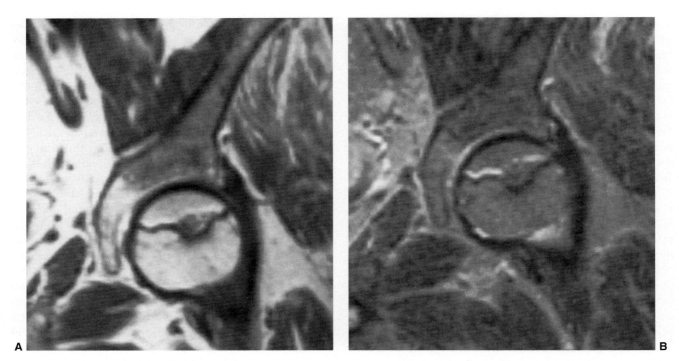

Figure 14-29   Marrow ischemia from avascular necrosis (AVN) in a 59-year-old man. A coronal, T1-weighted image (SE/600/20) of the left hip **(A)** demonstrates many features of ischemic marrow disease. A serpiginous line of decreased signal intensity defines the ischemic area in the superior portion of the femoral head. The marrow signal intensity within the ischemic region is comparable to the signal intensity of fatty marrow in the remainder of the femoral head. This pattern is associated with a less advanced stage of AVN. On a coronal T2-weighted image (SE 2,000/80) at the same location **(B)**, the "double-line sign" of AVN becomes evident as a band of high signal intensity seen to accompany the serpiginous dark line.

signal intensity on T1-weighted images (96,131–133) that makes them conspicuous within the higher signal intensity of surrounding fatty marrow (see Fig. 14-30). Melanoma, on the other hand, can demonstrate increased signal on T1-weighted images, presumably resulting from the paramagnetic effect of melanin. The mechanism by which myeloma can cause increased T1 signal is unclear.

T2 signal intensity behaviors of infiltrative processes are much more variable than their corresponding T1 signal intensity behaviors. While most infiltrative disorders demonstrate some prolongation of T2 relaxation that causes them to appear higher in signal intensity than surrounding marrow (see Fig. 14-31), many do not. This variability results not only from the unique tumor cell but also from its degree of cellularity, water content, and complicating or associated factors (sclerosis, fibrosis, necrosis, hemorrhage, and inflammatory debris) (134). On occasion, the cellularity and water fraction of an infiltrative process may approach that of hyperplastic or even normal red marrow. In these instances, T1 and T2 signal characteristics of normal and abnormal marrow regions can appear similar on spin-echo images. Other pulse sequences (e.g., STIR) may demonstrate subtle T1 and T2 relaxation differences not apparent on spin-echo images, yet even these sequences may not differentiate some neoplastic

cells from normal hematopoietic marrow. Newer techniques such as diffusion-weighted echo-planar imaging also appear to fall short in this regard and are statistically no more useful than fast STIR images for detecting marrow involvement (77). The use of dynamic contrast-enhanced MR imaging has shown some initial promise in differentiating normal red marrow from neoplastic disease when standard static MR imaging is unremarkable (41). Tumor neovascularity appears to be the basis on which this differentiation occurs. The technique will need to be validated in larger studies before it gains wide use. Currently, a combination of spin-echo T1-weighted and FSE STIR (or routine STIR) sequences appears to provide the highest sensitivity and specificity for detecting marrow infiltrative processes (77). Dynamic contrast-enhanced sequences could be added when the T1-weighted and STIR images yield equivocal, nondiagnostic, or clinically discrepant information (135).

The margins between infiltrative lesions and normal marrow may be indistinct or sharp based on the location of the lesion, the fraction of tumor cells present, the disease process itself, and signal characteristics of the abnormal cells. Infiltrative cells are more conspicuous against a background of fatty marrow as opposed to red marrow. Thus an infiltrative lesion that is sharply defined in the appendicular marrow

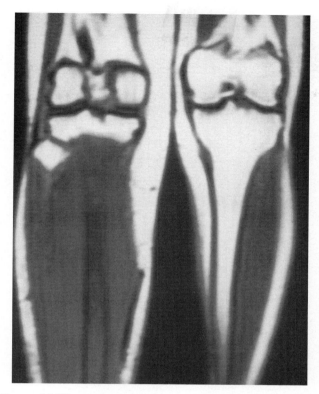

Figure 14-30   Marrow infiltration in Hodgkin lymphoma in a 38-year-old man. On a coronal, Tl-weighted image (SE 500/20) of the legs, localized lymphomatous marrow infiltration is apparent in the right tibia. Involved marrow demonstrates decreased signal intensity on the Tl-weighted image. The tumor extent can be readily identified in the high signal fatty marrow. Compare to the normal left side.

may appear indistinct in the axial skeleton where the red marrow fraction is higher. Similarly, when the fraction of tumor cells is low in a particular lesion, the margins of that lesion will be less sharp in the axial as opposed to the appendicular skeleton. By their nature, some infiltrative disorders involve marrow in a diffuse manner making them less conspicuous in the axial skeleton while others result in more focal lesions potentially increasing conspicuity. Monitoring specific sites can be helpful in identifying abnormal marrow. Disappearance of fat surrounding the basivertebral vein, particularly where it exits the vertebral body dorsally, has been described as one of the first signs of malignant bone marrow invasion in the spine (53). As expected, lesions with T1 and T2 values substantially different from normal red and yellow marrow would be expected to have more discrete margins than those lesions with T1 and T2 values closer to normal marrow. Other features of marrow lesions may also be helpful in discriminating infiltrative disorders. A rim of high signal intensity around a lower signal marrow lesion on T2-weighted images ("halo sign") excludes hematopoietic marrow as the cause and is a sign of metastatic disease (51). Presumably, this reflects fluid/edema/new bone formation in regions of peripheral trabecular destruction around metastatic lesions, most commonly those of prostate cancer.

However, due to substantial overlap in signal characteristics, reliable differentiation of neoplastic and nonneoplastic marrow lesions is not always possible without biopsy.

The skeletal distribution of neoplastic disorders tends to follow the pattern of normal red marrow distribution (136). This occurs for at least two reasons. First, many primary neoplasms (myeloma, leukemia, histiocytic lymphoma, Ewing sarcoma) are thought to originate in red marrow. Second, other disorders, such as metastases, spread hematogenously. These cells favor the rich vascularity of red marrow in contradistinction to the sparse vascularity of yellow marrow. These known patterns are of diagnostic and prognostic importance. For example, discovery of a metastatic lesion in the distal appendicular skeleton (where red marrow is generally sparse) may indicate extensive involvement of the axial skeleton by metastatic disease.

Although bone marrow biopsy/aspiration remains the most important diagnostic study in many infiltrative marrow disorders, the procedure suffers from recognized limitations of sampling errors and inability to estimate the extent of disease throughout the marrow compartment. Despite limitations in tissue characterization, most experience suggests that the local extent of marrow involvement by primary and metastatic tumors can be reliably determined by MR imaging (15,47,105,131,132,137). Similarly, "skip" lesions are readily identified. The information provided by MRI is valuable for staging purposes as a means for identification of potential biopsy sites, for determining high risk patients who may need rebiopsy (following an initial biopsy yielding unexpected negative results), and for assessment of response to therapy or disease progression. This information can also identify patients at increased risk for recurrence and thus direct the type and frequency of follow-up studies. All of these factors become critical when different therapeutic regimens are evaluated in the rapidly changing fields of hematology and oncology.

The MR features of many infiltrative disorders are known, yet their role in the management of patients with infiltrative marrow disorders is still evolving. With the exception of osteomyelitis, MRI currently has no role in the initial histologic determination of these processes. Once a diagnosis has been established, however, MR imaging can play an important role in staging and follow-up, as previously discussed. Many of these issues will be addressed for individual infiltrative marrow disorders.

Leukemias originate from clonal expansions of immature and mature white blood cell lines. Despite a common origin, they represent a heterogeneous group of infiltrative disorders with varying clinical and MRI features. Studies of leukemic patients (88,97,98,103,105,128) have detailed marrow alterations that occur before, during, and after treatment (138). Leukemic infiltration of marrow can be diffuse or spotty, dependending upon the extent of disease. MR studies of femoral marrow at the time of diagnosis in adults with acute leukemia typically identify uniform (41%), faint (31%), and scattered (28%) patterns of

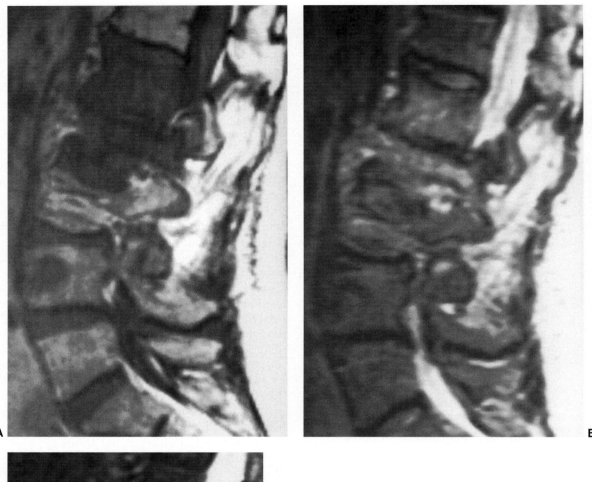

A

B

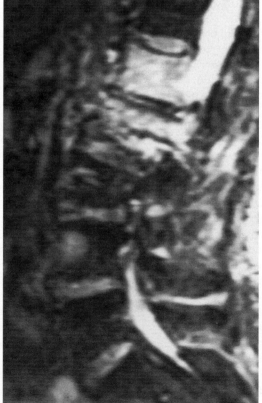

C

Figure 14-31   Marrow infiltration in metastatic disease in a 76-year-old woman. **A:** The expected appearance of metastatic disease is evident on this Tl-weighted sagittal image (SE 600/20) of the lumbar spine. Involved areas of the Ll, L2, and L4 vertebral bodies demonstrate decreased signal intensity. (Compression deformities of the L2 and L3 vertebral bodies are present). **B:** On a T2-weighted sagittal image (SE 2,000/80), the metastatic deposits demonstrate varying degrees of increase in signal intensity. The lesion in L4 is roughly isointense with surrounding marrow, while the lesions in L1 and L2 are higher in signal intensity than normal marrow. **C:** These same lesions become hyperintense and are much more conspicuous on a sagittal STIR image.

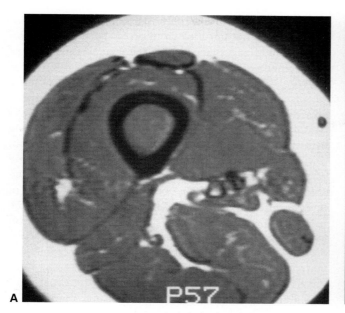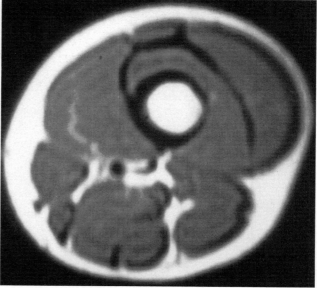

A   B

Figure 14-32 Marrow infiltration in leukemia in a 26-year-old woman. **A:** An axial, T1-weighted image (SE 500/20) of the right thigh demonstrates diffuse lowering of marrow signal intensity due to the prolonged T1 values of leukemic marrow. The marrow signal intensity is roughly comparable to that of muscle. Compare with normal marrow signal intensity at the same anatomic site in a similar age patient **(B).**

involvement (105). In the axial skeleton, due to the presence of larger red marrow fractions, distinct patterns are difficult to recognize. The most common MR finding observed in vertebral leukemic marrow is prolongation of T1-relaxation values (98,125,128,139) resulting in an overall lowering of marrow signal intensity on T1-weighted images (see Fig. 14-32). This usually results in signal intensities of the vertebral marrow appearing lower than that of intervertebral disks on T1-weighted images. Almost three fourths of patients with acute myeloid leukemia and nearly all patients with acute lymphoid leukemia have been shown to demonstrate this finding (140). There is a demonstrated difference between measured T1-relaxation values of affected marrow in patients with newly diagnosed and/or relapsed leukemia as compared with affected marrow in patients in remission or in unaffected marrow in normal age-matched controls (see Fig. 14-33). A measured T1 value less than 600 ms correlates with a disease-free state, while a T1 value greater than 750 ms correlates with leukemia (newly diagnosed or in relapse). Chemical shift imaging (37,129,141,142) and proton spectroscopy (143–147) may improve sensitivity for detecting marrow involvement. Even with these techniques, however, 10% of patients with acute myeloid leukemia, 41% of patients with chronic lymphocytic leukemia, and unknown percentages of patients with other leukemias have normal MR quantitative marrow analysis (138,143). Changes in T2-relaxation times of leukemic marrow are more variable. Although there may be some prolongation of T2 values, measured values show no statistically significant

difference from those of age-matched controls. Of the various types of leukemia, acute myelogenous leukemia (in adults), and acute lymphocytic leukemia (pretreatment or in relapse in children and adults) demonstrate the most profound marrow changes by MRI.

MRI of femoral marrow in patients with acute leukemia fails to identify significant responder or relapse rates at the time of diagnosis (148). Following therapy, however, femoral MR marrow patterns revert to normal fatty marrow in patients who achieve remission and remain abnormal in those who do not achieve remission (148). Therefore, patients with abnormal femoral marrow by MR imaging following therapy should be followed closely even despite a normal frequency of marrow blasts on bone marrow biopsy (148).

In chronic lymphocytic leukemia, patients who demonstrate prolonged T1-values on quantitative MR studies at the time of diagnosis have a poorer prognosis than those with normal range T1-values at presentation (129,149). Similarly, patients with chronic lymphocytic leukemia who display abnormal quantitative MR findings or abnormal marrow distribution patterns have significantly higher marrow and blood lymphocytosis (two criteria used to diagnose the disorder) (138).

Leukemic marrow often demonstrates regressive patterns by MRI following chemotherapy or radiation therapy for ablation of the leukemia. Acutely, the MR changes are consistent with edema and congestion of the marrow (103). After the acute alterations have resolved, MR findings reflect normocellular or hypocellular marrow with corresponding shortened T1 values and comparable increased signal

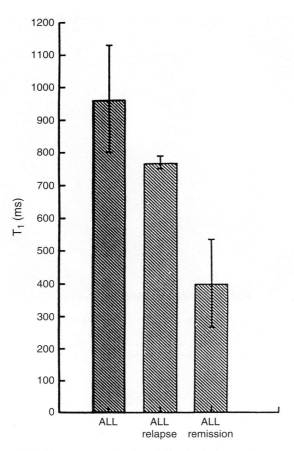

Figure 14-33 T1 relaxation times of vertebral bone marrow in patients with acute lymphocytic leukemia (ALL). Mean T1 relaxation times (+ standard deviation) of patients with newly diagnosed ALL, ALL in relapse, and ALL in remission are illustrated. Note that there is a significant difference between patients with disease and patients in a disease-free state. (Adapted from Moore SG, Gooding CA, Brash RC, et al. Bone marrow in children with acute lymphocytic leukemia: MR relaxation times. *Radiology* 1986;160:237–240.)

intensity on T1-weighted images. Following this, regeneration of normal marrow can be seen. Quantitative MR imaging is a potential tool to monitor marrow changes in patients with leukemia under management.

Other myeloproliferative disorders (chronic myelogenous leukemia, myelofibrosis, polycythemia vera, myelodysplastic syndromes, and mastocytosis) result from uncontrolled stem cell proliferation (150,151). These disorders have not been extensively studied to date. In the setting of chronic myelogenous leukemia (CML), MRI usually reveals a uniform pattern of marrow involvement (see Fig. 14-34). This uniform marrow pattern is observed to occupy the entire femur in CML patients with splenomegaly (adverse prognostic indicator) while only the proximal half of the femora tends to be involved in patients without splenomegaly (105). Following therapy, persistent abnormal femoral marrow patterns may indicate insufficient treatment despite normalization of white blood cell counts (88). In myelofibrosis (152), marrow space is replaced to a

variable degree by fibrosis. Fibrosis, along with hypercellularity, results in a lowering of marrow signal intensity on T1-weighted images (see Fig. 14-35). Due to the nature of replacement tissue (fibrous), marrow signal intensity is likewise diminished on T2-weighted images. In more advanced cases, where a larger amount of fibrous tissue is present, marrow signal intensity may be substantially lower than that of muscle on long TR/TE spin-echo images. Along with stem cell proliferation, polycythemia vera causes marrow reconversion with expected signal patterns on T1- and T2-weighted images. The reconverted marrow displays signal intensity lower than that of fat and higher than that of muscle on both opposed and nonopposed short TR/TE sequences (see Fig. 14-36A). The marrow appearance on long TR/TE images is much more variable. Reports describe decreased, normal, or increased signal intensity of involved marrow on T2-weighted sequences (see Fig. 14-36B) (134,152,153). Factors believed to affect the variable T2 appearance include the fraction of cellular marrow, the amount of fibrosis and the presence of hemosiderin from multiple transfusions. If present, fibrosis and siderosis would also be expected to lower T1 signal. The presence of nonfatty marrow in the femoral capital epiphysis and greater trochanter in patients with either myelofibrosis or polycythemia vera correlates with accepted clinical indicators of disease severity (high serum lactate dehydrogenase and low serum cholesterol) (154). Similarly, appendicular involvement in patients with polycythemia vera correlates with spleen size (an indicator of disease severity in these patients) (105). As in leukemia, MR evaluation of the femora appears to offer advantages over studying the spine in patients with myelodysplastic syndromes. Femoral MRI may prove useful in distinguishing hypoplastic myelodysplastic syndrome from aplastic anemia and in monitoring myelodysplastic patients for therapeutic response or evolution to leukemia (148). Abnormal proliferating mast cells are the cause of mastocytosis. Four clinical categories have been recognized to account for the wide spectrum of involvement and severity of the disease. These range from the mild indolent form (category I) to the aggressive form of mast cell leukemia (category IV). Higher categories of disease indicate poorer prognosis (150). Several MR signal patterns have been identified in patients with mastocytosis including normal fatty marrow, homogeneous and heterogeneous nonfatty marrow (low T1 signal and high STIR signal) and homogeneous and heterogeneous intermediate signal marrow (155). Although none of the MR signal patterns appears to correlate with disease category to any level of statistical significance, the normal marrow pattern has only been observed in category one disease. Presumably, variation in the histologic distribution of mast cells in the marrow of patients with mastocytosis (uniform dispersion, small focal lesions or larger aggregates) explains the diverse MR signal patterns.

Lymphomas arise from the lymphatic system and are classified as Hodgkin or non-Hodgkin varieties. Important

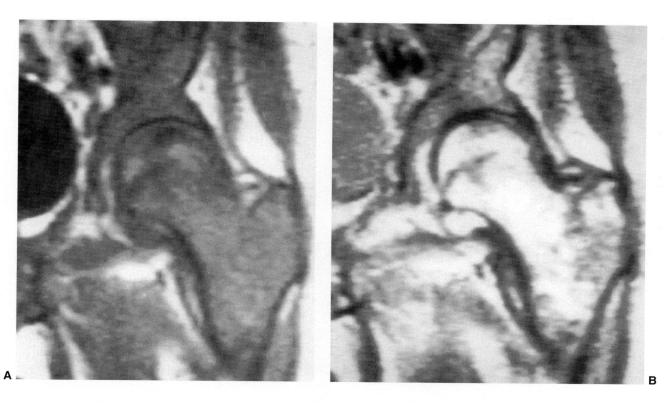

A   B

Figure 14-34 Marrow infiltration in chronic myelogenous leukemia (blast crisis) in a 66-year-old man. **A:** Diffuse lowering of marrow signal intensity is evident on this coronal, T1-weighted image (SE 525/32) of the left hip. **B:** The involved marrow demonstrates a marked increase in signal intensity on a T2-weighted image (SE 2,000/60). The marked increase in T2 signal intensity of leukemic marrow in this case may not be encountered in all forms of leukemia or even in different stages of the disease. (Courtesy of M.B. Desai, MD, New York.)

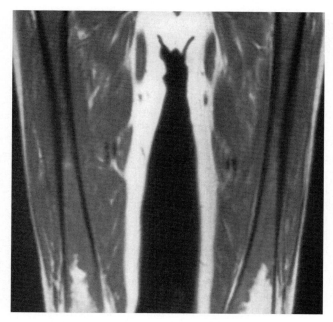

Figure 14-35 Marrow infiltration in myelofibrosis in a 66-year-old man. A coronal, Tl-weighted image (SE 500/20) of the thighs demonstrates infiltration/replacement of marrow in the femoral shafts by tissue that is low in signal intensity. This low signal intensity tissue indicates fibrotic marrow. The extent of involvement can be readily determined in this condition.

clinical and pathologic differences exist between these two types of lymphomas (156). Hodgkin disease is usually confined to lymph nodes and typically presents in a supra-diaphragmatic location. The disease generally spreads from one nodal group to another in a contiguous fashion. Extranodal involvement in Hodgkin disease is much less common than in non-Hodgkin lymphoma and indicates stage IV Hodgkin disease (except when the thymus and spleen are the only additional sites involved). These differences influence the appearance and role of MR imaging in each disease. In Hodgkin disease, treatment and prognosis are based on the extent of involvement of the lymphatic system at the time of diagnosis. In general, patients with stage IV disease require chemotherapy alone or in combination with general radiation therapy while patients with contiguous disease can be treated with local radiation therapy. With current therapies, Hodgkin disease is largely curable. Thus, the goals of treatment are to achieve a cure while limiting long-term therapeutic toxicity. Histologic evidence of bone marrow involvement has been reported in 5% to 32% of patients with Hodgkin disease regardless of patient age or extent of involvement at other sites (157). Bone destruction occurs with higher prevalence in patients with poorer prognosis based on unfavorable histologic findings (158). MRI has been reported to have sensitivities

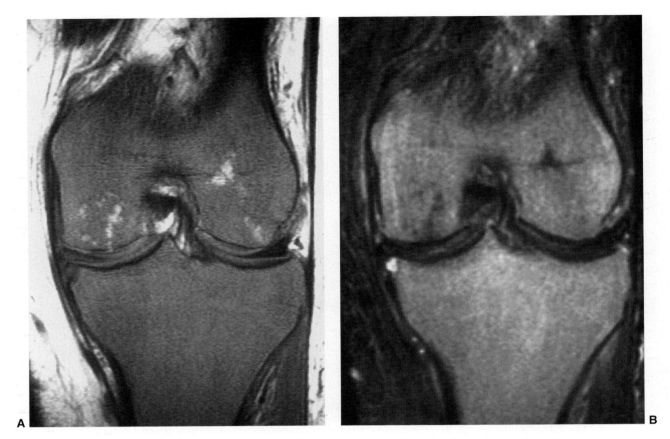

Figure 14-36   Marrow infiltration in polycythemia vera in a 63-year-old man. **A:** Nonfatty marrow occupies most of the visualized portions of the marrow cavity of the distal femur and proximal tibia on this T1-weighted coronal image (SE 600/20). This marrow probably represents proliferation of clone cells responsible for the patient's polycythemia vera in addition to some component of reconversion of yellow to red marrow. Although the signal intensities of this marrow are consistent with normal red marrow, this image can be recognized as abnormal due to the diffuse distribution throughout the epiphyses and metaphyses in this aged patient. **B:** The abnormal marrow displays increased signal intensity on this coronal T2-weighted image with fat saturation (SE 2200/80). (Case courtesy of Bruce Distell, MD, Fayetteville, NC.)

as high as 100%, specificities as high as 97% and very few or no false negatives for detecting bone marrow involvement in Hodgkin disease (77,133,159–161). These encouraging figures reflect the localized nature of bone marrow involvement in Hodgkin disease making it easier to identify on MR studies (Fig. 14-30). Hodgkin disease is more likely to produce focal lesions distant from the iliac crests (162). Osseous involvement can be the result of direct extension or hematogenous spread and typically is seen as a late manifestation of the disease (163,164). In decreasing order of frequency, osseous lesions are found at the following locations: thoracolumbar spine, pelvis, ribs, femora, and sternum. Primary lymphoma of bone (either Hodgkin or non-Hodgkin) is exceedingly rare (41,156). The vast majority of these cases are of the non-Hodgkin type. Primary lymphoma of bone typically presents as a solitary lesion in the metadiaphyseal region of a long bone with an accompanying soft-tissue mass (41). Multifocal primary lymphoma of bone accounts for only a very small percentage of all primary

osseous lymphoma. The focal nature of marrow involvement in Hodgkin disease hampers the ability of blind bone marrow biopsy to detect disease. Comparative studies between the two techniques (blind bone marrow biopsy and MRI) have shown MRI to be more sensitive at detecting marrow involvement (79,160,165). Because of this, bone marrow biopsy may falsely underestimate the stage in a patient with Hodgkin disease and is not systematically indicated as part of initial staging. Conversely, MRI is increasingly being recommended as part of initial staging (160). Patients with MR evidence of marrow involvement show higher relapse rates within 2 years of follow-up than patients without MR evidence of marrow involvement (160).

In non-Hodgkin lymphomas, histologic identification of the cell type assumes a more important role than extent of involvement in determining therapy and clinical course of disease. Bone marrow involvement is found in 20% to 40% of patients at the time of diagnosis (166–168). In low grade non-Hodgkin lymphoma, marrow involvement

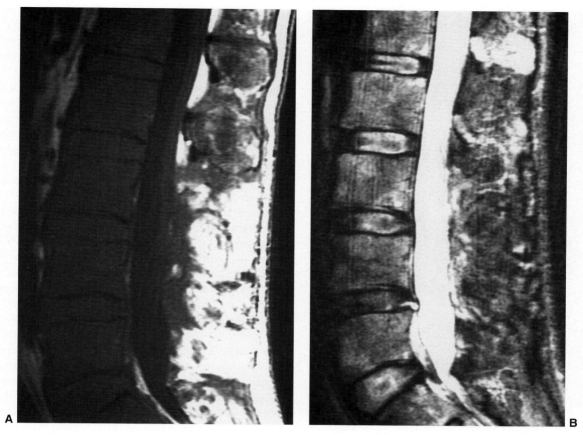

Figure 14-37 Marrow infiltration in non-Hodgkin lymphoma in a 33-year-old man. **A:** Diffuse abnormal marrow is evident throughout the visualized lumbar vertebrae on this T1-weighted image (SE 500/20). The marrow is lower in signal intensity than the intervertebral disks. **B:** With T2-weighting (FSE 2,800/98), the abnormal marrow displays inhomogeneous increased signal intensity. The diffuse nature of involvement is typical of low grade non-Hodgkin lymphoma.

tends to be diffuse (see Fig. 14-37). This lowers the sensitivity of MRI for detecting disease, particularly at sites where the red marrow fraction is high (spine) (143,165,169). In these instances, bone marrow biopsy has historically been deemed superior to MRI for detecting extent of disease. Dynamic gadolinium-enhanced MRI appears to significantly increase the sensitivity of MR for detecting marrow involvement in these cases and could ultimately replace bone marrow biopsy in these patients as well (84). The presumed basis for this improved sensitivity is the known angiogenesis properties of B-cell non-Hodgkin lymphoma (170). In the proximal femur (where the red marrow fraction is lower), MR imaging may prove to be superior to blind marrow biopsy even in patients with low-grade disease (167,171). Intermediate and high grades of non-Hodgkin lymphoma tend to have more focal marrow involvement. As in Hodgkin disease, marrow disease in these higher grades is better assessed with MR imaging than blind biopsy (79,143,162,165). Similarly, MRI appears to be more reliable in determining marrow involvement in patients with bone pain, elevated alkaline phosphatase or constitutional symptoms

(143). Protocols utilizing T1-weighted, FSE STIR and dynamic contrast-enhanced sequences appear to provide the highest sensitivities and specificities.

Myelomatous infiltration of bone marrow has no unique characteristic that distinguishes it from other infiltrating processes on MR images (133,139). The usual appearance of myeloma by MRI is nonspecific decreased signal intensity of involved bone marrow on T1-weighted images (see Fig. 14-38), although rarely, myeloma lesions may show increased signal intensity on T1-weighted images (10,130). The spine is the most common site of involvement (172). Affected sites show focal (see Fig. 14-39), spotty (see Fig. 14-40), or diffuse (see Fig. 14-41) involvement dependent upon the severity of the process (173). The focal and diffuse patterns correlate with abnormal values of serum hemoglobin and percentage of marrow plasmacytosis—factors associated with poorer prognosis.

Multiple myeloma exhibits nonspecific changes on T1-weighted images and in cases where the tumor burden is low can be difficult to distinguish from normal marrow. When patients are imaged on medium field-strength scanners, GRE T2*-weighted sequences have been found to be

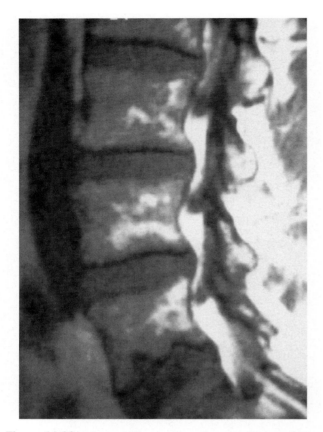

Figure 14-38 Marrow infiltration in myeloma in a 53-year-old man. A sagittal, T1-weighted image (SE 500/20) of the lumbar spine demonstrates patchy areas of decreased signal intensity throughout the visualized vertebral marrow. This appearance is not specific for myeloma, as it could occur in several other conditions. Nevertheless, the extent of marrow involvement is readily appreciated.

of value (121,174,175). These sequences improve the sensitivity of MR for detecting myelomatous lesions. At high-field strengths, however, trabecular bone causes local field inhomogeneities rendering the GRE sequences less useful. Detection of bone marrow myeloma on non-enhanced MR studies performed on high field units is best achieved with STIR or T2-weighted images with fat suppression (135). On these pulse sequences, untreated lesions are characterized by increased signal intensity. Untreated lesions also routinely show enhancement on T1-weighted images following the administration of gadolinium. However, this feature does not improve nondynamic contrast-enhanced T1-weighted image detection of myelomatous lesions as compared with T2-weighted or STIR images (152).

The combination of gadolinium-enhanced T1-weighted images, T2-weighted images with fat suppression and/or STIR/FSE STIR images holds promise for evaluation of response to therapy (see Fig. 14-42). Recognized patterns of therapeutic response to standard chemotherapy regimens include reduction in lesion size and number, conversion of diffuse to focal or normal marrow patterns, and conversion of enhancing to non-enhancing or rim-enhancing lesions (152,176). Lack of contrast enhancement has also been

reported as the main indicator of response to therapy on dynamic gadolinium-enhanced MR imaging (84). This is postulated to occur because of a five-fold decrease in microvessel surface area in myeloma patients in remission as compared to patients with active myeloma (177,178). This response to treatment can be seen as early as 2 to 4 months after initiation of conventional chemotherapy. Response to treatment with angiogenesis-inhibiting drugs has yet to be evaluated. In nonresponders there is no change in the pretreatment enhancement pattern or in the T2-weighted signal intensity of the lesions (152).

Whether employed to evaluate treated or untreated patients, MRI is currently the most sensitive imaging method available for detection of myelomatous marrow involvement (179). MRI of patients with myeloma demonstrates marrow involvement even when radionuclide bone scans and conventional radiographs are normal. Despite this, some patients with known myeloma will have normal MR studies. MRI has been shown to demonstrate evidence of marrow involvement in 25% to 50% of patients with stage I disease (Salmon and Durie classification) and 80% of myeloma patients with stage III disease (175,180–182). The remainder of patients in both groups will display normal MR studies. In this subset of patients with normal MR studies, however, dynamic gadolinium-enhanced MR imaging has been shown to improve detection of myeloma lesions (84). This improved detection relies on the angiogenesis properties of plasma cells creating increased vascularity in the myelomatous marrow. Reported sensitivity using this technique is 99%, however specificity is yet to be determined. Stage I patients with abnormal marrow on MRI appear to have a shorter time interval before more aggressive disease develops than stage I patients with normal MR studies (181,182). In stage III myeloma, the presence of a diffuse spinal marrow disease pattern on pretreatment MR studies is an indicator of a poor response to induction chemotherapy (174). Those stage III patients with diffuse spinal marrow disease have more severe alterations in hematologic parameters than patients with focal patterns or normal marrow. Also, patients with stage III myeloma and diffuse marrow involvement or greater than ten lesions on MR studies show an increased risk (six times) for developing compression fractures than do stage III patients with normal MR marrow patterns or less than ten foci of disease (183). Those patients with stage III disease and an abnormal MR appearance of spinal marrow who elect not to undergo therapy show shorter survival than patients with normal MR spinal studies (174).

At present, multiple myeloma remains an incurable disease with dismal median survival rates on the order of 3 years (99,171). Therapeutic options range from traditional combinations of melphalan and prednisone (38) to more recent myeloablative regimens in combination with marrow transplantation (64). As in other diseases, MR imaging could prove valuable in evaluating evolving therapeutic

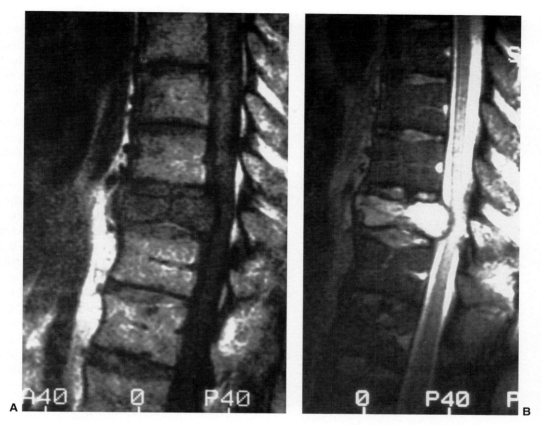

Figure 14-39 Focal marrow infiltration in myeloma (plasmacytoma) in a 49-year-old woman. **A:** On a sagittal T1-weighted image (SE 500/20) of the thoracic spine, diffuse low signal intensity is identified in a pathologic compression deformity of T-10. The abnormal low T1 signal displays increased signal intensity on the sagittal T2-weighted image (SE 2,000/80 with fat saturation) **(B).** This signal pattern, although nonspecific, is typical of untreated myeloma. Note also the convex posterior margin of the vertebral body, which is a finding associated with pathologic compression fractures.

regimens. Currently, however, the prognostic value of individual MR parameters of therapeutic response (decrease in the number or size of lesions, loss of enhancement with gadolinium, conversion of diffuse to focal or normal marrow patterns) is unclear. Evaluation of each parameter on pre- and posttreatment MR studies in patients undergoing myeloablative chemotherapy with bone marrow transplantation has shown that none have prognostic significance; however, an index based on all parameters does provide information relevant to overall survival (64). Work continues in this area.

Acquired immunodeficiency syndrome (AIDS) predisposes affected individuals to develop a variety of disorders and a spectrum of marrow signal intensity patterns. Among the disorders affecting bone marrow are osteomyelitis, AVN, non-Hodgkin lymphoma, and osseous Kaposi sarcoma (132,184–186). Osteomyelitis is frequently encountered in patients with AIDS. Multiple sites can be affected. Involved marrow displays signal patterns of infiltration by inflammatory tissue with low T1 and high T2 signal intensity. Osteonecrosis has a reported prevalence of roughly 5% and appears to be on the rise (187). Postulated reasons for AVN in this patient population include thromboembolic

phenomena and increased utilization of highly active antiretroviral therapy with its associated adverse effects (79,82). Non-Hodgkin lymphoma is the second most common tumor in adult AIDS patients (131,188) and considered as one of the diagnostic criteria for AIDS (189). Bone involvement is seen in up to 30% of patients with systemic disease (131,190,191). Favored sites include the spine, pelvis, lower extremities, and skull. MR signal patterns are indistinguishable from those of non-Hodgkin lymphoma in non-AIDS patients. Kaposi sarcoma is the most common tumor in the HIV-infected population, developing in up to 20% of cases (131,192). Osseous involvement, however, is rare (17,131,193) and thought to be the result of invasion from contiguous soft-tissue sources (17). MR findings of osseous Kaposi sarcoma include marrow invasion and edema with adjacent muscle/subcutaneous lesions and edema (17,192,193). All of these processes display expected MR features of infiltration from neoplastic/inflammatory cells.

Abnormal MR marrow patterns can also be found in AIDS patients without the local presence of neoplastic or inflammatory tissue. The most distinctive pattern

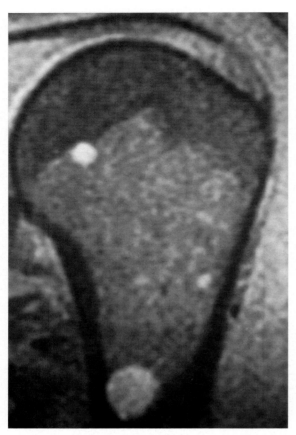

Figure 14-40 Spotty marrow infiltration in myeloma in a 53-year-old woman. A coronal proton density image (FSE 2,800/22 with fat saturation) of the humerus demonstrates the presence of spotty, rounded foci of increased signal intensity in the metaphyseal region. The morphologic appearance is representative of the spotty marrow pattern of myeloma. The increased signal intensity reflects the untreated status of this patient.

encountered is that of diffuse, uniform lowering of marrow signal intensity on both T1 and T2-weighted images (184,185) (see Fig. 14-43). Less commonly encountered is heterogeneous, mottled low signal intensity in the marrow. The degree to which these marrow patterns occur appears to be related to the quantity of extracellular marrow hemosiderin present (194). Reasons for marrow hemosiderin accumulation in AIDS patients are not clear. Multiple transfusions have been speculated as a cause, but iron deposition in AIDS patients occurs in the extracellular space as opposed to the reticuloendothelial system that is more typical of transfusion hemosiderosis. Anemia of chronic disease is presently considered to be the more likely etiology. AIDS patients with this anemia display low serum iron and total iron binding capacity despite increased marrow iron stores. Reticuloendothelial blockade is postulated as the cause of this phenomenon wherein iron release from macrophages is impaired. Increased bone marrow iron stores have been identified histologically in 65% of AIDS patients. The quantity of bone marrow iron correlates with a history of opportunistic infection and class 4 disease

(Centers for Disease Control and Prevention classification) (195). Similarly, an MR pattern of diffuse low signal on T1 and T2 images correlates with a history of opportunistic infection or neoplasia and a fall in CD4 count (184).

Lipidoses (Gaucher disease, Niemann-Pick disease) have received considerable attention. The most extensively studied is Gaucher disease (91,196–199). In this condition, glucocerebroside-laden cells (Gaucher cells) accumulate in various organs due to decreased activity of lysosomal glucocerebrosidase. The liver, spleen, lymph nodes, and bone marrow are most commonly affected. The type I variant of Gaucher disease is the most common phenotype. The most debilitating feature of type I disease is bone involvement, which can range from mild osteopenia with minimal symptoms to pathologic fractures and osteonecrosis (200,201). Involvement of bone marrow generally occurs in axial and proximal appendicular skeletal sites before peripheral sites are affected—probably reflecting the predilection of this disease for existing red marrow locations. In long bones, the disease starts in the metadiaphyses and ultimately spreads to the epiphyses and apophyses (196). As a result, epiphyses and apophyses are usually spared until late in the disease. Involved sites demonstrate focal or diffuse decreased signal intensity on both T1- and T2-weighted images (196) (see Fig. 14-44). In Gaucher-cell–laden marrow, marked shortening of the T2-relaxation time is the principal cause of diminished signal on both T1- and T2-weighted images. Theoretically, this T2 shortening is due to fast-exchanging protons in the glucocerebroside. Both homogeneous and inhomogeneous patterns of involvement are observed. An increase in T2 signal has been suggested as an indicator of active marrow disease such as infarction as it is observed more frequently in patients with bone pain (91,202,203) (Fig. 14-44). Marrow involvement is a dynamic process reflecting changing fractions of Gaucher cells, and hematopoietic and fat components. The fat fraction, as measured by Dixon quantitative chemical shift imaging, inversely correlates with the amount of Gaucher cells present and therefore severity of disease (204). Epiphyseal involvement also correlates with severe disease (202,205). MR studies are more sensitive than other imaging for detecting marrow involvement, often revealing extensive infiltration of Gaucher cells when conventional studies appear normal. As the burden of Gaucher cells increases, uninvolved marrow sites show progressive degrees of conversion of fatty to hematopoietic marrow (131).

Intramedullary osteonecrosis is a complication of Gaucher disease and, when present, produces expected alterations in the affected marrow. Identification of intramedullary or subperiosteal hemorrhage may be an important clue of acute or subacute episodes of infarction in these patients (91,165). Subacute intramedullary hemorrhage with its high T1 signal intensity would be expected to be more conspicuous against a background of low T1 signal Gaucher marrow. Marrow infarction and other

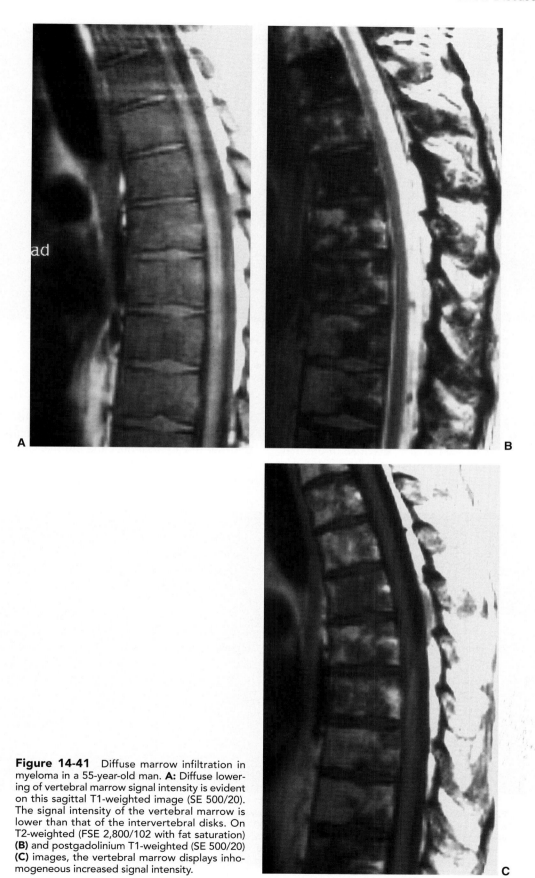

Figure 14-41 Diffuse marrow infiltration in myeloma in a 55-year-old man. **A:** Diffuse lowering of vertebral marrow signal intensity is evident on this sagittal T1-weighted image (SE 500/20). The signal intensity of the vertebral marrow is lower than that of the intervertebral disks. On T2-weighted (FSE 2,800/102 with fat saturation) **(B)** and postgadolinium T1-weighted (SE 500/20) **(C)** images, the vertebral marrow displays inhomogeneous increased signal intensity.

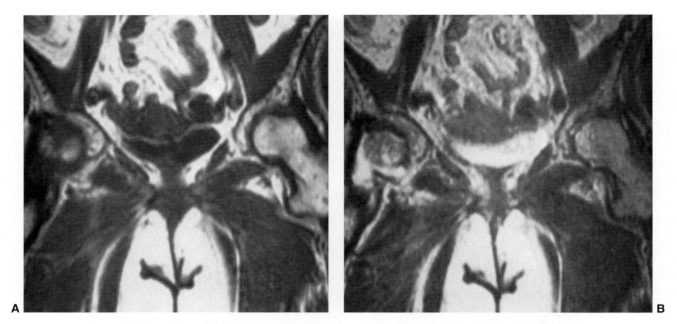

Figure 14-42 Marrow infiltration in myeloma in a 68-year-old man. Coronal images of the pelvis demonstrate the expected appearance of myeloma that has responded to therapy. Spotty areas of decreased signal intensity scattered throughout the marrow on a T1-weighted (SE 600/20) image **(A)**, remain low in signal intensity on long TR/TE sequences (SE 2,000/80) **(B)**.

osseous complications in patients with Gaucher disease directly correlate with the extent of marrow involvement as defined by MR imaging (91). A 10% decrease in the marrow fat fraction is associated with 85% increased risk of bone complications (204).

Enzyme replacement therapy with granulocyte stimulating factor is being used in patients with type I Gaucher disease to reduce the number of infections these patients experience (206,207). The therapy stimulates proliferation and differentiation of hematopoietic cells resulting in

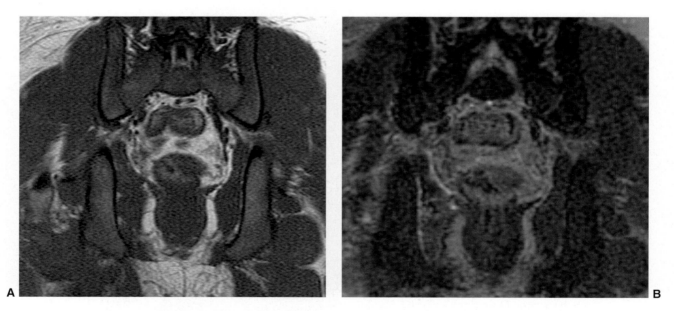

Figure 14-43 Abnormal marrow pattern in a 39-year-old man with AIDS. **A:** Coronal T1-weighted (SE 600/12) and **(B)** corresponding T2-weighted (SE 2400/ 80) images of the posterior pelvis. On the T1-weighted image, there is diffuse lowering of the marrow signal intensity. Fatty marrow should be present in a patient this age but none can be identified. On the T2-weighted image the marrow signal intensity becomes even darker as a result of increased marrow hemosiderin found in AIDS patients.

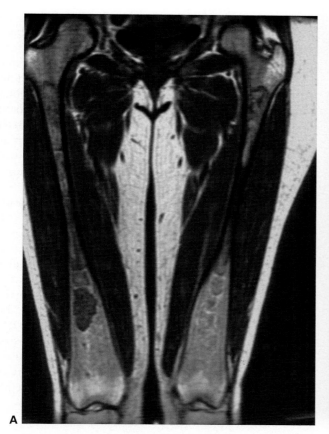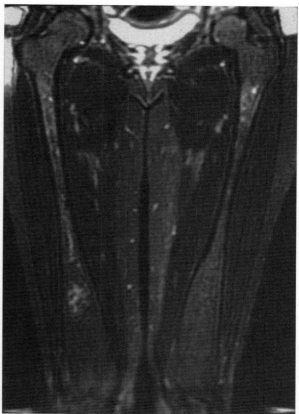

A   B

Figure 14-44   Marrow infiltration in Gaucher in a 40-year-old man. **A:** Coronal T1 (SE 600/18) and **(B)** T2-weighted (FSE 2,800/100 with fat saturation) images of the femora demonstrate several features of Gaucher disease. There is diffuse lowering of marrow signal in the femoral diaphyses and metaphyses on the T1-weighted image **A.** Generally men of this age will have predominately fatty marrow in the femoral diaphyses and distal metaphyses. The involved marrow becomes even lower in signal intensity on the T2-weighted image **B.** This effect is presumed to be due to the marked T2 shortening properties of Gaucher cells. Focal areas of increased T2 signal are identified in the proximal left femoral shaft and scattered throughout the right femoral shaft in **B.** Areas of high T2 signal in Gaucher marrow are associated with pain and active marrow disease, in this case evolving infarcts. These infarcts are the likely explanation for the pain the patient was experiencing at the time of the exam. Note the Erlenmeyer flask deformity of the distal femora also typical of Gaucher disease.

sustained elevation of circulating neutrophils (208). Treated patients demonstrate resolution of hepatosplenomegaly and hematopoietic reconstitution (67,136,209). Conventional and quantitative MR studies in a limited number of patients following therapy demonstrate normalization of T1 values and quantitative fat fractions (204,210). Visual patterns of marrow signal intensity and distribution can also return to normal (203). Some also show accompanying marrow reconversion/hyperplasia (131). These MR findings can be detected as early as 9 months after initiation of therapy (203). The response rate to this therapy approaches 86% in splenectomized patients (203). Focal marrow lesions with low signal intensity rims do not respond to therapy. Presumably these lesions represent infarcts.

Metastatic disease to bone marrow in adults is a common occurrence in some tumors. Among those studied with MR imaging, small cell lung carcinoma and female breast cancer have perhaps received the most attention.

Autopsy studies of lung cancer and breast cancer victims identify bone marrow involvement in approximately 50% of patients with small cell lung cancer and 85% of patients with breast cancer (78,211,212). Identification of bone marrow metastatic disease has important implications regarding staging, therapy, and prognosis. Using large fields of view (50 cm), MR screening from lumbar spine to proximal femora has revealed metastases in 25% of patients with small cell lung carcinoma who had no other signs of metastatic disease and 10% of patients classified as having limited disease (213). Marrow screening with MRI appears more sensitive at detecting metastases than all other imaging modalities and bone marrow biopsy (even when performed at multiple sites). This adds support for the use of MR marrow screening in patients with small cell carcinoma. Similarly, iliac crest biopsies are more rewarding when done with MR guidance. Although MRI is known to have overall limited specificity for marrow lesions, once a primary cancer has been identified, false positive MR marrow abnormalities are extremely low, probably because of the high likelihood of metastases compared with benign lesions in these settings (213). MRI in breast cancer patients with stage II to III disease shows good correlation between MR abnormal marrow and early development of clinical metastatic disease (214). Total-body echo-planar MR imaging provides a means for initial staging of breast cancer patients with accuracies equaling or exceeding multi-modality conventional methods (CT, scintigraphy, ultrasound, radiography) for detecting skeletal involvement (215). Additional benefits of patient convenience, cost, and time factors could allow MR imaging to replace other modalities in the staging of breast cancer.

Metastatic disease to bone marrow in young children is usually secondary to neuroblastoma (216). Neuroblastoma is the most common extracranial solid tumor in children. At the time of diagnosis, 79% of patients are below the age of 4 years (217) and nearly 70% of children have disseminated disease (15). The skeleton is the most common site of metastasis. Regionally limited disease is potentially resectable, while disseminated disease is not. MR studies of the femora in neuroblastoma patients identify two patterns of bony metastatic disease, nodular and diffuse (47). Involved sites display lowering of T1 signal intensity as compared to unaffected areas. On fat-saturated T2 and STIR sequences, the difference between normal and abnormal marrow is more conspicuous as metastatic disease becomes bright. Without fat saturation, however, differentiating normal from abnormal marrow can be difficult due to potential overlap of T2 signal intensities of neuroblastoma and combined hematopoietic/fatty marrow. Patients demonstrating the nodular pattern of marrow disease show better response to chemotherapy than those with the diffuse pattern. Following chemotherapy, patients with residual bone marrow metastases show significantly lower survival rates than those without residual metastases.

Inflammatory processes (infectious or noninfectious) replace or infiltrate normal marrow with inflammatory cells. In the case of infectious processes such as osteomyelitis, proliferating bacteria evoke an inflammatory response with resultant fluid accumulation in the marrow. Intramedullary pressure can increase and lead to marrow infarction. Increased water content and cellularity result in decreased marrow signal intensity on T1-weighted images and increased signal intensity on T2-weighted images (152,218). MR patterns may vary somewhat dependent upon the stage of osteomyelitis (152,196,218,219). Adjacent soft tissue edema and poorly marginated areas of involvement are features of acute, subacute, and recurrent osteomyelitis.

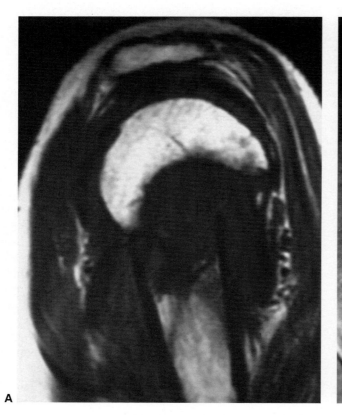 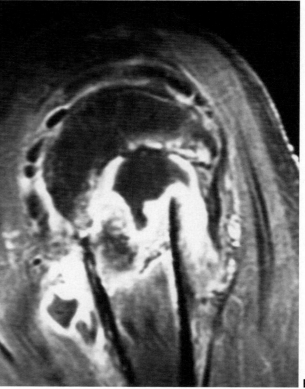

A B

Figure 14-45 Osteomyelitis with ring enhancement. T1-weighted images obtained before **(A)** (SE 500/20) and after **(B)** (SE 600/20 with fat saturation) administration of intravenous gadolinium demonstrate ring enhancement of an area of osteomyelitis in the proximal humeral metaphysis. When present, ring enhancement is a reliable sign of osteomyelitis.

Margins of involved sites are generally better defined in chronic osteomyelitis. Short TI inversion recovery and FSE–IR pulse sequences increase sensitivity for detecting osteomyelitis but tend to overestimate the true extent of infection as uninfected areas of marrow edema cannot be separated from infected regions with these sequences (155). This pitfall is particularly evident in settings of adjacent septic arthritis or neuropathic joint formation (220). The use of fat-suppressed, gadolinium-enhanced T1-weighted sequences results in significantly improved sensitivity and specificity as compared with either nonenhanced MR imaging or radionuclide bone scintigraphy for diagnosing osteomyelitis in all patients and particularly those with complicating clinical factors (221). Reliable patterns of osteomyelitis include rim enhancement (see Fig. 14-45) or enhancement of both soft tissue and bone marrow to a visually similar degree. Pre- and postcontrast, fat-suppressed images also better define the actual extent of infected marrow (222,223). Patients with septic or neuropathic joints again present potential pitfalls. In these settings, a small amount of subarticular enhancement may be present in the absence of infection making diagnosis of early osteomyelitis difficult. When more extensive involvement of the marrow space is present osteomyelitis is generally found. In all clinical settings, the diagnosis of osteomyelitis should not be suggested on MR studies without signal alterations on STIR, IR or fat-suppressed T2-weighted images coupled with marrow enhancement on postgadolinium T1-weighted images. Although most commonly confined to a single site, osteomyelitis can be multifocal in nature, particularly in infancy and childhood where up to 40% of cases have more than one site affected (113) (see Fig. 14-46) (224).

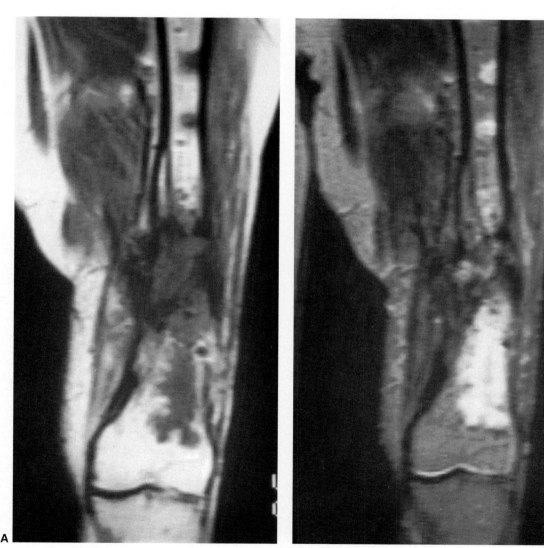

A   **B**

Figure 14-46 Marrow infiltration from multifocal infection in a 50-year-old man. Coronal T1- (SE 700/17) **(A)** and T2-weighted (SE 3,000/90) **(B)** images of the left femur demonstrate multiple foci of osteomyelitis throughout the medullary space. The foci demonstrate typical signal alterations encountered in osteomyelitis being low in signal intensity on Tl-weighted images and high in signal intensity on T2-weighted images.

In cases of infectious spondylitis, bone marrow signal alterations can be observed in vertebral bodies not involved with osteomyelitis (225). This phenomenon occurs in approximately 25% of patients with infectious spondylitis. The signal changes are nonspecific and mimic those encountered in patients with hyperplastic red marrow from other causes such as hematopoietic hyperplasia and hemolytic anemia (226). It is speculated that the decreased T1 signal intensity in this setting results from replacement of fat cells by nonneoplastic proliferating white blood cell precursors that are being stimulated to fight the ongoing infection. That being the case, the severity of marrow signal alteration would be expected to be influenced by the chronicity and gravity of the ongoing infection. Enhancement of this responding marrow following intravenous gadolinium can be documented quantitatively and often appreciated visually. The affected marrow would also be expected to show some degree of increased signal intensity on T2-weighted and inversion recovery imaging although in subtle cases the changes could prove difficult to appreciate visually. Since the pattern of marrow signal change is nonspecific, the possibility of an underlying marrow disorder would have to be considered if the marrow alterations did not return to a normal pattern following successful treatment of the spondylitis.

Chronic recurrent multifocal osteomyelitis (also referred to as chronic symmetric plasma cell osteomyelitis) (224,227,228) causes inflammatory marrow lesions at multiple skeletal locations. The disease shows a predilection for medial ends of clavicles and metaphyseal regions in lower extremities. Less commonly, other skeletal sites can be involved including the spine (229). Although these lesions mimic osteomyelitis, no definitive causative organism has been identified. The diagnosis is established through exclusion (230,231). The following criteria should be met before a diagnosis of chronic recurrent multifocal osteomyelitis is made: (i) two or more bone lesions identified clinically or on imaging studies; (ii) recurrent clinical symptoms (pain, swelling, and tenderness) lasting over 6 months with symptom-free intervals between attacks; (iii) 1 month of unsuccessful antibiotic therapy; (iv) typical lytic radiographic lesions (sometimes with intense sclerosis) that show increased uptake on bone scan; (v) no identifiable organism; (vi) no fistula, abscess, or sequestra formation; (vii) involvement of sites atypical of classical bacterial osteomyelitis such as the clavicles; (viii) nonspecific laboratory and histopathological findings consistent with osteomyelitis; and (ix) acne and palmoplantar pustulosis sometimes present (224,227). The disease is predominately found in children, with most patients presenting before 10 years of age. Many investigators believe that this disorder is closely related to SAPHO (synovitis, acne, pustulosis, hyperostosis, osteitis) syndrome (see below) in adults. MR findings at involved sites correlate with disease activity (224,232,233). In the active lytic phase, lesions display decreased T1 signal intensity and increased T2 signal intensity. As the lesions become more chronic and sclerotic radiographically, T1 and T2 signal intensity decline. Similarly, lesion enhancement with gadolinium is marked during active phases and decreases with declining lesion activity. Soft tissue involvement and abscess formation are lacking at affected sites in the appendicular skeleton and spine. Other characteristic features in the spine include multilevel involvement which usually skips vertebral bodies, a predilection for anterior vertebral involvement and varying degrees of vertebral collapse including vertebra plana.

SAPHO syndrome is another inflammatory process that produces marrow lesions at multiple skeletal locations (192,234,235). Patients display a variety of osseous and articular manifestations in association with chronic pustular skin lesions, particularly pustulosis palmaris et plantaris. Skeletal lesions are characterized by inflammation but no causative agent has been identified. Metaphyses of long bones are favored sites in children, while the anterior chest wall, including sternoclavicular, manubriosternal, and costosternal junctions, are most commonly affected in adults. Spinal involvement is increasingly being identified on MR studies in these patients. Thoracic vertebrae are most frequently affected followed by lumbar and then cervical vertebrae. MR findings in the spine correlate with recognized radiographic features of diffuse hyperostosis of the vertebral bodies, paravertebral ligamentous ossification, osteophyte/syndesmophyte formation and end-plate irregularities, erosions, and sclerosis (192). Focal and diffuse patterns of spinal marrow involvement have been identified on MRI (235). Focal lesions are typically located adjacent to end-plates or at the corners of the vertebral bodies and display low T1 signal intensity with hyperintense T2 signal intensity reflecting marrow changes associated with discitis. Other MR features of discitis, including hyperintense disc signal intensity on T2-weighted images and disc enhancement following intravenous gadolinium, may or may not be present. The differing presentations are presumed to reflect acute and chronic stages of discitis in this disorder. The diffuse pattern of signal abnormality is believed to signify the osteitis component of SAPHO syndrome. The marrow of several vertebral bodies and sometimes the posterior elements can be involved. Affected areas show low T1 and high T2 signal intensity. Signs of adjacent discitis need not be present. Paravertebral soft tissue swelling and signal changes have also been observed likely reflecting associated inflammatory response. MR findings at involved appendicular sites are identical to those seen in chronic recurrent multifocal osteomyelitis. Indeed, many authors believe that chronic recurrent multifocal osteomyelitis represents the childhood presentation of SAPHO syndrome.

Bone Marrow Edema

Most processes that produce a signal pattern of bone marrow edema (trauma, skeletal stress, reflex sympathetic dystrophy, regional migratory osteoporosis, transient osteoporosis, and bone marrow edema syndrome) are regionally limited, often affecting only one anatomic site (236,237). These focal processes are readily distinguished from diffuse marrow disorders. Confusion may arise, however, when a marrow edema process affects multiple sites. For example, in patients with insufficiency fractures of the pelvis, concurrent fractures can develop at sacral, parasymphyseal and the supraacetabular locations. The multiple abnormalities may raise suspicion of metastatic disease. However, when MR marrow abnormalities are encountered at these sites, the possibility of insufficiency fractures should be considered. In most cases, CT will resolve the issue by defining the fractures.

MR features of bone marrow edema include decreased marrow signal intensity on T1-weighted images and increased marrow signal intensity on T2-weighted images.

These findings reflect increased extracellular (interstitial) water. The amount of extra water controls the degree of signal intensity alteration, ranging from barely perceptible to quite conspicuous. Margins of the affected area are poorly defined and blend into adjacent normal marrow. Initiating, mediating, and controlling physiological factors of this edema are not clear. However, bone marrow edema is hypothesized to require hypervascularity or hyperperfusion (238).

Direct trauma can produce signal changes in bone marrow with or without associated complete fracture, insufficiency fracture, or stress fracture (239,240). These changes consist of irregular areas of low signal intensity on T1-weighted images that increase in signal intensity (greater than fat) on T2-weighted or STIR images (see Fig. 14-47). The degree of T1 and T2 signal intensity alteration

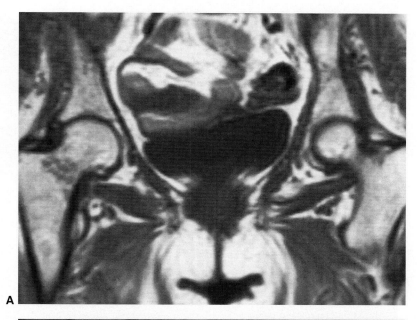

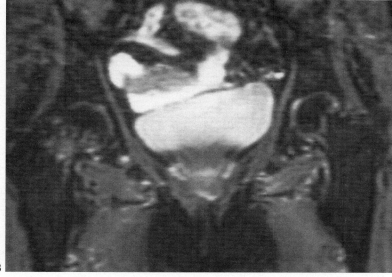

Figure 14-47 Marrow edema from stress fracture in a 69-year-old woman. An irregular band of decreased signal intensity is identified in the right femoral neck on this T1-weighted image (SE 600/20) **(A).** The involved area demonstrates increased signal intensity on a STIR image **(B).** This pattern presumably reflects marrow edema associated with a stress fracture of the femoral neck.

varies from subtle to profound, presumably reflecting the amount of edema present (see Fig. 14-48). Similarly, the extent of trauma-related marrow involvement can range from isolated foci intimately associated with the site of injury to diffuse regional marrow involvement. Although the MR signal patterns described above are consistent with increased tissue water, some contribution from hemorrhage may be present dependent upon the degree and time course of the injury. The contribution of hemorrhage remains unclear at present, as MR features of posttraumatic intraosseous hemorrhage have not been described experimentally or clinically, and time-related changes observed

in hemorrhage at other extracranial locations are yet to be observed in bone marrow injuries. In bone contusion, trabecular fractures, presumably present in most instances, typically are not apparent on MR studies, conventional radiographs, or CT.

Reflex sympathetic dystrophy (88,238) produces bone marrow changes through complex and poorly understood mechanisms, the net result of which appears to be accumulation of increased marrow water or edema. Factors associated with bone marrow edema such as mild inflammation, hyperemia, and increased bone turnover are sometimes evident on radionuclide studies and can be

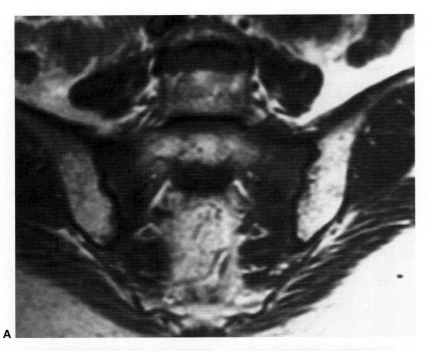

A

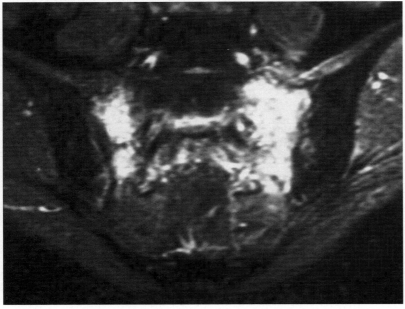

B

Figure 14-48 Marrow edema from sacral insufficiency fractures in a 72-year-old woman. **A:** Areas of low signal intensity are identified in the body of the sacrum and sacral ala on a coronal T1-weighted image (SE 600/20). The location of these signal changes is characteristic of sacral insufficiency fractures producing a distinctive "H" pattern. **B:** The regions of low T1 signal become bright on a coronal T2-weighted image (FSE 3,000/96 with fat saturation). The signal pattern is consistent with bone marrow edema associated with the insufficiency fractures.

shown histologically. MR abnormalities are inconsistently found (241). When present, increased tissue water produces expected MR signal patterns at involved sites. Regions of low signal intensity are evident on T1-weighted images and are correspondingly bright on T2-weighted images. The extent of marrow involvement is variable. MR signal patterns return to normal with resolution of the syndrome (88).

Transient osteoporosis is a condition of unknown cause characterized by spontaneous onset of self-limited pain and osteopenia. The pain may last up to 2 years before disappearing. Osteopenia of the involved site becomes radiographically evident within 8 weeks after the onset of pain and resolves over time (88,171,229,242,243). The proximal femur is by far the most common site involved; however, transient osteoporosis has been reported at several other locations, including the tarsus (244). A well-recognized clinical setting of transient osteoporosis of the hip occurs in women during the third trimester of pregnancy (245). In these patients, the left hip is almost exclusively involved. Hip involvement can also be seen in men and non-pregnant women, in which case either hip could be affected. MR imaging of transient osteoporosis reveals a bone marrow edema

pattern of low signal intensity on T1-weighted images and heterogeneous increased signal intensity on T2-weighted images. When present in the hip, the marrow edema extends from subarticular portions of the femoral head into the femoral neck and sometimes into the intertrochanteric region. Marrow involvement is usually diffuse, yet on occasion a portion of the femoral head may be spared (242). Mild acetabular involvement is variably present (246). MR findings generally precede radiographic changes.

A similar, and possibly related, syndrome of transient bone marrow edema occurs in major joints, typically the hip (236,238,246). As in the hip, knee involvement can occur spontaneously in healthy individuals but has also been described in the setting of patients receiving renal transplants (247). Involvement of the talus and other tarsal bones, although less common, has been reported (248,249). MR images of involved sites display signal intensity changes typical of marrow edema with diffuse low signal intensity on T1-weighted images and corresponding homogeneous high signal intensity on T2-weighted images (see Fig. 14-49). The process may involve only a portion of the epiphysis or the entire end of a long bone.

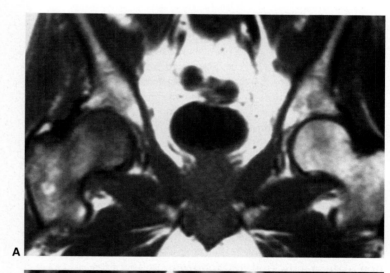

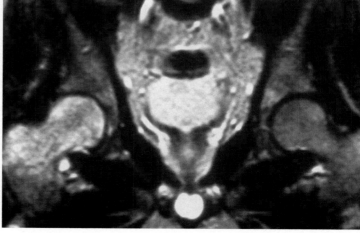

Figure 14-49 Marrow edema from transient bone marrow edema syndrome of the hip in a 48-year-old man. Signal changes are evident in the proximal right femur consistent with bone marrow edema. **A:** Diffuse, heterogeneous, low signal intensity is observed in the right femoral head and neck on a coronal T1-weighted image (SE 600/20). This area of signal abnormality displays increased signal intensity on a coronal T2-weighted image **(B)** (SE 2,000/80). Since the patient did not develop radiographically evident osteoporosis, the patient was believed to have transient bone marrow edema syndrome by exclusion.

Similarly, tarsal and carpal bones may show partial or diffuse involvement. Associated findings of joint effusion and periarticular soft tissue edema are generally present (248). Patients usually experience a protracted course of pain with limitation of motion. As with transient osteoporosis, the process is self-limited and repeat MR studies are normal. This entity is thought to differ from transient osteoporosis in that patients with true bone marrow edema syndrome fail to show radiographic evidence of osteopenia. Early AVN has been speculated as a possible etiology of this condition. Yet angiographic and scintigraphic studies reveal dilated nutrient arteries with increased perfusion of the involved bone (78) and follow-up imaging studies fail to reveal areas of marrow infarction. For these reasons, some investigators believe that the transient bone marrow edema syndrome should be considered a separate entity (246).

The MR pattern of bone marrow edema in the hip is not specific for any of the disorders previously discussed. Differential considerations in this setting include: (i) transient osteoporosis; (ii) transient bone marrow edema syndrome; (iii) early osteonecrosis; (iv) reflex sympathetic dystrophy; (v) osseous contusion or stress injury; (vi) infection; and (vii) infiltrating neoplasm (246). When subchondral marrow of the femoral head shows a homogeneous edema pattern on T2-weighted or contrast-enhanced T-1 weighted sequences, the cause has a high likelihood of being transient (250). When areas of low signal intensity exceeding 4 mm in width or 12 mm in length are identified on T2-weighted or contrast-enhanced T1-weighted sequences in addition to the marrow edema pattern, the etiology is more likely to be irreversible. High-resolution T2-weighted images have been suggested as a way to separate early osteonecrosis from transient osteoporosis and transient bone marrow edema syndrome by the presence of a focal subchondral defect (251); however, the presence of such a defect does not uniformly indicate osteonecrosis (250). Radiographically detectable osteopenia could be used to separate transient osteoporosis from transient bone marrow edema and osteonecrosis. Differentiating other causes would rely on the patient's clinical presentation, radiographic findings, follow-up radiographs, and possibly follow-up MR studies. When the diagnosis remains elusive, biopsy may be necessary.

The knee is also a frequent site of bone marrow edema. Most commonly, the edema is the result of trauma and reflects the presence of osseous contusion. Outside of trauma, many other processes can produce a bone marrow edema pattern in the knee, including rheumatologic conditions, septic arthritis, neuropathic joint formation, reflex sympathetic dystrophy, AVN, infiltrative neoplasm, transient osteoporosis, and transient bone marrow edema syndrome. The presence or absence of soft-tissue involvement becomes key in differentiating many of these disorders. Absent soft-tissue abnormalities, the leading differential considerations would be AVN, transient bone marrow

edema syndrome, transient osteoporosis, infiltrative neoplasm, and hematogenous infection (252). This list can be further narrowed in the same manner as it was in the setting of bone marrow edema of the hip. Additional discriminating features may be helpful. Patients with idiopathic osteonecrosis present with spontaneous onset of medial knee pain. Bone marrow edema in seen on MR images most commonly affecting the medial femoral condyle (143). Lateral femoral condyle or tibial involvement occurs infrequently (136). In hematogenous osteomyelitis, isolated involvement of the femur is more common than the tibia. Involvement of both should not be suspected unless there is concomitant joint involvement.

Bone marrow edema resembling the transient marrow edema syndrome has been described in the tibial diaphysis (253). It remains to be proven whether or not these marrow edema patterns are related to one another. A common initiating factor or causative agent has yet to be found. Nevertheless, it appears that transient marrow edema

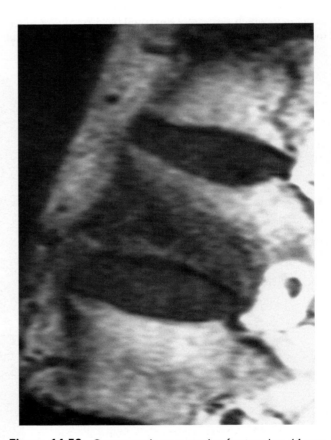

Figure 14-50 Osteoporotic compression fracture in a 64-year-old woman. A sagittal T1-weighted image (SE 500/20) of the spine demonstrates a mild compression deformity of T12. A transverse band of high signal intensity (normal fatty marrow) is present in the superior portion of the vertebral body. When present in a compression fracture, this or similar bands of fatty marrow are strong indicators that the fracture is of osteoporotic and not malignant origin. The low signal intensity in the inferior portion of the vertebral body likely reflects marrow edema related to the acute nature of the fracture.

occurs more commonly and in more forms than previously recognized.

PITFALLS

The pitfalls encountered in interpretation of MR studies in diffuse marrow disorders primarily relate to the distinction between normal hematopoietic marrow and pathologic processes in marrow. This distinction becomes extremely difficult when the pathologic tissue exhibits signal intensities similar to those of normal red marrow on both T1- and T2-weighted images. Disease processes most likely to present in this fashion include anemia (apart from aplastic anemia), metastatic disease, myeloma, lymphoma, and leukemia. At present, there is no reliable means to distinguish such disorders from red marrow through the use of MR imaging. MR spectroscopy, diffusion imaging, and dynamic contrast-enhanced imaging have potential to aid in the differentiation, but are, to date, unproven in large-scale clinical trials. In unclear cases, bone marrow aspiration or biopsy of MR abnormal marrow is necessary to establish a diagnosis (254,255).

Alterations in the expected distribution of red/yellow marrow throughout the skeleton further complicate MR bone marrow interpretation. This pitfall is common on MR examinations of the knee where persistent or reconverted red marrow is frequent. This focal red marrow presence is now recognized as physiologic in certain groups of patients as mentioned earlier (see section on reconversion). Among these are marathon runners (63), heavy smokers (greater than one pack/day), obese women who smoke, and patients under 39 years of age. Red marrow can also be influenced by menstruation, endurance activities, altitude, and various drug therapies (48,62,80,93,111,209,256). Persistent distal femoral red marrow requires further investigation when the patient's clinical history does not conform to one of the above situations or when the morphologic or signal pattern is atypical for normal hematopoietic marrow. The presence of red marrow in the epiphyseal regions of the knee is abnormal and requires further investigation.

Focal marrow processes are less often confused with diffuse marrow disease. Included among these processes is focal fat deposition in cellular marrow and degenerative changes about joints. Focal fat replacement demonstrates signal patterns of normal marrow fat on T1- and T2-weighted images

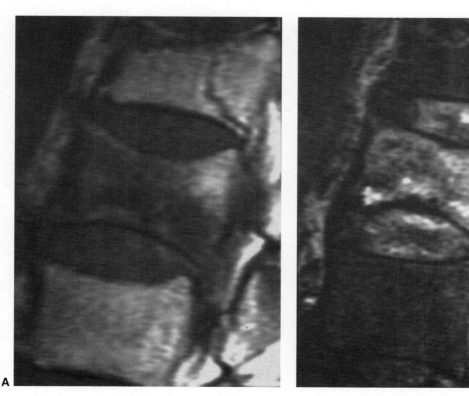

A **B**

Figure 14-51 Fluid sign of osteoporotic compression fracture in a 75-year-old woman. **A:** Sagittal T1 (SE 550/14) and **(B)** corresponding sagittal T2-weighted (FSE 2,800/105 with fat saturation) images of the lumbar spine demonstrate a compression deformity of L-2. Note the triangular and linear areas of fluid signal intensity adjacent to the compressed inferior endplate of L-2 on the T2-weighted image **B.** This sign is found predominately in osteoporotic compression fractures, as in this case.

and is typically found at certain locations in vertebral bodies (endplates, periphery, and about the central venous plexus). Vertebral marrow changes that occur in the setting of degenerative disc disease are generally characteristic and have been discussed earlier in this chapter. Degenerative changes at the margins of synovial articulations can also alter the MR appearance of subjacent bone marrow. Subchondral sclerosis can appear as focal decreased signal intensity on T1- and T2-weighted images. Subchondral cysts usually appear as foci of decreased signal intensity on T1-weighted images that become bright on T2-weighted images (following the signal pattern of synovial fluid). If not fluid-filled, these "cysts" will be less bright (or even low-signal intensity) on T2-weighted images. Usually, the MR findings associated with degenerative disease are explained with conventional radiographs of the region.

Diffuse lowering of marrow signal intensity on T1- and T2-weighted images in the absence of known systemic neoplastic disease can be an unexpected finding and potentially overlooked. When the signal changes are profound, identification of the abnormal marrow can be more reliably made than when signal changes are subtle. Absent clinically determining factors, only differential possibilities for the MR abnormalities can be suggested. Among these are chronic hemolytic anemias, AIDS, chronic inflammatory disease (e.g., rheumatoid arthritis), long-term chemotherapy, Gaucher, myelofibrosis, and patients with a history of multiple blood transfusions (90,199,257).

Separating benign from malignant vertebral compression fractures can be problematic in the acute setting (fractures of less than 2 months duration). The problem arises from edema, hemorrhage, and repair tissue that accompanies acute osteoporotic vertebral collapse (258,259). The resultant marrow signal changes can be difficult to differentiate from those seen in malignant compression fractures. Features favoring osteoporosis as the etiology include preservation of some normal marrow signal within the vertebral body (particularly in a horizontal bandlike pattern) (see Fig. 14-50), bandlike low signal intensity in the vertebral body on T1- and T2- weighted images (possibly representing compressed trabeculae and a fracture line), and retropulsion of a posterior bone fragment (53,121). The presence of a fluid collection within the vertebral body (fluid sign) can also be helpful in identifying osteoporotic compression fractures (17) (see Fig. 14-51). The fluid sign is described as being linear, triangular, or focal in configuration and displaying T1 and T2 signal equivalent to cerebrospinal fluid. The fluid collection is located adjacent to a fractured endplate. The finding can be present in roughly 25% of all fractures and up to 40% of osteoporotic fractures. There is an association between the severity of the fracture and the presence of a fluid sign. Histologically, the fluid collection corresponds to areas of osteonecrosis within the vertebral body. Radiographically, intravertebral vacuum clefts can be observed at involved

levels (17,260,261). Occasionally the fluid collection can become extensive and occupy most of the vertebral body (260). Although the MR fluid sign strongly suggests an osteoporotic fracture, the finding can rarely be encountered in malignant fractures (17). In these situations, histologic analysis has revealed areas of osteonecrosis adjacent to tumor. Signs suggesting malignant vertebral fractures include diffuse low T1 signal throughout the vertebral body and in the pedicles, epidural mass, encasing abnormal epidural tissue, focal paravertebral soft-tissue mass and convex posterior cortical margin of the vertebral body (see Fig. 14-52) (53,121). Controversy exists regarding other marrow signal patterns on noncontrast and contrast-enhanced pulse sequences in pathologic and acute benign compression fractures. Both display low signal intensity on T1-weighted sequences. On conventional T2-weighted images without fat suppression, some investigators have described osteoporotic fractures as being isointense and homogeneous (53,262). On FSE T2-weighted imaging without fat suppression others have described osteoporotic

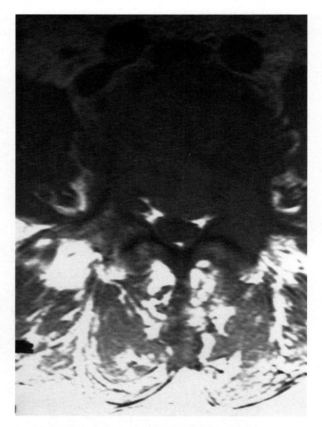

Figure 14-52 Malignant compression fracture from metastatic lung cancer in a 52-year-old man. An axial T1-weighted image (SE 500/20) of an L5 compression fracture demonstrates many of the features associated with malignant compression fractures. Note the presence of diffuse low signal intensity throughout the vertebral body extending into the pedicles and the presence of soft-tissue mass extending into the epidural and paraspinous soft tissues. These features are more typical of malignant compression fractures but can rarely be present in osteoporotic compression fractures.

fractures as having a spectrum of signal intensity ranging from low to hyperintense (121). Similarly, while some authors describe pathologic fractures as being hyperintense on conventional T2-weighted images without fat suppression, others describe a spectrum of low to hyperintense signal on FSE T2 images without fat suppression. This discrepancy may reflect interobserver variability and inherent differences between conventional and FSE sequences, particularly relating to the high signal displayed by fatty marrow on nonfat-saturated FSE T2 images. Variability in the types of tumors included in each study also probably contributes to observed differences in the signal patterns of pathologic fractures. Without fat saturation, gadolinium enhanced T1-weighted images show vertebral marrow returning to normal signal intensity in osteoporotic compression fractures (see Fig. 14-53) and displaying inhomogeneous enhancement in pathologic fractures (53). With fat saturation, gadolinium-enhanced T1-weighted sequences identify both homogenous and heterogeneous enhancement in benign and malignant compression fractures (53,121,263). These differences could relate to the presence or absence of fat saturation on the postcontrast

sequences. Even using these guidelines, some vertebral fractures remain problematic and sequential MR studies or biopsy may be necessary to determine the cause. This is particularly true in the setting of multiple myeloma, where some pathologic compression fractures occur in vertebrae that appear normal on MR imaging (183). Dynamic contrast-enhanced imaging and diffusion-weighted imaging appear promising as potential methods for resolving some of this confusion between benign and pathologic vertebral compression fractures (67,84,264).

Differentiating chronic osteoporotic compression fractures from most pathologic fractures is less problematic. Marrow signal intensity should return to normal in chronic osteoporotic compression fractures and any paravertebral soft tissue swelling/hemorrhage should resolve. Residual marrow signal alteration apart from fracture lines and discogenic changes requires explanation. As previously discussed, pathologic vertebral fractures from multiple myeloma can display normal-appearing marrow on routine MR examinations. Dynamic contrast-enhanced sequences could prove helpful in this setting, as these sequences have shown potential for identifying pathologic marrow before abnormalities are detectable on routine MR images (84).

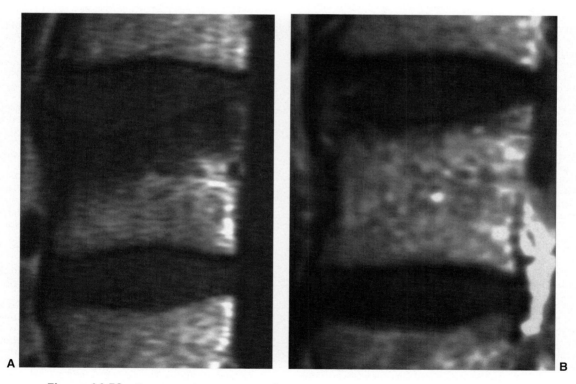

Figure 14-53 Osteoporotic compression fracture pre- and postgadolinium in a 74-year-old woman. Sagittal T1-weighted images (SE 500/15 without fat saturation) of L1 before **(A)** and after **(B)** the intravenous administration of gadolinium. On the precontrast image in **A** there is a band of low signal marrow subjacent to the compressed superior endplate of L1. Following the intravenous administration of gadolinium in **B,** the band of low signal shows homogeneous enhancement and becomes isointense with the remainder of the vertebral body. This pattern of enhancement is a good indicator of an osteoporotic compression fracture.

REFERENCES

1. Datz FL, Taylor A Jr. The clinical use of radionuclide bone marrow imaging. *Semin Nucl Med* 1985;15:239–259.
2. Daldrup-Link HE, Franzius C, Link TM, et al. Whole-body MR imaging for detection of bone metastases in children and young adults: comparison with skeletal scintigraphy and FDG PET. *AJR Am J Roentgenol* 2001;177:229–236.
3. Martin W, Delbeke W, Patton J, et al. Detection of malignancies with SPECT versus PET, with 2-[fluorine-18] fluoro-2-deosy-D-glucose. *Radiology* 1996;198:225–231.
4. Genant HK, Wilson JS, Bovill EG, et al. Computed tomography of the musculoskeletal system. *J Bone Joint Surg Am* 1980;62:1088–1101.
5. Vande Berg BC, Malghem J, Lecouvet FE, et al. Magnetic resonance imaging of the normal bone marrow. *Skeletal Radiol* 1998;27:471–483.
6. Trubowitz S, Davis S. *The bone marrow matrix. The human bone marrow: anatomy, physiology, and pathophysiology.* Boca Raton, FL: CRC, 1982:43–75.
7. Politis C, Karamerou A, Block M. Pathophysiologic aspects of the bone/marrow/fat relationship. *Lab Manage* 1983;21:40–55.
8. Snyder WS, Cook MH, Nasset ES, et al. *Report of the task group on reference man.* Oxford: Pergamon, 1974:79–98.
9. Tavossoli M, Houchin DB, Jacobs P. Fatty acid composition of adipose cells in red and yellow marrow: a possible determinant of haematopoietic potential. *Scand J Haematol* 1977;18:47–53.
10. Biermann A, Graf van Keyserlingk DG. Ultrastructure of reticulum cells in the bone marrow. *Acta Anat Basel* 1978;100:34–43.
11. Lichtman MA. The ultrastructure of the hemopoietic environment of the marrow: a review. *Exp Hematol* 1981;9:391–410.
12. Van Dyke D. Similarity in distribution of skeletal blood flow and erythropoietic marrow. *Clin Orthop* 1967;52:37–51.
13. Weiss L. The structure of bone marrow functional interrelationships of vascular and hematopoietic compartments in experimental hemolytic anemia: an electron microscopic study. *J Morphol* 1965;117:467–538.
14. Hartsock RJ, Smith EB, Petty CS. Normal variation with aging of the amount of hematopoietic tissue in bone marrow from the anterior iliac crest. *Am J Clin Pathol* 1965;43:326–331.
15. Bousvaros A, Kirks DR. Imaging of neuroblastoma: an overview. *Pediatr Radiol* 1986;16:89–106.
16. Emery JL, Follett GF. Regression of bone-marrow haemopoiesis from the terminal digits in the foetus and infant. *Br J Haematol* 1964;10:485–489.
17. Baur A, Stabler A, Arbogast S, et al. Acute osteoporotic and neoplastic vertebral compression fractures: fluid sign at MR imaging. *Radiology* 2002;225:730–735.
18. Hashimoto M. The distribution of active marrow in the bones of normal adults. *Kyushu J Med Sci* 1960;11:103–111.
19. Neumann E. Das gesetz der verbreitung des gelben und roten, markes in den extremitatenknochen. *Centralblatt Med Wiss* 1882;20:321–323.
20. Piney A. The anatomy of the bone marrow. *Br Med J* 1922;2:792–795.
21. Custer RP, Ahlfeldt FE. Studies on the structure and function of bone marrow. II. Variations in cellularity in various bones with advancing years of life and their relative response to stimuli. *J Lab Clin Med* 1932;17:960–962.
22. Koo KH, Dussault R, Kaplan P, et al. Age-related marrow conversion in the proximal metaphysis of the femur: evaluation with T1-weighted MR imaging. *Radiology* 1998;206:745–748.
23. Mirowitz SA. Hematopoietic bone marrow within the proximal humeral epiphysis in normal adults: investigation with MR imaging. *Radiology* 1993;188:689–693.
24. Richardson ML, Patten RM. Age-related changes in marrow distribution in the shoulder: MR imaging findings. *Radiology* 1994;192:209–215.
25. Vande Berg BC, Lecouvet FE, Moysan P, et al. MR assessment of red marrow distribution and composition in the proximal femur: correlation with clinical and laboratory parameters. *Skeletal Radiology* 1997;26:589–596.
26. Hashimoto M. Pathology of bone marrow. *Acta Haematol* 1962;27:193–216.
27. Vogler JB, Murphy WA. Bone Marrow Imaging. *Radiology* 1988;168:679–693.
28. Dunnill MS, Anderson JA, Whitehead R. Quantitative histological studies on age changes in bone. *J Pathol Bacteriol* 1967;94:275–291.
29. Huggins C, Blocksom BH Jr. Changes in outlying bone marrow accompanying a local increase of temperature within physiological limits. *J Exp Med* 1936;64:253–274.
30. Tribukait B. Experimental studies on the regulation of erythropoiesis with special reference to the importance of oxygen. *Acta Physiol Scand* 1963;58:1–48.
31. Custer RP. Studies on the structure and function of bone marrow. I. Variability of the hemopoietic pattern and consideration of method for examination. *J Lab Clin Med* 1932;17:951–959.
32. Jacobsen EM, Davis AK, Alpen EL. Relative effectiveness of phenylhydrazine treatment and hemorrhage in the production of an erythropoietic factor. *Blood* 1956;11:937–945.
33. Wehrli FW, MacFall JR, Shutts D, et al. Mechanisms of contrast in NMR imaging. *J Comput Assist Tomogr* 1984;8:369–380.
34. Laredo JD, Assouline E, Gelbert F, et al. Vertebral hemangiomas: fat content as a sign of aggressiveness. *Radiology* 1990;177:467–472.
35. Mitchell DG, Burk DL Jr, Vinitski S, et al. The biophysical basis of tissue contrast in extracranial MR imaging. *AJR Am J Roentgenol* 1987;149:831–837.
36. Rao VM, Fishman M, Mitchell DG, et al. Painful sickle cell crisis: bone marrow patterns observed with MR imaging. *Radiology* 1986;161:211–215.
37. Wismer GL, Rosen BR, Buxton R, et al. Chemical shift imaging of bone marrow: preliminary experience. *AJR Am J Roentgenol* 1985;145:1031–1037.
38. Alexanian R, Haut A, Khan AU, et al. Treatment for multiple myeloma: combination chemotherapy with different melphalan dose regimens. *JAMA* 1969;96:1680–1685.
39. Sebag GH, Dubois J, Tabet M, et al. Pediatric spinal bone marrow: assessment of normal age-related changes in the MRI appearance. *Pediatr Radiol* 1993;23:515–518.
40. Dwek JR, Shapiro F, Laor T, et al. Normal gadolinium-enhanced MR images of the developing appendicular skeleton: part 2. Epiphyseal and metaphyseal marrow. *AJR Am J Roentgenol* 1997;169:191–196.
41. Baur A, Stabler A, Bartl R, et al. MRI gadolinium enhancement of bone marrow: age-related changes in normals and in diffuse neoplastic infiltration. *Skeletal Radiol* 1997;25:414–418.
42. Chen W, Shih TT, Chen R, et al. Vertebral bone marrow perfusion evaluated with dynamic contrast-enhanced MR imaging: significance of aging and sex. *Radiology* 2001;220:213–218.
43. Saifuddin A, Bann K, Ridgway JP, et al. Bone marrow blood supply in gadolinium-enhanced magnetic resonance imaging. *Skeletal Radiol* 1994;23:455–457.
44. Montazel JL, Divine M, Lepage E, et al. Normal spinal bone marrow in adults: dynamic gadolinium-enhanced MR imaging. *Radiology* 2003;229:703–709.
45. Moore SG, Bisset GSI, Siegel MJ, et al. Pediatric musculoskeletal MR imaging. *Radiology* 1991;179:345–360.
46. Moore SG, Dawson KL. Red and yellow marrow in the femur: age-related changes in appearance at MR imaging. *Radiology* 1990;175:219–223.
47. Bohndorf K, Reiser M, Lochner B, et al. Magnetic resonance imaging of primary tumours and tumour-like lesions of bone. *Skeletal Radiol* 1986;15:511–517.
48. Caldemeyer KS, Smith RR, Harris A, et al. Hematopoietic bone marrow hyperplasia: correlation of spinal MR findings, Hematologic parameters, and bone mineral density in endurance athletes. *Radiology* 1996;198:503–508.
49. Schuck JE, Czarnecki DJ. MR detection of probable hematopoietic hyperplasia involving the knees, proximal femurs, and pelvis. *AJR Am J Roentgenol* 1989;143:655–656.
50. Levine CD, Schweitzer ME, Ehrlich SM. Pelvic marrow in adults. *Skeletal Radiol* 1994;23:343–347.
51. Schweitzer ME, Levine C, Mitchell DG, et al. Bull's-eyes and halos: useful MR discriminators of osseous metastases. *Radiology* 1993;188:249–252.

52. Ricci C, Cova M, Kang YS, et al. Normal age-related patterns of cellular and fatty bone marrow distribution in the axial skeleton: MR imaging study. *Radiology* 1990;177:83–88.

53. Algra PR, Bloem JL, Valk J. Disappearance of the basivertebral vein; a new MR imaging sign of bone marrow disease. *AJR Am J Roentgenol* 1991;157:1129–1130.

54. Dooms GC, Fisher MR, Hricak H, et al. Bone marrow imaging: magnetic resonance studies related to age and sex. *Radiology* 1985;155:429–432.

55. Genant HK, Cann CE. Quantitative computed tomography for assessing vertebral bone mineral. In: Genant HK, Chafetz H, Helms CA, eds. *Computed tomography of the lumbar spine.* San Francisco, CA: University of California, 1982:289–314.

56. Hajek PC, Baker LL, Goobar HE, et al. Focal fat deposition in axial bone marrow: MR characteristics. *Radiology* 1987;162: 245–249.

57. de Roos A, Kressel HY, Spritzer C, et al. MR imaging of marrow changes adjacent to end plates in degenerative lumbar disk disease. *AJR Am J Roentgenol* 1987;149:531–534.

58. Dawson KL, Moore SG, Rowland JM. Age-related marrow changes in the pelvis: MR and anatomic findings. *Radiology* 1992;183:47–51.

59. Duda SH, Laniado M, Schick F, et al. Normal bone marrow in the sacrum of young adults: differences between the sexes seen on chemical-shift MR imaging. *AJR Am J Roentgenol* 1995;164: 935–940.

60. Zawin JK, Jaramillo D. Conversion of bone marrow in the humerus, sternum, and clavicle: changes with age on MR images. *Radiology* 1993;188:159–164.

61. Waitches G, Zawin JK, Poznanski AK. Sequence and rate of bone marrow conversion in the femora of children as seen on MR imaging: are accepted standards accurate? *AJR Am J Roentgenol* 1994;162:1399–1406.

62. Wilson AJ, Hodge JC, Pilgram TK, et al. Prevalence of red marrow around the knee joint in adults as demonstrated on magnetic resonance imaging. *Acad Radiol* 1996;3:550–555.

63. Shellock FG, Morris E, Deutsch AL, et al. Hematopoietic bone marrow hyperplasia: high prevalence on MR images of the knee in asymptomatic marathon runners. *AJR Am J Roentgenol* 1992;158:335–338.

64. Barlogie B, Jagannath S, Vesole DH, et al. Superiority of tandem autologous transplantation over standard therapy for previously untreated multiple myeloma. *Blood* 1997;89:789–793.

65. Pal CR, Tasker AD, Ostlere SJ, et al. Heterogeneous signal in bone marrow on MRI of children's feet: a normal finding? *Skeletal Radiol* 1999;28:274–278.

66. Lazzarini KM, Troiana RN, Smith RC. Can running cause the appearance of marrow edema on MR images if the foot and ankle? *Radiology* 1997;202:504–542.

67. Baur A, Stabler A, Bruning R, et al. Diffusion-weighted MR imaging of bone marrow: differentiation of benign versus pathologic compression fractures. *Radiology* 1998;207:349–356.

68. Winkler ML, Ortendahl DA, Mille TC, et al. Characteristics of partial flip angle and gradient reversal imaging. *Radiology* 1988; 166:17–26.

69. Dixon WT. Simple proton spectroscopic imaging. *Radiology* 1984;153:189–194.

70. Disler DG, McCauley TR, Ratner LM, et al. In-phase and out-of-phase MR imaging of bone marrow: prediction of neoplasia based on the detection of coexistent fat and water. *AJR Am J Roentgenol* 1997;169:1439–1447.

71. Jones KM, Unger EC, Granstrom P, et al. Bone marrow imaging using STIR at 0.5 and 1.5 T. *Magn Reson Imaging* 1992;10:169–176.

72. Takagi S, Tanaka O. The role of magnetic resonance imaging in the diagnosis and monitoring of myelodysplastic syndromes or leukemia. *Leukemia and Lymphoma* 1996;23:443–450.

73. Lang PH, Fritz R, Majumdar S, et al. Hematopoietic bone marrow in the adult knee: spin-echo and opposed-phase gradient-echo mr imaging. *Skeletal Radiol* 1993;22:95–103.

74. Hendrick RE, Kneeland JB, Stark DD. Maximizing signal-to-noise and contrast-to-noise ratios in FLASH imaging. *Magn Reson Imaging* 1987;5:117–127.

75. Mirowitz SA, Apicella P, Reinus WR, et al. MR imaging of bone marrow lesions: relative conspicuousness on T1-weighted, fat-suppressed T2-weighted, and STIR images. *AJR Am J Roentgenol* 1994;162:215–221.

76. Pui MH, Goh PS, Choo HF, et al. Magnetic resonance imaging of musculoskeletal lesions: comparison of three fat-saturation pulse sequences. *Australas Radiol* 1997;41:99–102.

77. Yasumoto M, Nonomura Y, Yoshimura R, et al. MR detection of iliac bone marrow involvement by malignant lymphoma with various MR sequences including diffusion-weighted echo-planar imaging. *Skeletal Radiol* 2002;31:263–269.

78. Abrams HL, Spiro R, Goldstein N. Metastases in carcinoma: analysis of 1000 autopsied cases. *Cancer* 1950;3:336–340.

79. Allison GT, Bostrom MP, Glesby MJ. Osteonecrosis in HIV disease: epidemiology, etiologies, and clinical management. *AIDS* 2003;17:1–9.

80. Fletcher BD, Wall JE, Hanna SL. Effect of hematopoietic growth factors on MR images of bone marrow in children undergoing chemotherapy. *Radiology* 1993;189:745–751.

81. Ishizake H, Horikoshi H, Inoue T, et al. Bone marrow cellularity: quantification by chemical-shift misregistration in magnetic resonance imaging and comparison with histomorphometrical techniques. *Australas Radiol* 1995;39:411–414.

82. Monier P, Mckown K, Bronze MS. Osteonecrosis complicating highly active antiretroviral therapy in patients infected with human immunodeficiency virus. *Clin Infect Dis* 2000;31: 1488–1492.

83. Schick F, Einsele H, Kost R, et al. Hematopoietic reconstitution after bone marrow transplantation: assessment with MR imaging and H-1 localized spectroscopy. *J Magn Reson Imaging* 1994;4:71–78.

84. Rahmouni A, Montazel JL, Divine M, et al. Bone marrow with diffuse tumor infiltration in patients with lymphoproliferative diseases: dynamic gadolinium-enhanced MR imaging. *Radiology* 2003;229:710–717.

85. Moulopoulos LA, Maris TG, Papanikolaou N, et al. Detection of malignant bone marrow involvement with dynamic contrast-enhanced magnetic resonance imaging. *Ann Oncol* 2003;14: 152–158.

86. Vande Berg BC, Malghem J, Lecouvet FE, et al. Classification and detection of bone marrow lesions with magnetic resonance imaging. *Skeletal Radiol* 1998;27:529–545.

87. Sabin FR. Bone marrow. *Physiol Rev* 1928;8:191–244.

88. Bloem JL. Transient osteoporosis of the hip: MR imaging. *Radiology* 1988;167:753–755.

89. Tehranzadeh J, O'Malley P, Rafii M. The spectrum of osteoarticular and soft tissue changes in patients with human immunodeficiency virus (HIV) infection. *Crit Rev Diagn Imaging* 1996;37:305–347.

90. Tehranzadeh J, Ter-Oganesyan RR, Steinbach LS. Musculoskeletal disorders associated with HIV infection and AIDS. Part II: non-infectious musculoskeletal conditions. *Skeletal Radiol* 2004;33: 311–320.

91. Rosenthal DI, Scott JA, Barranger J, et al. Evaluation of Gaucher disease using magnetic resonance imaging. *J Bone Joint Surg Am* 1986;68:802–808.

92. Lanir A, Aghai E, Simon JS, et al. MR imaging in myelofibrosis. *J Comput Assist Tomogr* 1986;10:634–636.

93. Poulton TB, Murphy WD, Duerk JL, et al. Bone marrow reconversion in adults who are smokers: MR imaging findings. *AJR Am J Roentgenol* 1993;161:1217–1221.

94. Blomlie V, Rofstad EK, Skjonsberg A, et al. Female pelvic bone marrow: serial MR imaging before, during, and after radiation therapy. *Radiology* 1995;194:537–543.

95. Kaplan PA, Asleson RJ, Klassen LW, et al. Bone marrow patterns in aplastic anemia: observations with 1.5 T MR imaging. *Radiology* 1987;164:441–444.

96. Cohen MD, Klatte EC, Baehner R, et al. Magnetic resonance imaging of bone marrow disease in children. *Radiology* 1984; 151:715–718.

97. Kangarloo H, Dietrich RB, Taira RT, et al. MR imaging of bone marrow in children. *J Comput Assist Tomogr* 1986;10:205–209.

98. Olson DL, Shields AF, Scheurich CJ, et al. Magnetic resonance imaging of the bone marrow in patients with leukemia, aplastic anemia, and lymphoma. *Invest Radiol* 1986;21:540–546.

99. Amano Y, Hayashi H, Kumazaki T. Gd-DTPA enhanced MRI of reactive hematopoietic regions in marrow. *J Comput Assist Tomogr* 1994;18:214–217.

100. Kanwar VS, Wang WC, Winer-Muram HT, et al. Magnetic resonance imaging for evaluation of childhood aplastic anemia. *J Pediatr Hematol Oncol* 1995;17:284–289.

101. Carroll KW, Feller JF, Tirman PFJ. Useful internal standards for distinguishing infiltrative marrow pathology from hematopoietic marrow at MRI. *J Magn Reson Imaging* 1997;7:394–398.

102. Kricun ME. Red-yellow marrow conversion: its effect on the location of some solitary bone lesions. *Skeletal Radiol* 1985;14:10–19.

103. McKinstry CS, Steiner RE, Young AT, et al. Bone marrow in leukemia and aplastic anemia: MR imaging before, during, and after treatment. *Radiology* 1987;161:239–244.

104. Sugimura H, Kisanuki A, Tamura S, et al. Magnetic resonance imaging of bone marrow changes after irradiation. *Invest Radiol* 1994;29:35–41.

105. Aisen AM, Martel W, Braunstein EM, et al. MRI and CT evaluation of primary bone and soft tissue tumors. *AJR Am J Roentgenol* 1986;146:749–756.

106. Cavenagh EC, Weinberger E, Shae DW, et al. Hematopoietic marrow regeneration in pediatric patients undergoing spinal irradiation: MR depiction. *AJNR Am J Neuroradiol* 1995;16:461–467.

107. Otake S, Mayr NA, Ueda T, et al. Radiation-induced changes in MR signal intensity and contrast enhancement of lumbosacral vertebrae: do changes occur only inside the radiation therapy field? *Radiology* 2002;222:179–183.

108. Stevens SK, Moore SG, Kaplan ID. Early and late bone marrow changes following radiation: Magnetic resonance evaluation. *AJR Am J Roentgenol* 1990;154:745–750.

109. Casamassima F, Reggiero C, Caramella D, et al. Hematopoietic bone marrow recovery after radiation therapy: MRI evaluation. *Blood* 1989;73:1677–1681.

110. Kauczor HU, Dietl B, Brix G, et al. Fatty replacement of bone marrow after radiation therapy for Hodgkin disease: quantification with chemical shift imaging. *J Magn Reson Imaging* 1993;3:575–580.

111. Ryan SP, Weinberger E, White KS, et al. MR imaging of bone marrow in children with osteosarcoma: effect of granulocyte colony-stimulating factor. *AJR Am J Roentgenol* 1995;165:915–920.

112. Ojala AE, Lanning FP, Paakko EL, et al. Osteonecrosis in children treated for acute lymphoblastic leukemia; a magnetic resonance imaging study after treatment. *Med Ped Oncol* 1997;29:260–265.

113. Deely DM, Schweitzer ME. MR imaging of bone marrow disorders. *Radiol Clin North Am* 1997;35:193–212.

114. Lecouvet FE, Dechambre S, Malghem J, et al. Bone marrow transplantation in patients with multiple myeloma: prognostic significance of MR imaging. *AJR Am J Roentgenol* 2001;176:91–96.

115. Mitchell DG, Rao VM, Dalinka M, et al. Hematopoietic and fatty bone marrow distribution in the normal and ischemic hip: new observations with 1.5 T MR imaging. *Radiology* 1986;161:199–202.

116. Williams JL, Cliff MM, Bonakdarpour A. Spontaneous osteonecrosis of the knee. *Radiology* 1973;107:15–18.

117. Lotke PA, Ecker ML. Osteonecrosis-like syndrome of the medial tibial plateau. *Clin Orthop* 1983;176:148–152.

118. Totty WG, Murphy WA, Ganz WI, et al. Magnetic resonance imaging of the normal and ischemia femoral head. *AJR Am J Roentgenol* 1984;143:1273–1280.

119. Ehman RL, Berquist TH, McLeod RA. MR imaging of the musculoskeletal system: a 5-year appraisal. *Radiology* 1988;166:313–320.

120. Turner DA, Templeton AC, Selzer PM, et al. Femoral capital osteonecrosis: MR finding of diffuse marrow abnormalities without focal lesions. *Radiology* 1989;171:135–140.

121. Avrahami E, Tadmor R, Kaplinski N. The role of T2-weighted gradient echo in MRI demonstration of spinal multiple myeloma. *Spine* 1993;18:1812–1815.

122. Mitchell DG, Kressel HY, Arger PH, et al. Avascular necrosis of the femoral head: morphologic assessment by MR imaging, with CT correlation. *Radiology* 1986;161:739–742.

123. Ranade SE, Shah S, Advani SH, et al. Pulsed nuclear magnetic resonance studies of human bone marrow. *Physiol Chem Phys* 1977;9:297–299.

124. Zimmer WD, Berquist TH, McLeod RA, et al. Bone tumors: magnetic resonance imaging versus computed tomography. *Radiology* 1985;155:709–718.

125. Brady TJ, Gebhardt MC, Pykett IL, et al. NMR imaging of forearms in healthy volunteers and patients with giant-cell tumor of bone. *Radiology* 1982;144:549–552.

126. Cherryman GR, Smith FW. NMR scanning for skeletal tumours. *Lancet* 1984;1:1403–1404.

127. Sundaram J, McGuire MH, Herbold DR. Magnetic resonance imaging of osteosarcoma. *Skeletal Radiol* 1987;16:23–29 .

128. Moore SG, Gooding CA, Brasch RC, et al. Bone marrow in children with acute lymphocytic leukemia: MR relaxation times. *Radiology* 1986;160:237–240.

129. Thomsen C, Sorensen PG, Karle H, et al. Prolonged bone marrow T1-relaxation in acute leukemia: in vivo tissue characterization by magnetic resonance imaging. *Magn Reson Imaging* 1987;5:251–257.

130. Ross JS, Masaryk TJ, Modic MT, et al. Vertebral hemangiomas: MR imaging. *Radiology* 1987;165:165–169.

131. Biviji AA, Paiement GD, Steinbach LS. Musculoskeletal manifestations of human immunodeficiency virus infection. *J Am Acad Orthop Surg* 2002;10:312–320.

132. Boyko OB, Cory DA, Cohen MD, et al. MR imaging of osteogenic and Ewing's sarcoma. *AJR Am J Roentgenol* 1987;148:317–322.

133. Daffner RH, Lupetin AR, Dash N, et al. MRI in the detection of malignant infiltration of bvone marrow. *AJR Am J Roentgenol* 1986;146:353–358.

134. Fruehwald FXJ, Tscholakoff D, Schwaighofer B, et al. Magnetic resonance imaging of the lower vertebral column in patients with multiple myeloma. *Invest Radiol* 1988;23:193–199.

135. Rahmouni A, Divine M, Mathieu D, et al. Detection of multiple myeloma involving the spine: efficacy of fat-suppression and contrast-enhanced MR imaging. *AJR Am J Roentgenol* 1993;160:1049–1052.

136. Barton NW, Grady RO, Dambrosia JM. Treatment of Gaucher disease (letter). *N Engl J Med* 1993;328:1564–1565.

137. Pettersson H, Gillespy R III, Hamlin DJ, et al. Primary musculoskeletal tumors: examination with MR imaging compared with conventional modalities. *Radiology* 1987;164:237–241.

138. Lecouvet FE, Vande Berg BC, Michaux L, et al. Chronic lymphocytic leukemia: changes in bone marrow composition and distribution assessed with quantitative MRI. *J Magn Reson Imaging* 1998;8:733–739.

139. Nyman R, Rehn S, Glimelius B, et al. Magnetic resonance imaging in diffuse malignant bone marrow diseases. *Acta Radiol (Diagn)* 1987;28:199–205.

140. Vande Berg BC, Malghem J, Lecouvet FE. Leucemies et IRM. In: Sintzoff S, Laredo JD, Caroit M et al., eds. *Imagerie de l'os et de la moelle osseuse.* Montpellier: Sauramps Medical, 1995:173–184.

141. Gerard EL, Ferry JA, Amrein PC, et al. Compositional changes in vertebral bone marrow during treatment for acute leukemia: assessment with quantitative chemical shift imaging. *Radiology* 1992;183:39–46.

142. Rosen BR, Fleming DM, Kushner DC, et al. Hematologic bone marrow disorders: quantitative chemical shift MR imaging. *Radiology* 1988;169:799–804.

143. Bongers H, Schick F, Skalej M, et al. Localized in vivo 1H spectroscopy and chemical shift imaging of the bone marrow in leukemic patients. *Eur Radiol* 1992;2:350–356.

144. Jensen KE. Magnetic resonance imaging and spectroscopy of the bone marrrow in vivo—with special attention to the possibilities for tissue characterization in patients with leukemia. *Dan Med Bull* 1992;39:369–390.

145. Jensen KE, Jensen M, Grundtvig P, et al. Localized in vivo proton spectroscopy of the bone marrow in patients with leukemia. *Magn Reson Imaging* 1990;8:779–789.

146. Schick F, Einsele H, Bongers H, et al. Leukemic red bone marrow changes assessed by magnetic resonance imaging and localized 1H spectroscopy. *Ann Hematol* 1993;66:3–13.

147. Schick F, Einsele H, Lutz O, et al. Lipid selective MR imaging and localized 1H spectroscopy of bone marrow during therapy of leukemia. *Anticancer Res* 1996;16:1545–1551.

148. Takagi S, Tanaka O, Miura Y. Magnetic resonance imaging of femoral marrow in patients with myelodysplastic syndromes or leukemia. *Blood* 1995;86:316–322.

149. Lecouvet FE, Vande Berg BC, Michaux L, et al. Early chronic lymphocytic leukemia: prognostic value of quantitative bone marrow

MR imaging findings and correlation with hematologic variables. *Radiology* 1997;204:813–818.

150. Metcalfe DD. Classification and diagnosis of mastocytosis: current status. *J Invest Dermatol* 1991;96:2S–4S.

151. Dohner H, Guckel F, Knauf W, et al. Magnetic resonance imaging of bone marrow in lymphoproliferative disorders: correlation with bone marrow biopsy. *Br J Haematol* 1989;73:12–17.

152. Beltran J, Noto AM, McGhee RB, et al. Infections of the musculoskeletal system: high-field-strength MR imaging. *Radiology* 1987;164:449–454.

153. Jensen KE, Grube T, Thomsen C, et al. Prolonged bone marrow T1-relaxation in patients with polycythemia vera. *Magn Reson Imaging* 1988;6:291–296.

154. Kaplan KR, Mitchell DG, Steiner RM, et al. Polycythemia vera and myelofibrosis: correlation of MR imaging, clinical, and laboratory findings. *Radiology* 1992;183:329–334.

155. Avila NA, Ling A, Metcalfe DD, et al. Mastocytosis: magnetic resonance imaging patterns of marrow disease. *Skeletal Radiol* 1998;27:119–126.

156. Guermazi A, Brice P, de Kerviler E, et al. Extranodal Hodgkin disease: spectrum of disease. *Radiographics* 2001;21:161–179.

157. Papac RJ. Bone marrow metastases: a review. *Cancer* 1994;74:2403–2413.

158. Edeiken-Monroe B, Edeiken J, Kim EE. Radiologic concepts of lymphoma of bone. *Radiol Clin North Am* 1990;28:841–864.

159. Linden A, Zankovich R, Theissen P, et al. Malignant lymphoma: bone marrow imaging versus biopsy. *Radiology* 1989;173:335–339.

160. Varan A, Cila A, Buyukpamukcu M. Prognostic importance of magnetic resonance imaging in bone marrow involvement of Hodgkin disease. *Med Pediatr Oncol* 1999;32:267–271.

161. Tardivon AA, Munck JN, Shapeero LG, et al. Can clinical data help to screen patients with lymphoma for MR imaging of bone marrow? *Ann Oncol* 1995;6:795–800.

162. Hoane BR, Shields AF, Porter BA, et al. Detection of lymphomatous bone marrow involvement with magnetic resonance imaging. *Blood* 1991;78:728–738.

163. Gaudin P, Juvin R, Rozand Y, et al. Skeletal involvement as the initial disease manifestation in Hodgkin's disease: a review of 6 cases. *J Rheumatol* 1992;19:146–152.

164. Sandrasegaran K, Robinson PJ, Selby P. Staging of lymphoma in adults. *Clin Radiol* 1994;49:149–161.

165. Shields AF, Porter BA, Churchley S, et al. The detection of bone marrow involvement by lymphoma using magnetic resonance imaging. *J Clin Oncol* 1987;5:225–230.

166. Pond GD, Castellino RA, Horning S, et al. Non-Hodgkin lymphoma: influence of lymphography, CT, and bone marrow biopsy on staging and management. *Radiology* 1989;170:159–164.

167. Tsunoda S, Takagi S, Tanaka O, et al. Clinical and prognostic significance of femoral marrow magnetic resonance imaging in patients with malignant lymphoma. *Blood* 1997;89:286–290.

168. Krishnan A, Shirkhoda A, Tehranzadeh J, et al. Primary bone lymphoma: radiographic-MR imaging correlation. *Radiographics* 2003;23:1371–1387.

169. Richards MA, Webb JA, Jewell SE, et al. Low field strength magnetic resonance imaging of bone marrow in patients with malignant lymphoma. *Br J Cancer* 1988;57:412–415.

170. Ribatti D, Vacca A, Nico B, et al. Angiogenesis spectrum in the stroma of B-cell non-Hodgkin's lymphomas: an immunohistochemical and ultrastructural study. *Eur J Haematol* 1996;56:45–53.

171. Boccadoro M, Palumbo A, Argentino C, et al. Conventional induction treatments do not influence overall survival in multiple myeloma. *Br J Haematol* 1997;96:333–337.

172. Salmon SE, Cassady JR. Plasma cell neoplasms. In: De Vita VT, Hellman S, Rosenberg SA, eds. *Cancer: principles and practice in oncology*, 3rd ed. Philadelphia, PA: JB Lippincott, 1989:1853–1895.

173. Moulopoulos LA, Varma DGK, Dimopoulos MA, et al. Multiple myeloma: spinal MR imaging in patients with untreated newly diagnosed disease. *Radiology* 1992;185:833–840.

174. Lecouvet FE, Vande Berg BC, Michaux L, et al. Stage III multiple myeloma: clinical and prognostic value of spinal bone marrow imaging. *Radiology* 1998;209:653–660.

175. Vande Berg BC, Lecouvet FE, Michaux L, et al. Stage I multiple myeloma: value of MR imaging of the bone marrow in the determination of prognosis. *Radiology* 1996;201:243–246.

176. Moulopoulos LA, Dimopoulos MA, Alexanian R, et al. Multiple myeloma: MR patterns of response to treatment. *Radiology* 1994;209:441–446.

177. Rahmouni A, Divine M, Mathieu D, et al. MR appearance of multiple myeloma of the spine before and after treatment. *AJR Am J Roentgenol* 1993;160:1053–1057.

178. Rosenthal DI, Barton NW, McKusick KA. Quantitative imaging of Gaucher disease. *Radiology* 1992;185:841–845.

179. Gregory WM, Richards MA, Malpas JS. Combination chemotherapy versus melphalan and prednisolone in the treatment of multiple myeloma: an overview of published trials. *J Clin Oncol* 1992;10:334–342.

180. Libshitz HI, Malthouse SR, Cunningham D, et al. Multiple myeloma: appearance at MR imaging. *Radiology* 1992;182:833–837.

181. Moulopoulos LA, Dimopoulos MA, Smith TL, et al. Prognostic significance of magnetic resonance imaging in patients with asymptomatic multiple myeloma. *J Clin Oncol* 1995;13:251–256.

182. Vande Berg BC, Michaux L, Lecouvet FE, et al. Nonmyelomatous monoclonal gammopathy: correlation of bone marrow MR images with laboratory findings and spontaneous clinical outcome. *Radiology* 1997;202:247–251.

183. Lecouvet FE, Malghem J, Michaux L, et al. Vertebral compression fractures in multiple myeloma. Part II. Assessment of fracture risk with MR imaging of spinal marrow. *Radiology* 1997;204:201–205.

184. Eustace S, McGrath D, Albrecht M, et al. Clival marrow changes in AIDS: findings at MR imaging. *Radiology* 1994;193:623–627.

185. Steinbach L, Tehranzadeh J, Fleckenstein J, et al. Human immunodeficiency virus infection: musculoskeletal manifestations. *Radiology* 1993;186:833–838.

186. Krishna G, Chitkara RK. Osseous Kaposi's sarcoma. *JAMA* 2003;289:1106.

187. Miller KD, Masur H, Jones EC, et al. High prevalence of osteonecrosis of the femoral head in HIV-infected adults. *Ann Intern Med* 2002;137:17–25.

188. Clarke CA, Glaser SL. Epidemiologic trends in HIV-associated lymphomas. *Curr Opin Oncol* 2001;13:354–359.

189. Little RF, Gutierrez M, Jaffe ES, et al. HIV-associated non-Hodgkin lymphoma: incidence, presentation, and prognosis. *JAMA* 2001;285:1880–1885.

190. Safai B, Diaz B, Schwartz J. Malignant neoplasms associated with human immunodeficiency virus infection. *CA Cancer J Clin* 1992;42:74–95.

191. Wu CM, Davis F, Fishman EK. Musculoskeletal complications of the patient with acquired immunodeficiency syndrome (AIDS): CT evaluation. *Semin Ultrasound CT MR* 1998;19:200–208.

192. Boutin RD, Resnick D. The SAPHO syndrome: an evolving concept for unifying several idiopathic disorders of bone and skin. *AJR Am J Roentgenol* 1998;170:585–591.

193. Steinbach LS, Tehranzadeh J, Fleckenstein J, et al. Musculoskeletal manifestations of human immunodeficiency virus infection. *Radiology* 1993;186:833–838.

194. Geremia GK, Mcluney KW, Adler SS, et al. The magnetic resonance hypointense spine of AIDS. *J Comput Assist Tomogr* 1990;14:785–789.

195. Geller SA, Muller R, Greenberg ML, et al. Acquired immunodeficiency syndrome: distinctive features of bone marrow biopsies. *Arch Pathol Lab Med* 1985;109:138–141.

196. Berquist TH, Brown ML, Fitzgerald RH Jr, et al. Magnetic resonance imaging: application in musculoskeletal infection. *Magn Reson Imaging* 1985;3:219–230.

197. Hermann G, Pastores GM, Abdelwahab IF, et al. Gaucher disease: assessment of skeletal involvement and therapeutic responses to enzyme replacement. *Skeletal Radiol* 1997;26:687–696.

198. Scherer A, Engelbrecht V, Neises G, et al. MR imaging of bone marrow in glycogen storage disease type Ib in children and young adults. *AJR Am J Roentgenol* 2001;177:421–425.

199. Lanir A, Hadar H, Cohen I, et al. Gaucher disease: assessment with MR imaging. *Radiology* 1986;161:239–244.

200. Cremin BJ, Davey H, Golblatt J. Skeletal complications of type 1 Gaucher disease: the magnetic resonance features. *Clin Radiol* 1990;41:244–247.

201. Rourke JA, Heslin DJ. Gaucher's disease: roentgenologic bone changes over 20-year interval. *AJR Am J Roentgenol* 1965;94: 621–630.

202. Hermann G, Shapiro FS, Abdelwahab IF, et al. MR imaging in adults with Gaucher disease type I: evaluation of marrow involvement and disease activity. *Skeletal Radiol* 1993;22:247–251.

203. Poll LW, Koch J-A, vom Dahl S, et al. Magnetic resonance imaging of bone marrow changes in Gaucher disease during enzyme replacement therapy: first German long-term results. *Skeletal Radiol* 2001;30:496–503.

204. Maas M, Hollak CEM, Akkerman EM, et al. Quantification of skeletal involvement in adults with type I Gaucher disease: fat fraction measured by Dixon quantitative chemical shift imaging as a valid parameter. *AJR Am J Roentgenol* 2002;179:961–965.

205. Resnick D. Lipidoses, histiocytoses, and hyperlipoproteinemias. In: Resnick D, ed. *Diagnosis of bone and joint disorders*, 3rd ed. Philadelphia, PA: WB Saunders, 1995:2191–2203.

206. Pastores GM, Sibille AR, Grabowski GA. Enzyme therapy in Gaucher disease type I: dosage efficacy and adverse effect in 33 patients treated for 6 to 24 months. *Blood* 1993;82:408–416.

207. Figueroa ML, Rosenbloom BE, Kay AC, et al. A less costly regimen of alglucerase to treat Gaucher disease (see comments). *N Engl J Med* 1992;325:1632–1636.

208. Schroten H, Wendel U, Burdach S, et al. Colony-stimulating factors for neutropenia in glycogen storage disease IB. *Lancet* 1991;23:736–737.

209. Allison JW, James CA, Arnold GL, et al. Reconversion of bone marrow in Gaucher disease treated with enzyme therapy documented by MR. *Pediatr Radiol* 1998;28:237–240.

210. Maas M, van Kuijk C, Stoker J, et al. Quantification of bone involvement in Gaucher disease: MR imaging bone marrow burden score as an alternative to dixon quantitative chemical shift MR imaging-initial experience. *Radiology* 2003;229:554–561.

211. Coleman RE, Rubens RD. Bone metastases and breast cancer. *Cancer Treat Rev* 1985;12:251–270.

212. Ihde DC, Simms EB, Matthews MJ, et al. Bone marrow metastases in small cell carcinoma of the lung: frequency, description, and influence on chemotherapeutic toxicity and prognosis. *Blood* 1979;53:677–686.

213. Layer G, Steudel A, Schuller H, et al. Magnetic resonance imaging to detect bone marrow metastases in the initial staging of small cell lung carcinoma and breast carcinoma. *Cancer* 1999;85: 1004–1009.

214. Sanal SM, Flickinger FW, Caudell MJ, et al. Detection of bone marrow involvement in breast cancer with magnetic resonance imaging. *J Clin Oncol* 1994;12:1415–1421.

215. Horvath LJ, Burtness BA, McCarthy S, et al. Total-body echo-planar MR imaging in the staging of breast cancer: comparison with conventional methods-early experience. *Radiology* 1999; 211:119–128.

216. Tanabe M, Ohnuma N, Iwai J, et al. Bone marrow metastasis of neuroblastoma analyzed by MRI and its influence on prognosis. *Med Pediatr Oncol* 1995;24:292–299.

217. Brodeur GM, Castleberry RP. Neuroblastoma. In: Pizzo PA, Poplack DG, eds. *Principles and practices of pediatric oncology*, 3rd ed. Philadelphia, PA: Lippencott-Raven, 1997:761–797.

218. Fletcher BD, Scoles PV, Nelson AD. Osteomyelitis in children: detection by magnetic resonance. Work in progress. *Radiology* 1984;150:57–60.

219. Unger E, Moldofsky P, Gatenby R, et al. Diagnosis of osteomyelitis by MR imaging. *AJR Am J Roentgenol* 1988;150: 605–610.

220. Erdman WA, Tamburro F, Jayson HT, et al. Osteomyelitis: characteristics and pitfalls of diagnosis with MR imaging. *Radiology* 1991;180:533–539.

221. Morrison WB, Schweitzer ME, Bock GW, et al. Diagnosis of osteomyelitis: utility of fat-suppressed contrast-enhanced MR imaging. *Radiology* 1993;189:251–257.

222. Morrison WB, Schweitzer ME, Batte WG, et al. Osteomyelitis of the foot: relative importance of primary and secondary signs. *Radiology* 1998;207:625–631.

223. Morrison WB, Schweitzer ME, Book GW, et al. Diagnosis of osteomyelitis: utility of fat-suppressed contrast-enhanced MR imaging. *Radiology* 1993;189:251–257.

224. Jurik AG, Egund N. MRI in chronic recurrent multifocal osteomyelitis. *Skeletal Radiol* 1997;26:230–238.

225. Stabler A, Doma AB, Baur A, et al. Reactive bone marrow changes in infectious spondylitis: quantitative assessment with MR imaging. *Radiology* 2000;217:863–868.

226. Koo KH, Ahn IO, Kim R, et al. Bone marrow edema and associated pain in early stage osteonecrosis of the femoral head: prospective study with serial MR images. *Radiology* 1999;213: 715–722.

227. King SM, Laxer RM, Manson D, et al. Chronic recurrent multifocal osteomyelitis: a non-infectious inflammatory process. *Pediatr Infect Dis* 1987;6:907–911.

228. Weiner MD, Newbold RG, Merten DF. Chronic recurrent multifocal osteomyelitis. *AJR Am J Roentgenol* 1986;146:87–89.

229. Anderson SE, Heini P, Sauvain MJ, et al. Imaging of chronic recurrent multifocal osteomyelitis of childhood first presenting with isolated primary spinal involvement. *Skeletal Radiol* 2003;32:328–336.

230. Ippolito E, Farsetti P, Tudisco C. Vertebra plana. Long term follow-up in five patients. *J Bone Joint Surg Am* 1984;66:1364–1368.

231. Yu L, Kasser JR, O'Rourke E, et al. Chronic recurrent osteomyelitis. Association with vertebra plana. *J Bone Joint Surg Am* 1989;71:105–112.

232. Jurriaans E, Singh NP, Finlay K, et al. Imaging of chronic recurrent multifocal osteomyelitis. *Radiol Clin North Am* 2001;39:305–327.

233. Vanhoenacker FM, Baekelandt J, Vanwambeke K, et al. Chronic recurrent multifocal osteomyelitis. *JBR-BTR* 1998;81:84–86.

234. Chamot AM, Benhamou CL, Kahn MF, et al. Le syndrome acne pustulose hyperostose osteite (SAPHO). Resultats d'une enquete nationale. 85 observations. *Rev Rhum* 1987;54:187–196.

235. Nachtigal A, Cardinal E, Bureau NJ, et al. Vertebral involvement in SAPHO syndrome: MRI findings. *Skeletal Radiol* 1999;28: 163–168.

236. Takatori Y, Kokubo T, Ninomiya S, et al. Transient osteoporosis of the hip: magnetic resonance imaging. *Clin Orthop* 1991;271: 190–194.

237. Koo KH, Ahn IO, Song HR, et al. Increased perfusion of the femoral head in transient bone marrow edema syndrome. *Clin Orthop Relat Res* 2002;402:171–175.

238. Wilson AJ, Murphy WA, Hardy DC, et al. Transient osteoporosis: transient bone marrow edema? *Radiology* 1988;167:757–760.

239. Stafford SA, Rosenthal DI, Gebhardt MD, et al. MRI in stress fracture. *AJR Am J Roentgenol* 1986;147:553–556.

240. Yao L, Lee JK. Occult intraosseous fracture: detection with MR imaging. *Radiology* 1988;167:749–751.

241. Koch E, Hofer HO, Sialer G, et al. Failure of MR imaging to detect reflex sympathetic dystrophy of the extremities. *AJR Am J Roentgenol* 1991;156:113–115.

242. Hauzeur JP, Hanquinet S, Gevenois PA, et al. Study of magnetic resonance imaging in transient osteoporosis of the hip. *J Rheumatol* 1991;18:1211–1217.

243. Potter H, Moran M, Schneider R, et al. Magnetic resonance imaging in diagnosis of transient osteoporosis of the hip. *Clin Orthop* 1992;280:223–229.

244. Calvo E, Alvarez L, Fernandez-Yruegas D, et al. Transient osteoporosis of the foot: bone marrow edema in 4 cases studied with MRI. *Acta Orthop Scand* 1997;68:577–580.

245. Longstreth PL, Malinak LR, Hill CS Jr. Transient osteoporosis of the hip in pregnancy. *Obstet Gynecol* 1973;41:563–569.

246. Hayes CW, Conway WF, Daniel WW. MR imaging of bone marrow edema pattern: transient osteoporosis, transient bone marrow edema syndrome, or osteonecrosis. *Radiographics* 1993;13: 1001–1011.

247. Coates PT, Tie M, Russ GR, et al. Transient bone marrow edema in renal transplantation: a distinct post-transplantation syndrome with a characteristic MRI appearance. *Am J Transplant* 2002;2:467–470.

248. Gigena LM, Chung CB, Lektrakul N, et al. Transient bone marrow edema of the talus: MR imaging findings in five patients. *Skeletal Radiol* 2002;31:202–207.

249. Radke S, Vispo-Seara J, Walther M, et al. Transient bone marrow oedema of the foot. *Int Orthop* 2001;25:263–267.
250. Vande Berg BC, Malghem JJ, Lecouvet FE, et al. Idiopathic bone marrow edema lesions of the femoral head: predictive value of MR imaging findings. *Radiology* 1999;212:527–535.
251. Vande Berg BE, Malghem JJ, Labaisse MA, et al. MR imaging of avascular necrosis and transient marrow edema of the femoral head. *Radiographics* 1993;13:501–520.
252. Yu JS, Cook PA. Magnetic resonance imaging (MRI) of the knee: a pattern approach for evaluating bone marrow edema. *Crit Rev Diagn Imaging* 1996;37:261–303.
253. Reinus WR, Fischer KE, Ritter JH. Painful transient tibial edema. *Radiology* 1994;192:105–199.
254. Schellinger D, Lin CS, Fertikh D, et al. Normal lumbar vertebrae: anatomic, age, and sex variance in subjects at proton MR spectroscopy-initial experience. *Radiology* 2000;215:910–916.
255. Ballon D, Jakubowski AA, Tulipano PK, et al. Quantitative assessment of bone marrow hematopoiesis using parametric magnetic resonance imaging. *Magn Reson Med* 1998;39:789–800.
256. Tunaci M, Tunaci A, Engin G, et al. Imaging features of thalassemia. *Eur Radiol* 1999;9:1804–1809.
257. Soler R, Pombo F, Rodriquez E, et al. MR findings in hereditary spherocytosis. *Comput Med Imaging Graph* 1995;19:247–250.
258. Jung HS, Jee WH, McCauley TR, et al. Discrimination of metastatic from acute osteoporotic compression spinal fractures with MR imaging. *Radiographics* 2003;23:179–187.
259. Higer HP, Grimm J, Pedrosa P, et al. Transitorische osteoporose oder femurkopfnecrose: fruddiagnose mit der MRl. *Fortschr Rontgenstr* 1989;150:407–412.
260. Dupuy DE, Palmer WE, Rosenthal DI. Vertebral fluid collection associated with vertebral collapse. *AJR Am J Roentgenol* 1996;167:1535–1538.
261. Naul LG, Peet GJ, Maupin WB. Avascular necrosis of the vertebral body. *Radiology* 1989;172:219–222.
262. Cuenod CA, Laredo JD, Chevret S, et al. Acute vertebral collapse due to osteoporosis or malignancy: appearance on unenhanced and gadolinium-enhanced MR images. *Radiology* 1996;199:541–549.
263. Sugimura K, Yamasaki K, Kitagaki H, et al. Bone marrow diseases of the spine: differentiation with T1 and T2 relaxation times in MR imaging. *Radiology* 1987;165:541–544.
264. Spuentrup E, Buecker A, Adam G, et al. Diffusion-weighted MR imaging for differentiation of benign fracture edema and tumor infiltration of the vertebral body. *AJR Am J Roentgenol* 2001;176:351–358.

Miscellaneous Conditions

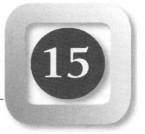

Thomas H. Berquist

As the techniques for magnetic resonance imaging (MRI) have improved, the applications have continued to expand (1–5). Many of these applications have been discussed in the previous pathologic and anatomic chapters. However, certain evolving applications or applications with overlap into multiple anatomic regions deserve mention here.

MYOPATHIES

The MR applications and characteristics of soft tissue infection, trauma, and neoplasms have been discussed in previous chapters. Early experience suggests MRI may also play a significant role in evaluation of other primary muscle and neuromuscular disorders. Both imaging and spectroscopy may be of value in this regard (2,6–21).

There are numerous overuse syndromes, inflammatory and metabolic myopathies, neural myopathies, and forms of muscular dystrophy that potentially could be studied with imaging techniques and/or MR spectroscopy (2,13,22,23). To date, none of these techniques have provided specific information for the exact histologic type of process or specific myopathy. Conventional imaging techniques provide limited information about nonneoplastic muscle diseases. Several authors have studied computed tomographic (CT) features of myopathy (20,24–26). Patterns of muscle replacement have been described using CT. Both localized and diffuse low density areas were noted in patients with pseudohypertrophic muscular dystrophy (20,24–27). Changes in selected muscle groups have been reported in Duchenne muscular dystrophy. Hawley et al. (24) demonstrated that CT scans of patients with neuromuscular diseases initially showed atrophy of muscles followed by decreased muscle density. Primary myopathies revealed similar changes but in reverse order, with decreased density preceding muscle atrophy. The low density areas in muscle seen on CT are likely due to fat and/or connective tissue replacement (24).

MRI has superior soft tissue contrast compared to CT. Therefore, detection of early muscle changes can be more easily accomplished. From an imaging standpoint, the findings seen on MRI may be no more specific than CT. However, certain important changes can be noted with MRI. The muscle groups can be easily distinguished and the extent of involvement determined by using multiple image planes. Using T1-weighted, T2-weighted, fat-suppressed, and short TI inversion recovery (STIR) sequences makes it possible to distinguish early edema or inflammation (high signal intensity on T2-weighted and STIR and low intensity on T1-weighted images) from fatty infiltration or replacement. Other changes, such as increase or decrease in muscle volume and fibrous replacement, can also be identified (see Figs. 15-1 and 15-2) (3,26,28).

Borghi et al. (7) studied T1 relaxation times. This group reported that T1 relaxation times were considerably reduced in patients with myopathy (normal 450 to 800 ms, myopathy ≤500ms). This is undoubtedly due to replacement of muscle with fat and fibrous tissue. Although further studies are needed, these data may be useful in differentiating myopathy from other pathology, such as neoplasms where T1 values are elevated (7).

Shellock et al. (29) studied T2 data on muscles during exercise that allowed differentiation between eccentric (lengthening or stretching) and concentric (shortening) of muscles with exercise. T2 relaxation times increase with exercise due to changes in intra- and extracellular water. Muscles performing eccentric activity have lower

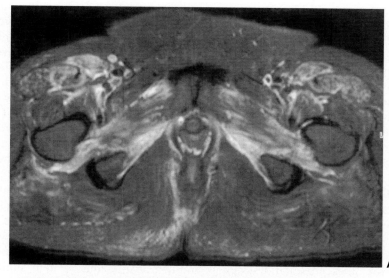

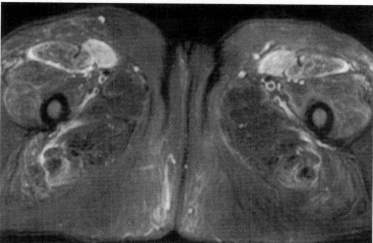

Figure 15-1 Axial fat-suppressed fast spin-echo T2-weighted images at the level of the ischial tuberosities **(A)** and the proximal thighs **(B)** demonstrating an infiltrative process in the adductor muscles and anterior musculature, predominantly the tensor fascia lata due to polymyositis.

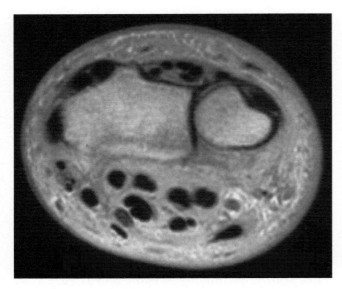

Figure 15-2 Axial proton density image of the wrist demonstrating complete fatty replacement of the muscles due to a chronic neuropathy.

T2 values than muscles performing concentric exercises (29,30).

The potential imaging role of MRI for evaluating myopathies include clearly defining the muscle groups involved, differentiating atrophy and fatty replacement for more acute inflammatory changes, following treatment phases and progression of disease, and localizing optimal sites for biopsy. The current use of imaging parameters alone does not obviate the need for clinical and histochemical studies to define the pathologic process completely.

Significant progress has been made in evaluating the utilization of spectroscopy for defining muscular and neuromuscular inflammatory diseases. With higher magnetic field strengths, imaging and spectroscopic studies with ^{31}P, ^{21}Na, ^{13}C, and other nuclei may be possible (11,31). Conditions such as inflammatory myopathies, metabolic myopathies, muscular dystrophies, and neuropathic muscular changes have been studied that demonstrate changes

in organic phosphate and phosphocreatine ratios as well as other phosphate metabolites. These studies may not only be useful in more specifically identifying the pathologic process, but also show potential in monitoring the response of patients to drug therapy (9,16,20,32). Further data are necessary before the role of spectroscopy in evaluating myopathies and neuromuscular disorders is completely understood (see Chapter 16).

In recent years, several articles have reviewed the role of MRI and MR spectroscopy in specific myopathies and muscular dystrophies. A review of these reports is warranted to demonstrate the current role of MRI in evaluating specific myopathies.

Duchenne Muscular Dystrophy

Diagnosis of Duchenne muscular dystrophy is generally accomplished using clinical and laboratory data. The disease most commonly affects young males (<5 years) who present with muscle weakness and markedly elevated serum creatine kinase levels (9,20,33). Diagnosis is confirmed with muscle biopsy (24,33).

Imaging has played a role in determining the extent of muscle involvement and following the progression of the disease process. Prior to MRI, CT was used to evaluate muscle volume and fatty degeneration (24,33). MRI, using axial and coronal or sagittal image planes with T2-weighted, fat-suppressed, T2-weighted, or STIR sequences, is a more sensitive technique due to its superior soft tissue contrast (3,34,35). Therefore, MRI has demonstrated utility in demonstrating the distribution and extent of muscle involvement (23,24). Liu et al. (33) demonstrated that certain muscles in the lower extremity were spared. The gracilis (100%), sartorius (83%), semitendinosus (69%), and semimembranosus (48%) were uninvolved most commonly (see Figs. 15-3 and 15-4). An MRI grading system was developed that correlated with the clinical (Brooke) system. The system was based on muscle involvement and the degree of fatty infiltration. The system, summarized in Table 15-1, was based on the number of muscles involved in the pelvis and thighs as well as

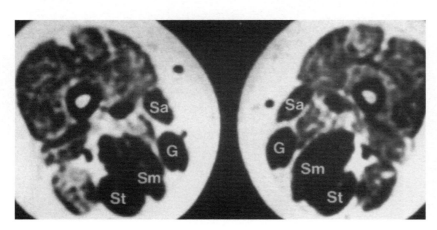

Figure 15-3 Axial image of the thigh (SE 400/20) in a patient with Duchenne muscular dystrophy demonstrating involvement of the muscles with sparing of the sartorius (*Sa*), gracilis (*G*), semimembranosus (*Sm*), and semitendinosus (*St*). (From Liu GC, Jong YJ, Chiang CH, et al. Duchenne muscular dystrophy: MR grading system with functional correlation. *Radiology* 1993; 186:475–480.)

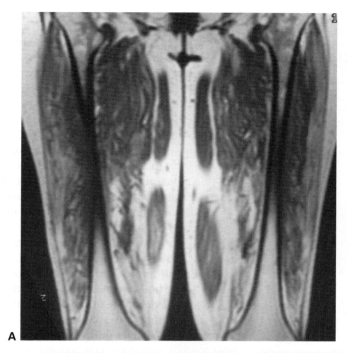

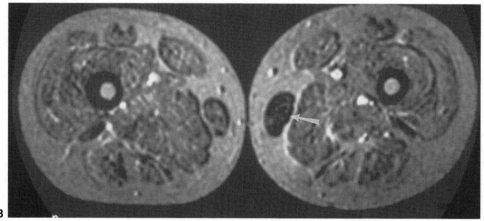

Figure 15-4   Duchenne muscular dystrophy. Coronal T1- **(A)** and axial T2-weighted **(B)** images in a patient with Duchenne muscular dystrophy. All muscles are involved except for partial sparing of the gracilis (*arrow*) on the left.

severity of fatty infiltration and increase in subcutaneous fat (33). The score correlated with disease progression and response to therapy (33).

Neurotrophic Myopathy

There are multiple causes of denervation myopathy, including spinal cord injury, nerve compression syndromes, Grave disease, and neuritis (23). MR evaluation of myopathies related to loss of motor neuron function has also been studied (35,36). MRI has been evaluated in acute and chronic conditions. Fleckenstein et al. (36) evaluated patients with acute neural injury and found MRI has little utility in the acute setting. Signal intensity

may remain normal for up to 15 days, but increased signal intensity on T2-weighted or STIR sequences is typically noted in 15 to 30 days. Signal intensity may remain increased for up to 1 year (35,36). Obviously, if the nerve injury or the cause for neuropathy is not corrected, one can expect fatty infiltration and atrophy of the involved muscles, sometimes before 1 year, which may overlap with changes described above. Fatty infiltration typically occurs as soon as 3 months after nerve injury (Fig. 15-2) (35).

We prefer axial T1-weighted and fat-suppressed fast spin-echo (FSE) T2-weighted or STIR images with comparison of both extremities. This allows subtle changes in muscle size or signal intensity to be more easily appreciated.

muscle involvement is probably underestimated because patients are often asymptomatic (47). Proximal limb muscle involvement is characteristically asymptomatic. Symptomatic muscle involvement only occurs in about 1.4% of patients (26,45). However, muscle biopsies demonstrate granulomas in 50% to 80% of patients (45).

Otake (26) reported two types of muscular involvement—nodular and myopathic. The former involves the extremities. Others consider three categories: palpable nodules, acute myositis, and chronic myopathy. Acute myositis causes inflammation with myalgia and tenderness. Muscle weakness and atrophy is common with chronic myositis (type 3) (40). Patients typically present with single or multiple palpable nodules. Nodules may be tender to palpation.

The myopathic type is symmetrical and presents with progressive weakness and muscle atrophy (26).

Imaging of sarcoid myopathy can be accomplished with CT, radionuclide scans, and MRI. Contrast-enhanced CT demonstrates peripherally enhancing lesions (47). Gallium-67 and technetium-99m scans have also been employed and provide the advantage of total body imaging to allow detection of multiple areas of involvement. Nodular lesions are demonstrated as focal areas of abnormal uptake compared to diffuse uptake of tracer with myopathic sarcoidosis (26). MRI features are useful with nodular lesions. Otake described stellate areas of low signal intensity with surrounding high signal intensity on T2-weighted or STIR sequences (see Fig. 15-6) (26). These

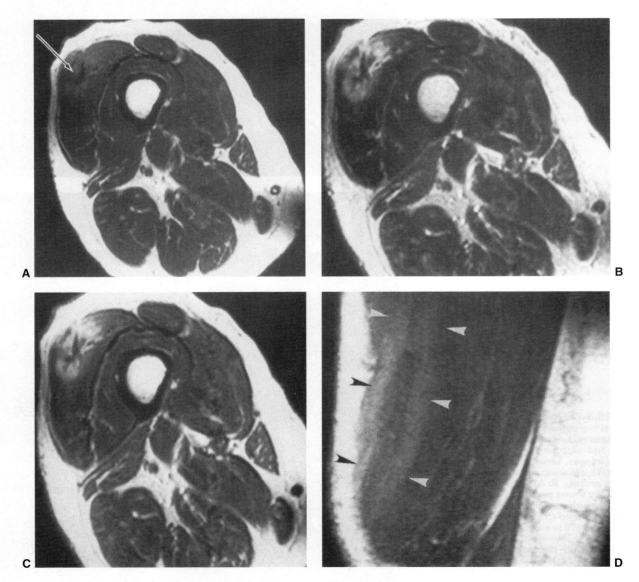

Figure 15-6 A 55-year-old female with nodular sarcoid involving the vastus lateralis. **A:** SE 550/30 axial shows a stellate low intensity region (*arrow*) with slight increased intensity at the margin. SE 1,800/50 **(B)** and SE 1,800/100 **(C)** images show more obvious increased intensity surrounding the low intensity region. Coronal SE 550/30 image **(D)** shows three stripes (*arrowheads*) with outer increased and central decreased signal intensity. (From Otake S. Sarcoidosis involving skeletal muscle: Imaging findings and relative value of imaging procedures. *AJR Am J Roentgenol* 1994;162:369–375.)

findings are not specific and can also be seen with fibromatosis or other local inflammatory and neoplastic lesions (44,47). Myopathic changes (types 2 and 3) have nonspecific MR features with diffuse increased signal intensity on T2-weighted or STIR sequences. Biopsy is required to confirm the diagnosis (26,40,44,47).

Diabetic Myopathy

Diabetic myopathy occurs in patients with poorly controlled diabetes mellitus (23). Diabetic myopathy or infarction most commonly involves the lower extremities. Patients present with acute pain and swelling of the involved extremity or extremities. Pain may be relieved by rest but returns with activity (8,23). The condition is most common in the lower extremities and may be bilateral in 38% to 43% of patients (48,49). The thigh muscles (vastus medialis, lateralis, and intermedius) are most commonly involved (81%) and the calf is involved in 19% of cases (48,49).

MRI should be accomplished using T1- and T2-weighted or STIR sequences (conventional or FSE) in two image planes to define the extent of involvement. Involved muscles are swollen and isointense on T1-weighted images. T2-weighted or fat-suppressed postgadolinium T1-weighted images are most useful to define areas of inflammation and tissue necrosis (see Fig. 15-7) (39,48,49). Involved areas have increased signal intensity on T2-weighted images. Areas of necrosis demonstrate peripheral enhancement similar to an abscess after intravenous contrast (3,48).

Infectious Myopathy

Myopathy may be related to bacterial, viral, mycobacterial, fungal, or parasitic organisms. Infections may be localized (pyomyositis, abscess, and gas gangrene) or generalized (40,50–52).

Pyomyositis is an acute infection usually due to *Staphylococcus aureus*. Other bacteria and mycobacteria are less common. Patients typically have underlying disease such as malignancy, diabetes, or AIDS. Patients present with pain, fever, and local swelling (40,52).

MR images demonstrate increased signal intensity in the involved muscle and subcutaneous tissues on T2-weighted or STIR sequences. Contrast-enhanced fat-suppressed T1-weighted images demonstrate peripheral enhancement (50,53).

Gas gangrene is diagnosed clinically. This is a rapidly progressive, potentially life-threatening clostridial infection. Onset is acute with severely ill patients. Crepitus is present on physical examination and gas is usually obvious on radiographs (40).

Generalized infectious myopathies are associated with HIV or related to rhabdomyolysis due to infections elsewhere (51,52).

Miscellaneous Myopathies

Granulomatous myositis has been described with sarcoidosis, but may also occur with Crohn disease or primary biliary cirrhosis. Patients with thymoma and myasthenia gravis may also develop granulomatous myositis (54). Granulomatous myositis has also been described with

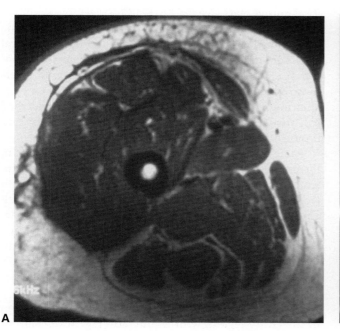
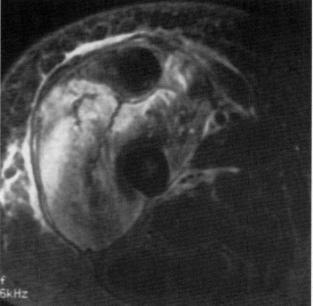

Figure 15-7 Diabetic muscle infarction. Axial T1- **(A)** and T2-weighted **(B)** images of the thigh show fascial, subcutaneous, and vastus muscle inflammation. Changes are more easily appreciated on the T2-weighted image in **B.**

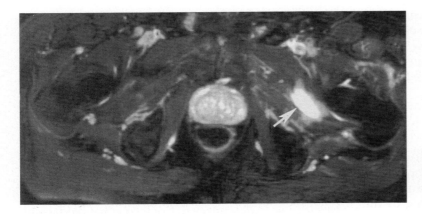

Figure 15-8 Adductor muscle tear. Axial fat-suppressed fast spin-echo T2-weighted image show a first- to second-degree strain with increased signal intensity involving nearly 50% of the cross-sectional area and a focal hematoma (*arrow*).

graft-versus-host disease (GVHD). This condition is seen in transplant patients. GVHD is reported in 25% to 40% of patients undergoing bone marrow transplant. Myositis of GVHD typically involves the proximal muscles of the extremity, but can involve distal muscles and the respiratory musculature (54).

Inclusion body myositis affects both the proximal and distal muscles. This condition leads to severe disability. Elderly patients are most often affected. The etiology is uncertain. However, one theory is accumulation of abnormal proteins in muscles. The condition is progressive, resulting in fatty replacement in the involved muscles. This is easily demonstrated on MR images (40,55).

Focal myositis is rare. This is considered a benign inflammatory pseudotumor. Etiology is unknown. MR features are not clearly defined. However, muscle swelling with inflammation and fatty infiltration has been reported. These changes are clearly demonstrated on STIR and T1-weighted images (40,56).

TRAUMA

Traumatic muscle and myotendinous injuries were discussed in anatomic chapters. However, the complexity of these injuries and the fact that they may have features similar to other myopathies indicate that we should include them in this section, as well. Injuries may be due to overuse resulting in microtrauma, rhabdomyolysis due to intense exercise, focal acute tears, or delayed-onset muscle soreness (DOMS) (28,30,57–62).

Muscle injuries are graded depending upon the extent of injury. First-degree strains result in injury of a few fibers. Second-degree injuries involve 50% of muscle fibers, and third-degree strains are complete disruptions of a muscle (see Fig. 15-8) (4,60,61). Minor injuries have excellent prognosis and usually are not imaged. Delayed-onset muscle soreness is muscle pain related to exertion that occurs hours to days after the initiating activity (57). This phenomenon is

associated with eccentric (lengthening) contraction that results in ultrastructure damage, elevated plasma proteins, and edema on T2-weighted MR images. The extent of edema correlates with pain levels and elevations in creatine kinase (57,61).

More significant injuries (second and third degree) are usually more acute (63). MR images using two planes and T2-weighted or STIR sequences permit the lesion to be accurately graded (see Figs. 15-8 and 15-9) (3,4). Hemorrhage or hematoma formation are more common in this setting. The appearance of hematomas depends upon the age, anatomic location, local tissue oxygenation, and hemoglobin breakdown products (See Chapter 2) (4). Hematomas tend to heal more slowly and may require evacuation if adjacent to neural structures (see Figs. 15-10 and 15-11) (3).

Rhabdomyolysis may be due to ethanol overdose, infection, crush injuries, collagen disease, or intense exercise. MR images typically show a more generalized process than local muscle tears (see Fig. 15-12) (3,62,64).

Calcific myonecrosis is a rare sequelae of muscle trauma (65). Knowledge of this condition is important, as clinical and radiographic features may mimic an aggressive neoplasm (66,67). Calcific myonecrosis occurs with cystic muscle degeneration. The process can occur 10 to 64 years after trauma and results in a painful, expansive, calcified soft tissue mass. A remote history of compartment syndrome is common (65,68).

Radiographs demonstrate plaque-like calcifications in the periphery of the mass. There may be adjacent bone erosion (66). Increased tracer accumulation is evident on technetium-99m bone scans. The fluid-filled mass with calcification is easily appreciated on CT studies. MRI demonstrates cystic changes on T1- and T2-weighted images. Calcifications may be more difficult to define if radiographs or CT are not available for comparison (65,66). Contrast enhancement does not facilitate the diagnosis (see Fig. 15-13) (65).

Treatment typically requires debridement and excision of the entire region, with wound coverage using skin or

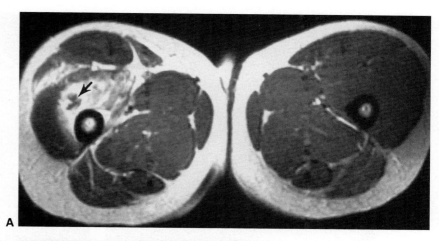

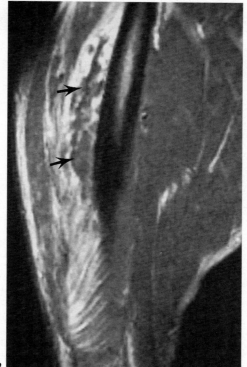

Figure 15-9 Second-degree muscle strain with extensive edema and hemorrhage and low intensity hematoma (*arrows*) seen on axial (**A**) and sagittal (**B**) images.

muscle flaps. Secondary infection following treatment is common (65,67).

Muscle hernias most frequently occur in the lower extremity. They are most common in athletes and soldiers. Hernias may be multiple and bilateral, with muscle protruding through the fascial defect. Muscle signal intensity is often normal on MRI. Though often palpable, it may be necessary to image muscle herniations with active muscle contraction. Therefore, fast scan techniques with motion studies or active muscle contraction may be required to confirm the diagnosis and exclude other soft tissue lesions (28).

EOSINOPHILIC FASCIITIS

Eosinophilic fasciitis is a relatively rare condition (69). Etiology is uncertain, but characterized by eosinophilia (63%), hypergammaglobulinemia (35%), elevated sedimentation rate (29%), and scleroderma-like skin findings (Table 15-3). Antinuclear antibodies are negative (70). Patients typically present with extremity edema and cutaneous induration. Symptoms of swelling, stiffness, and pain may be present acutely following strenuous exercise. Over time, contractures develop in 56% of patients. Joints most commonly affected in order of decreasing frequency include the elbow,

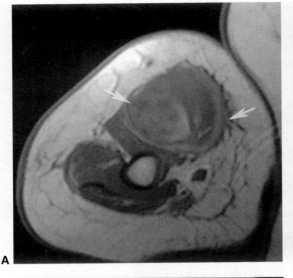

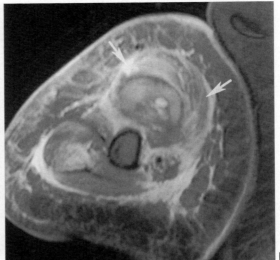

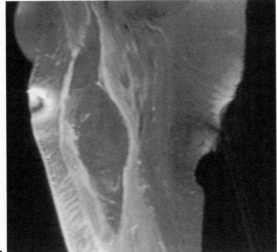

Figure 15-10 Biceps tear with a large hematoma. Axial T1- **(A)** and T2-weighted **(B)** images demonstrate a large hematoma (*arrows*) adjacent to the neurovascular structures. Sagittal contrast-enhanced T1-weighted image **(C)** shows the extent of the lesion with marginal enhancement.

TABLE 15-3

EOSINOPHILIC FASCIITIS VS. SCLERODERMA: COMMON USEFUL DISTINGUISHING FEATURES

	Eosinophilic Fasciitis	Scleroderma
Sex	Males = Females	Females
Symptoms with exercise	Common	Sometimes
Hand involvement	Uncommon	Common
Telangiectasia	Uncommon	Common
Visceral involvement	Rare	Common
ANA positive	Uncommon	Common
Fascial Bx	Inflammation	Normal

ANA, antinuclear antibodies; Bx, biopsy
Adapted from Lakhanpal S, Ginsburg WW, Michet CJ, et al. Eosinophilic fasciitis: clinical spectrum and therapeutic response in 52 cases. *Semin Arthritis Rheum* 1988;17:221–231.

wrist, ankle, and knees (70). Early diagnosis is important, as patients respond favorably to steroid therapy (69–71).

Diagnosis may be delayed due to misdiagnosis as scleroderma (Table 15-3) or even congestive heart failure (71). Until recently, imaging has not played a significant role in diagnosis of eosinophilic fasciitis. However, patients with active disease have characteristic MR features. These include fascial thickening, high signal intensity in the fascia on T2-weighted and STIR sequences, and enhancement following gadolinium administration (see Fig. 15-14) (71–74). These findings correlate with disease activity. Response to therapy and localization for biopsy are additional advantages of MRI features. Currently, definitive diagnosis requires biopsy of cutaneous and muscle tissue (71,72,74).

SARCOIDOSIS

Sarcoidosis is a multisystem disease (Table 15-2). Muscle involvement is symptomatic in 1.4% of patients, though

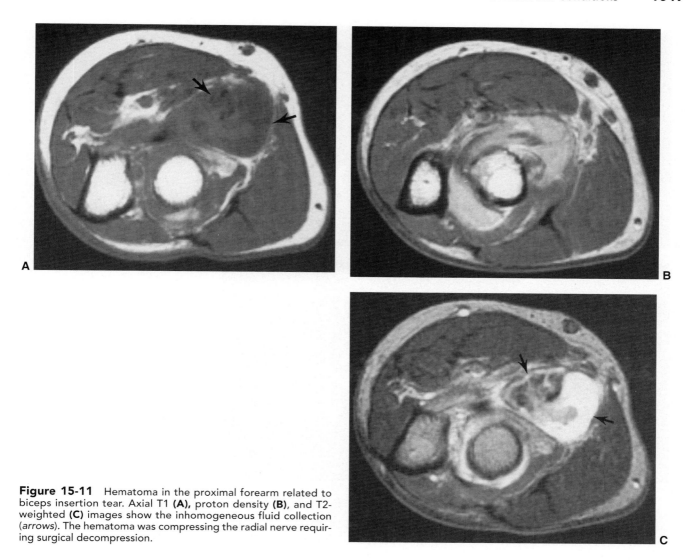

Figure 15-11 Hematoma in the proximal forearm related to biceps insertion tear. Axial T1 **(A)**, proton density **(B)**, and T2-weighted **(C)** images show the inhomogeneous fluid collection (*arrows*). The hematoma was compressing the radial nerve requiring surgical decompression.

muscle biopsies demonstrate granulomata in 50% to 80% of patients (45). Myopathy was discussed in a previous section. This section will focus on osseous and articular changes.

Inflammatory arthropathy is evident in up to 40% of patients with sarcoidosis (44). The knees, ankles, elbows, and wrists are most commonly involved. Lofgren syndrome is a well known feature of sarcoidosis. This consists of arthralgias, erythema nodosum, and bilateral hilar adenopathy. Arthralgias seen with Lofgren syndrome are likely related to circulating cytokines rather than granulomas. Arthralgias occur more commonly in women (44,45,75).

Patients present with pain and stiffness. Soft tissue swelling may be evident on radiographs, but osseous changes, except for osteopenia, are uncommon (75). Arthropathy at greater than 6 months typically involves two to three joints, including the knees, ankles, and phalanges of the hand. Sausagelike swelling of the fingers may be evident clinically and radiographically. Lacelike cystic changes may be evident in the phalanges (75).

MR features of arthropathy are nonspecific. Contrast-enhanced images may demonstrate synovial inflammation early. Tenosynovitis (see Fig. 15-15), tendonitis, and bursitis may also be present. Biopsy is required to establish the diagnosis (44,45,75).

Osseous involvement occurs in 5% to 13% of patients (40,44,45). The small bones of the hands and feet are classically involved. Cystic lacelike changes are characteristic. Deformities may result from pathologic fractures (75).

MRI is not required for diagnostic purposes. However, occult marrow lesions and cortical involvement can be identified that are not apparent radiographically. Changes are most conspicuous on T2- or proton density-weighted images (45,76). Osseous lesions in the long bones and axial skeleton are uncommon (44,77). Lesions may be painful or asymptomatic. Radiographs and radionuclide scans are not reliable as screening tools for sarcoidosis (45). Lesions may be lytic or permeative on radiographs. Vertebral lesions may be lytic or sclerotic (77).

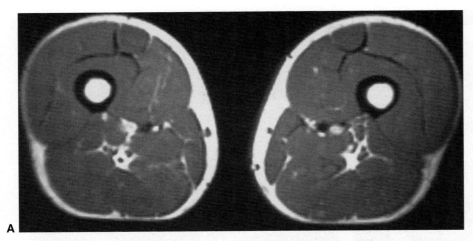

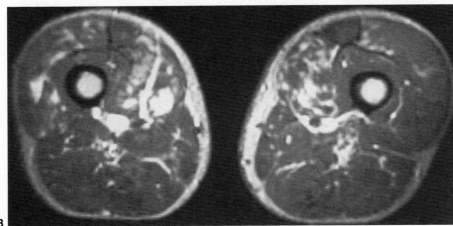

Figure 15-12 Bilateral rhabdomyolysis in an athlete. **A:** Axial T1-weighted (SE 500/20) image is normal. **B:** Axial T2-weighted image shows multiple areas of increased signal intensity in both thighs.

MR images may demonstrate well-defined or poorly marginated lesions in the marrow with or without cortical involvement. Though signal intensity varies, in most cases lesions are high signal intensity on T2- weighted or STIR sequences. Enhancement after contrast is inconsistent, does not make lesions more conspicuous, and, therefore, adds little to the diagnosis (see Fig. 15-16). Differential diagnosis includes metastasis, lymphoma, and myeloma. Lesions may appear fatty or fibrotic on follow-up (45).

ARTHROPATHIES

The role of MRI for evaluating specific arthropathies has been discussed briefly in each of the preceding anatomic chapters, specifically as they might apply to a given articular region. This section is intended to discuss in more detail the role of MRI for evaluating arthropathies. Infection was discussed in Chapter 13; therefore, joint space infection will not be re-evaluated here.

There are numerous arthropathies that may result in chronic disability, significant morbidity, and growing increases in cost for medical care (78–86).

Currently, diagnosis of arthropathies is based upon laboratory studies, clinical data, and radiographic features (87–94). Soft tissue changes occur prior to bony erosion and articular destruction. The superior soft tissue contrast of MRI provides the ability to differentiate cortical bone, articular cartilage, and the soft tissues in the joints, which allows improved early detection of inflammatory arthropathies. Though specificity of MRI is still being evaluated, new pulse sequences, utilization of gadolinium, and spectroscopy show promise for increasing the utility of MRI for detection and therapy monitoring of patients with arthropathy (95–100).

A review of the role of MRI in certain arthropathies, specifically conditions described in the MR literature in recent years, will help emphasize the current applications and limitations.

Osteoarthritis

Osteoarthritis (OA) results from mechanical and biological factors that interfere with the normal process of degeneration and synthesis of articular cartilage (84). Up to 85% of adults over age 75 years have OA. OA is second to cardiovascular

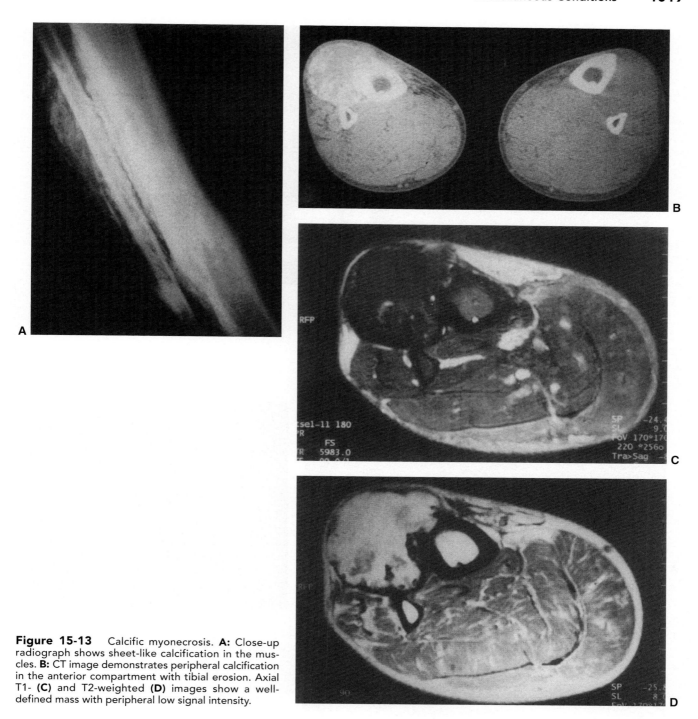

Figure 15-13 Calcific myonecrosis. **A:** Close-up radiograph shows sheet-like calcification in the muscles. **B:** CT image demonstrates peripheral calcification in the anterior compartment with tibial erosion. Axial T1- **(C)** and T2-weighted **(D)** images show a well-defined mass with peripheral low signal intensity.

disease in work-related disability. Treatment costs exceeded $58 billion in 1978, and are continuing to increase. New treatment methods require improved definition of the extent of disease and earlier detection to achieve optimal results (86,97,101).

The etiology of OA continues to be debated—genetic, metabolic, wear and tear, microtrauma, etc., but the radiographic hallmarks of joint space narrowing, sclerosis, and osteophyte formation are well known (72,84,102). Primary OA is most common in females, is familial, and affects the hands. Secondary OA affects the large joints, usually in the lower extremities and spine. This condition is more often referred to as degenerative joint disease or degenerative arthritis (72,84,102–106).

Clinical features and radiographs have been used for grading arthritic changes. Systems for the hip and knee

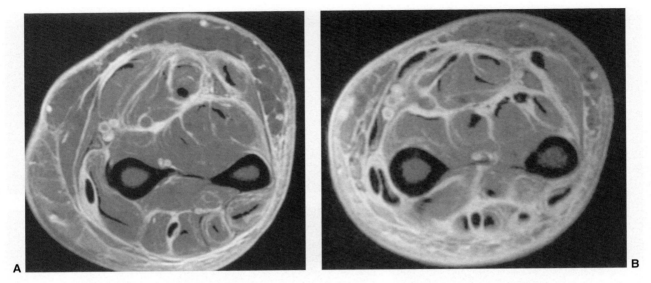

Figure 15-14   Eosinophilic fasciitis. Axial contrast enhanced fat-suppressed T1-weighted images **(A,B)** show marked enhancement of the fascia.

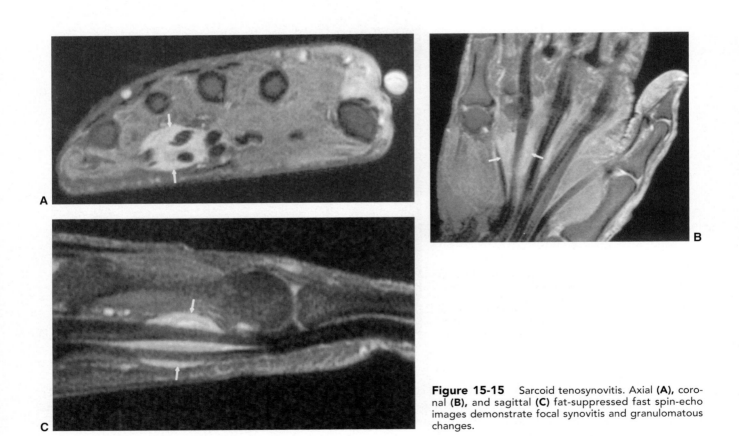

Figure 15-15   Sarcoid tenosynovitis. Axial **(A)**, coronal **(B)**, and sagittal **(C)** fat-suppressed fast spin-echo images demonstrate focal synovitis and granulomatous changes.

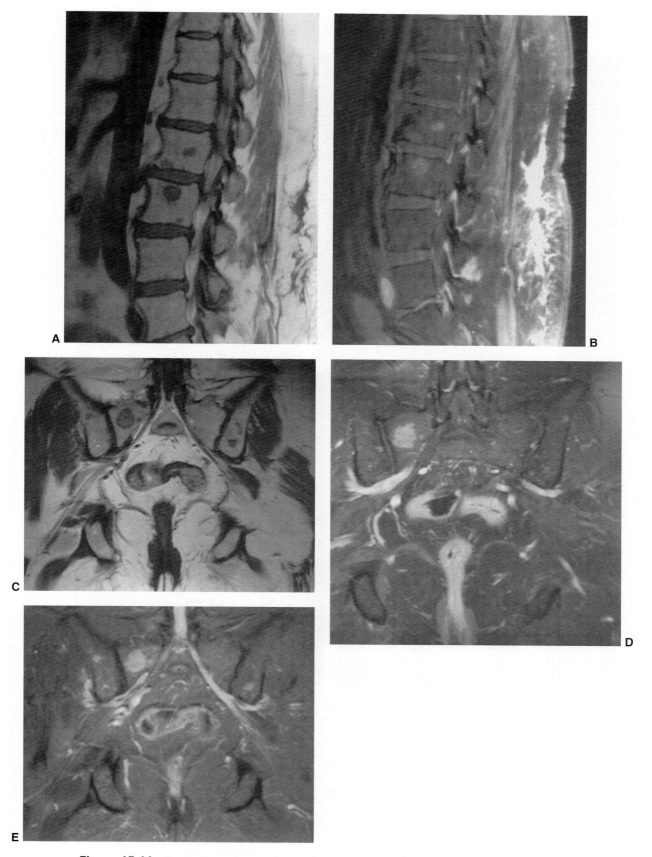

Figure 15-16 Osseous sarcoidosis. Sagittal T1- **(A)** and contrast-enhanced fat-suppressed T1-weighted **(B)** images of the spine and T1- **(C)**, T2-weighted **(D)** and contrast-enhanced **(E)** images of the posterior pelvis demonstrate multiple low signal intensity in **A,C** and high signal intensity in **D** lesions that enhance in **B,E**. Differentiation from metastasis would be difficult.

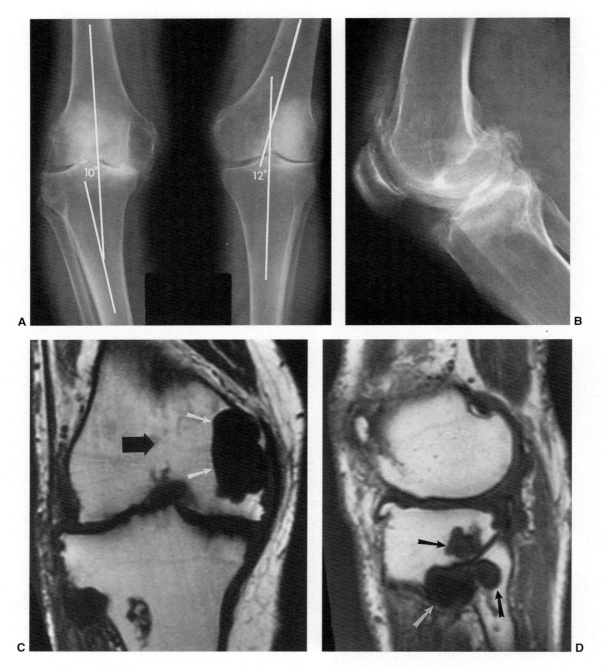

Figure 15-17   Anteroposterior standing (**A**) and lateral radiograph of the right knee (**B**) demonstrating advanced degenerative arthritis with marked joint space narrowing and medial subluxation on the right. The femorotibial angle is in 10° of varus. There is bilateral chondrocalcinosis, and the left knee demonstrates lateral compartment narrowing with a femorotibial angle of 12° valgus. MRI was performed to evaluate ligamentous support and bone loss prior to knee arthroplasty. Coronal (**C**) and sagittal (**D**) SE 400/10 images demonstrate medial femoral displacement (*large black arrow*) with joint space loss. The cartilage cannot be effectively evaluated with this pulse sequence. There is a large degenerative cyst or geode in the medial femur (*white arrows*) and also at the tibiofibular joint on the sagittal image (*arrows* in **D**). The former will require bone graft during implant positioning. Axial SE 2,000/80 images of the femur (**E**) and upper tibia (**F**) demonstrate the high signal intensity of the fluid in the cysts.

have been developed using standing radiographs and changes in the joint space, sclerosis, osteophyte formation, cystic change, and bone deformity (see Fig. 15-17) (84,102,107).

Clinical and radiographic grading systems have been commonly employed for evaluating patients with OA. The clinical scoring system most often used is the Western Ontario and McMaster University osteoarthritis index

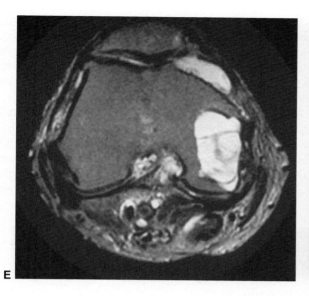
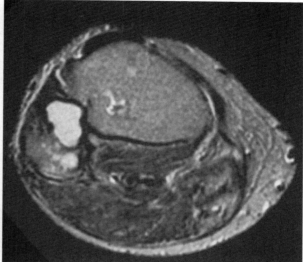

E   F

Figure 15-17   (continued)

(WOMAC) (108). This system measures pain, stiffness, and limitation of function. Pain and stiffness are graded on a five-point scale (0, none; 1, slight; 2, moderate; 3, severe; 4, extreme). Function focuses on mobility issues such as stair climbing, walking, rising from a supine or sitting position, and the ability to perform daily functions. The combined score can vary from 0 to 500 (97,108).

Radiographically, the Kellgren and Lawrence (KL) scale is commonly used by physicians (109). Marginal osteophytes,

joint space narrowing, and subchondral sclerosis are considered in this system. Scores can be simplified to five categories: 0, no evidence of OA; 1, doubtful with minute osteophytes; 2, osteophytes with joint space preserved; 3, moderate joint space narrowing with osteophytes; 4, severe osteophytes, marked joint space narrowing, and subchondral sclerosis.

From an imaging standpoint, MRI is more effective for detection of early cartilage abnormalities, subtle cystic or erosive changes, and synovial inflammation (see Fig. 15-18).

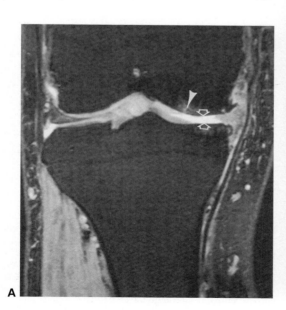
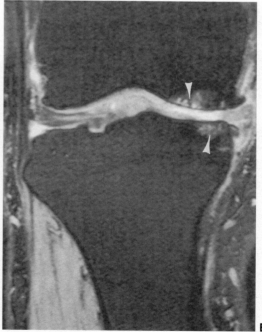

A   B

Figure 15-18   Coronal dual echo steady state (DESS) images **(A,B)** demonstrate grade IV cartilage loss in the medial compartment (*open arrows*), medial meniscal degeneration, marginal osteophytes and subchondral edema, and microgeode formation (*arrowheads*).

Bone marrow edema and damage to supporting structure can also be demonstrated. These changes contribute significantly to progression of OA. Link et al. (97) correlated clinical and radiographic staging with MR features. This effort and the work of others will be reviewed.

Most MRI studies have focused on evaluation of articular cartilage in patients with OA (102,105–107,110–115). Articular cartilage is avascular, has no neural supply, and is composed of extracellular matrix and chondrocytes. The extracellular tissue is composed of water, collagen, and proteoglycans (116). Water makes up 60% to 80% of the extracellular matrix (86,116).

Wayne et al. (117) used MRI to correlate cartilage function based upon biomechanical and biochemical composition. T2 was most useful to distinguish proteoglycan loss from cartilage loss. Gadolinium-enhanced T1-weighted studies show differences in T1 with and without contrast related to the degree of collagen and proteoglycan loss.

Ideally, the zones of articular cartilage described by Modl et al. (118) and McCauley and Disler (116) should be visible on MRI. The superficial zone is low signal intensity and corresponds to dense tangentially oriented collagen fibers (116,118,119). This accounts for about 10% of the thickness of articular cartilage (116). Just deep to the superficial layer

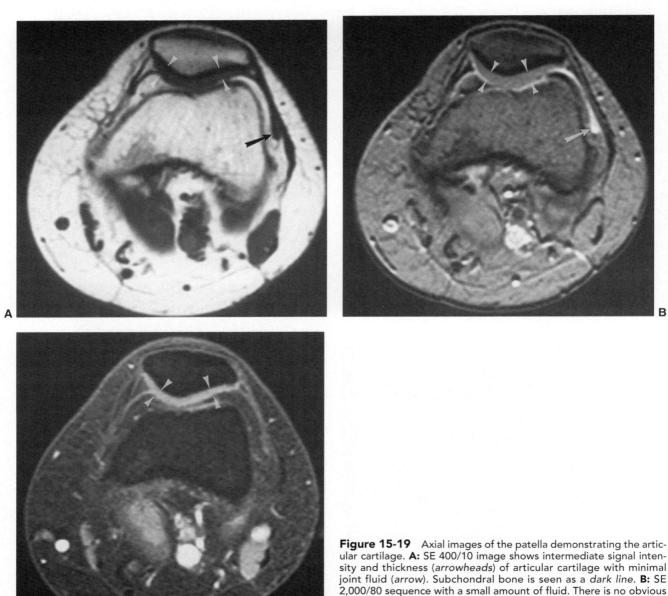

Figure 15-19 Axial images of the patella demonstrating the articular cartilage. **A:** SE 400/10 image shows intermediate signal intensity and thickness (*arrowheads*) of articular cartilage with minimal joint fluid (*arrow*). Subchondral bone is seen as a *dark line*. **B:** SE 2,000/80 sequence with a small amount of fluid. There is no obvious extension of fluid into cartilage. **C:** SPGR 55/5, flip angle 55° image with no effusion. Cartilage (*arrowheads*) is high signal intensity. Subchondral bone and marrow are both low signal intensity and are not clearly separable.

is a second layer of higher signal intensity that corresponds to the transitional cartilage zone. The collagen fibers in the transitional zone are obliquely oriented. The transitional zone makes up about 40% of the thickness of articular cartilage (116,118). The third layer is the radial zone, where collagen fibers are oriented perpendicular to the articular surface. Below this layer is a fourth deep layer of low intensity that corresponds to calcified cartilage and subchondral bone (118). The radial zone and calcified deep zone constitute about 50% of cartilage thickness (116).

When evaluating articular cartilage, MR features are conventionally compared to arthroscopic grading. Grade 0 indicates normal articular cartilage. Grade 1 demonstrates softening without cartilage loss; grade 2, shallow ulceration involving less than 50% of cartilage thickness; and grade 3, greater than 50% but not full thickness. Grade 4 changes include full thickness loss with exposed subchondral bone (Fig. 15-18) (120).

Proper selection of pulse sequence to permit optimal contrast to separate bone, articular cartilage, and joint fluid is essential. When there is no effusion, several sequences can be selected. However, this is often not known ahead of time (see Figs. 15-19 and 15-21). Therefore, a sequence that will increase contrast between joint fluid and cartilage is best for screening purposes (3,100,121–123). Numerous pulse sequences have been suggested but, to date, none are perfect (Table 15-4).

When a small or moderate amount of joint fluid is present, T1-weighted spin-echo sequences may be adequate to evaluate cartilage thickness. Cartilage fluid interfaces may be difficult to separate (see Fig.15-20) (122,128). Only about 70% of lesions are visible on T1-weighted sequences (86) (Table 15-4). T2-weighted spin-echo sequences using double echo techniques (SE 2,000 to 2,500/20 to 30, 60 to 90) are effective in patients with no fluid or a moderate effusion (Figs. 15-18 and 15-19). The proton density image (SE 2,000 to 2,500/20 to 30) can be used to evaluate thickness and the T2-weighted sequence with the higher signal intensity of the fluid demonstrates defects in cartilage. Proton density sequences provided better delineation of subchondral bone from cartilage compared to T2-weighted sequences (Fig. 15-20B) (86,116). Gradient-echo (GRE) sequences can be used in a similar fashion (400 to 700/13, 31, flip angle 30° to 45°) (122,127). GRE sequences with T2* weighting provide an arthrogram effect similar to T2-weighted spin-echo sequences (Table 15-4) (86,116). Using three-dimensional technique (60 1- to 1.5-mm contiguous sections) permits reformatting that may enhance lesion detection. Abnormal cartilage is demonstrated by morphologic defects or fluid extending into the cartilage (Fig. 16-20E) (116). Rose et al. (127) compared FSE sequences [2,000 to 4,200/20 to 80, 2 to 8 echo trains, 4- to 5-mm thick sections, 256 × 192 matrix and 10- to 14-cm field of view (FOV)] and found signal intensity increased in cartilage in patients with early chondromalacia (Fig. 15-21). We have found this sequence effective as well. Mohr found fat-suppressed proton density-weighted FSE sequences more effective that three-dimensional water excitation FLASH imaging (129).

Sonin et al. (130) used FSE proton density without fat suppression to evaluate articular cartilage. The sequence

---

TABLE 15-4

MR IMAGING OF ARTICULAR CARTILAGE

Pulse Sequence	Signal Intensity	Comments
T1-weighted spin-echo	Low–intermediate	Fast, good anatomic detail, fluid cartilage interface difficult to separate. 70% of lesions detected.
T2-weighted spin-echo	Intermediate	Fluid has arthrogram effect. Abnormal cartilage seen as ↑ signal from fluid in defect or abnormal cartilage.
GRE (T2*) (conventional or 3-D)	Intermediate	Thin sections. Reformatting with 3-D. Arthrogram effect. Abnormal cartilage seen as contour abnormality or fluid in defects.
Fat suppressed T2-weighted fast spin-echo	Intermediate	Early defects high signal intensity. Fast. Fluid and cartilage easily separated.
Fat-suppressed spoiled gradient-echo (3-D)	High	Fat suppression, ↑ dynamic range. 3-D reformatting.
DESS	High	Cartilage high intensity, subchondral bone and marrow low.
MR arthrography	Intermediate	Detects small defects.

From references 10, 86, 113, 115, and 122–127.

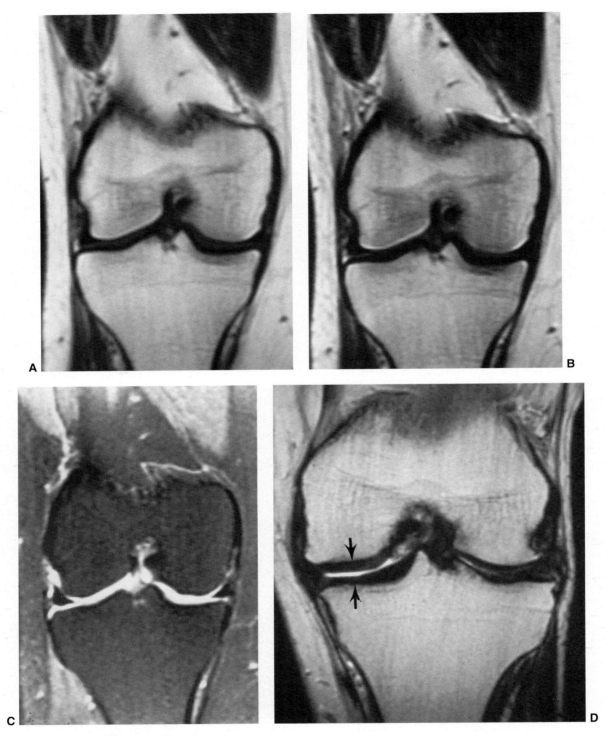

Figure 15-20 Coronal images of the knee with different pulse sequences and a varying amount of fluid in the knee. **A:** SE 316/11 T1-weighted image with a small amount of fluid. Articular cartilage defects and thickness are difficult to evaluate. **B:** Proton density SE 2,000/30 image does not clearly demonstrate the articular cartilage. **C:** Fat-suppressed SE 2,000/30 image shows high signal intensity fluid and cartilage that cannot be clearly separated. **D:** Fast spin-echo 4,200/30 image shows a small amount of high signal intensity fluid and cartilage thickness (*arrows*) is clearly demonstrated in the medial compartment **E:** GRE 700/31, flip angle 30°, show high intensity fluid and intermediate intensity cartilage (*arrow*). **F:** GRE 700/31, flip angle 40°, which is not optimally windowed. The cartilage is not clearly seen. There are osteophytes medially and laterally.

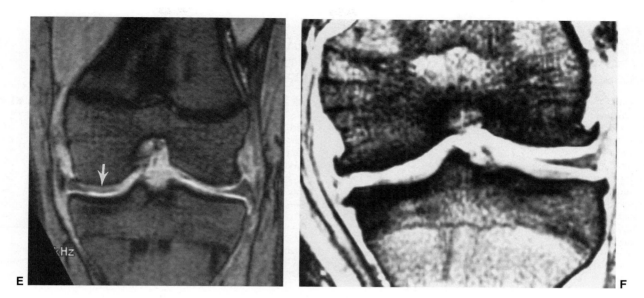

Figure 15-20 *(continued)*

has an additional advantage of providing effective evaluation of the menisci and ligaments. Cartilage on the patellar, femoral, and tibial surfaces was graded. Three reviewers compared MR findings to arthroscopic data and found MRI demonstrated sensitivities of 59% to 73.5%, specificities of 79% to 86%, and accuracies of 79% to 81%. Sensitivity was greater for the patella (80%) and lowest for the lateral tibial plateau (44%). Specificity was 75% for the patella and 95% for the lateral tibial plateau.

Fat-suppressed three-dimensional spoiled GRE (SPGR) sequences are very effective for evaluating articular cartilage (Tables 15-4 and 15-5) (116). Dynamic range is increased using fat suppression, and the advantages of thin section three-dimensional technique provide capability for reformatting (5,86).

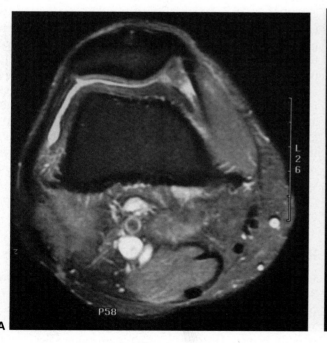
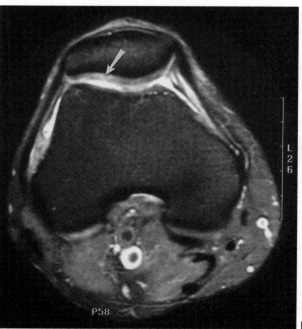

Figure 15-21 Axial fat-suppressed fast-spin echo proton density images of the knee **(A,B)** with a small effusion. There are early changes of chondromalacia seen as areas of high signal intensity *(arrow)* in the cartilage. Fluid and cartilage are clearly separable.

TABLE 15-5

EFFECTIVENESS OF MRI FOR CARTILAGE LESIONS

Imaging Technique	Specificity (%)	Sensitivity (%)	Accuracy (%)
Spin-echo	52–91	58–95	50–89
Gradient-echo	64–76	79–95	77–78
Fast-spin echo (fat suppressed)	73	98	98
Fat-suppressed spoiled gradient-echo (3-D)	86	97	91
MR arthography	80	98	94

From references 86, 113, 115, 122–124, 127, and 131.

TABLE 15-6

OSTEOARTHRITIS: MRI COMPARED TO KELLGREN-LAWRENCE

MR Feature	KL 1	KL 2	KL 3	KL 4
Cartilage (Grade III)	4	9	30	57
Marrow edema	75	37	73	83
Central osteophytes	22	14	14	50
Subchondral cysts	9	14	32	45
Popliteal cysts	6	13	25	56
Effusions	13	16	23	39
Meniscal tears	5	21	29	38
ACL tears	0	0	36	64

KL, Kellgren-Lawrence; ACL, anterior cruciate ligament.
Adapted from Link TM, Steinbach LS, Ghosh S, et al. Osteoarthritis MR image findings at different stages of disease and correlation with clinical findings. *Radiology* 2003;226:373–381.

To date, fat-suppressed FSE (Fig. 15-21) and three-dimensional SPGR or DESS sequences (Fig. 15-18) appear to be the most effective noncontrast techniques for evaluating articular cartilage (Table 15-5) (75,86,116,131,132).

Recently, Yoshioka et al. (100) reported the utility of MR microscopy for evaluating articular cartilage. Using conventional imagers and sequences it is difficult to evaluate the lamina consistently. Higher field strength (3 T) and microscopic techniques may be more effective. However, microscopic techniques used at different field strengths may not be comparable.

Intraarticular or intravenous gadolinium may be required to demonstrate subtle changes in articular cartilage consistently (100,119,133–137). However, errors in measurement of cartilage thickness have been reported (100).

Secondary changes of OA or degenerative arthritis include sclerosis or bony eburnation, osteophyte formation, and bone cysts or geodes (3,111,122). Sequences described above (Tables 15-4 and 15-5) are adequate for demonstrating these features. Both T1- and T2-weighted sequences are useful to help differentiate bone sclerosis from inflammation, necrosis, and cyst formation (see Figs. 15-17 and 15-22). MR arthrography does not add significant data for these changes.

Relating MR features to the clinical (WOMAC) and radiographic features (KL scale) is useful if the role of MRI is to be clearly defined for evaluating OA (97). Link et al. (97) evaluated 50 patients to compare MR features to the radiographic and clinical scales. There were 10 patients with a KL score of 1 (minute osteophytes), 11 with a score of 2 (osteophytes with normal joint space), 13 with a score of 3 (osteophytes with moderate joint space narrowing), and 16 with a score of 4 (severe arthrosis with marked joint space narrowing, osteophytes, and subchondral sclerosis). Cartilage damage increased with higher scores. All knees without cartilage lesions had scores of 1 to 2. Full-thickness lesions were evident in 13 of 16 patients with KL scores of 4.

Bone marrow edema (Fig. 15-18) was present in 60% of patients. Again, the majority had KL scores of 3 to 4. Popliteal cysts, subchondral cysts, meniscal tears, and central osteophytes were also more common with scores of 3 to 4. Anterior cruciate ligament tears were evident in 64% of patients with KL scores of 4 (Table 15-6). Clinical (WOMAC) scores did not compare to MR features in a similar manner (97).

Early diagnosis of OA, specifically cartilage abnormalities, is useful as new treatment approaches continue to evolve. Injured cartilage has limited healing potential, especially when defects exceed 2 to 4 mm in depth (101,138). Treatment options vary depending on the extent of damage and surgical preference. Attempts at surface restoration may include drilling and abrasion that rely upon recruiting pleuropotential stem cells to restore the articular surface. Redistribution of weight-bearing forces may be accomplished using osteotomy techniques. Various arthroplasty approaches (total joint replacement, hemiarthroplasty, interposition arthroplasty, allograft placement) are commonly used in advanced cases. Arthrodesis may be required when the above approaches fail or are contraindicated (138).

MRI provides useful information prior to and after therapy using the techniques described above (101,139).

Rheumatoid and Juvenile Rheumatoid Arthritis

Rheumatoid arthritis is a chronic destructive arthropathy affecting 1% to 2% of the population. The condition affects patients of all ages, but is most common in patients 22 to 55 years of age. Women are affected two to three times as frequently as men. The disease may progress slowly with periods of remission or present with rapid onset and progress to

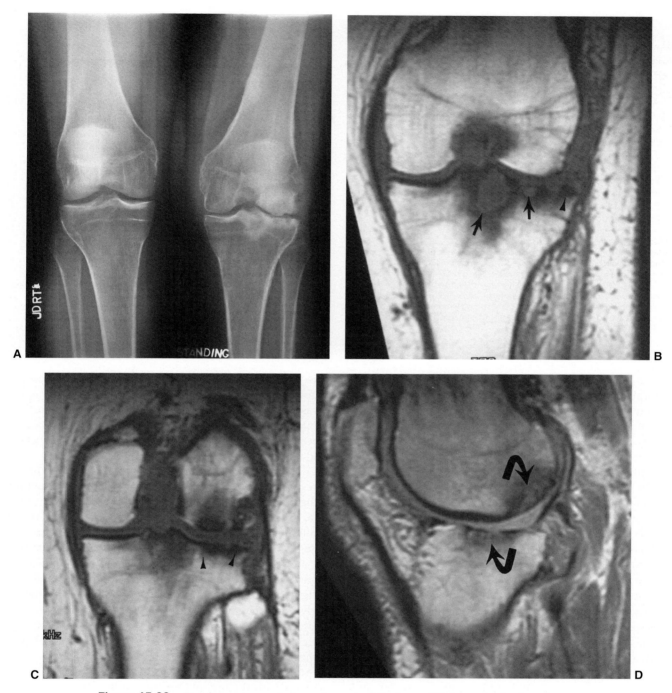

Figure 15-22   Standing anteroposterior radiograph of the knees **(A)** demonstrating lateral compartment degenerative disease on the left, with subchondral sclerosis and small bone defects in the tibia and femur. Coronal **(B,C)** SE 500/20 and sagittal **(D)** SE 2,000/20 images demonstrate subchondral cystic changes (*arrows*), bone sclerosis (*arrowheads*) and areas of mixed necrosis and repair (*curved arrows* in **D**).

severe disability and deformity. The clinical course is inconsistent with periods of remission in 10%, but the course is most often progressive (140). Permanent disability occurs in 10% to 20% of cases (40,140). As with other articular disorders, synovial proliferation and inflammatory soft tissue changes precede cartilage and bone changes by months to years (3,134,141,142). Clinical, laboratory, and radiographic findings have been used to monitor patients with both rheumatoid and juvenile rheumatoid arthritis. Clinical features of rheumatoid arthritis with peripheral

TABLE 15-7

CLINICAL DIAGNOSIS FOR RHEUMATOID ARTHRITIS: AMERICAN RHEUMATISM ASSOCIATION

1. Morning stiffness about joints lasting at least one hour[a]
2. Soft tissue swelling about three or more joints on physical examination[a]
3. Swelling of proximal interphalangeal, metacarpophalangeal, and wrist joints[a]
4. Symmetric swelling[a]
5. Rheumatoid nodules
6. Positive rheumatoid factor
7. Radiographic erosions hands and wrists

[a]Must be present 6 weeks or longer.
Adapted from references Taouli B, Zaim S, Peterfly CG, et al. Rheumatoid arthritis of the hand and wrist: comparison of three imaging techniques. *AJR Am J Roentgenol* 2004;182:937–943, Sugimoto H, Takida A, Masuyama J, et al. Early-stage rheumatoid arthritis: diagnostic accuracy of MR imaging, *Radiology* 1996; 1998:185–192, and Sugimoto H, Takeda A, Hyodok K. Early stage rheumatoid arthritis: prospective study of the effectiveness of MR imaging for diagnosis. *Radiology* 2000;210:569–575.

TABLE 15-8

RHEUMATOID ARTHRITIS STAGING

Stage	Symptoms/Signs	Image Features
1	None	None
2	Mild joint stiffness	Mild swelling, edema,or synovitis on MRI
3	Joint pain, swelling, morning stiffness, weakness Joints warm, ↓ ROM	Juxtaarticular osteopenia Synovial and soft tissue enhancement on MRI
4	More pronounced than stage 3	Early erosion, joint space narrowing
5	Loss of function, deformity, contractures	Progression with subluxation

ROM, range of motion
Adapted from Pope RM. Rheumatoid arthritis: pathogenesis and early recognition. *Am J Med* 1996;100(Suppl. 2A):35–95; and Harris ED Jr. Rheumatoid arthritis. Pathophysiology and implications for therapy. *N Engl J Med* 1990;322:1277–1289.

extremity involvement, usually symmetrical, are useful. The clinical diagnosis is facilitated by using the American Rheumatism Association criteria (Table 15-7), which are 91% to 94% sensitive and 89% specific when radiographic changes are present. Rheumatoid arthritis is diagnosed when four or more criteria are met. Criteria 1 through 4 must be present for 6 weeks or longer (99,140,143).

The problems are somewhat different with juvenile rheumatoid arthritis in that 80% of patients become symptomatic by age 7 and, therefore, bone changes may be difficult to evaluate with routine radiographs. Epiphyses may be incompletely ossified making evaluation more difficult with routine radiographs (93,113,120,144).

Marginal erosions at the synovial articular cartilage junction occur due to mechanical and enzymatic destruction of cartilage (95,96,140). Enzymatic destruction of proteoglycans weakens cartilage structure. Synovial pannus formation occurs due to inflammation leading to edema, hypervascularity, and cellular hyperplasia (140,145). Konig et al. (145) described three types of pannus that have implications for MRI. These categories include fibrous, hypervascular, and slightly hypervascular that can be roughly correlated with disease activity (133,145,146).

New treatment with combinations of disease-modifying antirheumatic drugs (DMARDS) have become effective at slowing progression. Therefore, early diagnosis is important (83). Pope (147) and Harris (148) described five pathologic stages of rheumatoid arthritidies (Table 15-8). Stage 1 is antigen exposure that is asymptomatic. Symptoms of stiffness and swelling begin in stage 2, though image features may be minimal (83,147,148). Synovial proliferation begins in stage 3. At this time, radiographs demonstrate juxtaarticular

osteopenia and contrast-enhanced MR images demonstrate synovial enhancement (see Fig. 15-23) (Table 15-8). Pannus invasion begins in stage 4, leading to marginal erosions and joint space narrowing. These changes progress to stage 5, where soft tissue imbalance and increased bone destruction lead to subluxation (Table 15-8) (83,149).

There have been numerous articles in the recent literature describing the utility of MRI in evaluating rheumatoid arthritis and juvenile rheumatoid arthritis (83,95,137,144, 146,150–152). MRI has demonstrated the capability for evaluating early soft tissue cartilage and bone changes in patients with rheumatoid and juvenile rheumatoid arthritis. The technique is also useful for monitoring disease activity and response to therapy. Initially, T1- and T2-weighted spin-echo sequences were employed to detect early bone (Fig. 15-20) and soft tissue changes. Synovial changes are usually more easily appreciated with T2-weighted FSE sequences, T2* GRE sequences or with MR arthrography (see Figs. 15-23 and 15-24) (83,153).

McQueen et al. (154) demonstrated erosions in 45% of patients with rheumatoid arthritis of less than 4 months' duration. Radiographs were positive in only 15%. The capitate was involved early, along with synovitis on the ulnar side of the wrist. Erosions were evident in 74% of patients after 1 year.

Patients with rheumatoid arthritis also have an increased incidence of extensor tendinitis (50% to 60%) (see Fig. 15-25) that leads to an increased incidence of tendon rupture. These findings can be easily evaluated with MRI or ultrasound (155).

Singson and Zaldieondo (153) noted irregular thickening of the synovium that was intermediate signal intensity

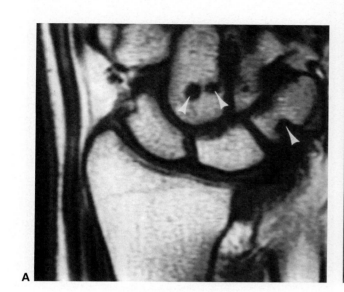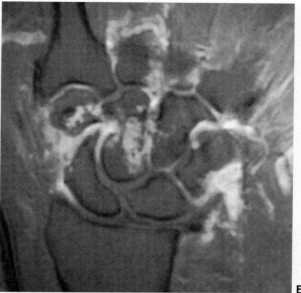

Figure 15-23 Rheumatoid arthritis. **A:** Coronal T1-weighted image demonstrates multiple erosions (*arrowheads*). **B:** Coronal contrast-enhanced image shows erosions in the capitate and synovial enhancement.

compared to darker fluid on T1-weighted sequences. Inflamed synovium or pannus was slightly lower intensity on T2-weighted spin-echo sequences. Pannus or hyperplastic synovium with hemosiderin was lower intensity on T2-weighted sequences. A similar or lower intensity could also be expected from fibrous synovial hypertrophy (145). Gadolinium demonstrates early synovial changes and erosions, and can differentiate subchondral pannus from eburnation (3,140,145,146,150). Reiser et al. (156) studied 34 joints pre- and post-gadolinium injection and found significant rapid enhancement of the proliferating inflamed synovium compared to the very minimal changes noted in bone and the adjacent soft tissues. This finding, though useful in early identification of inflammation, is not specific. Dynamic gadolinium studies with fast scan techniques and fat suppression are often used to improve postcontrast studies (119,140,145,157).

Spectroscopy may also play a role in identification of early and subtle soft tissue changes (158,159). To date, we most commonly use MRI with or without gadolinium to evaluate patients with indeterminate arthropathies, for early erosive and soft tissue changes, and for changes in the cervical spine region that are often associated with rheumatoid arthritis (see Fig. 15-26). Sagittal images with cervical spine flexion may improve evaluation of narrowing of the subarachnoid space (160). MRI may be particularly useful in children, where unossified cartilage and the monoarticular involvement, not uncommonly seen with juvenile rheumatoid arthritis, may make other imaging techniques less useful (see Fig. 15-27) (161).

In recent years, MRI has become a useful tool for evaluating response to therapy, measuring active synovial inflammation and pannus volume, and defining remissions (162–164). Dynamic enhancement techniques (SPGR sequence prior to and every 30 seconds after bolus injection) are useful to demonstrate more rapid synovial enhancement in patients with active disease (162,163). Patients with inactive disease show decreased synovial enhancement, decreased edema, and no new erosions (164). Serial MR studies in rheumatoid arthritis may provide more useful information regarding treatment and disease activity (154,164).

Pigmented Villonodular Synovitis

Pigmented villonodular synovitis (PVNS) is a relatively uncommon disorder characterized by synovial proliferation with hemosiderin deposition in the involved synovial tissues. The condition may involve joints, bursae, or tendon sheaths. There are diffuse forms (80% involve the knee) and localized forms such as giant cell tumor of the tendon sheath. Joint involvement is most common in the knee followed by the hip, ankle, shoulder, elbow, temporomandibular joint (TMJ), and spine (165,166). Pigmented villonodular synovitis occurs most commonly in the second through fifth decades with an age range of 10 to 90 years, though most patients are in their early 20s. The disease is usually monoarticular, which assists in diagnosis. Clinically, the involved joint is usually painful, and palpable soft tissue masses may be evident (165).

The etiology of PVNS is unknown. However, abnormal lipid metabolism, recurrent hemarthrosis, and neoplasm have all been considered (166,167). Histology

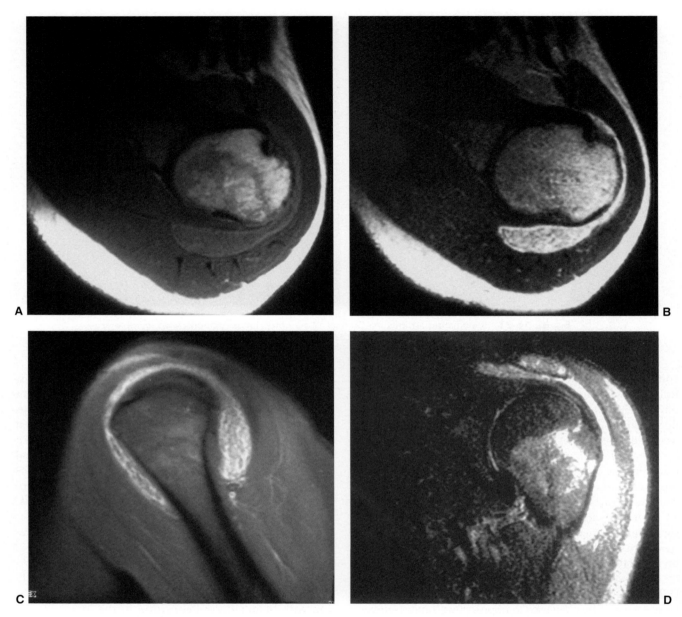

Figure 15-24 Rheumatoid arthritis with synovitis. Axial T1- **(A)**, T2-weighted **(B)** and fat suppressed T2-weighted sagittal **(C)** images demonstrate synovitis without bone involvement. Coronal T2-weighted image **(D)** demonstrates synovitis and marrow edema.

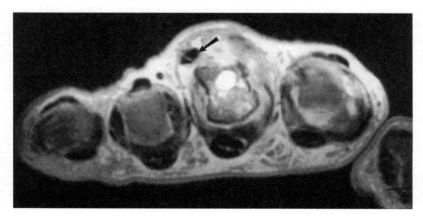

Figure 15-25 Axial T2-weighted image. Swelling and cystic change in the third metacarpophalangeal joint with extensor tendon subluxation (*arrow*).

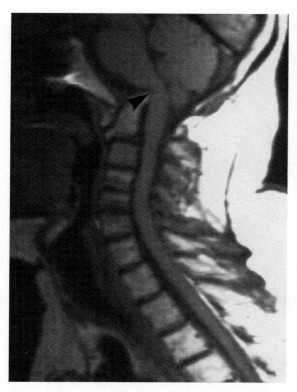

Figure 15-26 Sagittal SE 500/20 image of the cervical spine in a patient with rheumatoid arthritis. Note the position of the odontoid and brain stem compression (*arrowhead*).

demonstrates synovial hyperplasia with multinucleated giant cells, lipid-containing foam cells, increased vascularity, synovial fibrosis, and hemosiderin (165–167).

Radiographically, changes occur in approximately 80% of cases. The most common abnormality seen is soft tissue swelling and effusion. Increased density may be evident due to hemosiderin deposition. Cystic erosions occur in bone in up to 50% of patients (166). MR features of PVNS are fairly typical, allowing diagnosis of the condition in many cases, especially when coupled with the clinical findings. Both T1- and T2-weighted sequences are important to characterize the synovial changes and hemosiderin deposition accurately (see Fig. 15-28). The synovial nodules represent areas of proliferation containing hemosiderin or fibrosis, and they are demonstrated as large globular areas of low signal intensity on both T1- and T2-weighted sequences (165,167). Low signal intensity is even more obvious on high field (at least 1.5 T) GRE sequences. Areas of high signal intensity are related to synovial inflammation. Contrast-enhanced fat-suppressed T1-weighted images demonstrate irregular enhancement due to hypervascularity associated with synovial inflammation and proliferation (134). These findings are fairly specific in early cases when only subtle synovial changes are present. There are certain other conditions in which there is advanced synovial proliferation that can make diagnosis

more difficult. Patients with conditions such as synovial chondromatosis (see Fig. 15-30) and chronic long-standing infection (Fig. 15-27) may be difficult to differentiate from PVNS.

MRI is also useful for evaluating patients after synovectomy. Patients should be studied 3 months after surgery and/or radiation to provide a baseline for follow-up studies. This will permit detection of residual PVNS and provide more accurate data when recurrence is suspected. Recurrence rates are as high as 25% to 50% (166–168). MR parameters should be the same for all follow-up studies to assure ease of comparison. This includes T1- and T2-weighted sequences and contrast-enhanced studies in the appropriate imaging planes.

Gout

Clinical evaluation, laboratory data, and, after 6 to 8 years, radiographs provide sufficient data for diagnosis and management of patients with gout. MRI has not been commonly utilized for diagnosis. However, changes do appear earlier, the extent of involvement is more clearly defined, and so one must be familiar with the MR features (169,170).

Chronic tophaceous gout usually presents with asymmetric involvement of the feet, hands and wrists, elbows, and knees. Tophi may be periarticular or involve bursae, such as the olecranon bursa in the elbow (169). Radiographs demonstrate soft tissue masses or nodules near the joints. Bone erosions are classically well defined with overhanging edges. Patients with gout also have an increased incidence of avascular necrosis of the lunate and capitate (171).

MRI of patients with suspected gout should include T1, T2, and contrast-enhanced fat-suppressed T1-weighted images (170). Tophi are usually intermediate signal intensity on T1-weighted images. Signal intensity is variable on T2-weighted sequences. Inhomogeneous to low signal intensity is most common (169,170). Low signal intensity is more likely related to urate crystals and fibrosis than calcification (see Fig. 15-29). Radiographic comparison is very useful in this regard. Postcontrast images demonstrate enhancement related to granulation tissue and hypervascularity (170).

Synovial Chondromatosis/Osteochondromatosis

Primary synovial osteochondromatosis or chondromatosis (cartilage without ossification) is a disease of unknown etiology resulting in formation of synovial chondroma or osteochondromas due to synovial metaplasia (172). There are three phases of this process with differing radiographic presentation. The first phase presents with active intrasynovial metaplasia but no loose bodies. There is also a transitional phase with active synovial disease and loose bodies. In the third phase, loose bodies are present but there is no active synovial disease (172–174).

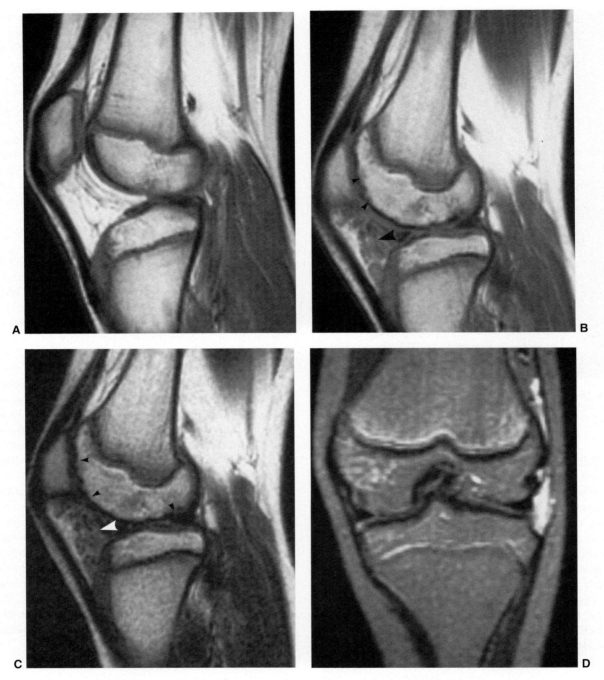

Figure 15-27   Juvenile rheumatoid arthritis. **A:** Sagittal SE 500/20 image of the normal knee. SE 500/20 **(B)** and SE 2,000/60 **(C)** images of the involved knee. There is irregularity of the epiphysis (*small arrowheads*) and decreased signal intensity in the infrapatellar fat on both sequences (*large arrowhead*) due to chronic synovial proliferation. Coronal SE 2,000/60 **(D)** image shows soft tissue inflammation and increased signal intensity in the femoral epiphysis due to hyperemia.

The condition affects males twice as commonly as females and usually occurs in the fifth decade. However, we have noted numerous cases of intrasynovial metaplasia in young females 20 to 30 years of age who present with unexplained hip pain and normal MR examinations. Subtle synovial changes are difficult to detect unless a significant effusion is present or intraarticular contrast is used (see Fig. 15-30). Most patients present with pain and decreased range of motion in the involved articulation. The hip is involved in more than 50% of cases. The other joints involved in this monoarticular disorder are the elbow, wrist, ankle, shoulder, TMJ, and hand (3,173).

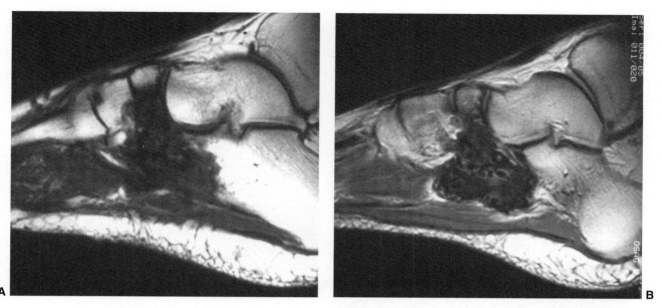

Figure 15-28   Sagittal T1- **(A)** and T2-weighted **(B)** images of the midfoot in a patient with PVNS. There is tarsal erosion and low signal intensity on both sequences due to synovial fibrosis and hemosiderin.

Routine radiographs are normal if nodules are not calcified or ossified. When nodules contain bone or calcium, the diagnosis is usually obvious because there are fairly uniform osteocartilaginous bodies with no evidence of degenerative arthritis, osteochondritis dissecans, or other articular disease to explain the loose bodies (172).

Diagnosis can be difficult with MRI during the active synovial phase when there are no loose bodies (Fig. 15-30 and Fig. 15-26). Conventional T1- and T2-weighted or T2*-weighted GRE images will demonstrate the process when there are loose bodies present. Cartilaginous loose bodies and calcified or ossified loose bodies are usually low signal

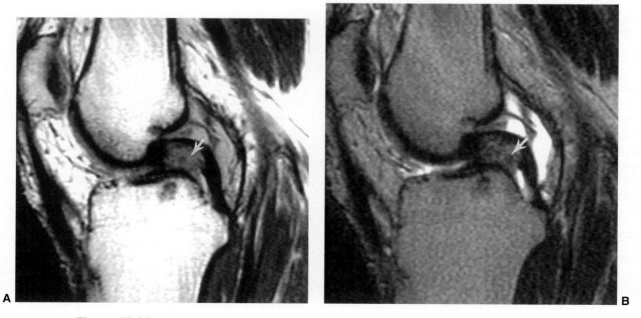

Figure 15-29   Gout. Sagittal proton density **(A)** and T2-weighted **(B)** images demonstrate an intraarticular tophus (*arrow*).

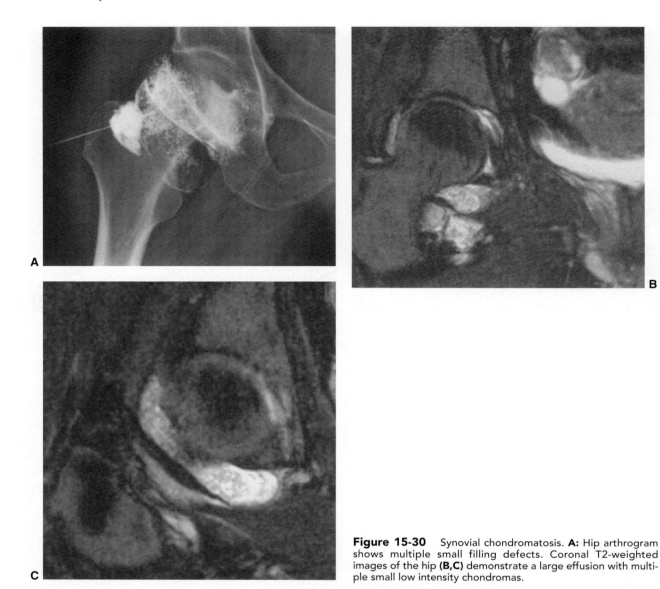

Figure 15-30 Synovial chondromatosis. **A:** Hip arthrogram shows multiple small filling defects. Coronal T2-weighted images of the hip **(B,C)** demonstrate a large effusion with multiple small low intensity chondromas.

intensity and easily appreciated against the high fluid signal intensity on T2-weighted sequences. Some loose bodies may actually contain fatty marrow and are easily identified on T1-weighted MR images (172,173). MR arthrograms may be best suited to evaluate this process (175) and other causes of intraarticular loose bodies. As noted above, the MR features may not be specific and difficult to differentiate from chronic (fibrotic) synovial proliferation and PVNS.

Amyloid Arthropathy

Dialysis-related amyloid arthropathy has recently been evaluated with MRI (176–178). This condition, which may be related to several factors, is attributed to long-term dialysis using cuprophan dialysis membranes. ß2-microglobulin is deposited with this form of amyloidosis (176).

Clinically, the condition is unusual if patients have been on dialysis less than 5 years, but occurs in 80% of patients on dialysis longer than 10 years. The arthropathy usually presents with pain and stiffness in the shoulders that spreads to the wrist and then to the joints of the lower extremities (176–178). Radiographs demonstrate osteopenia, lobulated soft tissue swelling, and subchondral cysts. The last may lead to pathologic fractures (178).

Clinical history and MR features are useful in diagnosis. Unlike most proliferative synovial disease (↑ signal on T2-weighted images), the intraosseous lesions of amyloid arthropathy have signal intensity between muscle and fibrous tissue regardless of the pulse sequence selected (see Fig. 15-31) (176). Though MR experience is still limited, this feature was reported in four patients by Cobby et al. (176) Synovial amyloid does not exhibit this effect

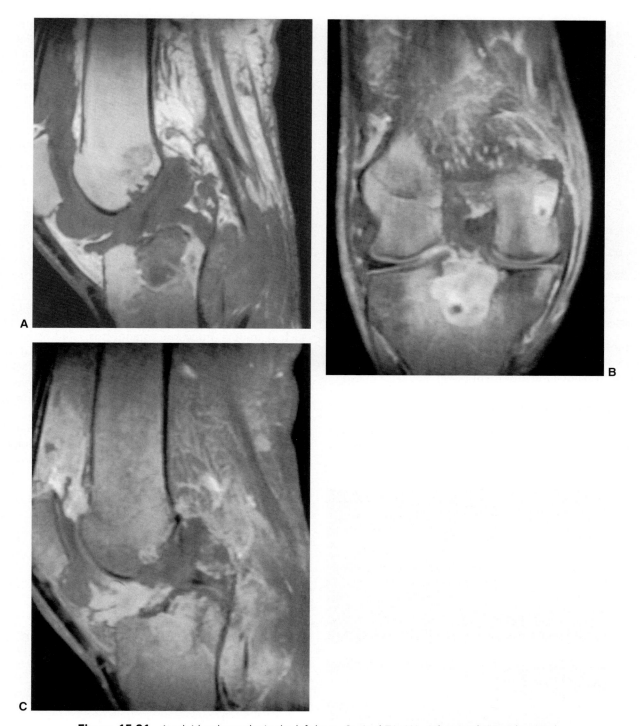

Figure 15-31 Amyloid arthropathy in the left knee. Sagittal T1- **(A)** and coronal **(B)** and sagittal T2-weighted **(C)** images demonstrate extensive cystic erosive changes with mixed signal intensity in the joint fluid.

on GRE sequences, which may be a useful feature for differentiating amyloid arthropathy from other conditions with hemosiderin deposition (98). Synovial thickening and joint and bursae fluid distention are common features (177). Thickening of the periarticular tendons is an

additional feature. Bone erosions not evident on radiographs are evident in 39% of patients on MR images (see Fig. 15-32) (178).

Rarely, amyloid deposits in dialysis patients may result in expansile lytic bone lesions (amyloidomas) that

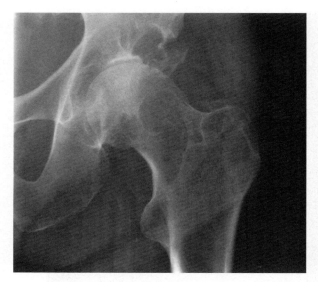

Figure 15-32 Amyloid arthropathy. Anteroposterior radiograph demonstrates large cystic erosions in the femoral neck and acetabulum.

resemble plasmacytoma. MR features are not well documented, but one would expect signal intensity changes similar to synovial involvement (179).

Miscellaneous Arthropathies

MRI features have also been described with hemochromatosis, sacroiliitis, hemophilia, and lipoma aborescens (94,180–183).

Features are generally not specific. One might assume that hemachromatosis should have some MR findings related to iron deposition. However, to date, MR features even in larger joints such as the knee have not been specific for this condition (180). Routine radiographs remain the most efficient screening technique for many arthropathies (3,180).

PEDIATRIC DISORDERS

Routine radiographs continue to play a major role in identification of congenital and pediatric disorders (184,185). MRI offers several potential advantages for the study of pediatric disorders, specifically as they relate to the growth plate and unossified epiphyses (136,181,184,186–191). Images of the extremities can be obtained in the axial plane as well as coronal, sagittal, and off-axis planes to define osseous and cartilaginous development and soft tissue structures better (see Fig. 15-33).

MRI of pediatric conditions has evolved rapidly (192). Many of the conditions described in the previous chapters such as trauma, infection, osteonecrosis and osteochondrosis, pediatric hip disorders (Chapter 6), and tarsal coalition (Chapter 8) are common applications for MRI in pediatric practice (187,193–199). These applications will not be reemphasized here. This section will focus on physeal abnormalities.

Growth plate deformities, specifically those related to trauma, are a common problem in pediatric orthopedic practice. Partial physeal arrest is particularly apt to cause

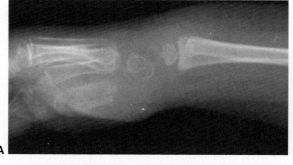

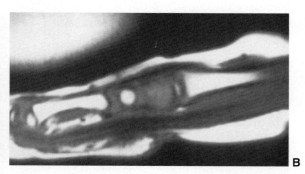

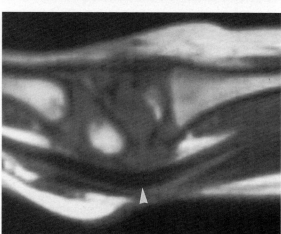

Figure 15-33 Three-year-old with pain and function loss in the wrist. **A:** Lateral radiograph shows swelling and incomplete ossification of the carpal bones. **B:** Sagittal SE 500/20 image of the normal wrist. **C:** Sagittal image of the involved wrist shows carpal collapse with shortening of the involved wrist. Note the volar displacement (*arrowhead*) of the flexor tendons.

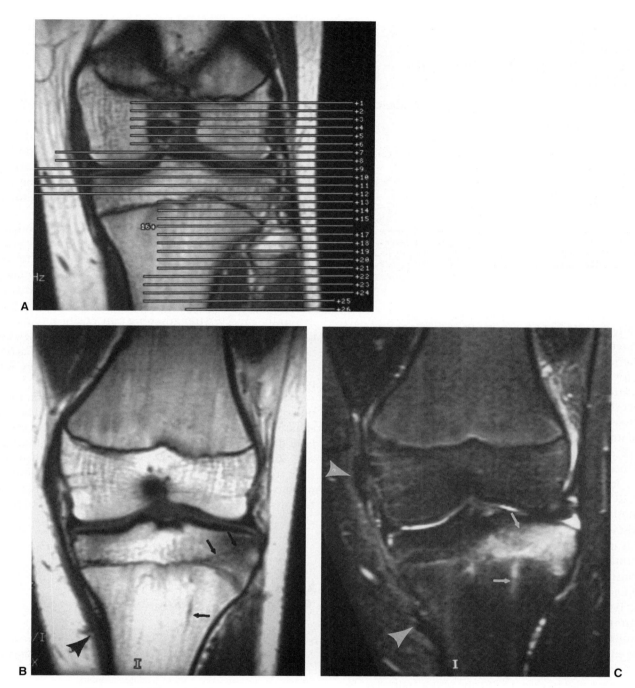

Figure 15-34 Adolescent male with valgus knee injury. **A:** Coronal SE 400/10 scout image demonstrates the irregular course of the tibial and femoral physes. No single axial image includes the growth plate in its entirety. Note the normal low signal intensity on T1-weighted images. Coronal SE 500/11 **(B)** and fat-suppressed T2-weighted **(C)** sequences demonstrate injuries to the medial collateral ligaments (*arrowheads*) and edema and fracture involving the tibial epiphysis and metaphysis (*arrows*). There is only a fine line of increased signal on the T2-weighted sequences **(C),** as the patient's physes were nearly mature.

problems. This is due to progressive angular deformity that occurs due to segmental growth of a portion of the growth plate while the injured portion is arrested. Though these changes are most often due to trauma, physeal arrest can also occur with infection, tumors, therapeutic radiation, burns, electrical injuries, and metabolic and hematologic abnormalities (191,200–204).

Histologically, the physis consists of a germinal zone adjacent to the epiphysis, a proliferating zone, a hypertrophic zone, and the fourth zone or zone of provisional

TABLE 15-9

SALTER-HARRIS CLASSIFICATION AND INCIDENCE OF INJURIES

Type	Definition	Incidence (%)
I	Fracture confined to the physis	6–8.5
II	Fracture through the physis extending into the metaphysis	73–75
III	Fracture through the physis extending into the epiphysis	6.5–8
IV	Fracture extends through metaphysis, physis, and epiphysis	10–12
V	Physeal crush injury	<1%

Adapted from Rogers LF, Pozanski AK. Imaging of epiphyseal injuries. *Radiology* 1994;191:297–308; and Salter RB, Harris WR. Injuries involving the epiphyseal plate. *J Bone Joint Surg* 1963;45A:587–622.

calcification near the metaphysis (204). The physes are typically irregular, which has significance in planning and interpreting MR images (see Fig. 15-34) (205–207).

The Salter-Harris classification (Table 15-9) is commonly used for growth plate fractures. Subtle injuries and unossified cartilage can be closely defined on MRI (Fig. 15-34). Proper classification is important for prognosis. Up to 30% of physeal injuries can result in measurable shortening or angulation. However, only a few (~2%) result in significant deformity (136,189,204).

Generally, imaging of growth plate abnormalities has been accomplished with routine radiographs or CT (202,204,209). These techniques usually are adequate for diagnosis and to assess the percentage of growth plate arrest or closure prior to consideration of surgical therapy.

It is important to determine the extent of growth plate abnormality (bony bar, fibrous bar, angular deformity) prior to considering surgical intervention (202,205–207,210). Type I growth arrest involves the periphery of the growth plate. Type II causes central closure with continued peripheral growth. Type III is more irregular, with variable angular deformity (202).

Recently, MRI has provided valuable information in evaluating patients with growth plate deformities. This is true for both preoperative (see Fig. 15-35) and postoperative (see Fig. 15-36) situations. MRI is particularly suited to situations where growth plate deformity is significant and tomographic or CT planes are difficult to obtain. Both T1- and T2-weighted or STIR sequences are useful to evaluate activity in the growth plate. However, T2-weighted spin-echo, FSE, GRE T2*, and STIR sequences are most useful to assess the normal increased signal intensity of an open physis (206,207, 210,211). Increased signal intensity is seen along growth plates with growth potential. Scar tissue has low signal intensity on both T1- and T2-weighted sequences. Bony bridges are seen as areas of sclerotic bone or have signal intensity similar to marrow (Fig. 15-35).

MRI can also be used to evaluate surgical closure (epiphyseodesis) of the uninjured extremity (212).

STRESS FRACTURES

Stress-related osseous injuries have become increasingly common due to increased activity and fitness initiatives. Stress fractures account for over 10% of sports medicine visits (213,214). Stress fractures have been traditionally grouped into two categories. Fatigue fractures occur when abnormal repetitive stress is applied to normal bone. An insufficiency fracture (see Chapter 6) results from normal stress applied to abnormal bone (214–216).

This section will be limited to discussion of stress fractures (fatigue fractures) and the role of MRI in their evaluation. The mechanism of injury may be multifactorial. Compressive, gravitational, and muscle forces all play a role in developing stress fractures (213,215,217). Muscle forces may affect bone in several ways. In the upper extremity muscle strengthening can create imbalance between muscle strength and bone resulting in stress fractures. Other factors include the specific type of activity (Table 15-10), training techniques, footwear, sex and patient age (214,217).

Clinical diagnosis may be difficult, depending on location of the injury. Stress fractures of the femur, tarsal bones, spine, sesamoids, pelvis, and tibial plateau may be particularly difficult to diagnose clinically (217). Longitudinal stress fractures of the tibia and femur are also problematic (215,216). The location is also important for treatment and prognosis, as certain fractures are more likely to become complete and displace. Examples include the femoral neck and diaphysis and the tibial shaft (213,214).

TABLE 15-10

COMMON STRESS FRACTURES

Location	Etiology
Metatarsals	Marching, running, ballet, prior surgery
Calcaneus	Jumping, running, marching
Tarsals	Long distance running
Sesamoids	Standing, cycling, skiing
Tibia	Running, ballet
Longitudinal	Soccer, running, cheerleading
Fibula	Running, parachute jumping
Patella	Hurdling
Femur	Running
Pelvis	Running, bowling, gymnastics
Spine	Lifting, golfing, ballet
Humerus	Baseball
Coracoid	Trap shooting
Ulna	Baseball, wheelchair patients
Hamate hook	Baseball, golf, tennis
Metacarpals	Weight lifting, gymnastics

From references 213–215, and 217.

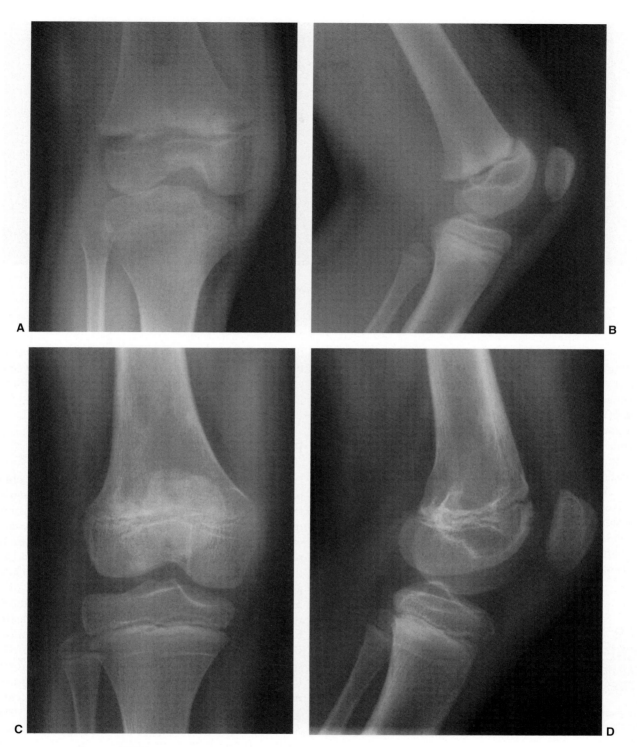

Figure 15-35   Anteroposterior **(A)** and lateral **(B)** radiographs demonstrate a slightly displaced Salter II fracture of the distal femoral growth plate. Radiographs 1 year later **(C,D)** show premature closure. The extent of physeal involvement is not clearly demonstrated Coronal T1- **(E)** and STIR **(F)** images show a small central bony bar (*arrows*). Evaluation is optimal on the STIR image as the open growth plate is high signal intensity.

Patients typically present with local pain related to activity that is reduced or relieved by rest. On physical examination there may be local tenderness, swelling, warmth and skin discoloration. Differential diagnosis varies to some extent with location. Table 15-11 summarizes conditions that may simulate stress fractures (213).

Multiple imaging techniques may be required for diagnosis. Radiographs are insensitive early (15%), but

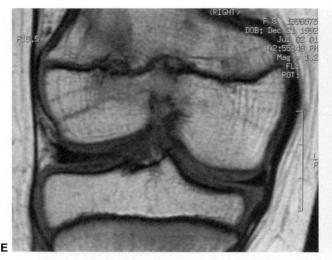

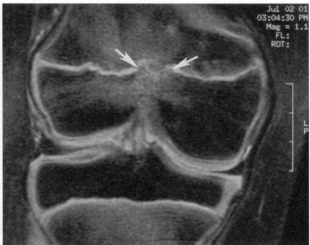

Figure 15-35   *(continued)*

usually become positive in several weeks (213,214,217). Radionuclide bone scans are sensitive early and can detect multiple fractures. Specificity is more problematic as other bone abnormalities can also result in a positive study (213,214). MRI is sensitive and can detect changes early, unlike radiographs. MRI can demonstrate marrow edema, cortical, periosteal, and soft tissue abnormalities. MRI is also useful for differentiating stress fractures from other conditions, especially when radiographs are normal (213–215).

T1-weighted sequences demonstrate marrow edema as low signal intensity (see Fig. 15-37). Fracture lines may be evident in the marrow but are less likely to be seen in the cortex. T2-weighted or STIR sequences provide more information regarding marrow, cortex, periostium, and

the soft tissues (see Fig. 15-38). Longitudinal stress fractures can also be evaluated with MRI. However, in certain cases, CT may more clearly demonstrate the fracture (215,216).

PAGET DISEASE

Paget disease is commonly encountered in the elderly population. The condition affects 3% to 4% of the population over age 40 (218). Paget disease is related to abnormal bone remodeling. Three phases have been described with varying radiographic and MR appearance. The lytic phase is predominantly osteoclastic. Large lytic areas in the skull (osteoporosis circumscripta) and the "blade of grass" appearance in the tibia are characteristic of this phase. The mixed phase results in cortical and trabecular thickening and bone enlargement. The osteoblastic or blastic phase results in areas of sclerosis. Distribution of skeletal involvement includes the skull (25% to 65%), spine (30% to 75%), pelvis (30% to 75%), and proximal long bones (25% to 30%). However, any osseous structure may be affected (218–221). Polyostotic disease occurs in 65% to 90% and isolated bone involvement in 10% to 35% (218). About 20% of patients are asymptomatic initially. Symptoms may include pain, increased warmth, increased bone size, bone deformity, kyphosis, and pathologic fractures (219,220).

Areas of involvement demonstrate marked increased tracer on technetium-99m bone scans. CT clearly demonstrates cortical and trabecular thickening as well as areas of sclerosis and fatty replacement. MR image features are now

---

TABLE 15-11

CLINICAL CONDITIONS SIMULATING STRESS FRACTURES

Neoplasms
Infections
Tendinitis
Periostitis
Ligament injury
Compartment syndrome
Gout
Pseudogout
Vascular occlusive disease

From references 213–215, and 217.

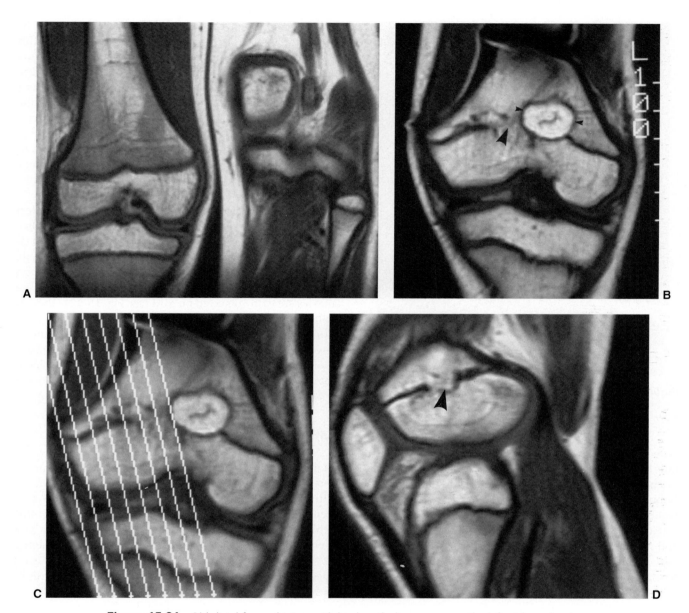

Figure 15-36 Old distal femoral injury with leg length discrepancy on the left. A bony bar has been resected and filled with a fat plug. SE 500/20 **(A)** image shows a normal right leg with increased signal in the normal growth plates on the right. The left leg is short. **B:** Coronal SE 500/20 image demonstrates the fat plug (*small arrowheads*) and a small bony bar (*large arrowhead*). Oblique sagittal images were selected **(C)** that allow a true sagittal view of the growth plate **(D)** which confirms only a small (<10%) bar (*arrowhead*).

more clearly defined (218–220). This is important because diagnosis may be confusing without radiographs or CT for comparison (see Fig. 15-39). In most cases, Paget disease is an incidental finding. Therefore, it is important to be aware of the uncomplicated MR features as well as potential complications.

Bone enlargement and cortical and trabecular thickening are seen as low signal intensity on MR images. Subtle

changes may be more conspicuous on CT. Three MRI patterns have been described for uncomplicated Paget disease. Fatty marrow signal intensity is maintained in the majority of longstanding cases (see Fig. 15-40) (222,223). Fatty marrow may be greater than that of uninvolved bone. In the late lytic or early mixed phase, the marrow has mixed low signal and fat signal on T1-weighted images. Marrow signal is inhomogenous high signal intensity on T2-weighted

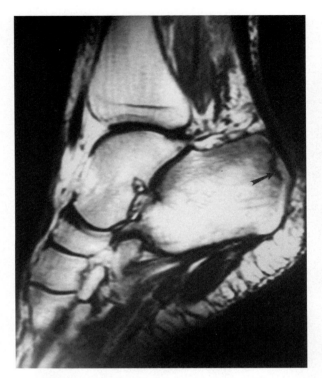

Figure 15-37 Sagittal T1-weighted image of the calcaneus demonstrates a low signal intensity stress fracture (*arrow*) with low signal intensity edema.

Malignant degeneration is rare (approximately 1%). The incidence may be higher (5% to 10%) in patients with severe polyostotic disease. Males are more commonly affected than females. The age range is 55 to 80 years. The pelvis, humerus, femur, and skull account for 80% of cases (224). Patients present with new focal pain and swelling (218,222,224). Tumors are usually high grade, with osteosarcoma being the most common (50% to 60%). Malignant fibrous histiocytoma or fibrosarcoma (20% to 25%) and lymphoma and angiosarcoma (1% to 3%) may also occur. Prognosis is poor, with 90% mortality in 3 years despite aggressive treatment (218,224).

Radiographs may demonstrate new lytic areas, cortical destruction, and soft tissue mass (219,220,222). Radiographic changes are useful for comparison with MR features. MRI demonstrates mass-like areas of intermediate signal intensity on T1- and increased signal intensity on T2-weighted sequences. Cortical destruction and soft tissue masses are easily detected on MRI (see Fig. 15-42). There is enhancement of nonnecrotic tissue after gadolinium injection. Lytic areas on radiographs may have low signal intensity or fat signal intensity on T1-weighted images. Malignancy is likely in the former. However, fat signal intensity need not be pursued and excludes malignancy if it compares to lucent or lytic areas in the bone (222,225).

MISCELLANEOUS BONE DISORDERS

Many of the bone disorders have been described in previous chapters, specifically Chapter 14. Certain marrow conditions, specifically metabolic disease (see Fig. 15-43), hemoglobinopathies, and infiltrative disorders are still typically evaluated with more conventional imaging techniques (94,104,169,181,226–232). Though imaging abnormalities are frequently nonspecific, new data using spectroscopy may be beneficial in certain metabolic conditions involving bone minerals (158).

sequence (see Fig. 15-41). The third pattern is seen in the late blastic phase, where sclerosis results in low signal intensity on all pulse sequences. Contrast enhancement is nonuniform but increased in hypervascular active disease regions (218,223).

Nonneoplastic complications include bowing, fractures, and neurologic symptoms. MRI is particularly useful in the last. Spinal stenosis, nerve compression, and the impact of basilar invagination are easily demonstrated with conventional MR techniques (218,224,225).

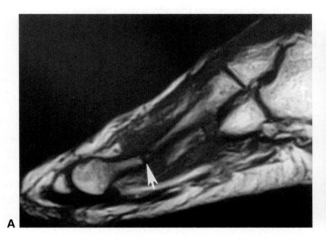

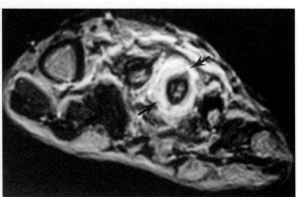

Figure 15-38 Third metatarsal stress fracture. **A:** Sagittal T1-weighted image demonstrates the fracture (*arrow*). **B:** Axial T2-weighted image shows high signal intensity in the periosteum and soft tissues (*arrows*) due to callus formation.

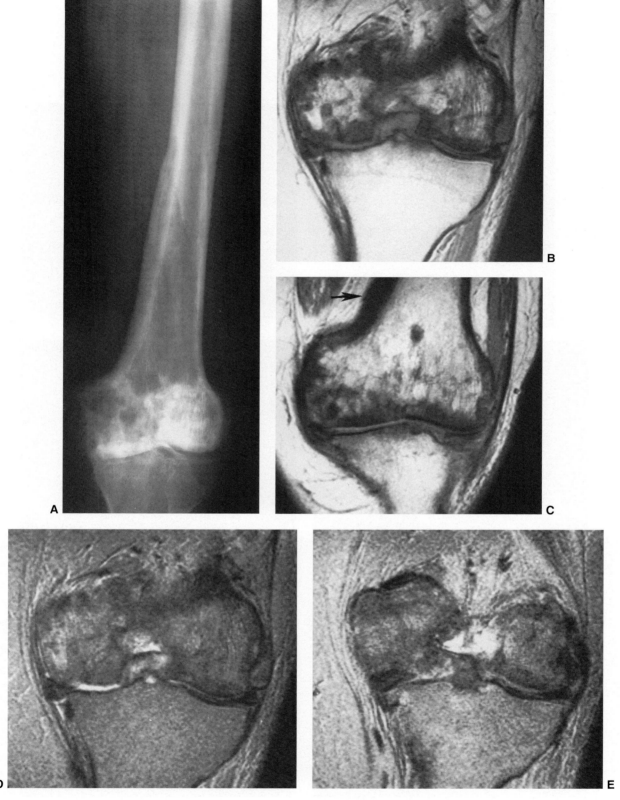

Figure 15-39 Anteroposterior radiograph of the femur **(A)** demonstrating cortical thickening, enlargement and sclerosis typical of Paget disease. Coronal SE 500/20 **(B,C)** and SE 2,000/80 **(D,E)** images show cortical thickening (*arrow* in **C**), prominent trabeculae and mixed areas of low and high signal intensity.

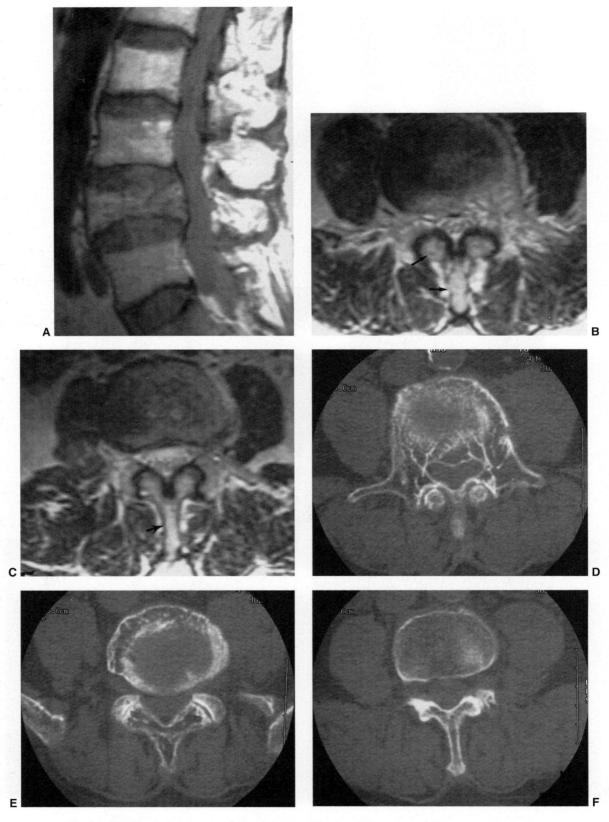

Figure 15-40   Paget disease of the spine with thin expanded cortex and fat in the marrow space. Sagittal **(A)** and axial **(B,C)** SE 500/20 images demonstrate vertebral compression with narrowing of the spinal canal. The posterior elements (*arrows*) are expanded and fatty tissue is present in the marrow. CT images **(D,E)** show typical features of Paget disease (compared to normal vertebra, **F**).

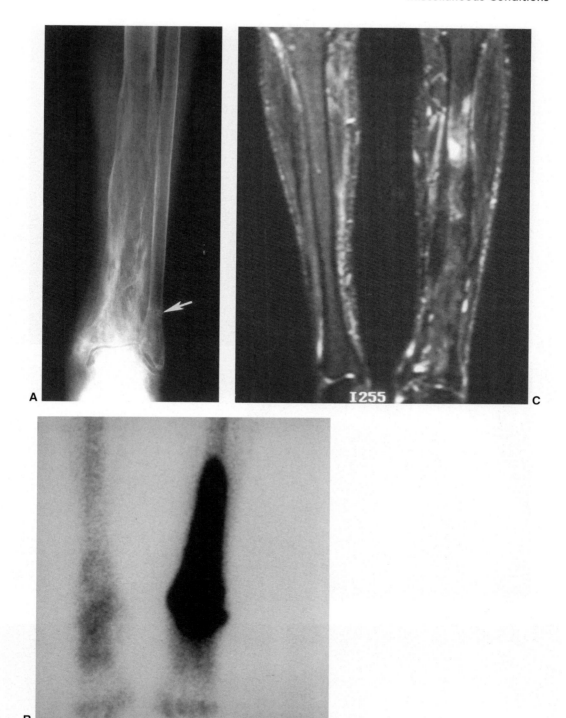

Figure 15-41 Mixed lytic and sclerotic Paget disease. **A:** Anteroposterior radiograph demonstrates lytic changes in the lower two thirds of the tibia. There are sclerotic changes distally. There is a subtle fibular stress fracture (*arrow*). **B:** Bone scan shows intense uptake in the area of involvement. **C:** Coronal T2-weighted image shows mixed fat, high signal intensity and low signal intensity distally due to bone sclerosis and trabecular thickening.

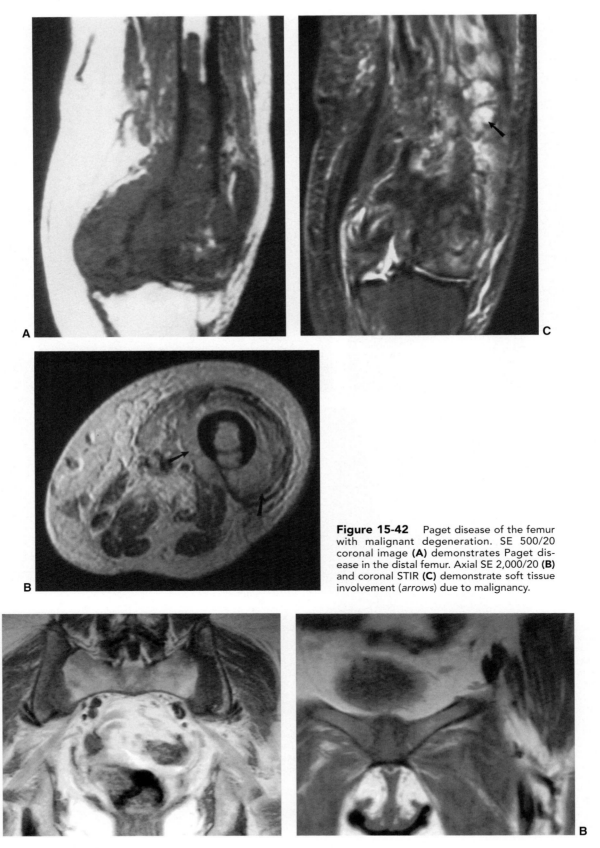

Figure 15-42 Paget disease of the femur with malignant degeneration. SE 500/20 coronal image **(A)** demonstrates Paget disease in the distal femur. Axial SE 2,000/20 **(B)** and coronal STIR **(C)** demonstrate soft tissue involvement (*arrows*) due to malignancy.

Figure 15-43 Renal osteodystrophy. Coronal T1-weighted images of the sacroiliac joints **(A)** and pubic symphysis **(B)** show joint irregularity and widening with intermediate signal intensity in the joint spaces.

REFERENCES

1. Baker DG, Schumacher HR, Wolf GL Jr. Nuclear magnetic resonance evaluation synovial fluid and articular tissues. *J Rheumatol* 1985;12:1062–1065.
2. Berfuss H, Fischer H, Hentschel D, et al. Whole-body MR imaging and spectroscopy with a 4-T system. *Radiology* 1988;169:811–816.
3. Berquist TH. Magnetic resonance techniques in musculoskeletal diseases. *Rheum Clin North Am* 1991;17:599–615.
4. Bush CH. The magnetic resonance imaging of musculoskeletal hemorrhage. *Skeletal Radiol* 2000;29:1–9.
5. Delfaut EM, Beltran J, Johnson G, et al. Fat suppression in MR imaging: techniques and pitfalls. *Radiographics* 1999;19:373–382.
6. Boeve WJ, Kamman RL, Mooyaart EL, et al. In vivo phosphorous magnetic resonance spectroscopy of bone and soft tissue tumors. Presented at: The Society of Magnetic Resonance in Medicine, Amsterdam, 1989.
7. Borghi L, Savoldi F, Scelsi R, et al. Nuclear magnetic resonance response of protons in normal and pathologic muscles. *Exp Neurol* 1983;81:89–96.
8. Delaney-Sathy LO, Fessell DP, Jacobson JA, et al. Sonography of diabetic muscle infarction with MR imaging, CT and pathologic correlation. *AJR Am J Roentgenol* 2000;174:165–169.
9. Dunn JF, Frostick S, Radda GK. Changes in high energy phosphate compounds associated with the primary defect in Duchenne's muscular dystrophy: a study of the MDX mouse. Presented at: The Society of Magnetic Resonance in Medicine, Amsterdam, 1989.
10. Edwards RHT, Dawson MJ, Griffith JR, et al. Nuclear magnetic resonance spectroscopy in research and clinical diagnosis. *Eur J Clin Invest* 1983;13:429–431.
11. Edwards RHT, Dawson MJ, Wilkie RE, et al. Clinical use of nuclear magnetic resonance in investigation of myopathy. *Lancet* 1982;1:725–731.
12. Jehenson P, Leroy-Willig A, deKeviler E, et al. MR imaging as a potential diagnostic test for metabolic myopathies: importance of variations in the T2 of muscle with exercise. *AJR Am J Roentgenol* 1993;161:347–351.
13. Jeneson JAL, Nederveen D, Bakker CJG. Dynamic exercise of the human forearm muscles: a combined IH MRI and 31P MRS study. Presented at: The Society of Magnetic Resonance in Medicine, Amsterdam, 1989.
14. Lanir A, Hadar H, Cohen I, et al. Gaucher disease: assessment with MR imaging. *Radiology* 1986;161:239–244.
15. Mancini DM, Ferraro N, Tuchler M, et al. Detection of abnormal calf muscle metabolism in patients with heart failure using phosphorus-31 nuclear magnetic resonance. *Am J Cardiol* 1988;62:1234–1240.
16. Matthews PM, Allaire C, Shoubridge E, et al. Phosphorus MRS in the clinical assessment of myopathies. Presented at: The Society of Magnetic Resonance in Medicine, Amsterdam, 1989.
17. Park JH, Vansant JP, Kumar NG, et al. Dermatomyositis correlative MR imaging and P-31 spectroscopy for quantitative characterization of inflammatory disease. *Radiology* 1990;177:473–479.
18. Peterson JJ, Kransdorf MJ, Bancroft LW, et al. Imaging characteristics of cystic adventitial disease of the peripheral arteries: presentation as a soft tissue mass. *AJR Am J Roentgenol* 2003;180:621–625.
19. Pollock L, Fullilove S, Shaw DG, et al. Proliferative myositis in a child. *J Bone Joint Surg Am* 1995;77A:132–134.
20. Rott HD, Briemesser FH, Rödl W. Imaging technics in muscular dystrophies. *J Génét Hum* 1985;33:397–403.
21. Tsai TS, Evans HA, Donnelly LF, et al. Fat necrosis after trauma. A benign cause of palpable lumps in children. *AJR Am J Roentgenol* 1997;169:1623–1626.
22. Feldman F, Zwass A, Staron RB, et al. MRI of soft tissue abnormalities: a primary cause of sickle cell crisis. *Skeletal Radiol* 1993;22:501–506.
23. May DA, Disler DG, Jones EA, et al. Abnormal signal intensity in skeletal muscle at MR imaging: patterns, pearls and pitfalls. *Radiographics* 2000;20:S295–S315.
24. Hawley RJ, Schllinger D, O'Doherty DS. Computed tomographic patterns of muscle in neuromuscular diseases. *Arch Neurol* 1984;41:383–387.
25. Metzler JP, Fleckenstein JL, White CL III, et al. MRI evaluation of amyloid myopathy. *Skeletal Radiol* 1992;21:463–465.
26. Otake S. Sarcoidosis involving skeletal muscle: imaging findings and relative value of imaging procedures. *AJR Am J Roentgenol* 1994;162:369–375.
27. O'Connell MJ, Powell T, Brennan D, et al. Whole-body MR imaging in the diagnosis of polymyositis. *AJR Am J Roentgenol* 2002;179:967–971.
28. Mellado JM, delPalomar LP. Muscle hernias of the lower leg: MRI findings. *Skeletal Radiol* 1999;28:465–469.
29. Shellock FG, Fukunaga T, Mink JH, et al. Acute effects of exercise on MR imaging of skeletal muscle: concentric vs. eccentric actions. *AJR Am J Roentgenol* 1991;156:765–768.
30. Shellock FG, Fukunaga T, Mink JH, et al. Exertional muscle injury: evaluation of concentric versus eccentric action with serial imaging. *Radiology* 1991;179:659–664.
31. Hands LJ, Bore PJ, Galloway G, et al. Muscle metabolism in patients with peripheral vascular disease investigated by 31P nuclear magnetic resonance spectroscopy. *Clin Sci* 1986;71:283–290.
32. Constantinides CD, Gillen JS, Boado FE, et al. Human skeletal muscle: sodium MR imaging and quantification-potential applications in exercise and disease. *Radiology* 2000;216:559–568.
33. Liu GC, Jong YJ, Chiang CH, et al. Duchenne muscular dystrophy: MR grading system for functional correlation. *Radiology* 1993;186:475–480.
34. Murphy WA, Totty WG, Carrol JE. MRI of normal and pathologic skeletal muscle. *AJR Am J Roentgenol* 1986;146:565–574.
35. Uetani M, Hayashi K, Matsunaga N, et al. Denervated skeletal muscle: MR imaging. *Radiology* 1993;198:511–515.
36. Fleckenstein JL, Watumull D, Conner KE, et al. Denervated human skeletal muscle: MR imaging evaluation. *Radiology* 1993;187:213–218.
37. Fraser DD, Frank JA, Dalakas MC. Inflammatory myopathies: MR imaging and spectroscopy. *Radiology* 1991;179:341–344.
38. Hernandez RJ, Sullivan DB, Chenevert TL, et al. MR imaging in children with dermatomyositis: finding and correlation with clinical and laboratory findings. *AJR Am J Roentgenol* 1993;161:359–366.
39. Hernandez RJ, Kein DR, Chenevert TL, et al. Fat-suppressed MR imaging of myositis. *Radiology* 1992;182:217–219.
40. Garcia J. MR of inflammatory myopathies. *Skeletal Radiol* 2000;29:425–438.
41. Bunch TW, O'Duffy JD, McLeod RA. Deforming arthritis of the hands in polymyositis. *Arthritis Rheum* 1976;19:243–248.
42. Jelinek JS, Mark AS, Barth WF. Sclerotic lesions of the cervical spine in sarcoidosis. *Skeletal Radiol* 1998;27:702–704.
43. Kazuyoski K, Shimizu H, Ogawa H, et al. MR and CT evaluation of sarcoid myopathy. *J Comput Assist Tomogr* 1991;15:1004–1007.
44. Koyama T, Ueda H, Togashi K, et al. Radiologic manifestations of sarcoidosis in various organs. *Radiographics* 2004;24:87–104.
45. Moore SL, Teirstein AE. Musculoskeletal sarcoidosis: spectrum of appearances at MR imaging. *Radiographics* 2003;23:1389–1399.
46. Nakamura Y, Jurihara N, Sato A, et al. Muscle sarcoidosis following malignant lymphoma: diagnosis by MR imaging. *Skeletal Radiol* 2002;31:702–705.
47. Kobayashi H, Kotoura Y, Sakahara H, et al. Solitary muscular sarcoidosis: CT, MRI and scintigraphic characteristics. *Skeletal Radiol* 1994;23:293–295.
48. Jelinek JS, Murphey MD, Aboulafia AJ, et al. Muscle infarction in patients with diabetes mellitus: MR imaging findings. *Radiology* 1999;211:241–247.
49. Khoury NJ, El-Khoury GY, Kathol MH. MRI diagnosis of diabetic muscle infarction: report of two cases. *Skeletal Radiol* 1997;26:122–127.
50. DeBoeck H, Noppen L, Desprechins B. Pyomyositis of the adductor muscles mimicking an infection of the hip. Diagnosis by magnetic resonance imaging. *J Bone Joint Surg Am* 1994;76A:747–750.
51. Steinbach LS, Tehranzadeh J, Fleckstein JL, et al. Human immune deficiency virus infection: musculoskeletal manifestations. *Radiology* 1993;186:833–838.
52. Tehranzadeh J, Ter-Oganesyan RR, Steinbach LS. Musculoskeletal disorders associated with HIV infection and AIDS. Part I: infectious musculoskeletal conditions. *Skeletal Radiol* 2004;33:249–259.

53. Gordon BA, Martinez S, Collins AJ. Pyomyositis: characteristics at CT and MR imaging. *Radiology* 1995;197:279–286.

54. Kaushik S, Flagg E, Wise CM, et al. Granulomatous myositis: a manifestation of chronic graft-versus-host disease. *Skeletal Radiol* 2002;31:226–229.

55. Adams SM, Chow CK, Prembiemar A, et al. The idiopathic infammatory myopathies: spectrum of MR imaging findings. *Radiographics* 1995;15:563–574.

56. Moskovic E, Fisher C, Westbury G, et al. Focal myositis, a benign inflammatory pseudotumor: CT appearances. *Br J Radiol* 1991;64:489–493.

57. Evans GFF, Haller RC, Wyrick PS, et al. Submaximal delayed-onset muscle soreness: correlations between MR imaging findings and clinical measures. *Radiology* 1998;208:815–820.

58. Lin J, Fessell DP, Jacobson JA, et al. An illustrated tutorial of musculoskeletal ultrasound: part 3, lower extremity. *AJR Am J Roentgenol* 2000;175:1313–1321.

59. Moore SG. Pediatric musculoskeletal imaging. In: Bradley WG, Start DD, eds. *Magnetic resonance imaging.* St. Louis, MO: Mosby–Year Book, 1992:2223–2331.

60. Palmer WE, Kuong SJ, Elmadbouh HM. MR imaging of myotendenous strain. *AJR Am J Roentgenol* 1999;173:703–709.

61. Pomeranz SJ, Heidt RS. MR imaging in the prognostication of hamstring injury. *Radiology* 1993;189:897–900.

62. Shintani S, Shiigai T. Repeat MRI in acute rhabdomyolsis: correlation with clinicopathological findings. *J Comput Assist Tomogr* 1993;17:786–791.

63. Ekman EF, Koman LA. Acute pain following musculoskeletal injuries and orthopedic surgery. *J Bone Joint Surg* 2004;86A:1316–1326.

64. Berquist TH. The elbow and wrist. *Top Magn Reson Imaging* 1989;1:15–27.

65. Holobinko JN, Damron TA, Scerpella PR, et al. Calcific myonecrosis. Keys to early recognition. *Skeletal Radiol* 2003;32:35–40.

66. Jansen DL, Connell DG, Vaisler BJ. Calcific myonecrosis of the calf manifesting as an enlarging soft tissue mass: imaging features. *AJR Am J Roentgenol* 1993;160:1072–1074.

67. Zohman GL, Pierce J, Chapman MW, et al. Calcific myonecrosis mimicking an invasive soft tissue neoplasm: a case report and review of the literature. *J Bone Joint Surg Am* 1998;80A:1193–1197.

68. Ogden JA. Current concepts review. The evaluation and treatment of partial physeal arrest. *J Bone Joint Surg* 1987;69A:1297–1302.

69. Michet CJ, Doyle JA, Ginsburg WW. Eosinophilic fasciitis: report of 15 cases. *Mayo Clin Proc* 1981;56:27–34.

70. Lakhanpal S, Ginsburg WW, Michet CJ, et al. Eosinophilic fasciitis: clinical spectrum and therapeutic response in 52 cases. *Semin Arthritis Rheum* 1988;17:221–231.

71. Moulton SJ, Kransdorf MJ, Ginsburg WW, et al. Eosinophilic fasciitis: specturm of MR imaging findings. Presented at: RSNA, Chicago, IL, Dec. 3, 2003.

72. Al-Shaikh A, Freeman C, Avruch L, et al. Use of magnetic resonance imaging in diagnosis of eosinophilic fasciitis. *J Rheumatol* 1994;37:1602–1608.

73. Imai T, Saitoh M, Matsumoto H. Eosinophilic fasciitis: MR evaluation. *Neurology* 2003;61:416.

74. Liou CH, Huang GS, Taylor JA, et al. Eosinophilic fasciitis in a military recruit: MR evaluation with clinical correlation. *Skeletal Radiol* 2003;32:52–57.

75. Visser H, Vosk H, Zanelle E, et al. Sarcoid arthritis: clinical characteristics, diagnostic aspects and risk factors. *Ann Rheum Dis* 2002;61:499–504.

76. Rayner CK, Barnet SP, McNeil JD. Osseous sarcoidosis-a magnetic resonance imaging diagnosis. *Clin Exp Rheumatol* 2002;20:546–548.

77. Poyanli A, Poyanli O, Sencer S, et al. Vertebral sarcoidosis: imaging findings. *Eur Radiol* 2000;10:92–94.

78. Beltran J, Caudill JL, Herman LA, et al. Rheumatoid arthritis: MR imaging manifestations. *Radiology* 1987;165:153–157.

79. Bergin D, Schweitzer ME. Indirect magnetic resonance arthrography. *Skeletal Radiol* 2003;32:551–558.

80. Chen CKH, Yeh LR, Pan H-B, et al. Intra-articular gouti tophi of the knee: CT and MR imaging in 12 patients. *Skeletal Radiol* 1999;28:75–80.

81. Choi J-A, Kim JE, Koh SH, et al. Arthropathy in Behcet disease: MR imaging findings in two cases. *Radiology* 2003;226:387–389.

82. Deutsch AL, Mink JH. Articular disorders of the knee. *Top Magn Reson Imaging* 1989;1:43–56.

83. Gaffney K, Cookson J, Blake D, et al. Quantification of rheumatoid synovitis by magnetic resonance imaging. *Arthritis Rheum* 1995;38:1610–1617.

84. Huch K, Kuettner KE, Dieppe P. Osteoarthritis in ankle and knee joints. *Semin Arthritis Rheum* 1997;26(4):667–674.

85. Otake S, Tsuruta Y, Yamana D, et al. Amyloid arthropathy of the hip joint: MR demonstration of presumed amyloid lesions in 152 patients with long-term dialysis. *Eur Radiol* 1998;8:1352–1356.

86. Recht MP, Resnick D. Magnetic resonance of articular cartilage: an overview. *Top Magn Reson Imaging* 1998;9(6):328–336.

87. Mitchell MJ, Sartoris DS, Resnick D. The foot and ankle. *Top Magn Reson Imaging* 1989;1:75–84.

88. Oloff-Solomon J, Solomon MA. Special radiographic techniques in the evaluation of arthritic disease. *Clin Podiatr Med Surg* 1988;5:25–36.

89. Sanchez RB, Quinn SF. MRI of inflammatory synovial processes. *Magn Reson Imaging* 1989;7:529–540.

90. Schweitzer ME, Falk A, Pathria MN, et al. MR imaging of the knee: can changes in the intracapsular fat pads be used as a sign of synovial proliferation in the presence of an effusion? *AJR Am J Roentgenol* 1993;160:823–826.

91. Smith DK, Totty WG. Articular disorders of the hip. *Top Magn Reson Imaging* 1989;1:29–41.

92. Vahlensieck M, Dombrowski F, Leutner C, et al. Magnetization transfer contrast (MTC) and MTC-subtraction: enhancement of cartilage lesions and intracartilaginous degeneration in vitro. *Skeletal Radiol* 1994;23:535–539.

93. Yulish BS, Lieberman JM, Newman AJ, et al. Juvenile rheumatoid arthritis: assessment with MR imaging. *Radiology* 1987;165:149–152.

94. Yulish BS, Lieberman JM, Strandjord SE, et al. Hemophilic arthropathy: assessment with MR imaging. *Radiology* 1987;164:759–762.

95. Bonel HM, Schneiner P, Seemann MD, et al. MR imaging of the wrist in rheumatoid arthritis using gadobenate dimeglumine. *Skeletal Radiol* 2001;30:15–24.

96. Jevtic V, Watt I, Rozman B, et al. Distinctive radiology features of small hand joints in rheumatoid arthritis and seronegative spondyloarthropathy demonstrated by contrast enhanced (Gd-DTPA) magnetic resonance imaging. *Skeletal Radiol* 1995;24:351–355.

97. Link TM, Steinbach LS, Ghosh S, et al. Osteoarthritis MR image findings at different stages of disease and correlation with clinical findings. *Radiology* 2003;226:373–381.

98. Narvaez JA, Narvaez J, Ortega R, et al. Hypointense synovial lesions on T2-weighted images: differential diagnosis with pathologic correlation. *AJR Am J Roentgenol* 2003;181:761–769.

99. Taouli B, Zaim S, Peterfly CG, et al. Rheumatoid arthritis of the hand and wrist: comparison of three imaging techniques. *AJR Am J Roentgenol* 2004;182:937–943.

100. Yoshioka H, Haishi T, Uematsu T, et al. MR microscopy of articular cartilage at 1.5 T: orientation and site dependence of laminar structures. *Skeletal Radiol* 2002;31:505–510.

101. Mosher TJ, Dardzinski BJ, Smith MB. Human articular cartilage: influence of aging and early symptomatic degeneration of the spatial variation of T2- preliminary findings at 3 T. *Radiology* 2000;214:259–266.

102. Fernandez-Madrid F, Karvonen RL, Teitge RA, et al. MR features of osteoarthritis of the knee. *Magn Reson Imaging* 1994;12:703–709.

103. Bongartz G, Bock E, Horbach T, et al. Degenerative cartilage lesions of the hip—magnetic resonance evaluation. *Magn Reson Imaging* 1989;7:179–186.

104. Brasch RC, Wesbey GE, Gooding CA, et al. Magnetic resonance imaging of transfusional hemosiderosis complicating thalassemia major. *Radiology* 1984;150:767–771.

105. Braunstein EM, Brandt KD, Albrecht M. MRI demonstration of hypertrophic articular cartilage repair in osteoarthritis. *Skeletal Radiol* 1990;19:335–339.

106. Broderick LS, Turner DA, Renfrew DL, et al. Severity of articular cartilage abnormality in patients with osteoarthritis: evaluation with fast spin-echo vs. arthroscopy. *AJR Am J Roentgenol* 1994; 162:99–103.

107. Li KC, Higgs J, Aisen AM, et al. MRI in osteoarthritis of the hip: gradations of severity. *Magn Reson Imaging* 1988;6:229–236.

108. Bellamy N, Buchanan WW, Goldsmith CH, et al. Vallidation of WOMAC: a health status instrument for measuring clinically important patient relevant outcomes to antirheumatic drug therapy in patients with osteoarthritis of the hip and knee. *J Rheumatol* 1988;15:1833–1840.

109. Kelgren J, Lawrence J. Radiological assessment of osteoarthritis. *Ann Rheum Dis* 1957;16:494–501.

110. Alexander CJ. Osteoarthritis: a review of old myths and current concepts. *Skeletal Radiol* 1990;19:327–333.

111. Bergman AG, Willeri HK, Lindstrand AL, et al. Osteoarthritis of the knee: correlation of subchondral MR signal abnormalities with histopathologic and radiographic features. *Skeletal Radiol* 1994;23:445–448.

112. Peterfly CG, Majundar S, Lang P, et al. MR imaging of the arthritic knee: improved discrimination of cartilage synovium and effusion with pulsed saturation transfer and fat suppressed T1 images. *Radiology* 1994;191:413–419.

113. Rubenstein JD, Kim JK, Heukelman RM. Effects of compression and recovery on bovine articular cartilage: appearance of MR images. *Radiology* 1996;201:843–850.

114. van der Linden E, Kroon HM, Doornbos J, et al. MR imaging of hyaline cartilage at 0.5 T: a quantitative and qualitative in vitro evaluation of three types of sequences. *Skeletal Radiol* 1998;27: 297–305.

115. Vasnawala SS, Pauly JM, Gold GE. MR imaging of knee cartilage with FEMR. *Skeletal Radiol* 2002;31:574–580.

116. McCauley TR, Disler DG. MR imaging of articular cartilage. *Radiology* 1998;209:629–640.

117. Wayne JS, Kraft KA, Shields KJ, et al. MR imaging of normal and matrix depleted cartilage: correlation with biomechanical function and biochemical composition. *Radiology* 2003;228: 493–499.

118. Modl JM, Sether LA, Haughton VM, et al. Articular cartilage: correlation of histologic zones with signal intensity at MR imaging. *Radiology* 1991;181:853–855.

119. Drapé JL, Thelen P, Gay-Depassier P, et al. Intra-articular diffusion of Gd-DOTA after intravenous injection in the knee: MR imaging evaluation. *Radiology* 1993;188:227–234.

120. Shahriaree H. Chondromalacia. *Contemp Orthop* 1985;11:27–39.

121. Goodwin DW, Dunn JF. High-resolution magnetic resonance imaging of articular cartilage: correlation with histology and pathology. *Top Magn Reson Imaging* 1998;9(6):337–347.

122. Hayes CW, Conway WF. Evaluation of articular cartilage: radiographic and cross sectional imaging techniques. *Radiographics* 1992;12:409–428.

123. Yeh LR, Kwak S, Kim YS, et al. Evaluation of articular cartilage thickness of the humeral head and glenoid fossa by MR arthrography: anatomic correlation in cadavers. *Skeletal Radiol* 1998; 27:500–504.

124. Bredella MA, Tirman PFJ, Peterfly CG, et al. Accuracy of T2-weighted fast spin-echo MR imaging with fat saturation in detecting cartilage defects in the knee. Comparison with arthroscopy in 130 patients. *AJR Am J Roentgenol* 1999;172: 1073–1080.

125. Disler DG, McCauley TR, Wirth CR, et al. Detection of knee hyaline cartilage defects using fat-suppressed three-dimensional spoiled gradient-echo MR imaging: comparison with standard MR imaging and correlation with arthroscopy. *AJR Am J Roentgenol* 1995;165:377–382.

126. Disler DG, McCauley TR. Clinical magnetic resonance imaging of articular cartilage. *Top Magn Reson Imaging* 1998;9(6):360–376.

127. Rose PM, Denloes TA, Szumoski J, et al. Chondromalacia patellae: fat-suppressed MR imaging. *Radiology* 1994;193:437–440.

128. Heuck AF, Steiger P, Stoller DW, et al. Quantification of knee joint fluid volume by MR imaging and CT using three-dimensional data processing. *J Comput Assist Tomogr* 1989;13:287–293.

129. Mohr A. The value of water excitation 3D FLASH and fat saturated PD weighted TSE MR imaging for detecting and grading articular cartilage lesions in the knee. *Skeletal Radiol* 2003;32: 396–402.

130. Sonin AH, Pensy RA, Mulligan ME, et al. Grading articular cartilage of the knee using fast spin-echo proton density weighted imaging without fat suppression. *AJR Am J Roentgenol* 2002;189:1159–1166.

131. Hodler J, Resnick D. Current status of imaging of articular cartilage. *Skeletal Radiol* 1996;25:703–709.

132. Hodler J, Loredo RA, Longo C, et al. Assessment of articular cartilage thickness of the humeral head: MR-anatomic correlation in cadavers. *AJR Am J Roentgenol* 1995;165:615–620.

133. Björhengren AG, Geborek D, Rydholm U, et al. MR imaging of the knee in acute rheumatoid arthritis: synovial uptake of gadolinium-DOTA. *AJR Am J Roentgenol* 1990;155:329–332.

134. Bollow M, Braun J, Hamm B, et al. Early sacroiliitis in patients with spondyloarthropathy: evaluation with dynamic gadolinium-enhanced MR imaging. *Radiology* 1995;194:529–536.

135. Brasch RC, Bennett HF. Consideration in the choice of contrast media for MR imaging. *Radiol* 1988;166:897–899.

136. Hajeck PC, Baker LL, Sartous DJ, et al. MR arthrography: anatomic-pathologic investigation. *Radiology* 1987;163:141–147.

137. Winalski CS, Aliabadi P, Wright RJ, et al. Enhancement of joint fluid with intravenously administered gadopentetate dimeglumine: technique, rationale and implications. *Radiology* 1993; 187:179–185.

138. O'Doherty DS, Schellinger D, Raptopoulos V. Computed tomographic patterns of pseudohypertrophic muscular dystrophy: preliminary results. *J Comput Assist Tomogr* 1977;14:482–486.

139. Gold GE, Bergman G, Pauley JM, et al. Magnetic resonance imaging of knee cartilage repairs. *Top Magn Reson Imaging* 1998; 9(6):377–392.

140. Sugimoto H, Takida A, Masuyama J, et al. Early-stage rheumatoid arthritis: diagnostic accuracy of MR imaging. *Radiology* 1996; 1998:185–192.

141. deLouge EE. Gadodiamide injection-enhanced magnetic resonance imaging of the body: results of a multicenter trial. *Acad Radiol* 1994;1:23–30.

142. Jevtic V, Kos-Golja M, Rozman B, et al. Marginal erosive discovertibral "Romanus" lesions in ankylosing spondylitis demonstrated by contrast enchanced Gd-DTPA magnetic resonance imaging. *Skeletal Radiol* 2000;29:27–33.

143. Sugimoto H, Takeda A, Hyodok K. Early stage rheumatoid arthritis: prospective study of the effectiveness of MR imaging for diagnosis. *Radiology* 2000;210:569–575.

144. Aisen AM, Marte W, Ellis JH, et al. Cervical spine involvement in rheumatoid arthritis: MR imaging. *Radiology* 1987;165: 159–163.

145. König H, Sieper J, Wolf KJ. Rheumatoid arthritis: evaluation of hypervascular and fibrous pannus with dynamic MR imaging enhanced with Gd-DTPA. *Radiology* 1990;176:473–477.

146. Poleksic L, Zdravkovic D, Jablanovic D, et al. Magnetic resonance imaging of bone destruction in rheumatoid arthritis: comparison with radiography. *Skeletal Radiol* 1993;22:577–580.

147. Pope RM. Rheumatoid arthritis: pathogenesis and early recognition. *Am J Med* 1996;100(Suppl. 2A):35–95.

148. Harris ED Jr. Rheumatoid arthritis. Pathophysiology and implications for therapy. *N Engl J Med* 1990;322:1277–1289.

149. Jevtic V, Watt I, Rozman B, et al. Contrast enhanced Gd-DTPA magnetic resonance imaging in the evaluation of rheumatoid arthritis during clinical trial with DMARDS. A prospective two year follow-up study on hand joints in 31 patients. *Clin Exp Rheumatol* 1999;15:151–156.

150. Adam G, Dammer M, Bohndorf K, et al. Rheumatoid arthritis of the knee. Value of gadopentetate dimeglumine-enhanced MR imaging. *AJR Am J Roentgenol* 1991;156:125–129.

151. Hervé-Somina CMP, Sebag GH, Prieur AM, et al. Juvenile rheumatoid arthritis of the knee: MR evaluation with Gd-DOTA. *Radiology* 1992;182:93–98.

152. Rominger MB, Bernreuter WK, Kinney PJ, et al. MR imaging of the hands in early rheumatoid arthritis: preliminary results. *Radiographics* 1993;13:37–46.

153. Singson RD, Zaldieondo FM. Value of unenhanced spin-echo MR imaging in distinguishing between synovitis and effusion of the knee. *AJR Am J Roentgenol* 1992;159:569–571.

154. McQueen FM, Stewart N, Crabbe J, et al. Magnetic resonance imaging of the wrist in early rheumatoid arthritis reveals a high prevalence of erosions at four months after symptom onset. *Ann Rheum Dis* 1998;57:530–536.

155. Swen WAA, Jacobs JWG, Hubach PCG, et al. Comparison of sonography and magnetic resonance imaging for diagnosis of partial tears of the extensor tendons in rheumatoid arthritis. *Rheumatology* 2000;39:55–62.

156. Reiser MF, Bongartz GP, Erlemann R, et al. Gadolinium-DTPA in rheumatoid arthritis and related disease: first results with dynamic magnetic resonance imaging. *Skeletal Radiol* 1989;18:591–597.

157. Yamato M, Tamai K, Yamagucki T, et al. MRI of the knee in rheumatoid arthritis: Gd-DTPA perfusion dynamics. *J Comput Assist Tomogr* 1993;17:781–785.

158. Blatter DD. Phosphorus-31 magnetic resonance spectroscopy of experimentally induced arthritis in rats. *Skeletal Radiol* 1987;16:183–189.

159. Terrier F, Hricak H, Revel D, et al. Magnetic resonance imaging and spectroscopy of periarticular inflammatory soft tissue changes in experimental arthritis of the rat. *Invest Radiol* 1985;20:813–823.

160. Reijnierse M, Breedveld FC, Kvoon HM, et al. Are magnetic resonance flexion views useful in evaluating cervical spine of patients with rheumatoid arthritis? *Skeletal Radiol* 2000;29:85–89.

161. Senac MO Jr, Deutsch D, Bernstein BH, et al. MR imaging in juvenile rheumatoid arthritis. *AJR Am J Roentgenol* 1988;150:873–878.

162. Goupille P, Roulot B, Akoka S, et al. Magnetic resonance imaging: a valuable method for detection of synovial inflammation in rheumatoid arthritis. *J Rheumatol* 2001;28:35–40.

163. Huh YM, Suh JS, Jeong FK, et al. Role of inflamed synovial volume of the wrist in re-defining remission of rheumatoid arthritis with gadolinium enhanced 3D-SPGR MR imaging. *J Magn Reson Imaging* 1999;10:202–208.

164. Lee J, Lee SK, Suh JS, et al. Magnetic imaging of the wrist in defining remission in rheumatoid arthritis. *J Rheumatol* 1997;24:1303–1308.

165. Mandelbaum BR, Grant AM, Hartzman S, et al. The use of MRI to assist in diagnosis of pigmented villonodular synovitis of the knee joint. *Clin Orthop* 1988;231:135–139.

166. Spritzer CE, Dalinka MK, Kressel HY. Magnetic resonance imaging of pigmented villonodular synovitis: a report of two cases. *Skeletal Radiol* 1987;16:316–319.

167. Jelinek JS, Kransdorf MJ, Utz JA, et al. Imaging of pigmented villonodular synovitis with emphasis on MR imaging. *AJR Am J Roentgenol* 1989;152:337–342.

168. Chin KR, Barr SJ, Winalski C. Treatment of advanced primary and recurrent diffuse pigmented villonodular synovitis of the knee. *J Bone Joint Surg Am* 2002;84A:2192–2202.

169. Popp JD, Bidgood WD, Edwards L. Magnetic resonance imaging of tophaceous gout in the hands and wrists. *Semin Arthritis Rheum* 1996;25:282–289.

170. Yu JS, Chung C, Recht M, et al. MR imaging of tophaceous gout. *AJR Am J Roentgenol* 1997;168:523–527.

171. Shin AY, Weinstein LP, Bishop AT. Kienbock's disease and gout. *J Hand Surg [Br]* 1999;24B:363–365.

172. Peh WCG, Shek TWH, Davies AM, et al. Osteochondroma and secondary synovial osteochondrom-atosis. *Skeletal Radiol* 1999;28:169–174.

173. Kramer J, Recht M, Deely DM, et al. MR appearance of idiopathic synovial osteochondromatosis. *J Comput Assist Tomogr* 1993;17:772–776.

174. Pitcher JD, Schofield TD, Youngberg R, et al. Synovial chondromatosis simulating neoplastic degeneration of osteochondroma: finding on MR and CT. *Skeletal Radiol* 1994;23:99–102.

175. Brossmann J, Preidler K-W, Daenen B, et al. Imaging of osseous and cartilaginous intra-articular bodies in the knee: comparison of MR imaging and MR arthrography with CT and CT arthrography in cadavers. *Radiology* 1996;200:509–517.

176. Cobby MJ, Adler RS, Swartz R, et al. Dialysis-related amyloid arthropathy: MR findings in four patients. *AJR Am J Roentgenol* 1991;157:1023–1027.

177. Escobedo EM, Hunter JC, Zuik-Brody GC, et al. Magnetic resonance imaging of dialysis-related amyloidosis of the shoulder and hip. *Skeletal Radiol* 1996;25:41–48.

178. Keller U, Oberhänsli R, Huber P, et al. Phosphocreatine content and intracellular pH of calf muscle measured by phosphorus NMR spectroscopy in occlusive arterial disease of the legs. *Eur J Clin Invest* 1985;15:382–388.

179. Rachbauer F, Krecy A, Bodner G. Amyloidoma of the clavicle. *AJR Am J Roentgenol* 2003;181:771–773.

180. Eustace S, Buff B, McCarthy C, et al. Magnetic resonance imaging of hemochromatosis arthropathy. *Skeletal Radiol* 1994;23:547–549.

181. Kulkarni MV, Drolshagen LF, Kaye JJ, et al. MR imaging of hemophiliac arthropathy. *J Comput Assist Tomogr* 1986;10:445–449.

182. Murphey MD, Wetzol LH, Bramble JM, et al. Sacroilitis: MR imaging findings. *Radiology* 1991;180:239–244.

183. Pettersson H, Gillespy T, Kitchens C, et al. Magnetic resonance imaging in hemophilic arthropathy of the knee. *Acta Radiol* 1987;28:621–625.

184. Bates DG, Hresko MT, Jaramillo D. Patellar sleeve fracture: demonstration with MR imaging. *Radiology* 1994;193:825–827.

185. Kristiansen LP, Gunderson RB, Steen H, et al. The normal development of tibial torsion. *Skeletal Radiol* 2001;30:519–522.

186. Barnewolt CE, Shapiro F, Jaramillo D. Normal gadolinium-enhanced MR images of the developing appendicular skeleton. Part 1. Cartilaginous epiphysis and physis. *AJR Am J Roentgenol* 1997;169:183–189.

187. Craig JG, Van Holsbeeck M, Zatz I. The utility of MRI in assessing Blount disease. *Skeletal Radiol* 2002;31:208–213.

188. Dwek JR, Shapiro F, Laor T, et al. Normal gadolinium-enhanced MR images of the developing appendicular skeleton: Part 2. Epiphyseal and metaphyseal marrow. *AJR Am J Roentgenol* 1997;169:191–196.

189. Eckland K, Jaramillo D. Patterns of premature physeal arrest: MR imaging in 111 children. *AJR Am J Roentgenol* 2002;178:967–972.

190. Futami T, Foster BK, Morris LL, et al. Magnetic resonance imaging of growth plate injuries: the efficacy and indications for surgical procedures. *Arch Orthop Trauma Surg* 2000;120:390–396.

191. White PG, Mali JY, Friedman L. Magnetic resonance imaging in acute physeal injuries. *Skeletal Radiol* 1994;23:627–631.

192. Dietrich RB. *Pediatric MRI*, 2nd ed. Philadelphia, PA: Lippincott Williams & Wilkins, 2002.

193. Johnson ND, Wood BP, Noh KS, et al. MR imaging anatomy of the infant hip. *AJR Am J Roentgenol* 1989;153:127–133.

194. Lee MS, Harcke HT, Kumar SJ, et al. Subtalar joint coalition in children: new observations. *Radiology* 1989;172:635–639.

195. Moore SG, Bissett GB III, Siegel MJ, et al. Pediatric musculoskeletal MR imaging. *Radiology* 1991;179:345–360.

196. Rush BH, Bramson RT, Ogden JA. Legg-Calvé-Perthes disease: detection of cartilaginous and synovial changes with MR imaging. *Radiology* 1988;167:473–476.

197. Scoles PV, Yoon YS, Makley JT, et al. Nuclear magnetic resonance imaging in Legg-Calvé-Perthes disease. *J Bone Joint Surg Am* 1984;66:1357–1363.

198. Siegel MJ. Magnetic resonance imaging of the pediatric pelvis. *Semin Ultrasound CT MR* 1991;12:475–505.

199. Toby EB, Koman LA, Bechtold RE. Magnetic resonance imaging of pediatric hip disease. *J Pediatr Orthop* 1985;5:665–671.

200. Chung T, Jaramillo D. Normal maturing distal tibia and fibula: changes with age at MR imaging. *Radiology* 1995;194:227–232.

201. Cohen MD. Magnetic resonance imaging of the pediatric musculoskeletal system. *Semin Ultrasound CT MR* 1991;12:506–523.

202. Havranek P, Lizler J. Magnetic resonance imaging in the evaluation of partial growth arrest after physeal injuries in children. *J Bone Joint Surg Am* 1991;73A:1234–1241.

203. O'Driscoll SW. The healing and regeneration of articular cartilage. *J Bone Joint Surg Am* 1998;80A:1795–1812.

204. Rogers LF, Pozanski AK. Imaging of epiphyseal injuries. *Radiology* 1994;191:297–308.

205. Harcke HT, Snyder M, Caro PA, et al. Growth plate of the normal knee: evaluation with MR imaging. *Radiology* 1992;183:119–123.

206. Jaramillo D, Hoffer FA, Shapiro F, et al. MR imaging of fractures of the growth plate. *AJR Am J Roentgenol* 1990;155:1261–1265.

207. Jaramillo D, Laor T, Zaleski DJ. Indirect trauma to the growth plate: results of MR imaging after epiphyseal and metaphyseal injury in rabbits. *Radiology* 1993;187:171–178.

208. Salter RB, Harris WR. Injuries involving the epiphyseal plate. *J Bone Joint Surg* 1963;45A:587–622.

209. Gabel GT, Peterson HA, Berquist TH. Premature partial physeal arrest. *Clin Orthop* 1991;272:242–247.

210. Jaramillo D, Hoffer FA. Cartilaginous epiphysis and growth plate. Normal and abnormal MR imaging findings. *AJR Am J Roentgenol* 1992;158:1105–1110.

211. Meyers SP, Weiner SN. Magnetic resonance imaging features of fractures using the short tau inversion recovery (STIR) sequence: correlation with radiographic findings. *Skeletal Radiol* 1991;20:499–507.

212. Synder M, Harcke HT, Bowen JR, et al. Evaluation of physeal behavior in response to epiphyseodesis with the use of serial magnetic resonance imaging. *J Bone Joint Surg Am* 1994;76A:224–229.

213. Berquist TH. *Imaging of orthopedic trauma*, 2nd ed. New York: Raven Press, 1992.

214. Daffner RH. Stress fractures. *Skeletal Radiol* 1978;2:221–229.

215. Craig JG, Widman D, Van Holsbeeck M. Longitudinal stress fracture: patterns of edema and the importance of the nutrient foramen. *Skeletal Radiol* 2003;32:22–27.

216. Williams M, Laredo J-D, Setbon S, et al. Unusual longitudinal stress fractures of the femoral diaphysis: report of 5 cases. *Skeletal Radiol* 1999;27:81–85.

217. Anderson MW, Greenspan A. Stress fractures. *Radiology* 1996;199:1–12.

218. Smith SE, Murphey MA, Motamedi K, et al. Radiologic spectrum of Paget disease of bone and its complications with pathologic correlation. *Radiographics* 2002;22:1191–1216.

219. Mirra JM, Brien EW, Tehranzadeh J. Paget's disease of bone: review with emphasis on radiographic features, part I. *Skeletal Radiol* 1995;24:163–171.

220. Mirra JM, Brien EW, Tehranzedeh J. Paget's disease of bone: review with emphasis on radiographic features, part II. *Skeletal Radiol* 1995;24:173–184.

221. Moore TE, Kathol MH, El-Koury GY, et al. Unusual radiologic features of Paget's disease of bone. *Skeletal Radiol* 1994;23:257–260.

222. Sundarum M, Khanna G, El-Khoury GY. T1-weighted MR imaging for distinguishing large osteolysis of Paget disease from sarcomatous degeneration. *Skeletal Radiol* 2001;30:378–383.

223. Vande Berg BC, Malghem J, Lecourvet FE, et al. Magnetic resonance appearance of uncomplicated Paget's disease of bone. *Semin Musculoskelet Radiol* 2001;5:69–77.

224. Boutin RD, Spitz DJ, Newman JS, et al. Complications of Paget disease at MR imaging. *Radiology* 1998;209:641–651.

225. Roberts MC, Kressel HY, Fallon MD, et al. Paget disease: MR imaging finding. *Radiology* 1989;177:341–345.

226. Blocklet D, Abramowicz M, Schoutens A. Bone. Bone marrow and MIBI scintigraphic findings in Gaucher's disease "bone crisis". *Clin Nucl Med* 2001;26A:765–769.

227. Helms CA. The use of fat suppression in gadolinium-enhanced MR imaging of the musculoskeletal system: a potential source of error. *AJR Am J Roentgenol* 1999;173:234–236.

228. Hill SM, Baker AR, Barton NW, et al. Sciatic nerve: paradoxic hypertrophy after amputation in young patients. *Radiology* 1997;205:559–562.

229. Kattapurum SV, Rosol MS, Rosenthal DI, et al. Magnetic resonance features of allografts. *Skeletal Radiol* 1999;28:383–389.

230. Krietner K-F, Kalden P, Neufang A, et al. Diabetes and peripheral arterial occlusive disease: prospective comparison of contrast enhanced three- dimensional MR angiography and conventional digital subtraction angiography. *AJR Am J Roentgenol* 2000;174:171–179.

231. Rao VM, Fishman M, Mitchell DG, et al. Painful sickle cell crisis: bone marrow patterns observed with MR imaging. *Radiology* 1986;161:211–215.

232. Sebes JI. Diagnostic imaging of bone and joint abnormalities associated with sickle cell hemoglobinopathies. *AJR Am J Roentgenol* 1989;152:1153–1159.

Clinical Spectroscopy

Thomas H. Berquist

Magnetic resonance spectroscopy (MRS) was developed prior to magnetic resonance imaging (MRI) (1,2). MRI provides excellent anatomic detail and clearly defines pathology due to its superior contrast and flexibility of image plane selection compared to computed tomography (CT) and other imaging techniques. MRS offers a noninvasive technique for evaluating biochemical changes *in situ* (3). Though MRS has progressed as a clinical tool, it is still not universally used clinically (1,3–5). Bottomly (3) described four challenges for MRS that needed to be accomplished before the technique becomes an accepted clinical tool. These challenges include providing technical feasibility in a clinical setting, interpreting and understanding the new chemical data in clinical medicine, obtaining adequate data on normal and pathologic tissues, and developing MRS into an efficacious diagnostic technique (3).

MRS continues to be an effective research tool (6). In recent years, more applications have evolved using hydrogen (^{1}H) and phosphorus (^{31}P) to study neurologic, cardiac, liver, breast, prostate, myopathies and bone, and soft tissue neoplasms (7–17). New techniques and higher field

strength whole body images (3 to 8 T) have contributed to the expanded utility of MRS (9,11,18–23).

This chapter will review current clinical applications and future potential. Certain basic principles will be reviewed primarily as they relate to clinical practice. An in-depth discussion of the physics of MRS is beyond the scope of this chapter.

BASIC PRINCIPLES OF MAGNETIC RESONANCE SPECTROSCOPY

Clinical MRS research has concentrated on ^{31}P, ^{1}H, carbon (^{13}C), sodium (^{23}Na), and fluorine (^{19}F) (1,4,24–30). ^{1}H and, to a lesser degree, ^{31}P are most commonly studied due to the need to obtain adequate signal-to-noise ratio (SNR) and clinically significant data (2,31,32). Though potentially useful, ^{13}C spectroscopy has also lagged behind due to significant modifications required for conventional clinical imaging systems (32).

Because of the improved spectra from smaller tissue volumes at clinical field strengths (1.5 T), much of the recent clinical research has shifted from phosphorus to hydrogen spectroscopy (32–34). New approaches may evolve with the increased use of higher (3 to 8 T) field strength magnets. However, to date there have been problems at higher field strength due to issues with shimming and T2 contraction (11,20).

When a given tissue sample is studied, the results depend upon the magnetic field strength, temperature, metabolic concentration, and sample size. Sensitivity and localization of the sample are critical. Even when coil selection is optimal, overlying tissue can reduce the signal (2).

To date, there is no consensus as to which localization technique is best. Six techniques have been commonly used (1,2,24,26): Rotating frame zeugmatography topical MR, depth-resolved surface coil spectroscopy, image-selected *in vivo* spectroscopy, one- to three-dimensional phase encoding or spectroscopic techniques, and chemical shift imaging. This group of techniques fall into three categories of spatial localization: spatial gradients in a radiofrequency field (i.e., rotating frame zeugmatography), static spatial gradients in the main magnetic field (i.e., topical MR), and pulsed spatial gradients at audio frequencies (i.e., depth-resolved surface coil spectroscopy, image-selected *in vivo* spectroscopy) (3).

In recent years, new techniques have been developed to improve clinical MRS. These include magnet designs, coils, sequences, and filters (7,18,19,21–23). New coil designs have significantly improved spatial resolution (21). Truncation effects for K-space sampling with two-dimensional MRS can be improved by using filters to improve image representation of the tissue being evaluated (23). New fast pulse sequences such as rapid acquisition with relaxation enhancement (RARE) have improved signal-to-noise ratios (18).

Also, from a practical standpoint, one should consider whether contrast enhancement, which is used much more commonly today, affects MRS data. A recent study suggests that there is no effect on MRS data (22).

Most clinical and research studies with *in vivo* spectroscopy have focused on ^{1}H, ^{31}P, and to a lesser degree, ^{13}C (1,4,25,27,30–33,35–37).

^{31}P is most often studied for its fundamental importance in energy metabolism and membrane construction (see Fig. 16-1) (1,13,16,17,38–41). Signal intensity is 1,000,000 times less than ^{1}H, so achieving adequate SNR can be difficult (1). Field strengths of ≥ 1.5 T are required.

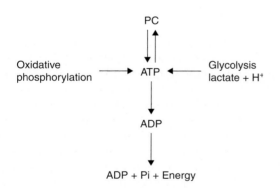

Glycolysis → ATP production and lactic acid production (33).

^{1}H spectroscopy is more often used than ^{31}P spectroscopy due to abundance, higher SNR, and performance at conventional MR field strengths of 1.5 T (3,9,12,14,15,42,43). Hydrogen spectroscopy demonstrates two large peaks (see Fig. 16-2); a water peak and CH_2 (methylene group) or fat peak (1). Though other ^{1}H moieties are present, they are usually not detected due to the strong fat and water peaks (1). Although ^{1}H has the highest sensitivity, the chemical shift range is narrow (see Chapter 1). Hydrogen spectroscopy provides *in vivo* data on glycolysis (lactate production and clearance, free amino acids, fatty acids, and neurotransmitters) (3,4,33,34).

^{13}C is a stable isotope of carbon with a weak but detectable MR signal and a large chemical shift range. The main utility of ^{13}C lies in lipid metabolism, predominantly triglycerides. Carbohydrate turnover can also be studied with ^{13}C spectroscopy (1,24).

CLINICAL APPLICATIONS

MRS of musculoskeletal disorders has included studies of anemia, ischemia, exercise, myopathies, muscular dystrophy, neoplasms, cartilage disorders, and metabolism (1,2, 6–9,16,42,44–49). Most clinical research has been concentrated on musculoskeletal neoplasms and metabolism. Attempts to improve lesion specificity (benign vs. malignant) and evaluate treatment and recurrence have been reported using MRI and MRI combined with MRS.

Musculoskeletal Neoplasms

MRI is the technique of choice for evaluating soft tissue masses and staging skeletal neoplasms. Though sensitive, MRI has not achieved outstanding specificity for differentiating benign from malignant tissues (13). Also, evaluating patients for recurrence after treatment is often difficult using conventional MRI techniques (5,50). Gadolinium and spectroscopy have been used to improve results when evaluating musculoskeletal neoplasms. Early experience with MRS and combined MRI–MRS examinations have demonstrated potential for spectroscopy (^{1}H and ^{31}P) (1,14,16,24,50–56).

Negendank et al. (5) studied 17 benign and 17 malignant bone and soft tissue tumors using combined MRI and ^{31}P MRS. Examinations were completed in 60 to 120 minutes, indicating the technique could be practical in the clinical environment. Hypocellular lesions could not be accurately studied due to low SNR in three patients (5). This work also suggested that tumors with hypocellularity such as desmoid tumors may not be easily studied with spectroscopy. Benign lesions demonstrated ^{31}P spectra similar to skeletal muscle. Malignant spectra differed in that there was a high phosphomonoester/nucleoside triphosphate (PMN/NTP) peak ratio. Though pH was higher in malignant lesions, the data were not statistically significant compared to pH in benign lesions (5,52). Okada et al. (14) demonstrated higher lactate levels in malignant lesions compared to benign lesions using proton (^{1}H) spectroscopy. In addition, choline compounds were only increased in solid neoplasms (14).

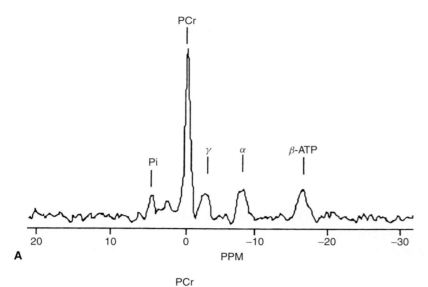

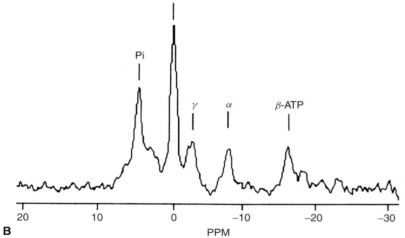

Figure 16-1 ^{31}P spectra from the calf at 1.5 T with a 14-cm coil. Two spectra were extracted from a set of 256 collected at 5-second intervals at rest **(A)** and 10 minutes into exercise **(B)**. α, β, and τ-ATP correspond to the three phosphorus moieties of adenosine triphosphate. (From Aisen AM, Chenevert TL: MR spectroscopy: Clinical perspective. *Radiology* 1989; 173:593–599.)

Other groups have reported similar results and also concluded that tumor specificity (benign vs. malignant) can be improved by combined MRI and MRS examinations (26,50,53–55,57,58). Zlatkin et al. (50) also examined histologic specificity as well as other practical aspects of combined MRI–MRS examinations of soft tissue tumors. Tumor size had a significant impact on spectra. Larger lesions (>500 cm^3), as measured with MR images, had less well-defined spectra (see Fig. 16-3). Tumor necrosis (high signal on T2-weight, low signal on T1-weight, unenhanced with gadolinium) was more often seen with larger histologically high-grade tumors (5,50). Although useful in defining the nature of lesions, tumor type was not possible to define, and contamination of spectra by adjacent muscle was also a problem. Though MRS offers improved specificity, further technical improvements are needed to refine technique, specifically coil and localization problems (50).

MRS has also been evaluated as a potential technique for evaluating tumor response to therapy and to differentiate post treatment changes from recurrent tumor (13,16,25, 37). Neoplasms typically demonstrate elevated inorganic phosphate, phosphomonoester (PME), and phosphodiester (PDE) peaks with lower phosphocreatine (PCr) compared to normal muscle. Additionally, pH values can be monitored (37). Changes in ^{31}P spectra noted in neoplasms described above can be monitored during and following treatment protocols to evaluate the response of lesions to treatment.

Data suggest spectral changes are more accurate than morphologic and signal intensity changes on MR images to determine therapeutic success and for detection of recurrent tumor (13,16,25,37). Maldonado et al. (39) evaluated treatment response using PME and PDE to adenosine triphosphate (ATP) ratios. These ratios (PME/ATP and PDE/ATP) were high in active tumors and were reduced in those patients who responded to therapy. Kettelhack et al. (13) evaluated ^{31}P data before and after therapy. Partial response was found in 47% demonstrated by decreased PME/PCR and PME/ATP ratios. ^{31}P spectroscopy was 94%

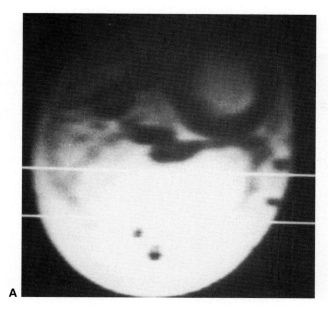

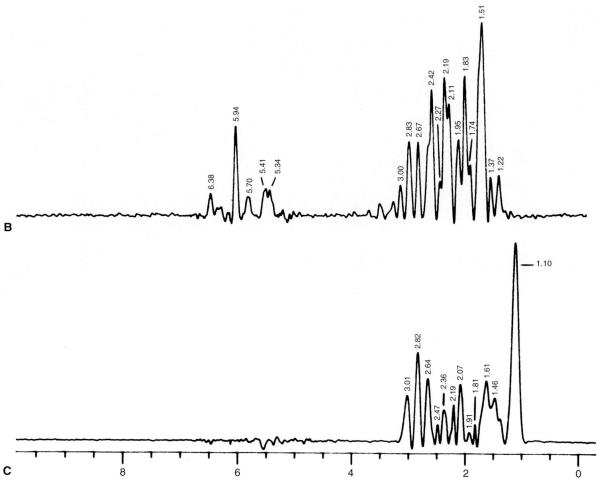

Figure 16-2 **A:** Axial image of the calf in a spina bifida patient with fatty replacement of muscle. Lines indicate the coronal section studied. **B:** Water-suppressed ^{1}H spectra from the gastrocnemius muscles of the abnormal leg. **C:** ^{1}H spectra from normal gastrocnemius muscles. Values are indicated in parts per million (ppm). Normal spectral **(C)** major resonance 1.10 ppm– (CH$_2$)n; –COCH$_2$CH$_2$–1.61 ppm; = CHCH$_2$–2.07 ppm; = COCH$_2$ – 2.64 ppm; = CH–CH$_2$–CH = 2.82 ppm; = NCH$_3$ – 3.01 ppm. Diseased muscle in **B** (CH$_2$)n – 1.15 ppm; with resonances from = CHCH$_2$ at 1.83, 2.11, 2.19, and 2.42 ppm. = CH = CH–aromatic region at 5.34, 5.41, 5.70, 5.94, and 6.38 ppm. (From Brny M, Langer BG, Glick RP, et al. In-vivo H-1 spectroscopy in humans at 1.5 T. *Radiology* 1988; 167:839–844.)

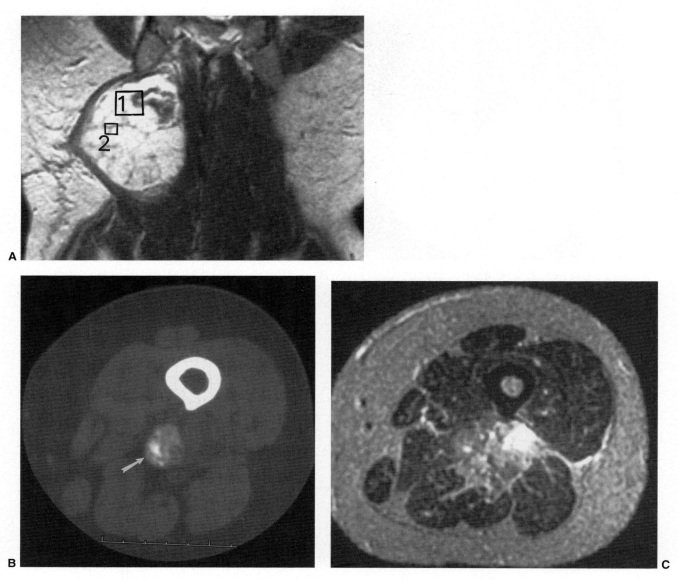

Figure 16-3 Soft tissue tumors with inhomogeneous signal intensity. Tumor cells and necrotic, fibrous, and other tissues could be included in the spectroscopy, some affecting results and reproducibility of data. **A:** Soft tissue chondrosarcoma with sample 1 including necrotic tissue and sample 2 fibrous septations. CT **(B)** and axial SE 2,000/80 MR image **(C)** demonstrating a calcified spindle cell sarcoma. The calcification (*arrow*) is obvious on CT but not easily appreciated on the MR section. How would this affect the spectrum?

specific and 68% sensitive for monitoring response or therapy.

MYOPATHIES AND MUSCLE DISORDERS

Muscle disorders including myopathies, muscular dystrophies, neuropathies, and exercise changes have been evaluated in several reports (7,8,33,38,40,43,46,59–66). Image features, ^{1}H, and ^{31}P MRS have provided interesting data in patients with normal metabolism and abnormal metabolic changes due to muscle disease.

Adenosine triphosphate (ATP) is a primary energy source for muscle metabolism. Therefore, comparison of normal spectra with spectral and pH changes during exercise can be useful for evaluating metabolic and muscular disorders (36,41,46,59,61,67–69). Changes in proton density and T2 relaxation time have been demonstrated in normal muscle with exercise. T2 relaxation time increases 20% to 44% and pH decreases from 0.35 to 1.1. These changes are probably related to acidosis and perfusion changes (59). With exercise, there is normally consumption of phosphocreatine (PCr), a decrease in pH, and increase in inorganic phosphate (Pi) (36,40,59). In patients with congestive heart failure, muscle

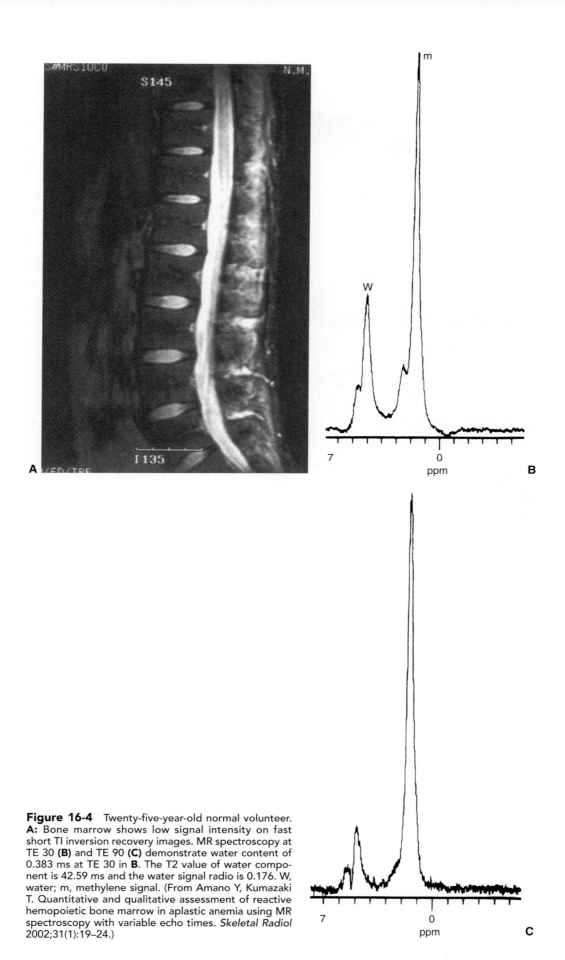

Figure 16-4 Twenty-five-year-old normal volunteer. **A:** Bone marrow shows low signal intensity on fast short TI inversion recovery images. MR spectroscopy at TE 30 **(B)** and TE 90 **(C)** demonstrate water content of 0.383 ms at TE 30 in **B**. The T2 value of water component is 42.59 ms and the water signal radio is 0.176. W, water; m, methylene signal. (From Amano Y, Kumazaki T. Quantitative and qualitative assessment of reactive hemopoietic bone marrow in aplastic anemia using MR spectroscopy with variable echo times. *Skeletal Radiol* 2002;31(1):19–24.)

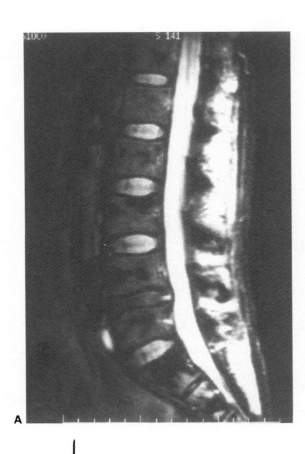

A

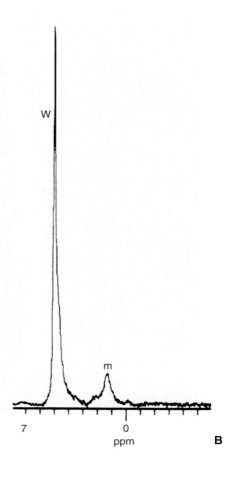

W

m

7   0

ppm

B

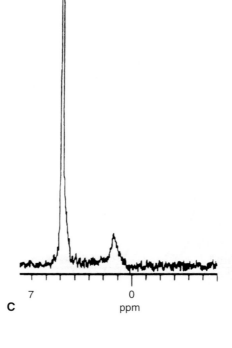

7   0

ppm

C

Figure 16-5 Fifty-three-year-old male with aplastic anemia. **A:** The reactive hemopoietic marrow in L1 was low intensity on T1-weighted spin-echo images and high intensity on fast STIR images. MR spectroscopy at TE 30 **(B)** and TE 90 **(C).** The water is larger than methylene at TE 30 in **B.** The water content was 0.716 compared to 0.383 in the normal volunteer. The T2 value of the water component was 69.46 ms and water signal ratio was 0.379, both significantly higher than the normal volunteer (Fig. 16-4, B and C). (From Amano Y, Kumazaki T. Quantitative and qualitative assessment of reactive hemopoietic bone marrow in aplastic anemia using MR spectroscopy with variable echo times. *Skeletal Radiol* 2002;31(1):19–24.)

PCr is nearly depleted with exercise (68). Conditions such as McArdle disease (myophosphorylase deficiency) and phosphofructokinase deficiency cause changes in spectra due to inability to break down glycogen. Therefore, lactate is not produced with exercise, and pH does not decrease compared to normal muscle with exercise (36,59,61,64).

Other myopathies may result in increase in fatty tissue which can be evaluated with either ^{1}H or ^{31}P MRS (7,33, 36,49). Funicello et al. (36) described low PCr/Pi ratio in patients with disc disease and muscle paresis. Patients with polymyositis and dermatomyositis demonstrate decreased choline/lipid and creatine/lipid ratios (35). ^{31}P MRS has demonstrated potential for evaluating many conditions affecting metabolism, mitochondrial lesions, muscular dystrophy, and muscle fatigue syndromes (3,43).

Sharma et al. (43) evaluated normal volunteers and patients with Duchenne muscular dystrophy using ^{1}H MRS. Concentrations of glycolytic substrate glucose, glutamine, and alanine were lower in patients with muscular dystrophy. In addition, there are also significantly lower levels of total creatine, choline, and acetate (43).

A noninvasive method of evaluating tissue viability, extent of muscle involvement, and exercise-related changes in ischemic disease could have a significant impact on patients with peripheral vascular disease, especially diabetes (70,71).

There have been several reports suggesting MRS may provide valuable information regarding muscle metabolism in patients with ischemic disease (61,72). Changes in ATP pathways, specifically Pi recovery after exercise and pH changes, can be related to tissue perfusion and correlated with the extent of vascular disease (72). Tissue viability is a particularly significant problem in diabetic patients. Ankle pressures, thermography, and transcutaneous oxygen measurements are indirect indications of tissue viability. MRS offers a noninvasive method to study high energy phosphates involved in oxidative metabolism. Increased Pi to PCr ratios may be useful for predicting soft tissue ischemia in diabetics (70).

OSSEOUS AND CARTILAGE DISORDERS

In recent years, MRS has been utilized with increased frequency to evaluate marrow abnormalities and changes in articular cartilage (10,42,44,45,48).

Amano et al. (45) have continued to evaluate marrow changes in aplastic anemia. Water content is higher in hemopoietic marrow using multiple echoes (TE 30,45,60,90) compared to normal marrow (see Figs. 16-4 and 16-5) (45). Age-related bone changes have also been evaluated, but studies are not conclusive at this point (10, 48).

Early studies evaluating water content, collagen, and proteoglycons may provide valuable information in patients with arthropathies (48).

MRS is an evolving technique that demonstrates proven or emergency utility for evaluating musculoskeletal pathology and metabolism. Both ^{31}P and ^{1}H spectra have been evaluated. The latter has been more frequently employed due to its abundance and ease of evaluation with 1.5 T clinical imagers. Combined MRI–MRS studies appear to be most useful and examination times (60 to 90 minutes) make these studies practical in a clinical setting.

Further studies in multiple environments, including new high field strength imagers (3 to 8 T), must be accomplished before MRS becomes a universally accepted clinical tool.

REFERENCES

1. Aisen AM, Chenevert TL. MR spectroscopy: clinical perspective. *Radiology* 1989;173:593–599.
2. Andrew ER, Bydder G, Griffiths J, et al. *Clinical magnetic resonance imaging and spectroscopy*. Chichester, John Wiley & Sons, 1990.
3. Bottomley PA. Human in vivo NMR spectroscopy in diagnostic medicine: clinical tool or research probe. *Radiology* 1989;170:1–15.
4. Bore PJ. The role of magnetic spectroscopy in clinical medicine. *Magn Reson Imaging* 1985;3:407–413.
5. Nedendank WG, Crowley MG, Ryan JR, et al. Bone and soft-tissue lesions: diagnosis with combined H-1 MR imaging and P-31 MR spectroscopy. *Radiology* 1989;173:181–188.
6. Shulman RG, Rothman DL. 13C NMR of intermediary metabolism: implications for systemic physiology. *Ann Rev Physiol* 2001;63:15–48.
7. Brechtel K, Jacob S, Machann J, et al. Acquired generalized lipoatrophy: highly selective MR lipid imaging and localized (1) H-MRS. *J Magn Reson Imaging* 2000;12(2):306–310.
8. Dort JC, Fan Y, McIntyre DD. Investigation of skeletal muscle denervation and reinnervation using magnetic resonance spectroscopy. *Otolaryngol Head Neck Surg* 2001;125(6):617–622.
9. Hu J, Jiang Q, Xia Y, et al. High spatial resolution *in-vivo* 2D (1) H magnetic resonance spectroscopic imaging of human muscles with band-selective technique. *Magn Reson Imaging* 2001;19(8):1091–1096.
10. Jung CM, Kugel H, Schulte O, et al. Proton-MR spectroscopy of the spinal bone marrow. An analysis of physiological signal behavior. *Radiologe* 2000;40(8):694–699.
11. Kantarci K, Reynolds G, Petersen RC, et al. Proton MR spectroscopy in mild cognitive impairment and Alzheimer's disease: comparison of 1.5 and 3 T. *AJNR Am J Neuroradiol* 2003;24(5):843–849.
12. Katz-Brull R, Lavin PT, Lenkinski RE. Clinical utility of proton magnetic resonance spectroscopy in characterizing breast lesions. *J Natl Cancer Inst* 2002;94(16):1197–1203.
13. Kettelhack C, Wickede MV, Vogl T, et al. 31 Phosphorus–magnetic resonance spectroscopy to assess histologic tumor response noninvasively after isolated limb perfusion of soft tissue tumors. *Cancer* 2002;94(5):1557–1564.
14. Okada T, Harada M, Matsceziak K, et al. Evaluation of female intrapelvic tumors by clinical proton MR spectroscopy. *J Magn Reson Imaging* 2001;13(6):912–917.
15. Schwartz AJ, Maisey NR, Collins DJ, et al. Early in vivo detection of metabolic response: a pilot study of 1H MR spectroscopy in extra cranial lymphoma and germ cell tumors. *Br J Radiol* 2002;75(9):959–966.
16. Shukla-Dave A, Poptani H, Loevner LA, et al. Prediction of treatment response of head and neck cancers with P-31MR spectroscopy from pretreatment phosphomonoester levels. *Acad Radiol* 2002;9(6):688–694.
17. Walecki J, Michalak MJ, Michalatz E, et al. Use of magnetic resonance spectroscopy in cardiology: state of the art. *Przegl Lek* 2002;59(8):601–605.
18. Dreher W, Leibfritz D. Fast proton spectroscopic imaging with high signal-to-noise radio: spectroscopic RARE. *Magn Reson Med* 2002;47(3):523–528.

19. Ebel A, Maudsley AA. Improved spectral quality for 3D MR spectroscopic imaging using a high spatial resolution acquisition strategy. *Magn Reson Imaging* 2003;21(2):113–120.

20. Gonen O. Higher field strength proton MR spectroscopy. *AJNR Am J Neuroradiol* 2003;24(5):781–782.

21. Lips O, Privalov AF, Dvinskikh SV, et al. Magnet design with high B(O) homogeneity for fast-field-cycling NMR applications. *J Magn Reson* 2001;149(1):22–28.

22. Smith JK, Kwock L, Castillo M. Effects of contrast material on single-volume proton MR spectroscopy. *AJNR Am J Neuroradiol* 2000;21(6):1084–1089.

23. Vikhoff-Baaz B, Starck G, Ljungberg M, et al. Effects of K-space filtering and image interpolation on image fidelity in (1) H MRSI. *Magn Reson Imaging* 2001;19(9):1227–1234.

24. Bachert P, Belleman ME, Layer G, et al. In vivo ^{1}H, ^{31}P –^{1}H and ^{13}C –^{1}H magnetic resonance spectroscopy of malignant histiocytoma and skeletal muscle tissue in man. *NMR Biomed* 1992;5:161–170.

25. Karczmar GS, Meyerhoff DJ, Boska MD, et al. P-31 spectroscopy study of response of superficial human tumors to therapy. *Radiology* 1994;179:149–153.

26. Lenkinski RE, Holland GA, Allman T, et al. Integrated MR imaging and spectroscopy with chemical shift imaging of P-31 at 1.5 T: initial clinical experience. *Radiology* 1988;169:201–206.

27. Merchant TE, Characiejus D, Kasimos JN, et al. Phosphodiesters in saponified extracts of human breast and colon tumors using 31P magnetic resonance spectroscopy. *Magn Reson Med* 1992;26:132–140.

28. Posse S, Schnuknecht B, Smith ME, et al. Short echo time proton spectroscopic imaging. *J Comput Assist Tomogr* 1993;17:1–14.

29. Sakuma H, Takeda K, Tagomi T, et al. 31-P spectroscopy in hypertrophic cardiomyopathy: comparison with Tl-201 myocardial perfusion imaging. *Am Heart J* 1993;125:1323–1328.

30. Schilling A, Gewiese B, Berger G, et al. Liver tumors: follow-up with P-31 MR spectroscopy after local chemotherapy and chemoembolization. *Radiology* 1992;182:877–890.

31. Nedendank WG, Brown TR, Evelhoch JL, et al. Proceedings of a national cancer institute workshop: MR spectroscopy and tumor cell biology. *Radiology* 1992;185:875–883.

32. Young IR. Review of modalities with future potential in radiology. *Radiology* 1994;192:307–317.

33. Bárány M, Langer BG, Glick RP, et al. In vivo H-1 spectroscopy in humans at 1.5 T. *Radiology* 1988;167:839–844.

34. Jelicks LA, Paul PK, O'Bryne E, et al. Hydrogen-1, Sodium-23, and carbon-13 MR spectroscopy of cartilage degeneration in vitro. *J Magn Reson Imaging* 1993;3:565–568.

35. Brix G, Heiland S, Bellemann ME, et al. MR imaging of fat-containing tissues: valuation of two quantitative imaging techniques in comparison with localized proton spectroscopy. *Magn Reson Imaging* 1993;11:977–991.

36. Funicello R, Barbirole B, Zanier P, et al. Energy metabolism in muscle paresis and recovery study by ^{31}P MR spectroscopy. *Ital J Neurol Sci* 1993;14:263–267.

37. Semmler W, Gademan G, Bachert-Baumann P, et al. Monitoring human tumor response to therapy by means of P-31 MR spectroscopy. *Radiology* 1988;166:533–539.

38. Boska MD, Nelson JA, Sripathi N, et al. ^{31}P MRS studies of exercising human muscle at high temporal resolution. *Magn Reson Med* 1999;41(6):1145–1151.

39. Maldonado X, Alonso J, Giralt J, et al. 31 phosphorus magnetic resonance spectroscopy in evaluation of head and neck tumors. *Int J Radiat Oncol Biol Phys* 1998;40(2):309–312.

40. Rossiter HB, Ward SA, Howe FA, et al. Dynamics of intramuscular 31P-MRS P(i) peak splitting and slow components of PCr and 02 uptake during exercise. *J Appl Physiol* 2002;93(6):2059–2069.

41. Smith SA, Montain SJ, Matott RP, et al. Effects of creatine supplementation on the energy cost to muscle: a 31-P MRS study. *J Appl Physiol* 1999;87(1):116–123.

42. Lendinara L, Accorsi C, Agostini C, et al. Proton magnetic relaxation in bone marrow related to age and bone mineral density: low-resolution *in vitro* studies. *Magn Reson Imaging* 2001;19(5):745–753.

43. Sharma U, Atri S, Sharma MC, et al. Skeletal metabolism in Duchenne muscular dystrophy (DMD): an *in vitro* proton NMR spectroscopic study. *Magn Reson Imaging* 2003;21(2):145–153.-

44. Amano Y, Kumazaki T. Proton MR imaging and spectroscopy evaluation of aplastic anemia: three bone marrow patterns. *J Comput Assist Tomogr* 1997;21(2):286–292.

45. Amano Y, Kumazaki T. Quantitative and qualitative assessment of reactive hemopoietic bone marrow in aplastic anemia using MR spectroscopy with variable echo times. *Skeletal Radiol* 2002;31(1):19–24.

46. Johansen L, Quistorff B. 31P-MRS characterization of sprint and endurance trained athletes. *Int J Sports Med* 2003;24(3):183–189.

47. Kwock L, Smith JK, Castillo M, et al. Clinical applications of proton MR spectroscopy in oncology. *Technol Cancer Res Treat* 2002;1(1):17–28.

48. Lattanzio PJ, Marshall KW, Damyanovich AZ, et al. Macro molecule and water magnetization exchange modeling in articular cartilage. *Magn Reson Med* 2000;44(6):840–851.

49. Lodi R, Muntoni F, Taylor J, et al. Correlative MR imaging and 31-P MR spectroscopy in sarcoglycan deficient limb girdle muscular dystrophy. *Neuromuscul Disord* 1997;7(8):505–511.

50. Zlatkin MB, Lenkinshi RE, Shinkwin M, et al. Combined MR imaging and spectroscopy of bone and soft tissue tumors. *J Comput Assist Tomogr* 1990;14:1–10.

51. Hoekstra HJ, Boeve WJ, Kamman RL, et al. Clinical applicability of human *in-vivo* phosphorus-31 magnetic resonance spectroscopy of bone and soft tissue tumors. *Ann Surg Oncol* 1994;1(6):504–511.

52. Nedendank WG. MR spectroscopy of musculoskeletal soft-tissue tumors. *Magn Reson Imaging Clin N Am* 1995;3(4):713–725.

53. Shinkwin MA, Lenkinski RE, Daly JM, et al. Integrated magnetic resonance imaging and phosphorus spectroscopy of soft tissue tumors. *Cancer* 1991;67:1849–1858.

54. Sostman HD, Charles HC, Rockwell S, et al. Soft-tissue sarcomas: detection of metabolic heterogeneity with P-31 MR spectroscopy. *Radiology* 1990;176:837–843.

55. Sostman HD, Prescott DM, Dewhirst MW, et al. MR imaging and spectroscopy for prognostic evaluation of soft tissue tumors. *Radiology* 1994;190:269–275.

56. Tráber F, Block W, Layer G, et al. Determination of 1H relaxation times of water in human bone marrow by fat-suppressed turbo spin-echo in comparison to MR spectroscopic methods. *J Magn Reson Imaging* 1996;6(3):541–548.

57. Schick F, Duda SH, Lutz O, et al. Lipids in bone tumors assessed by magnetic resonance: chemical shift and proton spectroscopy in-vivo. *Anticancer Res* 1996;16(3B):1569–1574.

58. Sijens PE, van der Bent MJ, Oudherk M. Phosphorus 31 chemical shift imaging of metastatic tumors located in the spine region. *Invest Radiol* 1997;32(6):344–380.

59. deKerviler E, Leroy-Willig A, Jehenson P, et al. Exercise-induced muscle modifications: study of healthy subjects and patients with metabolic myopathies with MR imaging and P-31 spectroscopy. *Radiology* 1991;181:259–264.

60. Fraiser DD, Frank JA, Dalakas MC. Inflammatory myopathies: MR imaging and spectroscopy. *Radiology* 1991;179:341–344.

61. Miller RG, Carson PJ, Moussovi RS, et al. The use of magnetic resonance spectroscopy to evaluate muscular fatigue and human muscle disease. *Appl Radiol* 1989;18:33–38.

62. Mountford CE, Lean CL, Hancock R, et al. Magnetic resonance spectroscopy detects cancer in draining lymph nodes. *Invasion Metastasis* 1993;13:57–71.

63. VanderGrond J, Crolla RMPH, Hove WT, et al. Phosphorus magnetic resonance spectroscopy of the calf muscle in patient with peripheral arterial occlusive disease. *Invest Radiol* 1993;29:104–108.

64. Roden M, Shulman GI. Applications of NMR spectroscopy to study glycogen metabolism in man. *Annu Rev Med* 1999;50:277–290.

65. Tráber F, Kaiser WA, Reiser MF, et al. MRI and MRS of the skeletal muscle. *Bildgebung* 1992;59:156–158.

66. Chung YL, Smith EC, Williams SC, et al. *In vivo* proton magnetic resonance spectroscopy in polymyositis and dermatomyositis. *Eur J Med Res* 1997;2(11):483–487.

67. Maidsley AA, Lin E, Weiner MW. Spectroscopic imaging display and analysis. *Magn Reson Imaging* 1992;10:471–485.

68. Okita K, Yonezawa K, Nishijima H, et al. Skeletal muscle metabolism limits exercise capacity in patients with chronic heart failure. *Circulation* 1998;98(18):1886–1891.

69. Sullivan MJ, Saltin B, Negro-Vilar R, et al. Skeletal muscle pH assessed by biochemical and 31-P MRS methods during exercise and recovery in man. *J Appl Physiol* 1994;77(5):2194–2200.

70. Brotzakis PZ, Sacco P, Jones DH, et al. 31P nuclear magnetic resonance spectroscopy of acutely ischemic limbs: the extent of changes and progress after reconstructive surgery. *Cardiovasc Surg* 1995;3(3):271–276.

71. Smith DG, Mills WJ, Steen RG, et al. Levels of high energy phosphate in the dorsal skin of the foot in normal and diabetic adults: the role of 31-P magnetic resonance spectroscopy and direct quantification with high pressure liquid chromatography. *Foot Ankle Int* 1999;20(4):258–262.

72. Williams DM, Fencil L, Chenevert TL. Peripheral arterial occlusive disease: P-31 MR spectroscopy of calf muscle. *Radiology* 1990;175:381–385.

Index

Page numbers followed by *f* indicate figures; page numbers followed by *t* indicate tables